Amyotrophic Lateral Sclerosis

Amyotrophic Lateral Sclerosis

edited by

Hiroshi Mitsumoto
Columbia Presbyterian Neurological Institute
New York, New York, U.S.A.

Serge Przedborski
Columbia Presbyterian Neurological Institute
New York, New York, U.S.A.

Paul H. Gordon
Columbia Presbyterian Neurological Institute
New York, New York, U.S.A.

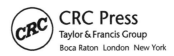

CRC Press
Taylor & Francis Group
Boca Raton London New York

CRC Press is an imprint of the
Taylor & Francis Group, an **informa** business
A TAYLOR & FRANCIS BOOK

CRC Press
Taylor & Francis Group
6000 Broken Sound Parkway NW Suite 300
Boca Raton, FL 33487-2742

First issued in paperback 2019

ISBN-13: 978-0-8247-2924-0 (hbk)
ISBN-13: 978-0-367-39184-3 (pbk)

Library of Congress Cataloging-in-Publication Data

Amyotrophic lateral sclerosis / edited by Hiroshi Mitsumoto, Serge Przedborski, Paul H. Gordon.
    p. cm. -- (Neurological disease and therapy ; 78)
   Includes bibliographical references and index.
   ISBN-13: 978-0-8247-2924-0 (alk. paper)
   ISBN-10: 0-8247-2924-2 (alk. paper)
   1. Amyotrophic lateral sclerosis. I. Mitsumoto, Hiroshi. II. Przedborski, Serge. III. Gordon, Paul H. IV. Series.

RC406.A24M58 2005
616.8'3--dc22   2005053812

**Visit the Taylor & Francis Web site at
http://www.taylorandfrancis.com**

**and the CRC Press Web site at
http://www.crcpress.com**

Foreword

Amyotrophic lateral sclerosis (ALS) is a motor system disease that primarily affects the final common motor pathways in the spinal cord and brain. However, ALS is a complex disorder that progresses at different rates in different people and is associated with a puzzling array of neurological and psychiatric symptoms that must arise in other "non-motor" regions of the nervous system. It is important, therefore, to take stock from time to time and assess progress from different perspectives. Among the perspectives that must be taken into account are the past history of the field; current concepts of pathophysiology, current hypotheses regarding genetic and environmental risk factors; and the most effective current therapies. It is also important to have a clear idea about modalities of supportive care available to ALS patients and their families. A more profound understanding of the quality of life predicaments faced by patients and patient advocates can lift the intensity of investigation from curiosity to urgency. This timely book touches on each of these issues.

We live in a medical community of extreme specialization. Laboratory science and clinical medicine are each so demanding that scientists and physicians learn about each others' advances from highly simplified summary presentations. There is little or no time to study subtle distinctions in subjects that lie beyond one's immediate area of expertise. Creativity in the laboratory can be enhanced by understanding the pathology of ALS, the natural history of the disease, and the spectrum of clinical manifestations. Likewise, the ability of physicians to appreciate variations in the usual clinical picture of ALS can be enhanced by a greater understanding of phenotypes caused by particular gene mutations and an appreciation of the effect of environmental toxins on gene expression. More refined diagnostic criteria based on molecular pathophysiology are needed to mark steps toward a cure. We must aim for molecular landmarks rather than complete reversal of the clinical picture to make incremental progress in therapeutics. Opportunities are missed, it seems to me, at the interfaces between basic research, clinical research, and patient care.

The chapters that follow illustrate why this is a time of great hope in the study and treatment of ALS. The first section of the book, "Overview of Clinical ALS," provides a remarkably complete description of the ALS phenotype. The second section, "Translational Research: Mechanisms Behind Therapy," brings the reader up to date regarding the major hypotheses of ALS pathogenesis. Novel approaches are spelled out in excellent chapters on ALS drug screening and on genetic causes and risk factors. The third section, "ALS Therapy: Care and Management," brings one up to date regarding current treatments and the best approaches to supportive care. It is the combination of these subjects that makes the book so compelling.

We know more about motor neurons than any other nerve cell in the central nervous system—how they initiate and conduct action potentials, when they are "born" and when they die, when they migrate from the germinal epithelium to their final positions within the spinal cord, how they extend axons to appropriate target muscles, and how they form functional neuromuscular synapses.

Distinctive patterns of transcription factor gene expression in subsets of motor neurons, sensory neurons, and the muscles they innervate have been described. Manipulation of these genes in vivo has shown that they play important roles in the organization of motor neuron pools and even in the formation of specific connections within the spinal cord and in the periphery. Such a molecular code will certainly provide new insights regarding neural circuits within the spinal cord. This information would greatly facilitate recovery of function and perhaps even true repair of damaged circuits.

We know when motor neurons die during development and during motor system diseases, but we don't know enough about how they die. Several hypotheses regarding mechanisms of neuronal loss in ALS are reviewed in the following chapters.

"Trophic" interactions have been uncovered that operate on a scale of hours to years. Proteins have been identified that may mediate trophic interactions between muscle and motor neurons in a retrograde (muscle to motor neuron) or anterograde (motor neuron to muscle) direction. Other trophic factors may mediate effects between neurons or glia and neurons within the same spinal cord segment. One or more of these proteins may play a role in the survival of neurons in ALS. The influence of muscle-derived factors has received support from the striking finding that insulin-like growth factor introduced into muscle and taken up by motor axons prolongs the survival of SOD1 mutant mice.

The discovery that mutations in SOD1 occur in certain families with ALS has been particularly important. Mice expressing mutant SOD1 have proved to be informative models of ALS. It is not clear why mutations in SOD1 cause death of motor neurons, but attention has focused on aggregates of mutant SOD1 protein. This begs the question, of course, but it places SOD1 and ALS on the list of "proteinopathies" that produce other neurodegenerative disorders-including the prion protein (Kuru, Creutzfeld/Jacob Disease, Gerstmann/Strassler Syndrome, and Familial Fatal Insomnia), synuclean (Parkinson's Disease), huntingtin (Huntington's Disease), and beta amyloid (Alzheimer's Disease).

Experiments in chimeric mice in which mutant SOD1 is expressed in some motor neurons and/or in some astrocytes have provided strong evidence that expression in motor neurons alone is not sufficient to cause disease. ALS is apparently not a motor neuron autonomous defect. Motor neurons may be the ultimate target, but other cells, including nearby glia, must express the mutant gene in order to affect the motor neurons.

These are important insights even though mutations in SOD1 have not been found in sporadic ALS. It is likely that other proteins contribute to the syndrome.

Hypotheses regarding the toxicity of glutamate and analogues and of free radicals have been revived. The discovery that the transport of glutamate is defective in ALS due to mutations in EAAT2 has led to specific testable hypotheses. Riluzole, the only medicine now approved for treatment of ALS by the FDA, is a glutamate receptor antagonist.

High-throughput screens of FDA-approved drugs using protein aggregation or motor neuron cell death are underway. This effort, funded by NINDS in collaboration with private ALS groups, has yielded unexpected and interesting results.

Despite the optimism of important insights described above, some caution must be expressed. First, ALS is a complex disease and we have a great deal to learn even about its most obvious aspects. Second, research in the next period of time will be conducted at a time of diminished resources and increasing constraints placed on the scientific enterprise. Recent years have seen the NIH budget level off – from annual increases of 12% to 15% to increases of 2% to 3%. This means, effectively, a real decrease in funding. Ongoing commitments coupled with the high rate of inflation in biomedical science will limit the number of new projects that can be funded. The percentage of "new" investigators under age 35 receiving grants has gone down every year over the past decade, and the average age at first independent funding from the NIH has crept up to 42. There is no evidence that these trends will be reversed in the near future even though there is universal agreement that we must capture young scientists in their most creative years. Philanthropic support is more critical now than ever before. We must bring more advocates to the field and we must help them understand more about ALS and how ALS is related to other CNS disorders.

We have been through difficult funding periods before. I believe that excellence will endure, and in the end it will win out. Even in the most difficult of times, we must not fail to stand by and promulgate the values of science. Open sharing of information, generosity of spirit, and reliance on objective, reproducible data are values inherent in the scientific method that have led to so many advances in biomedical science and that have relieved so much suffering. Constraints placed on science by political or religious considerations have been less discussed than the lack of funds, but in the long run they can be more damaging.

Gerald D. Fischbach, M.D.
Executive Vice President for Health and Biomedical Sciences
and Dean of the Faculty of Medicine
College of Physicians and Surgeons, Columbia University
New York, New York, U.S.A.

Preface

When one of the editors (HM) of this book began his neuromuscular research fellowship under the direction of Walter G. Bradley, D.M, F.R.C.P, at Tufts University in 1979, he bought a book on ALS published by the Academic Press, *Amyotrophic Lateral Sclerosis. Recent Research Trends*. The book was published in 1976 and, at that time, was the only book available on ALS. The book proved to be an important resource because the editor could quickly review recent advances in ALS research. In the 25 years since then, more than two dozen books on ALS have been published. The majority of the publications, however, were review summaries of results presented at ALS research conferences, most notably the two large volumes in the *Advances in Neurology* series published 10 years apart by Raven Press and edited by Dr. Lewis P. Rowland. Both were compilations of the state-of-the-art research presented at the Muscular Dystrophy Association International Conference on ALS.

Monographs and textbooks on ALS started appearing in the 1980s, and in the 1990s, a slow but steady flow of excellent multi-authored books were published, reflecting the surge of scientific knowledge on ALS. These multi-authored books tend to emphasize the progress in basic science research because, at the time, we still knew little about the causes and pathogenesis of the disease. A notable exception was a book on palliative care, published by Oxford University Press, addressing the ALS community's serious concern and need for information on end-of-life issues in ALS. Books on ALS written by a few authors are rare, although one of us (HM) is an author on such a book. *Amyotrophic Lateral Sclerosis*, published by Oxford University Press, recovered almost every aspect of ALS, clinically and scientifically; however, in-depth review of basic science had still been limited because the authors were primarily clinicians.

The recent progress in ALS research has become extraordinarily rapid, particularly in genetic and molecular areas and in translational research. Clinical research in ALS is advancing at an equally fast pace. For those of us still immersed in the search for a go-to source for the latest information, we theorized that this is the opportune time for a publication that thoroughly presents the cutting edge in ALS research and therapy. To accomplish this, we realized that we needed authors who were extremely knowledgeable and would be able to provide special expertise on different topics in ALS. We are especially fortunate to have found the authors best suited for each chapter in this book.

Conceptually, we divided the book into three sections: (i) Overview of Clinical ALS, (ii) Translational Research in ALS: Mechanisms behind Therapy, and (iii) ALS Therapy: Care and Management. In the "Overview," we cover knowledge needed for clinical practice, including history and epidemiology of the disease, how to evaluate patients and give the diagnosis, genetic disease (familial ALS), and dementia in ALS. This section essentially covers what one needs to know about ALS in daily neurology practice.

In the next section, "Translational Research in ALS," we cover a series of selected topics that were inspired by the intersection of neurobiology with clinical science. Less than two decades ago, it is fair to say that these two disciplines shared almost no tangible overlap. With the explosion and integration of molecular genetics and cell biology, research in the neurobiology of disease in ALS has become an endless source of new and exciting knowledge. Apart from being instrumental in improving our understanding of how and why certain cells such as motor neurons die in ALS, such research has also produced a growing number of reliable experimental models of ALS that are extensively used to preclinically evaluate new mechanisms of neurodegeneration and potential neuroprotective strategies. To provide the reader with a sense of exciting questions at the forefront of ALS neurobiology, topics such as protein aggregation, excitotoxicity, apoptosis, and inflammation are discussed. Admittedly, the areas covered in this section represent only a selection and not an exhaustive list of important subjects. However, we chose them with a idea of offering the reader a historical perspective, providing an accurate and up-to-date view of the main directions of research, and indicating the directions in which ALS research is evolving.

In the last section, "ALS Therapy," we discuss methods and techniques to maximize the quality of care and management. A multidisciplinary approach has become the standard of care for patients with ALS and is reflected in this section. The first chapter of this section describes how individual ALS multidisciplinary team clinics are run, pointing out their strengths and weaknesses or other issues. The ALS CARE Database and the American Academy of Neurology Practice Parameters, which provide recommendations for clinical practice in ALS, have become the driving force in improving the quality of ALS care and management. Intensive pharmacotherapy for symptomatic management, as well as pharmacotherapy in clinical trials are briefly described in the section. Key issues in nutritional and respiratory care are also briefly described. Finally, palliative care and end-of-life issues are discussed from a number of different perspectives.

In presenting the information with a broad perspective, we have tried to target a wide audience, particularly neurologists, neuromuscular experts, neuromuscular fellows, and residents. We are confident that neuroscientists who are interested in neurogeneration and ALS will find this book useful, too. Because it covers many areas of ALS in detail, we think that even ALS specialists will have a need for this book. Other health professionals who work with patients and families with ALS and deal with daily clinical issues are, needless to say, likely to find this book helpful as well.

We are deeply grateful to all of our contributors. Although they had many other commitments, they have provided exciting and highly informative chapters. Personally as the editors of this book, we enjoyed reading every chapter, each one reminding us what a joy it is to learn anew. Working with the individual authors was quite rewarding, resulting in new friendships and the discovery that we are comrades in the struggle to understand ALS and improve quality of care for our patients. We would also like to express our special thanks to the number of the faculty at Columbia University Medical Center. Gerald Fischbach, M.D., Dean and Executive Vice President of Health Affairs, graciously wrote the foreword to the book. His foreword is particularly well-suited and topical because he is a world-renowned researcher in motor neuron biology. Thomas Jessell, Ph.D., and Christopher Henderson, Ph.D., who lead the Neuroscience Institute and Motor Neuron Center at Columbia University, respectively, contributed outstanding chapters on motor neuron biology and screening of ALS drugs. Steve Albert, Ph.D., Clifton Gooch, M.D., Arthur Hays, M.D., Petra Kaufmann, M.D., M.S., Seth Pullman, M.D., Judy Rabkin, Ph.D., and Lewis Rowland, M.D., work closely with us here at Columbia. Such individuals make our institution truly great, and it is an honor to work with them.

We would like to express our special thanks to Ms. Jinnie Kim at Taylor & Francis, who has been with us from the initial planning to the final publication. She gave us her tireless support, continuous encouragement, and a superb effort in solving any issues that arose. We also acknowledge the hard work of her colleagues, Dana Bigelow, Joseph Stubenrauch, and Alan Kaplan for competently seeing the book through publication. We are deeply grateful to Dr. Lewis P. Rowland, who mentored all of us in neurology and ALS, and to Dr. Timothy A. Pedley who guided us as the Chairman of our department. Lastly, we would like to acknowledge the NIH, MDA, MDA Wings Over Wall Street, Project ALS, the Japan Foundation of Health and Aging, and the many other philanthropic supporters of the Eleanor and Lou Gehrig MDA/ALS Research Center.

Finally, we would like to dedicate this book to all our patients and their families who have come to our center. They have helped us in so many ways by participating in patient-oriented research and have taught us much about ALS and what it is like to be a patient with this disease. Our greatest hope is that the pathogenesis and causes of ALS are rapidly clarified and that much of the content described in this book quickly becomes obsolete, so that we can simply concentrate on providing effective therapy for patients with ALS.

Hiroshi Mitsumoto
Serge Przedborski
Paul H. Gordon

Contents

PART II: TRANSLATIONAL RESEARCH IN ALS: MECHANISMS BEHIND THERAPY

PART III: ALS THERAPY: CARE AND MANAGEMENT

Contributors

Loutfi S. Aboussouan Departments of Pulmonary Critical Care and Allergy, Cleveland Clinic Foundation Beachwood, Beachwood, Ohio, U.S.A.

Patrick Aebischer Integrative Biosciences Institute, Ecole Polytechnique Fédérale de Lausanne (EPFL), Lausanne, Switzerland

Steven M. Albert Department of Behavioral and Community Health Sciences, Graduate School of Public Health, University of Pittsburgh, Pittsburgh, Pennsylvania, U.S.A

Gabriele Almer Department of Neurology, Columbia University, New York, New York, U.S.A.

Fred Anderson Department of Surgery, Center for Outcomes Research, University of Massachusetts Medical School, Worcester, Massachusetts, U.S.A.

Stanley H. Appel Department of Neurology, Methodist Neurological Institute, Houston, Texas, U.S.A.

Joseph S. Beckman Linus Pauling Institute, Department of Biochemistry and Biophysics, Environmental Health Sciences Center, Oregon State University, Corvallis, Oregon, U.S.A.

Gian Domenico Borasio Interdisciplinary Center for Palliative Medicine and Department of Neurology, Motor Neuron Disease Research Group, Munich University Hospital, Grosshadern, Munich, Germany

Thierry Bordet Trophos, S.A., Marseille, France

Walter G. Bradley Department of Neurology, University of Miami School of Medicine, Miami, Florida, U.S.A.

Mark Bromberg Department of Neurology, University of Utah, Salt Lake City, Utah, U.S.A.

Benjamin R. Brooks Department of Neurology, University of Wisconsin Medical School, Madison, Wisconsin, U.S.A.

Gregory T. Carter   Department of Physical Medicine and Rehabilitation, University of Washington, Centralia, Washington, U.S.A.

David A. Chad   University of Massachusetts School of Medicine and UMass Memorial Health Care, Worcester, Massachusetts, U.S.A.

Laura Coker   Department of Public Health Sciences, Wake Forest University School of Medicine, Winston-Salem, North Carolina, U.S.A.

Valerie A. Cwik   Muscular Dystrophy Association, Tucson, Arizona, U.S.A.

Vanina Dal Bello-Haas   School of Physical Therapy, University of Saskatchewan, Saskatoon, Saskatchewan, Canada

Suzanne E. Danforth   Department of Speech Therapy, Massachusetts General Hospital, Boston, Massachusetts, U.S.A.

A. Dawson   Department of Clinical Neuroscience, Institute of Psychiatry, King's College London, London, U.K.

Maura L. Del Bene   Department of Neurology, New York University School of Medicine, New York, New York, U.S.A.

Lisa Dellefave   Department of Neurology and Clinical Neurosciences and Department of Cell and Molecular Biology, Northwestern University Feinberg School of Medicine, Chicago, Illinois, U.S.A.

Linda Boynton De Sepulveda   ALS Haven, Montecito, California, U.S.A.

Ian F. Dunn   Department of Neurosurgery, Brigham and Women's Hospital, Harvard Medical School, Boston, Massachusetts, U.S.A.

Jeffrey L. Elliott   University of Texas, Southwestern Medical Center, Dallas, Texas, U.S.A.

Alvaro G. Estévez   Department of Physiology, The University of Alabama at Birmingham, Birmingham, Alabama, U.S.A.

Robert M. Friedlander   Department of Neurosurgery, Brigham and Women's Hospital, Harvard Medical School, Boston, Massachusetts, U.S.A.

J. M. Gallo   Department of Clinical Neuroscience, Institute of Psychiatry, King's College London, London, U.K.

Linda Ganzini   Department of Psychiatry, Oregon Health & Science University, Portland, Oregon, U.S.A.

Angela L. Genge   Montreal Neurological Hospital, Montreal, Quebec, Canada

Clifton L. Gooch Department of Neurology, The Neurological Institute, Columbia University College of Physicians and Surgeons, New York, New York, U.S.A.

Paul H. Gordon Neurological Institute, Columbia University, New York, New York, U.S.A.

Neelam Gowda Department of Surgery, Center for Outcomes Research, University of Massachusetts Medical School, Worcester, Massachusetts, U.S.A.

Orla Hardiman Richmond Institute of Neurology, Beaumont Hospital, Dublin, Ireland

Arthur P. Hays Department of Pathology (Neuropathology), Columbia University Medical Center, Columbia University, New York, New York, U.S.A.

Paul R. Heath Academic Neurology Unit, Section of Neuroscience, University of Sheffield, Sheffield, U.K.

Terry Heiman-Patterson Neurology Control, Drexel University College of Medicine, Philadelphia, Pennsylvania, U.S.A.

Christopher E. Henderson Departments of Pathology and Neurology, Columbia University Medical Center, New York, New York, U.S.A.

Wei Huang Department of Surgery, Center for Outcomes Research, University of Massachusetts Medical School, Worcester, Massachusetts, U.S.A.

Carlayne E. Jackson Department of Medicine/Neurology, University of Texas Health Science Center, San Antonio, Texas, U.S.A.

Thomas M. Jessell Department of Biochemistry and Molecular Biophysics, Columbia University, New York, New York, U.S.A.

Wendy Johnston Neurology, University of Alberta, Alberta, Canada

Jean-Pierre Julien Department of Anatomy and Physiology, Research Centre of CHUQ, Quebec City, Quebec, Canada

Edward J. Kasarskis Department of Neurology, University of Kentucky, Lexington, Kentucky, U.S.A.

Petra Kaufmann Department of Neurology, The Neurological Institute, Columbia University College of Physicians and Surgeons, New York, New York, U.S.A.

Hitoshi Kikuchi Department of Neurology, Columbia University, New York, New York, U.S.A., and Department of Neurology, Neurological Institute, Graduate School of Medical Sciences, Fukuoka, Japan

Jiming Kong Department of Human Anatomy and Cell Science, University of Manitoba, Winnipeg, Manitoba, Canada

Lisa S. Krivickas   Department of Physical Medicine and Rehabilitation, Spaulding Rehabilitation Hospital and Harvard Medical School, Boston, Massachusetts, U.S.A.

Noah Lechtzin   Department of Medicine & Neurology, Johns Hopkins University School of Medicine, Baltimore, Maryland, U.S.A.

Peter Nigel Leigh   Department of Clinical Neuroscience, Institute of Psychiatry, King's College London, London, U.K.

Catherine Lomen-Hoerth   University of California, San Francisco, California, U.S.A.

Lan Chi T. Luu   Department of Nutritional Sciences and Neurology, University of Kentucky, Lexington, Kentucky, U.S.A.

Valerie McGuire   Division of Epidemiology, Department of Health Research and Policy, Stanford University School of Medicine, Stanford, California, U.S.A.

Jesse McLean   Department of Cell Biology, Robarts Research Institute, London, Ontario, Canada

Vincent Meininger   Fédération de Neurolgie Mazarin, Hôpital Salpétrière, Paris, France

Robert G. Miller   Department of Neurosciences, California Pacific Medical Center, San Francisco, California, U.S.A.

Hiroshi Mitsumoto   Eleanor and Lou Gehrig MDA/ALS Research Center, Department of Neurology, Columbia University Medical Center, The Neurological Institute, New York, New York, U.S.A.

Dan H. Moore   Research Institute, California Pacific Medical Center, San Francisco, California, U.S.A.

Brian Murray   Department of Neurology, Mater Misericordiae University Hospital, Dublin, Ireland

Makiko Nagai   Department of Neurology, Columbia University, New York, New York, U.S.A.

Lorene M. Nelson   Division of Epidemiology, Department of Health Research and Policy, Stanford University School of Medicine, Stanford, California, U.S.A.

Rebecca Pruss   Trophos, S.A., Marseille, France

Serge Przedborski   Departments of Neurology and Pathology and the Center for Neurobiology and Behavior, Columbia University, New York, New York, U.S.A.

Seth Pullman   Department of Neurology, The Neurological Institute, Columbia University College of Physicians and Surgeons, New York, New York, U.S.A.

Judith G. Rabkin   Department of Psychiatry, New York Psychiatric Institute, New York, New York, U.S.A.

A. Radunović   Department of Clinical Neuroscience, Institute of Psychiatry, King's College London, London, U.K.

Cédric Raoul   Integrative Biosciences Institute, Ecole Polytechnique Fédérale de Lausanne (EPFL), Lausanne, Switzerland

Steve Ringel   Department of Neurology, University of Colorado Health Sciences Center, Denver, Colorado, U.S.A.

Wim Robberecht   Department of Neurology, School of Medicine, University Hospital Gasthuisberg, University of Leuven, Leuven, Belgium

Jeffrey Rosenfeld   Division of Neurology, Carolinas Neuromuscular/ALS-MDA Center, Carolinas Medical Center, Charlotte, North Carolina, U.S.A.

Mark Ross   Department of Neurology, Mayo Clinic, Scottsdale, Arizona, U.S.A. and the ALS CARE Study Group

Lewis P. Rowland   Department of Neurology, Neurological Institute of New York, Eleanor and Lou Gehrig MDA/ALS Research Center, Columbia University Medical Center, New York, New York, U.S.A.

Toyokazu Saito   Departments of Neurology and Rehabilitation, Kitasato University Higashi Hospital and Kitasato University School of Allied Health Science, Sagamihara, Kanagawa, Japan

Silke Schmidt   Department of Medicine, Center for Human Genetics, Duke University Medical Center, Durham, North Carolina, U.S.A.

C. A. Shaw   Departments of Ophthalmology, Neuroscience, and Experimental Medicine, University of British Columbia, Vancouver, British Columbia, Canada

Pamela J. Shaw   Academic Neurology Unit, Section of Neuroscience, University of Sheffield, Sheffield, U.K.

Teepu Siddique   Department of Neurology and Clinical Neurosciences and Department of Cell and Molecular Biology, Northwestern University Feinberg School of Medicine, Chicago, Illinois, U.S.A.

Ericka P. Simpson   Department of Neurology, Methodist Neurological Institute, Houston, Texas, U.S.A.

Michael J. Strong   Department of Clinical Neurological Sciences, The University of Western Ontario, and Robarts Research Institute, London, Ontario, Canada

Nigel P. Sykes   St. Christopher's Hospice and King's College, University of London, London, U.K.

Rup Tandan   Department of Neurology, University of Vermont, Burlington, Vermont, U.S.A.

Jeffery M. Vance   Department of Medicine, Center for Human Genetics, Duke University Medical Center, Durham, North Carolina, U.S.A.

Markus Weber   Department of Neurology, Kantonsspital St. Gallen, St. Gallen, Switzerland

J. M. B. Wilson   Department of Neuroscience, University of British Columbia, Vancouver, British Columbia, Canada

Zuoshang Xu   Department of Biochemistry and Molecular Pharmacology, University of Massachusetts Medical School, Worcester, Massachusetts, U.S.A.

Albert A. Yen   Department of Neurology, Methodist Neurological Institute, Houston, Texas, U.S.A.

1

History of ALS

Paul H. Gordon
Neurological Institute, Columbia University, New York, New York, U.S.A.

HISTORY OF AMYOTROPHIC LATERAL SCLEROSIS: WHO'S WHO IN ALS?

There are several comprehensive historical accounts of amyotrophic lateral sclerosis (ALS) (1–4). Rather than recapitulate these, I have written a chronological "Who's Who" in ALS, giving brief biographies of those whose names are linked with the disorder or who have made substantial contributions to the understanding of ALS. As medical science progresses, breakthroughs are made at an even more rapid rate. The importance of recent discoveries, including the identification of genetic mutations underlying some familial forms of ALS and the subsequent advent of the transgenic mouse model, is considerable. This chapter is a historical accounting, however, and in order that none should be offended, I have not included contemporary contributions or biographies of living people. Below is a chronological listing of "Who is Who in ALS," illustrating the stories of those, now deceased, who contributed greatly to the way we view ALS.

FRANCOIS-AMILCAR ARAN (1817–1861)

Aran grew up, trained, and worked in Paris. His main interest was general medicine, particularly cardiology, but early in his career he worked closely with Duchenne, and he is credited with the first clinical descriptions of motor neuron disease (MND). In 1848, he reported a patient with progressive muscle weakness, and correctly suspected a neurogenic cause (5). In 1850, he published a series of 11 additional patients (6). He named the new syndrome progressive muscular atrophy (PMA), and separated it from other causes of weakness. In the later report, he recorded "fibrillary movements" of muscle, providing an early description of fasciculation, and wrote of the connection between fasciculation and spinal cord disorders. In describing case 8, Lecomte, a 33-year-old professional clown with weakness and muscle reactivity suggestive of hyperreflexia, Aran gave one of the earliest accounts of ALS. He was probably also the first to report familial MND in his description of case 7, whose sister and two maternal uncles were affected.

Aran acknowledged Duchenne in the 1850 paper: "I owe a thousand thanks to my friend Duchenne de Boulogne who freely put at my disposal all his material..." (6,7). So great was Duchenne's influence that in the 1850 paper, Aran reversed his earlier opinion and concluded that PMA was caused by muscle disease, Duchenne's principle area of research. Case 6 had shown changes in muscle at autopsy, which probably swayed the thinking of the two. In that article, Aran also discussed treatment with galvanic stimulation, another favorite of Duchenne, but offered little hope of success.

After Aran's publication, Duchenne asserted that he had reported the syndrome, which he considered of muscular origin, a year earlier, though there are no publications to support that claim. Duchenne later studied the autopsy of Lecomte and again concluded that PMA was a muscle disease. It was left to Jean Baptiste Cruveilhier (1791–1874) to show conclusively in 1853 that Lecomte died of disease in the spinal cord with atrophy of anterior nerve roots (8). Ten years later, Duchenne also finally agreed and accepted the view that PMA originated in the central nervous system. Credit for the description of PMA was given partly to Duchenne, and the syndrome was often referred to as Aran–Duchenne disease.

Thereafter, Aran's interest in and commitment to neurology waned. In 1858, he became "Professeur Agrégé" at the Hospital St. Antoine, where he published on a broad range of topics. His later career fell into obscurity, possibly because of his lifelong interest in general medicine, not only neurology, and also because he suffered from poor health. There are no existing pictures of Aran and few other details of his life are available (4).

GUILLAUME BENJAMIN ARMAND DUCHENNE DE BOULOGNE (1806–1875)

Duchenne was the son of a long line of fishermen and sea captains in the region of Boulogne-sur-Mer, France. He studied medicine at the University of Paris, where he graduated in 1831. He returned to Boulogne and took up private practice, but after his young wife died in childbirth, it is said that he lived only for his patients and his scholarship (7). Lonely and isolated, he returned to Paris in 1842 and began to investigate the function of skeletal muscle using Faradic current, which he employed both as a treatment and a diagnostic tool (9).

He had no permanent appointment in Paris, but instead cared for patients in hospitals all over the city. He questioned and examined his patients compulsively, often in their homes, relying on his own observations and rigorous neurological examination. Because of his lack of appointment, established physicians at times disregarded him, but his reputation grew slowly, particularly after he began to write in 1855 (9). He published his early work on Faradic currents in a book *De L'électrisation Localisée* (10).

Duchenne gained prominence in neurology because of his work on muscle disorders. He identified pseudohypertrophic muscular dystrophy as a primary muscle disease (11), invented the "harpoon" (tissue punch) that he employed to perform percutaneous muscle biopsies, and made original descriptions of photography in muscle histopathology, tabetic locomotor ataxia, and poliomyelitis, among others. Late in life, he concentrated more on the nervous system, particularly on histology.

Duchenne made several contributions to understanding MND. His view that PMA was myogenic held sway for some time, and he received part of the credit for the early descriptions. Even though Duchenne did not publish the first cases, Aran's reports contain some patients who had been studied by Duchenne, and the two worked closely together. In 1860, Duchenne described progressive bulbar palsy (PBP), distinguishing it from PMA by the rapidity and severity of bulbar symptoms (12). His own description of PMA was published in 1872 (10).

Duchenne was of middle height and thickset, and he spoke with a provincial accent. In his time, he was considered unworldly and inarticulate, which may explain why some of his contemporaries, such as Charcot, had more prominent careers. Charcot nevertheless regarded Duchenne highly, and Charcot's lectures contain frequent acknowledgment of his work (7,9). Duchenne's many contributions eventually culminated in election to medical societies throughout Europe. He died in Paris of a cerebral hemorrhage in 1875 at the age of 69.

JEAN-MARTIN CHARCOT (1825–1893)

Charcot, the eminent French neurologist, psychiatrist, and anatomist, was born in Paris, the son of a carriage-maker. In his youth, he was undecided about whether to pursue a career in medicine or art, but settled on medicine and graduated from the University of Paris in 1853. He interned at the Salpêtrière Hospital, where he became an attending physician in 1862. Over the next 30 years, he created an internationally famous school of neurology at the Salpêtrière. He was elected Professor of Pathological Anatomy in 1872, succeeding Alfred Vulpian (1826–1887), and 10 years later, a special Chair of Nervous Diseases was created for him (13).

In nineteenth century Paris, the Salpêtrière, so named because the buildings were once Louis XIIIth's gunpowder store, was an asylum for the mentally ill and the destitute, most of them women with chronic diseases. When Charcot arrived, he found innumerable unclassified conditions among the several thousand patients housed there (13). He followed patients clinically for years, documenting the symptoms and signs that he later compared with autopsy findings. He took notes, made drawings, collected published articles, and finally assembled autopsy and microscopic illustrations that enabled him to identify the pathological abnormalities associated with specific syndromes (14,15). Charcot's clinicoanatomic method made him renowned and also later became the hallmark of neurology as a whole.

He described and classified many conditions at the Salpêtrière, and in doing so, he established clinical neurology as an autonomous discipline. He differentiated multiple sclerosis from Parkinson's disease, naming the latter (16). He characterized the complications of tabes dorsalis and cerebral aneurysms, and defined peroneal muscular atrophy along with Pierre Marie and Tooth (13), generating a lasting eponym. In 1862, Charcot and Vulpian were the first to describe ankle clonus. Charcot's observations were not limited to neurology, but encompassed all of medicine, particularly rheumatic, abdominal, and pulmonary disorders.

Perhaps his greatest contribution was his work with MND, in which he demonstrated the involvement of both the anterior roots and the lateral columns. Prior to Charcot's descriptions, Sir Charles Bell (1774–1842), a British anatomist and surgeon, showed that the anterior nerve roots supply muscles. In 1830, Bell described a woman with muscle weakness whose anterior spinal cord had the "consistency of cream" at autopsy (17). Charcot knew of Bell's findings, and he had also credited both Aran and Duchenne with the clinical description of PMA, calling it the Aran–Duchenne type of progressive muscular weakness.

In 1865, Charcot reported a woman with hysterical attacks who had remitting and later permanent contractures (spasticity) of the limbs (18). Autopsy showed sclerosis of the lateral columns but normal cells in the gray matter of the spinal cord. This case became one of the sentinel descriptions of primary lateral sclerosis (the condition that is now recognized as PLS was described in detail in 1875 by Heinrich Erb), which was used by Charcot to associate lateral column disease with the upper motor neuron sign of spasticity. Charcot may have been the first to use the term "primary lateral sclerosis." In 1869, Charcot and Joffroy recorded two cases of PMA with similar degeneration of the posterolateral spinal cord (19). They emphasized that pathologic changes in the lateral columns and in the anterior horns of the spinal cord often occurred together.

Beginning in 1866, Charcot gave lectures on neurological subjects that became popular because of the inclusion of pathophysiology with the clinical demonstrations, and because of the theatricality of his presentations (13–15). At these sessions, the Tuesday Lectures, symptoms, diagnoses, and pathology were discussed focusing on patients brought in for demonstration. Those in attendance included his pupils, Marie and Babinski among others, and physicians from throughout Paris. His lectures were published in French and subsequently translated into English (20,21).

During a series of Tuesday Lectures up to and during 1874 using 20 patients and five autopsy studies, Charcot defined the clinical and pathological features of ALS (22). Not only did he demonstrate the association of weakness, fasciculation, and spasticity but also pointed out the prognosis and lack of treatment that still plagues us today. He separated ALS from PMA based on differing prognosis and the sparing of bulbar function and absence of rigidity in the latter (22–24). He referred to PMA as "protopathic," or primary, and conditions with both amyotrophy and spasticity as "deuteropathic," with the gray matter lesions occurring secondary to those in the white matter. By naming the disorder amyotrophic lateral sclerosis, he implied a propagation of disease from white to gray matter. Progressive bulbar palsy was recognized by Duchenne in 1861 and Dejerine connected it with MND in 1883, but Charcot was the first to characterize and name ALS, establishing it as a distinct condition.

Charcot has been described as austere and haughty (13,14). He presided over the Tuesday Lectures in his palatial Parisian home, which was open to socialites and scientists alike, with an air of sophistication. Toward the end of his career, he concentrated on studies of hysteria, laying much of the groundwork for Sigmund Freud, who worked under him at the Salpêtrière. While away on a vacation, Charcot died suddenly at the age of 68 of pulmonary edema, probably the consequence of cardiac ischemia. The next generation continued the Charcot tradition in identifying the neurological findings that became the modern neurological examination.

JOSEPH FRANCOIS FELIX BABINSKI (1857–1932)

Babinski, of Polish decent, was born in Paris and became "chef de clinique" under Charcot, following Pierre Marie and preceding Gilles de la Tourette. In 1879, he became a general medical intern, and subsequently published articles on the muscle spindle and the pathology of multiple sclerosis (25).

He began his career at the Salpêtrière Hospital at the height of Charcot's tenure. He participated in all of Charcot's major efforts, and his early work was linked to Charcot's success. In 1890, Babinski passed the examination for "Médecin des Hôpitaux" and his path to academic neurology seemed certain. By the time he qualified for "agrégé" or Associate Professor, however, Charcot's influence had waned. Both Babinski and Tourette failed the examination, apparently due to internal political subterfuge by Charles Bouchard (26). Charcot had trained Bouchard and their names are connected with the aneurysms that precede cerebral hypertensive hemorrhage, but after Bouchard became a professor of pathology in 1879, his relationship with Charcot deteriorated. Bouchard administered the examination for "professeur agrégé" when Babinski was an unsuccessful candidate. Babinski never attempted the examination again, and as a result, he never received a faculty position at the Salpêtrière. Instead, he became chief of service, which included neurology and neurosurgery, at the nearby Pitié Hospital, where he stayed until he retired in 1922.

In his time, Babinski was described as meticulous, logical, and conscientious (27). He was a discerning histopathologist, and he founded the Societe de Neurologie de Paris along with Brissaud, Pierre Marie, Dejerine, and others. His concept of hysteria, which he called "pithiatisme" (curable by suggestion), was that its manifestations were produced by suggestion and abolished by counter suggestion (25). Babinski noted that many of the symptoms and signs attributed to hysteria disappeared from the Salpêtrière after Charcot's death.

Although Charcot believed in close observation and accurate clinical documentation, he had relied more on history than examination, and rarely touched his patients (28). Babinski, consciously or unconsciously, distanced himself from his mentor by emphasizing the importance of physical signs to diagnosis, and developed a reputation for a painstaking neurological examination (27). He was an early proponent of the use of the reflex hammer.

In 1896 in France, new neurological discoveries were presented at the Biological Society of Paris. It was here that Duchenne presented cases of muscular dystrophy, and Broca cases of non-fluent aphasia (25). In February 22, 1896, two years and five months after Charcot's death, Babinski (29) made a short presentation that was summarized in 28 lines in the minutes of the society about the extensor toe sign, and linked it to the disorders of the central nervous system. In later publications, he stressed that the sign occurred with disease throughout the pyramidal tracts (30). He delineated not only the extensor toe sign, but also the fanning of the toes, emphasized that the sign did not occur in hysteria, and finally pointed out that it was usually seen along with exaggerated tendon reflexes. He further described the sign in the newborn, an association also depicted in medieval and renaissance paintings showing the infant Jesus' upward-pointing toe in response to stimulation (31).

Babinski was a large man with an austere manner, embodying his Polish heritage, which was unusual in the nineteenth century Paris (27). He remained a bachelor his entire life, and lived with his older brother Henri, who may have been more celebrated in French society because he was a gourmet chef. One story tells of Babinski interrupting ward rounds to return home after receiving word that one of Henri's soufflés was nearly done. They lived a quiet life in a large apartment in the fashionable neighborhood surrounding the Paris Opera.

Babinski was not the first to observe the extensor toe sign, but he is justifiably credited for its interpretation (32). Babinski received many awards, particularly outside France, and was even nominated for the Nobel Prize (25). Parkinson's disease marred the last years of his life. He died from complications of the illness in 1932, following Henri by a year.

WILHELM HEINRICH ERB (1840–1921)

Erb, the son of a forester from Bavaria, was an internist and neurologist. He graduated from Munich University and trained with Friedreich at Heidelberg University, succeeding him there as professor after some years spent both in Heidelberg and Leipzig. Erb became to Germany what Charcot was to France, and Gowers to England: her leading neurologist (33). He classified and described muscular dystrophies (34), which he distinguished from spinal muscular atrophies, upper brachial plexus palsy (Erb paralysis) (35), and myasthenia gravis (36). In 1892, he confirmed the syphilitic origin of tabes dorsalis (37).

In 1875, he gave one of the seminal reports of a spastic paraparesis, later named as PLS, and described the disorder in detail (38). He cited Charcot's case of 1865, but he was hesitant to use the term "lateral sclerosis" because the cause was still unclear. He also noted that one of his cases developed amyotrophy after six years, pointing out the late transition of PLS to ALS that still confounds us today (2).

Erb was also known for his work on the tendon reflexes, and he was one of the first to use a reflex hammer (39). In 1875, Erb and Carl Friedrich Otto Westphal (1883–1890) described the knee reflex in the same journal (40,41). Although they reported the reflex together for the first time, there is evidence that non-professionals were aware of it previously (42). While Westphal mistakenly looked at the knee jerk as a local muscle phenomenon, Erb saw it as a true reflex arc. The maneuver was quickly adopted as a part of the neurological examination in Europe and the United States, and appeared in the literature routinely within 10 years (43).

Erb was described as gentlemanly and immaculate in appearance. He was known to be detached, compulsive, and punctual and to have a strong temper. He had a large international practice, and treated both the poor and wealthy aristocrats. His later years were personally difficult because three of his four sons died, the last on the first day of World War I. Erb himself died in 1921 at the age of 81. On the way home from listening to *Beethoven's Eroica symphony*, he caught a cold, developed pneumonia, and died within a few days (42).

JOSEPH JULES DEJERINE (1849–1917)

Joseph Jules Dejerine was born and brought up in Geneva where his father was a carriage owner. He was athletic in school; he boxed and swam and fished on Lake Leman. In 1871, at 22 years of age, he moved to Paris to study medicine, and arrived during a time of turmoil created by the revolution. He became Vulpian's most distinguished pupil at the Salpêtrière, and eventually Professor of Diseases of the Nervous System, succeeding Charcot (44).

Dejerine described many new muscle and nerve disorders. He investigated alexia, cerebral localization, muscular dystrophy, Friedreich ataxia, hereditary neuropathy, olivopontocerebellar atrophy, and the thalamic pain syndrome (44). His contribution to MND came in 1883 when he integrated progressive bulbar palsy and ALS, describing the former as but one component of the latter (45). He showed that autopsy findings in the brainstems from patients with the two conditions were indistinguishable.

He married Augusta Marie Klumpke (1859–1927), an American physician he met at the Salpêtrière. She had studied medicine in Paris, and through intellect, courage, and persistence, became the first woman to receive the title of "interne des hôpitaux" at the Salpêtrière. When Dejerine died during World War I after becoming exhausted by his work in an army hospital, his wife carried on his clinical and research activities. She described a characteristic paralysis after brachial plexus lesions, assuring her place in eponymic fame, and she contributed to the understanding of neuroanatomy (46).

SIR WILLIAM RICHARD GOWERS (1845–1915)

William Richard Gowers, who was born in a small village in the north of London, was a founder of neurology in nineteenth century England. In 1870, he became a medical registrar at the National Hospital in Queen Square, London, which had been established 10 years earlier. He was house physician and then secretary to Jenner, before being appointed to the staffs of University College Hospital and the National Hospital in 1872. He later became Professor of Clinical Medicine at the University of London (47).

Gowers and his colleague, Hughlings Jackson, were largely responsible for building the National Hospital into one of the world's leading neurological institutions. His best known work was the two-volume *A Manual of Diseases of The Nervous System*, first published in 1886, in which he gathered the clinical knowledge of the time into a work that became known as the "bible of neurology" worldwide (48). It is still considered one of the most outstanding single-author textbooks of neurology ever written (49). He created numerous illustrations himself, and wrote many of the original drafts in shorthand, which he used to the point of obsession in his clinical work (50). He made especially important contributions to the understanding of muscle disease, epilepsy, and migraine headache.

By 1892, he postulated that PMA, progressive bulbar palsy, and ALS were parts of one single motor system degeneration. He stated in his textbook that all of his cases of PMA also had degeneration of the pyramidal tracts. He did not think Charcot's use of the term "ALS" was correct because it implied that atrophy of anterior horn cells was secondary to degeneration of the pyramidal tracts. Gowers concluded that PMA, PBP, and ALS were essentially one disease, and that the clinical manifestations were determined by the timing and extent of the motor neuron degeneration (51).

Gowers was an astute clinician and consummate observer, and his approach to patients helped define the modern neurological examination. He provided such clear illustrations of the method used by children with Duchenne dystrophy to rise from the ground to a standing position that it is still referred to as the "Gowers sign." He was a proponent of using the ophthalmoscope as part of the neurologist's examination, and he coined the term "knee jerk" (52). In the second (1893) edition of his textbook, Gowers described rigidity of the limbs, along with increased tendon jerks and clonus after a lesion of the pyramidal tracts (53).

Gowers was compulsive, philosophical, and passionate and was described as having a look between a Wise Man and the Ancient Mariner. He was knighted in 1897.

HIROSHI KAWAHARA (1858–1918)

Kawahara, who was born in April 5, 1858 in a small town near Nagasaki, became a pioneer of modern neurology in Japan. His great grandfather was a well-known haiku poet, but he chose to study medicine, and graduated from Tokyo Medical School, now called the University of Tokyo. He then assumed a professorship of pathology and internal medicine at the Aichi Medical School, now called Nagoya University School of Medicine, where he later became chair.

Throughout his career, his principal focus was neurology (54). He developed a systematic approach to the teaching and study of neurology, and published one of the first Japanese textbooks on clinical neurology in 1897 for which he had created many of the original drawings (55). He is credited with the first description of X-linked spinobulbar muscular atrophy, later called Kennedy disease, having published the clinical description and hereditary pattern in 1897 (56). He described the disease in two brothers and their maternal uncle.

Kawahara suffered from lifelong pulmonary tuberculosis. He retired in 1897 because of his illness, and died from it in 1918, at the age of 59 years.

KINNOSUKE MIURA (1864–1950)

Miura, a Japanese physician and pupil of Charcot, gave the first detailed description of ALS in Japan. Miura, the son of an ophthalmologist, was born on March 21, 1864, in Tominary Village in northern Japan. He graduated from the Medical College of Tokyo University and later accompanied the prince of Japan on a tour of Europe (57). At that time, medical education in Japan was given in German, in which Miura had written on the effect of ephedrine on the pupil (58). After traveling with the prince, he remained in Germany in 1891 to work with Erb, among others. He moved to Paris in 1893, where he studied neurology at the Salpêtrière.

It was in Paris, working under Charcot, that Miura developed his interest in MND. After returning to Japan, he became a professor at the University of Tokyo, where he described the first Japanese cases of ALS. He published a clinicopathological study of ALS (59), and in 1911 he was the first to report the high frequency of ALS in the Kii peninsula on the main island of Honshu (60).

Miura became fluent in English, French, German, Greek, and Latin. In 1903, he founded the Association for Psychiatry and Neurology in Japan, thus establishing neurology as an independent specialty. In 1949, he was awarded the Order of Cultural Merit, Japan's highest award for scientific contributions to the country.

Miura was widowed in 1927, and much of his estate was reportedly taken from him following World War II (61). He practiced until his last day. At age 87, while on his way to see a patient, he collapsed and was found unconscious in the street. An autopsy later showed that he died from a pontine hemorrhage.

W. RUSSELL BRAIN (1895–1966)

Lord Brain was a preeminent English neurologist. He trained at Oxford and at the London Hospital before entering neurology as a junior staff member at the Maida Vale Hospital for Nervous Diseases. He became a consultant at both hospitals and practiced at them for his entire professional life (62).

Lord Brain's research contributions were broad and largely clinical. He defined first, or most completely, carpal tunnel syndrome, dysthyroid ophthalmopahty, paraneoplastic syndromes, the dysphasias, cervical spondylotic myelopathy, limbic encephalitis, and Hashimoto encephalopathy. His two textbooks, *Diseases of the Nervous System* and *Clinical Neurology*, were written clearly and precisely, and both went into several editions (63). Following the lead of Gowers, he grouped PMA, PBP, and ALS into one disease. He conceived the term "motor neuron disease" in 1933, which is still used, rather than ALS particularly in England (64).

He guided public and political opinion in public health policy. His honors included the presidency of the Royal College of Physicians of London and of the Association of British Neurologists, Fellowship of the Royal Society, and honors bestowed by foreign institutions. He was editor of *Brain* from 1954 until his death in 1966. At the time of his death, he was acknowledged to be the foremost neurologist in England because of his contributions to so many diverse areas (62).

HENRY LOUIS GEHRIG (1903–1941)

Lou Gehrig was born in Manhattan on June 19, 1903 to German immigrant parents. He had three siblings who all died in infancy, and he grew up near poverty in part because his father drank heavily. He attended Columbia University on a football scholarship for two years before joining the New York Yankees baseball team in 1923 (65).

On June 1, 1925, "Columbia Lou" replaced injured first baseman Wally Pipp in the Yankee's starting lineup, where he played every day for the next 14 years. Known as the "Iron Horse," he played in 2130 consecutive games, and was never out of the lineup until May 2, 1939. He was not only one of the baseball's most durable athletes, but also became one of the game's greatest hitters. Gehrig was the cleanup hitter, where he batted behind Babe Ruth. He hit 300 or more in 12 consecutive seasons; drove in 100 or more runs in 13 consecutive seasons; batted in 150 or more runs in seven seasons; drove in an American League record 184 runs in 1931; hit 23 grand slam home runs, still a major league record; won the triple crown in 1934; won the Most Valuable Player award four times; and played in seven World Series (66). When he retired, his career batting average was 340, he had hit 493 homeruns, and had batted in 1995 runs. He was elected to the Baseball Hall of Fame in 1939, and the Yankees retired his number 4 Jersey, making him the first player to receive the honor.

By early 1939, Gehrig was no longer able to play baseball. He ended his consecutive game streak by taking himself out of the Yankees lineup at the age of 35. A testament to his durability and skill is that he probably played some of the 1937 season and the entire 1938 season with symptomatic ALS (67). In the winter following the 1937 season, Gehrig starred in a western film called *Rawhide*. In the movie, he appears to have atrophy of hand muscles and twice he arises from the ground using a partial Gowers maneuver. His batting average in 1938 was 295, 45 points below his career average. Following the 1938 season, his weakness became more noticeable. Eleanor, his wife, noticed that Lou, normally a strong ice skater, fell several times while skating. In the spring of 1939, teammates noticed Gehrig swing and miss 19 straight fastballs during batting practice and fall clumsily in the clubhouse (68). Once the season began, it was obvious he could no longer play. He had difficulty stooping for grounders and in getting to first base in time to receive throws. He batted less than 200, and on May 2, 1939, he benched himself. Later that summer, he was diagnosed with ALS.

In 1940, he worked for the City of New York as a parole commissioner. By the spring of 1941, however, Gehrig was confined to his home, and by May 1941, he was bedridden and barely able to move. He died on June 2, 1941, at the age of 37 years (68).

Lou was physically active and durable, as were other athletes who developed ALS. This has led to the hypothesis that athleticism may be a risk factor for ALS. Over the course of his consecutive game streak, Gehrig suffered a broken thumb, a broken toe, and back spasms. X-rays taken during his career showed 17 healed fractures in all (69).

Lou, typical of those with ALS, was also a quiet and noble person. He handled his illness the same way he conducted himself in health, seeing himself "not a mere victim of a form of paralysis but a symbol of hope for thousands of sufferers of the same disorder" (70). When he took himself out of the lineup and eventually died of ALS, he became an American folk hero. From that time forward, in the United States at least, ALS became widely known as Lou Gehrig's disease, one of only a few disorders to have derived its eponym from one of its victims.

Gehrig's contributions to ALS go beyond the association with his name. At the time of her death, his wife left part of their estate to the Columbia University Medical Center where the Eleanor and Lou Gehrig MDA/ALS Research Center is located. Permission to use the Gehrig name was gained with the approval of Mrs. Gehrig's lawyer, George Pollack. Proceeds of the sale of any merchandise with Gehrig's name or likeness are directed to charitable causes.

LEONARD T. KURLAND (1921–2001)

Leonard Kurland was born on December 24, 1921 in Baltimore, the youngest of 10 children of Russian immigrant parents. He obtained his bachelor's degree from Johns Hopkins University and MD degree from the University of Maryland. He received Masters and Doctorate of Public Health from Harvard and Johns Hopkins Universities, respectively (71).

He was the first Chief of the Epidemiology Branch of the National Institute of Neurological Diseases and Blindness, where he established the initial epidemiological studies of ALS. In 1964, he became the Chair of the Department of Medical Statistics and Population Genetics at the Mayo Clinic. There he helped develop epidemiological studies from the medical record system that contained lifelong records of the residents of Rochester and Olmsted County, Minnesota, a resource that has lead to over 1000 publications (71).

Kurland became known as the "father of neuroepidemiology." In his early career, he carried out population studies of multiple sclerosis and showed the geographical distribution of the disease (72). Some of his other works include epidemiologic studies of the effects of Agent Orange during the Vietnam War, the relationship between swine flu vaccine and Guillain-Barré syndrome (73), and the relationship between breast implants and connective tissue disorders (74).

With Donald Mulder, he organized the first epidemiological study of the Chamorro population of Guam, and helped characterize the ALS–Parkinson–Dementia complex (75,76). There had been mention of ALS on Mariana Island in a sanitary report as early as 1900 (77), and Okaya had described a case of Guamanian parkinsonism in 1936 (78). Harry Zimmerman (1901–1995), who was an Assistant Professor of Pathology at Yale before World War II and then a neuropathologist at the Montefiore Hospital in New York and later the first Dean of the Albert Einstein College of Medicine, was the first to report the high incidence of ALS on Guam (79). During the war, Zimmerman was part of a Navy research unit assigned to study tropical diseases (76). Zimmerman landed on Guam in mid-January 1945 and carried out autopsies at the local hospital. By May, he had examined at least seven cases of ALS. Two teams of naval physicians confirmed Zimmerman's observations and reported the results between 1952 and 1953. Kurland read the reports, recognized the opportunity, and visited Guam for the first time in 1953. In 1954, Mulder, Kurland, and colleagues were the first to report the combination of parkinsonism and ALS (75). The full extent of the clinical and pathological features of the Guamanian ALS–Parkinson–Dementia complex were later described by Asao Hirano, who followed Zimmerman as chief neuropathologist at Montefiore, and colleagues in 1961 (80). Kurland and Mulder also established the frequency of familial ALS at 5% to 10% (81). Kurland further studied the role of trauma in the pathogenesis of ALS (82), and together with Forbes Norris, he helped organize the first international symposium on ALS in 1969 (1,3).

His students considered Kurland a kind and remarkable human being, a great teacher, researcher, and writer (83). He died of heart attack at the age of 79 in 2001. He was survived by his wife who was 59 years old, five children, and eight grandchildren.

FORBES H. NORRIS (1928–1993)

Forbes Norris was born in Richmond, Virginia, to schoolteacher parents. His father had become a school superintendent (Dee H. Norris, personal communication). He attended public schools, followed by Harvard University and Medical School. He interned at Johns Hopkins University and did his neurology residency at the National Institutes of Health, where he studied clinical electrophysiology and neuromuscular disease with G. Milton Shy, and authored his first book *The EMG: A Guide and Atlas for Practical Electromyography* (84). He completed a senior fellowship at the Maida Vale Hospital of the University London under Lord Brain, and then became Associate Professor of Neurology at the University of Rochester, New York, before moving to the San Francisco area. He subsequently held positions in California academic institutions from 1966 to 1993, including associate professorships at the University of California, San Francisco, and at the University of the Pacific. He became Scientific Director and Vice President of the ALS and Neuromuscular Research Foundation at California Pacific Medical Center.

With Donald Mulder, Norris was one of the first clinical neurologists to restrict his research to ALS (Lewis P. Rowland, personal communication). He sponsored several landmark symposia that resulted in coeditorship of four books, including the *Remote Effects of Cancer on The Nervous System* (with Lord Brain) (85), *Motor Neuron Diseases* (with Leonard Kurland) (86), *Recent Advances of Toxicology and Epidemiology in ALS* (with F. C. Rose) (87), and *Practical Management of ALS* (with Hiroshi Mitsumoto) (88). He conducted studies of ALS based on his own observations, advocated the use of quantitative outcome measures for clinical trials (89), and developed the "Norris ALS Scale," one of the first functional rating scales for the disease. His interests also included the pathology of motor neuron diseases, the natural history of ALS, and respiratory treatment for patients with ALS (Robert G. Miller, personal communication).

Along with his wife and partner, Dee Holden Norris, he promoted aggressive symptomatic management of ALS. Although deemed idiosyncratic at the time, their ideas led to newly accepted approaches to the treatment of ALS. They helped pioneer the use of mechanical ventilation in patients with ALS, used feeding tubes before the development of the percutaneous endoscopic gastrostomy, coordinated home visits for ALS patients, and used the full continuum of health care for patients with ALS. Forbes Norris also made important epidemiologic contributions, collecting data about his own patients in the San Francisco area, and he was the first to emphasize the long duration of PMA.

He had a twinkle in his eye and a love for neurology that was palpable. He established deep and authentic relationships with patients and developed friendships with others in the field. Forbes Norris and his wife hosted ALS experts who visited California, and he was helpful to other clinicians and investigators around the world who looked to him to share his experience. Patients loved him deeply and both he and Dee were completely devoted to them.

He was recognized for his gentle humanity and was deemed a model for physicians to emulate for his compassionate approach to patients. When he died of colon cancer at the age of 65, the ALS Center at California Pacific Medical Center was renamed "The Forbes Norris MDA/ALS Research Center," a fitting tribute to the man who had devoted his career to helping those with the disease.

EDWARD H. LAMBERT (1915–2003)

Lambert was born in Minneapolis on August 30, 1915 to a second-generation Norwegian mother and a fourth-generation French-Scottish father. After his family moved to Chicago during the depression, he obtained his bachelors, masters, medical, and Ph.D. (physiology) degrees at the University of Illinois (90).

Early in his career, Lambert studied cardiovascular physiology. His doctoral thesis was on the effects of oxygen and carbon dioxide concentrations on blood flow and blood pressure. In 1943, he moved to the Mayo Clinic, where he later became Professor, to work in the Aero Medical Unit on acceleration-induced loss of consciousness in aviators. During World War II, he became a key investigator of in-flight testing, for which he was awarded the Presidential Certificate of Merit in 1947.

After the war, he began his pioneering work on the electrophysiology of neuromuscular diseases. Along with Lee M. Eaton and Douglas Rooke, he identified the myasthenic syndrome and used physiological criteria that distinguished it from myasthenia gravis (91). By 1969, he had also established electromyographical criteria for the diagnosis of ALS. Earlier papers had discussed the value of electrophysiology in the diagnosis of ALS, but Lambert's two publications firmly established the utility of EMG in the disease, assisting in the diagnosis and excluding other disorders (92,93). Lambert outlined features, since referred to as the "Lambert criteria," that he considered supportive of the diagnosis of ALS. He was careful to point out that the EMG findings in ALS are not pathognomonical, and also emphasized the importance of fasciculation potentials, which have been given less status in later diagnostic criteria (93). His reports on the electrophysiology of ALS are still considered unmatched for their broad description and deep insight (94).

He was the president of the American Association of Electromyography and Electrodiagnosis in 1956, and was awarded its lifetime achievement award. He was on the advisory board of *Muscle and Nerve,* and was an honorary member of the American Neurological Association. He died in Rochester at the age of 88 years. His fellow researcher and wife, Vanda Lennon, survived him.

CONCLUSION

I have outlined the histories of some of the founders in the field of ALS, those who laid the groundwork for what has now become a very active discipline. Each year sees an increasing amount of resources contributed to ALS. A search yielded 368 publications on ALS between 1970 and 1974. Between 2001 and 2004, there were over 2000 articles. Recent decades have also seen advances in patient care. In 1987, the Muscular Dystrophy Association appointed five specialized ALS Centers that were considered expert in the care and research of ALS. Today there are more than 30 centers across the United States. Similarly, the ALS Association, which began with four centers in 1994, now has 19 certified ALS Centers and another 39 ALS clinics. Most of these provide multidisciplinary care to patients, emphasizing means to improve the quality of life. At the same time, the ALS CARE database was developed and the American Academy of Neurology created practice parameters with the hope of standardizing the use of effective therapies for patients with ALS and tracking outcomes to raise the overall standard of care. Government support for clinical trials has also increased. The National Institutes of Health did not fund clinical trials in ALS until the late 1990s. Now there are several large studies funded every year.

The discovery of mutations in the superoxide dismutase gene underlying some familial forms of ALS, the subsequent advent of the transgenic mouse model, and FDA approval of the first treatment, riluzole, for ALS are recent major accomplishments. The work of our forbearers has been carried forward into our generation. Surely, the future will see even greater gains in areas of basic science research, translation to clinical trials, and in patient care, as we stand on the shoulders of our predecessors.

REFERENCES

1. Mitsumoto H, Chad DA, Pioro EP. History, terminology and classification of ALS. In: Mitsumoto H, Chad DA, Pioro EP, eds. Amyotrophic Lateral Sclerosis. Contemporary Neurology Series No. 49. New York: Oxford University Press, 1998:3–17.
2. Tyler HR, Shefner J. Amyotrophic lateral sclerosis. In: Vinken PJ, Bruyn GW, Klawans HL, eds. Diseases of the Motor System. New York: Elsevier, 1975:Vol. 59:169–215.
3. Norris RH. Adult spinal motor neuron disease. Progressive muscular atrophy (Aran' disease) in relation to amyotrophic lateral sclerosis. In: Vinken PJ, Bruyn GW, DeJong JMBV, eds. System Disorders and Atrophies Vol. 22. Amsterdam: North-Holland, 1975: 1–56.
4. Aran FA. Revue clinique des hopitaux et hospices. Un Med 1848; 2:553–554, 557–558.
5. Aran FA. Recherches sur une maladie non encore decrite du systeme musculaire (atrophie musculaire progressive). Arch Gen Med 1850; 24:15–35.
6. Pearce JMS. Some contributions of Duchenne de Boulogne (1806–75). J Neurol Neurosurg Psychiatry 1999; 67:322.
7. Cruveilhier J. Sur la paralysie musculaire progressive atrophique. Arch Gen Med 1853; 91:561–603.
8. Adams RD. Armand duchenne. In: Haymaker W, Schiller F, eds. The Founders of Neurology. 2nd ed. Springfield, IL: Charles C. Thomas, 1970:1–56.
9. Duchenne GBA. L'Electricisation Localisee. 3rd ed. 1872, pp. 486–563. Translated by GV Poore. Selections from the Clinical Works of Dr. Duchenne (de Boulogne). London: The New Sydenham Society, 1883:42–87.
10. Duchenne G, Joffroy A. De l'atrophie aigue et chronique des cellules nerveuses de la moelle et du bulbe rachidien. Propos d'une observation de paralysie labio-glosso-laryngee. Arch Physiol 1870; 3:499.

11. Duchenne GBA. Arch Gen Med (Paris) 1868; 11:5–25, 179–209, 305–312, 421–443, 552–588.
12. Wechsler IS. Jean martin charcot. In: Haymaker W, Schiller F, eds. The Founders of Neurology. Springfield, IL: Charles C Thomas, 1970.
13. Rowland LP. How amyotrophic lateral sclerosis got its name. The clinical-pathologic genius of Jean-Martin Charcot. Arch Neurol 2001; 58:512–515.
14. Goetz CG. Amyotrophic lateral sclerosis: early contributions of Jean-Martin Charcot. Muscle Nerve 2000; 23:336–343.
15. Charcot J-M. De la paralysie agitante. Oeuvres completes. Paris: Bureaux du Progres medical; Vol. 1; 1880, 155–189. (English translation: On paralysis agitans. In: Sigerson G, ed. Translator. Lectures on the disease of the nervous system. Philadelphia: HC Lea, 1881:247–260).
16. Bell C. The Nervous System of the Human Body. London: Longman, Rees, Orme, Brown and Green, 1830:132–136, 160–161.
17. Carcot JM. Sclerose des cordons lateraux de la moelle epiniere chez une femme hysterique atteinte de contracture permanente des quatres members. L'Union Med 1865; 25:451–461, 467–472.
18. Charcot JM, Joffroy A. Deux cas d'atrophie musculaire progressive. Arch Physiol 1869; 2:354–367.
19. Charcot JM. Charcot the Clinician: The Tuesday Lessons. In: Goetz CG, ed. Translator (with commentary). New York, Raven Press, 1987.
20. Charcot J-M. Charcot the Clinician: The Tuesday Lessons. In: Goetz CG, ed. Translator. New York, Raven Press, 1987.
21. Charcot JM. De la sclerose laterale amyotrophique. Prog Med 1874; 23:235–237, 24: 341–342, 29:453–455.
22. Charcot J-M. Amyotrophies spinales deuteropathiques sclerose laterale amyotrophique. In: Oeuvrews Completes. Paris: Bureaux du Progres Medical. Vol. 2, 1874:234–248 (Einglish translation: Deuteropathic spinal amyotrophies: amyotrophic lateral sclerosis. Sigerson G, ed. Translator. Lectures on diseases of the nervous system. London. New Sydenham Society, 1881:180–191.
23. Charcot JM. De la sclerose laterale amyotrophique. Prog Med 1874; 2:325–327, 341–342, 453–455.
24. Goetz CG. History of the extensor plantar response: Babinski and Chaddock signs. Semin Neurol 2002; 22:391–398.
25. Iragui VJ. The Charcot-Bouchard controversy. Arch Neurol 1986; 43:290–295.
26. Lance JW. The babinski sign. J Neurol Neurosurg Psychiatry 2002; 73:360–362.
27. Goetz CG, Bonduelle M, Gelfand T. Jean-Martin Charcot: Constructing Neurology. New York: Oxford University Press, 1995.
28. Babinski J. Sur le reflexe cutane plantaire dans certains affections organiques du systeme nerveux central. C R Soc Biol 1896; 48:207–208.
29. Babinski J. De l'abduction des orteils (signe de l' eventail). Rev Neurol (Paris) 1903; 11:728–729.
30. Massey WE, Sanders L. Babinski's sign in medieval, renaissance and baroque art. Arch Neurol 1989; 46:85–88.
31. Van Gijn J. The Babinski sign and the pyramidal syndrome. J Neurol Neurosurg Psychiatr 1975; 38:180–186.
32. Viets HR. Heinrich Erb. In: Haymaker W, Schiller F, eds. The Founders of Neurology. 2nd ed. Springfield, IL: Charles C. Thomas, 1970.
33. Erb WH, Schultze F. Arch Psychiat (Berlin) 1879; 9:369–388.
34. Erb WH. Verh Naturhist Med Verein (Heidelberg) 1877; 1:130–136.
35. Erb WH. Arch Psychiat (Berlin) 1879; 9:336–350.
36. Erb WH. Die Ätiologie der tabes. Samml Klin Vortr 1892; 53:515–542.
37. Erb WH. Uber einen wenig bekanten spinalen symptomen-complex. Berl klin Wochenschr 1875; 12:357–359.

38. Louis ED. Erb and Westphal: simultaneous discovery of the deep tendon reflexes. Semin Neurol 2002; 22:385–390.
39. Erb WH. Uber sehnenreflexe bei Gesunden und Ruckenmarkskranken. Archiv fur Psychiat und Nervenkrankh 1875; 5:792–802.
40. Westphal CO. Uber einige Bewegungs-Erscheinungen an gelahmten Gliedern. Arch fur Psychiat und Nervenkrankh 1875; 5:803–834.
41. McHenry LC. Garrison's History of Neurology. Springfield, IL: Charles C. Thomas, 1969.
42. Hamilton AM. The value of absent "tendon-reflex" as a diagnostic sign in locomotor ataxia, with an analysis of eight cases. Boston Med Surg J 1878; 99:781–788.
43. Zabriskie EG. Joseph Jules Dejerine. In: Haymaker W, Schiller F, eds. The Founders of Neurology. 2nd ed. Springfield, IL: Charles C. Thomas, 1970.
44. Dejerine J. Etude anatomique et clinique sur la paralysie labio-glosso-laryngee. Arch Physiol Norm Pathol 1883; 2:180–227.
45. Satran R. Augusta Dejerine-Klumpke. First woman intern in Paris hospitals. Ann Int Med 1974; 80:260–264.
46. Tyler KL. William Richard Gowers (1845–1915). J Neurol 2003; 250:1012–1013.
47. Gowers WR. A manual of diseases of the nervous system. 1–3rd ed. 1886–1899.
48. Critchley M. Sir William Gowers 1845–1915. London: Heinemann, 1949.
49. Tyler KL, Roberts D, Tyler RH. The shorthand publications of Sir William Richard Gowers. Neurology 2000; 55:289–293.
50. Gowers WR. A Manual of Diseases of the Nervous System. Vol. 1. 3rd ed. Philadelphia: Blakiston, 1899:531–558.
51. Foster Kennedy. William gowers. In: Haymaker W, Schiller F, eds. The Founders of Neurology. 2nd ed. Springfield IL: Charles C. Thomas, 1970.
52. Gowers CR. A manual of diseases of the nervous system. 2nd ed. Philadelphia: Blakiston, 1893:83.
53. Takahashi A. Hiroshi kawahara (1858–1918). J Neurol 2001; 248:241–242.
54. Kawahara H. Naiko-Iko (comprehensive Textbook of Internal Medicine). Vol. 1. Tokyo: Neurology, Handaya Medical publishers, 1897.
55. Kawahara H. A family of progressive bulbar palsy. Aichi Med J 1897; 16:3–4.
56. Iwata M. Kinnosuke miura (1864–1950). J Neurol 2000; 247:725–726.
57. Mirua K. Vorlaufige mitteilung uber ephedrine, ein neues mydriaticum. Berl Klin Wochschr 1887; 38:707.
58. Miura K. On amyotrophic lateral sclerosis. Sinkeigau Zasshi 1902; 1:1–15 (Japanese).
59. Miura K. Amyotrophische lateralsklerose unter dem bilde von sog. Bulbarparalyse. Neurol Jpn 1911; 10:366–369.
60. Katsunuma S. Memorial of late professor emeritus Kinnosuke Miura. Folia Psychiatr Neurol Jpn 1951; 4:371–373.
61. Lord Brain. Br Med J 1967; 1:56–57.
62. Brain WR. In: Diseases of the Nervous System. London: Oxford University Press, 1933.
63. Brain WR, Walton JN. Brain's Disease of the Nervous System. London: Oxford University Press, 1969:595–606.
64. Shampo MA, Kyle RA. Lou Gehrig—amyotrophic lateral sclerosis. Mayo Clin Proc 1993; 68:929.
65. Lou Gehrig Baseball Statistics by Baseball Almanac. http://www.baseball-almanac.com/players/player.php?p=gehrilo01
66. Kasarskis EJ, Winslow M. When did Lou Gehrig's personal illness begin? Neurology 1989; 39:1243–1245.
67. Cavicke D, O'Leary JP. Lou Gehrig's death. Am Surg 2001; 67:393–395.
68. Innes AM, Chudley E. Genetic landmarks through philately—Henry Louis 'Lou' Gehrig and amyotrophic lateral sclerosis. Clin Genet 1999; 56:425–427.
69. Kase M. World mourns deeply as death takes Lou Gehrig. Journal-American. From the Lou Gehrig file at the Baseball Hall of Fame, Cooperstown, NY. N Y J-Am 1941:18.
70. Whisnant JP, Mulder DW. Leonard T. Kurland: 1921–2001. Ann Neurol 2002; 51:663.

71. Kurland LT. Multiple sclerosis morbidity and mortality studies in the United States and Canada. Trans Am Neurol Assoc 1950; 75:264–267.
72. Langmuir AD, Bregman DJ, Kurland LT, et al. An epidemiologic and clinical evaluation of Guillain Barre syndrome reported in association with the administration of seine influenza vaccines. Am J Epidemiol 1984; 119:841–879.
73. Gabriel SE, O'Fallon WM, Kurland LT, et al. Risk of connective tissue disease and other disorders after breast implantation. N Engl J Med 1994; 330:1697–1702.
74. Kurland LT, Mulder DW. Epidemiologic investigations of amyotrophic lateral sclerosis: 1. Preliminary report on geographic distribution, with special reference to the Mariana Islands, including clinical and pathologic observations. Neurology 1954; 4:355–378, 438–448.
75. Rowland LP. NINDS at 50. New York: Demos Press, 2003:124–128.
76. Spencer PS. Guam ALS-Parkinsonism-Dementia: a long-latency neurotoxic disorder caused by "slow toxin(s)" in food? Can J Neurol Sci 1987; 14:347–357.
77. Okaya N. Gamu shimajima min chamoro-zoku (mikuronesyajin) ni okeru shinsen mahi no shorei (a case of paralysi agitans in a Chamorro, Micronesia, from Guam, US Territory). Tokyo Med j 1936; 2997:2517–2518.
78. Zimmerman HM. Monthly report to medical officer in command. U.S. Naval Medical Research unit No. 2, 1945.
79. Hirano A, Malamud N, Kurland L. Parkinsonism-dementia complex, an endemic disease on the Island of Guam. II Pathological features. Brain 1961; 84:662–679.
80. Kurland LT, Mulder DW. Epidemiologic investigations of amyotrophic lateral sclerosis. Familial aggregation indicative of dominant inheritance. Neurology 1955; 5:182–196.
81. Kurland LT, Radhakrishnan K, Smith GE, et al. Mechanical trauma as a risk factor in classic amyotrophic lateral sclerosis: lack of epidemiologic evidence. J Neurol Sci 1992; 113:133–143.
82. Radhakrishnan K. In memory of Leonard T. Kurland, the father of neuroepidemiology. Neurol India 2002; 50:377–378.
83. Norris FH. The EMG: A Guide and Atlas for Practical Electromyography. New York, London: Grune and Stratto, 1963.
84. Brain Lord, Norris FH. The Remote Effects of Cancer on the Nervous System. New York, London: Grune and Stratton, 1965.
85. Norris FH, Kurland LT. Motor Neuron Diseases. New york, London: Grune and Stratton, 1968.
86. Rose FC, Norris FH, eds. Amyotrophic Lateral Sclerosis: Recent Advances in Toxicology and Epidemiology. London: Smith-Gordon, 1990.
87. Amyotrophic Lateral Sclerosis: Comprehensive Management and Treatment. In: Mitsumoto H, Norris FT Jr, eds. New York: Demos Publisher, 1994:1–20.
88. ALS-From Charcot to the Present and into the Future. The Forbes H. Norris (1928–1993) Memorial Volume. In: Clifford Rose F, ed. Amyotrophic Lateral Sclerosis:3. Smith-Gordon/Nishimura (London) 1994.
89. Daube JR, Edward H. Lambert. Ann Neurol 2003; 54:690–691.
90. Simpson JA. Electrophysiology of neuromuscular junction disease: an appreciation of the contributions of Edward H. Lambert. Muscle Nerve 1982; 5:S6–S11.
91. Lambert EH, Mulder DW. Electromyographic studies in amyotrophic lateral sclerosis. Proc Staff Meet Mayo Clin 1957; 32:441–446.
92. Lambert EH. Electromyography in amyotrophic lateral sclerosis. In: Norris FH, Kurland LT, eds. Motor Neuron Diseases. New york: Grune and Stratton, 1969: 135–153.
93. Wilbourn AJ. Clinical neurophysiology in the diagnosis of amyotrophic lateral sclerosis: the Lambert and the el Escorial criteria. J Neurol Sci 1998; 160:S25–S29.

2
Epidemiology of ALS

Valerie McGuire and Lorene M. Nelson
Division of Epidemiology, Department of Health Research and Policy,
Stanford University School of Medicine, Stanford, California, U.S.A.

INTRODUCTION

Amyotrophic lateral sclerosis (ALS), or Lou Gehrig's disease, is the most common motor neuron disease. ALS is a late-onset rapidly deteriorating neurological disorder characterized by the selective death of motor neurons in the brain and spinal cord that innervate skeletal muscles, with clinical symptoms of progressive weakness, muscle wasting, and spasticity (1). The median survival with ALS is usually three years and the cause of death is respiratory failure, pneumonia, or cardiac arrhythmias. Scientific advancements have been made over the past several years to understand the Mendelian forms of ALS and other diseases of the motor neuron. The most significant advancement has been the identification of genes causing some forms of familial ALS (2,3), the spinal muscular atrophies (4,5), and frontotemporal dementia (6). The epidemiologic observation of specific patterns of familial aggregation in some individuals with motor neuron disease started the chain of events that led to the identification of the underlying genes. Despite exciting advances into understanding the molecular genetic basis of some Mendelian forms of the disease, however, the causes of sporadic (non-familial) ALS are still unknown, and the apparent selectivity for motor neurons remains unexplained.

EPIDEMIOLOGIC CLASSIFICATION OF FORMS OF ALS

On the basis of epidemiologic and genetic features, three major forms of ALS have been identified: (i) sporadic ALS, (ii) familial or hereditary ALS, and (iii) the Western Pacific (Mariana Islands) form. The latter was first described among the Chamorro people of Guam, and the ALS patients in this area acquire pathological characteristics similar to Parkinson's disease (PD) and Alzheimer's disease, referred to as ALS parkinsonism–dementia complex (PDC) (7,8). Two indigenous populations in Irian Jaya (western New Guinea) (9) and two areas in the Kii Peninsula of Japan also demonstrated an excess occurrence of ALS/PDC (10). ALS/PDC in the western Pacific in the 1950s is the best-known "geographic cluster" of ALS, and unfortunately, its causes remain unknown.

METHODOLOGICAL CONSIDERATIONS IN ALS RESEARCH

The correct classification of subjects with ALS is important to identify disease-associated risk factors. The importance of a universally accepted case definition for ALS was the result of two major consensus conferences, the first convened by the World Federation of Neurology (WFN) ALS Research Subcommittee (11), where disease definitions were developed, and a subsequent conference where case definition criteria were further refined (12). Table 1 summarizes the WFN "El Escorial" criteria for the diagnosis of ALS that require the presence, evolution, and progression of upper motor neuron (UMN) and lower motor neuron (LMN) findings at multiple levels. Progressive LMN signs alone may be accepted for the purpose of diagnosing ALS if the individual carries a gene for familial ALS and other causes have been excluded (13). Patients with ALS may be classified as definite, probable, possible, or suspected. Ross et al. (12) reported a method whereby using a combination of clinical, electrodiagnostic, and radiologic data, some patients would be classified as having "possible" ALS according to the WFN El Escorial criteria, and others would be considered as having "laboratory-supported definite ALS." However, many clinicians avoid this categorization by stating that a patient either has ALS or does not have ALS. The pathology and classification of ALS and other motor neuron diseases will be described in detail in later chapters.

Another methodologic challenge when conducting epidemiologic studies of ALS is case ascertainment, that is, the best method for finding patients to include in the study. In a case–control study, recruitment of ALS patients from referral-based centers such as specialized clinics or tertiary centers will be under-representative of the number of ALS cases available from the underlying population, resulting in referral bias. Older more debilitated patients or patients from lower socio-economic groups are less likely to be referred to specialized clinics. Yoshida et al. (14) noted that ALS patients from referral centers tend to be 10 years younger (mean age at diagnosis is 55 years) and have longer median survival (greater than three years) than do ALS patients recruited from defined populations such as residents of a well-defined geographic area (15,16). ALS patients recruited from referral centers

Table 1   El Escorial WFN Criteria for the Diagnosis of ALS

The diagnosis of ALS requires the presence of the following:
Signs of LMN degeneration by clinical, electrophysiological, or neuropathological
   examination in one or more of four regions (bulbar, cervical, thoracic, or lumbosacral).
Signs of UMN degeneration by clinical examination and progressive spread of signs within a
   region or other regions.
   Definite ALS: UMN and LMN signs in bulbar region and at least two of the other spinal
      regions *or* UMN and LMN signs in three spinal regions and signs of progression over a
      12-month period following diagnosis.
   Probable ALS: UMN and LMN signs in at least two regions with UMN signs rostral to a
      region with LMN signs *and* signs of progression over a 12-month period following diagnosis.
   Possible ALS: UNM and LMN signs in only one region *or* UNM signs in two or more
      regions (i.e., progressive bulbar palsy, primary lateral sclerosis).
   Suspected ALS: LMN signs in two or three regions (i.e., primary muscular atrophy).

Abbreviations: WFN, World Federation of Neurology; LMN, lower motor neuron; UMN, upper motor neuron; ALS, amyotrophic lateral sclerosis.
Source: Adapted from Refs. 11–13.

may be suitable for clinical trials or other experimental studies, but less than ideal for participating in studies to identify causal factors for the disease.

DESCRIPTIVE STUDIES

Incidence and Mortality Data

Excluding the western Pacific foci, the incidence of sporadic ALS in the United States is approximately 2 per 100,000 per year in population-based studies with near complete case ascertainment (14,15,17–19). Internationally, ALS is referred to as motor neuron disease (MND) and incidence rates for the disease worldwide ranges from 0.86 to 2.4 per 100,000 per year (20–26). With a median survival of three years, the prevalence ratio of ALS is approximately 6 per 100,000 per year or nearly three times the incidence rate. Since almost all patients with ALS die due to the disease, mortality rates for ALS should parallel incidence rates. However, the reported mortality rates for ALS in the United States are much lower than that for incidence rates (1.5 per 100,000 per year for all ages when compared to 2 per 100,000 per year). This phenomenon is probably due to underreporting of ALS on death certificates. The cumulative probability of developing the disease during a lifetime in the United States is about 1 in 1000 deaths for those reaching adulthood. The incidence and mortality rates for MND are also higher in recent decades than those previously reported in industrialized countries (18,23,24). This increase may be accounted for by improved ascertainment, better reporting, and loss of competing causes of mortality in a susceptible cohort (27–29).

The incidence of sporadic ALS is 20% to 60% higher in men than in women (19,22,25,30). Age-specific incidence rates appear to increase with age in population-based series peaking at ages 65 to 74 years (Fig. 1) (14,19,21). In contrast, the incidence of the disease peaks earlier at 55 to 60 years in referral-based studies (31,32).

Comparing age- and gender-specific rates among various studies is complicated by methodological differences in ascertaining ALS cases or assigning diagnostic criteria and different age distributions of the underlying populations. In order to make meaningful comparisons, the calendar years studied should be similar in all studies so that any differences in incidence rates are not due to changing rates over time. Chancellor and Warlow (33) compared the age- and gender-specific rates from eight surveys that were judged to have near complete case ascertainment and restricted the analysis to men and women aged 45 to 74 years (14,34–40). McGuire et al. (19) conducted a similar analysis and included the incidence rates from studies from western Washington State (19), Texas (41), and Scotland (42). A recent study from Italy added data from incidence studies conducted in Ireland, Sweden, and Italy (22,25,43–45). Table 2 shows the incidence of ALS in men and women from these 16 different studies, age-adjusted to the 1990 U.S. population for those 45 to 74 years old. Generally, the rates tend to be higher for northern latitudes than for southern latitudes, although the most recent survey in Piemonte Italy (25) shows rates that are similar to the studies in Washington State (19), Scotland (42), and Ireland (22). The lower incidence rates in earlier studies could reflect underascertainment of cases or differences in case-definition. In the three U.S. studies (14,19,41) and the Finnish study (39), the differences in rates are less striking between men and women than in the other twelve surveys. These differences may reflect the differences in case definition or case ascertainment, or differences in the prevalence of risk factors in certain populations.

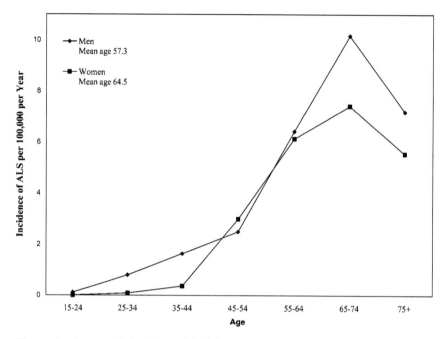

Figure 1 Age-specific incidence of ALS in men and women for western Washington State from April 1990 to March 1995. *Abbreviation*: ALS, amyotrophic lateral sclerosis. *Source*: From Ref. 19.

Table 2 Incidence of ALS in Men and Women in Different Studies Age-Adjusted to the 1990 U.S. Population for Those 45–74 Years of Age

Country	Years of survey	Latitude	Men	Women	Combined
Middle Finland (39)	1976–1981	66°	8.9	8.3	8.5
Northern Sweden (36)	1969–1980	66°	8.6	4.5	6.4
Middle Sweden (37)	1970–1981	60°	5.6	3.5	4.5
Scotland (42)	1988	56°	6.7	3.8	5.2
Denmark (38)	1974–1986	56°	4.2	2.9	3.5
Ireland (22)	1995–1997	53°	6.7	5.3	6.0
Washington, U.S.A. (19)	1990–1995	47°	5.8	5.3	5.5
Minnesota, U.S.A. (14)	1925–1984	45°	7.4	6.4	6.9
Southern Sweden (45)	1961–1990	45°	7.5	4.8	6.1
Reggio Emilia, Italy (44)	1985–1992	44°	6.7	4.5	5.5
Piemonte, Italy (43)	1966–1986	44°	3.4	2.2	2.7
Piemonte, Italy (25)	1995–1996	44°	6.1	4.7	5.4
Ontario, Canada (40)	1978–1982	44°	5.4	3.7	4.5
Sardinia (35)	1965–1974	40°	3.7	1.4	2.5
Israel (34)	1959–1974	32°	2.7	1.5	2.0
Texas, U.S.A. (41)	1985–1988	29°	3.7	3.6	3.6

Source: Adapted from Refs. 19, 25, and 33.

The incidence of ALS in racial or ethnic groups, other than Caucasians has not been well defined. A study by Annegers et al. (41), in Texas, reported an overall incidence rate of 1.5 per 100,000 for African American and Hispanics combined. However, the study did not achieve complete case ascertainment possibly due to differences in access to health care when compared to Caucasians and may have resulted in underestimation of the incidence of ALS in these groups. In the study in Western Washington State, the age-adjusted incidence rates were 0.74 per 100,000 per year for non-white men and 0.53 per 100,000 per year for non-white women (19). However, the number of non-white patients was small ($n = 10$), mainly comprised of African Americans. Future studies are thus needed to obtain estimates of the incidence of ALS in ethnic groups other than non-Hispanic Caucasians.

Mortality studies based on death certificate data have assessed racial and ethnic differences in death rates from ALS in the United States. These studies have shown that the rates for whites exceeded those for non-whites by 70%, and were higher among women and those older than 60 years (32,46). ALS mortality rates among African Americans were reported to be lower than mortality rates among U.S. Caucasians (47); however, using death certificates to identify ALS cases likely resulted in the under ascertainment of African American cases of ALS.

Epidemiology of Western Pacific ALS

The Western Pacific form of ALS was identified in the early 1950s, with incidence, prevalence, and mortality rates estimated to range from 50 per 100,000 per year to 100 per 100,000 per year (48,49). Males were twice as likely as females to be diagnosed with the disease and the median age at diagnosis was 44 years. Clusters of ALS, frequently in association with a PDC, were noted in three distinct geographic isolates (50): in Guam (Marianna Islands), in two villages of the Kii Peninsula of Japan, and among the Auyu and Jakai people in a small area of Irian Jaya (western New Guinea). The ALS/PDC clusters differed from community-identified clusters in two ways: (i) the 100-fold excess of occurrence (rather than two- or three-fold greater than the expected number of cases) and (ii) the continued excess incidence over time (51).

Familial aggregation of ALS/PDC was first recognized in Guam in the 1950s (48,52,53). However, the pattern of transmission does not follow simple Mendelian patterns of inheritance and suggests that an environmental agent may be associated with the disease. Plato et al. (54) examined the incidence and prevalence of ALS/PDC in Guam over the past 40 years and reported significantly higher rates for ALS and Parkinson's disease among relatives of ALS/PDC cases than in the general population of Guam. The rates were higher among siblings of patients with ALS and among the children of patients with PDC. However, excess risk for developing ALS or PD was also observed among wives, suggesting that ALS/PDC may be associated with an environmental factor and is not a Mendelian genetic disorder.

Another clue to the etiology of ALS/PDC is the prevalence of excessive neurofibrillary tangles in asymptomatic Chamorros. However, genetics alone do not explain the cause of Western Pacific ALS, given that people from three distinct geographic areas have high rates of ALS/PDC, and that Filipinos who emigrated to Guam at a young age also have high rates of ALS or PDC (55). Furthermore, age at diagnosis of ALS and PDC has been increasing in the southern villages of Guam over the past 30 years (51), a feature that would not be expected for a genetic disorder.

Two environmental hypotheses have been proposed to explain the epidemic of ALS/PDC in the western Pacific. The first hypothesis was centered on the possible deficiency of essential minerals in the soil, specifically calcium and magnesium (56,57). Subsequent studies on Guam, however, demonstrated that the food and water supply contained adequate concentrations of calcium and magnesium (58,59).

The second hypothesis regarding ALS/PDC suggests an environmental agent or toxicant. The epidemic occurrence of ALS/PDC in the western Pacific has focused attention on a related glutamate analog found in the seed of the *Cycas circinalis* cycad palm, β-N-methylamino-L-alanine (BMAA) (60). This toxin is released during the preparation of flour from the cycad and has been reported to induce upper and lower motor neuron death in macaque monkeys (61,62). However, this finding is controversial since the concentration of BMAA in the flour that had been washed is thought to be too low to induce disease (63).

Recently, Cox and Sacks (64) proposed that high concentrations of BMAA or its metabolites could have been ingested by the Chamorro people while consuming flying foxes (bats), which feed on the cycad nut. If biomagnification occurred, the bats would have high levels of BMAA. Although flying foxes are endangered today on Guam and the species thought to cause Western Pacific ALS is actually extinct, Banack and Cox (65) assessed museum specimens of these bats and reported that consuming a single bat could contribute 3751 mg of BMAA to the diet, which would be equivalent to eating 174 to 1014 kg of processed cycad flour. Whether consumption of flying foxes is associated with the etiology of the ALS/PDC remains to be answered.

The persistence of a high prevalence of neurodegenerative disease in some villages in Guam suggests the continued presence of an etiological mechanism, albeit in attenuated form. The changing spectrum may reflect improved case ascertainment or temporal differences between the interaction of environmental factors and genetic susceptibility among individuals at risk for ALS. The data are consistent with a constant level of exposure to an environmental toxin that peaked during World War II and has declined, but not completely disappeared. Age-specific incidence rates and mortality rates have decreased and age at onset has increased by 16 years for ALS and by 13 years for PDC (66). Individuals exposed to higher doses of toxin might develop ALS at a relatively early age, with or without associated PDC. Individuals exposed to a lesser dose might develop, at a later date, ALS with or without PDC, PDC alone, or dementia alone. However, a more recent report continues to suggest a possible genetic etiology (66). Environmental changes, especially in the diet of Chamorros, may have had a beneficial effect in a genetically susceptible population.

The Role of Clusters in ALS

Clusters arising from community reports of patients with ALS have yet to yield epidemiologically useful information about causes of ALS (67). Furthermore, very few suspected clusters are confirmed when rigorous criteria are applied and when multiple comparisons and chance findings are taken into account (67). To compensate for the effect of chance in assessing the potential significance of clusters arising from the community (68), Armon et al. (67) proposed that the value for the ratio of observed to expected cases that may be considered of epidemiological significance be increased. Precious resources could then be spent on clusters that, if confirmed, were not due to chance alone.

Mundt et al. (69) investigated an increase in mortality from ALS among the 32,000 civilian employees who had worked at Kelly Air Force Base in San Antonio, Texas. Patients and patient-interest groups joined forces with federal and state agencies, and external scientific advisors to evaluate the cluster. The study assessed ALS mortality in the context of overall mortality and other disease-specific mortality data. The investigators concluded that the scientific evidence did not support excess mortality from ALS; however, follow-up of this relatively young cohort continues, since only 10% of the civilian workers had died at the time of the investigation.

Reports from two studies suggest that the risk of ALS may be higher in young servicemen who were deployed to the Persian Gulf War (70,71). Both studies recruited cases via military and health records and publicity campaigns among military personnel. In one study, Haley (70) identified 20 cases of ALS diagnosed before the age of 45 and calculated the expected incidence of ALS from national mortality statistics. The investigator noted an excess risk of ALS. In the second study, two neurologists reviewed case records and supplemented their information with telephone and personal inquiries to confirm the cases of ALS (71). In addition, Horner et al. (71) compared the incidence of ALS in those who were deployed to the Gulf arena with those who were not deployed and found a two-fold increased risk of developing ALS. While analyzing the data according to the branch of service, the risk was significantly elevated in deployed personnel in the Air Force and the Army. A recent report from a cohort of men who were followed as part of an American Cancer Society study provided evidence that men who served in the military, regardless of branch of service or time period, were 60% more likely to die from ALS than those who did not serve (72). This cohort did not include Gulf War veterans. These findings raise the possibility that one or more exposures associated with military service in general may increase the risk of developing the disease. However, other studies are needed to confirm these findings and identify the reasons for the excess risk.

On the basis of the findings of Horner et al. (71), the Department of Veteran Affairs (VA) established a National Registry of Veterans with ALS. The primary goals of the registry are (i) to provide the VA with data on the current number and characteristics of veterans with ALS and to recruit newly diagnosed cases of ALS, (ii) to provide a mechanism to inform veterans with ALS about research studies and clinical trials for which they may be eligible to participate, and (iii) to establish a resource for the conduct of large-scale studies to identify epidemiological and genetic factors that may be associated with the disease.

EPIDEMIOLOGY OF FAMILIAL ALS

Only 5% to 10% of patients have one or more first degree relatives with ALS (1,14,73–76). Some cases with familial ALS have a Mendelian pattern of disease in their family, but many patients with familial ALS have no apparent Mendelian inheritance pattern. Familial ALS may be inherited in either an autosomal dominant, autosomal recessive, or X-linked recessive pattern (2,3). In the autosomal dominant cases, the gender ratio is close to 1:1. The most common form of inheritance is autosomal dominant (77,78). In only rare instances is the inheritance autosomal recessive (79).

Mutations at the SOD1 gene on chromosome 21 account for 20% of familial cases and are inherited as autosomal dominant with over 100 SOD1 mutations identified (77). Additional chromosomes implicated in autosomal recessive ALS are chromosome 15 (80) and chromosome 2 (78), as well as an X-linked gene (81). Patients with familial ALS are on average 15 to 20 years younger than patients diagnosed with sporadic ALS and tend to have distinctive phenotypes (82). Similar to mutation carriers with other diseases, not all carriers of SOD1 will develop ALS, suggesting that other unknown factors must be contributing to the penetrance of the SOD1 mutations. Chapter 3 provides more detail on the familial forms of ALS.

ANALYTIC STUDIES

Special Methodological Issues

The diagnosis of ALS generally occurs 12 months after the onset of clinical symptoms (14,21,83,84). Since muscle weakness accrues in a gradual manner, the disease must be biologically active long before the first clinical signs. Biological onset could predate clinical onset by three years or even longer. This assumption is based on two points: (i) 90% of the anterior horn cells have degenerated by the time of the patient's death, usually three years following the clinical onset of first symptoms, and (ii) ALS is diagnosed when at least half of the motor neurons have died (20).

A special consideration with regard to chronological relationship arises when trying to identify risk factors for ALS because the biological onset of the disease may precede its clinical manifestation by months or years. When conducting case–control studies to identify etiological risk factors that may be associated with the disease, the "reference date" should be one to five years prior to the date of diagnosis to exclude this preclinical period.

Types of Analytical Studies

The most appropriate scientific method to investigate the etiology of a rare disease such as ALS is the case–control design. Ideally, a prospective study design would allow the collection of risk factors before the disease occurs, but assembling a large cohort of patients, only a few of whom would develop ALS, takes years and is very costly. The cross-sectional study design would not be appropriate because the timing of exposure relative to the disease cannot be determined. If a case–control study revealed hypotheses, a retrospective cohort study might be utilized to follow up with regards to specific risk factors that have been measured in a cohort such as an occupational group (85). The chief disadvantages of case–control studies are the multiple sources of biases to which they are subjected (86) and the concern that testing multiple hypotheses may result in significant findings based on chance alone. Unfortunately, until recent years, most case–control studies of ALS have not been rigorously designed, usually relying on a small number of prevalent ALS cases from referral centers and choosing inappropriate control groups such as coworkers or spouses. Furthermore, publication bias is a major concern, since studies with positive findings are more likely to be published than studies with negative findings (87,88). For a more comprehensive review of the epidemiologic principles for the conduct of neurological studies, the readers should refer to Tanner and Ross (89) and Nelson and McGuire (90).

RISK FACTORS FOR ALS

ALS research has undergone exciting progress in the past decade, with evidence accumulating that injury caused by free radicals, exogenous neurotoxicants, excitotoxins, or a cumulative effect of all these factors may play an important role in the

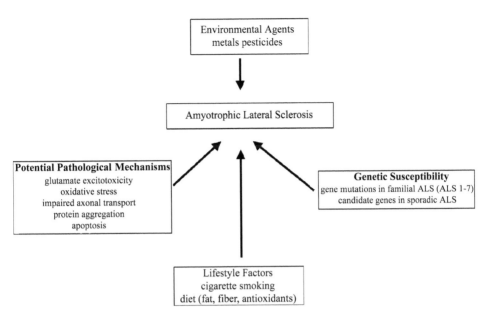

Figure 2 Etiological theories and pathogenic mechanisms for ALS. *Abbreviation*: ALS, amyotrophic lateral sclerosis.

pathogenesis of ALS (Fig. 2). Earlier theories purported that exposure to environmental toxicants, excessive physical activity, skeletal fractures, and electrical shock may play a role in the pathogenesis of ALS, and most epidemiologic studies have emphasized the investigation of these putative risk factors.

A notable limitation of previous case–control studies is that very few have examined risk factors for ALS among incident (newly diagnosed) cases, and almost all studies were conducted in referral centers with the exception of three studies that were conducted in population-based settings. A study in Scotland identified 103 incident cases from a motor neuron disease registry (91); however, this study was not a true incidence cohort because 39 of the incident ALS cases in the registry died prior to the initiation of the case–control study and the investigators did not collect information on the deceased subjects. A second study in New England included 109 ALS cases from two referral centers and recruited population-based control subjects using random digit dialing (92). A third population-based study from western Washington State identified incident cases (93). All other published case–control studies have used prevalent cases. This feature over-represents long-lived cases and makes it difficult for the investigators to distinguish etiological risk factors from prognostic factors. Selecting incident cases is extremely important, especially with a short duration disease such as ALS. A second limitation is that, with few exceptions (91,93,94), ALS case–control studies have not been conducted in defined populations, but in secondary study bases such as hospitals, referral centers, or ALS societies, where patients are not likely to be representative of ALS patients in the general population. A third limitation of previous studies is the small sample size (usually fewer than 100 cases of ALS), which affects the study's statistical power to detect associations.

Because of the methodological limitations noted above, case–control studies investigating risk factors for ALS have yielded conflicting results. The epidemiological evidence regarding risk factors is presented in Table 3.

Table 3 Risk Factors for ALS: Strength and Certainty of the Associations

	Strength of association
Known risk factors	
Age	↑↑↑
Disease-causing mutations (SOD1, alsin) in Mendelian ALS	↑↑↑
Gender (male > female)	↑ RR 1.2–1.4
Family history of ALS	↑ RR 3.0–4.0
Clusters (Persian Gulf War, Western Pacific ALS/PDC)	↑ RR 2.0–50+
Possible risk factors	
Neurotoxicant exposures	
Lead	
Mercury	
Pesticide exposure (insecticides, herbicides)	
Solvent exposure	
Certain occupation characteristics	
Electrical workers	
Farmers	
Industrial occupations	
Trauma	
Skeletal trauma, fractures	
Severe electrical shock (with unconsciousness)	
Vigorous physical activity	
Heavy manual labor	
Athleticism	
Lifestyle factors	
Cigarette smoking	
Alcohol intake	
Anthropometric measures (weight, body mass index)	
Diet	
High fat intake (saturated > monounsaturated)	
High glutamate intake	
Low fiber intake	
Low antioxidant intake	
Factors not widely investigated	
Infectious agents	
Medical history	
Other medical conditions	
Prescription and over-the-counter medication use	
Hormonal and reproductive factors (in women)	
Other exposures or lifestyle factors	
Caffeine intake	
Recreational drug use	
Hobbies, avocational exposures	
Residential chemical and pesticide exposure	
Residential proximity to industry	

Abbreviations: ALS, amyotrophic lateral sclerosis; SOD, superoxide dismutase; PDC, Parkinsonism–dementia complex.

Physical Trauma

Fractures

Several cases–control studies have identified physical trauma or limb injuries as risk factors for ALS, with odds ratios ranging from 1.3 to 10.0 (83,95–102). However, the overall excess of fractures occurred closer to the time of diagnosis. In a population-based case–control study in Scotland, the investigators found a significant association with fractures that occurred five years prior to date of diagnosis [odds ratio (OR) = 15.0, 95% confidence interval (CI) = 2.3–654], but reported no association with a lifetime history of fractures (91). A more recent study in western Washington State reported a similar finding with a lifetime history of previous fractures and only a weak association five years prior to date of diagnosis (103). Cases may be more prone to falls due to subclinical weakness prior to their diagnosis of ALS. A retrospective cohort study of ALS also showed no increased incidence of ALS in patients who had sustained head trauma (85).

*Electromagnetic Field (EMF) Exposure, Electrical Occupations, and
Electrical Shock*

EMF exposure has been the subject of several epidemiological investigations of ALS (104–107) and a recent review (108). Johansen and Olsen (105) conducted a large, retrospective cohort study among men employed in utility companies in Finland and reported a twofold increase in mortality from ALS. In another cohort study, Savitz et al. (106) reported a threefold increase in risk for ALS [relative risk (RR)= 3.1, 95% CI = 1.1–9.8] among men employed as electrical workers for 20 years or longer. Noonan et al. (107) used death certificate data for the years 1987 to 1996 to identify ALS cases in a case–control study conducted in Colorado. The investigators obtained a mean magnetic field index using a job–exposure matrix, and found no association between EMFs and ALS. However, individuals with a history of work in electrical occupations had a greater than twofold increased risk of ALS (OR = 2.30, 95% CI = 1.3–4.1). Two recent studies from Sweden reported conflicting results (109,110). Both studies addressed the association of EMF exposure with neurodegenerative diseases and used a job–exposure matrix to assess EMF exposure using death certificate data to ascertain cases and Census data to determine the person's occupation. Håkansson et al. (109) assessed a cohort of 538,221 engineering industry workers and found a greater than twofold increase in risk for ALS in cases with the highest exposure to EMF (OR = 2.2, 95% CI = 1.0–4.7). However, Feychting et al. (110) found no association with EMF exposure and risk of ALS in a cohort of nearly five million individuals in the 1980 Swedish Census, although they did report a 40% increase in risk for electrical or electronics workers.

The findings of elevated risk with EMF is intriguing because past case–control studies have also shown elevated risks associated with electrical shock (95,99,103,111–113), although many of the odds ratios were not statistically significant as the exposure to severe electrical shock was rare. Future studies are warranted to pursue the possibility that electrical occupations or EMF exposures are associated with ALS.

Physical Activity

Physical activity may affect the risk of ALS by modifying the extent of the exposure to a neurotoxicant, facilitating the toxin's transport to its target or making selective motor neurons more susceptible to injury by the neurotoxin (114). Several epidemiological studies reported that vigorous physical activity at work and during leisure time is associated with ALS (35,37,115–120), while two case–control studies did not report such an association (121,122). Workers engaged in heavy physical labor had a twofold increase in risk of developing ALS (115,120). ALS patients who had a history of athletic participation were significantly more likely to develop ALS.

In a population-based, case–control study of ALS conducted in Western Washington State, detailed information on lifetime physical activity, both at work and at leisure, was obtained from incident cases ($n = 174$) and population-based controls ($n = 348$) (122). The investigators measured physical activity at work as percent of time spent at each of five levels ranging from sedentary activities to doing heavy physical work. For leisure time activity, they assigned a value to each activity that reflected an estimate of the rate of energy as calories expended by the individual. In addition, the investigators examined physical activity in terms of indoor-outdoor and field–non-field sports. Neither overall physical activity nor vigorous activity either in workplace or leisure settings were associated with risk of ALS. The only significant result from the study was a 59% increase in risk for ALS among cases who participated in organized sports in high school. Compared with previous studies, this study was population-based, recruited a relatively large number of newly diagnosed cases of ALS, and collected very detailed quantitative information on lifetime physical activity from cases and their age- and sex-matched population-based controls subjects.

Recently, Chiò and Mora (123) analyzed mortality data among 24,000 Italian professional and semiprofessional soccer players who played between 1960 and 1997. During the study period, the investigators found a significant increase in mortality from ALS [standardized proportional mortality ratio (SPMR) = 11.6, 95% CI = 6.7–19.9]. As a result, a population-based, case–control study is currently underway in Italy to evaluate the association of professional sports activities with the risk of ALS (124). This study may add important new information to determine whether physical activity is associated with ALS.

Occupational

Metals

Several lines of investigation have linked ALS to heavy metal exposure, including (i) the linkage of several ALS-like syndromes to chronic lead or mercury exposure, suggesting that chronic metal toxicity can have a selective deleterious effect on motor neurons, (ii) studies finding increased metal content in tissues of ALS patients, and (iii) epidemiological studies finding significant associations between ALS and self-reported exposure to lead, mercury, and other heavy metals.

Several epidemiological studies have investigated the association of heavy metal exposure and ALS and have consistently reported elevated risk associated with exposure to lead (91,94,116,125,126), mercury (116,127), or heavy metals as a class (127,128). Control subjects were spouses, relatives, friends, and/or coworkers in all but three of the previous studies (91,94,126), possibly leading to overmatching of cases and controls with respect to metal exposure. The risk estimates associated with exposure to lead, mercury, or other heavy metals as a class ranged from 2.0 to 6.0 and were significant in all studies but two (95,128). Only three studies assessed duration of exposure to lead (91,94,126). Armon et al. (94) reported an increased risk of ALS among men exposed to greater than 200 cumulative lifetime hours of exposure to lead (OR = 5.5; 95% CI = 1.4–21.0). Similar results were reported in the study from Scotland for greater than 12 months of employment in occupations involving lead exposures (OR = 5.7; 95% CI = 1.6–30.0) (91). Kamel et al. (126) reported a significant trend with increasing lifetime days of lead exposure. Among subjects who reported more than 2000 lifetime days of lead exposure, the risk estimate was 2.3 (95% CI = 1.1–4.9) compared to subjects with no exposure to lead.

These studies relied on self-reporting and may be prone to recall bias. Cases are more likely to over-report certain exposures while control subjects may under-report exposures (101). In the study from western Washington State, McGuire et al. (93) illustrated the potential for recall bias. The investigators presented risk estimates based on subjects' self-reported exposure to lead and based on an industrial hygiene panel's assessment of lead exposure based on job history information. Compared to subjects who had never been exposed to lead, those who self-reported their lead exposure had a nearly two-fold increase in risk for ALS (OR = 1.9, 95% CI 1.0–3.6), while the expert panel's assessment showed no increase in risk for ALS [OR = 1.1 (95% CI 0.6–2.1)] (93).

Lead has been measured in bone in two epidemiological studies. A study in the early 1970s reported no association between bone lead and risk of ALS, following examination of lead concentration in bone from 25 ALS cases and from 17 autopsy controls (125). More recently, in a case–control study of ALS conducted in New England, blood and bone lead were measured in 107 cases and a subset of 41 population-based controls (126). Blood lead levels were significantly higher in ALS cases than controls, and measures of lead concentration in tibia and patella were somewhat higher among ALS cases than controls. The evidence from this study of a possible association between exposure to bone lead concentration and risk of ALS warrants further investigation.

The risk of ALS has been examined in occupations with the potential for exposure to metal. Three case-control studies reported an increased risk for ALS among welders (84,94,95); however, a fourth study noted no association with welding. Studies of metal working and metal casters also failed to observe any significant associations between these occupations and the risk of ALS (31,129,130).

Solvents

Organic solvents are widely used in occupational settings and are a health concern due to their neurotoxic properties. High-dose exposure to solvents shows clear evidence of dose-related acute neurologic deficits; however, longer-term, lower exposure to solvents is more difficult to quantify. Several epidemiologic studies have examined the role of exposure to solvents with the risk of ALS and the results have been inconsistent. Three studies reported a two- to three-fold increase in risk (91,113,120), while three other studies did not observe any association between solvent exposure and risk of ALS (84,97,102). A study from Western Washington state reported a 60% increase in risk for ALS when solvent exposure was self-reported (OR = 1.6, 95% CI, 1.1–2.5), but an expert panel's assessment of solvent exposure by reviewing job history information failed to show a significant association (OR = 1.2, 95% CI 0.8–1.9). However, the panel did observe significant associations between risk of ALS and exposure to specific groups of solvent chemicals including alcohols and ketones and degreasers (93).

As with metal exposure, epidemiologic studies have assessed employment in various occupations as a surrogate measure for exposure to solvents. Findings from two mortality studies in England and Wales found that leather workers were more likely to die from ALS than the general population (131,132). However, three other studies failed to show any significant associations between leather workers and risk of ALS (74,133–135). The study in Sweden also did not find any associations between ALS and shoemakers or tanners (135).

Paint products contain many types of solvents including hydrocarbons, alcohols and ketones, glycol ethers and esters, and terpenes. Several studies evaluated the association of paint with risk of ALS. A study in England of twin pairs discordant for disease and a case-control study in Italy found a greater than three-fold increase in risk for ALS among those with previous exposure to paint (100,130). However, a large population-based case-control study in Sweden reported no excess risk for ALS among painters (84), as did a smaller U.S. study with limited statistical power (102), and two studies in the United Kingdom (132,133).

Pesticides

Exposure to agricultural chemicals may be a risk factor for ALS although few studies have examined this relationship. Previous studies have observed an association between the risk of ALS and farming. In case-control studies conducted in Greece and Italy, agricultural workers and residents of rural areas were at increased risk for MND (83,100,136), and surveys in Sweden and Scotland reported that patients with MND were more likely to work in agrarian occupations compared to the general population (45,137). Investigators in the United States reviewed death certificates and noted that mortality rates for ALS were higher among farm residents (138). Despite these observations, many studies have found no association between risk of ALS and farming or rural living (96,97,102,103,121,132,133,139).

A few case-control studies have investigated the association between exposure to agricultural chemicals and risk of ALS. The most noteworthy finding was from a population-based study in Western Washington state that reported a two-fold increase in risk for ALS among men exposed to agricultural chemicals [OR and 95% CI=2.4 (1.2–4.8)], but not in women [OR and 95% CI = 0.9 (0.2–3.8)] (93), with a dose-response trend (p = 0.002). (93). These results were based on an industrial hygiene panel's assessment of exposure to agricultural chemicals. This study also examined the possible timing of agricultural chemical exposure and found that the highest risk occurred for the decade between age 22 and 32 years, lending support to the notion that injury to the motor neuron occurred years prior to the diagnosis of ALS (93). Two previous case-studies reported a two-fold increase in risk for ALS and exposure to pesticides, but the risk estimates were not statistically significant (95,113). Three other studies showed no association (84,91,120), although the study from Italy reported a weak, statistically significant association between rural residence and risk of ALS but no association with actual pesticide exposure (120).

There are numerous challenges to the accurate assessment of occupational exposures. Many of the exposures of interest are of low frequency so the risk estimates may be weak and not statistically significant. Other limitations include the lack of gold standards, open-ended questionnaires that are prone to recall bias and the inaccessibility of company records to verify job titles and tasks performed. The timing between exposure to a chemical agent and the onset of ALS is uncertain, making it unclear as to when the relevant exposures may have occurred. Biological samples and measurement methods may vary among studies making comparisons between studies problematic. Levels of chemical substances differ by country and vary by calendar period and job titles even within countries making it difficult to incorporate the industrial changes into the exposure assessment. Lastly, many studies rely on job titles and industries as surrogates for exposure to specific workplace exposures.

Lifestyle Risk Factors

To date, very few studies have investigated the association of ALS with lifestyle factors such as diet, cigarette smoking, and alcohol consumption.

Cigarette Smoking and Alcohol Consumption

Few studies have investigated the role of cigarette smoking and alcohol consumption in the etiology of ALS, despite the possibility that an environmental exposure may be associated with the disease (74,84,91,92,97,113,120,126,139–142). None of these studies reported an association with alcohol use. All but three of the studies (92,141,142) reported no association with cigarette smoking, possibly due to small sample size, use of prevalent cases, and hospital-based control subjects. Kamel et al. (92), in a case–control study conducted in New England, reported a nearly two-fold increase in risk for ALS among ever smokers (OR = 1.7, 95% CI = 1.0–2.8), although a dose response was not apparent for average number of cigarettes per day, years smoked, or pack-years. In a population-based, case–control study in Washington State, the investigators noted a similar result among subjects who had ever smoked cigarettes (alcohol-adjusted OR = 2.0, 95% CI = 1.3–3.2), with a greater than threefold increase in risk among current smokers (alcohol-adjusted OR = 3.5; 95% CI = 1.9–6.4) (141). A dose–response trend with increasing pack-years of smoking was significant. Weisskopf et al. (142) examined the association of tobacco use and ALS mortality among participants in the Cancer Prevention Study II cohort of the American Cancer Society. The authors reported a nearly 70% increase in ALS mortality among current smokers compared to never smokers (OR = 1.67, 95% CI = 1.24–2.24); however, this association was noted in women only.

Nelson et al. (141) proposed two mechanisms by which cigarette smoke could contribute to the risk of ALS. Cigarettes are comprised of thousands of chemical constituents, including pesticides, which may directly cause toxic injury to motor neuron cell components. A second possible mechanism is the formation of free radicals during the metabolism of the chemical constituents of cigarette smoke (143). As has been previously discussed, mutant superoxide dismutase enzyme has been postulated to induce cell death (144) or cause superoxide to bind with substrates such as nitric oxide that can lead to the production of damaging free radicals (145,146). One of the major exogenous constituents of cigarette smoke is nitric oxide (147). The hypothesis that cigarette smoking is associated with ALS warrants further investigation, ideally using studies that have a prospective design.

Diet

Very little is known about the association of ALS to diet. Four early case–control studies examined differences in consumption of a few food items (84,113,116,126). Only one case–control study used a food frequency questionnaire to assess nutrient intake (148). Dietary fat intake (>93 g/day compared with <42 g/day) was associated with a nearly threefold increase risk of ALS (education, smoking, fiber intake, and total energy intake adjusted OR = 2.7, 95% CI = 0.9–8.0; p for trend = 0.06).

Polyunsaturated fat, saturated fat, and linoleic acid all contributed to this positive association. The brain contains high concentrations of polyunsaturated fatty acids, especially linoleic acid, which makes the brain particularly vulnerable to oxidative damage (149–151). Since the membrane levels of polyunsaturated fatty acids are determined largely by dietary intake (149), the higher dietary consumption of polyunsaturated fatty acids could increase the amount of lipid substrate or cause changes in brain lipid composition, contributing to enhanced lipid peroxidation (150).

Dietary fiber intake (>18 g/day compared with <10 g/day) was associated with a 70% decrease in risk (fat-adjusted OR $= 0.3$, 95% CI $= 0.1$–0.7; p for trend $= 0.02$) (148). Two possible mechanisms may explain why dietary fiber may protect against the development of ALS. Dietary fiber has been shown to cause luminal dilution of potential carcinogens (152,153), which could potentially reduce absorption of a dietary toxin associated with ALS. Dietary fiber also shortens transit time in the large intestine (152) and could reduce the contact time and the absorption of a dietary toxin.

The investigators also found that glutamate (>15 g/day compared with <8.6 g/day) increased the risk for ALS (OR $= 3.2$, 95% CI $= 1.2$–8.0; p for trend < 0.02) (148). The positive association with glutamate intake is consistent with those etiological theories that suggest that glutamate excitotoxicity has a role in causing ALS. Glutamate is ubiquitous in the food supply, and it is possible that high levels of glutamate in the diet, combined with a disordered glutamate metabolism in the brain, could cause excitotoxic cell death of motor neurons.

Two studies have evaluated whether dietary antioxidants have a protective effect on the development of ALS in which free radicals play a role (148,154). A recent prospective study assessed the relationship between the use of Vitamin E, Vitamin C, Vitamin A, and multivitamin supplements and ALS mortality (154). Vitamin data were obtained from a cohort of a million people surveyed as participants in the American Cancer Society Prevention Study II. The investigators identified 525 deaths from ALS through linkage with the National Death Index. Subjects were classified as never users, occasional users (less than 15 times per month), and regular users (15 times or more per month). Regular users of Vitamin E supplements were at decreased risk of death from ALS. The investigators reported a dose–response trend with regular users of Vitamin E greater than 10 years decreasing their risk of death from ALS by 62% (age- and smoking-adjusted OR $= 0.38$, 95% CI $= 0.16$–0.92). Vitamin C, Vitamin A, and use of multivitamins had no apparent affect on the risk of ALS. This interesting finding has merit since animal studies have shown that transgenic mice over-expressing one of the SOD1 genes have delayed onset of motor neuron disease when given Vitamin E supplementation. However, in the population-based, case–control study from Washington State, the investigators did not find an association of antioxidant vitamin consumption, either in the diet or as a supplement, with the risk of ALS (148). Additional studies using comparable dietary methods are needed before firm conclusions are drawn regarding the role of diet in ALS.

FUTURE DIRECTIONS

The last two decades have seen significant advances in understanding the molecular genetic basis of some forms of familial ALS, and these advances hold great promise for identifying pathogenic mechanisms that may be involved in both familial and sporadic ALS. A goal of the future should be to identify the causes of ALS in 90%

to 95% of individuals for whom no cause is apparent. With a forward-looking per-spective, epidemiologists can build on the lessons learned from previous epidemio-logical investigations of ALS, which have yielded disappointingly few clues as to the etiology of the disease. Ideally, future case–control studies would attempt to avoid the methodological flaws of previous studies by: (i) conducting studies in well-defined populations that allow the inclusion of a large number of ALS cases and control subjects, (ii) recruiting incident rather than prevalent cases, to enable the identification of etiologic factors for the disease, (iii) increasing the sample size of ALS cases and controls to improve the statistical power to detect associations, (iv) including individuals from racial/ethnic groups other than Caucasian, (v) asses-sing exposures to environmental toxicants using the most rigorous and objective methods possible, including blinded exposure assessments and biological measures when possible, and (vi) collecting and storing genomic DNA for both ALS cases and controls for the future evaluation of candidate susceptibility genes.

The epidemiological study of ALS would benefit from seeking existing large cohort studies that have accumulated enough person-years of observation to identify an adequate number of ALS patients for study. Cohort studies collect information on risk factors prior to the development of the diseases and thus avoid recall bias, which can plague case–control studies. Even if such cohorts can be identified, how-ever, the investigation is limited to factors that have been measured in the back-ground study, which often have focused on behavioral risk factors such as cigarette smoking, alcohol consumption, and physical activity to the exclusion of factors that may be of particular interest in ALS research such as environmental toxicants and electrical injuries.

CONCLUSION

Given the methodological limitations of early studies, the epidemiological study of ALS is still in its infancy, and further research is needed to better understand genetic, behavioral, and environmental risk factors for this condition. Existing data on the incidence of ALS in different racial or ethnic groups are too incomplete to character-ize even crude differences between groups; therefore, further incidence studies that use comprehensive case ascertainment methods in racially diverse populations are needed. While advances have been made in identifying disease-causing genes for the Mendelian forms of ALS, very little is known about susceptibility genes or other risk factors for sporadic ALS, which comprises more than 90% of ALS cases.

The 1990s, the so-called "The Decade of the Brain," saw great strides in stan-dardizing the diagnosis, evaluation, and treatment of patients with ALS (11,13,155). The great strides in ALS research have been at the genetic and biochemical levels (156), with mechanism-based treatments based on the most recent discoveries yet to be developed and tested. With great effort, it may be possible to demonstrate within the next 10 years the biochemical chain of events by which genes for autoso-mal dominant ALS set the disease in motion, and the extent to which genetics play a role in sporadic ALS.

Epidemiology's chief contribution to ALS research has been in identifying the familial forms of the disease, and in providing the conceptual basis for requiring accuracy in case definition and the statistical tools to compare treatment outcomes of clinical trials. The methodological rigor of the best-designed population-based, case–control epidemiological studies has resulted in the debunking of many commonly held beliefs about the etiology of ALS, at the same time identifying new associations and raising new hypotheses.

REFERENCES

1. Williams DB, Windebank AJ. Motor neuron disease (amyotrophic lateral sclerosis). Mayo Clin Proc 1991; 66:54–82.
2. Hand CK, Rouleau GA. Familial amyotrophic lateral sclerosis. Muscle Nerve 2002; 25:135–159.
3. Majoor-Krakauer D, Willems PJ, Hofman A. Genetic epidemiology of amyotrophic lateral sclerosis. Clin Genet 2003; 63:83–101.
4. Harding AE. Inherited neuronal atrophy and degeneration predominantly of lower motor neurons. In: Dyck PJ, Thomas PK, eds. Peripheral Neuropathy. Philadelphia: WB Saunders Co, 1993:1051–1064.
5. Corcia P, Mayeux-Portas V, Khoris J, de Toffol B, Autret A, Muh JP, Camu W, Andres C. French ALS research group. Amyotrophic lateral sclerosis. Abnormal SMN1 gene copy number is a susceptibility factor for amyotrophic lateral sclerosis. Ann Neurol 2002; 51:243–246.
6. Hosler BA, Siddique T, Sapp PC, Sailor W, Huang MC, Hossain A, Daube JR, Nance M, Fan C, Kaplan J, et al. Linkage of familial amyotrophic lateral sclerosis with frontotemporal dementia to chromosome 9q21–q22. JAMA 2000; 284:1664–1669.
7. Hirano A, Kurland LT, Krooth RS, Lessell S. Parkinsonism-dementia complex, an endemic disease on the island of Guam. I. Clinical features. Brain 1961; 84:642–661.
8. Hirano A, Malamud N, Kurland LT. Parkinsonism-dementia complex, an endemic disease on the island of Guam. II. Pathological features. Brain 1961; 84:662–679.
9. Gajdusek DC, Salazar AM. Amyotrophic lateral sclerosis and parkinsonian syndromes in high incidence among the Auyu and Jakai people of West New Guinea. Neurology 1982; 32:107–126.
10. Shiraki H. The neuropathology of amyotrophic lateral sclerosis (ALS) in the Kii Peninsula and other areas of Japan. In: Norris FH Jr, Kurland LT, eds. Motor Neuron Diseases: Research on Amyotrophic Lateral Sclerosis and Related Disorders. New York: Grune & Stratton, 1969:80–84.
11. Brooks BR. El escorial world federation of neurology criteria for the diagnosis of amyotrophic lateral sclerosis. Subcommittee on motor neuron diseases/amyotrophic lateral sclerosis of the world federation of neurology research group on neuromuscular diseases and the el escorial "Clinical limits of amyotrophic lateral sclerosis" workshop contributors. J Neurol Sci 1994; 124:96–107.
12. Ross MA, Miller RG, Berchert L, Parry G, Barohn RJ, Armon C, Bryan WW, Petajan J, Stromatt S, Goodpasture J, McGuire D. Towards earlier diagnosis of amyotrophic lateral sclerosis: revised criteria. rhCNTF ALS Study Group. Neurology 1998; 50:768–772.
13. Brooks BR, Miller RG, Swash M, Munsat TL. El Escorial Revisited: Revised criteria for the diagnosis of amyotrophic lateral sclerosis. A consensus conference held at Airlie House, Warrenton, VI, 1998.
14. Yoshida S, Mulder DW, Kurland LT, Chu CP, Okazaki H. Follow-up study on amyotrophic lateral sclerosis in Rochester, Minnesota, 1925–1984. Neuroepidemiology 1986; 5:61–70.
15. Sorenson EJ, Stalker AP, Kurland LT, Windebank AJ. Amyotrophic lateral sclerosis in Olmsted County, Minnesota, 1925 to 1998. Neurology 2002; 59:280–282.
16. del Aguila MA, Longstreth WT Jr, McGuire V, et al. Prognosis in amyotrophic lateral sclerosis: a population-based study. Neurology 2003; 60:813–819.
17. Kurtzke JF. Which "neurodegenerative diseases" are on the rise? Health Environ Digest 1989; 3:3–8.

18. Lilienfeld DE, Perl DP. Projected neurodegenerative disease mortality in the United States, 1990–2040. Neuroepidemiology 1993; 12:219–228.
19. McGuire V, Longstreth WT Jr, Koepsell TD, van Belle G. Incidence of amyotrophic lateral sclerosis in three counties in western Washington state. Neurology 1996; 47:571–573.
20. Armon C, Kurland LT. Classic and western Pacific amyotrophic lateral sclerosis: epidemiologic comparisons. In: Hudson AJ, ed. Amyotrophic Lateral Sclerosis: Concepts in Pathogenesis and Etiology. Toronto: University of Toronto Press, 1989:144–165.
21. Christensen PB, Hojer-Pedersen E, Jensen NB. Survival of patients with amyotrophic lateral sclerosis in two Danish counties. Neurology 1990; 40:600–604.
22. Traynor BJ, Codd MB, Corr B, Forde C, Frost E, Hardiman O. Incidence and prevalence of ALS in Ireland, 1995–1997: a population-based study. Neurology 1999; 52: 504–509.
23. Seljeseth YM, Vollset SE, Tysnes OB. Increasing mortality from amyotrophic lateral sclerosis in Norway? Neurology 2000; 55:1262–1266.
24. Maasilta P, Jokelainen M, Loytonen, M Sabel CE, Gatrell AC. Mortality from amyotrophic lateral sclerosis in Finland, 1986–1995. Acta Neurol Scand 2001; 104:232–235.
25. Piemonte and Valle d'Aosta Register for Amyotrophic Lateral Sclerosis (PARALS). Incidence of ALS in Italy: evidence for a uniform frequency in Western countries. Neurology 2001; 56:239–244.
26. Mandrioli J, Faglioni P, Merelli E, Sola P. The epidemiology of ALS in Modena, Italy. Neurology 2003; 60:683–689.
27. Gompertz B. On the nature of the function expressive of the law of human mortality. Philos Trans R Soc London 1825; 115:513–585.
28. Riggs JE. Longitudinal Gompertzian analysis of amyotrophic lateral sclerosis mortality in the US, 1977–1986: evidence for an inherently susceptible population subset. Mech Ageing Dev 1990; 55:207–220.
29. Nielson S, Robinson I, Hunter M. Longitudinal Gompertzian analysis of ALS mortality in England and Wales, 1963–1989: estimate\es of susceptibility in the general population. Mech Ageing Dev 1992; 64:210–216.
30. Armon C. Motor neuron disease. In: Gorelick PB, Alter M, eds. Handbook of Neuroepidemiology. New York: Marcel Dekker Inc., 1994:407–456.
31. Gunnarsson L-G, Lindberg G, Soderfeldt B, Axelson O. Amyotrophic lateral sclerosis in Sweden in relation to occupation. Acta Neurol Scand 1991; 83:394–398.
32. Kurtzke JF. Risk factors in amyotrophic lateral sclerosis. Adv in Neurol 1991; 56: 245–270.
33. Chancellor AM, Warlow CP. Adult onset motor neuron disease: worldwide mortality, incidence and distribution since 1950. J Neurol Neurosurg Psychiatry 1992; 55: 1106–1115.
34. Kahana E, Zilber N. Changes in incidence of amyotrophic lateral sclerosis in Israel. Arch Neurol 1984; 41:157–160.
35. Rosati G, Pinna L, Granieri E, Aiello I, Tola R, Agnetti V, Pirisi A, de Bastiani P. Studies on epidemiological, clinical, and etiological aspects of ALS disease in Sardinia, Southern Italy. Acta Neurol Scand 1977; 55:231–244.
36. Forsgren L, Almay BG, Holmgren G, Wall S. Epidemiology of motor neuron disease in northern Sweden. Acta Neurol Scand 1983; 68:20–29.
37. Gunnarsson LG, Palm R. Motor neuron disease and heavy manual labor: an epidemiologic survey of Varmland County, Sweden. Neuroepidemiology 1984; 3:195–206.
38. Hojer-Pedersen E, Christensen PB, Jensen NB. Incidence and prevalence of motor neuron disease in two Danish counties. Neuroepidemiology 1989; 8:151–159.
39. Murros K, Fogelholm R. Amyotrophic lateral sclerosis in Middle-Finland: an epidemiological study. Acta Neurol Scand 1983; 67:41–47.
40. Hudson AJ, Davenport A, Hader WJ. The incidence of amyotrophic lateral sclerosis in southwestern Ontario, Canada. Neurology 1986; 36:1524–1528.

41. Annegers JF, Appel S, Lee JR, Perkins P. Incidence and prevalence of amyotrophic lateral sclerosis in Harris County Texas, 1985–1988. Arch Neurol 1991; 48:589–593.

42. Scottish Motor Neuron Disease Research Group. The Scottish motor neuron disease register: a prospective study of adult onset motor neuron disease in Scotland. Methodology, demography and clinical features of incident cases in 1989. J Neurol Neurosurg Psychiatry 1992; 55:536–541.

43. Chiò A, Tribolo A, Oddenino E, Schiffer D. A cross-sectional and cohort study of motor neuron disease in Piedmont, Italy. In: Clifford Rose F, ed. New Evidence in MND/ALS Research. London: Smith-Gordon, 1991:59–62.

44. Guidetti D, Bondavalli M, Sabadini R, Marcello N, Vinceti M, Cavalletti S, Marbini A, Gemignani F, Colombo A, Ferrari A, Vivoli G, Solime F. Epidemiological survey of amyotrophic lateral sclerosis in the province of Reggio Emilia, Italy: influence of environmental exposure to lead. Neuroepidemiology 1996; 15:301–312.

45. Gunnarsson LG, Lygner PE, Veiga-Cabo J, de Pedro-Cuesta J. An epidemic-like cluster of motor neuron disease in a Swedish county during the period 1973–1984. Neuroepidemiology 1996; 15:142–152.

46. Kurland LT, Kurtzke JF, Goldberg ID, Choi NW. Amyotrophic lateral sclerosis and other motor neuron disease. In: Kurland LT, Kurtzke JF, Goldberg ID. Epidemiology of Neurologic and Sense Organ Disorders (Vital and Health Statistics Monograph, American Public Health Association). Cambridge, MA: Harvard University Press, 1973:108–127.

47. Leone M, Chandra V, Schoenberg BS. Motor neuron disease in the United States, 1971 and 1973–1978: patterns of mortality and associated conditions at the time of death. Neurology 1987; 37:1339–1343.

48. Kurland LT, Mulder DW. Epidemiologic investigations of amyotrophic lateral sclerosis: 1. Preliminary report on geographic distribution, with special reference to the Mariana Islands, including clinical and pathologic observations. Neurology 1954; 4:355–378.

49. Kurland LT, Mulder DW. Epidemiologic investigations of amyotrophic lateral sclerosis. 2. Familial aggregations indicative of dominant inheritance. Neurology 1955; 5:182–258.

50. Kurland LT. Geographic isolates: Their role in neuroepidemiology. Adv Neurol 1978; 19:69–82.

51. Lavine L, Steele JC, Wolf N, Calne DB, O'Brien PC, Williams DB, Kurland LT, Schoenberg BS. Amyotrophic lateral sclerosis/parkinsonism dementia complex in southern Guam. Is it disappearing? In: Rowland LP, ed Advances in Neurology. New York: Raven Press, 1991:271–285.

52. Koerner DR. Amyotrophic lateral sclerosis on Guam: A clinical study and review of the literature. Ann Intern Med 1952; 37:1204–1220.

53. Arnold A, Edgren DC, Palladino VS. Amyotrophic lateral sclerosis: fifty cases observed on Guam. J Nerv Ment Dis 1953; 117:135–139.

54. Plato CC, Galasko D, Garruto RM, Plato M, Gamst A, Craig UK, Torres JM, Wiederholt W. ALS and PDC of Guam. Forty year follow-up. Neurology 2002; 58:765–773.

55. Garruto RM, Gajdusek DC, Chen K-M. Amyotrophic lateral sclerosis and Parkinsonism-dementia among Filipino migrants of Guam. Ann Neurol 1981; 10:341–350.

56. Gajdusek DC, Garruto RM, Salazar AM. Ecology of high incidence foci of motor neuron disease in Eastern Asia and Western Pacific and the frequent occurrence of the chronic degenerative neurological diseases in these foci. Tenth International Congress on Tropical Medicine and Malaria, Manila, Philippines, 1980:382.

57. Yase Y. (Motor neuron disease). Nippon Rinsho 1978; 35(suppl):1716–1717.

58. Zolon WJ, Ellis-Neill L. University of Guam Technical Report No. 64, 1986.

59. Armon C, Kurland LT, Smith GE, Steele JC. Sporadic and western pacific amyotrophic lateral sclerosis epidemiological implications. In: Smith RA, ed. Handbook of ALS. New York: Marcel Dekker Inc., 1992:93–131.

60. Whiting MG. Toxicity of cycads. Econ Bot 1963; 17:271–302.
61. Spencer PS, Nunn PB, Hugon J, Hugon J, Ludolph A, Roy DN. Motor neuron disease on Guam: possible role of a food toxin. Lancet 1986; 1:965.
62. Spencer PS. Guam ALS/Parkinsonism-dementia: a long-latency neurotoxic disorder caused by "slow toxin(s)" in food? Can J Neurol Sci 1987; 14:347–357.
63. Duncan MW. Beta-Methylamino-L-alanine (BMAA) and amyotrophic lateral sclerosis-parkinsonism dementia of the western Pacific. Ann NY Acad Sci 1992; 648:161–168.
64. Cox PA, Sacks OW. Cycad neurotoxins, consumption of flying foxes, and ALS-PDC disease in Guam. Neurology 2002; 58:956–959.
65. Banack SA, Cox PA. Biomagnefication of cycad neurotoxins in flying foxes. Neurology 2003; 61:387–389.
66. McGeer PL, Schwab C, McGeer EG, Haddock RL, Steele JC. Familial nature and continuing morbidity of the amyotrophic lateral sclerosis - parkinsonism dementia complex of Guam. Neurology 1997; 49:400–409.
67. Armon C, Daube JR, O'Brien PC, Kurland LT, Mulder DW. When is an apparent excess of neurologic cases epidemiologically significant? Neurology 1991; 41:1713–1718
68. Kurtzke JF. On statistical testing of prevalence studies. J Chron Dis 1966; 19:909–922.
69. Mundt DJ, Dell LD, Luippold RS, Sulsky SI, Skillings A, Gross R, Cox KL, Mundt KA. Cause-specific mortality among Kelly Air Force Base civilian employees, 1981–2001. J Occup Environ Med 2002; 44:989–996.
70. Haley RW. Excess incidence of ALS in young Gulf War veterans. Neurology 2003; 61:750–756.
71. Horner RD, Kamins KG, Feussner JR, Grambow SC, Hoff-Lindquist J, Harati Y, Mitsumoto H, Pascuzzi R, Spencer PS, Tim R, Howard D, Smith TC, Ryan MA, Coffman CJ, Kasarskis EJ. Occurrence of amyotrophic lateral sclerosis among Gulf War veterans. Neurology 2003; 61:742–749. Erratum in: Neurology 2003; 11; 61:1320.
72. Weisskopf M, O'Reilly E, McCullough M, Calle E, Thun M, Cudkowicz M, Ascherio A. Prospective study of military service and mortality from ALS. Neurology 2005; 64:32–37.
73. Mulder DW, Kurland LT, Offord KP, Beard CM. Familial adult motor neuron disease: amyotrophic lateral sclerosis. Neurology 1986; 36:511–517.
74. Li TM, Alberman E, Swash M. Comparison of sporadic and familial disease amongst 580 cases of motor neuron disease. J Neurol Neurosurg Psychiatry 1988; 51:778–784.
75. Williams DB, Floate DA, Leicester J. Familial motor neuron disease: differing penetrance in large pedigrees. J Neurol Sci 1988; 86:215–230.
76. Swash M, Leigh N. Criteria for diagnosis of familial amyotrophic lateral sclerosis. Neuromuscul Disord 1992; 2:7–9.
77. Siddique T, Figlewicz DA, Pericak-Vance MA, Haines JL, Rouleau G, Jeffers AJ, Sapp P, Hung WY, Bebout J, McKenna-Yasek D, Deng G, Horvitz HR, Gusella JK, Brown RH and Collaborators. Linkage of a gene causing familial amyotrophic lateral sclerosis to chromosome 21 and evidence of genetic-locus heterogeneity. N Engl J Med 1991; 324(20):1381–1384.
78. Siddique T, Nijhawan D, Hentati A. Familial amyotrophic lateral sclerosis. J Neural Transm Suppl 1997; 49:219–233.
79. Al-Chalabi A, Andersen PM, Chioza B, Shaw C, Sham PC, Robberecht W, Matthijs G, Camu W, Marklund SL, Forsgren L, Rouleau G, Laing NG, Hurse PV, Siddique T, Leigh PN, Powell JF. Recessive amyotrophic lateral sclerosis families with the D90A SOD1 mutation share a common founder: evidence for a linked protective factor. Hum Mol Genet 1998; 7:2045–2050.
80. Hentati A, Ouahchi K, Pericak-Vance MA, Nijhawan D, Ahmad A, Yang Y, Rimmler J, Hung W, Schlotter B, Ahmed A, Ben Hamida M, Hentati F, Siddique T. Linkage of a commoner form of recessive amyotrophic lateral sclerosis to chromosome 15q15–122 markers. Neurogenetics 1998; 2:55–60.

81. Buchanan DS, Malamud N. Motor neuron disease with renal cell carcinoma and post-operative neurologic remission. A clinicopathologic report. Neurology 1973; 23:891–894.
82. Chiò A, Brignolio F, Meineri P, Schiffer D. Phenotypic and genotypic heterogeneity of dominantly inherited amyotrophic lateral sclerosis. Acta Neurol Scand 1987; 75:277–282.
83. Granieri E, Murgia SB, Rosati G, Tola R, Pinna L, Paolino E, D'Agostini G. The frequency of amyotrophic lateral sclerosis among workers in Sardinia. IRCS Med Sci 1983; 11:898.
84. Gunnarsson LG, Bodin L, Soderfeldt B, Axelson O. A case-control study of motor neuron disease: its relation to heritability, and occupational exposures, particularly to solvents. Br J Ind Med 1992; 49:791–798.
85. Williams DB, Annegers JF, Kokmen E, O'Brien PC, Kurland LT. Brain injury and neurological sequelae: a cohort study of dementia, parkinsonism and amyotrophic lateral sclerosis. Neurology 1991; 41:1554–1557.
86. Schlesselman JJ. Case-Control Studies Design, Conduct, Analysis. New York: Oxford University Press, 1982 Inc.
87. Koren G, Klein N. Bias against negative studies in newspaper reports of medical research. JAMA 1991; 266:1824–1826.
88. Dickersin K, Min YI, Meinert CL. Factors influencing publication of research results. Follow-up of applications submitted to two institutional review boards. JAMA 1992; 267:374–378.
89. Tanner CM, Ross GW. Neuroepidemiology: Fundamental considerations. In: Nelson LN, Tanner CM, Van Den Eeden SK, McGuire VM, eds. Neuroepidemiology: From Principles to Practice. New York: Oxford University Press, 2004:1–22.
90. Nelson LN, McGuire VM. Study design, measures of effect, and sources of bias. In: Nelson LN, Tanner CM, Van Den Eeden SK, McGuire VM, eds. Neuroepidemiology: From Principles to Practice. New York: Oxford University Press, 2004:23–54.
91. Chancellor AM, Slattery JM, Fraser H, Warlow CP. Risk factors for motor neuron disease: a case-control study based on patients from the Scottish Motor Neuron Disease Register. J Neurol Neurosurg Psychiatry 1993; 56:1200–1206.
92. Kamel F, Umbach DM, Munsat TL, Shefner JM, Sandler DP. Association of cigarette smoking with amyotrophic lateral sclerosis. Neuroepidemiology 1999; 18:194–202.
93. McGuire V, Longstreth WT Jr, Nelson LM, Koepsell TD, Checkoway H, Morgan MS, van Belle G. Occupational exposures and amyotrophic lateral sclerosis. A population-based case-control study. Am J Epidemiol 1997; 145:1076–1088.
94. Armon C, Kurland LT, O'Brien PC, Mulder DW. Antecedent medical diseases in patients with amyotrophic lateral sclerosis: A population-based case-controlled study in Rochester, Minnesota, 1925–1987. Arch Neurol 1991; 48:283–286.
95. Deapen DM, Henderson BE. A case-control study of amyotrophic lateral sclerosis. Am J Epidemiol 1986; 123:790–799.
96. Kurtzke JF, Beebe GW. Epidemiology of amyotrophic lateral sclerosis: 1. A case-control comparison based on ALS deaths. Neurology 1980; 30:453–462.
97. Kondo K, Tsubaki T. Case-control studies of motor neuron disease. Association with mechanical injuries. Arch Neurol 1981; 38:220–226.
98. Angelini C, Armani M, Bresolin N. Incidence and risk factors in the Venice and Padua districts of Italy, 1972–1979. Neuroepidemiology 1983; 2:236–242.
99. Gallagher JP, Sanders M. Trauma and amyotrophic lateral sclerosis: a report of 78 patients. Acta Neurol Scand 1987; 75:145–150.
100. Chio A, Meineri P, Tribolo A, Schiffer D. Risk factors in motor neuron disease: a case-control study. Neuroepidemiology 1991; 10:174–184.
101. Kurland LT, Radhakrishnan K, Smith GE, Armon C, Nemetz PN. Mechanical trauma as a risk factor in classic amyotrophic lateral sclerosis: Lack of epidemiologic evidence. J Neurol Sci 1992; 113:133–143.
102. Strickland D, Smith SA, Dolliff G, Goldman L, Roelofs RI. Amyotrophic lateral sclerosis and occupational history: a pilot case-control study. Arch Neurol 1996; 53:730–733.

103. Cruz DC, Nelson LM, McGuire V, Longstreth WT Jr. Physical trauma and family history of neurodegenerative diseases in amyotrophic lateral sclerosis: a population-based case-control study. Neuroepidemiology 1999; 18:101–110.

104. Davanipour Z, Sobel E, Bowman JD, Qian Z, Will AD. Amyotrophic lateral sclerosis and occupational exposure to electromagnetic fields. Bioelectromagnetics 1997; 18:28–35.

105. Johansen C, Olsen JH. Mortality from amyotrophic lateral sclerosis, other chronic disorders, and electric shocks among utility workers. Am J Epidemiol 1998; 148:362–368.

106. Savitz DA, Checkoway H, Loomis DP. Magnetic field exposure and neurodegenerative disease mortality among electric utility workers. Epidemiology 1998; 9:398–404.

107. Noonan CW, Reif JS, Yost M, Touchstone J. Occupational exposure to magnetic fields in case-referent studies of neurodegenerative diseases. Scand J Work Environ Health 2002; 28:42–48.

108. Li C-Y, Sung F-C. Association between occupational exposure to power frequency electromagnetic fields and amyotrophic lateral sclerosis: a review. Am J Ind Med 2003; 43:212–220.

109. Håkansson N, Gustavsson P, Johansen C, Floderus B. Neurodegenerative diseases in welders and other workers exposed to high levels of magnetic fields. Epidemiology 2003; 14:420–426; discussion 427–428.

110. Feychting M, Jonsson F, Pedersen NL, Ahlbom A. Occupational magnetic field exposure and neurodegenerative disease. Epidemiology 2003; 14:413–419; discussion 427–428.

111. Gawel M, Zaiwalla Z, Rose FC. Antecedent events in motor neuron disease. J Neurol Neurosurg Psychiatry 1983; 46:1041–1043.

112. Sienko DG, Davis JP, Taylor JA, Brooks BR. Amyotrophic lateral sclerosis. A case-control study following detection of a cluster in a small Wisconsin community. Arch Neurol 1990; 47:38–41.

113. Savettieri G, Salemi G, Arcara A, Cassata M, Castiglione MG, Fierro B. A case-control study of amyotrophic lateral sclerosis. Neuroepidemiology 1991; 10:242–245.

114. Longstreth WT, Nelson LM, Koepsell TD, van Belle G. Hypotheses to explain the association between vigorous physical activity and amyotrophic lateral sclerosis. Med Hypotheses 1991; 34:144–148.

115. Breland AE, Currier RD. Multiple sclerosis and amyotrophic lateral sclerosis in Mississippi. Neurology 1967; 17:1011–1016.

116. Felmus MT, Patten BM, Swanke L. Antecedent events in amyotrophic lateral sclerosis. Neurology 1976; 26:167–172.

117. Palo J, Jokelainen M. Geographic and social distribution of patients with amyotrophic lateral sclerosis. Arch Neurol 1977; 34:724.

118. Bracco L, Antuono P, Amaducci L. Study of epidemiological and etiological factors of amyotrophic lateral sclerosis in the province of Florence, Italy. Acta Neurol Scand 1979; 60:112–124.

119. Roelofs-Iverson RA, Mulder DW, Elveback LR, Kurland LT, Molgaard CA. ALS and heavy metals: a pilot case-control study. Neurology 1984; 34:393–395.

120. Granieri E, Carreras M, Tola R, Paolino E, Tralli G, Eleopra R, Serra G. Motor neuron disease in the province of Ferrara, Italy in 1964–1982. Neurology 1988; 38:1604–1608.

121. Armon C, Kurland LT, Daube JR, O'Brien PC. Epidemiologic correlates of sporadic amyotrophic lateral sclerosis. Neurology 1991; 41:1077–1084.

122. Longstreth WT, McGuire V, Koepsell TD, Wang Y, van Belle G. Risk of amyotrophic lateral sclerosis and history of physical activity: a population-based case-control study. Arch Neurol 1998; 55:201–206.

123. Chiò A, Mora G. ALS and soccer: A methodological approach. Neuroepidemiology 2004; 23:155.

124. Beghi E, Chiò A, Hardiman O, Logroscino G, Mitchell JD, Swinger R. Amyotrophic lateral sclerosis and professional sports activities – A population-based case–control study. Neuroepidemiology 2004; 23:155.

125. Campbell AMG, Williams ER, Barltrop D. Motor neuron disease and exposure to lead. J Neurol Neurosurg Psychiatry 1970; 33:877–885.

126. Kamel F, Umbach DM, Munsat TL, Shefner JM, Hu H, Sandler DP. Lead exposure and amyotrophic lateral sclerosis. Epidemiology 2002; 13:311–319.

127. Pierce-Ruhland R, Patten BM. Repeat study of antecedent events in motor neuron disease. Ann Clin Res 1981; 13:102–107.

128. Gresham LS, Molgaard CA, Golbeck AL, Smith R. Amyotrophic lateral sclerosis and occupational heavy metal exposure: a case-control study. Neuroepidemiology 1986; 5:29–38.

129. Schulte PA, Burnett CA, Boeniger MF, Johnson J. Neurodegenerative diseases: occupational occurrence and potential risk factors, 1982 through 1991. Am J Public Health 1996; 86:1281–1288.

130. Graham AJ, Macdonald AM, Hawkes CH. British motor neuron disease twin study. J Neurol Neurosurg Psychiatry 1997; 62:562–569.

131. Hawkes CH, Fox AJ. Motor neuron disease in leather workers. Lancet 1981; 1:507.

132. Buckley J, Warlow C, Smith P, Hilton-Jones D, Irvine S, Tew JR. Motor neuron disease in England and Wales, 1959–1979. J Neurol Neurosurg Psychiatry 1983; 46:197–205.

133. Holloway SM, Mitchell JD. Motor neurone disease in the Lothian Region of Scotland 1961–1981. J Epidemiol Community Health 1986; 40:344–350.

134. Martyn CN. Motor neuron disease and exposure to solvents. Lancet 1989; 1:394.

135. Gunnarsson LG, Lindberg G. Amyotrophic lateral sclerosis in Sweden 1970–1983 and solvent exposure. Lancet 1989; 1:958.

136. Kalfakis N, Vassilopoulos D, Voumvourakis C, Ndjeveleka M, Papageorgiou C. Amyotrophic lateral sclerosis in southern Greece: an epidemiologic study. Neuroepidemiology 1991; 10:170–173.

137. Holloway SM, Emery AE. The epidemiology of motor neuron disease in Scotland. Muscle Nerve 1982; 5:131–133.

138. Bharucha NE, Schoenberg BS, Raven RH, Pickle LW, Byar DP, Mason TJ. Geographic distribution of motor neuron disease and correlation with possible etiologic factors. Neurology 1983; 33:911–915.

139. Provinciali L, Giovagnoli AR. Antecedent events in amyotrophic lateral sclerosis: do they influence clinical onset and progression? Neuroepidemiology 1990; 9:255–262

140. Mitchell JD, Davies RB, al-Hamad A, Gatrell AC, Batterby G. MND risk factors: an epidemiological study in the north west of England. J Neurol Sci 1995; 129(suppl):61–64.

141. Nelson LM, McGuire V, Longstreth WT, Matkin C. Population-based case-control study of amyotrophic lateral sclerosis in western Washington State. I. Cigarette smoking and alcohol consumption. Am J Epidemiol 2000b; 151:156–163.

142. Weisskopf MG, McCullough ML, Calle EE, Thun MJ, Cudkowicz M, Ascherio A. Prospective study of cigarette smoking and amyotrophic lateral sclerosis. Am J Epidemiol 2004; 160:26–33.

143. Howard DJ, Ota RG, Briggs LA, Hampton M, Pritsos CA, Environmental tobacco smoke in the workplace induces oxidative stress in employess, including increased production of 8-hydroxy-2'-deoxyguosine. Cancer Epidemiol Biomarkers Prev 1998; 7: 141–146.

144. Wiedau-Pazos M, Goto JJ, Rabizadeh S, Gralla EB, Roe JA, Lee MK, Valentine JS, Bredesen DE. Altered reactivity of superoxide dismutase in familial amyotrophic lateral sclerosis. Science 1996; 271:515–518.

145. Yim MB, Chock PB, Stadtman ER. Enzyme function of copper, zinc superoxide dismutase as a free radical generator. J Biol Chem 1993; 268:4099–4105.

146. Beckman JS, Carson M, Smith CD, Koppenol WH. ALS, SOD and peroxynitrite. Nature 1993; 364:584.

147. Eiserich JP, van der Vliet A, Handelman GJ, Halliwell B, Cross CE. Dietary antioxidants and cigarette smoke-induced biomolecular damage: a complex interaction. Am J Clin Nutr 1995; 62(suppl 6):1490S–1500S.

148. Nelson LM, Matkin C, Longstreth WT, McGuire V. Population-based case-control study of amyotrophic lateral sclerosis in western Washington State. II. Diet. Am J Epidemiol 2000a; 151:164–173.

149. Penzes L, Fischer HD, Noble RC. Some aspects on the relationship between lipids, neurotransmitters, and aging. Z Gerontol 1993; 26:65–69.

150. Bourre JM, Bonneil M, Clement M, Dumont O, Durand G, Lafont H, Nalbone G, Piciotti M. Function of dietary polyunsaturated fatty acids in the nervous system. Prostaglandins Leukot Essent Fatty Acids 1993; 48:5–15.

151. Liu D. The roles of free radicals in amyotrophic lateral sclerosis. J Mol Neurosci 1996; 7:159–167.

152. Hillemeier C. An overview of the effects of dietary fiber on gastrointestinal transit. Pediatrics 1995; 96:997–999.

153. Lupton JR, Turner ND. Potential protective mechanisms of wheat bran fiber. Am J Med 1999; 106:24S–27S.

154. Ascherio A, Weisskopf MG, O'Reilly E, Cudkowicz M, Jacobs E, McCullough M, Calle E, Thun M. Vitamin E intake and risk of amyotrophic lateral sclerosis. Ann Neurol 2005; 57:104–110.

155. Miller RG, Rosenberg JA, Gelinas DF, Mitsumoto H, Newman D, Sufit R, Borasio GD, Bradley WG, Bromberg MB, Brooks BR, Kasarskis EJ, Munsat TL, Oppenheimer EA. Practice parameter: the care of the patient with amyotrophic lateral sclerosis (an evidence-based review): report of the quality standards subcommittee of the american academy of neurology: ALS practice parameters task force. Neurology 1999; 52:1311–1323.

156. Shaw PJ. Science, medicine and the future: Motor neurone disease. BMJ 1999; 318:1118–1121.

3

The Pathology of Amyotrophic Lateral Sclerosis

Arthur P. Hays
Department of Pathology (Neuropathology), Columbia University Medical Center, Columbia University, New York, New York, U.S.A.

INTRODUCTION

The clinical diagnosis of probable or definite amyotrophic lateral sclerosis (ALS) based on El Escorial criteria (1) is probably correct in well over 95% of patients as determined by autopsy (2). The autopsy report helps us to reassure surviving family members that the diagnosis of the patient was correct during life in most instances and that clinical management was appropriate. As there is no available treatment to halt progression of ALS and prevent a fatal outcome, it is essential that new therapies be tested in clinical trials to eventually achieve success (3). Autopsy plays an important role in clinical trials by verifying the diagnosis of ALS in participating subjects and by detecting potentially adverse effects of treatment on tissue. Finally, autopsy shows an occasional unsuspected major disorder, such as an occult malignancy, that coexists with ALS.

The autopsy also offers important insights into the biology of ALS. This information allows investigators to generate hypotheses about underlying mechanisms that cause dysfunction and death of motor neurons. A major question has existed about ALS and other neurodegenerative disease for more than a century, namely, why are certain nerve cells targets of the disease and others are resistant (4,5)? Why are motor neurons of the ventral horn and hypoglossal nucleus vulnerable to ALS whereas nerve cells that control the movement of external eye muscles are spared? Recent research has begun to study the function and structure of these different populations of motor nerve cells in relation to ALS (6–9). Hopefully, knowledge about the molecular basis of resistance in motor neurons can eventually point to a therapeutic strategy to protect vulnerable cells. During the last 15 years, animal models of the human disease, particularly transgenic mice that express mutant Cu/Zn superoxide dismutase (SOD1), have provided remarkable advances in knowledge about the experimental disorder. These advances raise the important question of whether the animal models are valid for the human disease. The queries can be addressed, in part, by analysis of autopsy tissue. This investigation often requires use of frozen autopsy tissue that is stored at an institutional "bank" for future research after a surviving spouse or family members give proper consent for autopsy.

Biopsy of the nervous system presents the potential for making a definitive diagnosis of ALS early in the disease of patients, allowing them to participate in a clinical therapeutic trial before weakness is severe. However, removing even a small piece of spinal cord or the brain is not justified by the risk of serious complications. Biopsy of a nerve that supplies a redundant muscle, such as the gracilis muscle, is associated with no noticeable motor deficit and little risk of complication (10). The nerve of a clinically affected muscle demonstrates evidence of axonal degeneration with loss of large myelinated fibers (11). Unfortunately, these findings are not specific for ALS, and no specific pathological or other biomarker of the disorder in peripheral nerve is available yet. Currently, biopsy of nerve and muscle is limited to infrequent patients with atypical clinical features of ALS (1) to identify mimics of the disease, such as inclusion body myositis (12), a mitochondrial disorder (13), polyglucosan body disease (14), or multifocal motor neuropathy (MMN) (11). Because of the limitations of the biopsy, this chapter discusses chiefly the autopsy findings in ALS.

PATHOLOGY OF SPORADIC ALS

For over a century after the first detailed description of sporadic ALS (sALS) by Charcot in 1869 (15), the postmortem diagnosis rested on the finding of degeneration and loss of motor neurons in the precentral gyrus, brainstem, and spinal cord, attended by astrocytosis (proliferation of astrocytes and their cell processes or fibers) at the same sites (16–22). The interpretation included alterations ("degeneration") of surviving motor nerve cells, such as atrophy of the cell body and abundant lipofuscin, and secondary changes comprising pyramidal tract degeneration, loss of motor nerve fibers, and neurogenic abnormalities in skeletal muscle. None of these changes are specific for ALS, although the overall pattern supports the diagnosis.

In early studies, the brain and spinal cord often demonstrated mild pathological abnormalities of nerve cells other than motor neurons even though clinical findings were usually limited to the motor system. An example of non-motor pathological involvement in ALS was indicated historically by stains of myelin in the spinal cord, which often showed widespread myelin pallor within the lateral columns and anterior columns as a result of axonal degeneration and nerve cell death. This pallor and myelin breakdown products (Fig. 1) extend well beyond the crossed and uncrossed pyramidal tracts and clearly indicate subtle disorder of non-motor nerve cells (16,19,23). Involvement of other populations of nerve cells and tracts has been documented in numerous articles (16,19–22,24–30). Other parts of the nervous system are spared in sALS, as exemplified by the posterior columns (Fig. 1) in most cases (21,22,24) or motor cells that project to external eye muscles (16). These pathological findings oversimplify the state of the autopsy during this early period as clinical and pathological non-motor manifestations in ALS were documented in the literature, such as dementia and frontotemporal lobar degeneration of the brain or the Guamanian type of ALS, which is often accompanied by Parkinsonism and dementia (31–33). These more complex disorders presented a nosological conundrum. ALS and dementia, for example, were variously classified as atypical forms of ALS (20), unique entities (34,35), ALS with Creutzfeldt–Jakob disease (36), or the amyotrophic form of Creutzfeldt–Jakob disease (37,38).

Controversies about the pathological diagnosis of ALS and its variants have changed dramatically during the last 25 years and particularly during the last 15 years, with the recognition of intracytoplasmic inclusions that are nearly specific

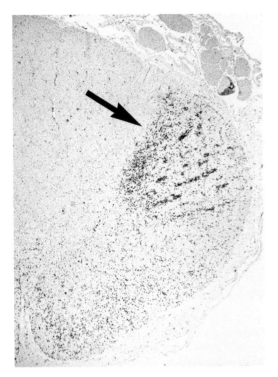

Figure 1 Transverse sections of a thoracic segment of the spinal cord in a patient with sALS. Numerous CD68-immunopositive macrophages and activated microglia are located in the pyramidal tract region (*arrow*). Fewer CD68-positive cells are present elsewhere in the lateral column and anterior columns. Immunoperoxidase stain of CD68, a macrophage/histiocyte marker. *Abbreviation*: sALS, sporadic amyotrophic lateral sclerosis.

for this disorder. These pathological markers of ALS have clarified nosology and have established that the disorder is more diverse than suspected. The inclusions have helped to confirm the nineteenth century notion (39) that ALS, progressive bulbar palsy, progressive muscular atrophy (PMA), and primary lateral sclerosis (PLS) are different manifestations of motor neuron disease (26,40). They have permitted recognition of a subclass of frontotemporal dementia as an infrequent expression of motor neuron disease (41–46). In addition, investigators have reported similar inclusions in the Guamanian type and certain forms of familial ALS (fALS) (47–50), suggesting that they share disease mechanisms with sALS. Finally, the inclusions can strongly support the diagnosis of ALS and its variants even when sampling is limited and loss of motor neurons is not documented by subjective or quantitative analysis.

Cytoplasmic Inclusions

Bunina Bodies

Bunina bodies (BBs) were reported in 1962 in two patients with fALS (51) but were subsequently identified in sALS (52). BBs are small, eosinophilic, hyaline inclusions within the cytoplasm of surviving motor neuronal cell bodies of the spinal cord and brain stem using the standard hematoxylin and eosin (H&E) stain (Fig. 2). Rarely,

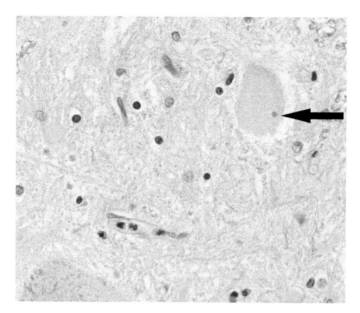

Figure 2 A Bunina body in a motor neuron of a ventral horn in sALS. The inclusion is located within abundant cytoplasmic lipofuscin of a nerve cell body. The structure is round, hyaline, and surrounded by an indistinct pale halo (*arrow*). The nucleus is not included within the plane of the tissue section (H&E). *Abbreviation*: sALS, sporadic amyotrophic lateral sclerosis.

they are found in dendrites (53,54). The inclusions are round or irregular in shape with dimensions that range from about 1 to 6 μm. They are often located within chromatolytic cells (see below), accompanied by abundant lipofuscin (40,55). Some of the inclusions are surrounded by a thin pale halo. The percentage of ALS patients with these inclusions varies from 65% to 95% in different autopsy surveys (40,56–62). Lack of BBs can often be attributed to a marked loss of nerve cells in many instances. When inclusions are seen, they are usually identified in a small minority of the surviving motor neurons, usually less than 10% of the cells, although higher values were reported (63). BBs are extremely rare in motor neurons of other disorders and are nearly pathognomonic of ALS.

The inclusions have been evaluated extensively by immunohistochemistry and electron microscopic examination, but these studies have not provided clues to the role of BBs in dysfunction and death of motor nerve cells. BBs express cystatin C (64–66), an inhibitor of lysosomal cathepsins (cysteine protease) (67). The inclusions usually do not express ubiquitin and are devoid of immunoreactive neurofilament (NF) protein and many other proteins (49,56,57,59,66). By electron microscopy, the inclusions were found to consist of electron dense granular material that completely or partially encloses large lucent areas and contains vesicular structures and a few filaments (50,62,68–73). The inclusions are surrounded by rough endoplasmic reticulum, other organelles, and abundant lipofuscin. BBs may be a consequence of degradation of cellular material within lysosomes (autophagy) (68), although the inclusions are not membrane-bound (40) and do not express acid phosphatase in contrast to lysosomes (61). Investigators have speculated that BBs arise from endoplasmic reticulum based on ultrastructural studies and spectrometry (72,74).

ALS patients infrequently demonstrate similar eosinophilic inclusions within Betz cells (56,75), motor neurons of the oculomotor nucleus (75), dorsal motor nucleus of the vagal nerve (69), and Onuf's nucleus (75–77). They have also been described in non-motor nerve cells including nerve cells of the subthalamic nucleus (78), locus ceruleus (79), the reticular formation of the medulla oblongata (80), Clarke's column (75,81), and dorsal root ganglia (69). The inclusions in some of these locations have characteristic ultrastructural features of BBs (72,75,76,79,80). However, the inclusions of the dorsal motor nucleus and dorsal root are not BBs but appear to be composed of melanin granules based on ultrastructure (69). In addition, the specificity of BBs in nerve cells for ALS is not well established apart from lower motor neurons. BBs have been observed in Betz cells of elderly individuals who did not have ALS (82). In our laboratory, we found similar inclusions by light microscopy within Betz cells of Parkinson's disease although they did not express cystatin C (D.K. Leung, G. Karlikaya, A.P. Hays, L.P. Rowland, 1999, unpublished observation). In contrast, BBs in motor neurons of the spinal cord and brainstem are highly specific for ALS, and they have been reported in most variants of the disorder, namely PMA, progressive bulbar palsy, PLS, ALS with frontotemporal lobe degeneration, Guamanian ALS, and rare types of fALS (83). BBs are not found in patients with fALS due to mutations of the *SOD1* gene (84) except for the recently reported G127X mutation (47).

Ubiquinated Inclusions

Ubiquinated inclusions of motor neurons of the spinal cord and brainstem are more important than BBs for diagnosis of ALS because they are observed in nearly 100% of patients and are highly specific for the disorder (49,56,57,62,85–88). Unlike BBs, ubiquinated inclusions are invisible or indistinct based on H&E and other standard stains.

There is one exception to this rule: occasional ubiquinated inclusions superficially resemble Lewy bodies of Parkinson's disease (Lewy body-like inclusions or LBLIs) (see below). Because most ubiquinated inclusions cannot be identified by H&E, they were not discovered by light microscopy until 1988 when investigators first used immunohistochemical analysis of the small protein, ubiquitin, in ALS (85,86).

Ubiquinated inclusions are composed of fibrils and are located in the cell body or, sometimes, in dendrites (Fig. 3). Some consist of a single intracytoplasmic fibril or a loosely arranged aggregate of fibrils and are known collectively as skein-like inclusions (SLIs). Others are round or irregular dense bodies with a homogeneous or fibrillary substructure and are termed dense or compact inclusions (CIs) (Table 1). These structures range from 5 to 25 μm in greatest dimension. A few CIs have typical histological features of LBLIs based on the H&E stain (Fig. 4A) and ubiquitin immunohistochemistry (Fig. 4B). The ultrastructure of SLIs and LBLIs is composed of filaments (about 15–20 nm in diameter) that are coated by a variable number of small granules, suggesting that these inclusions are closely related and composed of the same material (59,89–93). These filaments are thicker than NFs and express strongly immunoreactive ubiquitin (59,87,90,91).

In three studies of ALS, the average percent of surviving motor neurons bearing SLIs and CIs in spinal cords ranged from 8.5% to 27.8% (57,88,94). The higher value was based on immunofluorescence and may have been related, in part, to a higher resolution of that method than provided by immunoperoxidase, allowing better identification of single or sparse ubiquinated fibrils. SLIs are more numerous

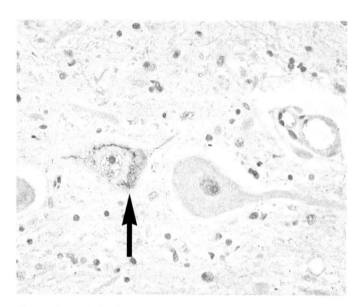

Figure 3   A skein-like inclusion in sALS. The inclusion consists of thin darkly stained fibrils (*arrow*) that are located in the cytoplasm of the cell body. Similar fibrils extend into two dendrites. Immunoperoxidase stain of ubiquitin. *Abbreviation*: sALS, sporadic amyotrophic lateral sclerosis.

than CIs in most cases of ALS. In one study, 21% of the surviving motor nerve cells contained SLIs and 6.8% had CIs (94). Of the CIs, only 0.5% of the surviving motor nerve cells displayed LBLIs. SLIs are also found in the nerve cells of Onuf's nucleus (76,77), Clarke's column (56), oculomotor nucleus (95), substantia nigra (96), and rarely elsewhere. Betz cells rarely contain SLIs (57) or CIs (97). Similar, but not identical, CIs appear in non-motor nerve cells of other cerebral structures, particularly

Table 1   Abbreviations

Term	Abbreviations
Basophilic inclusion	BI
Bunina body	BB
Cu/Zn superoxide dismutase	SOD1
Compact inclusion	CI
Familial amyotrophic lateral sclerosis	fALS
Hyaline conglomerate inclusion	HCI
Lewy body-like inclusion	LBLI
Mitogen-activated protein kinase	MAPK
Motor neuron disease-inclusion dementia	MNDID
Multifocal motor neuropathy	MMN
Neurofilament	NF
Primary lateral sclerosis	PLS
Progressive muscular atrophy	PMA
Skein-like inclusion	SLI
Superoxide dismutase gene	*SOD*1
Sporadic amyotrophic lateral sclerosis	sALS

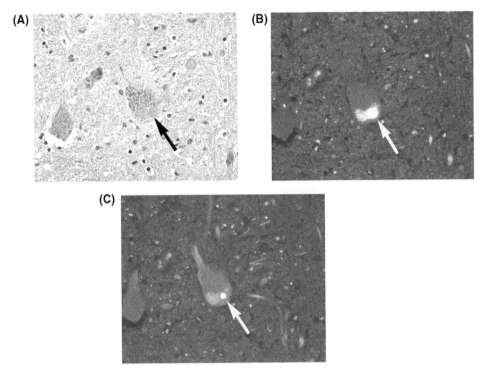

Figure 4 A Lewy body-like inclusion in sALS: (**A**) A faint, round, eosinophilic inclusion (*arrow*) is located within the cytoplasm of a motor nerve cell body. It is surrounded by an indistinct pale halo (H&E). (**B**) The same inclusion (*arrow*) is strongly immunoreactive for ubiquitin. Double label immunofluorescence stain, monoclonal antibody to ubiquitin. (**C**) Peripherin, an intermediate filament protein, is espressed in the core (*arrow*), but not the halo, of the inclusion. Double label immunofluorescence stain, polyclonal antibodies to peripherin. *Abbreviation*: sALS, sporadic amyotrophic lateral sclerosis.

the dentate gyrus of the hippocampal formation, cerebral cortex, striatum, and elsewhere (see below). In these cerebral locations, they are found in a minority of ALS patients but occur in most of those patients with ALS-frontotemporal dementia (44–46,62). Ubiquinated inclusions in motor neurons have been reported in nearly all variants of ALS except for sporadic juvenile ALS with basic inclusions (BIs) (see below).

Intense immunohistochemical analysis of ubiquinated inclusions has yielded little knowledge about the composition of ubiquinated inclusions since 1988 (28). Ubiquitin is a small protein that forms covalent bonds with other proteins to mark them for degradation through an ATP-dependent proteolytic system in a multimeric structure known as a proteasome. Ubiquinated inclusions are a common feature of neurodegenerative diseases and are subclassified by structure and composition. For example, the Lewy bodies of the substantia nigra in Parkinson's disease have a distinctive round hyaline appearance with a pale halo; they express ubiquitin, α-synuclein, NF subunits, and other proteins (98). Little is known about the composition of ubiquinated inclusions in ALS, but they express dorfin and NEDD8, proteins that participate in the ATP-dependent proteolytic system (99). These two proteins are also expressed in other ubiquinated inclusions such as the Lewy bodies of Parkinson's disease (100). The inclusions of ALS do not coexpress certain other proteins of this pathway, namely a ubiquitin hydrolase (PGP 9.5) (101) or markers of the proteasome (102,103).

LBLIs, but not SLIs, express several proteins in addition to ubiquitin and dorfin. These include epitopes of NF protein (56,104–108), peripherin (Fig. 4C) (94,109), 14-3-3 protein (a chaperone that recognizes phosphoserine-containing motifs) (110) and a cell cycle-dependent kinase, Cdk5 (111), an enzyme that catalyzes phosphorylation of NF subunits (112,113). LBLIs resemble Lewy bodies, but in sALS, they are less hyaline and do not express α-synuclein (94,96,106).

NF subunits and peripherin form the major intermediate filaments of motor neurons in adults and have an important role in structure and function, including axonal transport. Normally, middle- and high-molecular weight subunits of NF (NF-M, NF-H) become highly phosphorylated as the proteins move from the cell body into the axon. Both NF proteins and peripherin have been implicated in the pathogenesis of ALS based on studies of transgenic mice (114,115) and histological evidence that the proteins form aggregates in human disease (59,104,107,116–121). Moreover, mutations of the genes for the high-molecular weight subunit of NF protein (NF-H) (122,123) and peripherin (124,125) have been found in some patients with sALS. A mitogen-activated protein kinase, p38MAPK, has been identified in SLIs and CIs (126). The alpha form of this protein kinase phosphorylates NF subunits as well as other proteins (127). However, expression of p38MAPK was not seen in ubiquinated inclusions with a different set of commercially available antibodies to the protein (127).

Hyaline Conglomerate Inclusions

Hyaline conglomerate inclusions (HCIs) are located within the cell bodies of motor neurons and rarely Betz cells or other nerve cells of the brain and spinal cord. The inclusions are large with a smooth contour and irregular shape and have a pale, amphophilic, hyaline appearance (Fig. 5A). They are argyrophilic and express immunoreactive NF protein (Fig. 5B), peripherin (Fig. 5C), and SOD1 enzyme but have little detectable ubiquitin. HCIs are typical of fALS due to specific mutations of the SOD1 gene (see below). They are usually accompanied by cord-like swellings of axons in the ventral horn. Most sALS reports of these inclusions antedated the discovery of mutations in fALS, although some investigators suspected that it might be familial on the basis of histopathology, including HCIs and degeneration of the posterior columns and spinocerebellar tracts (128). Three different investigators reported that 3% to 7% of sALS patients have mutations of the SOD1 gene (129–131), and one autopsied patient with an I113T mutation demonstrated HCIs (48). This type of inclusion in motor neurons may be nearly specific for mutations of the gene (26,132). sALS with HCIs warrant sequencing of the SOD1 gene (94).

Basophilic Inclusions

BIs are intracytoplasmic inclusions of motor neurons that are seen in few patients with sALS (29,133–138). Most of the patients have been children or young adults with one form of juvenile ALS. The inclusions are round or irregular in contour and are several micrometers in greatest dimension. They showed argyrophilia in some reports (137–140), but not in others (136,141). A few inclusions have a speckled pattern of immunoreactive ubiquitin, but most are devoid of the protein. None express cytoskeletal proteins or other proteins tested by immunohistochemistry (136,139,140,142), although BIs contain RNA (137). The inclusions are distributed more widely than

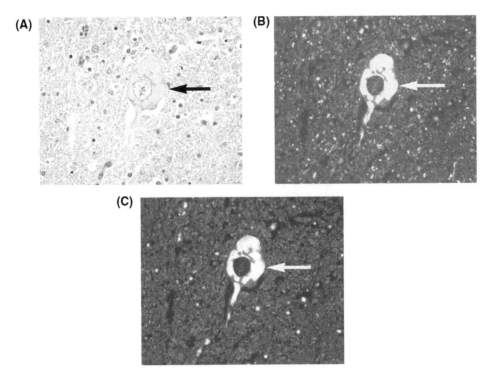

Figure 5 A hyaline conglomerate inclusion in sALS of a patient with an I113T mutation of *SOD*1 gene: (**A**) The inclusion fills the cytoplasm of a motor neuron (*arrow*) and extends into a dendrite. The structure is pale, slightly basophilic, and hyaline (H&E). (**B**) The heavy subunit of NF-is strongly expressed in the same inclusion (*arrow*). Double label immunofluorescence, monoclonal antibody to a phosphorylated epitope of NF-H. (**C**) The inclusion also shows immunoreactive peripherin. Double label immunofluorescence, polyclonal antibody to peripherin. *Abbreviations*: sALS, sporadic amyotrophic lateral sclerosis; NF-, neurofilament protein; SOD, superoxide dismutase.

other ALS inclusions and are commonly located in non-motor nerve cells of the basal ganglia, thalamus, substantia nigra, cerebellum, brainstem tegmentum, and others. Rare patients with BIs have non-motor clinical manifestations including dementia (136) and autonomic dysfunction (136,138). By electron microscopy, the inclusions are composed of a loosely arranged or compact meshwork of straight thick filaments coated by granular material (136,138–142). The filaments measure roughly 15 to 20 µm in diameters and the granules about 20 to 30 µm. These structures often are intermingled with a few NFs and sparse thick tubular filaments.

They do not exhibit rough endoplasmic reticulum except for a few profiles at the periphery. The ultrastructure of these inclusions resembles SLIs and LBLIs (141). However, this juvenile form of sALS does not exhibit BBs, SLIs or LBLIs. The findings suggest that the disorder is a distinct entity and are not seen with other forms of ALS.

Spheroids

Investigators first suspected a role for intermediate filaments in ALS in 1968, when neuropathologist Stirling Carpenter described large focal accumulations of NFs in axons of the ventral horn of the spinal cord (Fig. 6A) and brain stem (116). These axonal swellings are divided into large inclusions (spheroids) and smaller axonal swellings (globules). The inclusions are not useful for diagnosis because they occur in normal and neurological disease controls as well as in ALS. However, spheroids are more numerous in ALS patients than controls although not observed in all cases (104,116,118,121,143,144). These spheroids are located in the proximal part of the axon, particularly the initial segment or first internode of axon, arising from the motor neuron soma (75,116,145,146). In many instances, lack of these spheroids can be attributable to severe loss of motor nerve cells (also noted for inclusions of the cell body). By electron microscopy, the axonal swellings are composed of interwoven bundles of closely packed NFs and sparse mitochondria and smooth endoplasmic reticulum (116–118,121,143,144). This ultrastructure contrasts with the orderly parallel longitudinal arrangement of NFs in normal axons.

Spheroids strongly express all three subunits of NFs, heavy, light, and medium. The proteins include highly phosphorylated forms of NF-M and NF-H (Fig. 6B) resembling the phosphorylated state of these subunits in normal axons (107). The NF proteins of the cell body of normal nerve cells are less phosphorylated, but

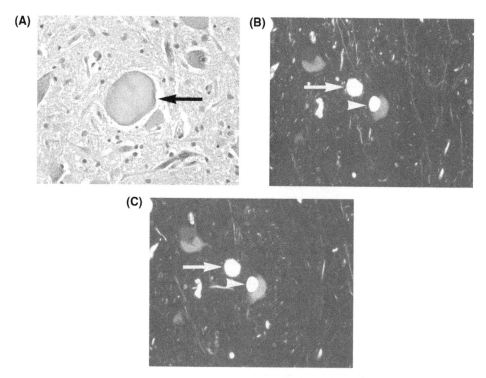

Figure 6 A large axonal swelling (spheroid) in sALS: (**A**) The spheroid is larger than motor neurons and has a pale, slightly basophilic structure with a finely fibrillar substructure (H&E). (**B**) A different spheroid expresses NF-H (*arrow*). A similar spheroid is present in cytoplasm of the cell body of a motor neuron (*arrowhead*), which also contains abundant granular, weakly autofluorescent lipofuscin. Double label immunofluorescence, monoclonal antibody to NF-H. (**C**) Peripherin is expressed in the same axonal spheroid (*arrow*) and the inclusion within the motor neuron (*arrowhead*). Double label immunofluorescence, polyclonal antibodies to peripherin. *Abbreviations*: sALS, sporadic amyotrophic lateral sclerosis; NF-H, neurofilament protein, heavy subunit.

the soma of motor neurons in ALS often abnormally expresses highly phosphorylated NF-M and NF-H (104,118). These perikaryal NFs are not organized into
discrete inclusions except as a minor component of LBLIs, but large inclusions
resembling spheroids (Fig. 6B,C) occur in a minority of ALS patients (104,117).
Axonal spheroids also express immunoreactive peripherin (Fig. 6C), STOP protein
(stable tubule on polypeptide), galectin-1, advanced glycated end products, and
several other proteins that are stained weakly and less constantly (108,119,147–154).
Little or no ubiquitin is detected in spheroids (56,59,85,86). Experimental studies of
similar axonal swellings of NFs in animals have demonstrated slowing of axonal transport, often associated with death of neurons (115,155,156). The molecular mechanisms
responsible for focal proliferation of NFs in axons and the relation between these
inclusions and motor neuron dysfunction and death are not understood, but research
on animal models suggests that spheroids could contribute to the pathogenesis of ALS
by interfering with axonal transport.

Chromatolytic Cells and Cell Death

A few surviving motor nerve cells in ALS have a rounded cell body with loss of Nissl
granules and a peripherally located nucleus (Fig. 7A). These morphological alterations resemble the "axonal reaction" or central chromatolysis seen in motor neurons
after nerve transection of experimental animals. The existence of chromatolytic cells
in ALS was initially controversial because one important autopsy survey reported no
central chromatolysis (20). Other investigators found infrequent chromatolytic cells
in ALS patients (16,157,158), but similar cells were reported in a comparable number
of controls (158). The controversy has gradually subsided over the last 20 years,
owing to the recognition of numerous chromatolytic cells in rare ALS patients.
These cells tend to be more numerous in patients who have progressed rapidly to
death within a few months after onset of symptoms (55,76,104,159–161). Structural
differences exist between these cells and true central chromatolysis (see below) and
may be responsible, in part, for the disagreement.

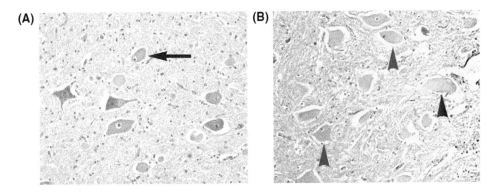

Figure 7 Central chromatolysis of motor neurons: (**A**) A motor neuron shows loss of Nissl
bodies and a peripherally located nucleus of a patient with sALS (*arrow*). These chromatolytic
cells are often smaller than their counterparts in motor neuropathy (see **B**) (H&E). (**B**) Three
motor neurons show typical central chromatolysis in a patient with a motor neuropathy and
Waldenström's macroglobulinemia (H&E). *Abbreviation*: sALS, sporadic amyotrophic lateral
sclerosis. *Source*: From Ref. 236.

True central chromatolysis of motor neurons is triggered by axonal transection and reflects complex modifications of the cell from a transmitting function to a growth mode to effect axonal regeneration (162,163). The structure of the cell body shifts from a concave contour between dendrites and the axon to a rounded shape and usually an increase of volume (163,164). The Nissl granules undergo dissolution (chromatolysis) in the center of the cell whereas they tend to be retained at the periphery. These changes are attended by prominent Golgi profiles, a disordered pattern of the rough endoplasmic reticulum and an increase of polyribosomes, mitochondria, and lysosomes. The increase and redistribution of ribosomal RNA transforms the motor neuron to a cell body with centrally located "dust-like" or "powdery" basophilic cytoplasm as judged by light microscopy (40,164,165). At the same time, the nucleus moves from the center to the periphery, and it and the nucleolus becomes larger (164,166). Synapses are lost or displaced from the surface of the cell body and dendrites by microglial cells (163). Within hours of axonal transection, the cell shows a dramatic change in gene expression (162,163). During this process, NFs become less numerous in the axons but are increased in the soma with a shift of NF proteins to a higher phosphorylated state (167). In adult animals, the soma of the neuron returns to a normal state if the regenerating axon reaches the muscle and reinnervates myofibers. However, if regeneration is unsuccessful or the site of axonal transection is close to the cell body, then the neuron may die. This is exemplified by experimentally induced avulsion of the sciatic nerve and attached nerve roots of adult rats, which results in chromatolysis and apoptosis of motor neurons. In this model, loss of 30% of the nerve cells is observed 21 days after axons are disrupted (168).

The chromatolytic cells of ALS have some of the same features of true central chromatolysis but the cell body tends to be smaller (25,55,169–172). The nucleus and nucleolus are smaller than normal and show less RNA and fewer ribosomes. Nissl bodies disappear centrally but may be retained at the periphery of the soma. The past literature reports large abnormal masses of Nissl-like material in some of these cells (40,157). However, many of the chromatolytic cells are devoid of Nissl granules or other basophilic material and are sometimes called "achromatic" cells. They are filled with abundant lipofuscin and often express a high-phosphorylated state of NF protein (104,118,121). The cells exhibit loss of synapses as observed in central chromatolysis (172) but are accompanied by severe atrophy of the dendrites and axons (170). By electron microscopy, the initial segment of the axon emanating from the cell body has a marked reduction of NFs and organelles, possibly a consequence of impaired axonal transport from the cell body. The abnormal structural features of chromatolytic cells of ALS are often highlighted by the presence of intracytoplasmic inclusions including BBs, ubiquinated inclusions, BIs, and HCIs (55,59,139,160, 172–176). Many of these features are unlike true central chromatolysis.

The significance of chromatolytic cells in ALS is not known, but limited structural and molecular cytopathology suggests a dysfunctional cell and a prelude to cell death. Some investigators have postulated a pathway that starts with chromatolysis and progresses to atrophy of the cell body and dendrites (175,177). The penultimate stage is a shrunken and rounded cell body with indistinct neurites and a condensed cytoplasm and nucleus. This alteration resembles apoptosis structurally and presumably leads to disintegration of the cell. The characteristic dense chromatin clumps of neuronal apoptosis have not been reported convincingly in ALS despite careful search. Some investigators detected DNA fragmentation in cells by terminal deoxy-nucleotidyltransferase-mediated dUTP-biotin nick-end labeling (TUNEL) in tissue sections (178,179), but others did not (180,181). DNA cleavage heralds cell death in experimental animals, but the finding in autopsy tissue is difficult to interpret because DNA degradation may be caused by terminal hypoxemia, postmortem autolysis, and other variables. Despite these technical problems, M. J. Martin concluded that DNA fragmentation is present in cells during the stage of somatodendritic atrophy and apoptotic-like transformation but not in chromatolysis. In addition, tissue levels of cell death regulatory proteins were found to be altered in ALS tissue in a pattern that facilitates apoptosis. These molecular and progressive structural changes in motor neurons closely resemble apoptosis and cell death in experimental animals. If this sequence from chromatolytic cells to cell death in ALS is supported by further investigation, it could permit molecular and structural analysis of isolated motor neurons at early and terminal stages of cell injury.

Ventral Spinal Roots and Peripheral Nerves

Morphological studies of motor nerve fibers have provided an incomplete view of the alterations in ALS at different levels of axons as they extend from the motor neuron through the spinal cord, ventral roots, nerves, nerve terminals, and motor end plates. This view is limited technically by lack of a practical method to analyze the structure of a whole motor unit, which comprises motor neuron, motor axon, and the many muscle fibers supplied by the same nerve cell. This limitation is compounded by the problem of distinguishing between motor fibers and other large diameter myelinated fibers of mixed nerves in disease states although immunohistochemical methods can make this distinction in healthy animals (182–185). As a result, investigation of ALS patients has not provided a clear picture of how motor axons die and whether injured axons are capable of regeneration. The concepts regarding the lower motor neurons in this discussion are based on limited morphological data and are supplemented by knowledge about the functional aspects of motor units in ALS.

Electrophysiological analysis of ALS patients using motor unit number estimates indicate that they progressively disappear with a constant rate of 50% every six months during most of the course (186,187). This rate of depletion must vary widely in different muscles because autopsies have suggested a widely varying degree of motor neuron loss and neurogenic atrophy in muscle at different sites. The findings in even the most severely affected muscles imply that less than 1% of motor neurons die each day. As the cell body dies, motor axons in the ventral roots and peripheral nerves degenerate and are accompanied by secondary breakdown of myelin sheaths and a loss of the large diameter myelinated fibers. Analysis of teased myelinated fibers in one study showed that roughly 40% of fibers consisted of a series of myelin ovoids (breakdown products) indicating axonal degeneration (188). This percentage probably reflects axonal degeneration that has taken place over a period of a few weeks as myelin debris is cleared slowly.

Axonal atrophy and a dying-back form of axonal degeneration typify many toxic and metabolic disorders of peripheral nerves, but the mode of degeneration of nerves in ALS has received little investigation. Bradley et al. (188) evaluated proximal and distal segments of the phrenic nerve and found distal axonal atrophy but not proximal. The initial segment of axon, which arises from the motor neuron soma, also exhibits some atrophy (170). In addition, the sizes of myelinated fibers tend to shift from large-caliber fibers to a smaller size in ventral roots (189,190), phrenic nerve (188), and intramuscular nerves (191). This result may be caused by atrophy of axons (190) although other investigators have proposed that the change in size may reflect axonal regeneration (188,189).

In ALS, the average density of large diameter myelinated fibers (number of fibers/transverse area of endoneurium) of the distal part of the phrenic nerve were 18% less than in the proximal segment (188). This pattern suggests a dying-back component but is only a minor aspect of overall axonal degeneration. This interpretation is supported by teased myelinated fiber analysis, which did not demonstrate difference in the rate of axonal degeneration in proximal and distal segments of the nerve. This pattern implies that the axons between the two sites degenerate nearly simultaneously and again minimizes the importance of dying-back. This type of analysis is based on only one study and does not exclude a prominent dying-back disorder within intramuscular nerve fibers or other nerves (192).

Two major forms of axonal regeneration occur in peripheral nerve. One form consists of collateral reinnervation of muscle fibers provided by neighboring intact nerve terminals that are capable of sprouting and replacing the original nerve supply of a denervated fiber. This process gradually expands the number of muscle fibers in each motor unit and is thought to provide the basis for enlarged compound muscle action potentials in ALS although collateral reinnervation appears to be less efficient in comparison to other disorders (193). The reinnervation is supported by morphological analysis of nerve terminals, which exhibit signs of increased sprouting and innervation of adjacent muscle fibers (194–196).

The other type of regeneration occurs within the nerve roots and the main trunks of the peripheral nerves if the distal part of the axon degenerates. The proximal segment of a transected axon in a healthy experimental animal sprouts into one or more axons and grows within the residual basal lamina toward the muscle fiber. When these regenerating axons eventually become remyelinated, they can appear as a closely packed cluster of myelinated fibers. In addition, teased fibers of regenerating axons typically exhibit uniformly shortened internodes. Neither regenerative clusters (11,188) nor uniformly shortened internodes are prominent in ALS (11,188,197). These findings suggest that "healthy" motor neurons in ALS are capable of sprouting terminally within the muscle and can provide collateral reinnervation of myofibers but that degenerating nerve cells are unable to sprout and grow significantly within the nerve roots or nerve trunks. Biopsies of a "motor" nerve branch that supplies a nearby skeletal muscle might demonstrate numerous regenerative clusters or onion bulbs in a motor neuropathy, a finding that helps to distinguish the disorder from motor neuron disease (11,198–201).

Other

Two other pathological aspects of ALS have been the focus of investigation during the last 15 years. One consists of fragmentation of the Golgi apparatus in the Betz cells and motor neurons (202–204). This abnormality is found in ALS and certain variants including Guamanian ALS (205), juvenile ALS with BIs (139), and fALS with mutations of *SOD*1 (206). The alteration is not specific for ALS but is known to be one of the earliest abnormalities in the transgenic mouse model of motor neuron disease caused by mutant SOD1 enzyme (207,208). A fundamental defect of microtubules may be responsible for both the Golgi fragmentation (209) and early impairment of axonal transport in this model (210–213).

The other pathological aspect of ALS consists of a marked inflammatory response in the pyramidal tracts as indicated by numerous activated microglia and macrophages (214–217). Similar but lesser numbers of these cells are found in the vicinity of motor neurons in the precentral gyrus, brain stem, and ventral horns and certain other structures such as the lateral columns and anterior columns (apart from the pyramidal tracts). These cells are accompanied by smaller numbers of dendritic cells and T cells, chiefly CD8-positive cytotoxic T cells (214,215,218,219). The degree of inflammatory cell infiltration of the affected tissues exceeds inflammation observed in cerebral infarcts where the cells are thought to have a solely scavenger function.

In addition, activated microglia are located throughout the pyramidal tracts, in contrast to myelin breakdown and pallor where the changes are most prominent distally in spinal cord levels. These findings argue also against a purely scavenger role for the inflammatory cells. Intense investigations of inflammation in ALS and mouse models of the disease have not provided a clear explanation for the inflammation but suggest that the inflammatory process participates in motor neuron degeneration (216,220,221). This idea fits with increased survival of mutant SOD1 transgenic mice in response to therapeutic agents that suppress microglial activation (222–224), or inhibit activity of inducible cyclooxygenase 2 (225).

PROGRESSIVE MUSCULAR ATROPHY AND MULTIFOCAL MOTOR NEUROPATHY

The clinical syndrome of PMA resembles ALS but lacks upper motor neuron signs (spasticity, tendon reflexes, Babinski reflexes, or Hoffmann signs) (2). At autopsy, up to about half of the patients have pathological evidence of ALS including pyramidal tract degeneration (16,18,20,58,62,226–230). Most of the remaining patients do not have pathological indicators of upper motor neuron involvement but exhibit BBs or ubiquinated inclusions in the soma of lower motor neurons suggesting that PMA is a variant of ALS (226).

The clinical differential diagnosis of PMA includes MMN, inclusion body myositis, Kennedy syndrome, hexosaminidase deficiency, paraneoplastic motor neuron disease, chronic inflammatory demyelinating polyneuropathy, and others. MMN is rare but perhaps is the most important of this group clinically because the patients often respond to immunosuppressive therapy or intravenous immunoglobulin (IVIG) (2,231–233). They usually have electrodiagnostic abnormalities (motor nerve conduction slowing and conduction block) and may have high-titer antibodies to GM1 gangliosides. Motor and cutaneous nerve biopsies of patients have pathological evidence of either a demyelinating or an axonal neuropathy (11,199,234). Recently, Taylor et al. (201) studied fascicular nerve biopsies taken for diagnostic purposes from eight forearm or arm nerves at the site of the conduction block in seven patients with typical MMN. Abnormalities were seen in seven of eight nerves, including a varying degree of multifocal fiber (axonal) degeneration and loss, segmental remyelination, and prominent regenerating fiber clusters. There were no segmental demyelination or onion bulbs. Small epineurial perivascular inflammatory infiltrates were observed in two nerves. Irrespective of the mechanism underlying the fiber changes, the investigators concluded that the pathological findings explain the observed weakness, muscle wasting, and alterations of motor unit potentials. Discrete multifocal axonal degeneration may also explain why the functional abnormalities remain unchanged for long periods. The biopsies in these patients were performed two years or more after the onset of symptoms. The authors suggest that intervention may be more effective in an earlier stage when conduction block is not accompanied by substantial axonal degeneration.

There are only eight autopsies with motor neuropathies of suspected autoimmune etiology (Table 2) (235–242). The series includes two patients who had

Table 2 Reported Autopsy Pathology of Patients with Motor Neuropathy of Suspected Autoimmune Etiology

Case	Age of onset/ gender	Disease duration (months)	Conduction abnormality	Anti-GM1 antibodies	Therapy	Response	Death	Motor neuron loss	Inclusions	Chroma- tolysis	Peripheral nerve roots and nerves	References
1	52/M	~2	Slowing/ block	Yes	CHOP for lymphoma	None	Multiorgan failure	No	NR	NR	MFL	235
2	48/M	14	Marked slowing	NR	Chlorambucil for Waldenström's, plasma exchange	None	Possible cardiac dysrrhythmia	No	No	Many	MFL	236
3	82/M	9	Mild slowing	No	IVIG	Transient	Ventilatory failure	No	NR	Few	MFL, lymphocytes	237
4	44/F	3	Normal	Yes	Plasma exchange	None	Broncho- pneumonia	Yes	SLIs	Many	Paranodal demyelination	238
5	64/M	~6	Marked slowing	NR	Prednisone	Transient	Ventilatory failure	Yes	No	Few	MFL, onion bulbs	239
6	71/M	72	Block	Yes	Chlorambucil	None	NR	Yes	No	Yes	MFL	240
7	64/M	~60	Slowing/ block	No	Prednisone	Minimal	Ventilatory failure	Yes	BBs	None	Paranodal & segmental demyelination, lymphocytes	241
8	53/F	19	Block	Yes	Cyclophosphamide	None	Ventilatory failure	Yes[a]	BBs	Few	Focal demyelination	242

[a]The spinal cord also had pyramidal tract degeneration.

Abbreviations: CHOP, cyclophosphamide, doxorubicin, vincristine, and prednisone; IVIG, intravenous immunoglobulin; NR, not reported; MFL, myelinated fiber loss; BB, Bunina body; SLI, Skein-like inclusions.

electrodiagnostic studies but were not tested for conduction block or anti-GM1 antibodies (236,239). The pathological studies are limited because of variation in scope and methodology, but they raise questions about the relationship of neuropathy and ALS or PMA (235–242). Three patients had no loss of motor neurons (235–237). Central chromatolysis motor neurons were found in two (236,237) and were numerous in one (236). The reports did not state whether ALS-type inclusions were present or absent, but the autopsy case of Rowland et al. (236) was subsequently re-examined and did not show any BBs, SLIs, or LBLIs (A. P. Hays, 2001, unpublished observation). The chromatolytic cells had typical features of axonal reaction (Fig. 7B) and tended to be larger than similar cells found in ALS (Fig. 7A). Routine histology of nerves of paraffin sections showed loss of myelinated fibers, and one case had lymphocytic infiltrates (237). Two patients had a demyelinating neuropathy based on electrodiagnostic findings (235,236), and the other was axonal (237). These autopsy findings have typical features of a neuropathy.

In contrast, the central nervous system of five other patients had moderate to severe loss of motor neurons (238–242); three had SLIs or BBs (238,241,242); three displayed chromatolytic cells (238,240,242); one showed pyramidal tract degeneration (242). Although the pathology suggests PMA or ALS, the nerves of all five patients demonstrated evidence of a chronic demyelinating neuropathy. All eight autopsied patients progressed clinically with little or no response to immunosuppressive agents or IVIG (235–242). The clinical findings, electrodiagnostic studies and the autopsy suggest a combination of PMA or ALS and a neuropathy. Alternatively, the neuropathy may begin in the peripheral nervous system with secondary changes in the motor neurons. This alternative may be clarified by more detailed autopsy studies in neuropathies using modern methods to detect motor neuron inclusions.

PRIMARY LATERAL SCLEROSIS

Primary lateral sclerosis (PLS) is a rare disorder of upper motor neurons. The major clinical features of this disorder have been refined during the last 15 years (243–248) spurred, in part, by the discovery of a rare juvenile form of PLS caused by mutations of the *ALS2* gene. Symptoms begin with insidious progressive spasticity and survival is often for 10 years or more. The disorder is usually sporadic and begins in the fifth decade. Similar disorders are excluded by laboratory testing including electromyography (EMG), magnetic resonance imaging of the spinal cord, and methods to evaluate upper motor neurons and tracts (243–245,249–252). The clinical diagnosis of PLS is made only after four years of clinical onset if EMG is normal (243).

Autopsy helps to confirm the diagnosis by excluding other disorders that can mimic PLS such as multiple sclerosis, a multi-infarct state, corticobasal degeneration, progressive supranuclear palsy, or tropical spastic paraparesis (HTLV-1 infection).

There is no consensus about the pathological criteria for making the diagnosis of PLS because autopsies are rare and insufficiently studied to generalize about morphological findings (245,253–264). Pyramidal tract degeneration with little or no involvement of the lower motor neurons is the only constant feature of these cases. Most of the patients showed atrophy of the precentral gyrus and loss of Betz cells, but others did not (263). Only four autopsied patients with PLS have been worked up pathologically using modern methods to detect ubiquinated inclusions (26,255,256,262); three demonstrated ubiquinated inclusions (SLIs or CIs) in lower motor neurons; a fourth case showed ubiquinated inclusions in cortical neurons of the motor neuron disease type (see below), but no abnormalities of lower motor neurons (26). Although the data are insufficient to draw conclusions about the pathological basis of PLS, they suggest that the disorder is a variant of ALS. A close relationship between PLS and ALS is suggested by rare patients with longstanding PLS who later develop clinical features of lower motor neuron dysfunction (ALS) (265). In addition, electrophysiological and pathological evidence of minor involvement of lower motor neurons occurs in this disorder (20,243,244,263,266).

PLS may also involve non-motor nerve cells as suggested by finding cognitive impairment in eight of nine patients with PLS (267). Four other autopsied patients with PLS had dementia (20,260,261,268). Two of these patients exhibited frontotemporal or generalized gyral atrophy and both exhibited BBs and SLIs in lower motor neurons. One of these patients also had ubiquinated inclusions of the motor neuron disease type in nerve cells of the dentate gyrus and frontotemporal cortex.

A fifth patient had a clinical syndrome of PLS and Parkinsonism with similar pathology including inclusions within dentate and cortical neurons (259). These observations fit with the idea that these disorders are different manifestations of ALS based on the unifying features of the autopsy (26).

Although the autopsy of patients with the syndrome of PLS can confirm the clinical diagnosis, it raises a semantic issue. Should a PLS patient with BBs, SLIs or CIs in the motor neurons be classified as ALS based on pathology even though no evidence of lower motor neuron dysfunction existed during life and no loss of the nerve cells was detected by autopsy? A sensible solution is to preserve the term PLS with the qualifier that it represents a variant of motor neuron disease if the pathology is supportive. In addition, it is not clear whether the pathological diagnosis of PLS can be distinguished from other rare disorders, such as hereditary spastic paresis (269,270), alsinopathies (271–273), lathyrism (274,275), or Konzo (276,277). This problem arises from lack of knowledge about the underlying pathology of these disorders using modern autopsy methods to detect and define inclusions.

ALS-DEMENTIA

There are several syndromes of ALS and dementia with differing pathological findings (247,278), but one type is considered to be a form of motor neuron disease with non-motor involvement of the cortical neurons (34,279–282). The ALS patients typically have frontotemporal dementia, which may begin with progressive aphasia (46,283). Motor neuron disease can precede, follow, or coincide with the onset of dementia and it may be autosomal dominant (45,284,285).

Autopsy demonstrates loss of motor neurons in hypoglossal nucleus and spinal cord. BBs, SLIs, and LBLIs are present in surviving motor nerve cells (41,45,46, 261,286–289). Pyramidal tract degeneration is usually present and varies from mild to marked. Rarely, patients with dementia exhibit clinical and pathological features of PLS (259–261).

The substantia nigra often demonstrates loss of nerve cells; the surviving cells exhibit ubiquinated inclusions that differ from Lewy bodies (290). The cerebral cortex typically displays loss of neurons, rare ballooned cells, astrocytosis, and superficial spongiform change (21,35,36,41,45,46,279,282,286). The alterations predominate in the frontal and temporal lobes. The spongy changes resemble the spongiform encephalopathy of Creutzfeldt–Jakob disease. However, the changes do not

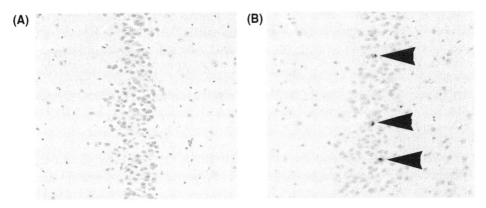

Figure 8 Ubiquinated neuronal inclusions in ALS-dementia: (**A**) The neurons of the dentate gyrus appear to be normal in a patient with ALS and frontotemporal degeneration (H&E). (**B**) Three neurons from the same area of the dentate gyrus exhibit small round or elliptical ubiquinated inclusions within cytoplasm. These inclusions do not express tau, α-synuclein, or neurofilament protein (not shown). Immunoperoxidase stain, polyclonal antibody to ubiquitin. *Abbreviation*: ALS, amyotrophic lateral sclerosis.

affect the deeper layers of the cortex or other gray matter structures, and the disorder is not transmissible (38) with one exception (291,292).

Distinctive ubiquinated inclusions are found in the cytoplasm of granule cell neurons of the dentate gyrus (Fig. 8B) and, less commonly, in the neocortex (43,45,46,286,293). They resemble CIs and a similar ultrastructure (43,294) but often have an elliptical or rod-like shape. They are invisible in H&E (Fig. 8A) and silver stains and do not express tau, α-synuclein or other proteins by immunohistochemistry with the exception of the proteins, p62 (295,296) and NEDD8 (297). The p62 protein is expressed in other ubiquinated inclusions and are thought to be involved in the ubiquitin pathway whereas the structure and function of NEDD8 resemble that of ubiquitin. The inclusions are accompanied by cortical ubiquinated neurites, and both express the same proteins. Similar but less frequent ubiquinated inclusions and neurites are found in the brain of a minority of ALS patients with no cognitive impairment.

Some patients have frontotemporal dementia with no clinical evidence of motor neuron disease but demonstrate a similar cerebral pathology including ubiquinated inclusions in non-motor neurons (286,289,298–306). One report described intranuclear ubiquinated inclusions in neurons of the dentate gyrus and cerebral cortex. This type of frontotemporal dementia has been given the name, motor neuron disease-inclusion dementia (MNDID) (301).

The motor neurons in the spinal cord and brainstem are normal in most patients but a few cases showed BBs, SLIs, LBLIs, or fragmentation of the Golgi apparatus (286,299,305,306) suggesting that MNDID is closely related to ALS–dementia. In addition, ALS, ALS–dementia, and MNDID have occurred in members of the same family supporting the idea that these syndromes represent different manifestations of the same disease.

FAMILIAL ALS

About 10% of patients have fALS. Most are autosomal dominant, and about 20% of fALS are caused by mutations of the *SOD*1 gene. Publications about research on the mouse model of ALS induced by mutant human SOD1 protein emphasize the clinical similarities between fALS and sALS (103,307,308), but it is worthwhile to highlight differences in intracytoplasmic inclusions. First, HCIs are distinctive inclusions that are nearly specific for fALS with rare exceptions (309). Over 100 different mutations affect the gene, but HCIs have been linked to only four different *SOD*1 mutations: A4V (310), A4T (311), H48Q (312), and I113T (48,313,314). Second, BBs have not been detected in SOD1-ALS with one exception (47). Third, many of the mutations are associated with round hyaline inclusions that resemble Lewy bodies (47,103,315–317,320). These inclusions resemble the LBLIs of sALS, but they are much more hyaline and show subtle ultrastructural differences including more entrapped NFs and other organelles (319). They strongly express SOD1 enzyme but do not exhibit immunoreactive NF protein. Fourth, hyaline inclusions are found in astrocytes in some fALS of long duration (317–321). The pathogenetic significance of the inclusions in ALS are not known, but pathological differences between fALS and the common sporadic form raise the possibility that the underlying disease mechanisms are dissimilar.

The gene responsible for most other patients with fALS is not known, but genetic analysis has identified an increasing number of gene loci linked to the syndromes, known as ALS1-8.

Mutations of ALS2 (alsinopathy) (272,273), ALS4 (322), and ALS8 genes (323) have been identified. No autopsies have been reported yet in patients with ALS2 or ALS8 disorders, but two ALS4 patients are described in detail (324). They showed pathological findings of ALS consisting of marked loss of motor neurons and pyramidal tract degeneration in the spinal cord. There were no detectable BBs or ubiquinated inclusions in the motor nerve cells although nerve cell loss was severe. In addition, the abnormalities included loss of neurons in dorsal root ganglia, axonal degeneration of nerves roots and nerves, and myelin pallor in posterior columns. Atypical ubiquinated spheroids were located in ventral horns, nerve roots, and peripheral nerves. They were composed of small membrane bound organelles or vesicles but no accumulations of NFs. The protein encoded by the gene has a DNA/RNA helicase domain, but it is not clear how the mutation leads to fALS.

CLOSING REMARKS

Immunohistochemical studies of the protein ubiquitin defined ubiquinated inclusions in motor nerve cells of ALS over 15 years ago. The abnormality is highly specific for the disorder, and it has solidified the classification of motor neuron disease and its variants including ALS-dementia. The ubiquinated inclusions are also expressed in motor neurons of fALS caused by mutations of the *SOD*1 gene. The pathological similarities among the different forms of motor neuron disease suggest shared features of pathogenesis. These observations promise further insights into the nature of the sporadic disorder as the molecular mechanisms are elucidated by future investigation.

REFERENCES

1. Brooks BR, Miller RG, Swash M, Munsat TL. El Escorial revisited: revised criteria for the diagnosis of amyotrophic lateral sclerosis. Amyotroph Lateral Scler Other Motor Neuron Disord 2000; 1:293–299.

2. Rowland LP. Diagnosis of amyotrophic lateral sclerosis. J Neurol Sci 1998; 160(suppl 1): S6–S24.
3. Mitsumoto H. Clinical trials: present and future. Amyotroph Lateral Scler Other Motor Neuron Disord 2001; 2(suppl 1):S10–S14.
4. Kaminski HJ, Richmonds CR, Kusner LL, Mitsumoto H. Differential susceptibility of the ocular motor system to disease. Ann N Y Acad Sci 2002; 956:42–54.
5. Shaw PJ, Eggett CJ. Molecular factors underlying selective vulnerability of motor neurons to neurodegeneration in amyotrophic lateral sclerosis. J Neurol 2000; 247(suppl 1): I17–I27.
6. Shaw PJ, Chinnery RM, Ince PG. Non-NMDA receptors in motor neuron disease (MND): a quantitative autoradiographic study in spinal cord and motor cortex using [3H]CNQX and [3H]kainate. Brain Res 1994; 655:186–194.
7. Ince P, Stout N, Shaw P, Slade J, Hunziker W, Heizmann CW, Baimbridge KG. Parvalbumin and calbindin D-28k in the human motor system and in motor neuron disease. Neuropathol Appl Neurobiol 1993; 19:291–299.
8. Alexianu ME, Ho BK, Mohamed AH, La Bella V, Smith RG, Appel SH. The role of calcium-binding proteins in selective motoneuron vulnerability in amyotrophic lateral sclerosis. Ann Neurol 1994; 36:846–858.
9. Williams TL, Day NC, Ince PG, Kamboj RK, Shaw PJ. Calcium-permeable alpha-amino-3-hydroxy-5-methyl-4-isoxazole propionic acid receptors: a molecular determinant of selective vulnerability in amyotrophic lateral sclerosis. Ann Neurol 1997; 42:200–207.
10. Abouzahr MK, Lange DJ, Latov N, Olarte M, Rowland LP, Hays AP, Corbo M. Diagnostic biopsy of the motor nerve to the gracilis muscle. Technical note. J Neurosurg 1997; 87:122–124.
11. Corbo M, Abouzahr MK, Latov N, Iannaccone S, Quattrini A, Nemni R, Canal N, Hays AP. Motor nerve biopsy studies in motor neuropathy and motor neuron disease. Muscle Nerve 1997; 20:15–21.
12. Dabby R, Lange DJ, Trojaborg W, Hays AP, Lovelace RE, Brannagan TH, Rowland LP. Inclusion body myositis mimicking motor neuron disease. Arch Neurol 2001; 58:1253–1256.
13. Finsterer J. Mitochondriopathy mimicking amyotrophic lateral sclerosis. Neurologist 2003; 9:45–48.
14. McDonald TD, Faust PL, Bruno C, DiMauro S, Goldman JE. Polyglucosan body disease simulating amyotrophic lateral sclerosis. Neurology 1993; 43:785–790.
15. Charcot JM, Joffroy A. Deux cas d'atrophy musculaire progressive avec lésions de la substance grise et des faisceaux antérolatéraux de la moelle épinière. Arch Physiol Neurol Pathol 1869; 2:785–790.
16. Holmes G. The pathology of amyotrophic lateral sclerosis. Rev Neurol Psychiatry 1909; 7:693–725.
17. Hirano A, Arumugasamy N, Zimmerman HM. Amyotrophic lateral sclerosis. A comparison of Guam and classical cases. Arch Neurol 1967; 16:357–363.
18. Lawyer T Jr, Netsky MG. Amyotrophic lateral sclerosis. AMA Arch Neurol Psychiatry 1953; 69:171–192.
19. Smith MC. Nerve fibre degeneration in the brain in amyotrophic lateral sclerosis. J Neurol Neurosurg Psychiatry 1960; 23:269–282.
20. Brownell B, Oppenheimer DR, Hughes JT. The central nervous system in motor neurone disease. J Neurol Neurosurg Psychiatry 1970; 33:338–357.
21. Castaigne P, Lhermitte F, Cambier J, Escourolle R, Le Bigot P. Neuropathological study of 61 cases of amyotrophic lateral sclerosis. Nosological discussion. Rev Neurol (Paris) 1972; 127:401–414.
22. Hughes JT. Pathology of amyotrophic lateral sclerosis. Adv Neurol 1982; 36:61–74.
23. Ikuta F, Makifuchi T, Ohama E, Takeda S, Oyanagi K, Nakashima S, Motega T. Tract degeneration of the human spinal cord: some observations on amyotrophic lateral

sclerosis and hemispherectomized humans. Shinkei Kenkyu No Shinpo 1982; 26: 710–736.

24. Chou SM. Pathology—light microscopy of amyotrophic lateral sclerosis. In: Smith RA, ed. Handbook of Amyotrophic Lateral Sclerosis. New York: Marcel Dekker Inc., 1992:133–181.

25. Hirano A. Cytopathology of amyotrophic lateral sclerosis. In: Rowland LP, ed. Amyotrophic Lateral Sclerosis and Other Motor Neuron Diseases Vol. 56. New York: Raven Press, 1991:91–101.

26. Ince PG, Lowe J, Shaw PJ. Amyotrophic lateral sclerosis: current issues in classification, pathogenesis and molecular pathology. Neuropathol Appl Neurobiol 1998; 24:104–117.

27. Tandan R, Bradley WG. Amyotrophic lateral sclerosis: Part 1. Clinical features, pathology, and ethical issues in management. Ann Neurol 1985; 18:271–280.

28. Wharton S, Ince PG. Pathology of motor neuron disorders. In: Shaw PJ, Strong MJ, eds. Motor Neuron Disorders Vol. 28. Philadelphia, PA: Butterworth-Heinemann, 2003:17–49.

29. Mizutani T, Sakamaki S, Tsuchiya N, Kamei S, Kohzu H, Horiuchi R, Ida M, Shiozawa R, Takasu T. Amyotrophic lateral sclerosis with ophthalmoplegia and multisystem degeneration in patients on long-term use of respirators. Acta Neuropathol (Berl) 1992; 84:372–377.

30. Hayashi H, Kato S. Total manifestations of amyotrophic lateral sclerosis. ALS in the totally locked-in state. J Neurol Sci 1989; 93:19–35.

31. Hirano A, Kurland LT, Krooth RS, Lessell S. Parkinsonism-dementia complex, an endemic disease on the island of Guam. I. Clinical features. Brain 1961; 84:642–661.

32. Hirano A, Malamud N, Ku Rland LT. Parkinsonism-dementia complex, an endemic disease on the island of Guam. II. Pathological features. Brain 1961; 84:662–679.

33. Malamud N, Hirano A, Kurland LT. Pathoanatomic changes in amyotrophic lateral sclerosis on Guam. Special reference to the occurrence of neurofibrillary changes. Arch Neurol 1961; 5:401–415.

34. Mitsuyama Y. Presenile dementia with motor neuron disease in Japan: clinicopathological review of 26 cases. J Neurol Neurosurg Psychiatry 1984; 47:953–959.

35. Wikstrom J, Paetau A, Palo J, Sulkava R, Haltia M. Classic amyotrophic lateral sclerosis with dementia. Arch Neurol 1982; 39:681–683.

36. Myrianthopoulos NC, Smith JK. Amyotrophic lateral sclerosis with progressive dementia and with pathologic findings of the Creutzfeldt-Jakob syndrome. Neurology 1962; 12: 603–610.

37. Allen IV, Dermott E, Connolly JH, Hurwitz LJ. A study of a patient with the amyotrophic form of Creutzfeldt-Jakob disease. Brain 1971; 94:715–724.

38. Salazar AM, Masters CL, Gajdusek DC, Gibbs CJ Jr. Syndromes of amyotrophic lateral sclerosis and dementia: relation to transmissible Creutzfeldt-Jakob disease. Ann Neurol 1983; 14:17–26.

39. Dejerine J. Étude anatomique et clinique sur la paralysie labio-glosso-larngée. Arch Physiol Norm Path 1883; 2(Série 3):188–270.

40. Chou SM. Pathognomony of intraneuronal inclusions in ALS. In: Tsubaki T, Toyokura Y, eds. Amyotrophic Lateral Sclerosis. Proceedings of the International Symposium on Amyotrophic lateral sclerosis. Baltimore: University Park Press, 1979:135–176.

41. Kusaka H, Imai T. Pathology of motor neurons in amyotrophic lateral sclerosis with dementia. Clin Neuropathol 1993; 12:164–168.

42. Jackson M, Lowe J. The new neuropathology of degenerative frontotemporal dementias. Acta Neuropathol (Berl) 1996; 91:127–134.

43. Okamoto K, Hirai S, Yamazaki T, Sun XY, Nakazato Y. New ubiquitin-positive intraneuronal inclusions in the extra-motor cortices in patients with amyotrophic lateral sclerosis. Neurosci Lett 1991; 129:233–236.

44. Okamoto K, Murakami N, Kusaka H, Yoshida M, Hashizume Y, Nakazato Y, Matsubara E, Hirai S. Ubiquitin-positive intraneuronal inclusions in the extramotor

cortices of presenile dementia patients with motor neuron disease. J Neurol 1992; 239: 426–430.

45. Wightman G, Anderson VE, Martin J, Swash M, Anderton BH, Neary D, Mann D, Luthert P, Leigh PN. Hippocampal and neocortical ubiquitin-immunoreactive inclusions in amyotrophic lateral sclerosis with dementia. Neurosci Lett 1992; 139:269–274.

46. Yoshida M. Amyotrophic lateral sclerosis with dementia: the clinicopathological spectrum. Neuropathology 2004; 24:87–102.

47. Jonsson PA, Ernhill K, Andersen PM, Bergemalm D, Brannstrom T, Gredal O, Nilsson P, Marklund SL. Minute quantities of misfolded mutant superoxide dismutase-1 cause amyotrophic lateral sclerosis. Brain 2004; 127:73–88.

48. Ince PG, Tomkins J, Slade JY, Thatcher NM, Shaw PJ. Amyotrophic lateral sclerosis associated with genetic abnormalities in the gene encoding Cu/Zn superoxide dismutase: molecular pathology of five new cases, and comparison with previous reports and 73 sporadic cases of ALS. J Neuropathol Exp Neurol 1998; 57:895–904.

49. Matsumoto S, Hirano A, Goto S. Ubiquitin-immunoreactive filamentous inclusions in anterior horn cells of Guamanian and non-Guamanian amyotrophic lateral sclerosis. Acta Neuropathol (Berl) 1990; 80:233–238.

50. Wada M, Uchihara T, Nakamura A, Oyanagi K. Bunina bodies in amyotrophic lateral sclerosis on Guam: a histochemical, immunohistochemical and ultrastructural investigation. Acta Neuropathol (Berl) 1999; 98:150–156.

51. Bunina TL. On intracellular inclusions in familial amyotrophic lateral sclerosis. Zh Nevropatol Psikhiatr Im S S Korsakova 1962; 62:1293–1299.

52. Hirano A. Pathology of amyotrophic lateral sclerosis. In: Alpers MP, Gajdusek DC, Gibbs CJ, National Institutes of Health (U.S.), eds. Slow, Latent, and Temperate Virus Infections. NINDB Monograph No. 2. Washington: U.S. National Institute of Neurological Diseases and Blindness (for sale by the Supt. of Docs. U.S. Govt. Print. Off.), 1965:23–37.

53. Kusaka H. Neuropathology of the motor neuron disease—Bunina body. Rinsho Shinkeigaku 1999; 39:65–66.

54. Kuroda S, Ishizu H, Kawai K, Otsuki S. Bunina bodies in dendrites of patients with amyotrophic lateral sclerosis. Acta Med Okayama 1990; 44:41–45.

55. Wakayama I. Morphometry of spinal motor neurons in amyotrophic lateral sclerosis with special reference to chromatolysis and intracytoplasmic inclusion bodies. Brain Res 1992; 586:12–18.

56. Bergmann M. Motor neuron disease/amyotrophic lateral sclerosis—lessons from ubiquitin. Pathol Res Pract 1993; 189:902–912.

57. Leigh PN, Whitwell H, Garofalo O, Buller J, Swash M, Martin JE, Gallo JM, Weller RO, Anderton BH. Ubiquitin-immunoreactive intraneuronal inclusions in amyotrophic lateral sclerosis. Morphology, distribution, and specificity. Brain 1991; 114:775–788.

58. Leung DK, Hays A, Karlikaya G, Del Bene ML, Rowland LP. Diagnosis of ALS: Clinicopathologic analysis of 76 autopsies. Neurology 1999; 52:A164.

59. Murayama S, Mori H, Ihara Y, Bouldin TW, Suzuki K, Tomonaga M. Immunocytochemical and ultrastructural studies of lower motor neurons in amyotrophic lateral sclerosis. Ann Neurol 1990; 27:137–148.

60. Nakano I, Donnenfeld H, Hirano A. A neuropathological study of amyotrophic lateral sclerosis. With special reference to central chromatolysis and spheroid in the spinal anterior horn and some pathological changes of the motor cortex. Shinkei Naika (Neurol Med [Tokyo]) 1983; 18:136–144.

61. Okamoto K, Morimatsu M, Hirai S, Ishida Y. Intracytoplasmic inclusions (Bunina bodies) in amyotrophic lateral sclerosis. Acta Pathol Jpn 1980; 30:591–597.

62. Piao YS, Wakabayashi K, Kakita A, Yamada M, Hayashi S, Morita T, Ikuta F, Oyanagi K, Takahashi H. Neuropathology with clinical correlations of sporadic amyotrophic lateral sclerosis: 102 autopsy cases examined between 1962 and 2000. Brain Pathol 2003; 13:10–22.

63. Tomonaga M. Selective appearance of Bunina bodies in amyotrophic lateral sclerosis. A study of the distribution in midbrain and sacral cord. J Neurol 1980; 223:259–267.

64. Okamoto K, Hirai S, Amari M, Watanabe M, Sakurai A. Bunina bodies in amyotrophic lateral sclerosis immunostained with rabbit anticystatin C serum. Neurosci Lett 1993; 162:125–128.

65. Matsumoto S, Kusaka H, Ito H, Shibata N, Asayama T, Imai T. Sporadic amyotrophic lateral sclerosis with dementia and Cu/Zn superoxide dismutase-positive Lewy body-like inclusions. Clin Neuropathol 1996; 15:41–46.

66. van Welsem ME, Hogenhuis JA, Meininger V, Metsaars WP, Hauw JJ, Seilhean D. The relationship between Bunina bodies, skein-like inclusions and neuronal loss in amyotrophic lateral sclerosis. Acta Neuropathol (Berl) 2002; 103:583–589.

67. Mason RW, Sol-Church K, Abrahamson M. Amino acid substitutions in the N-terminal segment of cystatin C create selective protein inhibitors of lysosomal cysteine proteinases. Biochem J 1998; 330(pt 2):833–838.

68. Hart MN, Cancilla PA, Frommes S, Hirano A. Anterior horn cell degeneration and Bunina-type inclusions associated with dementia. Acta Neuropathol (Berl) 1977; 38:225–228.

69. Hirano A. Aspects of the ultrastructure of amyotrophic lateral sclerosis. In: Rowland LP, ed. Human Motor Neuron Diseases Vol. 36. New York: Raven Press, 1982:75–88.

70. Tomonaga M, Saito M, Yoshimura M, Shimada H, Tohgi H. Ultrastructure of the Bunina bodies in anterior horn cells of amyotrophic lateral sclerosis. Acta Neuropathol (Berl) 1978; 42:81–86.

71. Takahashi H, Ikuta F. Bunina body in amyotrophic lateral sclerosis. No to Shinkei. Brain Nerve 1992; 44:525–532.

72. Takahashi H, Ohama E, Ikuta F. Are bunina bodies of endoplasmic reticulum origin? An ultrastructural study of subthalamic eosinophilic inclusions in a case of atypical motor neuron disease. Acta Pathol Jpn 1991; 41:889–894.

73. Sasaki S, Maruyama S. Ultrastructural study of Bunina bodies in the anterior horn neurons of patients with amyotrophic lateral sclerosis. Neurosci Lett 1993; 154:117–120.

74. Yoshida S, Mitani K, Wakayama I, Kihira T, Yase Y. Bunina body formation in amyotrophic lateral sclerosis: a morphometric-statistical and trace element study featuring aluminum. J Neurol Sci 1995; 130:88–94.

75. Okamoto K, Hirai S, Shoji M, Harigaya Y, Fukuda T. Widely distributed Bunina bodies and spheroids in a case of atypical sporadic amyotrophic lateral sclerosis. Acta Neuropathol (Berl) 1991; 81:349–353.

76. Okamoto K, Hirai S, Ishiguro K, Kawarabayashi T, Takatama M. Light and electron microscopic and immunohistochemical observations of the Onuf's nucleus of amyotrophic lateral sclerosis. Acta Neuropathol (Berl) 1991; 81:610–614.

77. Pullen AH, Martin JE. Ultrastructural abnormalities with inclusions in Onuf's nucleus in motor neuron disease (amyotrophic lateral sclerosis). Neuropathol Appl Neurobiol 1995; 21:327–340.

78. Takahashi H, Ohama E, Ikuta F, Tokiguchi S. An autopsy case of atypical motor neuron disease with Bunina bodies in the lower motor and subthalamic neurons. Acta Pathol Jpn 1991; 41:46–51.

79. Iwanaga K, Wakabayashi K, Honma Y, Takahashi H. Amyotrophic lateral sclerosis: occurrence of Bunina bodies in the locus ceruleus pigmented neurons. Clin Neuropathol 1997; 16:23–26.

80. Nakano I, Hashizume Y, Tomonaga T. Bunina bodies in neurons of the medullary reticular formation in a case of amyotrophic lateral sclerosis. Acta Neuropathol (Berl) 1990; 79:689–691.

81. Takahashi H, Oyanagi K, Ohama E, Ikuta F. Clarke's column in sporadic amyotrophic lateral sclerosis. Acta Neuropathol (Berl) 1992; 84:465–470.

82. Sasaki S, Iwata M. Ultrastructural study of Betz cells in the primary motor cortex of the human brain. J Anat 2001; 199:699–708.

83. Tsuchiya K, Shintani S, Nakabayashi H, Kikugawa K, Nakano R, Haga C, Nakano I, Ikeda K, Tsuji S. Familial amyotrophic lateral sclerosis with onset in bulbar sign, benign clinical course, and Bunina bodies: a clinical, genetic, and pathological study of a Japanese family. Acta Neuropathol (Berl) 2000; 100:603–607.
84. Kato S, Shaw P, Wood-Alum C, Leigh PN, Shaw C. Amyotrophic lateral sclerosis. In: Dickson D, ed. Neurodegeneration: The Molecular Pathology of Dementia and Movement Disorders. Basel: ISN Neuropath Press, 2003:350–368.
85. Leigh PN, Anderton BH, Dodson A, Gallo JM, Swash M, Power DM. Ubiquitin deposits in anterior horn cells in motor neurone disease. Neurosci Lett 1988; 93:197–203.
86. Lowe J, Lennox G, Jefferson D, Morrell K, McQuire D, Gray T, Landon M, Doherty FJ, Mayer RJ. A filamentous inclusion body within anterior horn neurones in motor neurone disease defined by immunocytochemical localisation of ubiquitin. Neurosci Lett 1988; 94:203–210.
87. Kato T, Katagiri T, Hirano A, Kawanami T, Sasaki H. Lewy body-like hyaline inclusions in sporadic motor neuron disease are ubiquitinated. Acta Neuropathol 1989; 77:391–396.
88. Schiffer D, Autilio-Gambetti L, Chio A, Gambetti P, Giordana MT, Gullotta F, Migheli A, Vigliani MC. Ubiquitin in motor neuron disease: study at the light and electron microscope. J Neuropathol Exp Neurol 1991; 50:463–473.
89. Lowe J, Blanchard A, Morrell K, Lennox G, Reynolds L, Billett M, Landon M, Mayer RJ. Ubiquitin is a common factor in intermediate filament inclusion bodies of diverse type in man, including those of Parkinson's disease, Pick's disease, and Alzheimer's disease, as well as Rosenthal fibres in cerebellar astrocytomas, cytoplasmic bodies in muscle, and Mallory bodies in alcoholic liver disease. J Pathol 1988; 155:9–15.
90. Migheli A, Autilio-Gambetti L, Gambetti P, Mocellini C, Vigliani MC, Schiffer D. Ubiquitinated filamentous inclusions in spinal cord of patients with motor neuron disease. Neurosci Lett 1990; 114:5–10.
91. Migheli A, Attanasio A, Schiffer D. Ubiquitin and neurofilament expression in anterior horn cells in amyotrophic lateral sclerosis: possible clues to the pathogenesis. Neuropathol Appl Neurobiol 1994; 20:282–289.
92. Mizusawa H, Nakamura H, Wakayama I, Yen SH, Hirano A. Skein-like inclusions in the anterior horn cells in motor neuron disease. J Neurol Sci 1991; 105:14–21.
93. Nakano I, Shibata T, Uesaka Y. On the possibility of autolysosomal processing of skein-like inclusions Electron microscopic observation in a case of amyotrophic lateral sclerosis. J Neurol Sci 1993; 120:54–59.
94. He CZ, Hays AP. Expression of peripherin in ubiquinated inclusions of amyotrophic lateral sclerosis. J Neurol Sci 2004; 217:47–54.
95. Okamoto K, Hirai S, Amari M, Iizuka T, Watanabe M, Murakami N, Takatama M. Oculomotor nuclear pathology in amyotrophic lateral sclerosis. Acta Neuropathol (Berl) 1993; 85:458–462.
96. Su M, Yoshida Y, Ishiguro H, Hirota K. Nigral degeneration in a case of amyotrophic lateral sclerosis: evidence of Lewy body-like and skein-like inclusions in the pigmented neurons. Clin Neuropathol 1999; 18:293–300.
97. Lowe J, Aldridge F, Lennox G, Doherty F, Jefferson D, Landon M, Mayer RJ. Inclusion bodies in motor cortex and brainstem of patients with motor neurone disease are detected by immunocytochemical localisation of ubiquitin. Neurosci Lett 1989; 105:7–13.
98. Jellinger KA, Mizuno Y. Parkinson's disease. In: Dickson D, ed. Neurodegeneration: The Molecular Pathology of Dementia and Movement Disorders. Basel: ISN Neuropath Press, 2003:159–187.
99. Niwa J, Ishigaki S, Doyu M, Suzuki T, Tanaka K, Sobue G. A novel centrosomal ring-finger protein, dorfin, mediates ubiquitin ligase activity. Biochem Biophys Res Commun 2001; 281:706–713.
100. Hishikawa N, Niwa J, Doyu M, Ito T, Ishigaki S, Hashizume Y, Sobue G. Dorfin localizes to the ubiquitylated inclusions in Parkinson's disease, dementia with Lewy bodies,

multiple system atrophy, and amyotrophic lateral sclerosis. Am J Pathol 2003; 163: 609–619.

101. Lowe J, McDermott H, Landon M, Mayer RJ, Wilkinson KD. Ubiquitin carboxyl-terminal hydrolase (PGP 9.5) is selectively present in ubiquitinated inclusion bodies characteristic of human neurodegenerative diseases. J Pathol 1990; 161:153–160.

102. Ii K, Ito H, Tanaka K, Hirano A. Immunocytochemical co-localization of the proteasome in ubiquitinated structures in neurodegenerative diseases and the elderly. J Neuropathol Exp Neurol 1997; 56:125–131.

103. Watanabe M, Dykes-Hoberg M, Culotta VC, Price DL, Wong PC, Rothstein JD. Histological evidence of protein aggregation in mutant SOD1 transgenic mice and in amyotrophic lateral sclerosis neural tissues. Neurobiol Dis 2001; 8:933–941.

104. Munoz DG, Greene C, Perl DP, Selkoe DJ. Accumulation of phosphorylated neurofilaments in anterior horn motoneurons of amyotrophic lateral sclerosis patients. J Neuropathol Exp Neurol 1988; 47:9–18.

105. Shibata N, Hirano A, Kobayashi M, Sasaki S, Kato T, Matsumoto S, Shiozawa Z, Komori T, Ikemoto A, Umahara T, Asayama K. Cu/Zn superoxide dismutase-like immunoreactivity in Lewy body-like inclusions of sporadic amyotrophic lateral sclerosis. Neurosci Lett 1994; 179:149–152.

106. Sasaki S, Maruyama S. Immunocytochemical and ultrastructural studies of hyaline inclusions in sporadic motor neuron disease. Acta Neuropathol 1991; 82:295–301.

107. Schmidt ML, Carden MJ, Lee VM, Trojanowski JQ. Phosphate dependent and independent neurofilament epitopes in the axonal swellings of patients with motor neuron disease and controls. Lab Invest 1987; 56:282–294.

108. Wong NK, He BP, Strong MJ. Characterization of neuronal intermediate filament protein expression in cervical spinal motor neurons in sporadic amyotrophic lateral sclerosis (ALS). J Neuropathol Exp Neurol 2000; 59:972–982.

109. Robertson J, Julien JP. Cytoskeletal abnormalities in amyotrophic lateral sclerosis/motor neuron disease. In: Shaw PJ, Strong MJ, eds. Motor Neuron Disorders. Vol. 28. Philadelphia, PA: Butterworth-Heinemann, 2003:315–339.

110. Kawamoto Y, Akiguchi I, Nakamura S, Budka H. 14-3-3 proteins in Lewy body-like hyaline inclusions in patients with sporadic amyotrophic lateral sclerosis. Acta Neuropathol (Berl) 2004; 108:531–537.

111. Nakamura S, Kawamoto Y, Nakano S, Ikemoto A, Akiguchi I, Kimura J. Cyclin-dependent kinase 5 in Lewy body-like inclusions in anterior horn cells of a patient with sporadic amyotrophic lateral sclerosis. Neurology 1997; 48:267–270.

112. Sun D, Leung CL, Liem RK. Phosphorylation of the high molecular weight neurofilament protein (NF-H) by Cdk5 and p35. J Biol Chem 1996; 271:14,245–14,251.

113. Shetty KT, Link WT, Pant HC. cdc2-like kinase from rat spinal cord specifically phosphorylates KSPXK motifs in neurofilament proteins: isolation characterization. Proc Natl Acad Sci USA 1993; 90:6844–6848.

114. Julien JP. Amyotrophic lateral sclerosis. Unfolding the toxicity of the misfolded. Cell 2001; 104:581–591.

115. Julien JP, Beaulieu JM. Cytoskeletal abnormalities in amyotrophic lateral sclerosis: beneficial or detrimental effects? J Neurol Sci 2000; 180:7–14.

116. Carpenter S. Proximal axonal enlargement in motor neuron disease. Neurology 1968; 18:841–851.

117. Hirano A, Donnenfeld H, Sasaki S, Nakano I. Fine structural observations of neurofilamentous changes in amyotrophic lateral sclerosis. J Neuropathol Exp Neurol 1984; 43:461–470.

118. Manetto V, Sternberger NH, Perry G, Sternberger LA, Gambetti P. Phosphorylation of neurofilaments is altered in amyotrophic lateral sclerosis. J Neuropathol Exp Neurol 1988; 47:642–653.

119. Migheli A, Pezzulo T, Attanasio A, Schiffer D. Peripherin immunoreactive structures in amyotrophic lateral sclerosis. Lab Invest 1993; 68:185–191.

120. Toyoshima I, Yamamoto A, Masamune O, Satake M. Phosphorylation of neurofila-
     ment proteins and localization of axonal swellings in motor neuron disease. J Neurol
     Sci 1989; 89:269–277.
121. Sobue G, Hashizume Y, Yasuda T, Mukai E, Kumagai T, Mitsuma T, Trojanowski JQ.
     Phosphorylated high molecular weight neurofilament protein in lower motor neurons in
     amyotrophic lateral sclerosis and other neurodegenerative diseases involving ventral
     horn cells. Acta Neuropathol (Berl) 1990; 79:402–408.
122. Figlewicz DA, Krizus A, Martinoli MG, Meininger V, Dib M, Rouleau GA, Julien JP.
     Variants of the heavy neurofilament subunit are associated with the development of
     amyotrophic lateral sclerosis. Hum Mol Genet 1994; 3:1757–1761.
123. Al-Chalabi A, Andersen PM, Nilsson P, Chioza B, Andersson JL, Russ C, Shaw CE,
     Powell JF, Leigh PN. Deletions of the heavy neurofilament subunit tail in amyotrophic
     lateral sclerosis. Hum Mol Genet 1999; 8:157–164.
124. Gros-Louis F, Lariviere R, Gowing G, Laurent S, Camu W, Bouchard JP, Meininger V,
     Rouleau GA, Julien JP. A frameshift deletion in peripherin gene associated with amyo-
     trophic lateral sclerosis. J Biol Chem 2004; 279:45,951–45,956.
125. Leung CL, He CZ, Kaufmann P, Chin SS, Naini A, Liem RK, Mitsumoto H, Hays AP.
     A pathogenic peripherin gene mutation in a patient with amyotrophic lateral sclerosis.
     Brain Pathol 2004; 14:290–296.
126. Bendotti C, Atzori C, Piva R, Tortarolo M, Strong MJ, DeBiasi S, Migheli A. Activated
     p38MAPK is a novel component of the intracellular inclusions found in human amyo-
     trophic lateral sclerosis and mutant SOD1 transgenic mice. J Neuropathol Exp Neurol
     2004; 63:113–119.
127. Ackerley S, Grierson AJ, Banner S, Perkinton MS, Brownlees J, Byers HL, Ward M,
     Thornhill P, Hussain K, Waby JS, Anderton BH, Cooper JD, Dingwall C, Leigh PN,
     Shaw CE, Miller CC. p38alpha stress-activated protein kinase phosphorylates neurofila-
     ments is associated with neurofilament pathology in amyotrophic lateral sclerosis. Mol
     Cell Neurosci 2004; 26:354–364.
128. Hughes JT, Jerrome D. Ultrastructure of anterior horn motor neurones in the Hirano-
     Kurland-Sayre type of combined neurological system degeneration. J Neurol Sci 1971;
     13:389–399.
129. Andersen PM, Nilsson P, Keranen ML, Forsgren L, Hagglund J, Karlsborg M,
     Ronnevi LO, Gredal O, Marklund SL. Phenotypic heterogeneity in motor neuron dis-
     ease patients with CuZn-superoxide dismutase mutations in Scandinavia. Brain 1997;
     120(pt 10):1723–1737.
130. Jackson M, Al-Chalabi A, Enayat ZE, Chioza B, Leigh PN, Morrison KE. Copper/zinc
     superoxide dismutase 1 and sporadic amyotrophic lateral sclerosis: analysis of 155 cases
     and identification of a novel insertion mutation. Ann Neurol 1997; 42:803–807.
131. Jones CT, Swingler RJ, Brock DJ. Identification of a novel SOD1 mutation in an appar-
     ently sporadic amyotrophic lateral sclerosis patient and the detection of Ile113Thr in
     three others. Hum Mol Genet 1994; 3:649–650.
132. Ince PG, Shaw PJ, Slade JY, Jones C, Hudgson P. Familial amyotrophic lateral sclerosis
     with a mutation in exon 4 of the Cu/Zn superoxide dismutase gene: pathological and
     immunocytochemical changes. Acta Neuropathol (Berl) 1996; 92:395–403.
133. Wohlfart G, Swank RL. Pathology of amyotrophic lateral sclerosis: fiber analysis of the
     ventral roots and pyramjidal tracts of the spinal cord. Arch Neurol Psychiatry 1941;
     46:783–799.
134. Berry RG, Chambers RA, Duckett S, Terrero R. Clinicopathological study of juvenile
     amyotrophic lateral sclerosis. Neurology 1969; 19:312.
135. Kusaka H, Matsumoto S, Imai T. An adult-onset case of sporadic motor neuron disease
     with basophilic inclusions. Acta Neuropathol (Berl) 1990; 80:660–665.
136. Matsumoto S, Kusaka H, Murakami N, Hashizume Y, Okazaki H, Hirano A. Basophilic
     inclusions in sporadic juvenile amyotrophic lateral sclerosis: an immunocytochemical and
     ultrastructural study. Acta Neuropathol (Berl) 1992; 83:579–583.

137. Nelson JS, Prensky AL. Sporadic juvenile amyotrophic lateral sclerosis. A clinicopatho-logical study of a case with neuronal cytoplasmic inclusions containing RNA. Arch Neurol 1972; 27:300–306.

138. Oda M, Akagawa N, Tabuchi Y, Tanabe H. A sporadic juvenile case of the amyo-trophic lateral sclerosis with neuronal intracytoplasmic inclusions. Acta Neuropathol (Berl) 1978; 44:211–216.

139. Fujita Y, Okamoto K, Sakurai A, Kusaka H, Aizawa H, Mihara B, Gonatas NK. The Golgi apparatus is fragmented in spinal cord motor neurons of amyotrophic lateral sclerosis with basophilic inclusions. Acta Neuropathol (Berl) 2002; 103:243–247.

140. Hilton DA, McLean B. December 2001: rapidly progressive motor weakness, starting in pregnancy. Brain Pathol 2002; 12:267–269.

141. Sasaki S, Toi S, Shirata A, Yamane K, Sakuma H, Iwata M. Immunohistochemical and ultrastructural study of basophilic inclusions in adult-onset motor neuron disease. Acta Neuropathol (Berl) 2001; 102:200–206.

142. Aizawa H, Kimura T, Hashimoto K, Yahara O, Okamoto K, Kikuchi K. Basophilic cytoplasmic inclusions in a case of sporadic juvenile amyotrophic lateral sclerosis. J Neurol Sci 2000; 176:109–113.

143. Delisle MB, Carpenter S. Neurofibrillary axonal swellings and amyotrophic lateral sclerosis. J Neurol Sci 1984; 63:241–250.

144. Leigh PN, Swash M. Cytoskeletal pathology in motor neuron diseases. Adv Neurol 1991; 56:115–124.

145. Sasaki S, Maruyama S, Yamane K, Sakuma H, Takeishi M. Swellings of proximal axons in a case of motor neuron disease. Ann Neurol 1989; 25:520–522.

146. Sasaki S, Kamei H, Yamane K, Maruyama S. Swelling of neuronal processes in motor neuron disease. Neurology 1988; 38:1114–1118.

147. Corbo M, Hays AP. Peripherin and neurofilament protein coexist in spinal spheroids of motor neuron disease. J Neuropathol Exp Neurol 1992; 51:531–537.

148. Toyoshima I, Sugawara M, Kato K, Wada C, Hirota K, Hasegawa K, Kowa H, Sheetz MP, Masamune O. Kinesin and cytoplasmic dynein in spinal spheroids with motor neu-ron disease. J Neurol Sci 1998; 159:38–44.

149. Shibata N, Asayama K, Hirano A, Kobayashi M. Immunohistochemical study on superoxide dismutases in spinal cords from autopsied patients with amyotrophic lateral sclerosis. Dev Neurosci 1996; 18:492–498.

150. Sasaki S, Iwata M. Immunoreactivity of beta-amyloid precursor protein in amyotrophic lateral sclerosis. Acta Neuropathol (Berl) 1999; 97:463–468.

151. Letournel F, Bocquet A, Dubas F, Barthelaix A, Eyer J. Stable tubule only polypeptides (STOP) proteins co-aggregate with spheroid neurofilaments in amyotrophic lateral sclerosis. J Neuropathol Exp Neurol 2003; 62:1211–1219.

152. Kikuchi S, Ogata A, Shinpo K, Moriwaka F, Fujii J, Taniguchi N, Tashiro K. Detec-tion of an Amadori product, 1-hexitol-lysine, in the anterior horn of the amyotrophic lateral sclerosis and spinobulbar muscular atrophy spinal cord: evidence for early invol-vement of glycation in motoneuron diseases. Acta Neuropathol (Berl) 2000; 99:63–66.

153. Kato T, Kurita K, Seino T, Kadoya T, Horie H, Wada M, Kawanami T, Daimon M, Hirano A. Galectin-1 is a component of neurofilamentous lesions in sporadic and famil-ial amyotrophic lateral sclerosis. Biochem Biophys Res Commun 2001; 282:166–172.

154. Doherty MJ, Bird TD, Leverenz JB. Alpha-synuclein in motor neuron disease: an immunohistologic study. Acta Neuropathol (Berl) 2004; 107:169–175.

155. Lee MK, Marszalek JR, Cleveland DW. A mutant neurofilament subunit causes massive, selective motor neuron death: implications for the pathogenesis of human motor neuron disease. Neuron 1994; 13:975–988.

156. Liem RK, Leung CL. Neuronal intermediate filament overexpression and neurodegen-eration in transgenic mice. Exp Neurol 2003; 184:3–8.

157. Bertrand I, Van Bogaert L. La scléroses latérale amyotrophique (Anatomie Pathologi-que). Rev Neurol 1925; 32:779–806.

158. Sobue G, Hashizume Y, Sahashi K, Takahashi A, Mukai E, Matsuoka Y, Mukoyama M. Amyotrophic lateral sclerosis. Lack of central chromatolytic response of motor neurocytons corresponding to active axonal degeneration. Arch Neurol 1983; 40:306–309.

159. Inoue K, Hirano A. Early pathological changes of amyotrophic lateral sclerosis: autopsy findings of a case of 10 months' duration. Shinkei Naika [Neurol Med (Tokyo)] 1979; 11:448–455.

160. Kusaka H, Imai T, Hashimoto S, Yamamoto T, Maya K, Yamasaki M. Ultrastructural study of chromatolytic neurons in an adult-onset sporadic case of amyotrophic lateral sclerosis. Acta Neuropathol (Berl) 1988; 75:523–528.

161. Hirano A. In pursuit of the early pathological alterations in ALS. In: Tsubaki T, Toyokura Y, eds. Amyotrophic Lateral Sclerosis. Amsterdam: Elsevier Science Publishers B.V., 1988:193–198.

162. Fu SY, Gordon T. The cellular and molecular basis of peripheral nerve regeneration. Mol Neurobiol 1997; 14:67–116.

163. Kreutzberg GW. Reaction of the neuronal cell body to axonal damage. In: Stys PK, Waxman SG, Kocsis JD, eds. The Axon: Structure, Function, and Pathophysiology. New York: Oxford University Press, 1995.

164. Lieberman AR. The axon reaction: a review of the principal features of perikaryal responses to axon injury. Int Rev Neurobiol 1971; 14:49–124.

165. Hirano A. Pathology of motor neurons with special reference to amyotrophic lateral sclerosis and related diseases. In: Tsubaki T, Toyokura Y, eds. Amyotrophic Lateral Sclerosis: Proceedings of the International Symposium on Amyotrophic Lateral Sclerosis. Baltimore: University Park Press, 1979:107–133.

166. Sears TA. Structural changes in intercostal motoneurones following axotomy. J Exp Biol 1987; 132:93–109.

167. Rosenfeld J, Dorman ME, Griffin JW, Gold BG, Sternberger LA, Sternberger NH, Price DL. Distribution of neurofilament antigens after axonal injury. J Neuropathol Exp Neurol 1987; 46:269–282.

168. Martin LJ, Kaiser A, Price AC. Motor neuron degeneration after sciatic nerve avulsion in adult rat evolves with oxidative stress and is apoptosis. J Neurobiol 1999; 40:185–201.

169. Kusaka H, Hirano A. Morphometric study of central chromatolysis in amyotrophic lateral sclerosis. Shinkei Naika [Neurol Med (Tokyo)] 1985; 22:246–251.

170. Nakano I, Hirano A. Atrophic cell processes of large motor neurons in the anterior horn in amyotrophic lateral sclerosis: observation with silver impregnation method. J Neuropathol Exp Neurol 1987; 46:40–49.

171. Sasaki S, Maruyama S. Synapse loss in anterior horn neurons in amyotrophic lateral sclerosis. Acta Neuropathol (Berl) 1994; 88:222–227.

172. Sasaki S, Iwata M. Ultrastructural study of the synapses of central chromatolytic anterior horn cells in motor neuron disease. J Neuropathol Exp Neurol 1996; 55:932–939.

173. Hirano A, Kurland LT, Sayre GP. Familial amyotrophic lateral sclerosis. A subgroup characterized by posterior and spinocerebellar tract involvement and hyaline inclusions in the anterior horn cells. Arch Neurol 1967; 16:232–243.

174. Hirano A, Nakano I, Kurland LT, Mulder DW, Holley PW, Saccomanno G. Fine structural study of neurofibrillary changes in a family with amyotrophic lateral sclerosis. J Neuropathol Exp Neurol 1984; 43:471–480.

175. Martin LJ. Neuronal death in amyotrophic lateral sclerosis is apoptosis: possible contribution of a programmed cell death mechanism. J Neuropathol Exp Neurol 1999; 58:459–471.

176. Kato T, Katagiri T, Hirano A, Sasaki H, Arai S. Sporadic lower motor neuron disease with Lewy body-like inclusions: a new subgroup?. Acta Neuropathol (Berl) 1988; 76:208–211.

177. Kikuchi H, Doh-ura K, Kawashima T, Kira J, Iwaki T. Immunohistochemical analysis of spinal cord lesions in amyotrophic lateral sclerosis using microtubule-associated protein 2 (MAP2) antibodies. Acta Neuropathol (Berl) 1999; 97:13–21.

178. Yoshiyama Y, Yamada T, Asanuma K, Asahi T. Apoptosis related antigen, Le(Y) and nick-end labeling are positive in spinal motor neurons in amyotrophic lateral sclerosis. Acta Neuropathol (Berl) 1994; 88:207–211.

179. Ekegren T, Grundstrom E, Lindholm D, Aquilonius SM. Upregulation of Bax protein and increased DNA degradation in ALS spinal cord motor neurons. Acta Neurol Scand 1999; 100:317–321.

180. He BP, Strong MJ. Motor neuronal death in sporadic amyotrophic lateral sclerosis (ALS) is not apoptotic. A comparative study of ALS and chronic aluminium chloride neurotoxicity in New Zealand white rabbits. Neuropathol Appl Neurobiol 2000; 26:150–160.

181. Migheli A, Cavalla P, Marino S, Schiffer D. A study of apoptosis in normal and pathologic nervous tissue after in situ end-labeling of DNA strand breaks. J Neuropathol Exp Neurol 1994; 53:606–616.

182. Szabolcs MJ, Kopp M, Schaden GE. Carbonic anhydrase activity in the peripheral nervous system of rat: the enzyme as a marker for muscle afferents. Brain Res 1989; 492:129–138.

183. Szabolcs MJ, Windisch A, Koller R, Pensch M. Axon typing of rat muscle nerves using a double staining procedure for cholinesterase and carbonic anhydrase. J Histochem Cytochem 1991; 39:1617–1625.

184. Rende M, Giambanco I, Buratta M, Tonali P. Axotomy induces a different modulation of both low-affinity nerve growth factor receptor and choline acetyltransferase between adult rat spinal and brainstem motoneurons. J Comp Neurol 1995; 363:249–263.

185. Kou SY, Chiu AY, Patterson PH. Differential regulation of motor neuron survival and choline acetyltransferase expression following axotomy. J Neurobiol 1995; 27:561–572.

186. Shefner JM, Gooch CL. Motor Unit Number Estimation in Neurologic Disease In: Pourmand R, Harati Y, eds., Neuromuscular Disorders. Vol. 13. London: Lippincott Williams and Wilkins, 2002:349.

187. Dantes M, McComas A. The extent and time course of motoneuron involvement in amyotrophic lateral sclerosis. Muscle Nerve 1991; 14:416–421.

188. Bradley WG, Good P, Rasool CG, Adelman LS. Morphometric and biochemical studies of peripheral nerves in amyotrophic lateral sclerosis. Ann Neurol 1983; 14:267–277.

189. Hanyu N, Oguchi K, Yanagisawa N, Tsukagoshi H. Degeneration and regeneration of ventral root motor fibers in amyotrophic lateral sclerosis. Morphometric studies of cervical ventral roots. J Neurol Sci 1982; 55:99–115.

190. Kawamura Y, Dyck PJ, Shimono M, Okazaki H, Tateishi J, Doi H. Morphometric comparison of the vulnerability of peripheral motor and sensory neurons in amyotrophic lateral sclerosis. J Neuropathol Exp Neurol 1981; 40:667–675.

191. Rosales RL, Osame M, Madriaga EP, Navarro JC, Igata A. Morphometry of intramuscular nerves in amyotrophic lateral sclerosis. Muscle Nerve 1988; 11:223–226.

192. Fischer LR, Culver DG, Tennant P, Davis AA, Wang M, Castellano-Sanchez A, Khan J, Polak MA, Glass JD. Amyotrophic lateral sclerosis is a distal axonopathy: evidence in mice and man. Exp Neurol 2004; 185:232–240.

193. Eisen A, Swash M. Clinical neurophysiology of ALS. Clin Neurophysiol 2001; 112: 2190–2201.

194. Bjornskov EK, Norris FH Jr, Mower-Kuby J. Quantitative axon terminal and end-plate morphology in amyotrophic lateral sclerosis. Arch Neurol 1984; 41:527–530.

195. Telerman-Toppet N, Coers C. Motor innervation and fiber type pattern in amyotrophic lateral sclerosis and in Charcot-Marie-Tooth disease. Muscle Nerve 1978; 1:133–139.

196. Wohlfart G. Collateral regeneration from residual motor nerve fibers in amyotrophic lateral sclerosis. Neurology 1957; 7:124–134.

197. Sobue G, Matsuoka Y, Mukai E, Takayanagi T, Sobue I. Pathology of myelinated fibers in cervical and lumbar ventral spinal roots in amyotrophic lateral sclerosis. J Neurol Sci 1981; 50:413–421.

198. Bradley WG, Bennett RK, Good P, Little B. Proximal chronic inflammatory polyneuropathy with multifocal conduction block. Arch Neurol 1988; 45:451–455.
199. Kaji R, Oka N, Tsuji T, Mezaki T, Nishio T, Akiguchi I, Kimura J. Pathological findings at the site of conduction block in multifocal motor neuropathy. Ann Neurol 1993; 33:152–158.
200. Auer RN, Bell RB, Lee MA. Neuropathy with onion bulb formations and pure motor manifestations. Can J Neurol Sci 1989; 16:194–197.
201. Taylor BV, Dyck PJ, Engelstad J, Gruener G, Grant I. Multifocal motor neuropathy: pathologic alterations at the site of conduction block. J Neuropathol Exp Neurol 2004; 63:129–137.
202. Mourelatos Z, Adler H, Hirano A, Donnenfeld H, Gonatas JO, Gonatas NK. Fragmentation of the Golgi apparatus of motor neurons in amyotrophic lateral sclerosis revealed by organelle-specific antibodies. Proc Natl Acad Sci USA 1990; 87:4393–4395.
203. Gonatas NK, Stieber A, Mourelatos Z, Chen Y, Gonatas JO, Appel SH, Hays AP, Hickey WF, Hauw JJ. Fragmentation of the Golgi apparatus of motor neurons in amyotrophic lateral sclerosis. Am J Pathol 1992; 140:731–737.
204. Fujita Y, Okamoto K, Sakurai A, Amari M, Nakazato Y, Gonatas NK. Fragmentation of the Golgi apparatus of Betz cells in patients with amyotrophic lateral sclerosis. J Neurol Sci 1999; 163:81–85.
205. Mourelatos Z, Hirano A, Rosenquist AC, Gonatas NK. Fragmentation of the Golgi apparatus of motor neurons in amyotrophic lateral sclerosis (ALS). Clinical studies in ALS of Guam and experimental studies in deafferented neurons and in beta, beta′-iminodipropionitrile axonopathy. Am J Pathol 1994; 144:1288–1300.
206. Fujita Y, Okamoto K, Sakurai A, Gonatas NK, Hirano A. Fragmentation of the Golgi apparatus of the anterior horn cells in patients with familial amyotrophic lateral sclerosis with SOD1 mutations and posterior column involvement. J Neurol Sci 2000; 174:137–140.
207. Mourelatos Z, Gonatas NK, Stieber A, Gurney ME, Dal Canto MC. The Golgi apparatus of spinal cord motor neurons in transgenic mice expressing mutant Cu, Zn superoxide dismutase becomes fragmented in early, preclinical stages of the disease. Proc Natl Acad Sci USA 1996; 93:5472–5477.
208. Stieber A, Gonatas JO, Gonatas NK. Aggregation of ubiquitin and a mutant ALS-linked SOD1 protein correlate with disease progression and fragmentation of the Golgi apparatus. J Neurol Sci 2000; 173:53–62.
209. Strey CW, Spellman D, Stieber A, Gonatas JO, Wang X, Lambris JD, Gonatas NK. Dysregulation of stathmin, a microtubule-destabilizing protein, and up-regulation of Hsp25, Hsp27, and the antioxidant peroxiredoxin 6 in a mouse model of familial amyotrophic lateral sclerosis. Am J Pathol 2004; 165:1701–1718.
210. Williamson TL, Cleveland DW. Slowing of axonal transport is a very early event in the toxicity of ALS-linked SOD1 mutants to motor neurons. Nat Neurosci 1999; 2:50–56.
211. Warita H, Itoyama Y, Abe K. Selective impairment of fast anterograde axonal transport in the peripheral nerves of asymptomatic transgenic mice with a G93A mutant SOD1 gene. Brain Res 1999; 819:120–131.
212. Borchelt DR, Wong PC, Becher MW, Pardo CA, Lee MK, Xu ZS, Thinakaran G, Jenkins NA, Copeland NG, Sisodia SS, et al. Axonal transport of mutant superoxide dismutase 1 and focal axonal abnormalities in the proximal axons of transgenic mice. Neurobiol Dis 1998; 5:27–35.
213. Zhang B, Tu P, Abtahian F, Trojanowski JQ, Lee VM. Neurofilaments and orthograde transport are reduced in ventral root axons of transgenic mice that express human SOD1 with a G93A mutation. J Cell Biol 1997; 139:1307–1315.
214. Lampson LA, Kushner PD, Sobel RA. Major histocompatibility complex antigen expression in the affected tissues in amyotrophic lateral sclerosis. Ann Neurol 1990; 28: 365–372.

215. Kawamata T, Akiyama H, Yamada T, McGeer PL. Immunologic reactions in amyotrophic lateral sclerosis brain and spinal cord tissue. Am J Pathol 1992; 140:691–707.
216. McGeer PL, McGeer EG. Inflammatory processes in amyotrophic lateral sclerosis. Muscle Nerve 2002; 26:459–470.
217. Troost D, Van den Oord JJ, Vianney de Jong JM. Immunohistochemical characterization of the inflammatory infiltrate in amyotrophic lateral sclerosis. Neuropathol Appl Neurobiol 1990; 16:401–410.
218. Engelhardt JI, Tajti J, Appel SH. Lymphocytic infiltrates in the spinal cord in amyotrophic lateral sclerosis. Arch Neurol 1993; 50:30–36.
219. Henkel JS, Engelhardt JI, Siklos L, Simpson EP, Kim SH, Pan T, Goodman JC, Siddique T, Beers DR, Appel SH. Presence of dendritic cells, MCP-1, and activated microglia/macrophages in amyotrophic lateral sclerosis spinal cord tissue. Ann Neurol 2004; 55:221–235.
220. Minghetti L. Cyclooxygenase-2 (COX-2) in inflammatory and degenerative brain diseases. J Neuropathol Exp Neurol 2004; 63:901–910.
221. Almer G, Guegan C, Teismann P, Naini A, Rosoklija G, Hays AP, Chen C, Przedborski S. Increased expression of the pro-inflammatory enzyme cyclooxygenase-2 in amyotrophic lateral sclerosis. Ann Neurol 2001; 49(2):176–185.
222. Zhu S, Stavrovskaya IG, Drozda M, Kim BY, Ona V, Li M, Sarang S, Liu AS, Hartley DM, Wu du C, et al. Minocycline inhibits cytochrome c release and delays progression of amyotrophic lateral sclerosis in mice. Nature 2002; 417:74–78.
223. Van Den Bosch L, Tilkin P, Lemmens G, Robberecht W. Minocycline delays disease onset and mortality in a transgenic model of ALS. Neuroreport 2002; 13:1067–1070.
224. Kriz J, Nguyen MD, Julien JP. Minocycline slows disease progression in a mouse model of amyotrophic lateral sclerosis. Neurobiol Dis 2002; 10:268–278.
225. Drachman DB, Frank K, Dykes-Hoberg M, Teismann P, Almer G, Przedborski S, Rothstein JD. Cyclooxygenase 2 inhibition protects motor neurons and prolongs survival in a transgenic mouse model of ALS. Ann Neurol 2002; 52:771–778.
226. Ince PG, Evans J, Knopp M, Forster G, Hamdalla HH, Wharton SB, Shaw PJ. Corticospinal tract degeneration in the progressive muscular atrophy variant of ALS. Neurology 2003; 60:1252–1258.
227. Iwanaga K, Hayashi S, Oyake M, Horikawa Y, Hayashi T, Wakabayashi M, Kondo H, Tsuji S, Takahashi H. Neuropathology of sporadic amyotrophic lateral sclerosis of long duration. J Neurol Sci 1997; 146:139–143.
228. Sasaki S, Iwata M. Immunocytochemical and ultrastructural study of the motor cortex in patients with lower motor neuron disease. Neurosci Lett 2000; 281:45–48.
229. Sasaki S, Iwata M. Motor neuron disease with predominantly upper extremity involvement: a clinicopathological study. Acta Neuropathol (Berl) 1999; 98:645–650.
230. Tsuchiya K, Shintani S, Kikuchi M, Kondo H, Kamaya T, Ohbu S, Kato S, Hayashi H, Ikeda K, Nakano I. Sporadic amyotrophic lateral sclerosis of long duration mimicking spinal progressive muscular atrophy: a clinicopathological study. J Neurol Sci 1999; 162:174–178.
231. Pestronk A. Multifocal motor neuropathy: diagnosis and treatment. Neurology 1998; 51:S22–S24.
232. Nobile-Orazio E, Terenghi F, Carpo M, Bersano A. Treatment of multifocal motor neuropathy. Neurol Sci 2003; 24(suppl 4):S251–S255.
233. Latov N, Chaudhry V, Koski CL, Lisak RP, Apatoff BR, Hahn AF, Howard JF Jr. Use of intravenous gamma globulins in neuroimmunologic diseases. J Allergy Clin Immunol 2001; 108:S126–S132.
234. Santoro M, Uncini A, Corbo M, Staugaitis SM, Thomas FP, Hays AP, Latov N. Experimental conduction block induced by serum from a patient with anti-GM1 antibodies. Ann Neurol 1992; 31:385–390.

235. Noguchi M, Mori K, Yamazaki S, Suda K, Sato N, Oshimi K. Multifocal motor neuropathy caused by a B-cell lymphoma producing a monoclonal IgM autoantibody against peripheral nerve myelin glycolipids GM1 and GD1b. Br J Haematol 2003; 123:600–605.
236. Rowland LP, Defendini R, Sherman W, Hirano A, Olarte MR, Latov N, Lovelace RE, Inoue K, Osserman EF. Macroglobulinemia with peripheral neuropathy simulating motor neuron disease. Ann Neurol 1982; 11:532–536.
237. Gorson KC, Ropper AH, Adelman LS, Raynor EM, Saper CB. Chronic motor axonal neuropathy: pathological evidence of inflammatory polyradiculoneuropathy. Muscle Nerve 1999; 22:266–270.
238. Cai Z, Blumbergs PC, Koblar SA, Cash K, Manavis J, Ghabriel MN, Thompson PD. Peripheral nervous system and central nervous system pathology in rapidly progressive lower motor neuron syndrome with immunoglobulin M anti-GM1 ganglioside antibody. J Peripher Nerv Syst 2004; 9:79–91.
239. Ghatak NR, Campbell WW, Lippman RH, Hadfield MG. Anterior horn changes of motor neuron disease associated with demyelinating radiculopathy. J Neuropathol Exp Neurol 1986; 45:385–395.
240. Adams D, Kuntzer T, Steck AJ, Lobrinus A, Janzer RC, Regli F. Motor conduction block and high titres of anti-GM1 ganglioside antibodies: pathological evidence of a motor neuropathy in a patient with lower motor neuron syndrome. J Neurol Neurosurg Psychiatry 1993; 56:982–987.
241. Oh SJ, Claussen GC, Odabasi Z, Palmer CP. Multifocal demyelinating motor neuropathy: pathologic evidence of "inflammatory demyelinating polyradiculoneuropathy." Neurology 1995; 45:1828–1832.
242. Veugelers B, Theys P, Lammens M, Van Hees J, Robberecht W. Pathological findings in a patient with amyotrophic lateral sclerosis and multifocal motor neuropathy with conduction block. J Neurol Sci 1996; 136:64–70.
243. Gordon PH, Katz BA, Pinto M, Hays AP, Mitsumoto H, Rowland LP. The natural history of primary lateral sclerosis. In press.
244. Strong MJ, Gordon PH. Primary lateral sclerosis, hereditary spastic paraplegia and amyotrophic lateral sclerosis—discrete entities or spectrum? Amyotroph Lateral Scler Other Motor Neuron 2005; 6:8–16.
245. Pringle CE, Hudson AJ, Munoz DG, Kiernan JA, Brown WF, Ebers GC. Primary lateral sclerosis. Clinical features, neuropathology, and diagnostic criteria. Brain 1992; 115(pt 2):495–520.
246. Rowland LP. Primary lateral sclerosis: disease, syndrome, both or neither? (Comment). J Neurol Sci 1999; 170:1–4.
247. Rowland LP. Research advances in amyotrophic lateral sclerosis (ALS): a personal view. Neurol Neurochair Pol 2005; 39:1–8.
248. Swash M, Desai J, Misra VP. What is primary lateral sclerosis? (See comment). J Neurol sci 1999; 170:5–10.
249. Zhai P, Pagan F, Statland J, Butman JA, Floeter MK. Primary lateral sclerosis: a heterogeneous disorder composed of different subtypes? Neurol 2003; 60:1258–1265.
250. Ulug AM, Grunewald T, Lin MT, Kamal AK, Filippi CG, Zimmerman RD, Beal ML. Diffusion tensor imaging in the diagnosis of primary lateral sclerosis. J Magn Reson Imaging 2004; 19:34–39.
251. Kaufmann P, Pullman SL, Shungu DC, Chan S, Hays AP, Del Bene ML, Dover MA, Vukic M, Rowland LP, Mitsumoto H. Objective tests for upper motor neuron involvement in amyotrophic lateral sclerosis (ALS). Neurology 2004; 62:1753–1757.
252. Chan S, Kaufmann P, Shungu DC, Mitsumoto H. Amyotrophic lateral sclerosis and primary lateral sclerosis: evidence-based diagnostic evaluation of the upper motor neuron. Neuroimaging Clin N Am 2003; 13:307–326.
253. Beal MF, Richardson EP Jr. Primary lateral sclerosis: a case report. Arch Neurol 1981; 38:630–633.

254. Kato S, Hirano A, Llena JF. Primary lateral sclerosis: a case report. Shinkei Naika 1990; 32:501–506.

255. Koga H, Ozeki T, Makiura Y. Sporadic motor neuron disease with marked fronto-temporal atrophy: an autopsied case mimicking primary lateral sclerosis. Shinkei Byourigaku (Neuropathology) 2003; 23:A40.

256. Konogaya M, Sakai M, Matsuoka Y, Konagaya Y, Hashizume Y. Upper motor neuron predominant degeneration with frontal and temporal lobe atrophy. Acta Neuropathol (Berl) 1998; 96:532–536.

257. Kuzuhara S, Namural G, Inomata H, Toyokura Y, Tomonaga A. A case with marked atrophy in the frontotemporal lobe similar to Pick's disease in addition to the clinical as well as pathological features of primary lateral sclerosis. Shinkei Byourigaku (Neuro-pathology) 1985; 6:295–296.

258. Imai H, Furukawa Y, Sumino S, Mori H, Ueda G, Shirai T, Kondo T, Mizuno Y. (A 65-year-old woman with dysarthria, dysphagia, weakness, and gait disturbance) No to Shinkei. Brain Nerve 1995; 47:399–410.

259. Mochizuki A, Komatsuzaki Y, Iwamoto H, Shoji S. Frontotemporal dementia with ubiquitinated neuronal inclusions presenting with primary lateral sclerosis and parkin-sonism: clinicopathological report of an autopsy case. Acta Neuropathol (Berl) 2004; 107:377–380.

260. Sugihara H, Horiuchi M, Kamo T, Fujisawa K, Abe M, Sakiyama T, Tadokoro M. A case of primary lateral sclerosis taking a prolonged clinical course with dementia and having an unusual dendritic ballooning. Neuropathology 1999; 19:77–84.

261. Tan CF, Kakita A, Piao YS, Kikugawa K, Endo K, Tanaka M, Okamoto K, Takahashi H. Primary lateral sclerosis: a rare upper-motor-predominant form of amyotrophic lateral sclerosis often accompanied by frontotemporal lobar degeneration with ubiquiti-nated neuronal inclusions? Report of an autopsy case and a review of the literature. Acta Neuropathol 2003; 105:615–620.

262. Watanabe R, Iino M, Honda M, Sano J, Hara M. Primary lateral sclerosis. Neuro-pathology 1997; 17:220–224.

263. Younger DS, Chou S, Hays AP, Lange DJ, Emerson R, Brin M, Thompson H Jr, Rowland LP. Primary lateral sclerosis. A clinical diagnosis reemerges. Arch Neurol 1988; 45:1304–1307.

264. Fisher CM. Pure spastic paralysis of corticospinal origin. Can J Neurol Sci 1977; 4: 251–258.

265. Bruyn RP, Koelman JH, Troost D, de Jong JM. Motor neuron disease (amyotrophic lateral sclerosis) arising from longstanding primary lateral sclerosis. J Neurol Neurosurg Psychiatry 1995; 58:742–744.

266. Le Forestier N, Maisonobe T, Spelle L, Lesort A, Salachas F, Lacomblez L, Samson Y, Bouche P, Meininger V. Primary lateral sclerosis: further clarification. J Neurol Sci 2001; 185:95–100.

267. Caselli RJ, Smith BE, Osborne D. Primary lateral sclerosis: a neuropsychological study. Neurology 1995; 45:2005–2009.

268. Tsuchiya K, Arai M, Matsuya S, Nishimura H, Ishiko T, Kondo H, Ikeda K, Matsush-ita M. Sporadic amyotrophic lateral sclerosis resembling primary lateral sclerosis: report of an autopsy case and a review of the literature. Neuropathology 1999; 19:71–76.

269. Fink JK. Progressive spastic paraparesis: hereditary spastic paraplegia and its relation to primary and amyotrophic lateral sclerosis. Semin Neurol 2001; 21:199–207.

270. Wharton SB, McDermott CJ, Grierson AJ, Wood JD, Gelsthorpe C, Ince PG, Shaw PJ. The cellular and molecular pathology of the motor system in hereditary spastic parapar-esis due to mutation of the spastin gene. J Neuropathol Exp Neurol 2003; 62:1166–1177.

271. Eymard-Pierre E, Lesca G, Dollet S, Santorelli FM, di Capua M, Bertini E, Boespflug-Tanguy O. Infantile-onset ascending hereditary spastic paralysis is associated with mutations in the alsin gene. Am J Hum Genet 2002; 71:518–527.

272. Hadano S, Hand CK, Osuga H, Yanagisawa Y, Otomo A, Devon RS, Miyamoto N, Showguchi-Miyata J, Okada Y, Singaraja R, et al. A gene encoding a putative GTPase regulator is mutated in familial amyotrophic lateral sclerosis 2. Nat Genet 2001; 29:166–173.
273. Yang Y, Hentati A, Deng HX, Dabbagh O, Sasaki T, Hirano M, Hung WY, Ouahchi K, Yan J, Azim AC, et al. The gene encoding alsin, a protein with three guanine-nucleotide exchange factor domains, is mutated in a form of recessive amyotrophic lateral sclerosis. Nat Genet 2001; 29:160–165.
274. Hirano A, Llena JF, Streifler M, Cohn DF. Anterior horn cell changes in a case of neurolathyrism. Acta Neuropathol (Berl) 1976; 35:277–283.
275. Striefler M, Cohn DF, Hirano A, Schujman E. The central nervous system in a case of neurolathyrism. Neurology 1977; 27:1176–1178.
276. Tshala-Katumbay D, Eeg-Olofsson KE, Kazadi-Kayembe T, Tylleskar T, Fallmar P. Analysis of motor pathway involvement in konzo using transcranial electrical and magnetic stimulation. Muscle Nerve 2002; 25:230–235.
277. Spencer PS. Food toxins, ampa receptors, and motor neuron diseases. Drug Metab Rev 1999; 31:561–587.
278. Rowland LP. Ten central themes in a decade of ALS research. In: Rowland LP, ed. Amyotrophic Lateral Sclerosis and Other Motor Neuron Diseases. Vol. 56. New York: Raven Press, 1991:3–23.
279. Morita K, Kaiya H, Ikeda T, Namba M. Presenile dementia combined with amyotrophy: a review of 34 Japanese cases. Arch Gerontol Geriatr 1987; 6:263–277.
280. Neary D, Snowden JS, Mann DM, Northen B, Goulding PJ, Macdermott N. Frontal lobe dementia and motor neuron disease. J Neurol Neurosurg Psychiatry 1990; 53: 23–32.
281. Hudson AJ. Amyotrophic lateral sclerosis and its association with dementia, parkinsonism and other neurological disorders: a review. Brain 1981; 104:217–247.
282. Horoupian DS, Thal L, Katzman R, Terry RD, Davies P, Hirano A, Deteresa R, Fuld PA, Petito C, Blass J, Ellis JM. Dementia and motor neuron disease: morphometric, biochemical, and Golgi studies. Ann Neurol 1984; 16:305–313.
283. Strong MJ, Lomen-Hoerth C, Caselli RJ, Bigio EH, Yang W. Cognitive impairment, frontotemporal dementia, and the motor neuron diseases. Ann Neurol 2003; 54(suppl 5): S20–S23.
284. Rosso SM, Kamphorst W, de Graaf B, Willemsen R, Ravid R, Niermeijer MF, Spillantini MG, Heutink P, van Swieten JC. Familial frontotemporal dementia with ubiquitin-positive inclusions is linked to chromosome 17q21–22. Brain 2001; 124:1948–1957.
285. Hosler BA, Siddique T, Sapp PC, Sailor W, Huang MC, Hossain A, Daube JR, Nance M, Fan C, Kaplan J, et al. Linkage of familial amyotrophic lateral sclerosis with frontotemporal dementia to chromosome 9q21-q22. JAMA 2000; 284:1664–1669.
286. Bergmann M, Kuchelmeister K, Schmid KW, Kretzschmar HA, Schroder R. Different variants of frontotemporal dementia: a neuropathological and immunohistochemical study. Acta Neuropathol (Berl) 1996; 92:170–179.
287. Tsuchiya K, Ikeda K, Mimura M, Takahashi M, Miyazaki H, Anno M, Shiotsu H, Akabane H, Niizato K, Uchihara T, et al. Constant involvement of the Betz cells and pyramidal tract in amyotrophic lateral sclerosis with dementia: a clinicopathological study of eight autopsy cases. Acta Neuropathol (Berl) 2002; 104:249–259.
288. Tsuchiya K, Ikeda K, Haga C, Kobayashi T, Morimatsu Y, Nakano I, Matsushita M. Atypical amyotrophic lateral sclerosis with dementia mimicking frontal Pick's disease: a report of an autopsy case with a clinical course of 15 years. Acta Neuropathol (Berl) 2001; 101:625–630.
289. Ikeda K, Tsuchiya K. Motor neuron disease group accompanied by inclusions of unidentified protein signaled by ubiquitin. Neuropathology 2004; 24:117–124.

290. Al-Sarraj S, Maekawa S, Kibble M, Everall I, Leigh N. Ubiquitin-only intraneuronal inclusion in the substantia nigra is a characteristic feature of motor neurone disease with dementia. Neuropathol Appl Neurobiol 2002; 28:120–128.

291. Connolly JH, Allen IV, Dermott E. Transmissible agent in the amyotrophic form of Creutzfeldt-Jakob disease. J Neurol Neurosurg Psychiatry 1988; 51:1459–1460.

292. Worrall BB, Rowland LP, Chin SS, Mastrianni JA. Amyotrophy in prion diseases. Arch Neurol 2000; 57:33–38.

293. Wilson CM, Grace GM, Munoz DG, He BP, Strong MJ. Cognitive impairment in sporadic ALS: a pathologic continuum underlying a multisystem disorder. Neurology 2001; 57:651–657.

294. Okamoto K, Hirai S, Amari M. Electron microscopy of ubiquitin-positive intraneuronal inclusions in the extra-motor cortices of amyotrophic lateral sclerosis. Shinkei Byourigaku (Neuropathology) 1996; 16:112–116.

295. Nakano T, Nakaso K, Nakashima K, Ohama E. Expression of ubiquitin-binding protein p62 in ubiquitin-immunoreactive intraneuronal inclusions in amyotrophic lateral sclerosis with dementia: analysis of five autopsy cases with broad clinicopathological spectrum. Acta Neuropathol (Berl) 2004; 107:359–364.

296. Arai T, Nonaka T, Hasegawa M, Akiyama H, Yoshida M, Hashizume Y, Tsuchiya K, Oda T, Ikeda K. Neuronal and glial inclusions in frontotemporal dementia with or without motor neuron disease are immunopositive for p62. Neurosci Lett 2003; 342:41–44.

297. Mori F, Nishie M, Piao YS, Kito K, Kamitani T, Takahashi H, Wakabayashi K. Accumulation of NEDD8 in neuronal and glial inclusions of neurodegenerative disorders. Neuropathol Appl Neurobiol 2005; 31:53–61.

298. Furukawa Y, Iseki E, Hino H, Kanai A, Odawara T, Kosaka K. Ubiquitin and ubiquitin-related proteins in neurons and dendrites of brains of atypical Pick's disease without Pick bodies. Neuropathology 2004; 24:38–45.

299. Holton JL, Revesz T, Crooks R, Scaravilli F. Evidence for pathological involvement of the spinal cord in motor neuron disease-inclusion dementia. Acta Neuropathol (Berl) 2002; 103:221–227.

300. Iseki E, Li F, Odawara T, Hino H, Suzuki K, Kosaka K, Akiyama H, Ikeda K, Kato M. Ubiquitin-immunohistochemical investigation of atypical Pick's disease without Pick bodies. J Neurol Sci 1998; 159:194–201.

301. Jackson M, Lennox G, Lowe J. Motor neurone disease-inclusion dementia. Neurodegeneration 1996; 5:339–350.

302. Kovari E, Gold G, Giannakopoulos P, Bouras C. Cortical ubiquitin-positive inclusions in frontotemporal dementia without motor neuron disease: a quantitative immunocytochemical study. Acta Neuropathol (Berl) 2004; 108:207–212.

303. Munoz DG, Dickson DW, Bergeron C, Mackenzie IR, Delacourte A, Zhukareva V. The neuropathology and biochemistry of frontotemporal dementia. Ann Neurol 2003; 54(suppl 5):S24–S28.

304. Odawara T, Iseki E, Kanai A, Arai T, Katsuragi T, Hino H, Furukawa Y, Kato M, Yamamoto T, Kosaka K. Clinicopathological study of two subtypes of Pick's disease in Japan. Dement Geriatr Cogn Disord 2003; 15:19–25.

305. Toyoshima Y, Piao YS, Tan CF, Morita M, Tanaka M, Oyanagi K, Okamoto K, Takahashi H. Pathological involvement of the motor neuron system and hippocampal formation in motor neuron disease-inclusion dementia. Acta Neuropathol (Berl) 2003; 106:50–56.

306. Uchihara T, Sato T, Suzuki H, Ikeda K, Akiyama H, Takatori T. Bunina body in frontal lobe dementia without clinical manifestations of motor neuron disease. Acta Neuropathol (Berl) 2001; 101:281–284.

307. Cleveland DW, Rothstein JD. From Charcot to Lou Gehrig: deciphering selective motor neuron death in ALS. Nat Rev Neurosci 2001; 2:806–819.

308. Bruijn LI, Miller TM, Cleveland DW. Unraveling the mechanisms involved in motor neuron degeneration in ALS. Annu Rev Neurosci 2004; 27:723–749.
309. Bigio EH, Johnson NA, Rademaker AW, Fung BB, Mesulam MM, Siddique N, Dellefave L, Caliendo J, Freeman S, Siddique T. Neuronal ubiquinated intranuclear inclusions in familial and non-familial frontotemporal dementia of the motor neuron disease type associated with amyotrophic lateral sclerosis. J Neuropathol Exp Neurol 2004; 63:801–811.
310. Shibata N, Hirano A, Kobayashi M, Siddique T, Deng HX, Hung WY, Kato T, Asayama K. Intense superoxide dismutase-1 immunoreactivity in intracytoplasmic hyaline inclusions of familial amyotrophic lateral sclerosis with posterior column involvement. J Neuropathol Exp Neurol 1996; 55:481–490.
311. Takahashi H, Makifuchi T, Nakano R, Sato S, Inuzuka T, Sakimura K, Mishina M, Honma Y, Tsuji S, Ikuta F. Familial amyotrophic lateral sclerosis with a mutation in the Cu/Zn superoxide dismutase gene. Acta Neuropathol (Berl) 1994; 88:185–188.
312. Shaw CE, Enayat ZE, Powell JF, Anderson VE, Radunovic A, al-Sarraj S, Leigh PN. Familial amyotrophic lateral sclerosis. Molecular pathology of a patient with a SOD1 mutation. Neurology 1997; 49:1612–1616.
313. Kokubo Y, Kuzuhara S, Narita Y, Kikugawa K, Nakano R, Inuzuka T, Tsuji S, Watanabe M, Miyazaki T, Murayama S, Ihara Y. Accumulation of neurofilaments and SOD1-immunoreactive products in a patient with familial amyotrophic lateral sclerosis with I113T SOD1 mutation. Arch Neurol 1999; 56:1506–1508.
314. Rouleau GA, Clark AW, Rooke K, Pramatarova A, Krizus A, Suchowersky O, Julien JP, Figlewicz D. SOD1 mutation is associated with accumulation of neurofilaments in amyotrophic lateral sclerosis. Ann Neurol 1996; 39:128–131.
315. Tan CF, Piao YS, Hayashi S, Obata H, Umeda Y, Sato M, Fukushima T, Nakano R, Tsuji S, Takahashi H. Familial amyotrophic lateral sclerosis with bulbar onset and a novel Asp101Tyr Cu/Zn superoxide dismutase gene mutation. Acta Neuropathol (Berl) 2004; 108:332–336.
316. Kadekawa J, Fujimura H, Ogawa Y, Hattori N, Kaido M, Nishimura T, Yoshikawa H, Shirahata N, Sakoda S, Yanagihara T. A clinicopathological study of a patient with familial amyotrophic lateral sclerosis associated with a two base pair deletion in the copper/zinc superoxide dismutase (SOD1) gene. Acta Neuropathol (Berl) 1997; 94: 617–622.
317. Kato S, Shimoda M, Watanabe Y, Nakashima K, Takahashi K, Ohama E. Familial amyotrophic lateral sclerosis with a two base pair deletion in superoxide dismutase 1: gene multisystem degeneration with intracytoplasmic hyaline inclusions in astrocytes. J Neuropathol Exp Neurol 1996; 55:1089–1101.
318. Takehisa Y, Ujike H, Ishizu H, Terada S, Haraguchi T, Tanaka Y, Nishinaka T, Nobukuni K, Ihara Y, Namba R, et al. Familial amyotrophic lateral sclerosis with a novel Leu126Ser mutation in the copper/zinc superoxide dismutase gene showing mild clinical features and Lewy body-like hyaline inclusions. Arch Neurol 2001; 58:736–740.
319. Ohi T, Nabeshima K, Kato S, Yazawa S, Takechi S. Familial amyotrophic lateral sclerosis with His46Arg mutation in Cu/Zn superoxide dismutase presenting characteristic clinical features and Lewy body-like hyaline inclusions. J Neurol Sci 2004; 225:19–25.
320. Kato S, Takikawa M, Nakashima K, Hirano A, Cleveland DW, Kusaka H, Shibata N, Kato M, Nakano I, Ohama E. New consensus research on neuropathological aspects of familial amyotrophic lateral sclerosis with superoxide dismutase 1 (SOD1) gene mutations: inclusions containing SOD1 in neurons and astrocytes. Amyotroph Lateral Scler Other Motor Neuron Disord 2000; 1:163–184.
321. Kato S, Hayashi H, Nakashima K, Nanba E, Kato M, Hirano A, Nakano I, Asayama K, Ohama E. Pathological characterization of astrocytic hyaline inclusions in familial amyotrophic lateral sclerosis. Am J Pathol 1997; 151:611–620.

322. Chen YZ, Bennett CL, Huynh HM, Blair IP, Puls I, Irobi J, Dierick I, Abel A, Kennerson ML, Rabin BA, et al. DNA/RNA helicase gene mutations in a form of juvenile amyotrophic lateral sclerosis (ALS4). Am J Hum Genet 2004; 74:1128–1135.

323. Nishimura AL, Mitne-Neto M, Silva HC, Richieri-Costa A, Middleton S, Cascio D, Kok F, Oliveira JR, Gillingwater T, Webb J, et al. A mutation in the vesicle-trafficking protein VAPB causes late-onset spinal muscular atrophy and amyotrophic lateral sclerosis. Am J Hum Genet 2004; 75:822–831.

324. Rabin BA, Griffin JW, Crain BJ, Scavina M, Chance PF, Cornblath DR. Autosomal dominant juvenile amyotrophic lateral sclerosis. Brain 1999; 122(pt 8):1539–1550.

4

The Causes of Sporadic Amyotrophic Lateral Sclerosis

Lewis P. Rowland

Department of Neurology, Neurological Institute of New York, Eleanor and Lou Gehrig MDA/ALS Research Center, Columbia University Medical Center, New York, New York, U.S.A.

INTRODUCTION

Much is known about the *pathogenesis* of amyotrophic lateral sclerosis (ALS); that is, how the disease comes about in molecular terms. Virtually all the information has come from studies of the transgenic mouse bearing mutations of superoxide dismutase 1 (SOD1). The process seems to be similar in mice and humans. In contrast, little is known about the *etiology* of non-genetic or sporadic human ALS. Bruijn et al. (1) suggest that the cause sets off the same cascade of pathophysiology in the SOD1 transgenic mouse and in humans, differing only in that one cause is a mutation and other causes are not yet clearly identified.

In ALS and other age-related neurodegenerative diseases, it is assumed that there must be genetic susceptibility factors to explain why ALS is so rare; only a few people have the permissive genomic structure. Then, environmental factors are invoked to explain how the disease arises in a susceptible person. We know little about the susceptibility factors and even less about possible environmental agents. However, the topic is not a total void and I will here review what is known about the etiology of sporadic ALS.

GENETIC SUSCEPTIBILITY TO ALS

It may seem to be an oxymoron to state that unrecognized mutations may explain why some people have ALS. Nevertheless, when a new mutation is recognized as a cause of ALS, surveys of sporadic cases turn up some with a pathogenic mutation in that gene (2). In Italy, 3 of 48 sporadic cases proved to have SOD1 mutations (3). Andersen (4) gave similar figures of 3% in England, 4% in Scandinavia, and 7% in Scotland. Also, incomplete penetrance of some SOD1 mutations could explain why mutations are found in some people with apparently sporadic disease (5). In one of the sporadic cases, the occurrence of a new mutation was documented because it was not present in the patient's parents (6). Similarly, mutations of other genes for familial ALS have been found in apparently sporadic ALS (7,8). SOD1 mutations are thought to account for 20% of all familial ALS, so new discoveries of mutations in other genes are likely to be uncovered for some time to come. There are already eight forms of familial motor neuron diseases (9) and three new gene products were identified in 2004.

As for susceptibility genes, one of the first to be examined was the SMN1 gene, where mutations cause spinal muscular atrophy of childhood and adolescence. It seemed reasonable to wonder whether this gene could contribute to the development of adult-onset ALS, but the first studies of SMN1 (10,11) found no mutations in patients with ALS. Later, Corcia et al. (12) found that "16% of ALS patients had an abnormal copy number of the SMN1 gene (one or three copies), compared with 4% of controls." They concluded that abnormalities in the SMN1 gene locus might be a susceptibility factor for ALS. Unique sites may determine susceptibility to ALS-frontotemporal dementia (13). Mutations in the gene for vascular endothelial growth factor (VEGF) render a person twice as likely to develop ALS (14,15).

Majoor-Krakauer et al. (16) noted 12 susceptibility genes for ALS. In contrast, however, Veldink et al. (17) surveyed 17 possible susceptibility factors and deemed as almost all of them "unlikely," "non-significant," or "possible but (only a) single study." They also found homozygous deletions of SM2 (the centromeric form of the protein) in 16% of patients and 4% of controls; patients with the homozygous mutation had a shorter mean survival time. They concluded that the SMN2 gene might be a phenotypic modifier (18). Neurofilament gene mutations have been noted but seem to be of uncertain influence (15). The Hfe gene was mutated in hemochromatosis and, in one study (19), was mutated in 31% of patients with sporadic ALS and 14% of controls.

Scarmeas et al. (20) found that patients with ALS tend to be naturally slim and more of them than controls had been varsity athletes in high school or college, but past studies had been inconsistent on this point. Others have noticed the unusual prevalence of athletes with ALS (21,22). In 2003, professional soccer players seemed to have excess risk in Italy (23). It is uncertain whether the hard labor of athletics is the risk factor (24); we have not noted an unusual prevalence of laborers in our urban ALS center. An alternative explanation for the prominence of athletes is that slimness and athletic talent are non-specific genetic markers of susceptibility to ALS. That is, the genetic basis of athleticism could be linked to genetic susceptibility genes. Similarly, many clinicians believe that most patients with ALS are "nice" people, which could also be a genetic risk factor (25). Similarly, the frequent association of ALS with parkinsonism might be a manifestation of shared genetic susceptibility, but that has not been proven (26).

However, if genetic susceptibility is a crucial element in the causation of sporadic ALS, there is still a need to document the genes involved.

TRANSMISSIBLE AGENTS IN ALS

Prions: D. Carleton Gajdusek won the Nobel Prize in Medicine in 1976. The award was given for the demonstration that we now call as "age-related neurodegenerative diseases" could be transmitted to primates by injecting CNS tissues from affected humans into an animal. For a while they focused on ALS-dementia and concluded that it was not transmissible. That conclusion may not have been warranted and the story deserves retelling.

Gajdusek surely deserved the prize, but he was assisted by many others, especially Clarence Joseph Gibbs, his veterinarian-virologist partner, who did the injections, cared for the animals, and studied the tissues. Others included almost-anonymous French scientists who, in 1936, had demonstrated that scrapie, a disease of sheep, could be transmitted to other sheep; their report was greeted with skepticism but the finding was confirmed by William Gordon in Scotland in 1939; the latent period from the time of injection to the onset of symptoms could be more than one year.

Vincent Zigas migrated from Estonia to Australia during World War II and became a public health officer in New Guinea. There he introduced Gajdusek to "kuru," which means "trembling" in the native language and had become the name for a lethal neurological disease. Cannibalism had been implicated by anthropologists Robert and Shirley Glasse (she was later Shirley Lindenbaum). Gajdusek and Zigas reported the disease in 1958. They sent the postmortem brain specimens to Igor Klatzo, a neuropathologist at the National Institute of Neurological Diseases and Blindness, and he recognized the similarity of brain pathology in kuru to that of Creutzfeldt–Jakob disease (CJD). Meanwhile, William Hadlow, an American veterinary neuropathologist, was working on scrapie in England. He saw an exhibition on kuru prepared by Gajdusek for a London showing. Hadlow was impressed by the "uncanny" similarity of pathology of kuru to scrapie, recalled the transmission of scrapie, and sent a letter in 1959 to the editor of *Lancet* with a copy to Gajdusek; in the letter Hadlow suggested experiments for primate transmission. Their efforts at NINDB were abetted by another virologist-administrator, Joseph Smadel, who assured them the needed facilities. The first injections by Gajdusek and Gibbs were achieved in 1963 and, two years later, Gibbs reported that two of the four chimpanzees injected with kuru had come down with the disease (27,28).

Gajdusek deserved the prize, but he had lot of help (29) and there was more to come. Gajdusek and his partners demonstrated transmission of CJD and the Gerstmann–Scheinker–Sträussler disease. Nevertheless, they were confronted by mysteries of the causal agent—not only the prolonged non-virus-like latency, but also lack of DNA and surprising resistance to heat, radiation, and chemicals that kill viruses. The terms they used included "atypical viruses," "slow viruses," and "persistent viral infection."

A second Nobel prize in 1997 for work on these rare diseases was given to Stanley Prusiner, who identified the agents as "prions" (pronounced by Prusiner as "pree-on," *not* rhyming with Zion). He heretically defined a novel form of life composed of a self-replicating protein without nucleic acids. He too was assisted by ingenious and skilled colleagues, but Prusiner was the one who was criticized and even vilified until his evidence, summarized in 1982 (30), was finally accepted. A key element was the discovery of the prion gene (PrP) and the discovery that familial cases of CJD were linked to mutations of that gene.

Why consider prions in a discussion of ALS? Early, there had been literature on the "amyotrophic form of CJD (31)." However, Gajdusek's group never transmitted ALS itself; they later transmitted ALS-dementia in only 2 of 33 cases and dismissed those two as "atypical" (32). They abjured the term "amyotrophic CJD" and it more or less disappeared from the literature. However, one more of the 33 attempted transmissions succeeded after a long latent period (33), making the total transmission success rate almost 10%—and failure meant only that the particular attempt failed; under other circumstances some of the others might have been successful. Moreover, the "atypical' features did not exclude either diagnosis—ALS or CJD (34).

Worrall et al. (35) described a mother with ALS and iatrogenic CJD (from treatment with human growth hormone from pituitary extracts); they sought but did not find evidence of shared genetic susceptibility to both diseases. In reviewing the literature, Worrall found 50 cases in which there was either clinical or EMG evidence of lower motor neuron disease in proven sporadic or familial prion disease (36). Cases of peripheral neuropathy or amyotrophy are still being reported, some with both visible fasciculation and sensory loss, and others with purely lower motor neuron syndromes (37–39). The abnormal prion protein may be deposited in peripheral nerves, but dementia may overshadow symptoms of a neuropathy (40). One patient with dementia, wasted hands, and fasciculations (both visible and in the EMG) also had periodic complexes in the EEG, but proved at autopsy to have frontotemporal dementia with ubiquitinated inclusions, not a prion disease (41).

Viral Diseases

Paralytic poliomyelitis is no longer a problem in industrialized countries, but the affinity of that virus for motor neurons was an early stimulus for the belief that ALS could be caused by a virus, especially after Gajdusek provided the evidence for long latency and persistent infections of the nervous system that were attributed to "slow viruses." Unfortunately, all efforts failed to uncover a role for poliovirus in ALS (42–44). Reports in the past few years have led to controversy, but provided no consistent evidence of poliovirus or other enterovirus in postmortem spinal cord of patients with ALS (45–47).

In the meantime, another virus has shown affinity for the motor neuron, the West Nile virus, which can be demonstrated in humans by magnetic resonance imaging (48). Although meningitis and encephalitis are common syndromes, acute flaccid paralysis without sensory loss is the motor neuron syndrome. Recovery may be incomplete but long-term progression has not been described (49).

We have described a syndrome of persistent motor neuron disorder—benign fasciculation and cramp—which was seen in two patients after complete recovery from poliomyelitis and another with a purely motor idiopathic myelitis, presumably viral (50). All three were observed for three years after the onset of fasciculations, with no new weakness or atrophy. The following is a previously unpublished example of the postpolio fasciculation-cramp syndrome of Foley and Denny-Brown.

> In 1946, at age 8, the patient had a stiff neck and fever during an epidemic of poliomyelitis. He later recalled no paralysis during that episode and later, in high school he played varsity football. In 1993, he had idiopathic thrombotic thrombocytopenic purpura. In 1994, at age 57, he had cramps and visible fasciculation in the gastrocnemius muscles. Examined in 2003, he still had symptoms but neurological examination was normal except for the fasciculation and EMG showed no abnormality except for the fasciculation.

These cases suggest that viral infections can cause persistent motor neuron syndromes in humans, but do not provide evidence that any particular virus causes ALS. Currently, attention is directed to two major considerations of specific transmissible agents as possible causes of motor neuron disorders: Lyme disease (51) and HIV infection.

HIV Infection

The major neurological complication of HTLV-1 infection is myelopathy with back pain and urinary symptoms, but some patients show features of ALS (52). In HIV, however, there have been only five autopsies of HIV-positive patients who had both upper and lower motor neuron signs in life. None of them had a typical clinical course or typical findings of ALS. One patient with HIV had signs consistent with ALS as well as an IgM kappa gammopathy and anti-GM1 antibodies; autopsy confirmed the diagnosis of ALS (53,54).

In 2000, however, HIV-positive patients with upper and lower motor neuron signs were reported to have responded to treatment with either nucleoside anti-HIV agents or protease inhibitors (55–58). These syndromes differed from ALS in several features: rapidity of progression, CSF pleocytosis, and, in two patients, MRI changes in the spinal cord. The patients recovered so there were no autopsies. Later, a drug–responsive case was linked to the HIV-1 clade C (59). In three similar cases, however, antiretroviral therapy failed (60–62).

Therefore, there seem to be two kinds of motor neuron disorders in HIV-positive people, one suggesting a subacute viral myelitis that may respond to antiviral therapy, and the other, ALS of the usual lethal variety. Neurologists who direct the patients to the HIV Centers think that ALS is too rare at the age of their patients to carry out formal tests that would determine whether being HIV-positive is a risk factor for ALS. An example of concomitant but independent ALS and HIV follows:

> In 1999, at age 53, this woman was found to be HIV-positive, infected by her husband. She was immediately given highly active anti-retroviral therapy (HAART). The viral load decreased and she remained asymptomatic until March 2001, when she noted dysarthria, gait disorder, and weak hands. In June 2002, findings included fasciculation of the tongue, dysarthria, weak and wasted hands, hyperreflexia, and Hoffmann signs but no Babinski sign. Her neurological disability became progressively worse as viral load disappeared, demonstrating that ALS and HIV infection were independent coincidences.

Transgenic mice carrying the HIV-1 genome develop either a vacuolar myelopathy (63) or an axonal neuropathy (64), but not with the histopathological stigmata of motor neuron disease. Reverse transcriptase enzyme activity has been found in the blood of 59% of 59 ALS patients, compared to 5% of 58 controls (65). The investigators later found similar enzyme activity in relative, suggesting inheritance of the transcriptase (65a). There was no reverse transcriptase activity, however, for HIV-1, HIV-2, or HTLV-1 or 2. Instead, the evidence pointed to some unknown retrovirus. There is little or no information about the molecular basis of motor neuron disease in either HTLV-1 disease or HIV.

Lyme Disease (Neuroborreliosis)

In regions where Lyme disease is endemic, there is a persistent hope among patients that this curable disease will be held responsible for the manifestations of ALS, but a review of the literature yields only three possible cases (66–68). The following patient, reported by Hemmer et al. (66), provides the most convincing evidence that the organism can cause a progressive disease of motor neurons.

> A 33-year-old man noted weakness of both hands and his gait became abnormal, with no paresthesias or bladder symptoms. With the finding of high serum titers of Lyme antibodies, the patient was treated with doxycycline and then cefotaxime but the neurological symptoms persisted. Fifteen months after symptom-onset and six months after antibiotic treatment, examination showed weak, wasted hands and a mild spastic paraparesis. Muscle stretch reflexes were not mentioned. EMG showed active denervation in hand muscles, anterior tibials, and masseters.

Central conduction was prolonged but peripheral nerve conduction studies showed no neuropathy and evoked potential studies gave normal results. Borrelia antibody titers were slightly elevated in serum and "clearly raised" in the CSF. The CSF cell count was 5—after antibiotic therapy had started—and CSF synthesis rates were high for IgG. He was treated with ceftriaxone intravenously for two weeks and oral prednisone for 10 weeks, improving continuously. Eighteen months after the treatment the patient had returned to work without "physical impairment."

Comment: The neurological disorder in this patient was described incompletely. Nevertheless, there was a clear description of amyotrophy that progressed for more than one year and was reversed after antibiotic therapy and a decline of antibody titers for Borrelia. The above case and the other two patients, although often-cited as examples of ALS caused by Borrelia, did not meet the criteria set by the American Academy of Neurology for the diagnosis of neuroborreliosis (69), which requires at least one of the following: typical rash, unequivocal evidence of exposures, and proof of the causative organism by culture, histology, or polymerase chain reaction. Either the condition was not ALS (because of CSF pleocytosis) or it was not borreliosis. Two cases lacked history of tick bite, typical rash, and data on antibodies. In one of the cases, the CNS disease progressed after the antibodies disappeared with treatment, so demonstrating the presence of Lyme antibodies in a person with ALS does not mean that the neurological disorder has been caused by infection. Many asymptomatic people test positive for Lyme antibodies. Many patients with ALS have had long-term antibiotic therapy for Lyme disease without any effect on the neurological disorder.

Reversible Motor Neuron Disease

Tucker et al. (70) described 10 patients who had syndromes of ALS and recovered completely without special treatment. Tsai et al. (71) added another. These 11 patients all had weakness, wasting, fasciculation, and hyperreflexia. The time from symptom-onset to maximal loss varied from 6 weeks to 14 months, and the time to recovery was from 5 months to 24 months. None had bulbar symptoms. Only one of the eight so far studied had high CSF protein content and none had CSF pleocytosis. The cause of this variant of motor neuron disease is totally unknown, but the time course raises the possibility of a viral infection.

AUTOIMMUNITY IN ALS

Like the viral theory of ALS, the role of autoimmunity has never been proven, but casts a shadow over clinical observations that include paraneoplastic syndromes, monoclonal gammopathy, lymphoproliferative disease, Kikuchi disease, and a spontaneous disease of wild mice.

In 1989, Pestronk et al. (72) reported that 78% of patients with ALS had antibodies to the GM1 ganglioside. Largely on the basis of that observation, Drachman and Kuncl (73) postulated that ALS might be an "unconventional" autoimmune disease, unconventional because the target tissue showed no lymphocytic infiltration and that the antiganglioside had not been proven to be involved in pathogenesis. They postulated that the antibodies might be carried by retrograde transport to the cell body of the motor neuron. Since previously administered immunotherapy had failed in ALS, they treated patients with the most powerful immune therapy, total lymphoid irradiation—and failed again (74).

In that paper (74), they listed Drachman's criteria needed to identify a disease as autoimmune: (i) antibody is present in patients with the disease, (ii) antibody interacts with the target antigen, (iii) passive transfer of the antibody reproduces features of the disease, (iv) immunization with the antigen produces a model disease, and (v) reduction of the antibody titer ameliorates the disease.

By that time, their studies show that the prevalence of GM1 antibodies dropped from 78% to less than 15% (75), a figure closer to those of others (76,77).

In the meantime, Stanley Appel and his associates had dramatically met criterion No. 4 by inducing an autoimmune motor neuron disease by sensitizing recipient guinea pigs with injections of bovine gray matter (78). Later, they summarized their evidence (79). They rejected the argument that failure of immunotherapy excluded autoimmunity by citing the failure of such treatment to affect type-1 diabetes mellitus, which is believed to be autoimmune. They had found a high prevalence of thyroid disease and thyroid antibodies in patients with ALS; many patients with one autoimmune disease have others of that class and may have several different types of autoantibodies. They found deposits of immunoglobulins in ALS motor neurons. They found anti-GM1 antibodies in 14% of ALS patients and 15% of normal controls. Instead, they found calcium channel antibodies of skeletal muscle L type. In passive transfer experiments, these antibodies killed cultured motor neurons and increased miniature end plate potential frequency at the neuromuscular junction.

These observations were presented at an international meeting and were answered by Drachman along with Angel Vincent and others (80). Inhibition of the calcium L-channels should inhibit neuromuscular transmission and there was no evidence of antibodies to the N-type or P-type, which they considered more relevant. The transfer experiments showed an effect on nerve terminals but no loss of motor neurons.

Five years later, Appel was emphasizing inflammation in ALS and was still interested in autoimmunity, including observations of a decremental response to repetitive stimulation of patients with sporadic ALS (81).

In the past five years, there have been no major attempts to develop immunotherapy for an autoimmune sporadic ALS. However, a novel concept, stimulation of innate protective autoimmunity, has led to the use of glatiramer acetate (82). Nevertheless, other aspects of autoimmunity continue to engage interest—for some, if not all patients.

Paraneoplastic ALS

The term "paraneoplastic neurological disorder" implies that a neurological syndrome is causally related to the associated tumor in the absence of metastases to the central or peripheral nervous system and the neurological disorder is not a complication of radiotherapy or chemotherapy. Autoimmunity has come to be the favored theory of paraneoplastic neurological diseases.

The concept of paraneoplastic pathology is attributed to Denny-Brown (83), who described sensory neuropathy in a patient with lung cancer. The same patient was also reported by Wyburn-Mason (84). They did not mention autoimmunity, a concept yet to emerge. The main proponent of that theory was Lord Brain, who published several papers on the subject in the 1950s; by 1965, British investigators had described paraneoplastic sensory neuropathy, sensorimotor neuropathy, cerebellar degeneration, and progressive multifocal leucoencephalopathy. Brain also believed that there was an excessive number of cancers among patients with motor neuron disease (85); early adherents included G. Milton Shy, W. King Engel, and

Forbes H. Norris. In 1964, Brain and Norris (86) organized a meeting on paraneoplastic syndromes. There, Norris and Engel (87) reported that 11 of 140 ALS
patients had malignant neoplasms of diverse nature; the frequency of almost 8%
was deemed excessive. Two of the 11 had lymphomas.

However, Raymond Adams (88) commented that this was not his personal
experience, and I (89) noted that there had been only one carcinoma among 80
autopsy-proven cases of ALS in the series of the renowned neuropathologist, Harry
Zimmerman, at Montefiore Hospital in New York. The concept of paraneoplastic
motor neuron disease virtually dropped from view for the next two decades.

Later, Zisfein and Caroscio (90) found an annual incidence of 0.57% of cancers
among 347 patients with ALS, almost the same as the rate found in the general
population, and Kondo (91) found no increase of cancer among patients with
ALS in an autopsy series in Japan. In 1989, Rosenfield and Posner (92) also found
no evidence of increased frequency of cancer among patients with MND, merely the
occasional concurrence of two diseases affecting people in the same age group.
Similarly, there was association with malignancy other than melanoma in a survey
of 1.9 million cancer survivors (29a). The excessive numbers at NIH and London
Hospital could have been due to ascertainment bias, the investigators attracting
patients with disorders of special interest at the particular medical center.

There has not yet been a formal case–control series and only one population
study has been reported to reduce ascertainment bias. Gubbay et al. (93) found that
10% of all the patients with MND in Israel had a malignancy, a frequency at least
four times more than expected. However, Chiò et al. (94), similarly, ascertained all
cases in a region in Italy and found no excess incidence of cancer in patients with
MND. Vigliani et al. (95) noted no paraneoplastic antibodies in 14 patients with
ALS and cancers and they found no improvement with treatment of the tumor; it
was the ALS that was lethal in these patients, not the tumor.

Nevertheless, the subject has not disappeared because of anecdotal reports of
neurological benefit when a tumor was excised (96–102). Also, an association of
motor neuron disease with lymphoma became evident in 1963 (103) and has become
increasingly recognized (104) as described below. Other observations suggest a
possible link to motor neuron disorders, such as neuromyotonia (105), or a spinal
cord syndrome that includes fasciculation and myoclonus (106). Neuromyotonia
has been seen in patients with thymoma or lung cancer, with myasthenia gravis
(107,108) or with Morvan syndrome, a combination of neuromyotonia with antibodies
to potassium channels in patients with thymoma or lung cancer and manifest by severe
insomnia, hallucinations, and weight loss (109,110).

Most reports concerned syndromes of either mixed upper and lower motor neuron disorders (ALS) or those confined to lower motor neurons [progressive muscular
atrophy (PMA)]. However, Forsyth et al. (111) described three patients with elements
of ALS among other multiple CNS findings, as previously reported for paraneoplastic
encephalomyelitis; all three had anti-Hu antibodies. The anti-Hu antibodies placed
this syndrome at the top of a small list of well-supported autoimmune motor neuron
diseases. The same antibodies have also been found in paraneoplastic sensory neuropathy and mixed CNS syndromes but in only one patient with an uncomplicated
motor neuron disease that included both lower and upper motor neuron signs
(112). Patients with ALS and no tumor do not show anti-Hu antibodies (113). Anti-
Hu antibodies were found in one patient with ALS and carcinoma of the ovary (114).

In addition to the anti-Hu cases, Forsyth et al. (111) also described five women
with carcinoma of the breast and the upper motor neuron syndrome of primary

lateral sclerosis (PLS). However, other women had breast cancer and typical ALS. One of them had an IgA monoclonal gammopathy with antineuronal antibodies that reacted with neurofilaments (115) or other neuronal antigens (116), but several such patients lacked those antibodies when tested in the laboratory of Norman Latov.

Among other reported patients with presumed PLS, two possible cases at autopsy were associated with malignant neoplasms, one myeloma (117) and the other lung cancer (118). PLS may turn into ALS after months or years and three of the five cases of Forsyth et al. (111) ultimately developed lower motor neuron signs, implying that they actually had ALS, but other patient had signs of PLS for six years before breast cancer was discovered (119). It has not been proven that this association with breast cancer occurs more often than by chance; a case–control or population study would be necessary. Nevertheless, the findings of Forsyth et al. (111) make it necessary to evaluate the possibility of breast cancer in any woman with what seems to be PLS. There have been other cases of breast cancer with typical ALS (120) and some had paraneoplastic antibodies (121,122).

Renal cancer is another malignancy with a special relationship to ALS because there is hope that removal of the tumor will reverse the motor neuron disease. Buchanan and Malamud (96) described a man who had only lower motor neuron signs at first, later developed Babinski signs, improved after removal of a clear cell carcinoma, was neurologically "nearly normal" for four years, and then died of metastases. Autopsy showed loss of motor neurons and gliosis without change in the corticospinal tracts or peripheral nerves. Evans et al. (97) described a similar case. We were therefore hopeful when we encountered a man with ALS, IgM monoclonal paraproteinemia, and renal cancer. Removal of the tumor, however, did not reverse progression of the neurological disease and he died of metastatic disease (123). Unraveling the relationship between motor neuron diseases and malignant tumors should be a fruitful field for molecular or epidemiologic research.

ALS and Lymphoma

My interest in lymphoproliferative disease and motor neuron diseases began more than 40 years ago, when Houston Merritt asked me to write a review of paraneoplastic syndromes. By good fortune, Stuart Schneck was then a neuropathology fellow with Abner Wolf in the Columbia Division of Neuropathology. Together, we set out to find examples of the several syndromes. We found two young women with motor neuron disease and lymphoma (124). Walton et al. (125) described a clinically similar case, but his showed CNS inflammation that was not seen in our cases. The literature lay dormant thereafter except for occasional case reports.

Our interest was revived in 1981 when we encountered a 42-year-old man who had widespread weakness and wasting with visible fasciculation, no upper motor neuron signs, slow motor nerve conduction velocities, high CSF protein content, and IgM monoclonal gammopathy. He died within two years. No lymphoma was found at autopsy. There was postmortem evidence of peripheral neuropathy and chromatolysis of motor neurons was deemed a retrograde change. The case was reported as "peripheral neuropathy simulating motor neuron disease" (126). Since then, however, chromatolysis has been seen in patients with clinically and pathologically typical ALS. The above case remains as an example of the problem of separating a motor neuron disease from a motor neuropathy; some patients may have both disorders.

In contrast to the uncertainty about the association of motor neuron diseases with cancers, there has been interest in the link of ALS to lymphoproliferative diseases, including Waldenström macroglobulinemia, chronic lymphocytic leukemia, Hodgkin disease, and other lymphomas (127–129). There has been no case–control study to prove that the association is more than a chance relationship, but there are now at least 65 reported cases (128,130). In one series of patients with Hodgkin disease, the prevalence of MND was 1%, which was 1000 times more than in population figures (132).

Although it was once thought that the neurological disorder is primarily the one affecting the lower motor neuron (a neuronopathy), more than half of reported cases have upper motor neuron signs in life and the corticospinal tracts have been affected in more than half of the autopsy cases. Either the lymphomatous disease or the motor neuron disease can appear first or the two may occur together. When the lymphoma occurs first, the interval may be as long as 25 years before the neurological disorder starts, which makes it unlikely that the lymphoma is producing an antineuronal antibody to cause the motor neuron disease. The neurological disorder is usually responsible for disability or death, but the outcome in not easily predicted. In the series of Oppenshaw and Slatkin (131), 4 of 393 patients with Hodgkin disease had a lower motor neuron syndrome. One patient died within three years and another saw all neurological symptoms disappear in one year. Gordon et al. (127) noted that 23 patients had been treated with immunosuppressive drugs, but only three of them responded. Individual case experience still has an impact, as illustrated by the following:

> At age 36 in 1996, this woman first had symptoms of a purely lower motor neuron disorder. Normal results were found in nerve conduction studies, immunofixation electrophoresis (no monoclonal protein), tests for anti-GM1, anti-myelin associated glycoprotein, paraneoplastic antibodies, HIV, CSF examination, or search for occult neoplasm (including positron emission tomography). Treatment with plasmapheresis, intravenous immunoglobulins, or cyclophosphamide gave no benefit. In 1998, a tonsillar mass appeared and was biopsied. Instead of the suspected lymphoma the mass proved to be histiocytic necrotizing lymphadenitis or Kikuchi disease (132). This is a benign condition that must be differentiated from lymphoma histologically because it is self-limited and complete spontaneous recovery is the rule, as it was in this case. However, respiratory failure supervened and she died without autopsy in 2004.

Monoclonal Gammopathy (Plasma Cell Dyscrasia) and ALS/MND

Although cases had been recorded earlier, experience with one patient set us off on a decade of observations about monoclonal proteins in patients with ALS/MND. The patient, described above, was a 48-year-old man with a lower motor neuron syndrome and IgM gammopathy. Michael Shy and associates then found that 5% of ALS patients and 1% of controls had a monoclonal protein (133). Immunofixation gave higher figures and, in subsequent analyses, 5% to 10% of patients showed a monoclonal paraprotein, usually an IgM globulin (in contrast to the IgG monoclonal proteins found in asymptomatic elderly people). Studies in Belgrade also gave a figure of 10% (134). In Scotland, however, Willison found no difference between ALS patients and controls (135), which could result from studying different populations. However, the M-protein does not always have antibody activity and, if it does, the reactive antigens have included GM1, GD1b, chondroitin sulfate, and neurofilament protein. At one time, some investigators thought there were anti-GM1 antibodies in most patients with ALS, but that soon faded to a number less than 15%. Currently, it seems that this antibody is often found in patients with multifocal motor neuropathy, but only rarely in patients with upper motor neuron signs. No animal model with motor neuron disease and gammopathy has been produced. Injections of an M-protein with anti-GM1 activity led to conduction block and demyelination. Immunosuppressive treatment of ALS patients with monoclonal gammopathy, with or without antibody activity, has not ameliorated the ALS/MND. Although patients with monoclonal paraproteinemia have been excluded from many therapeutic trials for ALS, the clinical pattern is no different from "ordinary" ALS.

> Another instructive case was recorded by Simpson et al. An HIV-positive 45-year-old man developed weakness, atrophy, fasciculation, and hyperreflexia. Electromyography showed a pure motor axonal neuropathy. Immunoelectrophoresis identified an IgM kappa gammopathy and the titer of antibodies to asialo-GM1 was 1:3200 (normal <1:800). In the days before protease inhibitors, he did not respond to zidovudine, intravenous immunoglobulins, or prednisone. He died four years after onset of neurological symptoms. Autopsy showed degeneration of lower motor neurons and corticospinal tracts.

Comment: This case binds several themes together, including persistent viral infection and monoclonal gammopathy with antiganglioside activity in a patient with autopsy-proven ALS. How could it come about? It might be possible to think of a scenario in which the motor neuron disease somehow causes lymphoproliferation, which in turn leads to monoclonal gammopathy with an antibody attack on motor neurons, or the virus might cause lymphoproliferation directly and the antineuronal monoclonal could attack the cells.

A spontaneous disease of mice might provide the clue. The virus causes lymphoma, monoclonal gammopathy, and motor neuron disease. That theory is attractive but the murine disease has been known for more than 30 years (136,137) and the molecular biology of the virus has been known for 15 years (138). Still, there has been no demonstration of any mechanism like this in humans.

CONCLUSIONS

Anecdotal evidence keeps the viral theory of ALS causation alive, and prions may cause a transmissible motor neuron disease. Autoimmunity has been difficult to prove as a general cause of sporadic ALS and epidemiologic studies have not shown an excessive frequency of motor neuron disease in patients with cancers. However, there have been 10 reports of motor neuron syndromes that disappeared when a tumor was excised and in some patients antineuronal antibodies have been identified. Moreover, there are at least 65 known cases of motor neuron diseases (including upper motor neuron signs) in patients with lymphoproliferative diseases, suggesting that there may be a paraneoplastic form of MND, and there seems to be an excess of monoclonal gammopathy in patients with ALS. Reports of increased incidence of lymphomas, breast cancer, and carcinoma of the lung with MND require documentation by case-control studies. These clues lead to a continuing search for the causes of sporadic ALS.

ACKNOWLEDGMENTS

The author is indebted to Hiroshi Mitsumoto, Director of the Eleanor and Lou Gehrig MDA/ALS Research Center, for his support and to associates engaged in

ALS research and patient care: Steven Albert, Steven Chan, Maura Del Bene, Clifton Gooch, Paul Gordon, Sheila Hayes, Arthur P. Hays, Petra Kaufmann, Alexander Khandji, Dale J. Lange, Norman Latov, Dora Leung, Elan D. Louis, Robert E. Lovelace, Dominique Majoor-Krakauer, D Peregrine Murphy, Elliott F. Osserman, Ruth Ottman, Judith Rabkin, Saud Sadiq, Keith Sanders, William B. Sherman, Neil Shneider, Dikoma Shungu, Michael Shy, Werner Trojaborg, Bradford Worrall, and David S. Younger.

REFERENCES

1. Bruijn LI, Miller TM, Cleveland DW. Unraveling the mechanisms involved in motor neuron degeneration in ALS. Annu Rev Neurosci 2004; 27:723–749.
2. Orrell RW, Habgood J, Rudge P, Lane RJ, de Belleroche JS. Difficulties in distinguishing sporadic from familial amyotrophic lateral sclerosis. Ann Neurol 1996; 119:1153–1172.
3. Gellera C. Genetics of ALS in Italian families. ALS and other motor neuron disorders 2001; 2(suppl 1):S43–S46.
4. Andersen PM. Genetics of sporadic ALS. ALS Other Motor Neuron Disord 2001; 2(suppl 1):S37–S41.
5. Rexania K, Yan J, Delliefave L, Deng H-X, Siddique N, Pascussi RT, Siddique T, Roos RP. A rare Cu/Zn superoxide dismutase mutation causing familial amyotrophic lateral sclerosis with variable age at onset, incomplete penetrance, and a sensory neuropathy. ALS and other motor neuron disorders 2003; 2(suppl):S43–S46.
6. Alexander MD, Traynor BJ, Miller N, Corr B, Frost E, McQuaid S, Brett FM, Green A, Hardiman O. "True" sporadic ALS associated with a novel SOD-1 mutation. Ann Neurol 2002; 52(5):680–683.
7. Gros-Louis F, Lariviere R, Gowing G, Laurent S, Camu W, Bouchard JP, Meininger V, Rouleau GA, Julien JP. A frameshift deletion in peripherin gene associated with amyotrophic lateral sclerosis. J Biol Chem 2004; 279(44):45951–45956. Epub 2004 Aug 17.
8. Munch C, Sedlmeier R, Meyer T, Homberg V, Sperfeld AD, Kurt A, Prudlo J, Peraus G, Hanemann CO, Stumm G, et al. Point mutations of the p150 subunit of dynactin (DCTN1) gene in ALS. Neurology 2004; 63(4):724–726.
9. Kunst CB. Complex genetics of amyotrophic lateral sclerosis. Am J Hum Genet 2004; 75:933–942.
10. Moulard B, Salachas F, Chassande B, Briolotti V, Meininger V, Malafosse A, Camu W. Association between centromeric deletions of the SMN gene and sporadic adult-onset lower motor neuron disease. Ann Neurol 1998; 43(5):640–644.
11. Parboosingh JS, Figlewicz DA, Krizus A, Meininger V, Azad NA, Newman DS, Rouleau GA. Spinobulbar muscular atrophy can mimic ALS: the importance of genetic testing in male patients with atypical ALS. Neurology 1997; 49(2):568–572.
12. Corcia P, Mayeux-Portas V, Khoris J, de Toffol B, Autret A, Muh JP, Camu W, Andres C. French ALS Research Group. Ann Neurol 2002; 51:243–246.
13. Prudlo J, Alber B, Kalscheuer VM, Roemer K, Martin T, Dullinger J, Sittinger H, Niemann S, Heutink P, Ludolph AC, et al. Chromosomal translocation t(18;21) (q23;q22.1) indicates novel susceptibility loci for frontotemporal dementia with ALS. Ann Neurol 2004; 55(1):134–138.
14. Lambrechts D, Storkebaum E, Morimoto M, Del-Favero J, Desmet F, Marklund SL, Wyns S, Thijs V, Andersson J, van Marion I, Al-Chalabi A, Bornes S, Musson R, Hansen V, Beckman L, Adolfsson R, Pall HS, Prats H, Vermeire S, Rutgeerts P, Katayama S, Awata T, Leigh N, Lang-Lazdunski L, Dewerchin M, Shaw C, Moons L, Vlietinck R, Morrison KE, Robberecht W, Van Broeckhoven C, Collen D, Andersen PM, Carmeliet P. VEGF is a modifier of amyotrophic lateral sclerosis in mice

and humans and protects motoneurons against ischemic death. Nat Genet 2003; 34(4):383–394.

15. Storkebaum E, Lambrechts D, Carmeliet P. VEGF: once regarded as a specific angiogenic factor, now implicated in neuroprotection. Bioessays 2004; 26(9):943–954.

16. Majoor-Krakauer D, Willens PJ, Hofman A. Genetic epidemiology of amyotrophic lateral sclerosis. Clin Genet 2003; 63:83–101.

17. Veldink JH, Van Den Berg LH, Wokke JH. The future of motor neuron disease. The challenge is in the genes. J Neurol 2004; 251(4):491–500.

18. Veldink JH, van den Berg LH, Cobben JM, Stulp RP, De Jong JM, Vogels OJ, Baas F, Wokke JH, Scheffer H. Homozygous deletion of the survival motor neuron 2 gene is a prognostic factor in sporadic ALS. Neurology 2001; 56(6):749–752.

19. Wang X-S, Lee S, Simmons Z, Boyer P, Scott K, Liu W, Connor J. Increased incidence of the Hfe mutation in amyotrophic lateral sclerosis and related cellular consequences. J Neurol Sci 2004; 227:27–33.

20. Scarmeas N, Shih T, Stern, Y, Ottman R, Rowland LP. Premorbid weight, body mass, and athletics in ALS and related syndromes. Neurology 2002; 59:773–775.

21. Critchley M. Discussion on motor neurone disease. Proc R Soc Med 1962; 55:1066.

22. Felmus MT, Patten BM, Swanke L. Antecedent events in amyotrophic lateral sclerosis. Neurology 1976; 26:167–172.

23. Beretta S, Carri MT, Beghi E, Chio A, Ferrarese C. The sinister side of Italian soccer. Lancet Neurol 2003; 2(11):656–657.

24. Longstreth WT, Nelson LM, Koepsell TD, Van Belle G. Hypotheses to explain the association between vigorous physical activity and amyotrophic lateral sclerosis. Med Hypoth 1991; 34:144–148.

25. Wilbourn AJ, Mitsumoto H. Why are patients with amyotrophic lateral sclerosis so nice? Proceedings of the 9th International Symposium ALS/MND, Munich, 1998.

26. Majoor-Krakauer D, Ottman R, Johnson WG, Rowland LP. Familial aggregation of amyotrophic lateral sclerosis, dementia, and Parkinson's disease: evidence of shared genetic susceptibility. Neurology 1994; 44:1872–1877.

27. Gibbs CJ Jr, Gajdusek DC. Attempts to demonstrate a transmissible agent in kuru, amyotrophic lateral sclerosis, and other subacute, and chronic progressive nervous system degenerations of man. In: Gajdusek DC, Gills CJ Jr, Alpers M, eds. Slow, Latent, and Temperate Virus Infection, Government Printing Office, 1965:39–49.

28. Gajdusek DC, Gibbs CJ Jr, Alpers M. Experimental transmission of a kuru-like syndrome to chimpanzees. Nature 1966; 209:794–796.

29. Rowland LP. NINDS at 50. New York: Demos Press, 2003:183–192.

30. Prusiner S. Novel proteinaceous infectious particles cause scrapie. Science 1982; 216: 136–144.

31. Allen IV, Dermott E, Connolly JH, Hurwitz LJ. A study of a patient with the amyotrophic form of Creutzfeldt-Jakob disease. Brain 1971; 94(4):715–724.

32. Salazar AM, Masters CL, Gajdusek DC, Gibbs CJ Jr. Syndromes of amyotrophic lateral sclerosis and dementia; relation to transmissible Creutzfeldt-Jakob disease. Ann Neurol 1983; 14:17–26.

33. Connolly JH, Allen IV, Dermott E. Transmissible agent in the amyotrophic form of Creutzfeldt-Jakob disease. J Neurol Neurosurg Psychiatry 1988; 51:1459–1460.

34. Rowland LP. Diagnosis of ALS. J Neurol Sci 1998; 160:S6–S24.

35. Worrall BB, Rowland LP, Del Bene M, Leung D, Chin SS. Mother with amyotrophic lateral sclerosis and daughter with Creutzfeldt-Jakob disease: coincidence or genetic risk factor for both diseases?. Arch Neurol 1999; 56:1502–1504.

36. Worrall BB, Rowland LP, Chin SS-M, Mastrianni JA. Amyotrophy in prion disease. Arch Neurol 2000; 57:33–39.

37. Nowacki P, Kulczycki J, Narolewska A, Grzelec H. Amyotrophic form of Creutzfeldt-Jakob disease with rapid course in 82-year-old man. Folia Neuropathologica 2000; 38(4):161–163.

38. Niewiadomska M, Kulczycki J, Wochnik-Dyjas D, Szpak GM, Rakowicz M, Lojkowska W, Niedzielska K, Inglot E, Wieclawska M, Glazowski C, Tarnowska-Dziduszko E. Impairment of the peripheral nervous system in Creutzfeldt-Jakob disease. Arch Neurol 2002; 59(9):1430–1436.

39. Kovacs T, Aranyi Z, Szirmai I, Lantos PL. Creutzfeldt-Jakob disease with amyotrophy and demyelinating polyneuropathy. Arch Neurol 2002; 59(11):1811–1814.

40. Favereaux A, Quadrio I, Perret-Liaudet A, Vital C, Ouallet JC, Brochet B, Biacabe AG, Petry KG, Kopp N, Vital A. Prion protein accumulation involving the peripheral nervous system in a sporadic case of Creutzfeldt-Jakob disease. Neuropathol Appl Neurobiol 2003; 29(6):602–605.

41. Esteban JC, Atares B, Zarranz JJ, Velasco F, Lambarri I. Dementia, amyotrophy, and periodic complexes on the electroencephalogram: a diagnostic challenge. Arch Neurol 2001; 58(10):1669–1672.

42. Jubelt B. Motor neuron diseases and viruses: poliovirus, retroviruses, and lymphomas. Curr Op Neurol Neurosurg 1992; 5(5):655–658.

43. Viola MV, Myers JC, Gann KL, Gibbs JC Jr, Roos RP. Failure to detect poliovirus genetic information in amyotrophic lateral sclerosis. Ann Neurol 1979; 5(4):402–403.

44. Swanson NR, Fox SA, Mastaglia FL. Search for persistent infection with poliovirus or other enteroviruses in amyotrophic lateral sclerosis-motor neurone disease. Neuromusc Disord 1995; 5(6):457–465.

45. Walker MP, Schlaberg R, Hays AP, Bowser R, Lipkin WI. Absence of echovirus sequences in brain and spinal cord of amyotrophic lateral sclerosis patients. Ann Neurol 2001; 49(2):249–253.

46. Berger MM, Kopp N, Vital C, Redl B, Aymard M, Lina B. Detection and cellular localization of enterovirus RNA sequences in spinal cord of patients with ALS. Neurology 2000; 54(1):20–25.

47. Nix WA, Berger MM, Oberste MS, Brooks BR, McKenna-Yasek DM, Brown RH Jr, Roos RP, Pallansch MA. Failure to detect enterovirus in the spinal cord of ALS patients using a sensitive RT-PCR method. Neurology 2004; 62(8):1372–1377.

48. Li J, Loeb JA, Shy ME, Shah AK, Tselis AC, Kupski WJ, Lewis RA. Asymmetric flaccid paralysis: a neuromuscular presentation of West Nile virus infection. Ann Neurol 2003; 53(6):703–710.

49. Tyler KL. West Nile virus infection in the United Stated. Arch Neurol 2004; 61:1190–1195.

50. Fetell MR, Smallberg G, Lewis LD, Lovelace RE, Hays AP, Rowland LP. A benign motor neuron disorder: delayed cramps and fasciculation after poliomyelitis or myelitis. Ann Neurol 1982; 11(4):423–427.

51. Halperin JJ, Kaplan GP, Brazinsky S, Tsai TF, Cheng T, Ironside A, Wu P, Delfiner J, Golightly M, Brown RH, et al. Immunologic reactivity against Borrelia burgdorferi in patients with motor neuron disease. Arch Neurol 1990; 47(5):586–594.

52. Matsuzaki T, Nakagawa M, Nagai M, Nobuhara Y, Usuku K, Higuchi I, Takahashi K, Moritoyo T, Arimura K, Izumo S, Akiba S, Osame M. HTLV-I-associated myelopathy (IHAM)/tropical spastic paraparesis (TSP) with amyotrophic lateral sclerosis-like manifestations. J Neurovirol 2000; 6:544–548.

53. Simpson DM, Morgello S, Citak K, Corbo M, Latov N. Motor neuron disease associated with HIV and anti-sialo GM1 antibody. Muscle Nerve 1994: 17:1091 (abstract).

54. Simpson DM, Tagiati M. Neuromuscular syndromes in HIV disease. In: Berger J, Levy RM, eds. AIDS and the Nervous System. 2nd ed. Philadelphia: Lippincott-Raven, 1997:189–221.

55. MacGowan DJ, Scelsa SN, Waldron M. An ALS-like syndrome with new HIV infection and complete response to antiretroviral therapy. Neurology 2001; 57(6):1094–1097.

56. Moulignier A, Moulonguet A, Pialoux G, Rozenbaum W. Reversible ALS-like disorder in HIV infection. Neurology 2001; 57:995–1001.

57. Nishio M, Koizumi K, Moriwaka F, Koike T, Sawada K. Reversal of HIV-associated motor neuron syndrome after highly active antiretroviral therapy. J Neurol 2000; 248:233–234.

58. Calza L, Manfredi R, Freo E, Farneti B, Tampellini L, d'Orsi G, Chiodo F. Transient reversal of HIV-associated motor neuron disease following the introduction of highly active antiretroviral therapy. J Chemother 2004; 16(1):98–101.

59. Sinha S, Mathews T, Arunodaya GR, Siddappa NB, Ranga U, Desai A, Ravi V, Taly AB. HIV-1 clade-C-associated "ALS"-like disorder: first report in India. J Neurol Sci 2004; 224:97–100.

60. Zoccolella S, Carbonara S, Minerva D, Palagano G, Bruno F, Ferrannini E, Iliceto G, Serlenga L, Lamberti P. A case of concomitant amyotrophic lateral sclerosis and HIV infection. Eur J Neurol 2002; 9(2):180–182.

61. Sastre-Garriga J, Tintoré M, Raguer N, Ruíz I, Montalban X, Codina A. Lower motor neuron disease in an HIV-2 infected woman. J Neurol 2000; 247:718–719.

62. Galassi G, Gentilini M, Ferrari S, Ficarra G, Zonari P, Mongiardo N, Tommelleri G, Di Rienzo B. Motor neuron disease and HIV-1 infection in a 30-year-old HIV-positive heroin abuser: a causal relationship?. Clin Neuropathol 1998; 17(3):131–135.

63. Goudreau G, Carpenter S, Beaulieu N, Jolicoeur P. Vacuolar myelopathy in transgenic mice expressing human immunodeficiency virus type 1 proteins under the regulation of the myelin basic protein gene promoter. Nat Med 1996; 2(6):655–661.

64. Thomas FP, Chalk C, Lalonde R, Robitaille Y, Jolicoeur P. Expression of human immunodeficiency virus type 1 in the nervous system of transgenic mice leads to neurological disease. J Virol 1994; 68(11):7099–7107.

65. Andrews WD, Tuke PW, Al-Chalabi A, Gaudin P, Ijaz S, Parton MJ, Garson JA. Detection of reverse transcriptase activity in the serum of patients with motor neuron disease. J Med Virol 2000; 61(4):527–532.

65a. Steele AJ, Al-Chalabi A, Ferrante K, Cudkowicz ME, Brown RH Jr, Garson JA. Detection of serum reverse transcriptase activity in patients with ALS and unaffected blood relatives. Neurology 2005; 64(3):454–458.

66. Hemmer B, Glocker FX, Kaiser R, Lucking CH, Deuschl G. Generalised motor neuron disease as an unusual manifestation of Borrelia burgdorferi infection. J Neurol Neurosurg Psychiatry 1997; 63:257–258.

67. Deibener J, Kaminsky P, Debouverie M, Aubrun P, Maurer P, Gerard A, Duc M. Syndrome du motorneurone et maladie de Lyme. Lien de causalite ou association fortuite? Presse Med 1997: 26:1144 (letter).

68. Hansel Y, Ackerl M, Stanek G. ALS-ähnlicher Krankheitsverlauf bei chronischer Neuroborreliose. Wien Med Wchnschr 1995; 145:186–188.

69. Halperin JJ, Logigian EL, Finkel MF, Pearl RA. Practice parameters for the diagnosis of patients with nervous system Lyme borreliosis (Lyme disease). Quality standards subcommittee of the American Academy of Neurology. Neurology 1996; 46(3):619–627.

70. Tucker T, Layzer RB, Miller RG, Chad D. Subacute, reversible motor neuron disease. Neurology 1991; 41(10):1541–1544.

71. Tsai CP, Ho HH, Yen DJ, Wang V, Lin KP, Liao KK, Wu ZA. Reversible motor neuron disease. Eur Neurol 1993; 33(5):387–389.

72. Pestronk A, Adams RN, Cornblath D, Kuncl RW, Drachman DB, Clawson L. Patterns of serum IgM antibodies to GM1 and GD1a gangliosides in amyotrophic lateral sclerosis. Ann Neurol 1989; 25(1):98–102.

73. Drachman DB, Kuncl RW. Amyotrophic lateral sclerosis: an unconventional autoimmune disease? Ann Neurol 1989; 26:269–274.

74. Drachman DB, Chaudhry V, Cornblath D, et al. Trial of immunosuppression in amyotrophic lateral sclerosis using total lymphoid irradiation. Ann Neurol 1994; 35:142–150.

75. Pestronk A. Invited review: motor neuropathies, motor neuron disorders, and antiglycolipid antibodies. Muscle Nerve 1991; 14:927–936.

76. Sanders KA, Rowland LP, Murphy PL, et al. Motor neuron diseases and amyotrophic lateral sclerosis: GM1 antibodies and paraproteinemia. Neurology 1993; 43:418–420.

77. Nobile-Orazio E, Carpo M, Meucci N. Are there immunologically treatable motor neuron diseases? Amyotroph Lateral Scler Other Motor Neuron Disord 2001; 2(suppl 1): S23–S30.

78. Engelhardt JI, Appel SH, Killian JM. Experimental autoimmune motor neuron disease. Ann Neurol 1989; 26:368–376.

79. Appel SH, Smith RG, Alexianu MF, Engelhardt JI, Stefani JE. Autoimmunity as an etiological factor in sporadic amyotrophic lateral sclerosis. In: Serratrice F, Munsat T, eds. Pathogenesis and Therapy of Amyotrophic Lateral Sclerosis. Philadelphia: Lippincott-Raven Publishers; Adv Neurol 1995; 68:47–57.

80. Drachman DB, Fishman PS, Rothstein Jd, Motomura M, Lang B, Vincent A, Mellits ED. Amyotrophic lateral sclerosis. An autoimmune disease? In: Serratrice F, Munsat T, eds. Pathogenesis and Therapy of Amyotrophic Lateral Sclerosis. Philadelphia: Lippincott-Raven Publishers; Adv Neurol 1995; 68:59–65.

81. Smith RG, Appel SH. Immunosuppression and anti-inflammatory agents in ALS. ALS and other motor neuron disorders 2000; 1(suppl 4):33–43.

82. Angelov DN, Waibel S, Guntinas-Lichius O, Lenzen M, Neiss WF, Tomov TL, Yoles E, Kipnis J, Schori H, Reuter A, Ludolph A, Schwartz M. Therapeutic vaccine for acute and chronic motor neuron diseases: implications for amyotrophic lateral sclerosis. Proc Natl Acad Sci USA 2003; 100(8):4790–4795.

83. Denny-Brown DE. Primary sensory neuropathy with muscular changes associated with carcinoma. J Neurol Neurosurg Psychiatry 1948; 11:73–87.

84. Wyburn-Mason R. Bronchial carcinoma presenting as polyneuritis. Lancet 1948; 1: 203–206.

85. Brain WR, Croft PB, Wilkinson M. Motor neurone disease as a manifestation of neoplasm (with a note on the course of classical motor neurone disease). Brain 1965; 88: 479–500.

86. Lord Brain, Norris FH Jr, eds. The Remote Effects of Cancer on the Nervous System. New York: Grune and Stratton, 1965.

87. Norris FH Jr, Engel WK. Carcinomatous amyotrophic lateral sclerosis. In: Ref. 86, 24–34.

88. Adams RD. Discussion of Ref. 87, page 39.

89. Rowland LP. Discussion of Ref. 84, page 40.

90. Zisfein J, Caroscio JT. No association of amyotrophic lateral sclerosis with cancer. Mt Sinai J Med 1988; 55:159–161.

91. Kondo K. Motor neuron disease and Parkinson's disease are not associated with other disorders at autopsy. Neuroepidemiology 1984; 3:182–194.

92. Rosenfield D, Posner JB. Motor neuron disease and malignant tumors. In: Rowland LP, ed. Amyotrophic Lateral Sclerosis and other Motor Neuron Diseases. New York: Raven Press, 1991:445–462.

92a. Freedman DM, Travis LB, Gridley G, Kuncl RW. Amyotrophic lateral sclerosis mortality in 1.9 million U.S. cancer survivors. Neuroepidemiology 2005; 25(4):176–180. [Epub ahead of print.]

93. Gubbay SS, Kahana E, Zilber N, Cooper G, Pintov S, Leibowitz Y. Amyotrophic lateral sclerosis. A study of its presentation and prognosis. J Neurol 1985; 232:295–300.

94. Chiò A, Brignoplio F, Meineri P, Russo MG, Tribolo A, Schiffer D. Motor neuron disease and malignancies: results of a population study. J Neurol 1988; 235:374–375.

95. Vigliani MC, Polo P, Chio A, Giometto B, Mazzini L, Schiffer D. Patients with amyotrophic lateral sclerosis and cancer do not differ clinically from patients with sporadic amyotrophic lateral sclerosis. J Neurol 2000; 247(10):778–782.

96. Buchanan DS, Malamud N. Motor neurone disease with renal cell carcinoma and postoperative neurological remission. Neurology 1973; 28:891–894.

97. Evans BS, Fagan C, Arnold T, Dropcho EJ, Oh SJ. Paraneoplastic motor neuron disease and renal cell carcinoma; improvement after nephrectomy. Neurology 1990; 40: 960–963.

98. Gerling GM, Woolsey RM. Paraneoplastic motor neuron disease. Mo Med 1967; 64:503–506.

99. Mitchell DM, Olczak SA. Remission of a syndrome indistinguishable from motor neuron disease after resection of bronchial carcinoma. BMJ 1979; 2:176–177.

100. Stephens TW, Rougas A, Ghose MK. Pure motor neuropathy complicating carcinoma of the bronchus recovered after surgery. Brit J Dis Chest 1966; 60:107–109.

101. Barron KD, Rodichok LD. Cancer and disorders of motor neurons. In: Rowland LP, ed. Human Motor Neuron Diseases. New York: Raven Press, 1982:267–272.

102. Yamada M, Shintani S, Mitani K, Kametani H, Wada Y, Furukawa T, Tsukagoshi H, Ozaki K, Eishi Y, Hatakeyama S. Peripheral neuropathy with predominantly motor manifestations in a patient with carcinoma of the uterus. J Neurol 1988; 235:368–370.

103. Rowland LP, Schneck S. Neuromuscular disorders associated with malignant neoplastic disease. J Chron Dis 1963; 16:777–795.

104. Schold SC, Cho ES, Sonasundaram M, Posner JP. Subacute motor neuronopathy; a remote effect of lymphoma. Ann Neurol 1979; 5:271–287.

105. Caress JB, Abend WK, Preston DC, Logigian EL. A case of Hodgkin's lymphoma producing neuromyotonia. Neurology 1997; 49:258–259.

106. Roobol TH, Kazzaz BA, Vallejo CJ. Segmental rigidity and spinal myoclonus as a paraneoplastic syndrome. J Neurol Neurosurg Psychiatry 1987; 50:628–631.

107. Mygland A, Vincent A, Newsom-Davis J, Kaminski H, Zorzato F, Agius M, Gilhus NE, Aarli JA. Autoantibodies in thymoma-associated myasthenia gravis with myositis or neuromyotonia. Arch Neurol 2000; 57(4):527–531.

108. Cottrell DA, Blackmore KJ, Fawcett PRW, Birchall D, Vincent A, Barnard S, Walls TJ. Sub-acute presentation of Morvan's syndrome after thymectomy. J Neurol Neurosurg Psychiatry 2004; 75(10):1504–1505.

109. Hart IK, Maddison P, Newsom-Davis J, Vincent A, Mills KR. Phenotypic variants of autoimmune peripheral nerve hyperexcitability. Brain 2002; 125(pt 8):1887–1895.

110. Liguori R, Vincent A, Clover L, Avoni P, Plazzi G, Cortelli P, Baruzzi A, Carey T, Gambetti P, Lugaresi E, Montagna P. Morvan's syndrome: peripheral and central nervous system and cardiac involvement with antibodies to voltage-gated potassium channels. Brain 2001; 24(12):2417–2426.

111. Forsyth PA, Dalmau J, Graus F, Cwik V, Rosenblum MK, Posner JB. Motor neuron syndromes in cancer patients. Ann Neurol 1997; 41:722–730.

112. Verma A, Berger JR, Snodgrass S, Petito C. Motor neuron disease: a paraneoplastic process associated with anti-Hu antibody and small cell lung carcinoma. Ann Neurol 1996; 40:112–116.

113. Kiernan JA, Hudson AJ. Anti-neurone antibodies are not characteristic of amyotrophic lateral sclerosis. Neuroreport 1993; 4:427–430.

114. Khawaja S, Sripathi N, Ahmad BK, Lennon VA. Paraneoplastic motor neuron disease with type 1 Purkinje cell antibodies. Muscle Nerve 1998; 21:943–945.

115. Hays AP, Roxas A, Sadiq SA, Vallejos H, D'Agati V, Thomas FP, Torres R, Sherman WH, Bailey-Braxton D, Hays AG, Rowland LP, Latov N. A monoclonal IgA in a patient with amyotrophic lateral sclerosis reacts with neurofilaments and surface antigen on neuroblastoma cells. J Neuropathol Exp Neurol 1990; 49:383–398.

116. Ferracci F, Fassetta G, Butler MH, Floyd S, Solimena M, De Camilli P. A novel anti-neuronal antibody in a motor neuron syndrome associated with breast cancer. Neurology 1999; 53(4):852–855.

117. Brownell B, Trevor-Hughes J. Central nervous system in motor neuron disease. J Neurol Neurosurg Psychiatry 1970; 33:338–357.

118. Younger DS, Chou S, Hays AP, Lange DJ, Emerson R, Brin M, Thompson H Jr, Rowland LP. Primary lateral sclerosis: a clinical diagnosis reemerges. Arch Neurol 1988; 45:1304–1307.

119. Corcia P, Honnorat J, Geunnoc AM, de Toffol B, Autret A. Sclérose latérale primitive et cancer du sein: syndrome neologique paranéoplasique ou association fortujite? Rev Neurol (Paris) 2000; 156:1020–1022.

120. Kijima Y, Yoshinaka H, Higuchi I, Owaki T, Aikou T. A case of amyotrophic lateral sclerosis and breast cancer. Breast Cancer 2005; 12(1):57–59.

121. Rojas-Marcos I, Rousseau A, Keime-Guibert F, Rene R, Cartalat-Carel S, Delattre JY, Graus F. Spectrum of paraneoplastic of paraneoplastic neurologic disorders in women with breast and gynecologic cancer. Medicine (Baltimore) 2003; 82(3):216–223.

122. Berghs S, Ferracci F, Maksimova E, Gleason S, Leszczynski N, Butler M, DeCamilli P, Solimena M. Autoimmunity to beta IV spectrin in paraneoplastic lower motor neuron syndrome. Proc Natl Acad Sci USA 2001; 98(12):6945–6950.

123. Rowland LP. Diagnosis of amyotrophic lateral sclerosis. J Neurol Sci 1998; 160:S6–S24.

124. Rowland LP, Schneck SA. Neuromuscular disorders associated with malignant neoplastic disease. J Chron Dis 1963; 16:777–795.

125. Walton JN, Tomlinson BE, Pedru GW. Subacute "poliomyelitis" and Hodgkin's disease. J Neurol Sci 1968; 6:435–445.

126. Rowland LP, Defendini R, Sherman W, Hirano A, Olarte MR, Latov N, Lovelace RE, Inoue K, Osserman EF. Macroglobulinemia with peripheral neuropathy simulating motor neuron disease. Ann Neurol 1982; 11:532–536.

127. Gordon PH, Rowland LP, Younger DS, Sherman WH, Hays AP, Louis ED, Lange DJ, Trojaborg W, Lovelace RE, Murphy PL, Latov N. Lymphoproliferative disorders and motor neuron disease. Neurology 1997; 48:1671–1678.

128. Rowland LP, Gordon PH, Younger DS, Sherman WH, Hays AP, Louis ED, Lange DJ, Trojaborg W, Lovelace RE, Murphy PL, Latov N. Lymphoproliferative disorders and motor neuron disease. Neurology 1998; 50:576.

129. Leone KV, Phillips LH. Lymphoproliferative disorders and motor neuron disease. Neurology 1998; 50:576 (letter).

130. Case Records of the Massachusetts General Hospital Case 16–1999. Lymphoplasmacytic lymphoma with motor neuronopathy and Waldenström macroglobulinemia. Discussed by D. Chad. N Engl J Med 1999; 340:1661–1669.

131. Openshaw H, Slatkin E. Motor neuron disease in Hodgkin's lymphoma. Neurology 1998; 50:A31.

132. Bosch X, Guilabert A, Miquel R, Campo E. Enigmatic Kikuchi-Fujimoto disease: a comprehensive review. Am J Clin Pathol 2004; 122(1):141–152.

133. Shy ME, Rowland LP, Smith T, Trojaborg W, Latov N, Sherman W, Pesce MA, Lovelace RE, Osserman EF. Motor neuron disease and plasma cell dyscrasia. Neurology 1986; 36:1429–1436.

134. Rowland LP. Amyotrophic lateral sclerosis with paraproteins and autoantibodies. In: Serratrice G, Munsat TL, eds. Pathogenesis and Therapy of Amyotrophic Lateral Sclerosis. Philadelphia: Lippincott-Raven, 1995:93–105.

135. Willison HJ, Chancellor AM, Paterson G, Veitch J, Singh S, Whitelaw J, Kennedy PG, Warlow CP. Antiglycolipid antibodies, immunoglobulins and paraproteins in motor neuron disease: population-based case control study. J Neurol Sci 1993; 114:209–215.

136. Gardner MB, Henderson BE, Officer JE, Rongey RW, Parker JC, Oliver C, Estes JD, Huebner RJ. A spontaneous lower motor neuron disease apparently caused by indigenous type-C RNA virus in wild mice. J Natl Cancer Inst 1973; 51(4):1243–1254.

137. Gardner MB, Rasheed S, Klement V, Rongey RW, Brown JC, Dworsky R, Henderson BE. Lower motor neuron disease in wild mice caused by indigenous type C virus and search for a similar etiology in human amyotrophic lateral sclerosis. UCLA Forum Med Sci 1976; 19:217–234.

138. Paquette Y, Hanna Z, Savard P, Brousseau R, Robitaille Y, Jolicoeur P. Retrovirus-induced murine motor neuron disease: mapping the determinant of spongiform degeneration within the envelope gene. Proc Natl Acad Sci USA 1989; 86(10):3896–3900.

5
ALS Clinical Motor Signs and Symptoms

Valerie A. Cwik

Muscular Dystrophy Association, Tucson, Arizona, U.S.A.

INTRODUCTION

Amyotrophic lateral sclerosis (ALS) is a progressive degenerative disease of the motor system, comprising a combination of upper motor neuron (UMN) and lower motor neuron (LMN) symptoms and signs in the four central nervous system regions: brainstem, cervical, thoracic, and lumbosacral. At any given stage of the disease, the clinical manifestations of ALS depend on the regional combinations of UMNs and LMNs involved. Since there is no single biologic marker or investigative test that establishes or confirms a diagnosis of ALS, the identification of the disorder is heavily dependent on clinical recognition of the signs and symptoms.

According to the El Escorial and revised Airlie House diagnostic criteria for ALS, the diagnosis of clinically definite ALS requires the presence of both UMN and LMN signs in three body regions (1,2). Clinical, laboratory, and neuropathological criteria have also been established for less definitive categories. The clinical features of ALS will be reviewed in detail in this chapter; the classification, diagnosis, and presentation of diagnosis will be discussed in a later chapter.

UPPER MOTOR NEURON FEATURES

Although required for a diagnosis of definite ALS, the clinical manifestations of the UMN lesions in ALS are not as well studied as those of the LMNs and are not systematically reported in published studies of ALS. This likely results from the fact that quantification of abnormalities of the UMNs is quite insensitive when compared with LMNs, and that the UMN lesions in ALS are not responsible for the major disabilities that occur in this disorder.

Lesions of the UMN may cause two general problems: (i) impaired ability to activate motor neurons rapidly and selectively, and (ii) alterations in segmental reflex activity (3). These two types of problems are manifest, clinically, by a variety of UMN signs and symptoms.

Impaired activation of motor neurons, or reduced central motor drive, results in diminished firing rates and reduced recruitment of motor units (4). The clinical consequence is diminished muscle activation, which results in slowed repetitive movements and weakness. Rates of finger tapping and foot tapping, in a defined period of time, are easily performed and may be used to quantify this deficit. However, the weakness due to UMN loss in ALS is often difficult to quantify clinically, as it is overshadowed by the weakness due to LMN lesions.

Changes in segmental reflex activities are the second consequence of UMN impairment. Lesions of the corticospinal tracts may produce the classic UMN signs of spastic tone, clasp-knife response, and hyperreflexia with spread or clonus, which are easily assessed in the cervical and lumbar regions. Other focal signs are elicitable in each of the four central nervous system regions.

In the bulbar region, lesions of the corticobulbar tracts are responsible for an exaggerated or clonic jaw jerk, a hyperactive gag reflex, forced yawning, and a suck or snout reflex. Rapid alternating movements of the tongue may be slowed, and there may be associated synkinetic horizontal deviations of the jaw.

Loss of inhibition for the complex motor acts of laughter and crying, which causes emotional lability or the pseudobulbar affect, may also be seen in ALS. Laughing and crying are thought to depend on a number of neural pathways involved in emotion, respiration, vocalization, and facial movements; involved structures include the orbitofrontal cortex, subcortical and brainstem structures, and the cerebellum (5). While the pseudobulbar effect may result from lesions in a variety of locations, such as combined bilateral internal capsule and basal ganglia damage, or lesions of the substantia nigra, cerebral peduncles, and hypothalamus, emotional lability in ALS is likely to occur from lesions of the corticobulbar tracts (6).

More dubious brainstem UMN signs include the palmomental reflex and the corneomandibular response. The palmomental reflex is an involuntary contraction of the mentalis muscle of the chin caused by stroking the thenar eminence. While it is an easy and a rapid test to perform, this reflex may be elicited in more than 50% of normal adults, and its prevalence increases with advancing age (7–9). A strong, sustained, and easily reproducible response is more likely to indicate UMN pathology. However, in general, the clinical utility of the palmomental sign is of uncertain significance.

Similarly, the corneomandibular has been advocated as a useful indicator for UMN loss affecting the corticotrigeminal tract (10). When this reflex is present, stimulation of the cornea produces lateral deviation of the jaw. In a study of 42 patients with ALS, the corneomandibular response was the most prevalent UMN response, present in 71%, compared to extensor plantar responses in 36%, pseudobulbar palsy in 33%, Hoffmann's sign in 29%, and exaggerated jaw jerk in 22% (10). In contrast, the corneomandibular response was present in only 6% of 110 patients with cerebrovascular disease. When present, the response is usually unilateral in cerebrovascular disease, and bilateral in ALS. While Okuda and colleagues suggest that the corneomandibular reflex is the most sensitive indicator of UMN degeneration in ALS, others suggest that it is a normal phenomenon in a significant proportion of the healthy population (7).

Evidence for UMN loss specific to the thoracic region is limited to the loss of superficial abdominal reflexes. While they are rarely reported in the published studies of ALS, Mulder has commented that the abdominal reflexes usually remain brisk (11).

As noted above, abnormalities of tone and reflexes are readily identified in the extremities. Preserved reflexes in a weak and wasted limb also constitute UMN findings, sometimes called probable upper motor neuron (PUMN) signs. In the upper extremities one may elicit Hoffmann's sign in one or both hands. In the lower extremities, an extensor plantar response, or Babinski sign, is a classic UMN sign.

Plantar stimulation may also produce a few quick contractions of the tensor fascia lata on the lateral aspect of the thigh, without any displacement of the leg at the hip. It must be noted that abnormalities in the various reflexes do not necessarily occur together, even within a single region.

The most commonly reported UMN sign in ALS is the extensor plantar response, present in 28% to 50% of the individuals in several large series (10,12–15). However, hyperreflexia may occur more frequently, identified in 47% and 87% of ALS patients in two large series (12,16).

Care must be taken to be certain that the responses to reflex testing are correctly interpreted either as pathologic or as normal. For example, brisk tendon reflexes and Hoffmann's signs may be sometimes seen in the normal state, particularly in persons who are anxious. On the other hand, the Babinski response is at times absent when other pyramidal signs are present. The extensor plantar response is actually a combination of extensor hallucis longus and hallux flexor movements; in the case of significant weakness of the extensor hallucis longus muscle, either the response may be absent or it may demonstrate a flexor movement (17). In yet other cases, there may be fragmentation of the Babinski response, with an up-going great toe without fanning of the others, or vice versa.

UMN dysfunction is not typically the problem that brings the individual to medical attention. Stiffness occurs as the initial symptom in only a small minority of ALS patients (1.3–6%) (12,13). However, marked spasticity in the legs may produce functional disability and initiate the diagnostic process. Upright quiet stance is generally unaffected in ALS, but balance may be poor due to stiffness of the legs and slowed reaction times to postural shifts, as may occur when pushed or bumped (18). The gait may be slow and labored.

While weakness due to UMN dysfunction or loss may occur in any region of the body, it is generally mild and difficult to examine, and is often overshadowed by or inseparable from the weakness due to LMN lesions. In the legs, in particular, marked spasticity may also make UMN weakness impossible to detect.

LOWER MOTOR NEURON FEATURES

While disability in ALS is due to a combination of UMN and LMN dysfunction or loss, for most individuals it is the LMN problems that dominate and necessitate medical attention. The stigmata of LMN loss, weakness and atrophy, along with the associated symptoms of cramps and fasciculations, may occur in any of the four central nervous system regions. As mentioned previously, the presence of both LMN and UMN findings in three body regions establishes the definitive diagnosis of ALS. However, when symptoms and signs are restricted to a single limb or region, ALS may be overlooked, initially, as a potential diagnosis.

Initial Symptoms

Weakness is the initial symptom in the majority of the individuals with ALS, reportedly occurring in 58% to 63% in several large series (12–14). Typically, the weakness is asymmetric, and the distribution of weakness is in a segmental pattern, rather than a peripheral nerve distribution, corresponding to the degeneration of anterior horn cells in the spinal cord. As noted in Table 1, weakness and/or atrophy starting in the limbs, occurring in 51% to 81%, is more common than bulbar onset ALS (12–15,19,20).

Table 1 Initial Clinical Features/Site of Onset in ALS

	Gubbay (12) n=201	Jokelainen (13) n=255	Li (14) n=560	Caroscio (15) n=269	Traynor (19) n=388	Haverkamp (20) n=831
Weakness/Motor	63.2	58	63			71.1
Arm(s)	10.7*			27.1*	18**	35.8**
Both arms	8.5			4.5		
Leg(s)	11.9*			22.7*	29.1**	34.9**
Both legs	19.8			13.4		
Hemiparesis	3.8					
Combined arms and legs	8.5				10.6	4.4
Difficulty walking			16			
Bulbar symptoms	22	28	19#	25.3	35.3	25
Dysphagia/choking		5			9.8	1.2
Dysarthria		23	23#		25.5	23.8
Cramps/pain	8.8	4		1.5		
Stiffness/clumsiness	1.3	6				
Fasciculations	3.5	3		5.5		
Atrophy	9.7		11			
Sensory symptoms	3.5					3.9

*Unilateral limb symptoms.
**Unspecified unilateral or bilateral.
#Authors report that 23% of patients reported difficulty in speaking as the first symptom, and that the disease started in the bulbar muscles in 19%.
(Due to variations in reporting initial site of onset, symptoms and signs in the different studies, totals do not always add to 100%.)

With limb onset, symptoms begin in the arms and legs with about equal frequency (12,13,15,19). In the upper extremities, symptoms are typically unilateral initially, but may be bilateral in a small percentage of patients (less than 10%) (12,15). In the legs, the problems are more commonly bilateral than in the arms at initial presentation (12,15).

Occasionally disease onset may be generalized (7%) or occur simultaneously in both an arm and leg (11%) (19). Presentation with hemiparesis is unusual, but does occur in ALS. In such cases it is important to exclude another cause for the symptomatology, such as a unilateral brain or spinal cord lesion. Fasciculations or cramps are rarely the presenting complaint, reported in only 3% to 6% and 2% to 9% of patients, respectively (12,13,15).

In the early stages of ALS, individual LMN lesions may not produce substantial disability; however, the lesions accumulate over time and become progressively more disabling.

Cramps

A muscle cramp is an involuntary contraction of a skeletal muscle that produces significant pain and a hard bulge or knot in the muscle. Cramps are commonly brought on by contraction of the muscle, and stretching often provides relief. Cramps are common in normal individuals, typically occurring under conditions such as pregnancy, sports, sleep, and during strong voluntary contractions. When associated with disease, cramps are not limited to ALS; e.g., they may occur in other types of acquired or hereditary neuropathies, in renal failure, or due to electrolyte disturbances. Muscle contractures that occur with metabolic disorders such as McArdle's disease may simulate a cramp, but are electrophysiologically distinct. Therefore, cramps are a common and annoying problem, and they are not specific to ALS.

However, cramps are a common feature of ALS occurring in up to 10% of patients as the initial presenting symptom, and in up to 50% of all persons who develop ALS (15). Cramps tend to predominate in the leg muscles, but also occur, frequently, in the hand and forearm muscles. Cramps in the abdominal muscles may develop spontaneously, but are often precipitated by twisting, bending, or stretching movements. In the neck muscles, cramps may be brought on by yawning. While muscle cramps tend to be problematic early in the course of ALS and in muscles that are in the early stages of involvement, they tend to diminish and even disappear as the disease progresses.

Fasciculations

A fasciculation is a spontaneous discharge of a single motor unit that causes a brief contraction of a portion of a muscle, and may be documented by clinical observation, by electromyographic (EMG) testing, or both. Like cramps, fasciculations are a non-specific feature of ALS; they also may occur in acquired and hereditary neuropathies and in systemic conditions such as hyperthyroidism, or may occur unrelated to any identifiable disorder.

Rarely are fasciculations the single presenting problem in ALS, occurring in only approximately 3% to 6% of persons with ALS (12,13,15). However, they are frequently present in the earliest stages of the disease. Like cramps, fasciculations tend to diminish in the later stages of the ALS, when muscle wasting is severe. Up to 90% of individuals with ALS are reported to have fasciculations at some point in their disease course (12,15,16). Fasciculations in ALS typically occur as single twitches, but may also appear in pairs or triplets. Their frequency ranges from rare to nearly continuous, and their distribution may be focal, scattered, or generalized.

Although they may occur in any voluntary muscle, fasciculations are more commonly observed in the upper extremities in ALS (12,13). While they are readily observed in the lower legs, intrinsic hand, and forearm muscles, as well as in the biceps, triceps, and deltoid muscles of the upper arms, fasciculations are not invariable in any of these locations. It may be necessary to have the patient undress to observe fasciculations in the pectoralis and shoulder girdle muscles of the upper trunk and back, and in the quadriceps muscles of the thigh. In the face, fasciculations may be observed in the orbicularis oris muscle and the mentalis muscle of the chin.

With bulbar symptoms, fasciculations of the tongue are a common occurrence. Fasciculations of the tongue should be looked for with the tongue at rest in the mouth; they are similar in appearance, although somewhat smaller than fasciculations in limb muscles. With protrusion of the tongue, one often sees quivering movements, which should not be confused with true fasciculations.

Fasciculations, in and of themselves, are not necessarily a sign of serious disease. They are a normal and common phenomenon, experienced by up to 70% of the population (21). They may occur without known cause, or may be precipitated or exacerbated by emotional or physical stress, fatigue, lack of sleep, excessive caffeine intake, medications such as β-agonists and thyroxine, smoking, cold, or hyperthyroidism (21,22). The most common location for fasciculations in a healthy population is the arms, particularly the deltoid and intrinsic hand muscles. The orbicuralis oculi muscle ("eye twitch") is also a common location for benign fasciculations. In one large study, participants reported fasciculations in the legs only 6% of the time (21).

Benign fasciculations occur in all age groups, and most commonly start in the second and third decades. The interval between episodes of fasciculations varies from daily in a small percentage to greater than six months. In a study of 121 individuals with fasciculations, Blexrud et al. (22) noted that 19 individuals had experienced an acute infectious illness, suggestive of a viral syndrome, in the month preceding the onset of the fasciculations.

The appearance of fasciculations in an otherwise healthy person may be a cause for great anxiety. Prior to the Internet age, this phenomenon was generally restricted to medical personnel and medical students who were well aware of the association of widespread fasciculations with motor neuron disease. However, in this age of electronic information that is readily accessible 24 hours a day, more non-medical individuals are aware that fasciculations may portend ALS, prompting evaluation by a neurologist. In such cases, the person may be quite distressed. If other signs and symptoms of the disease are lacking, they should be strongly reassured of the improbability of ALS. Fasciculations without atrophy or weakness, or without electrophysiologic evidence for denervation, are very unlikely to be the first sign of ALS. Follow-up of 121 individuals with fasciculations 2 to 32 years after their onset failed to demonstrate the development of ALS in any (22). However, there are scattered reports of fasciculations as the presenting sign in ALS. In an early case report, there was striking evidence for active denervation on the initial EMG study; in this case, clinical weakness and atrophy were not noted for four years (23). Very recently there has been a report of seemingly benign fasciculations, associated with cramps and myalgias, in an individual with a normal neurological examination, who developed motor neuron disease more than a year later (24). Again, the initial

EMG examination was abnormal, demonstrating rare fibrillation potentials, and a muscle biopsy demonstrated a few angulated fibers. These examples reinforce the fact that fasciculations may be considered benign only in the presence of a normal neurological examination and a normal EMG (except for fasciculations). However, these cases were atypical in that clinical weakness and atrophy were delayed in appearance. In most cases of new-onset fasciculations that progress to ALS, weakness and atrophy usually appear within several months of the onset of fasciculations.

Bulbar Lower Motor Neuron Symptoms and Signs

Bulbar symptoms and signs may be the presenting problem in ALS, or may occur later in the course of the disease. Approximately 19% to 35% of patients with ALS have onset of symptoms in the bulbar region; these individuals are more likely to be female and to be somewhat older than those with limb onset ALS (12–15,19). While limb findings in ALS are typically asymmetric, the oral and facial findings are characteristically bilateral and symmetric.

With bulbar onset ALS, dysarthria generally develops prior to dysphagia. Both UMN and LMN lesions may contribute to the speech difficulty. The UMN speech tends to be slow and effortful, with poor enunciation, and a harshness and a strained quality to the voice. Neuronal loss in the brainstem may also cause slow and effortful speech, with breathiness of the voice and slurring of consonants (25). Velopharyngeal incompetence may result in air leakage through the nose and lend a hypernasal quality to the voice. Because of the overlap of symptoms, it is not always possible to completely distinguish the UMN components from the LMN components of dysarthria. In fact, dysarthria in ALS is usually due to combined UMN and LMN dysfunction.

Early speech problems are due, typically, to tongue weakness, leading to difficulty with production of words containing the lingual and dental consonants, such as "D," "T," and "L." However, the speech problems do not necessarily correlate with severity of the tongue weakness, as jaw movements may help to compensate for the tongue weakness (26). Other factors that contribute to the dysarthria include lip and palate strength, pulmonary function, and vocal cord movement. As a rule, loss of tongue and lip function has more effect on speech quality and articulation than respiratory and jaw factors. It has been estimated that the tongue and lips use about 10% to 30% of their maximum contractile force for speech production, while less than 2% of respiratory and jaw functions are related to this activity (27).

Dysarthria and dysphonia inevitably progress. As the vocal cords, respiratory muscles, and posterior pharyngeal muscles weaken, the voice may become hypernasal, hypophonic, hoarse and/or breathy, and there may be difficulty with gutteral sounds, such as "G" and "K." Eventually, there may be total anarthria.

Swallowing problems are sometimes reported as an early bulbar symptom. Initially, the problem is with moving a bolus of food from the front to the back of the oropharynx due to tongue weakness, rather than an actual problem with the pharyngeal muscles involved in swallowing. Early on there may also be pocketing of food between the cheek and gum; weakness of the tongue necessitates dislodging the food with a sweeping movement of the finger. Over time, difficulty with thin liquids and difficulty managing foods that fragment, such as rice, ground beef, and crackers, may be other commonly reported problems.

In the later stages of bulbar weakness, the masseter muscles may become involved, producing difficulty in chewing and, in the most severe situations, inability to close the mouth, producing a slack-jaw appearance to the face. As the pharyngeal muscles weaken, swallowing becomes increasingly more difficult, leading to choking and aspiration. Bilateral palatal weakness may allow diversion of food and, especially, fluids into the nasal cavity; i.e., nasal regurgitation. Warm thin water is the most difficult consistency to swallow due to its rapid transit from the mouth to pharyngolarynx; patients learn early on that thicker consistencies are more easily swallowed. Patients learn also, or should be taught, that tucking the chin when swallowing will help lower the risk of aspiration. As swallowing ability worsens, food and fluid intake diminishes. There may be failure to thrive and a need for insertion of a feeding tube.

Weakness of the facial muscles typically is not severe at any stage, but may lead to evasion of the lower lip and difficulty pursing the lips. Inability to whistle, food spillage, and inability to use a straw appear as the facial weakness progresses. Drooling is a particularly distressing problem for some patients and caregivers; it tends to occur later in the course of bulbar symptoms, and is due to a combination of incompetence of lip closure and difficulty with oral transport and swallowing of saliva. Pooling of saliva in the posterior oropharynx may also lead to "wet" or gurgled speech production.

Spasmodic stridorous breathing, especially with coughing, results from paradoxical adduction of the vocal cords leading to glottal narrowing and the stridorous sound. These episodes, called paroxysmal laryngeal spasms, may be very frightening to patients and caregivers when they first occur. For the most part, the spasms are self-limited, and patients learn that quiet breathing through the nose may help abort or reduce the severity of an attack of stridor. Rarely these episodes may be prolonged, requiring medical assessment and intervention (Chapter 10).

Bulbar Examination

The physical findings in bulbar onset ALS relate to the stage of the disease. Early on, when symptoms are mild, inspection of the tongue may reveal fasciculations along with scalloping of the edges of the tongue or frank atrophy. In addition to the normal midline tongue furrow, there may be an additional furrow on either side of the tongue (Fig. 1). While the individual may be able to protrude the tongue fully in the midline, early weakness of the tongue may be detected by asking the patient to forcefully push the tongue into the side of the cheek, resisting the examiner's finger placed outside the cheek.

With disease progression, inability to protrude the tongue past the lips is often associated with significant dysarthria; inability to protrude the tongue past the incisors correlates with a need to alter the diet to very soft foods or thick liquids (28). Eventually the tongue is markedly atrophic and lies immobile in the mouth. As a rule, there is more tongue weakness than jaw and lip weakness in patients with either bulbar-onset or limb-onset ALS.

Weakness of the facial muscles tends to involve the lower face. To assess lip competence, the examiner can check for lip closure strength with the lips pursed. Additional tests for lip strength include sucking the gloved finger of the examiner and holding a seal while puffing out the cheeks with a breath.

As bulbar weakness progresses into the middle stages, the palate, muscles of mastication, pharyngeal constrictor muscles, and buccinators may become involved. Examination may reveal impaired or absent palatal elevation with a prolonged "ah." The gag reflex may be hyperactive or absent. The examiner should listen for changes in the voice such as breathiness, hoarseness, or hypernasality. The patient should be asked to repeat various syllables: "ma" or "pa" to assess lip function; "la," "ta," or

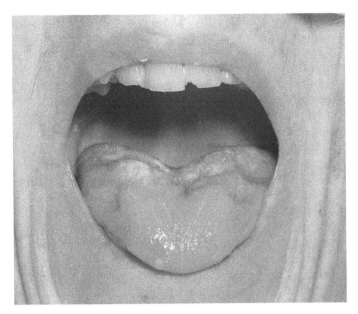

Figure 1 Moderate tongue atrophy with development of new furrows lateral to midline.

"da" for tongue function, and "ga" or "ka" for palatal function. Alternatively, all three types of sounds may be assessed with repetition of the syllables "pa-ta-ka." Swallowing can be assessed in the clinic by having the individual drink some warm water; the examiner should listen for sputtering or even frank coughing with the swallow, or for a gurgling sound as the person attempts to talk. Check masseter bulk with jaw clenching; pterygoid strength is testing by having the person move the jaw side-to-side.

Vocal cord paralysis may produce a strained, strangled voice. On examination, the vocal cords may show limited abduction, with full adduction.

Upper Extremity Lower Motor Neuron Symptoms and Signs

When the onset of symptoms is in the upper extremities, weakness may first appear in the hand, in the forearm, or in the upper arm or shoulder girdle muscles. With onset in the hand, the patient may complain of loss of finger dexterity and have difficulty picking up small objects, writing, turning keys, and fastening buttons. On examination there is wasting and weakness of the intrinsic hand muscles which may occur in a focal or a generalized pattern. In some individuals the lateral hand muscles associated with the thenar side of the hand are preferentially affected. In such cases, there is painless atrophy and weakness of the abductor pollicis brevis and first dorsal interosseous muscles of the hand, preventing adduction and opposition of the thumb. The hypothenar muscles, which are innervated by the same myotome, are relatively spared. This pattern of weakness is characteristic for ALS, as well as for other forms of anterior horn cell disease, and has been called the split hand syndrome (29). In rare instances, the reverse pattern is seen, with severe involvement of the hypothenar musculature and relative sparing of the thenar group (30). In many, however, the wasting and weakness is more or less uniform over the entire hand, particularly in advanced stages of the disease.

As weakness of the interossei and lumbrical muscles progresses, a claw hand deformity develops (Fig. 2). The fingers are extended at the MCP joints, and flexed at the proximal and distal interphalangeal joints. Both weakness and atrophy typically ascend up the arm prior to spreading to the contralateral hand and arm. Some patients may experience early unilateral finger and wrist drop, due to weakness of the extensor muscles of the hand and wrist. Weakness of these and other forearm muscles leads to difficulty with stabilization of the hand, causing problems with activities such as opening jars or lifting items with the hand in the pronated position. Bracing of the wrist and/or fingers may lead to a more functional posture.

Weakness of the biceps and other arm muscles may have significant functional consequences due to the dependence on elbow flexion for activities of daily living. Initially, patients may have difficulty in carrying heavy items, such as shopping bags or heavy cooking utensils. As elbow flexor weakness progresses, lifting the hand to the face or mouth for activities such as eating, drinking, shaving, and tooth-brushing becomes problematic. When weakness begins in the muscles of the arm, the elbow extensors tend to remain relatively strong.

In some patients, weakness of the muscles of the shoulder girdle is the first complaint. Biceps muscle weakness often is an early accompaniment to the shoulder girdle weakness. In such cases, strength in the hand and forearm muscles is preserved initially. Patients complain of difficulty in using the arms over the head, such as for lifting items from a high shelf or washing the hair. With progression to the contralateral shoulder girdle muscles, the arms hang limply and completely pronated at the sides and swing without control during ambulation, a syndrome that, variously, has been called the dangling-arm syndrome, man-in-a-barrel syndrome, or brachial amyotrophic diplegia (31). Patients use a characteristic flinging movement of the arm to raise the arm at the shoulder. In some cases, this presentation may portend a slower and more benign disease.

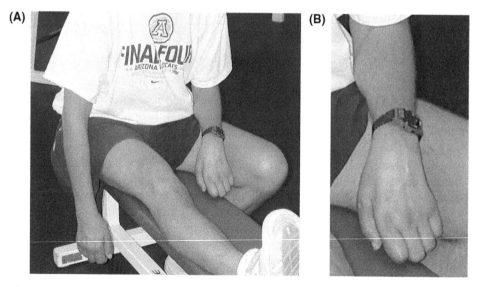

Figure 2 (**A**) Asymmetric hand weakness and atrophy. Note the claw-hand deformity of the left hand. (**B**) Close-up of A, demonstrating wasting of the interosseous muscles, especially the first dorsal interosseous.

Complications of Arm Weakness

While muscle weakness in the shoulder, arm, and hand muscles may produce significant disability, the loss of muscle strength may also lead to other problems. With increasing immobility of particular muscle groups, contractures of the joints may occur. The common sites at which these occur are the fingers and the shoulders. Flexion contractures of the fingers, when mild, may actually aid in functional activities that require a gripping action. However, with progression, the hand may develop a fixed flexion posture with the fingernails digging into the palms.

Contractures at the shoulders may produce a particularly painful condition called adhesive capsulitis or frozen shoulder. Patients with significant deltoid muscle weakness are most at risk because of their inability to raise the arm at the shoulder. Initial tightness occurs with posterior flexion of the arm at the shoulder; as the shoulder tightness develops, there is increasing difficulty with abduction of the arm at the shoulder. This is a very painful condition which is preventable, at least in large part, by the performance of active or passive range of motion exercises. Once a frozen shoulder has developed, it may require shoulder injections, combined with physical therapy, to resolve.

Purplish discoloration and swelling of the hand, due to the development of dependent edema when the arm hangs limply, is sometimes distressing and uncomfortable for patients. This is easily relieved by elevating the hand and arm.

Weakness of Axial and Trunk Musculature

Weakness of the axial musculature leads to two characteristic presentations: head drop and kyphosis. Many patients also experience problems due to abdominal muscle weakness.

In ALS, head drop may occur at any stage of the illness. Weakness of the neck extensor muscles is the causative problem. Symptoms of mild to moderate neck extensor weakness include difficulty in raising the head from a flexed position, as might occur when one bends forward over the sink while brushing the teeth. At the same time, patients may complain of problems controlling the head while riding in a car, particularly when coming to a stop. In such cases, the head will fling forward with the chin coming to rest on the chest. It may be difficult to return the head to the upright position. Although ALS is not considered a painful disease, cervical pain is a common feature of neck muscle weakness.

Bilateral weakness of the sternocleidomastoid muscles produces difficulty in lifting the head from the pillow when lying in the supine position. In such cases, turning onto one side and then sitting up allows one to attain the upright posture. When weakness of the sternocleidomastoid and neck extensor muscles occurs simultaneously, the head may be particularly unstable on the neck and difficult to control. For many individuals with neck weakness, a lightweight, adjustable neck brace is useful for riding in the car or keeping the head in a comfortable position while reading.

Weakness of the paraspinal muscles in the thoracic and upper lumbar regions may produce changes in posture, including a kyphosis or an "S"–shaped posture of the spine, when viewed from the side. Functional consequences of such weakness include difficulty in straightening the spine from a "bent-forward" posture, such as trying to pick up something from the ground or floor. Difficulty in rolling over in bed becomes increasingly difficult as truncal and limb muscle weakness progress.

The abdominal muscles may also weaken, producing difficulty with sitting up from a supine position. Reduced abdominal strength may contribute to a weak cough, difficulty in having a bowel movement, and increased abdominal girth. Some individuals complain of an uncomfortable bloating or increase in the size of the abdomen after eating.

Lower Extremity Lower Motor Neuron Signs and Symptoms

Weakness and atrophy in the lower extremities often begins in the distal leg muscles, more commonly in the dorsiflexors, evertors, and invertors of the ankle than in the muscles for plantarflexion. As a result, tripping over the toes and foot-drop are common complaints. While weakness in the legs may start unilaterally, not uncommonly problems are reported in both legs simultaneously (13–20%) (12,15). As the weakness ascends up the leg, there may be progressive difficulty going up or down stairs, stepping up or down a curb, or arising from a chair. Eventually, walking, standing, and bearing weight for transfers may become impossible.

Complications of Leg Weakness

Complications of leg weakness are primarily twofold: falls and dependent edema. In the early stages, falls may be due to tripping over the toes from foot-drop. With progressive leg, thigh, and hip girdle weakness, walking becomes more difficult at first, then precarious. Bone fractures and face and head injuries due to falls are not uncommon occurrences in those with significant leg weakness.

Dependent edema more commonly occurs in the feet and distal legs than in the arms. The cause of the edema relates to the lack of muscle contraction to assist in venous blood return to the heart. The feet may become discolored, cool, and swollen. Patients complain that shoes are difficult to fit and are uncomfortable to wear. Compression stockings, applied before getting out of bed in the morning, may help keep the edema in check. Elevation of the feet periodically during the day may also reduce some of the swelling and discomfort.

Deep vein thrombosis (DVT) is not commonly reported in ALS, but may occur more frequently than recognized. In a single published report, only 1 of 97 ALS control subjects in a clinical trial of topiramate developed DVT over the 12 month duration of the study (32). However, it is possible that DVTs, with or without pulmonary embolism, may go unrecognized, especially in the later stages of the disease.

Contractures in the joints of the legs usually do not occur in ALS.

Respiratory Features

Respiratory problems associated with ALS will be described in full detail in a later chapter, and only brief mention will be made here. Shortness of breath or other respiratory symptoms are not commonly reported as the initial problem in ALS. However, respiratory failure due to diaphragmatic weakness and pulmonary complications of bulbar paralysis (i.e., aspiration pneumonia) are the most common causes of death in ALS. In general, respiratory muscle involvement in ALS is related to the stage of the disease, but not to onset in the upper versus lower extremities (33). Respiratory insufficiency or failure is typically a late manifestation of the disease; in most patients with respiratory symptoms, at least moderate limb or bulbar weakness is already present. However, there are occasional reports of individuals presenting with respiratory failure (34,35). In such cases, there are often clues to the underlying diagnosis of ALS either clinically (fasciculations, wasting, weakness, and/or UMN signs), or by nerve conduction and EMG studies. Patients presenting with respiratory failure may be evaluated first by a pulmonologist or in the intensive care unit, often causing a delay in the diagnosis of ALS.

Baseline pulmonary function may range from supernormal to below normal. In a study of 36 patients, at diagnosis 31 (86%) had evidence of respiratory muscle weakness as measured by reduction in vital capacity, negative inspiratory pressure, or positive expiratory pressure (36). However, only seven patients complained of shortness of breath at the time of presentation.

UNCOMMON FEATURES

Eye Movement Abnormalities in ALS

In the older literature, it has been reported that the eyelids and extraocular muscles are always spared in ALS (11,37). In more recent years, there have been occasional reports of ophthalmoplegia in ALS. However, even with advanced brainstem disease, ophthalmoplegia is rare and pathologic documentation of involvement of the oculomotor nuclei is sparse.

There are occasional reports of ophthalmoplegia in patients on respirators, and at least one report of ophthalmoparesis, and eventual ophthalmoplegia, occurring in the middle stages of bulbar onset ALS, when disability was only moderate (38,39). Autopsy in this case demonstrated striking neuronal loss in the oculomotor nuclei, as well as the fourth and sixth cranial nuclei, along with other brainstem nuclei. In some cases there may be supranuclear impairment of eye movements, with the preservation of oculocephalic reflexes (40).

There are also rare reports of other types of eye movement abnormalities in ALS, including nystagmus, defective saccades, apraxia of gaze to lateral pursuit, and breakdown of smooth tracking pursuits into saccadic motions (41–43). Inability to close the eyelids on voluntary command has been reported and has been confirmed, pathologically, as a supranuclear palsy in some (44). This phenomenon typically occurs in those with spastic bulbar palsy, also a supranuclear problem.

Sphincter Involvement

In individuals with ALS, LMN control of the bladder and bowel sphincters usually remains normal, even in advanced stages of the disease. There are only sparse reports of sphincter weakness in ALS; in a series of 255 patients, one had rectal sphincter weakness, one had bladder sphincter weakness, and one had weakness of both sphincters (12,13). The relative paucity of sphincter disturbance correlates with the pathological findings in the spinal cord. In Onuf's nucleus, the neurons which inner-vate the muscles of the pelvic floor demonstrate a resistance to degeneration. How-ever, inclusions that are typical for ALS are observed in a small percentage of these neurons: Bunina bodies, Lewy body-like inclusions, and conglomerate inclusions (45–48).

Although not generally reported in the ALS literature, many patients will com-plain of urinary urgency, which responds well to antispasmodic agents, suggesting an UMN cause for the symptoms.

Cognitive Dysfunction

Although not a motor symptom or sign, brief mention of cognitive dysfunction in ALS will be made here; detailed information may be found in Chapter 10. Traditionally, patients with ALS have been told that cognitive function remains normal over the course of the disease. While clinically significant dementia remains uncommon, recent studies involving detailed cognitive testing have revealed deficits in frontal executive function in up to 50% of ALS patients (49).

PROGRESSION OF SYMPTOMS

Progression of signs and symptoms in ALS relates to cumulative motor neuron loss within a given region as well as anatomic spread of the disease. The pattern of dissemination of symptoms shows that ALS typically advances from one focal region to involve other regions that are anatomically contiguous. Caroscio and Brooks both report that regional spread, from one to the other arm (cervical to cervical region) or from one to the other leg (lumbar to lumbar), occurs prior to vertical spread in the spinal cord or from the cervical spinal cord into the brainstem (15,50). Caudal to rostral spread, either within the spinal cord or from the spinal cord to the brainstem, occurs at a faster rate than rostral to caudal spread. When onset is in the arm, spread to involve the brainstem occurs faster than propagation from the leg to the brainstem (50).

Clinical worsening of disease severity reflects, primarily, progressive LMN loss. Although there is considerable variability in deterioration rates between ALS patients, most will demonstrate a striking linear decline when megascores or composite scores for various testing measures are analyzed (15,16,27,51,52). However, in one small study, 25% of patients achieved a plateau in rate of progression lasting for nine months or more (15). As a rule, decline in strength in the upper extremities occurs at a faster rate than in the lower extremities, and bulbar function appears to deteriorate more slowly than limb function or respiratory function (16,50–52).

Respiratory failure or other pulmonary complications are the usual cause of death in ALS. For those patients in the United States who opt against tracheostomy and ventilator use, median survival is generally three to five years, although a substantial number may live longer than five and ten years (29% and 16%, respectively, in one series) (12). For those who choose invasive ventilation, care must be taken to preserve communication and prevent development of the locked-in state (53).

CONCLUSION

Despite advances in technology over the past couple of decades, ALS is still diagnosed by history and clinical examination, with supporting evidence from laboratory studies. In the advanced stages, the diagnosis of ALS is not difficult. However, in the early stages, particularly when symptoms and signs may be restricted to only a portion of a single body region, clinical acumen and a heightened index of suspicion are the keys to arriving at the correct diagnosis. The first descriptions of ALS appeared in the mid-19th century, yet many gaps remain in our knowledge of its clinical manifestations. Some clinical symptomatology is still not fully explained and there is limited published information about the complications of ALS. Further clinical studies can make an important contribution to the study of ALS.

REFERENCES

1. Brooks BR. El Escorial World Federation of Neurology criteria for the diagnosis of amyotrophic lateral sclerosis: subcommittee on Motor Neuron Diseases/Amyotrophic Lateral Sclerosis of the World Federation of Neurology Research Group on Neuromuscular Diseases and the El Escorial "Clinical Limits of Amyotrophic Lateral Sclerosis" workshop contributors. J Neurol Sci 1994; 124(suppl):96–107.
2. Miller RG, Munsat TL, Swash M, Brooks BR. For the World Federation of Neurology Committee on Research Consensus guidelines for the design and implementation of clinical trials in ALS. J Neurol Sci 1999; 169:2–12.
3. Ashby P, Mailis A, Hunter J. The evaluation of "Spasticity". Can J Neruol Sci 1987; 14:497–500.
4. Kent-Braun JA, Walker CH, Weiner MW, Miller RG. Functional significance of upper and lower motor neuron impairment in amyotrophic lateral sclerosis. Muscle Nerve 1998; 21:762–768.
5. Haymaker W, Hartwif K. Disorders of the brainstem and its cranial nerves. In: Baker AB, Joynt RJ, eds. Clinical Neurology. Vol. 3. Chap. 40. Philadelphia: JB Lippincott Company, 1988:15.
6. Masdeu JC. The localization of lesions affecting the cerebral hemispheres. In: Brazis PW, Masdeu JC, Biller J, eds. Localization in Clinical Neurology. Boston: Little Brown and Company, 1985.
7. Jacobs L, Gossman MD. Three primitive reflexes in normal adults. Neurology 1980; 30:184–188.
8. Otomo E. The palmomental reflex in the aged. Geriatrics 1965; 20:901–905.
9. Owen G, Mulley GP. The palmomental reflex: a useful clinical sign? J Neurol Neurosurg Psychiatry 2002; 73:113–115.
10. Okuda B, Kodama N, Kawabata K, Tachibana H, Sugita M. Corneomandibular reflex in ALS. Neurology 1999; 52:1699–1703.
11. Mulder DW. Amyotrophic lateral sclerosis: clinical syndrome and differential diagnosis. Med Clin North America 1960; 44:1013–1024.
12. Gubbay SS, Kahana E, Zilber N, Cooper G, Pintov S, Leibowitz Y. Amyotrophic lateral sclerosis. A study of it presentation and prognosis. J Neurol 1985; 232:295–300.
13. Jokelainen M. Amyotrophic lateral sclerosis in Finland II. Clinical characteristics. Acta Neurol Scandinav 1977; 56:194–204.
14. Li T-M, Alberman E, Swash M. Clinical features and associations of 560 cases of motor neuron disease. J Neurol Neurosurg Psychiatry 1990; 53:1043–1045.
15. Caroscio JT, Mulvihill MN, Sterling R, Abrams B. Amyotrophic lateral sclerosis: its natural history. Neurol Clin 1987; 5:1–8.
16. Ringel SP, Murphy JR, Alderson MK, Bryan W, England JD, Miller RG, Petajan JH, Smith SA, Roelofs RI, Ziter F, et al. The natural history of amyotrophic lateral sclerosis. Neurology 1993; 43:1316–1322.
17. Landau WM, Clare MH. The plantar reflex in man, with special reference to some conditions where the extensor response is unexpectedly absent. Brain 1959; 82:321–355.
18. Nardone A, Galante M, Lucas B, Schieppati M. Stance control is not affected by paresis and reflex hyperexcitability: the case of spastic patients. J Neurol Neurosurg Psychiatry 2001; 70:635–643.
19. Traynor BJ, Codd MB, Corr B, Forde C, Frost E, Hardiman OM. Clinical features of amyotrophic lateral sclerosis according to the El Escorial and Airlie House diagnostic criteria: a population-based study. Arch Neurol 2000; 57:1171–1176.
20. Haverkamp LJ, Appel V, Appel SH. Natural history of amyotrophic lateral sclerosis in a database population: validation of a scoring system and a model for survival prediction. Brain 1995; 118:707–719.
21. Reed DM, Kurland LT. Muscle fasciculations in a healthy population. Arch Neurol 1963; 9:363–367.

22. Blexrud MC, Windebank AJ, Daube JR. Long-term follow-up of 121 patients with benign fasciculations. Ann Neurol 1993; 34:622–625.

23. Fleet WS, Watson RT. From benign fasciculations and cramps to motor neuron disease. Neurology 1986; 36:997–998.

24. De Carvalho M, Swash M. Cramps, muscle pain, and fasciculations. Not always benign? Neurology 2004; 63:721–723.

25. Hillel A, Dray T, Miller R, Yorkston K, Konikow N, Strande E, Browne J. Presentation of ALS to the otolaryngologist/head and neck surgeon: getting to the neurologist. Neurology 1999; 53(suppl 5):S22–S25.

26. DePaul R, Abbs JH, Caligiuri M, Gracco VL, Brooks BR. Hypoglossal, trigeminal and facial motoneuron involvement in amyotrophic lateral sclerosis. Neurology 1988; 38: 281–283.

27. DePaul R, Abbs JH. Manifestations of ALS in the cranial motor nerves: dynametric, neuropathologic, and speech motor data. Neurol Clin 1987; 5:231–250.

28. Hillel A, Miller R. Bulbar amyotrophic lateral sclerosis: patterns of progression and clinical management. Head Neck 1989; 11:51–59.

29. Wilbourn AJ, Sweeney PJ. Dissociated wasting of medial and lateral hand muscles with motor neuron disease. Can J Neurol Sci 1994; 21(suppl 2):S9.

30. Wilbourn AJ. The "Split Hand Syndrome." Muscle Nerve 2000; 23:138

31. Katz JS, Wolfe GI, Andersson PB, Saperstein DS, Elliot JL, Nations SP, Bryan WW, Barohn RJ. Brachial amyotrophic diplegia: a slowly progressive motor neuron disorder. Neurology 1999; 53:1071–1076.

32. Cudkowicz ME, Shefner JM, Schoenfeld DA, Brown RH, Johnson H, Qureshi M, Jacobs M, Rothstein JD, Appel SH, Pascuzzi RM, et al. For the Northeast ALS Consortium. A randomized, placebo-controlled trial of topiramate in amyotrophic lateral sclerosis. Neurology 2003; 61:456–464.

33. Marti-Fabregas J, Dourado M, Sanchis J, Miralda R, Pradas J, Illa I. Respiratory function detrioration is not time-linked with upper-limb onset in amyotrophic lateral sclerosis. Acta Neurol Scand 1995; 92:261–264.

34. Fromm GB, Wisdom PJ, Block AJ. Amyotrophic lateral sclerosis presenting with respiratory failure: diaphragmatic paralysis and dependence on mechanical ventilation in two patients. Chest 1977; 71:612–614.

35. Scelsa SN, Yakubov B, Salzman SH. Dyspnea-fasciculation syndrome: early respiratory failure in ALS with minimal motor signs. Amyotroph Later Scler Other Motor Neuron Disord 2002; 3:239–243.

36. Schiffman PL, Belsh JM. Pulmonary function at diagnosis of amyotrophic lateral sclerosis. Chest 1993; 103:508–513.

37. Rowland LP. Motor neuron diseases: the clinical syndromes. In: Mulder DW, ed. The Diagnosis and Treatment of Amyotrophic Lateral Sclerosis. Boston, MA: Houghton Mifflin Professional Publishers, 1980:7–27.

38. Mizutani T, Aki M, Shiozawa R, Unakami M, Nozawa T, Yaima K, Tanabe H, Hara M. Development of ophthalmoplegia in amyotrophic lateral sclerosis during long-term use of respirators. J Neurol Sci 1990; 99:311–319.

39. Harvey DG, Torack RM, Rosenbaum HE. Amyotrophic lateral sclerosis with ophthalmoplegia. A clinicopathologic study. Arch Neurol 1979; 36:615–617.

40. Hayashi H, Kato S, Kawada T, Tsubaki T. Amyotrophic lateral sclerosis: oculomotor function in patients in respirators. Neurology 1987; 37:1431–1432.

41. Kushner MJ, Parrish M, Burke A, Behrens M, Hays AP, Frame B, Rowland LP. Nystagmus in motor neuron disease: clinicopathological study of two cases. Ann Neurol 1984; 16:71–77.

42. Leveille A, Kiernan J, Goodwin JA, Antel J. Eye movements in amyotrophic lateral sclerosis. Arch Neurol 1982; 39:684–686.

43. Jacobs L, Bozian D, Heffner RR, Barron SA. An eye movement disorder in amyotrophic lateral sclerosis. Neurology 1981; 31:1282–1287.

44. Sunohara M, Mukoyama M, Funamoto H, Kamei N, Tomi H, Satoyoshi E. Supranuclear paralysis preventing lid closure in amyotrophic lateral sclerosis. Jpn J Med 1989; 28: 515–519.

45. Kihira T, Yoshida S, Uebayashi Y, Yase Y, Yoshimasu F. Involvement of Onuf's nucleus in ALS: demonstration of intraneuronal conglomerate inclusions and Bunina bodies. J Neurol Sci 1991; 104:119–128.

46. Kihira T, Mizusawa H, Tada J, Namikawa T, Yoshida S, Yase Y. Lewy body-like inclusions in Onuf's nucleus from two cases of sporadic amyotrophic lateral sclerosis. J Neurol Sci 1993; 115:51–57.

47. Kihira T, Yoshida S, Yoshimasu F, Wakayama I, Yase Y. Involvement of Onuf's nucleus in amyotrophic lateral sclerosis. J Neruol Sci 1997; 147:81–88.

48. Bergmann M, Volpel M, Kuchelmeister K. Onuf's nucleus is frequently involved in motor neuron disease/amyotrophic lateral sclerosis. J Neurol Sci 1995; 129:141–146.

49. Lomen-Hoerth C, Murphy J, Langmore S, Kramer JH, Olney RK, Miller B. Are amyotrophic lateral sclerosis patients cognitively normal? Neurology 2003; 60:1094–1097

50. Brooks BR. Natural history of ALS: symptoms, strength, pulmonary function and disability. Neurology 1996; 47(suppl 2):S71–S82.

51. Munsat TL, Andres PL, Finison L, Conlon T, Thibodeau L. The natural history of motoneuron loss in amyotrophic lateral sclerosis. Neurology 1988; 38:409–413.

52. Pradas J, Finison L, Andres PL, Thornell B, Hollander D, Munsat TL. The natural history of amyotrophic lateral sclerosis and the use of natural history controls in therapeutic trials. Neurology 1993; 43:751–755.

53. Hayashi H, Kato S. Total manifestations of amyotrophic lateral sclerosis. ALS in totally locked-in state. J Neurol Sci 1989; 93:19–35.

6

Frontotemporal Dysfunction in Amyotrophic Lateral Sclerosis

Catherine Lomen-Hoerth
University of California, San Francisco, California, U.S.A.

Michael J. Strong
Department of Clinical Neurological Sciences, The University of Western Ontario, and Robarts Research Institute, London, Ontario, Canada

INTRODUCTION AND TERMINOLOGY

Although historically amyotrophic lateral sclerosis (ALS) has been considered to be a disorder restricted to the motor system, an association between dementia and ALS was first noted in the late 1800s and studies dating back to the 1930s documented dementia syndromes in ALS (1). In an extensive review of dementia with either ALS or Parkinson's disease, Hudson concluded that dementia was indeed rarely associated with ALS (2). Subsequently, dementia in association with motor neuron disease (MND) was described by Mitsuyama and colleagues as a presenile dementia with executive dysfunction that later progressed to ALS (3,4). In 1994, the Lund and Manchester groups introduced the term frontotemporal dementia (FTD) with MND, to describe an entity in which MND was associated with ubiquitin-positive, tau-negative inclusions in the hippocampus, entorhinal cortex, and frontal neocortex (5). Until very recently, considerable debate surrounded the incidence, clinical, and neuroimaging features of dementia in ALS, with different terminologies utilized to describe the entity of ALS with frontotemporal lobar degeneration (FTLD). In part, this confusion arose due to the reliance upon Alzheimer's disease (AD)-based dementia criteria for the assessment of cognition in the ALS population (6). These tools emphasize memory and orientation dysfunction, and are insensitive to the most common dementia associated with ALS in which the core features are executive dysfunction, behavioral disorders, and language impairment, reflective of a FTLD.

While the basis of any FTLD is a disease process involving the progressive degeneration of frontal or anterior temporal lobe neurons, the clinical manifestations are varied. The core features, however, are consistent, and include alterations in behavior, executive, and/or language functions with relative sparing of episodic memory. The current clinical diagnostic criteria divide FTLD into three clinical categories: (i) FTD, which is characterized primarily by personality changes, behavioral problems, emotional blunting, and loss of insight, (ii) non-fluent progressive aphasia (NFPA), which presents with non-fluent speech, and (iii) semantic dementia (SD), characterized by fluent speech with significant semantic memory loss. Although these categories may be excessively restrictive when applied to the FTLDs associated with MND and have been expanded to include a variety of neuropathological characteristics, they do more precisely capture patients with cognitive impairments in the setting of ALS (7,8). When ALS patients are studied with a focus on behavioral, executive, and language changes, ALS dementia rates increase (8–10). Thus, while some studies report rates of dementia as low as 3% in sporadic ALS and 15% in familial cases (11), recent studies using neuropsychological measures sensitive to disturbances in frontal lobe function have documented dementia rates as high as 28% to 48% (10,12–14). In a recent study of 100 ALS patients screened for dementia, 50% of those patients with definite ALS were found to have executive function deficits, with most of this subpopulation meeting the Neary research criteria for FTLD (15). In this latter study, ALS patients with FTLD tended to be older, had a family history of dementia, and have a lower FVC when compared to patients without dementia. The converse is also true in that the prevalence of MND is higher in patients with an isolated FTLD than previously believed, with one study reporting 15% meeting the criteria for probable ALS and an additional 36% meeting criteria for possible ALS (16). Hence, the occurrence of FTLD in association with ALS is significant.

The cerebral, neuropsychological, and pathological deficits associated with ALS are increasingly recognized to exist on a spectrum. Many non-demented ALS patients will exhibit deficits on verbal and design fluency (17–19), verbal reasoning, visual attention (17), initiation of random movements (20), and problem solving (21,22). Behaviorally, ALS patients also vary with regards to the severity of their frontotemporal lobar impairment. Many meet full Neary criteria for FTLD (7,23,24); others have mild or moderate levels of behavioral or executive dysfunction, while still others appear normal (25). The difficulty thus rests in classifying the cognitive dysfunction of ALS solely as a dementia. In this sense, the existing terminology fails to reflect the nature of what is believed to be a spectrum, both clinically and neuropathologically. For instance, in an unselected ALS cohort, we observed a spectrum of frontal lobe dysfunction in half of the ALS patients studied (Lomen-Hoerth et al., current submission). The cognitive and behavioral abnormalities varied in severity with 22% meeting Neary criteria for FTLD, 17% demonstrating more subtle behavioral disturbances and 9% exhibiting subtle cognitive dysfunction. While all ALS patients with cognitive and behavioral abnormalities also had frontal atrophy on their MRI scans, a few ALS patients without any cognitive or behavioral abnormalities also had frontal atrophy (Murphy et al., current submission). Given this, and in the absence of an internationally agreed upon terminology for describing the range of frontotemporal deficits that can occur in ALS, we have adopted an approach that attempts to reconcile aspects of both the clinical and neuropathological features of FTLD in association with motor neuron degeneration (Table 1).

CLINICAL FEATURES

As described above, there is a considerable spectrum of cognitive and behavioral deficits reflective of frontotemporal dysfunction among the ALS population. Those ALS patients with cognitive dysfunction (ALSci) have significant impairment in executive function with preservation of long-term memory and spatial skills.

Table 1 Terminology

Terminology	Existing, synonymous terms within the literature	Characteristics
ALS		A pure motor system disorder as defined by the El Escorial criteria; no clinical evidence of frontotemporal dysfunction
ALSci		Deficits in one or more of verbal and design fluency, verbal reasoning, visual attention, initiation of random movements, and problem solving, but insufficient to meet the Neary criteria for FTD
ALSbi		Behavioral or executive dysfunction in association with ALS
ALS-FTD	ALS-dementia (ALS-D), FTD-MND	ALS patient meeting Neary criteria for FTD
FTD-MND-like		Cases of FTLD in which there is neuropathological evidence of motor neuron degeneration, but insufficient to be classified as ALS
ALS-dementia		ALS with dementia, not typical of FTLD

Abbreviations: ALSci, ALS with cognitive impairment; ALSbi, ALS with behavioral impairment; FTD, frontotemporal dementia; FTLD, frontotemporal lobar degeneration.

Affected individuals typically perform worse on tests of phonemic fluency, abstract problem solving, response inhibition, category fluency, and naming, despite there being no group differences in terms of presence of pseudobulbar affect, level of depression, gender, education level, or disease progression. Those ALS patients with neurobehavioral deficits (ALSbi) are more disinhibited and irritable than ALS patients without frontotemporal dysfunction. These findings could not be explained by depression in that if the cognitive or neurobehavioral abnormalities were due simply to clinical depression associated with disease progression, one would have anticipated similar features across all the ALS patients and a correlation with the degree of depression. In fact, no group differences were observed between ALS patients with or without frontotemporal dysfunction when measuring depression by NPI interview or by self-report on the Geriatric Depression Scale.

Given this, it was of considerable interest that both ALS groups (with or without frontotemporal dysfunction) demonstrated cortical atrophy by neuroimaging, including significant bilateral atrophy of the frontal, temporal, and parietal lobes. In addition, the ALS subgroup with frontotemporal dysfunction had significantly more left frontal atrophy, consistent with the observation that several of the five impaired neuropsychological tests have been shown to be reflective of left frontal lobe dysfunction. The degree of atrophy was similar among ALS-FTD and behaviorally and cognitively impaired patients, suggesting that this group as a whole may form a distinct subtype of ALS patients. However, even the cognitively and behaviorally intact ALS patients had greater frontal atrophy than an age-matched control group, suggesting that most ALS patients have frontal lobe degeneration. This critical observation is fundamentally at odds with our conceptualization of ALS as a motor system selective or specific disorder, and hence longitudinal studies are needed to determine whether the subgroup of ALS patients with frontal lobe atrophy in the absence of neuropsychological or behavioral deficits develops cognitive or behavioral dysfunction over time. The shortened lifespan of the ALS patients makes it difficult to know if enough time will pass for those cognitively or behaviorally normal patients to develop abnormalities. Pathology and imaging may be more sensitive tools to measure the extent of extra motor involvement in ALS.

The hypothesis that ALS is associated with a continuum of slowly developing and variable frontal lobe abnormalities is suggested by the large proportions of patients classified as cognitively "uncertain" in prior work (8). Many investigators have reported that neuropsychological performance in ALS patients is not uniform across all patient groups, with some patients performing normally and others abnormally (13,17,24,26). Although many studies have documented the presence of verbal fluency deficits, poor sustained attention, impaired set-shifting, poor response inhibition, and poor problem solving and judgment in cognitively impaired ALS patient (13,19,24,26–28), the same pattern of deficits can be seen in otherwise normal ALS patients, albeit to a milder degree. Whether there is a single etiology for cognitive impairment in ALS or whether there are distinctive subtypes of ALS related to frontal lobe dysfunction is not known. Future pathological and genetic studies are required to answer this question.

NEUROIMAGING CORRELATES

Few studies have analyzed patterns of brain atrophy, metabolism, and blood flow in ALS patients (24,29–33). Most of these studies did not make a distinction between ALS patients with or without cognitive or behavioral impairments. Mild to moderate cerebral atrophy in the parietal, frontal, temporal, occipital lobes, and the insulae is seen in ALS patients (34). The ALS patients have pronounced reductions in rCBF in frontal and anterior temporal cortices, primary motor cortices, and anterior cingulate on PET (24). Similar findings can be observed using the CT cerebral blood flow studies (Fig. 1). Investigations using SPECT reveal that ALS patients have metabolic reduction in the frontal lobes (35). A limited number of investigators did separate those patients with unspecified dementia from non-demented ALS patients or those patients with or without deficits on neuropsychological testing. ALS patients with verbal fluency deficits showed the same but more severe pattern of cerebral blood flow impairment on PET studies (26). PET investigations on ALS patients with dementia also showed decreased uptake in the frontal lobe and additional abnormalities in the temporal, parietal, and right thalamic regions (14,19,20,36). Both SPECT and functional MR imaging studies of ALS patients with neuropsychological dysfunction have abnormal anterior cingulate metabolism compared with cognitively normal ALS patients (33) and have frontal hypoperfusion (12).

The pattern of atrophy in FTLD patients without ALS also involves the frontal and temporal lobes, corresponding to the clinical areas of dysfunction (37,38). New methods for assessing atrophy have been recently developed both with and without the use of standard templates for comparing patients. Voxel-based morphometry (VBM) studies have been used to identify regions associated with atrophy in various neurodegenerative diseases but have not been previously applied in ALS. VBM involves statistical comparisons between groups that are performed on a voxel by voxel basis, and those voxels that are significantly different between the groups

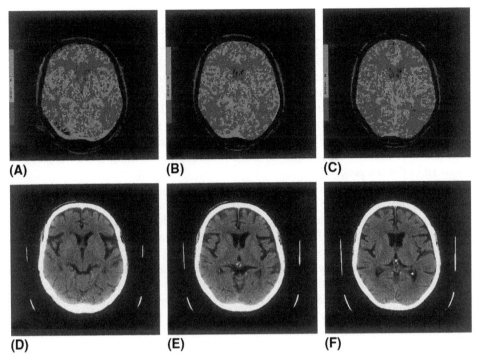

Figure 1 CT cerebral blood flow studies of an individual with both ALS and cognitive impairment consistent with a frontotemporal degeneration (FTD). In these images, black coloration represents the lowest measurable values, while gray is the maximal value. The static CT images (**D–F**) demonstrate a moderate degree of frontotemporal atrophy. The blood flow (**A**) and blood volume (**B**) maps show striking decreases in the frontal and temporal/parietal regions indicated by the predominance of black coloration as compared to the transverse sinuses (*red*) and the thalamic nuclei (*green*). Reductions in the cerebral blood flow are most marked in the anterior frontal regions. However, the decrease in blood volume in these regions is less marked. As a result, the increase in mean transit time is more prominent (**C**). (*See color insert.*)

are noted. Recent comparisons of FTLD patients without ALS compared with normal controls identified atrophy of the right dorsolateral frontal cortex and left premotor cortex in FTD patients, atrophy of the anterior temporal cortex in patients with semantic dementia, and atrophy of the left frontal cortex in NFPA patients (39). Applying new techniques such as these to ALS may help further define ALS subtypes of cognitive impairment.

GENETICS OF FTD AND ALS

An additional constellation of symptoms associated with the ALS was first reported after World War II in Guam among native Chamorros and termed the ALS-parkinsonism dementia complex of Guam (40,41). Close to 50% of the siblings of these patients developed parkinsonism and dementia, 25% developed ALS, and 5% of the siblings had parkinsonism, dementia, and ALS (42,43). Still idiopathic in etiology, the incidence of this syndrome has dropped dramatically, but still occurs in Guam (44). Of relevance to this discussion, the co-occurrence of ALS and FTLD has also been described in families outside Guam as the disinhibition–dementia–parkinsonism–amyotrophy complex (45,46). In the most extensively studied family (Mo family), personality and behavioral changes were the first symptoms in 12 of 13 affected patients (46). Symptom onset was around age 45 years on average and the mean duration to death was 13 years. There was early memory loss, anomia, and poor construction with later involvement of orientation, speech, and calculations. All affected members had rigidity, bradykinesia, and postural instability. On neuropathology, there was atrophy and spongiform change in the frontotemporal cortex, and neuronal loss and gliosis in the substantia nigra and amygdala. Two individuals had anterior horn cell loss and one subject had fasciculations and muscle wasting. There were no Lewy bodies, neurofibrillary tangles (NFT), or amyloid plaques. The genetic locus was linked to chromosome 17q21–22 and a mutation found in the intron adjacent to exon 10 in the tau gene.

More than 13 kindreds of families with FTLD and linkage to chromosome 17 have been described (47,48). Corticospinal disturbances, muscle wasting, and fasciculations were found in four of these 13 families, and there were occasional patients with dysphagia and dysarthria. Mutations in the tau gene, located on chromosome 17, were found in many of these families, particularly those with extrapyramidal disturbances; however, few FTLD-ALS cases are caused by known tau mutations (49–52). Subsequently 25 different mutations have been identified in the tau genes that are presumed to cause FTLD symptoms. Although the findings of ALS have been reported in only a few of the familial FTLD cases, few of the patients have ever been examined by individuals with neuromuscular expertise.

Not all chromosome 17-linked pedigrees with ALS and FTD are clearly linked to the tau gene. An example of this is the recent description of linkage to a non-tau locus on chromosome 17 of "San Francisco Family-B" (Fig. 2) in which several family members had ALS, FTD, or ALS-FTD (53). Approximately half of the living first-degree relatives of affected individuals over the age of 20 had evidence of impaired executive function and frontal atrophy on MRI examination in the absence of reduction of motor unit counts or symptoms of amyotrophy. Of the eight family members with FTD who underwent electrophysiological evaluation, one had definite ALS. An additional patient without FTD but a definitive diagnosis of ALS declined electrophysiological evaluation. Genotyping is underway for all the available microsatellite markers in this region. The multipoint LOD score is 3.5. A series of genes

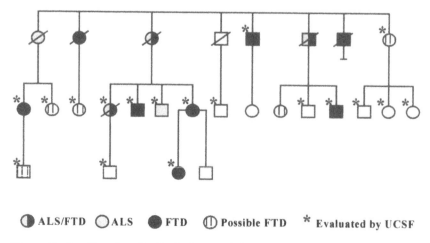

Figure 2 San Fransisco family B. *Source*: Adapted from Ref. 53.

have been found in the chromosome 17 region that could be hypothesized to cause neurodegeneration by affecting clearance of proteins targeted for destruction (53). In addition, another FTLD-ALS family has been localized to chromosome 9q21-q22 (54). Similar to the above family, patients either had ALS, FTLD, or both, suggesting the presence of modifying genes influencing the phenotype of these patients.

There is little evidence to date that sporadic ALS with FTLD degeneration is associated with chromosome 17 linked tau (55).

MOLECULAR NEUROPATHOLOGY OF FRONTOTEMPORAL DEGENERATION IN ALS

As with the clinical phenomenon noted above, a plethora of terms has been applied to the neuropathology of cognitive impairment in the ALS. In part, this is because it is not yet known whether classical ALS with a florid FTD [variably known as ALS-dementia (ALS-D), ALS-FTD, or FTD-MND] is the natural consequence of the more subtle deficits of frontal executive function or behavioral impairment that are the hallmarks of the earliest aspects of frontotemporal dysfunction in ALS. Similarly, it is not entirely clear that the florid FTD described to precede the occurrence of ALS in the Japanese literature is the same process (3,56). Twenty-five percent of the Mitsuyama cases (3) had severe dementia onsetting on average 29 months prior to the onset of ALS. The remaining cases demonstrated more frontal than temporal neuronal loss, slight to moderate levels of dementia symptoms, and a more recent dementia onset of 10 months preceding the ALS symptoms. However, among the North American population, the occurrence of severe dementia antedating the development of motor dysfunction is rarely described, with the more common process seeming to be the development of a frontotemporal syndrome after the onset of motor system degeneration (6).

The natural history studies to define this are just now in process using contemporary clinical, neuropathological, and neurochemical measures. In addition, the recently introduced terminology of FTD-MND-like, meant to include those cases in which the neuropathological features are consistent with a motor neuron degeneration but not diagnostic of ALS, further increases the spectrum of potential overlap among motor neuron degeneration and FTD. At the moment, however, the clinical phenomenology and neuroimaging correlates strongly suggest that ALS with either cognitive dysfunction or behavioral impairment, or with dementia, are reflective of frontotemporal lobar degeneration. The fact that the diagnosis of these entities is based first and foremost upon the clinical and neuropathological evidence of the ALS renders them sufficiently distinct from the remaining FTD syndromes to justify their inclusion as unique categories within the current classification of the FTDs (Table 2).

Classical Neuropathology of ALS

At the core of neuropathology of ALS associated with a FTLD remains the classical neuropathological features of ALS. At minimum, there must be evidence of motor system degeneration that includes the loss of anterior horn cells (AHC), brainstem motor nuclei, and of the descending supraspinal pathways involved in motor function (57). The degenerative process is accompanied by a wide array of neuropathological

Table 2 Molecular Characterization of the Frontotemporal Dementias (FTDs)

	Pathology[c]						Inclusion immunostaining characteristics[d]					Unique features
	Gross frontal & temporal atrophy	Microvacuolar pathology[a]	Hippocampal inclusions[b]	Cytoplasmic inclusions	Intranuclear inclusions	Motor neuron degeneration	Ubiquitin	Tau	PHF-1	α-synuclein	Neurofilament	
1. Pick's Disease	++	++	++	++	?	--	++	++	++	++	++	Pick body, PHF-1 immunoreactive, ballooned neurons more commonly seen
2. Chromosome 17 linked												
a. FTDP-17, tau linked	++	++	++	++	?	+/-	++	++	?	--	--	Frontotemporal dementia with parkinsonism and linkage to tau gene; prominent pathology of substantia nigra (129)
b. FTD-17, non tau linked	++	++	++	++	?	++	+/-	++	?	++	?	San Francisco family A; typical features of ALS; predominantly 4R/0N insoluble tau isoforms; prominent tau and α-synuclein immunoreactive inclusions (53)
3. FTLD (DLDH)	++	++			--	--	--	--	--	--	--	Neuronal loss consistent with FTD pattern
4. FTD-MND (MNDID).												
sporadic	++	++			--	+/-	++	--	--	--	--	FTD with motor neuron disease, not ALS by definition
familial	++	++				++	+/-	--	--	--	--	

										Comment
5. FTLD-U	++	++	++	– –	– –	++	– –	– –	– –	– –	FTLD with ubiquitin only immunoreactive changes; requires the absence of motor neuron degeneration (46)
6. NIBD	++	++	++	+/–	+/–	++	+/–	– –	– –	++	
7. CBD	++	– –	– –	– –	– –	?	++	?	– –	+	Early onset dementia, pyramidal and extrapyramidal signs, achromatic ballooned neurons immunoreactive to phosphorylated neurofilament and αB-crystallin (130,133–135)
8. ALS											
a. ALS	– –	– –	– –	– –	++	++	– –	– –	– –	++	Conforms to El Escorial criteria for diagnosis of ALS; clinical and neuropathological evidence restricted to degeneration of the UMNs and LMNs
b. ALSci	++	++	++	– –	++	++	++	+/–	– –	++	Predominant manifestation of a frontal dysexecutive syndrome
c. ALS-D	++	++	++	– –	++	++	++	+/–	– –	++	Florid characteristics of FTD; lower motor neuron predominant (131,132)
d. ALS/PD of Guam	++	++	++	?	++	++	++	++	++	++	Widespread NFT formation

a Microvacuolar degeneration affecting layers II and III, predominantly temporal and frontal, consistent with a pathological diagnosis of FTD.

b Hippocampal dentate granule cells with intraneuronal ubiquitinated inclusions.

c Pathology commonly observed (++), rarely observed; (+/–), never observed; (– –), not stated or examined for (?).

d Immunostaining for most representative type of inclusions overlap exists amongst individual syndromes.

Abbreviations: CBD, corticobasal degeneration; DLHD, dementia lacking distinct histopathology; FTDP, frontotemporal dementia with parkinsonism; FTLD, frontotemporal lobar degeneration; MNDID, motor neuron disease inclusion dementia; NIBD, neurofilament inclusion body dementia; NFT, neurofibrillary tangle.

features in which both cortical upper motor neurons (UMN) and either brainstem motor neurons or AHC lower motor neurons (LMN) are involved. This is important when one then begins to consider the appropriate classification of the FTLDs in which motor system degeneration is found at autopsy. Among the neuropathological hallmarks of ALS are a variety of intracellular inclusions, the nomenclature of which is somewhat confusing. However, as suggested by Ince and colleagues (58), only three broad groups of inclusions should be considered consistent with the diagnosis of ALS. These include Bunina bodies, ubiquitinated inclusions or skein-like structures, and hyaline conglomerates (59–63).

Bunina bodies, intensely eosinophilic small inclusions (<2–$3 \mu m$), are considered pathognomic of ALS. Ultrastructurally, these aggregates are electron dense masses surrounded by vesicular and tubular structures (64). They are immunoreactive with cystatin C (65), and to date, have not been seen in disorders other than ALS. They are not, however, seen in all cases of ALS. The second type of inclusion consists of ubiquitinated inclusions that may take the form of either serpinginous skein-like structures or intensely immunoreactive intracellular aggregates (66,67). When the latter are discrete and surrounded by a clear halo, they have been termed "Lewy body-like inclusions," a terminology which is misleading in that these structures do not contain α-synuclein–a key component of true Lewy bodies of Parkinson's disease. Ultrastructurally, ubiquitin immunoreactive skeins are composed primarily of bundles of filaments, 10 to 15 nm in diameter, that are believed to be the aggregation of ubiquitin with protein targeted for degradation (68,69). The final grouping of intracellular aggregates are neurofilamentous in origin and appear either as densely argentophilic masses, replacing much of the perikaryal contents, or as glassy hyaline cytoplasmic clearings seen on routine hematoxylin and eosin staining. Both are intensely immunoreactive to neurofilament proteins, but particularly to the highly phosphorylated high molecular weight neurofilament.

In addition to these neuropathological features of motor system degeneration and intracellular inclusion formation, microglial proliferation and activation is a prominent component of ALS, as is astrocytic gliosis. Not unexpectedly, degenerating motor tracts (i.e., the corticospinal tracts) contain an abundant number of large, protoplasmic microglial cells, almost certainly involved in the clearance of myelin debris of the degenerating tract. Microglial proliferation is prominent in the regions of the degenerating motor neuron and may take the appearance of satellitosis in which the motor neuron is surrounded and appearing to be engulfed by microglial (by definition >5 microglia per neuron). In this scenario, it has been postulated that the microglial cell is playing a more direct role in mediating neuronal injury (70).

Neuropathology of Frontotemporal Degeneration in ALS

In addition to these typical features of ALS, the neuropathological characteristics of both frontotemporal lobar degeneration concurrent with ALS is typical of that observed among the larger grouping of FTD (71,72). This includes the presence of spongiform degeneration in frontal and precentral gyrus cortical layers II and III with diffuse subcortical gliosis (3,72–84). In addition to reduced neuronal density in the anterior cingulate gyrus, neuronal loss is also evident in the substantia nigra and amygdala (85). Activated microglia, readily detected with HLA DR3 immunostaining are also evident throughout the affected neocortex. Ubiquitin immunoreactive dystrophic neurites are evident in the extramotor cortices, but with a predominance of involvement in the frontal, temporal, and hippocampal cortex. While ubiquitin immunoreactive intraneuronal inclusions are often observed within the dentate granule cells, the superficial frontal and temporal cortical layers, and in the entorhinal cortex, these are not specific to cognitively impaired ALS cases and can be observed in other forms of neurodegeneration (83,86–88). However, these ubiquitin immunoreactive inclusions are unique in lacking immunoreactivity to either microtubule associated protein tau or α-synuclein (3,83,86,87,89,90). Neuropathological criteria for the diagnosis of ALS-D, encapsulating many of these features, have been recently proposed (Table 3) (72).

As will be seen, these are best viewed as core features. The key issue remains the extent to which alterations in tau protein metabolism, ubiquitous among the remaining FTLDs, also occurs in cognitively impaired patients with ALS. It is clear, however, that it can no longer be stated that tau-immunoreactive structures are absent in ALS. Noda et al. (73) first described three cases of late adult on-setting ALS in which tau immunoreactive thread-like structures were observed in the neuropil and in glial cells (as coiled bodies) in the hippocampus, parahippocampal gyrus, and amygdala. In two of the three cases, the neuropil and glial tau immunoreactive structures occurred in the absence of pathology typical of Alzheimer's disease. These features can also be seen in cognitively intact ALS patients, although considerably less extensive than observed in cognitively impaired ALS cases, consistent with the previous hypothesis based on neuroimaging data that ALS and ALS with frontotemporal lobar degeneration may form a disease continuum (56,71,91–94).

In a detailed neuropathological study of cognitively impaired ALS patients, the authors have observed that tau immunoreactive intracellular aggregates are present in both astrocytes and oligodendroglial cells, in addition to those observed in degenerating neurons (Fig. 3). While the presence of tau-immunoreactive neuronal positive inclusions was not restricted to cognitively impaired ALS cases, but was also observed in cognitively intact patients, in the former tau immunostaining was more intense and more likely to replace the cytoplasm. Characteristics of the cognitively

Table 3 Core Neuropathological Criteria for the Diagnosis of ALS with Frontotemporal Lobar Degeneration

---

Gross changes
  Mild to moderate frontotemporal cortical atrophy
Microscopic changes in the frontotemporal cortices
  Mild to moderate neuronal loss and gliosis, affecting predominantly layers II and III with spongiosis
  Subcortical gliosis of the frontotemporal lobe
  Degeneration of the substantia nigra and amygdala
Motor neuron system
  Involvement of both upper and lower motor neurons including the hypoglossal nuclei, consistent with ALS
Immunohistochemical features
  Ubiquitin-positive and tau- and α-synuclein negative intraneuronal inclusions and dystrophic neurites in both neurons and extra-motor small neurons of the frontotemporal cortices, amygdala, striatum, and hippocampal dentate granular cells
  Tau immunoreactive fibrillary pathology in frontotemporal cortex (neuronal, astrocytic, extraneuronal neuritic threads)

Source: Modified from Ref. 72.

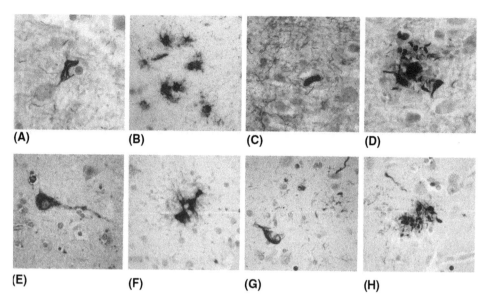

Figure 3 Tau protein aggregation characteristic of frontotemporal lobar degeneration in ALSci. Archival, paraffin-embedded tissue taken at the level of the anterior cingulate gyrus, was either stained with the Gallyas-Braak silver stain sensitive to tau aggregation (**A–D**) or with a mouse monoclonal antibody recognizing phosphorylated tau protein (**E–H**). Tau aggregation was observed within neurons (**A,E**), astrocytes (**B,F**), as extraneuronal neuritic threads (**C,G**), and as aggregations with the appearance of plaques (**D,H**). In the latter, no evidence of B-amyloid deposition was found (data not shown) and the density of such plaques was always less than that observed in Alzheimer's disease (magnification before reproduction 40 times). (*See color insert.*)

impaired ALS cases was the presence of intense tau immunoreactivity within neurons in layers II and III. This latter finding was reminiscent of the distribution of NFT in Guamanian ALS/parkinsonism–dementia (95). Both the cognitively impaired and cognitively intact ALS cases possessed tau-immunoreactive astrocytic inclusions within cortical layer I, deep cortical layers, and subcortical white matter. Control cases were free of tau pathology. We also observed astrocytic proliferation, a feature previously described by others (96–98). In addition to these findings, and unique to the cognitively impaired ALS patients, extraneuronal tau-immunoreactive aggregates were observed. These were the most evident utilizing the Gallyas-Braak silver staining, sensitive to aberrant tau deposition (99), and assumed a number of morphologies, including curvilinear neuropil threads, rare argyrophilic granules, and dense rounded aggregates with irregular fibrillary margins.

The presence of ubiquitin immunoreactive intraneuronal inclusions has been considered by some to be pathognomic of frontotemporal degeneration in ALS. Such inclusions are readily observed within the dentate gyrus, and generally are large, crescentic, and ubiquitin immunoreactive aggregates. Recently, intranuclear ubiquitin immunoreactive aggregates have been described in cases of FTD with motor neuron degeneration, predominantly but not exclusively in the familial FTD variants (100,101). Typically, however, clear documentation of ALS has not been provided, and in many cases, the classification of FTD-MND type is applied. Thus, the role of intranuclear ubiquitin immunoreactive inclusions in the diagnostic armatarium for frontotemporal lobar degeneration in ALS remains to be defined.

ALS, FTD, AND THE DEGENERATIVE TAUOPATHIES

The evidence cited above raises the distinct possibility that the frontotemporal degeneration of ALS is a tauopathy (94). The prototypical example of abnormal tau metabolism in ALS is that of the ALS/parkinsonism–dementia complex of the western Pacific. As described above, this variant of ALS remains as the only known hyperendemic variant of ALS (102–105). An intriguing aspect of the western Pacific variant of ALS is the co-occurrence of the neurofilamentous pathology of ALS with NFT morphologically identical to those observed in Alzheimer's disease (106–110). Severe cortical atrophy and widespread NFT formation are hallmarks of this disorder, with the NFTs bearing the immunohistochemical and ultrastructural characteristics of Alzheimer disease NFTs (106,107,111–113). In contrast to Alzheimer's disease, the hyperphosphorylated, highly insoluble, tau triplet protein (the fundamental constituent of the NFT) is more widely distributed in both cortical and subcortical structures in the western Pacific variant of ALS (114). Lewy-like bodies containing accumulations of α-synuclein and typical of those observed in Parkinson's disease are also observed predominantly with neurons of the amygdala (115,116).

Tau Metabolism

The primary function of tau protein is to bind to the microtubules and to both promote their assembly and enhance their stability in a polymerized state. Hyperphosphorylated tau, as observed in a number of tauopathies, is a highly insoluble protein that will polymerize in the somatodendritic neuronal compartment and form NFTs. Six alternatively spliced tau isoforms exist in the adult human nervous system, containing either three (3R) or four (4R) microtubule-binding domains, with the additional microtubule-binding domain encoded by exon 10 (E10) (Fig. 4). Mutations in the tau gene appear to cause tau protein accumulations by at least two broad mechanisms (117). In one group, intronic mutations adjacent to the $3'$ end of the E10 can lead to an increased expression of the E10 encoded domain, producing a predominance of the 4R tau isoform and thus a greater predominance of the four microtubule-binding domain tau isoforms. An example of such a mutation is the $^{N}279^{K}$ mutation that strengthens the expression of an exon-splicing enhancer, leading to increased E10 expression. In contrast, the $\Delta280^{K}$ mutation results in a loss of the exon-splicing enhancer and a loss of E10 expression, leading to a predominance of the 3R tau isoform (with less avid microtubule-binding). Within E10 is another regulatory element, the "exon splicing silencer," which is abolished with the $^{L}284^{L}$ mutation and which thus leads to increased E10 expression. Intronic mutations immediately $5'$ adjacent to E10 also appear to result in an increased E10 expression. In the second group of tau mutations, the mutations are associated with abnormalities of tau protein function leading to a reduction in tau affinity and binding to microtubules (e.g., $^{G}272^{V}$, $^{V}337^{M}$, and $^{R}406^{W}$ mutations).

Thus, tau mutations can give rise to a number of specific effects on tau metabolism, including impairments in tau function, the promotion of tau filament formation, or perturbations in tau gene splicing (47). The latter can give rise to a number of unique tau aggregates. The neuropathological observation of prominent intracellular aggregation of tau proteins is the predominant feature that links together the degenerative tauopathies, including Alzheimer's disease. This recognition that different perturbations in tau metabolism can give rise to seemingly unique tau pathology

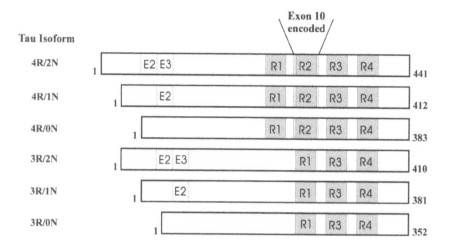

18 - amino acid microtubule binding repeats

Figure 4 Six human tau isoforms are generated by alternative splicing of the tau gene which includes 16 exons. Alternative splicing of the E2, E3, and E10 exons produce the six isoforms, with E10 encoding an 18 amino acid microtubule-binding repeat. The isoforms range from 352 to 441 amino acids in length.

has led to the concept that a "signature" tau neuropathology can be developed for the individual tauopathies. For example, corticobasal degeneration (CBD), a disorder characterized by progressive motor dysfunction with postural abnormalities, can be characterized by the deposition of hyperphosphorylated tau as filamentous inclusions in neurons and glia, with 4R-tau as the predominant isoform (118). The sarkosyl-insoluble tau fraction in both the gray and white matter contained predominantly the hyperphosphorylated 4R-tau isoforms, with the isoforms recognized by the monoclonal antibody AT8 (recognizing phosphorylation at Ser-202/Thr-205) specifically increased in the white matter. This is in distinction to Pick's disease, an uncommon FTD marked by prominent frontotemporal degeneration clinically, and neuropathologically by discrete frontal and anterior temporal cortical atrophy with achromatic neurons (Pick cells) and intraneuronal argentophilic inclusions (Pick bodies). The biochemical "signature" of this tauopathy is the accumulation of both 3R and 4R-tau isoforms within both gray and white matter sarkosyl-insoluble fraction (119). At the level of the immunohistochemical analysis of the intraneuronal aggregates, both CBD and progressive supranuclear palsy (PSP) can be differentiated from Pick's disease by the observation of 4R-tau immunostaining of intraneuronal aggregates, a feature not observed in Pick's neuronal aggregates (although observed within glial aggregates) (120). A similar process can be adopted for a number of the remaining tauopathies, including argryophilic grain disease, dementia lacking distinctive histopathology (DLDH), and AD (121–124).

FTD Associated with Motor Neuron Degeneration

What to do then with the cases of FTD in which motor neuron degeneration is observed at neuropathological examination? The FTDs are a heterogeneous group of diseases, sharing common features of frontotemporal lobar degeneration (Table 1). The difficulty of defining ALS within the context of the currently accepted terminology of the FTDs occurs at several levels. First, within the rubric of the FTDs are multiple disease entities with considerable overlap in neuropathological features—in many instances, it is the extent to which such features are present or absent that differentiates one entity from another. Second, the concept of motor neuron degeneration is used extremely liberally such that the reader is often left uncertain as to the extent to which a neuropathological or clinical diagnosis of ALS is appropriate, as opposed to a simple amyotrophy of isolated LMN syndrome. Third, the use of the terminology of MND within the classification of the FTDs is less concise than might have occurred if the initial crafting of terminologies was undertaken by those with a focus on the peripheral nervous system, rather than those with a primary focus on cognition. Finally, the classification of the FTDs is a work in evolution, modified by newer neurochemical studies, and by newer immunohistochemical markers. To highlight this, in a recent analysis of 29 cases derived from a brain bank which had been previously classified neuropathologically as FTD, the majority of cases were nontauopathies, with the most common diagnosis that of FTLD with ubiquitin-only immunoreactive neuronal changes (125). Other diagnoses included Pick's disease, FTD with parkinsonism linked to chromosome 17 (FTDP-17), FTLD (also known as dementia lacking distinctive histopathology—DLDH), FTLP with MND (FTLD-MND), and neurofilament inclusion body disease (NIBD).

The finding of motor neuron ubiquitin-immunoreactive aggregates in the presence of the pathological features of a FTD but in the absence of overt clinical features of MND has led to the concept of a unique FTD termed "motor neuron disease inclusion dementia" (MNDID) (126). Of interest, has been the observation of ubiquitinated intranuclear inclusions (Ub-INI) in the striatum of patients with familial MNDID only. Ub-INI had previously been described in nine cases of MNDID, none of whom had ALS (127). Of these, one has subsequently developed ALS. It is not clear whether this is the same entity as described by MacKenzie and Feldman in which intranuclear ubiquitin immunoreactive inclusions were observed in the majority of familial FTD MND-like cases (101). It is likely, however, that these inclusions can be seen in both ALS-D and FTDs with motor neuron degeneration not typical of ALS (the FTD-MND-like rubric) (100).

A conceptually important and novel entity is the recent description of FTD with NIBD. The index case demonstrated features of florid FTD, both clinically and neuropathologically, with MND, with tau-negative, neurofilament immunoreactive inclusions (128). Although some of the inclusions had the morphology of Pick bodies, they were not immunoreactive to PHF-1 immunostaining. Unfortunately, the autopsy was limited to the brain only and hence the extent to which this overlaps with ALS or ALS-D remains uncertain. It is likely, however, based on the observation of anterior horn neuronal loss with neurophagia in the upper cervical cord that was available for examination, that this was indeed a crossover case of FTD with ALS in which neurofilament aggregates outside of the motor neurons were evident.

FRONTOTEMPORAL DYSFUNCTION IN ALS: CLINICAL IMPACT AND PROGNOSIS

While the preceding discussion has focused on the molecular and neuropathological consequences of frontotemporal degeneration in ALS, this entity is also of clinical relevance. Cognitive and behavioral impairments in ALS may have a significant impact on survival. Over the past two years we have carefully tracked our 100 patient ALS cohort described above, collecting clinical information and survival data. Several patients underwent additional or repeat testing. Twenty-eight of the original 100 patients now meet research criteria for FTLD based on neurobehavioral interviews and formal neuropsychological testing. Nineteen patients are borderline in their behavior or language function and have not consented to detailed evaluation, and 53 patients are not suspected to have cognitive abnormalities based on word generation testing, behavioral observation, or, in nearly half, formal evaluation. Patients with a bulbar onset were more than twice as likely to have received an FTLD diagnosis, 14 of 30 (47%), as compared with only 14 of 69 (20%) of the limb onset patients receiving a dementia diagnosis (the twenty-third patient had respiratory onset of ALS and was not included in this analysis). Additionally among patients with obvious upper motor neuron signs, 23 of 68 (34%) had FTLD, in contrast to only 5 of 32 (16%) having FTLD in those with only soft upper motor neuron signs. Family history of a neurodegenerative disease increased the risk of ALS-FTLD, suggesting that those patients with ALS-FTLD may be more likely to have genetic influences over the disease than ALS only patients.

The comorbid diagnosis of FTLD may be associated with an adverse effect on survival. The median survival from symptom onset of ALS was two years four months for those with FTLD and three years three months for the 53 with normal executive and behavioral function. The 28 patients with ALS-FTLD had a significantly shorter survival than the 53 ALS patients with normal executive and behavioral function (log rank $\chi^2 = 5.14$, $p < 0.03$). To test our clinical impression that poor compliance with treatment recommendations by ALS-FTLD patients may be a factor influencing shorter survival, we set criteria for compliance with non-invasive positive pressure ventilation (NPPV) and percutaneous endoscopic gastrostomy (PEG) recommendations and determined the frequency of compliance among the ALS and ALS-FTLD patients based on retrospective chart review. Compliance with recommendations for NPPV occurred in fewer patients with ALS-FTLD (5 of 18 or 28%) than in patients with ALS and normal behavioral function (14 of 23 or 61%), a significant difference ($z = 2.22$, one-tail $p < 0.02$). Similarly compliance with recommendations for PEG occurred in fewer patients with ALS-FTLD (4 of 16, or 25%) than in patients with ALS and normal behavioral function (8 of 12, or 67%), a significant difference ($z = 2.01$, one-tail $p < .03$). However, bulbar onset and older age at onset are also associated with shorter survival and these two characteristics are more common in ALS-FTLD than in ALS alone, so larger cohorts of both groups are necessary to distinguish the effects of FTLD, bulbar onset, age, and compliance on survival.

Cognitive and behavioral involvement in ALS has significant caregiver implications in addition to implications regarding disease mechanism discussed in detail later in this chapter. For example, caregivers are likely to benefit from hearing that their loved-ones' personality and behavior changes have a biological basis. In addition, caregivers require education in how to manage behavior change, plan for support services for patients, and cope with increase dependency as patients are less able to participate in making judgments about their care. Caregivers should be alerted to identify those patients who have exhibited the classic depression, anxiety, and disinhibition symptoms of early frontotemporal dementia or the language impairment of semantic dementia or progressive non-fluent aphasia several years prior to their ALS onset. This group is more likely to have the more severe dementia that will complicate their care and are likely to require psychiatric medication and behavior management consultation to provide adequate care.

CONCLUSIONS

The premise that cognitive and behavioral dysfunction in ALS is rare can no longer be substantiated. The critical issue, however, and one which engenders a great deal of controversy, is whether cognitive impairment is a ubiquitous accompaniment of ALS. At this point in time, there is no evidence that would support such a statement, and hence one is left considering ALS as a syndrome in which ALS may exist as a unique entity reflective as a degenerative process of the motor system, and in which degeneration of the frontotemporal lobar type can occur. When present, the latter can behave in a florid fashion, bearing all of the hallmarks of a frontotemporal degeneration (ALS-FTD). In its more subtle manifestations, either a frontal dysexecutive syndrome or behavioral syndrome may occur, or both. It is intriguing, however, that frontal, temporal, and parietal cortical atrophy, observed on neuroimaging, and disproportionate to that observed in age-matched controls, are seen across all ALS patients. The observation of alterations in tau solubility also cut across boundaries of cognitively intact and cognitively impaired ALS patients, being present in approximately 75% of all ALS patients. This latter number is concordant with more recent studies of the prevalence of either cognitive dysfunction in the ALS population, in which approximately 75% of all ALS patients have some degree of cognitive dysfunction (Appel, personal observation). Both of these data suggest that the "pure" phenotype of ALS in which the disease process is restricted to the motor neurons is in fact rare, and that the more common variant is a more complicated phenotype in which the neurodegeneration extends well outside of the boundaries of the motor system. There are biological implications to such a conclusion. There seems little doubt that classical ALS, in addition to the myriad of neurochemical abnormalities that are currently being catalogued, can be considered a disorder of abnormal protein aggregation (61). Having accepted this premise, it is only left to determine whether some variants of ALS then fall into the broader categorization of the degenerative tauopathies in which the constellation of motor system degeneration (as opposed to only LMN degeneration), frontotemporal lobar degeneration, neurofilamentous aggregates and ubiquitin immunoreactive aggregates marks it as a unique entity or whether ALS fits within the wider spectrum of the FTLDs. The most recent consensus terminology for the FTDs is already out of date, and does not speak to the issue of ALS and FTD. Placing ALS within this spectrum will likely require advances in our understanding of the biochemistry of the tauopathy of ALS.

Finally, consensus terminology is required in order to bring some order to what is becoming an increasingly complex picture. Approaching the same entity with an interest in cognition yields a terminology reflective of a FTD, with little critical emphasis on the nature of the motor neuron degeneration. Approaching as a peripheral nerve disorder, the FTD tends to be loosely described. It is also not clear that the phenomenology is appropriately described. Is the frontotemporal dysexecutive syndrome with verbal praxis deficits most commonly observed in the ALS population properly considered a FTD, or should the latter be reserved for those with a florid frontotemporal syndrome typical of the FTDs? Answering all of these issues will be the focus of much discussion in the immediate future.

REFERENCES

1. Neary D, Snowden JS, Mann DM. Cognitive change in motor neurone disease /amyotrophic lateral sclerosis MND/ALS. J Neurol Sci 2000; 180:15–20.
2. Hudson AJ. Amyotrophic lateral sclerosis and its association with dementia, parkinsonism and other neurological disorders: A review. Brain 1981; 194:217–247.
3. Mitsuyama Y. Presenile dementia with motor neuron disease in Japan: clinico-pathological review of 26 cases. J Neurol Neurosurg Psychiat 1984; 47:953–959.
4. Mitsuyama Y, Takamiya S. Presenile dementia with motor neuron disease in Japan. A new entity? Arch Neurol 1979; 36:592–593.
5. Brun AEB, Gustafson L, Passant U, Mann DM, Neary D, Snowden JS. Consensus statement: clinical and neuropathological criteria for frontotemporal dementia. Lund and Manchester groups. J Neurol Neurosurg Psychiat 1994; 57:416–418.
6. Strong MJ, Grace GM, Orange JB, Leeper HA. Cognition, language and speech in amyotrophic lateral sclerosis: A review. J Clin Exp Neuropsych 1996; 18(2):291–303.
7. Neary D. Dementia of frontal lobe type. J Am Geriatr Soc 1990; 38:71–72.
8. Barson FP, Kinsella GJ, Ong B, Mathers SE. A neuropsychological investigation of dementia in motor neurone disease MND. J Neurol Sci 2000; 180(107):113.
9. Snowdon DA, Kemper SJ, Mortimer JA, Greiner LH, Wekstein DR, Markesbery WR. Linguistic ability in early life and cognitive function and Alzheimer's disease in late life. Findings from the Nun Study. JAMA 1996; 275(7):528–532.
10. Rakowicz WP, Hodges JR. Dementia and aphasia in motor neuron disease: an under-recognised association? J Neurol Neurosurg Psychiat 1998; 65:881–889
11. Hudson AJ. Amyotrophic lateral sclerosis/parkinsonism/dementia: clinico-pathological correlations relevant to Guamanian ALS/PD. Can J Neurol Sci 1991; 18(387):389.
12. Portet F, Cadilhac C, Touchon J, Camu W. Cognitive impairment in motor neuron disease with bulbar onset. ALS and other motor neuron disorders 2001; 2:23–29.
13. Massman PJ, Sims J, Cooke N, Haverkamp LJ, Appel V, Appel SH. Prevalence and correlates of neuropsychological deficits in amyotrophic lateral sclerosis. J Neurol Neurosurg Psychiat 1996; 61:450–455.
14. Abe K, Fujimura H, Toyooka K, Sakoda S, Yorifuji S, Yanagihara T. Cognitive function in amyotrophic lateral sclerosis. J Neurol Sci 1997; 148:95–100.
15. Lomen-Hoerth C, Murphy J, Langmore S, Kramer JH, Olney RK, Miller B. Are amyotrophic lateral sclerosis patients cognitively normal? Neurology 2003; 60:1094–1097
16. Lomen-Hoerth C, Anderson T, Miller B. The overlap of amyotrophic lateral sclerosis and frontotemporal dementia. Neurology 2002; 59:1077–1079.
17. Gallassi R, Montagna P, Ciardulli C, Lorusso S, Mussato V, Stracciari A. Cognitive impairment in motor neurone disease. Acta Neurol Scand 1985; 71:480–484.
18. Gallassi R, Montagna P, Morreale A, Lorusso S, Tinuper P, Daidone R, Lugaresi E. Neuropsychological, electroencephalogram and brain computed tomography findings in motor neuron disease. Eur Neurol 1989; 29:115–120.
19. Ludolph AC, Langen KJ, Regard M, Herzog H, Kemper B, Kuwert T, Bottger IG, Feinendegen L. Frontal lobe function in amyotrophic lateral sclerosis: A neuropsychological and positron emission tomography study. Acta Neurol Scand 1992; 85:81–89.
20. Abrahams S, Leigh PN, Kew JJM, Goldstein LH, Lloyd CML, Brooks DJ. A positron emission tomography study of frontal lobe function verbal fluency in amyotrophic lateral sclerosis. J Neurol Sci 1995; 129(suppl):44–46.
21. David AS. Neuropsychological measures in patients with amyotrophic lateral sclerosis. Acta Neurol Scand 1987; 75:284.
22. Abrahams S, Goldstein LH, Lloyd CM, Brooks DJ, Leigh PN. Cognitive deficits in non-demented amyotrophic lateral sclerosis patients: a neuropsychological investigation. J Neurol Sci 1995; 129(suppl):54–55.
23. Neary D, Snowden JS, Northen B, Goulding P. Dementia of the frontal lobe type. J Neurol Neurosurg Psychiat 1988; 51:353–361.

24. Talbot PR, Goulding PJ, Lloyd JJ, Snowden JS, Neary D, Testa HJ. Inter-relation between "classic" motor neuron disease and frontotemporal dementia: neuropsychological and single photon emission computed tomography study. J Neurol Neurosurg Psychiat 1995; 58:541–547.

25. Cavalleri F, DeRenzi E. Amyotrophic lateral sclerosis with dementia. Acta Neurol Scand 1994; 89:391–394.

26. Kew JJM, Goldstein LH, Leigh PN, Abrahams S, Cosgrave N, Passingham RE, Frackowiak RSJ, Brooks DJ. The relationship between abnormalities of cognitive function and cerebral activation in amyotrophic lateral sclerosis. Brain 1993; 116:1399–1423.

27. Abe K, Takanashi M, Watanabe Y, Tanaka H, Fujita N, HirabukI N, Yanagihara T. Decrease in N-acetyoaspartate/creatine ratio in the motor area and the frontal lobe in amyotrophic lateral sclerosis. Neuroradiology 2001; 43:537–541.

28. Hartikainen P, Helkala EL, Soininen H, Riekkinen P Sr. Cognitive and memory deficits in untreated Parkinson's disease and amyotrophic lateral sclerosis patients: a comparative study. J Neurol Transm Park Dement Sect 1993; 6:127–137.

29. Ohnishi T, Hoshi H, Nagamachi S, Futami S, Watanabe K, Mitsuyama Y. Regional cerebral blood flow study with ^{123}I-IMP in patients with degenerative dementia. Am J Neuroradiol 1991; 12:513–520.

30. Ludolph AC, Elger CE, Böttger IW, Kuttig AG, Lottes G, Brune GG. N-isopropyl-p-^{123}I-amphetamine single photon emission computer tomography in motor neuron disease. Eur Neurol 1989; 29:255–260.

31. Waldemar G, Varstrup S, Jensen TS, Johnsen A, Boysen G. Focal reductions in cerebral blood flow in amyotrophic lateral sclerosis: A [^{99m}Tc]-d,l-HMPAO SPECT study. J Neurol Sci 1992; 107:19–28.

32. Dalakas MC, Hatazawa J, Brooks RA, Di Chiro G. Lowered cerebral glucose utilization in amyotrophic lateral sclerosis. Ann Neurol 1987; 22:580–586.

33. Strong MJ, Grace GM, Orange JB, Leeper HA, Menon R, Aere C. A prospective study of cognitive impairment in ALS. Neurology 1999; 53:1665–1670.

34. Poloni M, Capitani E, Mazzini L, Ceroni M. Neuropsychological measures in amyotrophic lateral sclerosis and their relationship with CT scan-assessed cerebral atrophy. Acta Neurol Scand 1986; 74:257–260.

35. Abe K. Autosomal dominant ALS. Ryoikibetsu Shokogun Shirizu 1999; 27(2):320–322.

36. Kew JJM, Leigh PN, Playford ED, Passingham RE, Goldstein LH, Frackowiak RSJ, Brooks DJ. Cortical function in amyotrophic lateral sclerosis. Brain 1993; 116:655–680.

37. Poloni M, Patrini C, Rocchelli B, Rindi G. Thiamin monophosphate in the CSF of patients with amyotrophic lateral sclerosis. Arch Neurol 1982; 39:507–509.

38. Kew JJ, Leigh N. Dementia with motor neurone disease. Baillieres Clin Neurol 1992; 1:611–626.

39. Rosen HJ, Gorno-Tempini ML, Goldman WP, Perry RJ, Schuff N, Weiner M, Feiwell R, Kramer JH, Miller BL. Patterns of brain atrophy in frontotemporal dementia and semantic dementia. Neurology 2002; 58:198–208.

40. Hirano A, Kurland LT, Krooth RS, Lessell S. Parkinsonism-dementia complex, an endemic disease on the island of Guam. I. Clinical features. Brain 1961; 84:642–661.

41. Hirano A, Malamud N, Kurland LT. Parkinsonism-dementia complex, an endemic disease on the island of Guam. II. Pathological features. Brain 1961; 84:662–679.

42. Plato CC, Reed DM, Elizan TS, Kurland LT. Amyotrophic lateral sclerosis/Parkinsonism-dementia complex of Guam. IV. Familial and genetic studies. Am J Hum Genet 1967; 19:617–632.

43. McGeer PL, Schwab C, McGeer EG, Haddock RL, Steele JC. Familial nature and continuing morbidity of the amyotrophic lateral sclerosis-parkinsonism dementia complex of Guam. Neurology 1997; 47:400–409.

44. Garruto RM, Yanagihara R, Gajdusek DC. Disappearance of high-incidence amyotrophic lateral sclerosis and parkinsonism-dementia on Guam. Neurology 1985; 35: 193–198.

45. Gilbert JJ, Kish SJ, Chang L-J, Morito C, Shannak K, Hornykiewicz O. Dementia, parkinsonism and motor neuron disease: neurochemical and neuropathological correlates. Ann Neurol 1988; 24:688–691.

46. Lynch T, Sano M, Marder KS, Bell KL, Foster NL, Defendini RF, Sima AAF, Keohane C, Nygaard TG, Fahn S, Mayeux R, Rowland LP, Wilhelmsen KC. Clinical characteristics of a family with chromosome 17-linked disinhibition-dementia-parkinsonism-amyotrophy complex. Neurology 1994; 44:1878–1884.

47. Lee VMY, Goedert M, Trojanowski JQ. Neurodegenerative tauopathies. Ann Rev Neurosci 2001; 24:1121–1159.

48. Foster NL, Wilhelmsen K, Sima AAF, Jones MZ, D'Amato CJ, Gilman S, and conference participants. Frontotemporal dementia and parkinsonism linked to chromosome 17: A consensus conference. Ann Neurol 1997; 41:706–715.

49. Clark LN, Poorkaj P, Wszolek Z, Geschwind DH, Nassreddine ZS, Miller B, Li D, Payami H, Awert F, Markopoulou K, Andreadis A, D'Souza I, Lee VM, Reed L, Trojanowski JQ, Zhukareva V, Bird T, Schellenberg G, Wilhelmsen KC. Pathogenic implications of mutations in the tau gene in pallido-ponto-nigral degeneration and related neurodegenerative disorders linked to chromosome 17. Proc Natl Acad Sci USA 1998; 95(22):13,103–13,107.

50. Hutton M, Lendon CL, Rizzu P, Baker M, Froelich S, Houlden H, Pickering-Brown SM, Chakraverty S, Isaacs A, Grover A, Hackett J, Adamson J, Lincoln S, Dickson D, Davies P, Petersen RC, Stevens M, de Graaff E, Wauters E, van Baren J, Hillebrand M, Joosse M, Kwon JM, Nowotny P, Heutink P. Association of missense and 5″-splice-site mutations in tau with the inherited dementia FTDP-17. Nature 1998; 393(6686): 702–705.

51. Spillantini MG, Goedert M. Tau protein pathology in neurodegenerative diseases. TINS 1998; 21:428–433.

52. Poorkaj P, Bird TD, Wijsman E, Nemens E, Garruto RM, Anderson L, Andreadis A, Wiederholt WC, Raskind M, Schellenberg GD. Tau is a candidate gene for chromosome 17 frontotemporal dementia. Ann Neurol 1998; 43(6):815–825.

53. Wilhelmsen KC, Forman MS, Rosen HJ, Alving LI, Goldman J, Feiger J, Lee JV, Segall SK, Kramer JH, Lomen-Hoerth C, Rankin KP, Johnson J, Feiler HS, Weiner MW, Lee VMY, Trojanowski JQ, Miller BL. 17q-Linked frontotemporal dementia-amyotrophic lateral sclerosis without tau mutations with tau and α-synuclein inclusions. Arch Neurol 2004; 61:398–406.

54. Hosler BA, Siddique T, Sapp PC, Sailor W, Huang MC, Daube JR, Nance M, Fan C, Kaplan J, Hung W-Y, McKenna-Yasek D, Haines JL, Pericak-Vance MA, Horvitz HR, Brown RH, Jr. Linkage of familial amyotrophic lateral sclerosis with frontotemporal dementia to chromosome 9q21–q22. JAMA 2000; 284(13):1664–1669.

55. Levchenko A, Robitaille Y, Strong MJ, Rouleau GA. Tau mutations are not a predominant cause of frontotemporal dementia in Canadian patients. Can J Neurol Sci 2004; 31(3):363–367.

56. Kishikawa M, Nakamura T, Iseki M, Ikeda T, Shimokawa I, Tsujihata M, Nagasato K. A long surviving case of amyotrophic lateral sclerosis with atrophy of the frontal lobe: a comparison with the Mitsuyama type. Acta Neuropathol 1995; 89:189–193.

57. World Federation of Neurology Research Group on Neuromuscular Disease. El Escorial World Federation of Neurology criteria for the diagnosis of amyotrophic lateral sclerosis. J Neurol Sci 1994; 124(suppl):96–107.

58. Wharton S, Ince PG. Pathology of motor neuron disorders. In: Shaw PJ, Strong MJ, eds. Motor Neuron Disorders. Philadelphia: Butterworth Heinemann, 2003:17–50.

59. Migheli A, Pezzulo T, Attanasio A, Schiffer D. Peripherin immunoreactive structures in amyotrophic lateral sclerosis. Lab Invest 1993; 68(2):185–191.

60. Wong N, He BP, Strong MJ. Characterization of neuronal intermediate filament protein expression in cervical spinal motor neurons in sporadic amyotrophic lateral sclerosis ALS. J Neuropathol Exp Neurol 2000; 59(11):972–982.

61. Strong MJ. Neurofilament metabolism in sporadic amyotrophic lateral sclerosis. J Neurol Sci 1999; 169:170–177.

62. Leigh PN, Dodson A, Swash M, Brion J-P, Anderton BH. Cytoskeletal abnormalities in motor neuron disease. An immunohistochemical study. Brain 1989; 112:521–535.

63. van Welsem ME, Hogenhuis JA, Meininger V, Metsaars WP, Hauw JJ, Seilhean D. The relationship between Bunina bodies, skein-like inclusions and neuronal loss in amyotrophic lateral sclerosis. Acta Neuropathol 2002; 103:583–589.

64. Sasaki S, Murayama S. Ultrastructural study of Bunina bodies in the anterior horn neurons of patients with motor neuron disease. Neurosci Lett 1993; 154:117–120.

65. Okamato K, Hirai S, Amari M, Watanabe M, Sakurai A. Bunina bodies in amyotrophic lateral sclerosis immunostained with rabbit anti-cystatin C serum. Neurosci Lett 1993; 162:125–128.

66. Leigh PN, Anderton BH, Dodson A, Gallo J-M, Swash M, Power DM. Ubiquitin deposits in anterior horn cells of motor neuron disease. Neurosci Lett 1988; 93:197–203.

67. Lowe J, Lennox G, Jefferson D, Morrell K, McQuire D, Gray T, Landon M, Doherty FJ, Mayer RJ. A filamentous inclusion body within anterior horn neurones in motor neurone disease defined by immunocytochemical localisation of ubiquitin. Neurosci Lett 1988; 94:203–210.

68. Sasaki S, Murayama S. Ultrastructural study of skein-like inclusions in the anterior horn neurons of patients with motor neuron disease. Neurosci Lett 1992; 147:121–124.

69. Schiffer D, Autilio-Gambetti L, Chio A, Gambetti P, Giordana MT, Gullotta F, Migheli A, Vigliani MC. Ubiquitin in motor neuron disease: Study at the light and electron microscope. J Neuropathol Exp Neurol 1991; 50:463–473.

70. Strong MJ. The basic aspects of therapeutics in amyotrophic lateral sclerosis. Pharmacol Ther 2003; 983:379–414.

71. Wilson CM, Grace GM, Munoz DG, He BP, Strong MJ. Cognitive impairment in sporadic ALS. A pathological continuum underlying a multisystem disorder. Neurology 2001; 57:651–657.

72. Yoshida M. Amyotrophic lateral sclerosis with dementia: The clinicopathological spectrum. Neuropathology 2004; 24:87–102.

73. Noda K, Katayama S, Watanabe C, Yamamura Y, Nakamura S. Gallyas- and tau-positive glial strucutres in motor neuron disease with dementia. Clin Neuropath 1999; 18(5):218–225.

74. Morris HR, Khan MN, Janssen JC, Brown JM, Perez-Tur J, Baker M, Ozansoy M, Hardy J, Hutton M, Wood NW, Lees AJ, Revesz T, Lantos P, Rossor MN. The genetic and pathological classification of familial frontotemporal dementia. Arch Neurol 2001; 58:1813–1816.

75. Caselli RJ, Windebank AJ, Petersen RC, Komori T, Parisi JE, Okazaki E, Iverson R, Dinapoli RP, Graff-Radford NR, Stein SD. Rapidly progressing aphasic dementia and motor neuron disease. Ann Neurol 1993; 33:200–207.

76. Ferrer I, Roig C, Espino A, Peiro G, Matias Guiu X. Dementia of frontal lobe type and motor neuron disease. A Golgi study of the frontal cortex. J Neurol Neurosurg Psychiat 1991; 54:932–934.

77. Kato S, Oda M, Hayashi H, Kawata A, Shimizu T. Participation of the limbic system and its associated areas in the dementia of amyotrophic lateral sclerosis. J Neurol Sci 1994; 126:62–69.

78. Kawashima T, Kikuchi H, Takita M, Doh-ura K, Ogomori K, Oda M, Iwaki T. Skein-like inclusions in the neostriatum from a case of amyotrophic lateral sclerosis with dementia. Acta Neuropathol 1998; 96:541–545.

79. Munoz DG. The pathology of Pick complex. In: Kertesz A, Munoz DG, eds. Pick's disease and Pick complex. New York: John Wiley and Sons, 1998:211–239.

80. Horoupian DS, Katzman R, Terry RD, Davies P, Hirano A, DeTersa R, Fuld PA, Petito C, Blass J, Ellis JM. Dementia and motor neuron disease: morphometric, biochemical and golgi studies. Ann Neurol 1984; 16:305–313.

81. Brun A, Passant U. Frontal lobe degeneration of non-Alzheimer type. Acta Neurol
     Scand 1996; 168:28–30.
82. Giannakopoulos P, Hof PR, Bouras C. Dementia lacking distinctive histopathology:
     clinicopathological evaluation of 32 cases. Acta Neuropathol Berl 1995; 89:346–355.
83. Jackson M, Lowe J. The new neuropathology of degenerative frontotemporal demen-
     tias. Acta Neuropathol 1996; 91:127–134.
84. Neary D, Snowden J. Fronto-temporal dementia: nosology, neuropsychology, and
     neuropathology. Neurology 1998; 51:1546–1554.
85. Soni W, Luthert PJ, Leigh PN, Mann DMA. A morphometric study of the neuropatho-
     logical substrate of dementia in patients with motor neuron disease. Neuropathol Appl
     Neurobiol 1993; 19:203.
86. Okamoto K, Hirai S, Yamazaki T, Sun X, Nakazato Y. New ubiquitin-positive intra-
     neuronal inclusions in the extra-motor cortices in patients with amyotrophic lateral
     sclerosis. Neurosci Lett 1991; 129:233–236.
87. Wightman G, Anderson VER, Martin J, Swash M, Anderton BH, Neary D, Mann D,
     Luthert P, Leigh PN. Hippocampal and neocortical ubiquitin-immunoreactive inclu-
     sions in amyotrophic lateral sclerosis with dementia. Neurosci Lett 1992; 139:269–274.
88. Lowe J, Blanchard A, Morrell K, Lennox G, Reynolds L, Billett M, Landon M, Mayer
     RJ. Ubiquitin is a common factor in intermediate filament inclusion bodies of diverse
     type in man, including those of Parkinson's disease, Pick's disease, and Alzheimer's dis-
     ease, as well as Rosenthal fibres in cerebellar astrocytomas, cytoplasmic bodies in mus-
     cle, and mallory bodies in alcoholic liver disease. J Pathol 1988; 155:9–15.
89. Ikemoto A, Hirano A, Akiguchi I, Kimura J. Comparative study of ubiquitin immunor-
     eactivity of hippocampal granular cells in amyotrophic lateral sclerosis with dementia,
     Guamanian amyotrophic lateral sclerosis and Guamanian parkinsonism-dementia com-
     plex. Acta Neuropathol 1997; 93:265–270.
90. Lowe J. New pathological findings in amyotrophic lateral sclerosis. J Neurol Sci 1994;
     124(suppl):38–51.
91. Hayashi H, Kato S. Total manifestations of amyotrophic lateral sclerosis. J Neurol Sci
     1989; 93:19–35.
92. Hayashi H, Kato S, Kawada A. Amyotrophic lateral sclerosis patients living beyond
     respiratory failure. J Neurol Sci 1991; 105:73–78.
93. Mizutani T, Aki A, Shiozawa R, Unakami M, Nozawa T, Yajima K, Tanabe H, Hara
     M. Development of ophthalmoplegia in amyotrophic lateral sclerosis during long-term
     use of respirators. J Neurol Sci 1990; 99:311–319.
94. Yang W, Sopper MM, Leystra-Lantz C, Strong MJ. Microtubule-associated tau protein
     positive neuronal and glial inclusions in amyotrophic lateral sclerosis. Neurology 2003;
     61(12):1766–1773.
95. Buée-Scherrer V, Buée L, Hof PR, Leveugle B, Gilles C, Loerzel AJ, Perl DP, Dela-
     courte A. Neurofibrillary degeneration in amyotrophic lateral sclerosis/parkinsonism-
     dementia complex of Guam. Immunochemical characterization of tau proteins. Am J
     Pathol 1995; 146(4):924–932.
96. Berry RW, Quinn B, Johnson N, Cochran EJ, Ghoshal N, Binder LI. Pathological glial
     tau accumulations in neurodegenerative disease: review and case report. Neurochem Int
     2001; 39:469–479.
97. Cruz-Sanchez FF, Moral A, Tolosa E, de Belleroche J, Rossi ML. Evaluation of neu-
     ronal loss, astrocytosis and abnormalities of cytoskeletal components of large motor
     neurons in the human anterior horn in aging. J Neural Trans 1998; 105:689–701.
98. Ikeda K, Akiyama H, Arai T, Nishimura T. Glial tau pathology in neurodegenerative
     diseases: their nature and comparison with neuronal tangles. Neurobiol Aging 1998;
     19(15):S85–S91.
99. Munoz DG. Stains for the differential diagnosis of degenerative dementias. Biotech
     Histochem 1999; 74(6):311–320.

100. Bigio EH, Johnson NA, Rademaker AW, Fung BB, Mesulam M-M, Siddique N, Dellefave L, Caliendo J, Freeman S, Siddique T. Neuronal ubiquitinated intranuclear inclusions in familial and non-familial frontotemporal dementia of the motor neuron disease type associated with amyotrophic lateral sclerosis. J Neuropathol Exp Neurol 2004; 63(8):801–811.

101. Mackenzie IRA, Feldman H. Neuronal intranuclear inclusions distinguish familial FTD-MND type from sporadic cases. Dement Geriatr Cogn Disord 2004; 17:333–336.

102. Reed DM, Brody JA. Amyotrophic lateral sclerosis and parkinsonism-dementia on Guam 1945–1972. I. Descriptive epidemiology. Am J Epidemiol 1975; 101:287–301.

103. Garruto RM, Gajdusek DC, Chen KM. Amyotrophic lateral sclerosis among Chamorro migrants from Guam. Ann Neurol 1980; 8:612–619.

104. Torres J, Iriarte LLG, Kurland LT. Amyotrophic lateral sclerosis among Guamanians in California. California Medicine 1957; 86(4):385–388.

105. Yanagihara RT, Garruto RM, Gajdusek DC. Epidemiological surveillance of amyotrophic lateral sclerosis and parkinsonism-dementia in the Commonwealth of the Northern Mariana Islands. Ann Neurol 1983; 13:79–86.

106. Hirano A, Arumugasamy N, Zimmerman HM. Amyotrophic lateral sclerosis. A comparison of Guam and classical cases. Arch Neurol 1967; 16:357–363.

107. Hirano A. Neuropathology of amyotrophic lateral sclerosis and parkinsonism-dementia complex on Guam. In: Luthy L, Bischoff A, eds. Proceedings of the fifth international congress of neuropathology. Amsterdam: Excerpta Medica, 1966:190–194.

108. Malamud N, Hirano A, Kurland LT. Pathoanatomic changes in amyotrophic lateral sclerosis on Guam. Arch Neurol 1961; 5:401–415.

109. Oyanagi K, Makifuchi T, Ohtoh T, Chen K-M, van der Schaff T, Gajdusek DC, Chase TN, Ikuta F. Amyotrophic lateral sclerosis of Guam: the nature of the neuropathological findings. Acta Neuropathol 1994; 88:405–412.

110. Kuzuhara S, Kokubo Y, Sasaki R, Narita Y, Yabana T, Hasegawa M, Iwatsubo T. Familial amyotrophic lateral sclerosis and Parkinsonism-dementia complex of the Kii Peninsula of Japan: clinical and neuropathological study and tau analysis. Ann Neurol 2001; 49:501–511.

111. Rodgers-Johnson P, Garruto RM, Yanigahara R, Chen KM, Gajdusek DC, Gibbs CJ, Jr. Amyotrophic lateral sclerosis and parkinsonism-dementia on Guam: A 30-year evaluation of clinical and neuropathological trends. Neurology 1986; 36:7–13.

112. Shankar SK, Yanagihara R, Garruto RM, Grundke-Iqbal I, Kosik KS, Gajdusek DC. Immunocytochemical characterization of neurofibrillary tangles in amyotrophic lateral sclerosis and Parkinsonism-Dementia of Guam. Ann Neurol 1989; 25:146–151.

113. Hirano A, Dembitzer HM, Kurland LT, Zimmerman HM. The fine structure of some intraganglionic alterations: neurofibrillary tangles, granulovacuolar bodies, and "rodlike" structures in Guam amyotrophic lateral sclerosis and parkinsonism-dementia complex. J Neuropathol Exp Neurol 1968; 27:167–182.

114. Buée-Scherrer V, Buée L, Hof PR, Leveugle B, Gilles C, Loerzel AJ, Perl DP, Delacourte A. Neurofibrillary degeneration in amyotrophic lateral sclerosis/parkinsonism-dementia complex of Guam. Am J Pathol 1995; 68(4):924–932.

115. Yamazaki M, Arai Y, Baba M, Iwatsubo T, Mori O, Katayama Y, Oyanagi K. Alpha-synuclein inclusions in amygdala in the brains of patients with the parkinsonism-dementia complex of guam. J Neuropathol Exp Neurol 2000; 59:585–591.

116. Forman MS, Schmidt ML, Kasturi S, Perl DP, Lee VMY, Trojanowski JQ. Tau and α-synuclein pathology in amygdala of Parkinsonsim-dementia complex patients of Guam. Am J Pathol 2002; 1605:1725–1731.

117. D'Souza I, Poorkaj P, Hong M, Nochlin D, Lee VMY, Bird TD, Schellenberg GD. Missense and silent tau gene mutations cause frontotemporal dementia with parkinsonism-chromosome 17 type, by affecting multiple alternative RNA splicing regulatory elements. Proc Natl Acad Sci USA 1999; 96:5598–5603.

118. Forman MS, Zhukareva V, Bergeron C, Chin SSM, Grossman M, Clark C, Lee VMY, Trojanowski JQ. Signature tau neuropathology in gray and white matter in corticobasal degeneration. Am J Pathol 2002; 160(6):2045–2053.

119. Zhukareva V, Mann D, Pickering-Brown SM, Uryu K, Shuck T, Shah K, Grossman M, Miller BL, Hulette CM, Feinstein SC, Trojanowski JQ, Lee VMY. Sporadic Pick's disease: a tauopathy characterized by a spectrum of pathological τ isoforms in gray and white matter. Ann Neurol 2002; 51:730–739.

120. Arai T, Ikeda K, Akiyama H, Shikamoto Y, Tsuchiya K, Yagishita S, Beach T, Rogers J, Schwab C, McGeer PL. Distinct isoforms of tau aggregated in neurons and glial cells in brains of patients with Pick's disease, corticobasal degeneration and progressive supranuclear palsy. Acta Neuropathol 2001; 101:167–173.

121. Tolnay M, Sergeant N, Ghestem A, Chalbot S, de Vos RAI, Jansen Steur ENH, Probst A, Delacourte A. Argyrophilic grain disease and Alzheimer's disease are distinguished by their different distribution of tau protein isoforms. Acta Neuropathol 2002; 104:425–434.

122. Bussière T, Hof PR, Mailliot C, Brown CD, Caillet-Boudin ML, Perl DP, Buée L, Delacourte A. Phosphorylated serine422 on tau proteins is a pathological epitope found in several diseases with neurofibrillary degeneration. Acta Neuropathol 1999; 97:221–230.

123. Zhukareva V, Vogelsberg-Ragaglia V, Van Deerlin VMD, Bruce J, Shuck T, Grossman M, Clark CM, Arnold SE, Masliah E, Galasko D, Trojanowski JQ, Lee VMY. Loss of brain tau defines novel sporadic and familial tauopathies with frontotemporal dementia. Ann Neurol 2001; 49:165–175.

124. Zhukareva V, Shah K, Uryu K, Braak H, Del Tredici K, Sundarraj S, Clark C, Trojanowski JQ, Lee VMY. Biochemical analysis of τ proteins in argyrophilic grain disease, Alzheimer's disease, and Pick's disease. A comparative study. Am J Pathol 2002; 161(4):1135–1141.

125. Josephs KA, Holton JL, Rossort MN, Godbolt AK, Ozawa T, Strand K, Khan N, Al-Sarraj S, Revesz T. Frontotemporal lobar degeneration and ubiquitin immunohistochemistry. Neuropathol Appl Neurobiol 2004; 30:369–373.

126. Jackson M, Lennox G, Lowe J. Motor neuron disease-inclusion dementia. Neurodegeneration 1996; 5:339–350.

127. Woulfe J, Kertesz A, Munoz DG. Frontotemporal dementia with ubiquitinated cytoplasmic and intranuclear inclusions. Acta Neuropathol 2001; 102:94–100.

128. Bigio EH, Lipton AM, White CL III, Dickson DW, Hirano A. Frontotemporal and motor neurone degeneration with neurofilament inclusion bodies: additional evidence for overlap between FTD and ALS. Neuropathol Appl Neurobiol 2003; 29:239–253.

129. Sima AA, Defendi R, Keohane C, D'Amato C, Foster NL, Parchi P, Gambetti P, Lynch T, Wilhelmsen KC. The neuropathology of chromosome 17-linked dementia. Ann Neurol 1996; 396:734–743.

130. Wenning GK, Litvan I, Jankovic J, Giranata R, Mangone CA, McKee A, Poewe W, Jellinger K, Chaudhuri KR, D'Olhaberriague L, Pearce RKB. Natural history and survival of 14 patients with corticobasal degeneration confirmed at postmortem examination. J Neurol Neurosurg Psychiat 1998; 64:184–189.

131. Nakano I. Frontotemporal dementia with motor neuron disease amyotrophic lateral sclerosis with dementia. Neuropathology 2000; 20(1):68–75.

132. Kusaka H, Imai T. Pathology of motor neurons in amyotrophic lateral sclerosis with dementia. Clin Neuropathol 1993; 12(3):164–168.

133. Uchihara T, Shibuya K, Nakamura A, Yagishita S. Siver stains distinguish tau-positive structures in corticobasal degeneration/progressive supranuclear palsy and in Alzheimer's disease - comparison between gallyas and Campbell-Switzer methods. Acta Neuropathol 2005; 109:299–305.

134. Mott RT, Dickson DW, Trojanowski JQ, Zhukareva V, Lee VM, Forman M, Van Deerlin V, Ervin JF, Wang D-S, Schmechel DE, Hulette CM. Neuropathological, biochemical, and molecular characterization of the forntotemporal dementias. J Neuropathol Exp Neurol 2005; 64(5):420–428.

135. Wakabayashi K, Takahashi H. Pathological heterogeneity in progressive supranuclear palsy and corticobasal degeneration. Neuropathology 2004; 24:79–86.

7

Familial ALS and Genetic Approaches to ALS

Teepu Siddique and Lisa Dellefave
Department of Neurology and Clinical Neurosciences and Department of Cell and Molecular Biology, Northwestern University Feinberg School of Medicine, Chicago, Illinois, U.S.A.

ALS BACKGROUND

It has been known since the late 1800s that ALS can be an inherited disease. One of the earliest descriptions of ALS pedigrees was published by Osler (1) in 1880. He described 13 individuals in two generations of the Farr family from Vermont with the progressive muscular atrophy (PMA) variant of ALS. PMA is a common phenotype in superoxide dismutase 1 (SOD1) gene-linked ALS. Mutation analysis of affected descendants of the Farr family has revealed an A4V mutation in the SOD1 gene. Later, multigenerational ALS families were described by others (2–5).

GENETIC APPLICATION TO ALS

Approximately 90% of ALS cases occur in individuals with no family history of ALS and are said to have sporadic ALS (SALS) (5). Approximately 10% of individuals with ALS have at least one affected family member and are classified as having familial ALS (FALS). As the majority of cases are sporadic, ALS was considered to be a non-genetic disease. However, as genetic technology and statistical tools became advanced, it became possible to address the genetic contribution in familial subgroups of largely sporadic disorders. Most FALS cases have a Mendelian pattern of inheritance, as has been shown in 20% of FALS families who have mutations in the SOD1 gene as the cause of disease (6,7). Understanding the basis of genetic locus heterogeneity in ALS and the etiopathogenesis in other motor neuron diseases (Table 1) provides multiple starting points in search of possible common intersections in molecular pathways.

APPROACHES TO MENDELIAN INHERITED ALS

Single genes that cause Mendelian inherited disease are generally more penetrant than genes that cause disease through multifactorial inheritance and are more easily identified. The SOD1 locus for ALS (8) was identified through the new commonly employed

Table 1a Categories of Disorders of the Motor Neuron: Lower Motor Neuron Involvement Only

Motor neuron disease	Inheritance	Gene	Protein	Clinical features of disease	Reference
Spinal muscular atrophy (SMA) 1	AR	Survival motor neuron (SMN)	SMN protein	Onset in utero to six months. Presents with hypotonia and weakness; problems with sucking, swallowing, and breathing. Never able to sit	87
SMA2	AR	SMN	SMN protein	Onset between 3 and 15 months. Proximal leg weakness, fasciculations, and fine hand tremor. Never able to stand. Facial muscles spared	87
SMA3	AR, AD	SMN	SMN protein	Onset 15 months to teen years. Proximal leg weakness, delayed motor milestones	87
SMA4	AR	SMN	SMN protein	Onset is median age of 37 years. Proximal weakness; variable within families	87
	AD	VAPB	Vesicle-associated/synaptobrevin-associated membrane protein B	Late-onset SMA Finkel type atypical ALS in seven families	58
Distal spinal muscular atrophy (SMA5)	AR	IGHMP2	Immunoglobulin mu binding protein 2	Infantile onset. Distal muscle atrophy and weakness with severe respiratory involvement	88
	AR	Loci: 11q13.3	Unknown	Childhood onset. Distal muscle atrophy and weakness	89
	AR	Loci: 9p21.1-p12	Unknown	Childhood onset with pyramidal features	90
	AD	GARS	Glycyl tRNA synthase	Adult onset. Slowly progressive distal amyotrophy, upper limb predominant	91

Disease	Inheritance	Locus/Gene	Gene product	Description	Ref
Distal SMA	AD	BSCL2	Seipin	Adult onset. Slowly progressive distal amyotrophy	92
	AD	Loci: 12q2-q24	Unknown	Congenital, non-progressive with contractures	93
	AD	Loci: 2q14	Unknown	Adult onset. Slowly progressive distal amyotrophy with vocal cord paralysis	94
	AD	Loci: 12q24.3	Unknown	Adult onset. Slowly progressive distal amyotrophy	95
	X-linked recessive	Loci: Xq13.1-q21	Unknown	Childhood onset pes cavus or varus. Gait instability with distal amyotrophy	96
Spinal bulbar muscular atrophy	X-linked recessive	AR	Androgen receptor	Onset teens to adulthood. Proximal muscle weakness, muscle atrophy, and fasciculations	97
Spinal bulbar muscular atrophy	AD	DCTN1	Dynactin	Onset is early adulthood. Progressive weakness of facial muscles, hands, and distal lower extremities without sensory symptoms. Respiratory muscles involved. Single family identified	66

Table 1b Categories of Disorders of the Motor Neuron: Upper Motor Neuron Involvement Only

Motor neuron disease	Inheritance	Gene	Protein	Clinical features of disease	Reference
Juvenile primary lateral sclerosis JPLS1 (ALS2)[a]	AR	ALS2	Alsin	Progressive ascending UMN disorder starting in infancy with lower extremities and eventually involving the arms and bulbar regions	10, 98
Hereditary spastic paraplegia (HSP) pure	AD			In general, symptoms of pure AD HSP are: Onset varies intra and interfamily. Bilateral lower extremity spastic weakness often with urinary bladder disturbance	
		SPG3A: SPG3A gene	Atlastin	Symptom onset may be earlier (less than 11 years). Typical features of AD HSP	99
		SPG4: SPG4 gene	Spastin	Symptom onset may be later (after 20 years). Cognitive impairment in some cases	100
		SPG6: NIPA1 gene	Non-imprinted Prader-Willi syndrome 1	Symptom onset may be later (after 20 years). Typical features of AD HSP	101
		SPG8: 8q23-q24	Unknown	Symptom onset may be later (after 20 years). Typical features of AD HSP	102
		SPG10: KIF5A gene	Neuronal kinesin heavy chain protein	Symptom onset may be earlier (less than 11 years). Typical features of AD HSP	103
		SPG12: 19q13	Unknown	Symptom onset may be earlier (less than 11 years). Typical features of AD HSP	104

Inheritance	Locus/Gene	Protein	Clinical features	Ref
	SPG13: HSPD1 gene	60 kDa heat shock protein	Symptom onset may be later (after 20 years). Typical features of AD HSP	105
	SPG19: 9q33-q34	Unknown	Symptom onset may be later (after 20 years). Typical features of AD HSP.	106
AR	SPG5A: 8p12-q13	Unknown	Childhood onset. Spasticity of lower limbs, abnormally active tendon reflexes, dysfunction of bladder spincter	107
	SPG11: 15q13-q15	Unknown	Hereditary spastic paraparesis with thin corpus callosum	108
	SPG24: 13q14	Unknown	Hereditary spastic paraparesis with sensorineural deafness	109
HSP complicated AD	SPG9: 10q23.3-q24.1	Unknown	Mean age of onset, third decade. Spastic paraplegia with cataracts, gastrointestinal reflux, motor neuronopathy	110
	SPG17: Silver syndrome 11q12-q24	Unknown	Onset juvenile or adult. Spastic paraplegia with amyotrophy—spasticity of lower limbs accompanied by weakness and wasting of small hand muscles	111
	SAX1: 12p13	Unknown	Spasticity, ataxia, dysarthria, dysphagia, and eye movement abnormalities	112
AR	SPG7: SPG7 gene	Paraplegin	Mean age of onset is 25 years. Progressive lower extremity weakness spasticity, hyperreflexia, dysarthria, dysphagia, optic disc pallor, optic atrophy, axonal	113

(Continued)

Table 1b Categories of Disorders of the Motor Neuron: Upper Motor Neuron Involvement Only (*Continued*)

Motor neuron disease	Inheritance	Gene	Protein	Clinical features of disease	Reference
		SPG15: 14q22-q24	Unknown	neuropathy, and evidence of vascular lesions on MRI Spasticity with pigmented maculopathy, distal amyotrophy, dysarthria, and mental retardation	114
		Troyer syndrome: SPG20 gene	Spartin	Onset is childhood. Spastic tetraplegia dysarthria, with distal muscle wasting, short stature, learning difficulties, delay in motor milestones, emotional lability	57
		SPG21: SPG21 gene	Maspardin	Young adult onset. Spasticity with cognitive decline. MRI shows cerebral, cerebellar, corpus callosum atrophy with white matter hyperintensity	115
		ARSACS: SACS gene	Sacsin	Absent sensory nerve conduction, reduced motor-nerve velocity, hypermyelination of retinal-nerve fibers. High carrier frequency in descendents of Charlevoix-Saguenay-Lac-Saint-Jean region of Quebec	116
	X-linked	SPG1: L1CAM gene	Neural cell adhesion molecule L1 protein	Mutations in L1CAM can cause a variety of phenotypes: Spastic paraplegia with mental retardation and adducted thumbs; X-linked hydrocephalus; MASA syndrome; CRASH syndrome	117

SPG2: PLP gene	Myelin proteolipid protein	Mutations in PLP can cause a variety of phenotypes ranging from Pelizaeus-Merzbacher to SPG2. SPG2 manifests as spastic paraparesis similar to uncomplicated AD-HSP		118
SPG16: Xq11.2-q23	Unknown	Phenotype similar to SPG2 however do not have mutations in PLP gene		119
Primary lateral sclerosis	Sporadic		Onset adulthood. Lower and upper extremity spasticity and weakness	120

[a]can also present as UMN-predominant ALS (Table 2).

Abbreviations: AD, autosomal dominant; AR, autosomal recessive.

strategy of positional cloning. High consanguinity lends itself to homozygosity mapping (9) and was successfully used to identify loci for ALS2 (10) and ALS5 (8). These strategies use genotyping of highly polymorphic markers at average distances of 20, 10, or 5 centiMorgans (cm). Recently, use of microsatelite markers and restriction fragment length polymorphisms has been reported with very dense arrays of single nucleotide polymorphisms placed on chips or beads for very rapid genotyping.

The application of DNA genotyping and statistical genetic technique was first demonstrated in FALS in 1988 (5) and was then used to identify genetic locus heterogeneity in FALS and linkage to the SOD1 locus on chromosome 21q22 (11). Tight linkage of FALS to markers on chromosome 21q22 just 25 megabases from the SOD1 gene lead to the identification of mutations in SOD1 and was established as the first causative gene for ALS (6,7). Subsequently, six additional genetic loci for FALS and seven loci for related motor neuron degenerations were identified (Tables 2 and 3). Thus, locus genetic heterogeneity was established as a multi-etiologic basis of FALS, hence scleroses rather than sclerosis is a more accurate appellation, and is also probably true of SALS (first publicly articulated by Stanley Appell).

Once the causative gene for a disease is identified, the primary goal is to identify the mechanism by which the disease is caused. This usually includes the development of genetically modified animal models. The gene mutation may result in the loss of a normal function (homozygous or dominant negative effect), a haploinsufficiency, or the gain of a completely novel and toxic function. The latter is especially true in many dominantly inherited disorders of neurodegeneration such as ALS (SOD1), Huntington disease, Alzheimer disease, Parkinson disease, and Spinocerebellar Ataxia.

Mendelian Inherited ALS

Mendelian inherited ALS accounts for a minority of ALS cases (10%), but provides an important resource to identify the etiopathogenesis of motor neuron degeneration. FALS can be transmitted as a dominant or a recessive trait, but it is usually inherited as an adult-onset disorder with an autosomal dominant inheritance

Table 2 ALS Genes and Loci

Percentage of patients with familial	Locus name	Inheritance	Disease name	Gene	Locus	Product	Reference
20%	ALS1	AD	FALS	SOD1	21q22.1	Superoxide Dismutase (Cu-Zn)	6, 7, 11
Rare	ALS2	AR	Juvenile ALS type 3	ALS2	2q33	Alsin	10, 98, 121
Single family	ALS3	AD	FALS		18q21	Unknown	122
Rare	ALS5	AR	Juvenile ALS type 1		15q15.1-q21.1	Unknown	8
Three families	ALS6	AD	FALS		16q12	Unknown	123–125
Single family	ALS7	AD	FALS		20ptel	Unknown	125
Single family	XALS	X-linked dominant	FALS		X	Unknown	12

Table 3 ALS Related Motor Neuron Disorders, Genes and Loci with Both UMN and LMN Involvement

Percentage of patients with familial	Locus name	Inheritance	Disease name	Gene	Locus	Product	Reference
Rare	ALS4[a]	AD		SETX	9q34	Senataxin	63, 126
Rare	ALS8[b]	AD		VAPB	20q13	VAPB	58
Rare (<1%)	FTD/ALS	AD	ALS with FTD		9q21-q22	Unknown	127
Rare	FTD/ALS	AD			17q	Unknown	128
	SPG17	AD	Silver syndrome	SPG20	11q12-q14	Unknown	111
	SPG20	AR	Troyer syndrome		13q12.3	Spartin	57
		AD	IBMPFD[c]	VCP	9p21.1-p12	Valosin containing protein	62

[a]Never have bulbar involvement. Slow progression, long duration, distal wasting with pyramidal signs and sensory loss (previously called hereditary motor neuropathy with spasticity). Mutations in Senataxin have also been identified in a different disorder of ataxia and oculomotor apraxia (AOA2).
[b]This is a disorder that appears to be proximal SMA IV (Finkel type) with some UMN findings.
[c]Inclusion body myopathy associated with Paget disease of bone and FTD.

pattern. Autosomal recessive inheritance is rare and limited to juvenile onset ALS or to those persons with a double dose of the D90A or N86S mutations in the SOD1 gene. Interestingly, an X-linked dominantly inherited ALS has also been described (12), a rarely observed phenomenon in neurogenetics. In view of the genetic heterogeneity demonstrated in ALS, it is hoped that each additional disease-causing gene identified will contribute to the understanding of the multiple etiologies of ALS.

Understanding ALS Pathophysiology Through Mendelian Inherited ALS

Human Studies in SOD1 Linked ALS. A usual presentation of FALS, especially SOD1-linked ALS, is one of monomelic weakness without significant loss of muscle bulk. This state may persist for many months before significant weakness or muscle wasting is noted at the site of initial presentation or in other regions. Recognition of this presentation prompted revision (13) in the El Escorial Criteria of 1994 (14); a qualification was made for those with FALS. The FALS distinction was made with the designation of "Clinically Definite FALS—Laboratory Supported" such that if the pathogenic mutation has been determined (e.g., mutations in the SOD1 gene), the diagnosis may be upgraded when the clinical manifestations of ALS present with progressive upper and/or lower motor neuron signs in at least a single region (in the absence of another cause for the abnormal neurological signs). In practice, LMN features predominate in FALS, especially those linked to mutations in the SOD1 gene. The calf muscles may be the very initial site of LMN symptom of weakness accompanied by a loss of the Achilles reflex (T. Siddique, unpublished observation). The S1 Achilles reflex is a monosynaptic reflex thought to be modulated by glutamate. Absence of this reflex in a muscle with strength of 4/5 on the MRC scale or greater is a common observation in FALS, and argues against excess glutamate as the primary mechanism of disease in FALS.

Certain phenotypic features may be typical of SOD1-linked FALS, but they are non-specific and, therefore, not distinct enough to make a clinical diagnosis of SOD1 FALS versus FALS caused by a different gene. Human ALS caused by SOD1 has been identified as having a mean age of onset of 45.5 ± 8.9 years; lower extremity onset being more common than upper extremity, and even less frequently bulbar onset; these symptoms occur without gender bias (15). The duration of disease may vary by SOD1 mutation, but not onset; the age of onset of symptoms for those with SOD1 mutations ranges from 15 to 81 years (15,16). The rate of progression of the disease has been correlated to specific SOD1 gene mutations. For example, the A4V mutation, present in approximately 50% of all North American families, has been consistently associated with a rapid disease course of 1.0 ± 0.4 years (15). In sharp contrast, there are mutations that confer a significantly longer mean duration of disease of at least 10 years, such as the G37R (18.7 ± 11.4 years; $n = 8$, one family), G41D (17.0 ± 6.3 years; $n = 7$, one family), H46R (17.4 ± 6.4 years; $n = 5$, a Japanese family; a second North America family had similar duration of disease), and G93C (10.1 ± 6.2 years; $n = 7$, one family) (15,17). Extensive variability in progression has been documented for patients with the I113T mutation (2.5–20 years) (18), G93R mutation (2–12 years) (18), and G85R mutation (16 months–13 years) (T. Siddique, unreported) versus less variability with the E100G mutation (5–8 years) (18). This variability is suggestive of additional genetic and/or environmental influences.

Penetrance of SOD1 mutations is variable and is based on each specific mutation. The penetrance of some SOD1 mutations is reduced in comparison to other SOD1 mutations; most notable is the significantly reduced penetrance of the

I113T and D90A mutations (18,19). This is in contrast to a generally high penetrance of the A4V mutation.

The dosage of certain SOD1 mutations appears to have an effect on the onset of ALS. An example of this is of an affected Pakistani girl of consanguineous parents with a homozygous N86S mutation of the SOD1 gene (16). Her disease onset was at the age of 13, while her uncle (a presumed heterozygote for the mutation) did not begin to manifest symptoms until the age of 32 (16). The second and more common example of dosage and SOD1 gene mutations is that of the homozygous D90A mutation identified in more than 80 cases belonging to 40 apparently independent sporadic and FALS pedigrees (20). Most of the cases are from northern Scandinavia where the D90A allele frequency is 2.7% (21). D90A heterozygous individuals typically do not develop ALS when they are of Scandinavian origin, thus the D90A mutation has an autosomal recessive inheritance pattern in those of northern Scandinavian ethnicity. In contrast, a slowly progressive form of the disease has been described in affected individuals, who are D90A homozygotes, originating from United States, France, United Kingdom, Belgium, and Byelorussia, and present as apparent SALS. In addition, dominant pedigrees have also been identified (20–23). Thus, in ethnic backgrounds other than northern Scandinavian, the D90A mutation could be inherited as autosomal recessive or dominant. It is therefore prudent to test SALS cases of northern Scandinavian or Swedish background with lower extremity onset and slow progression for the D90A mutation and with presentation of a slowly progressive disorder for the I113T mutation. The benign nature of the D90A mutation in individuals of Scandinavian origin is thought to be mediated by a genetic factor acting in *cis* close to the SOD1 locus (24).

Cu, Zn Superoxide Dismutase 1 Gene

The SOD1 gene is around 11 kb in size containing five exons and four introns with several alternatively spliced forms (25). The SOD1 protein consists of 153 highly conserved amino acids with copper and zinc binding sites (6). Over 100 mutations, predominantly missense, have been found in 68 of the 153 codons, spread over all five exons; of these, seven were detected in exon 3 (26–31) (www.alsod.org).

Function of the Normal SOD1 Protein.   The superoxide dismutases are a group of three isoenzymes that play a key role in reducing free-radical-induced cellular damage. They scavenge the superoxide (O_2^-) free radicals produced as a by product of oxidative respiration and the cytochrome P450 system:

$$O_2^- + Enz - Cu^{2+} + H^+ \rightarrow O_2^- + Enz - Cu^+, \tag{1}$$

$$O_2^- + Enz - Cu^+ + H^+ \rightarrow H_2O_2 + Enz - Cu_2, \tag{2}$$

$$O_2^- + H^+ \rightarrow H_2O_2 + O_2. \tag{3}$$

SOD1 is primarily a cytosolic enzyme (32), but is also present in small amounts in mitochondria and other organelles (33,34). Manganese SOD (SOD2) is present in the mitochondria and it's gene is located on chromosome 6q27 (26). Extracellular SOD, (SOD3) also contain copper and zinc and its gene is coded on chromosome 4p (26). No mutations have been described in SOD2 or SOD3 in ALS patients.

SOD1 is a 320 kDa homodimeric protein. Each monomer has a Greek key β-barrel fold and binds to one copper and one zinc ion (35). The dimer interface is stabilized by hydrophobic interactions, and dimerization doubles the dismutase activity of SOD1. An electrostatic channel guides superoxide ions to the active site, which contains Cu^{2+}.

The channel is lined by the amino acids Lys 122, Lys 134, and Arg 143, which provide positive charges (35). Four cysteine residues are present in human SOD1, two are free (C_6, C_{111}) and the other two are oxidized as a sulphydryl bridge (C_{57}, C_{146}). The zinc ion provides stability and increases its melting temperature, as does the cysteine bridge C_{57}–C_{146}. The rate of the dismutase reaction is very rapid, 2×10^9/M/sec, which probably indicates that the rate of the reaction is limited only by substrate availability (36). Access to the active site is size and charge selective, and thus specifically allows the negatively charged superoxide ion, while excluding larger and positively charged ions (35).

The mechanisms by which mutations in SOD1 cause FALS are not fully understood. Transgenic mice or rats over-expressing ALS associated mutant SOD1 develop an ALS-like phenotype, while transgenic mice over-expressing wild type SOD1 (wtSOD1) remain unaffected; SOD1 knockout mice show axonal damage but do not show motor neuron degeneration (37–43), suggesting that the 100 plus SOD1 mutants associated with ALS have a toxic property that triggers motor neuron degeneration in ALS.

Much research on the pathogenesis of ALS originally focused on a highly reactive copper atom in the SOD1 protein. Investigations of mutant SOD1 as a generator of H_2O_2 and its reaction with the product of superoxide with nitric oxide have failed to elucidate the basic mechanism of disease (44) because removal of copper, essential for these reactions, by using copper chaperone of SOD (CCS) or copper chelators failed to ameliorate ALS in mutant SOD1 transgenic mice (45). Similarly, antiapoptotic agents (46) and upregulators of the $EAAT_2$ transporter (47) have marginal effect on survival of transgenic SOD1 mice. Recent focus has been on astrocytes (glia) (48–50), microglia, and mitochondria (T. Siddique, unpublished observation).

Etiopathogenesis of SOD1 ALS. Genetically modified mouse models are an important resource to understand the biochemical and cellular pathology at various stages of the disease, not possible in humans. A mouse model overexpressing the G93A mutation in SOD1 was made on the heels of the discovery of SOD1 mutations in 1994 (37) and replicated with other SOD1 mutations (38,39,41,43). A large proportion of the literature (350 papers since 1994) on the etiopathogenesis of ALS report using these models.

Even though ALS is a disorder of people (or mice) and does not occur in cell culture, cell, or organotypic models, they are used to understand the basic mechanism of disease at the cellular level. The mutant gene can be transfected into the cells and the interaction of the mutant protein with other proteins, its cellular localization, and predisposition to aggregate formation can be studied. For example, individual organelles of the cell containing the mutant protein can be separated and studied for the inimical effects of the mutant protein on the organelles such as damage to energy homeostasis due to the toxic effect of mutant protein inside mitochondria.

Onset Related to Expression of Protein in Mice. In human disease, SOD1 enzyme activity level does not correlate with disease severity. For example, mutations with marginally reduced enzyme activity such as D90A, H46R, G85R, and G93D (21,51) do produce the disease. In animal models, transgenic mice over-expressing wtSOD1 do not develop ALS, but do show ultrastructural vacuolar pathology in the spinal cord and motor axons. When transgenic mice over-expressing wtSOD1 are cross-bred with transgenic mice over-expressing mutant SOD1, the ALS phenotype and pathology appear earlier. This has been noted with G93A and L126Z transgenic mice (52). In addition, deposits of wtSOD1 can be identified in spinal cords of clinically asymptomatic L126Z mice. The wtSOD1 can also convert over-expressing A4V transgenic mice to an ALS phenotype. A4V transgenic mice, on their own, do not develop ALS. In addition, G93A mice cross-bred with SOD1 knockout demonstrate a small but measurable delay in onset of disease (HX. Deng and T. Siddique, unpublished observation). Possible explanations for these observations include increased load in the mutant SOD1 clearing system or conversion of wtSOD1 to a toxic variety. It should be pointed out that mutant SOD1 may itself have to undergo a conformational change to be toxic. Thus both wild type and SOD1 may exist as both non-toxic and toxic forms. It may be energetically economical to convert the mutant form to a highly stable toxic variety than the wild type form, but the mutant could possibly chaperone such a change in wtSOD1. Alternatively, an increase in SOD1 load may relate to an overburdened RNA turnover system (HX. Deng et al., unpublished observation 2004).

Site of Pathology (Spinal Cord and Brainstem) Relates to Increased Accumulation of SOD1 with Age and Age at Onset. In-spite of the varied pathology described in animals with ALS over-expressing mutant SOD1 (37–39,41,53), the central lesson has been that onset of disease correlates with the levels of expression of protein, which in turn is related to copy number of the transgene. This has been demonstrated by correlating RNA or protein expression to onset in transgenic mouse lines carrying the same mutation or by engineering homozygotes for the mutations (53).

We (N. Cole and T. Siddique, unpublished) have shown that SOD1 protein levels are highest in the spinal cord of the G93A animal model for ALS with levels diminishing in the brain and liver and the least amount in the kidneys; the accumulation of the toxic protein correlates with age. These studies, taken together, suggest that the targeted region, viz the spinal cord and brainstem, are unable to effectively deal with the mutant protein load leading to the region specific pathology and dysfunction noted in ALS mice, and probably in humans.

Toxicity of Protein Aggregates. Aggregates of SOD1, like mutant prion aggregation in other neurodegenerative disorders, have been proposed as mechanism of toxicity for ALS. Transgenic mouse models have identified mutant SOD1 protein aggregates in the brain and spinal cord. Inspite of intense effort, the function of these aggregates, of both SOD1 and other aggregated proteins within the brain and spinal cord, is not fully understood. It is debated that the aggregates could be a mechanism of detoxification or toxicity, depending on their cellular location. As the ubiquitin-proteosome is a major protein disposal system, protein aggregation suggests problems in the pathway for this system. However, very little mutant SOD1 has been shown to be ubiquinated in the transgenic mouse models of ALS (54). In order to explain the aggregation, it has been reasoned that a component of the ubiquitin-proteosome system such as an E3 enzyme may be impaired. Niwa et al. identified Dorfin, a RING finger E3 utiquitin ligase localized to the inclusion bodies of motor neurons of human FALS patients with SOD1 mutations, SALS patients as well as mutant SOD1 transgenic mice (55). Dorfin is involved in the ubiquitylation and targeted degradation of mutant SOD1, however, wtSOD1 does not appear to be the substrate for Dorfin (55). Recently, valosin containing protein (VCP) has been shown to interfere with E3 ligase activity of Dorfin (56).

Etiopathogenesis of the ALSIN Gene

Mutations in ALSIN are a rare experiment of nature that results in severe and progressive dysfunction of the corticospinal tract. The ALSIN gene encodes the protein product alsin and is associated with juvenile onset PLS and UMN-predominant ALS (10). The ALSIN gene makes two transcripts of the protein by alternate splicing, a short and a long form. It is hypothesized that the homozygous loss of the long-form results in the phenotype of juvenile onset PLS, whereas a homozygous loss of both short form and long forms results in the phenotype of juvenile onset ALS (10). The specific function of alsin is not fully known, but it is believed to be a guanine nucleotide exchange factor involved in membrane transport events in the neuron. The vacuolar protein sorting or other motifs associated with endosomal trafficking have been implicated in other motor neuron disorders besides ALS2 [Troyer syndrome (SPG20 gene) (57), ALS8 (Finkel SMA/SMA4) (VAPB gene) (58)] as well as in other neurodegenerative diseases [chorea-acanthocytosis (CAC gene) (59) and Niemann-Pick type C1 (NPC1) (60)]. Knockout models of the ALSIN gene do not exhibit a robust phenotype of motor neuron degeneration, but special copper–silver staining methods show distal axonal degeneration in the corticospinal tracts of knockout mice (HX. Deng and T. Siddique, unpublished data). The corticospinal tracts in rodents are small and lie behind the central cord, raising the concern about rodents as appropriate models of UMN disease and spinal cord injury.

Pathway of SOD1 and ALSIN Neurodegeneration

Cross-breeding experiments using G93A mice and Alsin knock-out mice did not alter the onset or survival of G93A (mutant SOD1) mice (HX. Deng and T. Siddique, unpublished data). This observation may indicate that UMN neurodegeneration (Alsin related) could utilize a different pathway than SOD1 related neurodegeneration (predominantly UMN). In vitro experiments are at variance with observations, and instead suggest a protective role for Alsin in SOD1 linked cell death (61).

Locus Heterogeneity

Although, the bulk of current information about ALS pathogenesis is derived from the SOD1 gene, SOD1 gene mutations account for only a minority of FALS. With two ALS genes and five ALS loci identified, it is apparent that virtually identical clinical and pathological phenotypes can arise from multiple causes (Table 2). It is therefore very important that additional ALS genes and loci be identified to further the understanding of the multiple pathways involved in the pathogenesis of ALS.

Etiopathogenesis of Other Genes Identified in ALS Related Motor Neuron Disorders with Both UMN and LMN Involvement. Inclusion body myopathy associated with Paget disease of bone and frontotemporal dementia (IBMPFD) features adult onset proximal and distal muscle weakness, early onset Paget disease of bone and premature frontotemporal dementia. IBMPFD is caused by the gene encoding VCP, which is associated with cellular activities including cell cycle control, membrane fusion, and the ubiquitin-proteosome degradation pathway (62). Finkel type SMA is an adult-onset autosomal dominant SMA caused by mutations in the VAPB gene, which has been shown to act during ER-golgi transport and secretion (58). Troyer syndrome, characterized by spastic paraparesis with dysarthria, distal amyotrophy, mild developmental delay, and short stature, is caused by mutations in the SPG20 gene encoding the protein spartin, which may be involved in endosomal trafficking (57). ALS4, also known as distal hereditary motor neuropathy with pyramidal features, is a rare childhood or adolescent onset form of ALS characterized by slow disease progression, limb weakness, severe muscle wasting, and pyramidal signs. ALS4 is caused by mutations in the SETX gene encoding the protein

Senataxin, which contains a DNA/RNA helicase domain with a possible role in RNA processing (63). Curiously, mutations in SETX have been known to cause a recessively inherited disorder of oculomotor apraxia and cerebellar ataxia (AOA2) (63) (Table 3).

Related Motor Neuron Disorders. Axonal transport is very important to neuronal health and relies on the kinesin (anterograde) and dynein (retrograde) motors. Studies suggest that defects in axonal transport may play a role in motor neuron degeneration. In transgenic mice expressing human $SOD1^{G37R}$ and $SOD1^{G85R}$ mutants, slow axonal transport was evident at least six months prior to the onset of clinical signs of disease; however no changes were demonstrated in fast axonal transport (64). Dynein, the molecular motor responsible for unidirectional retrograde vesicle transport along microtubules, is associated in a multiprotein complex with dynactin that activates its motor function. The cramping 1 (Cra1) and legs at odd angles mice (65), both heterozygous for mutations in dynein (DNCHC1), when bred with the G93A mice, delay onset of symptoms in the G93A mice, suggesting an axonal component in the pathogenesis of SOD1 linked ALS. A mutation in the DCTN1 gene encoding the p150 subunit of the transporter protein dynactin has been identified in a family with slowly progressive autosomal dominant form of lower motor neuron disease without sensory symptoms (66), further solidifying the role of axonal transport in motor neuron disease.

APPROACHES TO SALS AS A GENETICALLY COMPLEX OR MULTIFACTORIAL DISORDER

Approximately, 90% of ALS patients belong to the SALS subgroup (5). SALS is believed to be a multifactorial disease (multiple genes interacting with environmental factors). SALS and its multiple etiologies remain to be elucidated. Complex genetic diseases characteristically do not show a Mendelian pattern of inheritance, but a genetic component contributes to disease susceptibility. Identification of susceptibility genes provide clues to the pathogenesis and may point to intersecting environmental factors.

The human genome project and advances in large scale genotyping, statistical genetics, and bioinformatics have made it possible to investigate genes and DNA variations that confer disease susceptibility in disorders such as SALS. Some polymorphisms may not influence susceptibility but may affect onset, severity, and duration, thus influencing the phenotype. Susceptibility genes can be analyzed for their association between a specific allele and a disease in a large population. Successful gene mapping in complex diseases depends on many factors, which include study design, adequate statistical power of a large sample size, extent of genetic heterogeneity, and appropriate mechanisms for verification of the susceptibility genes.

Association Studies in SALS

Association studies focus on whether a specific allele of a genetic marker is found with increased frequency in individuals with the disease as compared to the frequency of the marker in individuals without the disease. Association studies can be conducted with population based case–control samples or family-based samples.

Population-based association studies involve recruitment of individual subjects, both affected cases and controls. Population-based studies are more efficient in terms of time, resources, and logistics; however, the limitation is that cases and controls may not be well matched, resulting in confounding data. As a rule of thumb, the cases and controls should be matched by ethnicity, age, and gender and some investigators advocate a ratio of 1:2, cases versus controls.

Family-based association studies involve recruitment of the affected individual in addition to their unaffected parents (called a trio) or an unaffected sibling (called a sib-pair). An advantage of family-based studies is that the affected samples and control samples have the same genetic background and are therefore well matched. The limitation of family-based studies is the difficulty of acquiring enough parents and siblings for the necessary statistical power. This can especially be the case in late-onset disorders, such as ALS, where collecting samples from both parents may not be possible because one or both parents are frequently deceased and as such, the ascertained population is skewed towards younger individuals.

Association studies have been utilized in identifying potential susceptibility genes in ALS.

APOE

The Apolipoprotein E (APOE) gene was initially shown to be associated with late-onset AD (LOAD) and subsequently shown to have an effect on onset of LOAD (67). The effect of APOE polymorphisms on onset, rather than causation of disease, has lead to it being tested in many neurological disorders, including ALS. The APOE gene polymorphisms comprising of alleles 2, 3, and 4 have been the focus of at least five association studies with ALS (68–72). A recent study identified the E∗2 allele as protective against an early onset of ALS (73); this is the first study to subclassify the role of the APOE polymorphism in ALS.

SMN

The survival motor neuron (SMN) gene was screened in association studies of ALS because both SMA and ALS are caused by motor neuron degeneration. LMN-dominant ALS is an especially enticing subgroup of SALS to study, because it resembles adult-onset SMA, even though SMA is usually proximal in onset. The SMN region contains two, almost identical, copies of SMN, called SMN1 (or SMNt for telomeric) and SMN2 (or SMNc for centromeric); SMN1 and SMN2 are highly homologous. The SMN2 copy number is known to be a modifying gene to SMN1. Several studies have been performed in SALS patients attempting to correlate the SMN2 copy number or deletions within the SMN1 gene to ALS disease (74–76). Some studies showed a modest difference in SMN2 copy number in SALS patients; the data has not been reproduced to confirm a genetic susceptibility of SMN to be associated with ALS.

VEGF

The vascular endothelial growth factor (VEGF) gene is another potential susceptibility gene because it has been shown to promote growth of blood vessels, and is a neuronal growth factor. In addition, when the promoter region of VEGF was knocked out in genetically modified mice, a subgroup of mice survived and developed motor neuron-like disease. An association study between SNP in the VEGF promoter and ALS showed ALS to be associated with susceptibility haplotypes of the VEGF promoter responsible for decreased VEGF product (77). Additional studies in SALS patients are necessary to confirm these results.

Intermediate Filaments

Peripherin (78) is a type-III intermediate neurofilament protein expressed predominantly in the peripheral nervous system. Neurofilaments have been implicated in the pathogenesis of motor neuron diseases based on mouse models (79), their presence in inclusions within motor neurons (80–82) and reported association of polymorphisms in the neurofilament heavy chain (NFH) (83–85). A frameshift mutation was identified in peripherin in one individual with ALS; additional studies of ALS patients are therefore necessary to confirm these results (78).

GENETIC TESTING AND COUNSELING IN ALS

Currently, the SOD1 gene is the only known gene to cause adult-onset ALS that meets the El Escorial criteria, other genes with mutations that cause ALS related motor neuron disease are usually very rare and may not meet the El Escorial criteria for ALS (Table 2). Other genes should be tested if the patient's phenotype resemble the phenotype associated with mutations in these other genes. For example, mutations in the SETX gene are associated with a slowly progressive motor neuron degeneration with both LMN and UMN involvement confined to the upper and lower extremities; bulbar involvement has not been described. On the contrary, the Alsin gene is predominantly an UMN disorder with occasional involvement of LMN, but importantly no adult-onset cases have been reported with mutations in ALSIN (Table 3).

FALS

SOD1 Gene Testing

SOD1 gene testing is usually performed using single strand conformation polymorphism analysis, which has 80% sensitivity and by sequencing it has greater than 99% sensitivity and specificity (specificity data based on unpublished data from T. Siddique et al.). Genetic testing for the SOD1 gene is indicated in individuals with a diagnosis of ALS who have at least one family member affected with ALS. Apparent SALS patients are tested if they have typical clinical profiles of the D90A mutation or slowly progressive ALS consistent with I113T. It would be expected that 20% of FALS individuals would have a mutation within the SOD1 gene.

No SOD1 Mutation Identified. Those FALS patients who do not have an SOD1 mutation as the cause of their ALS are considered to have non-SOD1 type FALS based on their family history, for which the disease-causing gene(s) have not been identified. Other motor neuron disease genes could be considered on the basis of phenotype. Genetic testing cannot be offered to other family members.

SOD1 Mutation Identified. An SOD1 mutation is indicative of being the cause of the ALS in the affected individual and in other affected family members.

Presymptomatic Genetic Testing. For affected individuals with an SOD1 gene mutation, presymptomatic genetic testing can be provided to other at-risk family members. Presymptomatic genetic testing can have a significant impact on the person undergoing testing, therefore following a presymptomatic genetic testing protocol should be followed. A presymptomatic genetic testing protocol, utilizing data from numerous studies of at-risk individuals who underwent testing, has been developed for Huntington Disease (HD) (86). The protocol consists of pre-test consultations with a genetic counselor, neurologist, and psychologist as well as in-person results disclosure with the neurologist and/or genetic counselor. The HD protocol has since been adapted for other adult-onset fatal neurogenetic diseases. In addition to offering presymptomatic genetic testing to at-risk individuals of SOD1 mutation families, prenatal testing, or preimplantation genetic diagnosis can also be performed;

however, due to the ethical considerations with these decisions, consultation with a genetic counselor is essential.

SALS

Indications for SOD1 genetic testing in an apparently SALS patient are: lower extremity onset, LMN predominant monomelic presentation, early onset disease, Scandinavian ancestry, or slow progression of disease. Genetic testing for affected individuals with a diagnosis of SALS is possible; however, it should only be performed with appropriate patient consultation. Two to three percent of apparently SALS patients will have a mutation within the SOD1 gene. When a mutation is identified in an apparently SALS patient, the risk assessment for other family members changes substantially. This is because the lifetime risk for SALS is 1:800 for women and 1:600 for men, whereas at-risk family members of SOD1 mutation patients would inherit the mutation with a risk of 1:2. When low penetrant SOD1 mutations, like I113T, are identified in apparent SALS, risk assessment of other family members becomes imprecise.

REMAINING QUESTIONS TO BE ANSWERED

Obviously, there is much to be learned about the pathophysiology of ALS. Identification of additional FALS genetic loci and genes will provide the means to develop additional cellular and animal models to study the disease process. The genetic models of familial disease will be the main stay of research until the cause(s) of sporadic disease is/are identified and replicated, therefore, the current task of identifying causative genes requires urgent attention. ALS is a multietiologic disease and many genes are involved in causing ALS (both FALS and SALS); a major priority will be to elucidate the pathways by which these genes cause disease. A wider understanding will be obtained when the points of intersection of these pathways and the disease processes are identified. These nodal points will be important queries for environmental factors that may trigger interactions between genes and environment in causing SALS.

ACKNOWLEDGMENTS

Acknowledgments of this work to: The National Institute of Neurological Disorders and Stroke (NS050641, NS046535), Les Turner ALS Foundation, Vena E. Schaff ALS Research Fund, Harold Post Research Professorship, Herbert and Florence C. Wenske Foundation, the Muscular Dystrophy Association of America, Ralph and Marian Falk Medical Research Trust, Abbott Labs Duane and Susan Burnham Professorship, and The David C. Asselin MD Memorial Fund.

REFERENCES

1. Osler W. Heredity in progressive muscular atrophy as illustrated in Farr family of Vermont. Arch Med 1880; 4:316–3207.
2. Engel WK, Kurland LT, Klatzo I. An inherited disease similar to amyotrophic lateral sclerosis with a pattern of posterior column involvement. An intermediate form? Brain 1959; 82:203–220.

3. Mulder DW, Kurland LT, Offord KP, Beard CM. Familial adult motor neuron disease: amyotrophic lateral sclerosis. Neurology 1986; 36(4):511–517.

4. Horton WA, Eldridge R, Brody JA. Familial motor neuron disease. Evidence for at least three different types. Neurology 1976; 26(5):460–465.

5. Siddique T, Pericak-Vance MA, Brooks BR, Roos RP, Hung WY, Antel JP, Munsat TL, Phillips K, Warner K, Speer M, et al. Linkage analysis in familial amyotrophic lateral sclerosis. Neurology 1989; 39(7):919–925.

6. Deng HX, Hentati A, Tainer JA, Iqbal Z, Cayabyab A, Hung WY, Getzoff ED, Hu P, Herzfeldt B, Roos RP, et al. Amyotrophic lateral sclerosis and structural defects in Cu,Zn superoxide dismutase. Science 1993; 261(5124):1047–1051.

7. Rosen DR, Siddique T, Rouleau G, Brown RH. Mutations in Cu/Zn superoxide dismutase gene are associated with familial amyotrophic lateral sclerosis. Nature 1993; 364(6435):362.

8. Hentati A, Ouahchi K, Pericak-Vance MA, Nijhawan D, Ahmad A, Yang Y, Rimmler J, Hung W, Schlotter B, Ahmed A, et al. Linkage of a commoner form of recessive amyotrophic lateral sclerosis to chromosome 15q15-q22 markers. Neurogenetics 1998; 2(1): 55–60.

9. Lander ES, Schork NJ. Genetic dissection of complex traits. Science 1994; 265(5181): 2037–2048.

10. Yang Y, Hentati A, Deng HX, Dabbagh O, Sasaki T, Hirano M, Hung WY, Ouahchi K, Yan J, Azim AC, et al. The gene encoding alsin, a protein with three guanine-nucleotide exchange factor domains, is mutated in a form of recessive amyotrophic lateral sclerosis. Nat Genet 2001; 29(2):160–165.

11. Siddique T, Figlewicz DA, Pericak-Vance MA, Haines JL, Rouleau G, Jeffers AJ, Sapp P, Hung WY, Bebout J, McKenna-Yasek D, et al. Linkage of a gene causing familial amyotrophic lateral sclerosis to chromosome 21 and evidence of genetic-locus heterogeneity. N Engl J Med 1991; 324(20):1381–1384.

12. Hong S BB, Siddique T. X-linked dominant locus for late-onset familial amyotrophic lateral sclerosis. Soc Neurosci Abst 1998; 24:478.

13. Brooks BR, Miller RG, Swash M, Munsat TL. El Escorial revisited: revised criteria for the diagnosis of amyotrophic lateral sclerosis. Amyotroph Lateral Scler Other Motor Neuron Disord 2000; 1(5):293–299.

14. Brooks BR. El Escorial World Federation of Neurology criteria for the diagnosis of amyotrophic lateral sclerosis. Subcommittee on Motor Neuron Diseases/Amyotrophic Lateral Sclerosis of the World Federation of Neurology Research Group on Neuromuscular Diseases and the El Escorial "Clinical limits of amyotrophic lateral sclerosis" workshop contributors. J Neurol Sci 1994; 124(suppl):96–107.

15. Juneja T, Pericak-Vance MA, Laing NG, Dave S, Siddique T. Prognosis in familial amyotrophic lateral sclerosis: progression and survival in patients with glu100gly and ala4val mutations in Cu, Zn superoxide dismutase. Neurology 1997; 48(1):55–57.

16. Hayward C, Brock DJ, Minns RA, Swingler RJ. Homozygosity for Asn86Ser mutation in the CuZn-superoxide dismutase gene produces a severe clinical phenotype in a juvenile onset case of familial amyotrophic lateral sclerosis. J Med Genet 1998; 35(2):174.

17. Cudkowicz ME, McKenna-Yasek D, Sapp PE, Chin W, Geller B, Hayden DL, Schoenfeld DA, Hosler BA, Horvitz HR, Brown RH. Epidemiology of mutations in superoxide dismutase in amyotrophic lateral sclerosis. Ann Neurol 1997; 41(2):210–221.

18. Orrell RW, Habgood JJ, Gardiner I, King AW, Bowe FA, Hallewell RA, Marklund SL, Greenwood J, Lane RJ, deBelleroche J. Clinical and functional investigation of 10 missense mutations and a novel frameshift insertion mutation of the gene for copper–zinc superoxide dismutase in UK families with amyotrophic lateral sclerosis. Neurology 1997; 48(3):746–751.

19. Jones CT, Swingler RJ, Simpson SA, Brock DJ. Superoxide dismutase mutations in an unselected cohort of Scottish amyotrophic lateral sclerosis patients. J Med Genet 1995; 32(4):290–292.

20. Andersen PM, Spitsyn VA, Makarov SV, Nilsson L, Kravchuk OI, Bychkovskaya LS, Marklund SL. The geographical and ethnic distribution of the D90A CuZn-SOD mutation in the Russian Federation. Amyotroph Lateral Scler Other Motor Neuron Disord 2001; 2(2):63–69.

21. Sjalander A, Beckman G, Deng HX, Iqbal Z, Tainer JA, Siddique T. The D90A mutation results in a polymorphism of Cu,Zn superoxide dismutase that is prevalent in northern Sweden and Finland. Hum Mol Genet 1995; 4(6):1105–1108.

22. Khoris J, Moulard B, Briolotti V, Hayer M, Durieux A, Clavelou P, Malafosse A, Rouleau GA, Camu W. Coexistence of dominant and recessive familial amyotrophic lateral sclerosis with the D90A Cu,Zn superoxide dismutase mutation within the same country. Eur J Neurol 2000; 7(2):207–211.

23. Jackson M, Al-Chalabi A, Enayat ZE, Chioza B, Leigh PN, Morrison KE. Copper/zinc superoxide dismutase 1 and sporadic amyotrophic lateral sclerosis: analysis of 155 cases and identification of a novel insertion mutation. Ann Neurol 1997; 42(5):803–807.

24. Al-Chalabi A, Andersen PM, Chioza B, Shaw C, Sham PC, Robberecht W, Matthijs G, Camu W, Marklund SL, Forsgren L, et al. Recessive amyotrophic lateral sclerosis families with the D90A SOD1 mutation share a common founder: evidence for a linked protective factor. Hum Mol Genet 1998; 7(13):2045–2050.

25. Hirano M, Hung WY, Cole N, Azim AC, Deng HX, Siddique T. Multiple transcripts of the human Cu,Zn superoxide dismutase gene. Biochem Biophys Res Commun 2000; 276(1):52–56.

26. Boukaftane Y, Khoris J, Moulard B, Salachas F, Meininger V, Malafosse A, Camu W, Rouleau GA. Identification of six novel SOD1 gene mutations in familial amyotrophic lateral sclerosis. Can J Neurol Sci 1998; 25(3):192–196.

27. Siddique T, Nijhawan D, Hentati A. Molecular genetic basis of familial ALS. Neurology 1996; 47(4 suppl 2):S27–S34; discussion S34–S25.

28. Shaw CE, Enayat ZE, Chioza BA, Al-Chalabi A, Radunovic A, Powell JF, Leigh PN. Mutations in all five exons of SOD-1 may cause ALS. Ann Neurol 1998; 43(3):390–394.

29. Garcia-Redondo A, Bustos F, Juan YSB, Del Hoyo P, Jimenez S, Campos Y, Martin MA, Rubio JC, Canadillas F, Arenas J, et al. Molecular analysis of the superoxide dismutase 1 gene in Spanish patients with sporadic or familial amyotrophic lateral sclerosis. Muscle Nerve 2002; 26(2):274–278.

30. Segovia-Silvestre T, Andreu AL, Vives-Bauza C, Garcia-Arumi E, Cervera C, Gamez J. A novel exon 3 mutation (D76V) in the SOD1 gene associated with slowly progressive ALS. Amyotroph Lateral Scler Other Motor Neuron Disord 2002; 3(2):69–74.

31. Andersen PM, Sims KB, Xin WW, Kiely R, O'Neill G, Ravits J, Pioro E, Harati Y, Brower RD, Levine JS, et al. Sixteen novel mutations in the Cu/Zn superoxide dismutase gene in amyotrophic lateral sclerosis: a decade of discoveries, defects and disputes. Amyotroph Lateral Scler Other Motor Neuron Disord 2003; 4(2):62–73.

32. Fridovich I. Superoxide dismutases. Annu Rev Biochem 1975; 44:147–159.

33. Okado-Matsumoto A, Fridovich I. Amyotrophic lateral sclerosis: a proposed mechanism. Proc Natl Acad Sci USA 2002; 99(13):9010–9014.

34. Okado-Matsumoto A, Fridovich I. Subcellular distribution of superoxide dismutases (SOD) in rat liver: Cu,Zn-SOD in mitochondria. J Biol Chem 2001; 276(42):38,388–38,393.

35. Getzoff ED, Tainer JA, Stempien MM, Bell GI, Hallewell RA. Evolution of CuZn superoxide dismutase and the Greek key beta-barrel structural motif. Proteins 1989; 5(4):322–336.

36. Klug D, Rabani J, Fridovich I. A direct demonstration of the catalytic action of superoxide dismutase through the use of pulse radiolysis. J Biol Chem 1972; 247(15):4839–4842.

37. Gurney ME, Pu H, Chiu AY, Dal Canto MC, Polchow CY, Alexander DD, Caliendo J, Hentati A, Kwon YW, Deng HX, et al. Motor neuron degeneration in mice that express a human Cu,Zn superoxide dismutase mutation. Science 1994; 264(5166):1772–1775.

38. Wong PC, Pardo CA, Borchelt DR, Lee MK, Copeland NG, Jenkins NA, Sisodia SS, Cleveland DW, Price DL. An adverse property of a familial ALS-linked SOD1

mutation causes motor neuron disease characterized by vacuolar degeneration of mito-chondria. Neuron 1995; 14(6):1105–1116.

39. Ripps ME, Huntley GW, Hof PR, Morrison JH, Gordon JW. Transgenic mice expressing an altered murine superoxide dismutase gene provide an animal model of amyotrophic lateral sclerosis. Proc Natl Acad Sci USA 1995; 92(3):689–693.

40. Reaume AG, Elliott JL, Hoffman EK, Kowall NW, Ferrante RJ, Siwek DF, Wilcox HM, Flood DG, Beal MF, Brown RH Jr, et al. Motor neurons in Cu/Zn superoxide dismutase-deficient mice develop normally but exhibit enhanced cell death after axonal injury. Nat Genet 1996; 13(1):43–47.

41. Bruijn LI, Becher MW, Lee MK, Anderson KL, Jenkins NA, Copeland NG, Sisodia SS, Rothstein JD, Borchelt DR, Price DL, et al. ALS-linked SOD1 mutant G85R mediates damage to astrocytes and promotes rapidly progressive disease with SOD1-containing inclusions. Neuron 1997; 18(2):327–338.

42. Ho YS, Gargano M, Cao J, Bronson RT, Heimler I, Hutz RJ. Reduced fertility in female mice lacking copper–zinc superoxide dismutase. J Biol Chem 1998; 273(13):7765–7769.

43. Nagai M, Aoki M, Miyoshi I, Kato M, Pasinelli P, Kasai N, Brown RH Jr, Itoyama Y. Rats expressing human cytosolic copper–zinc superoxide dismutase transgenes with amyotrophic lateral sclerosis: associated mutations develop motor neuron disease. J Neurosci 2001; 21(23):9246–9254.

44. Beckman JS, Chen J, Crow JP, Ye YZ. Reactions of nitric oxide, superoxide and peroxynitrite with superoxide dismutase in neurodegeneration. Prog Brain Res 1994; 103:371–380.

45. Subramaniam JR, Lyons WE, Liu J, Bartnikas TB, Rothstein J, Price DL, Cleveland DW, Gitlin JD, Wong PC. Mutant SOD1 causes motor neuron disease independent of copper chaperone-mediated copper loading. Nat Neurosci 2002; 5(4):301–307.

46. Li M, Ona VO, Guegan C, Chen M, Jackson-Lewis V, Andrews LJ, Olszewski AJ, Stieg PE, Lee JP, Przedborski S, et al. Functional role of caspase-1 and caspase-3 in an ALS transgenic mouse model. Science 2000; 288(5464):335–339.

47. Guo H, Lai L, Butchbach ME, Stockinger MP, Shan X, Bishop GA, Lin CL. Increased expression of the glial glutamate transporter EAAT2 modulates excitotoxicity and delays the onset but not the outcome of ALS in mice. Hum Mol Genet 2003; 12(19):2519–2532.

48. Pramatarova A, Laganiere J, Roussel J, Brisebois K, Rouleau GA. Neuron-specific expression of mutant superoxide dismutase 1 in transgenic mice does not lead to motor impairment. J Neurosci 2001; 21(10):3369–3374.

49. Lino MM, Schneider C, Caroni P. Accumulation of SOD1 mutants in postnatal moto-neurons does not cause motoneuron pathology or motoneuron disease. J Neurosci 2002; 22(12):4825–4832.

50. Gong YH, Parsadanian AS, Andreeva A, Snider WD, Elliott JL. Restricted expression of G86R Cu/Zn superoxide dismutase in astrocytes results in astrocytosis but does not cause motoneuron degeneration. J Neurosci 2000; 20(2):660–665.

51. Esteban J, Rosen DR, Bowling AC, Sapp P, McKenna-Yasek D, O'Regan JP, Beal MF, Horvitz HR, Brown RH Jr. Identification of two novel mutations and a new poly-morphism in the gene for Cu/Zn superoxide dismutase in patients with amyotrophic lateral sclerosis. Hum Mol Genet 1994; 3(6):997–998.

52. Deng HX, Fu R, Siddique T. Overxpression of Normal SOD1 in ALS mice expressing mutant SOD1 leads to earlier onset of disease and shorter life-span of mice. American Journal of Human Genetics 1998; 63(4):A357.

53. Dal Canto MC, Gurney ME. A low expressor line of transgenic mice carrying a mutant human Cu,Zn superoxide dismutase (SOD1) gene develops pathological changes that most closely resemble those in human amyotrophic lateral sclerosis. Acta Neuropathol (Berl) 1997; 93(6):537–550.

54. Jonsson PA, Ernhill K, Andersen PM, Bergemalm D, Brannstrom T, Gredal O, Nilsson P, Marklund SL. Minute quantities of misfolded mutant superoxide dismutase-1 cause amyotrophic lateral sclerosis. Brain 2004; 127(Pt 1):73–88.

55. Niwa J, Ishigaki S, Hishikawa N, Yamamoto M, Doyu M, Murata S, Tanaka K, Taniguchi N, Sobue G. Dorfin ubiquitylates mutant SOD1 and prevents mutant SOD1-mediated neurotoxicity. J Biol Chem 2002; 277(39):36793–36798.

56. Ishigaki S, Hishikawa N, Niwa J, Iemura S, Natsume T, Hori S, Kakizuka A, Tanaka K, Sobue G. Physical and functional interaction between Dorfin and Valosin-containing protein that are colocalized in ubiquitylated inclusions in neurodegenerative disorders. J Biol Chem 2004; 279(49):51376–51385.

57. Patel H, Cross H, Proukakis C, Hershberger R, Bork P, Ciccarelli FD, Patton MA, McKusick VA, Crosby AH. SPG20 is mutated in Troyer syndrome, an hereditary spastic paraplegia. Nat Genet 2002; 31(4):347–348.

58. Nishimura AL, Mitne-Neto M, Silva HC, Richieri-Costa A, Middleton S, Cascio D, Kok F, Oliveira JR, Gillingwater T, Webb J, et al. A mutation in the vesicle-trafficking protein VAPB causes late-onset spinal muscular atrophy and amyotrophic lateral sclerosis. Am J Hum Genet 2004; 75(5):822–831.

59. Rampoldi L, Dobson-Stone C, Rubio JP, Danek A, Chalmers RM, Wood NW, Verellen C, Ferrer X, Malandrini A, Fabrizi GM, et al. A conserved sorting-associated protein is mutant in chorea-acanthocytosis. Nat Genet 2001; 28(2):119–120.

60. Carstea ED, Morris JA, Coleman KG, Loftus SK, Zhang D, Cummings C, Gu J, Rosenfeld MA, Pavan WJ, Krizman DB, et al. Niemann-Pick C1 disease gene: homology to mediators of cholesterol homeostasis. Science 1997; 277(5323):228–231.

61. Kanekura K, Hashimoto Y, Niikura T, Aiso S, Matsuoka M, Nishimoto I. Alsin, the product of ALS2 gene, suppresses SOD1 mutant neurotoxicity through RhoGEF domain by interacting with SOD1 mutants. J Biol Chem 2004; 279(18):19247–19256.

62. Watts GD, Wymer J, Kovach MJ, Mehta SG, Mumm S, Darvish D, Pestronk A, Whyte MP, Kimonis VE. Inclusion body myopathy associated with Paget disease of bone and frontotemporal dementia is caused by mutant valosin-containing protein. Nat Genet 2004; 36(4): 377–381.

63. Chen YZ, Bennett CL, Huynh HM, Blair IP, Puls I, Irobi J, Dierick I, Abel A, Kennerson ML, Rabin BA, Nicholson GA, Auer-Grumbach M, Wagner K, De Jonghe P, Griffin JW, Fischbeck KH, Timmerman V, Cornblath DR, Chance PF. DNA/RNA helicase gene mutations in a form of juvenile amyotrophic lateral sclerosis (ALS4). Am J Hum Genet 2004; 74(6):1128–1135.

64. Williamson TL, Cleveland DW. Slowing of axonal transport is a very early event in the toxicity of ALS-linked SOD1 mutants to motor neurons. Nat Neurosci 1999; 2(1):50–56.

65. Hafezparast M, Klocke R, Ruhrberg C, Marquardt A, Ahmad-Annuar A, Bowen S, Lalli G, Witherden AS, Hummerich H, Nicholson S, Morgan PJ, Oozageer R, Priestley JV, Averill S, King VR, Ball S, Peters J, Toda T, Yamamoto A, Hiraoka Y, Augustin M, Korthaus D, Wattler S, Wabnitz P, Dickneite C, Lampel S, Boehme F, Peraus G, Popp A, Rudelius M, Schlegel J, Fuchs H, Hrabe de Angelis M, Schiavo G, Shima DT, Russ AP, Stumm G, Martin JE, Fisher EM. Mutations in dynein link motor neuron degeneration to defects in retrograde transport. Science 2003; 300(5620):808–812.

66. Puls I, Jonnakuty C, LaMonte BH, Holzbaur EL, Tokito M, Mann E, Floeter MK, Bidus K, Drayna D, Oh SJ, Brown RH Jr., Ludlow CL, Fischbeck KH. Mutant dynactin in motor neuron disease. Nat Genet 2003; 33(4):455–456.

67. Corder EH, Saunders AM, Strittmatter WJ, Schmechel DE, Gaskell PC, Small GW, Roses AD, Haines JL, Pericak-Vance MA. Gene dose of apolipoprotein E type 4 allele and the risk of Alzheimer's disease in late onset families. Science 1993; 261(5123):921–923.

68. Mui S, Rebeck GW, McKenna-Yasek D, Hyman BT, Brown RH, Jr. Apolipoprotein E epsilon 4 allele is not associated with earlier age at onset in amyotrophic lateral sclerosis. Ann Neurol 1995; 38(3):460–463.

69. Al-Chalabi A, Enayat ZE, Bakker MC, Sham PC, Ball DM, Shaw CE, Lloyd CM, Powell JF, Leigh PN. Association of apolipoprotein E epsilon 4 allele with bulbar-onset motor neuron disease. Lancet 1996; 347(8995):159–160.

70. Moulard B, Sefiani A, Laamri A, Malafosse A, Camu W. Apolipoprotein E genotyping in sporadic amyotrophic lateral sclerosis: evidence for a major influence on the clinical presentation and prognosis. J Neurol Sci 1996; 139(suppl):34–37.

71. Smith RG, Haverkamp LJ, Case S, Appel V, Appel SH. Apolipoprotein E epsilon 4 in bulbar-onset motor neuron disease. Lancet 1996; 348(9023):334–335.

72. Siddique T, Pericak-Vance MA, Caliendo J, Hong ST, Hung WY, Kaplan J, McKenna-Yasek D, Rimmler JB, Sapp P, Saunders AM, Scott WK, Siddique N, Haines JL, Brown RH. Lack of association between apolipoprotein E genotype and sporadic amyotrophic lateral sclerosis. Neurogenetics 1998; 1(3):213–216.

73. Li Y, Pericak-Vance M, Haines J, Siddique N, McKenna-Yasek D, Hung W, Sapp P, Allen C, Chen W, Hosler BA, Saunders AM, Dellefave L, Brown RH, Siddique T. Age at onset modulates the effect of apolipoprotein E in amyotrophic lateral sclerosis. Neurogenetics 2004; 5(4):209–213.

74. Parboosingh JS, Meininger V, McKenna-Yasek D, Brown RH Jr, Rouleau GA. Deletions causing spinal muscular atrophy do not predispose to amyotrophic lateral sclerosis. Arch Neurol 1999; 56(6):710–712.

75. Veldink JH, van den Berg LH, Cobben JM, Stulp RP, De Jong JM, Vogels OJ, Baas F, Wokke JH, Scheffer H. Homozygous deletion of the survival motor neuron 2 gene is a prognostic factor in sporadic ALS. Neurology 2001; 56(6):749–752.

76. Corcia P, Mayeux-Portas V, Khoris J, de Toffol B, Autret A, Muh JP, Camu W, Andres C. Abnormal SMN1 gene copy number is a susceptibility factor for amyotrophic lateral sclerosis. Ann Neurol 2002; 51(2):243–246.

77. Lambrechts D, Storkebaum E, Morimoto M, Del-Favero J, Desmet F, Marklund SL, Wyns S, Thijs V, Andersson J, van Marion I, Al-Chalabi A, Bornes S, Musson R, Hansen V, Beckman L, Adolfsson R, Pall HS, Prats H, Vermeire S, Rutgeerts P, Katayama S, Awata T, Leigh N, Lang-Lazdunski L, Dewerchin M, Shaw C, Moons L, Vlietinck R, Morrison KE, Robberecht W, Van Broeckhoven C, Collen D, Andersen PM, Carmeliet P. VEGF is a modifier of amyotrophic lateral sclerosis in mice and humans and protects motoneurons against ischemic death. Nat Genet 2003; 34(4):383–394.

78. Gros-Louis F, Lariviere R, Gowing G, Laurent S, Camu W, Bouchard JP, Meininger V, Rouleau GA, Julien JP. A frameshift deletion in peripherin gene associated with amyotrophic lateral sclerosis. J Biol Chem 2004; 279(44):45951–45956.

79. Beaulieu JM, Nguyen MD, Julien JP. Late onset of motor neurons in mice overexpressing wild-type peripherin. J Cell Biol 1999; 147(3):531–544.

80. Carpenter S. Proximal axonal enlargement in motor neuron disease. Neurology 1968; 18(9):841–851.

81. Corbo M, Hays AP. Peripherin and neurofilament protein coexist in spinal spheroids of motor neuron disease. J Neuropathol Exp Neurol 1992; 51(5):531–537.

82. Migheli A, Pezzulo T, Attanasio A, Schiffer D. Peripherin immunoreactive structures in amyotrophic lateral sclerosis. Lab Invest 1993; 68(2):185–191.

83. Figlewicz DA, Krizus A, Martinoli MG, Meininger V, Dib M, Rouleau GA, Julien JP. Variants of the heavy neurofilament subunit are associated with the development of amyotrophic lateral sclerosis. Hum Mol Genet 1994; 3(10):1757–1761.

84. Al-Chalabi A, Andersen PM, Nilsson P, Chioza B, Andersson JL, Russ C, Shaw CE, Powell JF, Leigh PN. Deletions of the heavy neurofilament subunit tail in amyotrophic lateral sclerosis. Hum Mol Genet 1999; 8(2):157–164.

85. Tomkins J, Usher P, Slade JY, Ince PG, Curtis A, Bushby K, Shaw PJ. Novel insertion in the KSP region of the neurofilament heavy gene in amyotrophic lateral sclerosis (ALS). Neuroreport 1998; 9(17):3967–3970.

86. Guidelines for the molecular genetics predictive test in Huntington's disease. International Huntington Association (IHA) and the World Federation of Neurology (WFN) Research Group on Huntington's Chorea. Neurology 1994; 44(8):1533–1536.

87. Lefebvre S, Burglen L, Reboullet S, Clermont O, Burlet P, Viollet L, Benichou B, Cruaud C, Millasseau P, Zeviani M, et al. Identification and characterization of a spinal muscular atrophy-determining gene. Cell 1995; 80(1):155–165.

88. Grohmann K, Schuelke M, Diers A, Hoffmann K, Lucke B, Adams C, Bertini E, Leonhardt-Horti H, Muntoni F, Ouvrier R, Pfeufer A, Rossi R, Van Maldergem L, Wilmshurst JM, Wienker TF, Sendtner M, Rudnik-Schoneborn S, Zerres K, Hubner C. Mutations in the gene encoding immunoglobulin mu-binding protein 2 cause spinal muscular atrophy with respiratory distress type 1. Nat Genet 2001; 29(1):75–77.

89. Viollet L, Zarhrate M, Maystadt I, Estournet-Mathiaut B, Barois A, Desguerre I, Mayer M, Chabrol B, LeHeup B, Cusin V, Billette De Villemeur T, Bonneau D, Saugier-Veber P, Touzery-De Villepin A, Delaubier A, Kaplan J, Jeanpierre M, Feingold J, Munnich A. Refined genetic mapping of autosomal recessive chronic distal spinal muscular atrophy to chromosome 11q13.3 and evidence of linkage disequilibrium in European families. Eur J Hum Genet 2004; 12(6):483–488.

90. Christodoulou K, Zamba E, Tsingis M, Mubaidin A, Horani K, Abu-Sheik S, El-Khateeb M, Kyriacou K, Kyriakides T, Al-Qudah AK, Middleton L. A novel form of distal hereditary motor neuronopathy maps to chromosome 9p21.1-p12. Ann Neurol 2000; 48(6):877–884.

91. Antonellis A, Ellsworth RE, Sambuughin N, Puls I, Abel A, Lee-Lin SQ, Jordanova A, Kremensky I, Christodoulou K, Middleton LT, Sivakumar K, Ionasescu V, Funalot B, Vance JM, Goldfarb LG, Fischbeck KH, Green ED. Glycyl tRNA synthetase mutations in Charcot-Marie-Tooth disease type 2D and distal spinal muscular atrophy type V. Am J Hum Genet 2003; 72(5):1293–1299.

92. Auer-Grumbach M, Loscher WN, Wagner K, Petek E, Korner E, Offenbacher H, Hartung HP. Phenotypic and genotypic heterogeneity in hereditary motor neuronopathy type V: a clinical, electrophysiological and genetic study. Brain 2000; 123(Pt 8): 1612–1623.

93. van der Vleuten AJ, van Ravenswaaij-Arts CM, Frijns CJ, Smits AP, Hageman G, Padberg GW, Kremer H. Localisation of the gene for a dominant congenital spinal muscular atrophy predominantly affecting the lower limbs to chromosome 12q23-q24. Eur J Hum Genet 1998; 6(4):376–382.

94. McEntagart M, Norton N, Williams H, Teare MD, Dunstan M, Baker P, Houlden H, Reilly M, Wood N, Harper PS, Futreal PA, Williams N, Rahman N. Localization of the gene for distal hereditary motor neuronopathy VII (dHMN-VII) to chromosome 2q14. Am J Hum Genet 2001; 68(5):1270–1276.

95. Timmerman V, De Jonghe P, Simokovic S, Lofgren A, Beuten J, Nelis E, Ceuterick C, Martin JJ, Van Broeckhoven C. Distal hereditary motor neuropathy type II (distal HMN II): mapping of a locus to chromosome 12q24. Hum Mol Genet 1996; 5(7): 1065–1069.

96. Takata RI, Speck Martins CE, Passosbueno MR, Abe KT, Nishimura AL, Da Silva MD, Monteiro A Jr, Lima MI, Kok F, Zatz M. A new locus for recessive distal spinal muscular atrophy at Xq13.1-q21. J Med Genet 2004; 41(3):224–229.

97. La Spada AR, Roling DB, Harding AE, Warner CL, Spiegel R, Hausmanowa-Petrusewicz I, Yee WC, Fischbeck KH. Meiotic stability and genotype-phenotype correlation of the trinucleotide repeat in X-linked spinal and bulbar muscular atrophy. Nat Genet 1992; 2(4):301–304.

98. Hadano S, Hand CK, Osuga H, Yanagisawa Y, Otomo A, Devon RS, Miyamoto N, Showguchi-Miyata J, Okada Y, Singaraja R, Figlewicz DA, Kwiatkowski T, Hosler BA, Sagie T, Skaug J, Nasir J, Brown RH Jr, Scherer SW, Rouleau GA, Hayden MR, Ikeda JE. A gene encoding a putative GTPase regulator is mutated in familial amyotrophic lateral sclerosis 2. Nat Genet 2001; 29(2):166–173.

99. Zhao X, Alvarado D, Rainier S, Lemons R, Hedera P, Weber CH, Tukel T, Apak M, Heiman-Patterson T, Ming L, Bui M, Fink JK. Mutations in a newly identified GTPase

gene cause autosomal dominant hereditary spastic paraplegia. Nat Genet 2001; 29(3):326–331.

100. Hazan J, Fonknechten N, Mavel D, Paternotte C, Samson D, Artiguenave F, Davoine CS, Cruaud C, Durr A, Wincker P, Brottier P, Cattolico L, Barbe V, Burgunder JM, Prud'homme JF, Brice A, Fontaine B, Heilig B, Weissenbach J. Spastin, a new AAA protein, is altered in the most frequent form of autosomal dominant spastic paraplegia. Nat Genet 1999; 23(3):296–303.

101. Rainier S, Chai JH, Tokarz D, Nicholls RD, Fink JK. NIPA1 gene mutations cause autosomal dominant hereditary spastic paraplegia (SPG6). Am J Hum Genet 2003; 73(4):967–971.

102. Hedera P, Rainier S, Alvarado D, Zhao X, Williamson J, Otterud B, Leppert M, Fink JK. Novel locus for autosomal dominant hereditary spastic paraplegia, on chromosome 8q. Am J Hum Genet 1999; 64(2):563–569.

103. Reid E, Kloos M, Ashley-Koch A, Hughes L, Bevan S, Svenson IK, Graham FL, Gaskell PC, Dearlove A, Pericak-Vance MA, Rubinsztein DC, Marchuk DA. A kinesin heavy chain (KIF5A) mutation in hereditary spastic paraplegia (SPG10). Am J Hum Genet 2002; 71(5):1189–1194.

104. Reid E, Dearlove AM, Osborn O, Rogers MT, Rubinsztein DC. A locus for autosomal dominant "pure" hereditary spastic paraplegia maps to chromosome 19q13. Am J Hum Genet 2000; 66(2):728–732.

105. Hansen JJ, Durr A, Cournu-Rebeix I, Georgopoulos C, Ang D, Nielsen MN, Davoine CS, Brice A, Fontaine B, Gregersen N, Bross P. Hereditary spastic paraplegia SPG13 is associated with a mutation in the gene encoding the mitochondrial chaperonin Hsp60. Am J Hum Genet 2002; 70(5):1328–1332.

106. Valente EM, Brancati F, Caputo V, Bertini E, Patrono C, Costanti D, Dallapiccola B. Novel locus for autosomal dominant pure hereditary spastic paraplegia (SPG19) maps to chromosome 9q33-q34. Ann Neurol 2002; 51(6):681–685.

107. Hentati A, Pericak-Vance MA, Hung WY, Belal S, Laing N, Boustany RM, Hentati F, Ben Hamida M, Siddique T. Linkage of 'pure' autosomal recessive familial spastic paraplegia to chromosome 8 markers and evidence of genetic locus heterogeneity. Hum Mol Genet 1994; 3(8):1263–1267.

108. Winner B, Uyanik G, Gross C, Lange M, Schulte-Mattler W, Schuierer G, Marienhagen J, Hehr U, Winkler J. Clinical progression and genetic analysis in hereditary spastic paraplegia with thin corpus callosum in spastic gait gene 11 (SPG11). Arch Neurol 2004; 61(1):117–121.

109. Hodgkinson CA, Bohlega S, Abu-Amero SN, Cupler E, Kambouris M, Meyer BF, Bharucha VA. A novel form of autosomal recessive pure hereditary spastic paraplegia maps to chromosome 13q14. Neurology 2002; 59(12):1905–1909.

110. Seri M, Cusano R, Forabosco P, Cinti R, Caroli F, Picco P, Bini R, Morra VB, De Michele G, Lerone M, Silengo M, Pela I, Borrone C, Romeo G, Devoto M. Genetic mapping to 10q23.3-q24.2, in a large Italian pedigree, of a new syndrome showing bilateral cataracts, gastroesophageal reflux, and spastic paraparesis with amyotrophy. Am J Hum Genet 1999; 64(2):586–593.

111. Windpassinger C, Wagner K, Petek E, Fischer R, Auer-Grumbach M. Refinement of the Silver syndrome locus on chromosome 11q12-q14 in four families and exclusion of eight candidate genes. Hum Genet 2003; 114(1):99–109.

112. Meijer IA, Hand CK, Grewal KK, Stefanelli MG, Ives EJ, Rouleau GA. A locus for autosomal dominant hereditary spastic ataxia, SAX1, maps to chromosome 12p13. Am J Hum Genet 2002; 70(3):763–769.

113. Casari G, De Fusco M, Ciarmatori S, Zeviani M, Mora M, Fernandez P, De Michele G, Filla A, Cocozza S, Marconi R, Durr A, Fontaine B, Ballabio A. Spastic paraplegia and OXPHOS impairment caused by mutations in paraplegin, a nuclear-encoded mitochondrial metalloprotease. Cell 1998; 93(6):973–983.

114. Hughes CA, Byrne PC, Webb S, McMonagle P, Patterson V, Hutchinson M, Parfrey NA. SPG15, a new locus for autosomal recessive complicated HSP on chromosome 14q. Neurology 2001; 56(9):1230–1233.

115. Simpson MA, Cross H, Proukakis C, Pryde A, Hershberger R, Chatonnet A, Patton MA, Crosby AH. Maspardin is mutated in mast syndrome, a complicated form of hereditary spastic paraplegia associated with dementia. Am J Hum Genet 2003; 73(5): 1147–1156.

116. Engert JC, Berube P, Mercier J, Dore C, Lepage P, Ge B, Bouchard JP, Mathieu J, Melancon SB, Schalling M, Lander ES, Morgan K, Hudson TJ, Richter A. ARSACS, a spastic ataxia common in northeastern Quebec, is caused by mutations in a new gene encoding an 11.5-kb ORF. Nat Genet 2000; 24(2):120–125.

117. Jouet M, Rosenthal A, Armstrong G, MacFarlane J, Stevenson R, Paterson J, Metzenberg A, Ionasescu V, Temple K, Kenwrick S. X-linked spastic paraplegia (SPG1), MASA syndrome and X-linked hydrocephalus result from mutations in the L1 gene. Nat Genet 1994; 7(3):402–407.

118. Willard HF, Riordan JR. Assignment of the gene for myelin proteolipid protein to the X chromosome: implications for X-linked myelin disorders. Science 1985; 230(4728): 940–942.

119. Starling A, Rocco P, Cambi F, Hobson GM, Passos Bueno MR, Zatz M. Further evidence for a fourth gene causing X-linked pure spastic paraplegia. Am J Med Genet 2002; 111(2):152–156.

120. Pringle CE, Hudson AJ, Munoz DG, Kiernan JA, Brown WF, Ebers GC. Primary lateral sclerosis. Clinical features, neuropathology and diagnostic criteria. Brain 1992; 115(Pt 2):495–520.

121. Hentati A, Bejaoui K, Pericak-Vance MA, Hentati F, Speer MC, Hung WY, Figlewicz DA, Haines J, Rimmler J, Ben Hamida C, Hamida MB, Brown RH, Siddique T. Linkage of recessive familial amyotrophic lateral sclerosis to chromosome 2q33-q35. Nat Genet 1994; 7(3):425–428.

122. Hand CK, Khoris J, Salachas F, Gros-Louis F, Lopes AA, Mayeux-Portas V, Brewer CG, Brown RH, Jr., Meininger V, Camu W, Rouleau GA. A novel locus for familial amyotrophic lateral sclerosis, on chromosome 18q. Am J Hum Genet 2002; 70(1):251–256.

123. Ruddy DM, Parton MJ, Al-Chalabi A, Lewis CM, Vance C, Smith BN, Leigh PN, Powell JF, Siddique T, Meyjes EP, Baas F, de Jong V, Shaw CE. Two families with familial amyotrophic lateral sclerosis are linked to a novel locus on chromosome 16q. Am J Hum Genet 2003; 73(2):390–396.

124. Abalkhail H, Mitchell J, Habgood J, Orrell R, de Belleroche J. A new familial amyotrophic lateral sclerosis locus on chromosome 16q12.1–16q12.2. Am J Hum Genet 2003; 73(2):383–389.

125. Sapp PC, Hosler BA, McKenna-Yasek D, Chin W, Gann A, Genise H, Gorenstein J, Huang M, Sailer W, Scheffler M, Valesky M, Haines JL, Pericak-Vance M, Siddique T, Horvitz HR, Brown RH Jr. Identification of two novel loci for dominantly inherited familial amyotrophic lateral sclerosis. Am J Hum Genet 2003; 73(2):397–403.

126. Chance PF, Rabin BA, Ryan SG, Ding Y, Scavina M, Crain B, Griffin JW, Cornblath DR. Linkage of the gene for an autosomal dominant form of juvenile amyotrophic lateral sclerosis to chromosome 9q34. Am J Hum Genet 1998; 62(3):633–640.

127. Hosler BA, Siddique T, Sapp PC, Sailor W, Huang MC, Hossain A, Daube JR, Nance M, Fan C, Kaplan J, Hung WY, McKenna-Yasek D, Haines JL, Pericak-Vance MA, Horvitz HR, Brown RH, Jr. Linkage of familial amyotrophic lateral sclerosis with frontotemporal dementia to chromosome 9q21-q22. JAMA 2000; 284(13):1664–1669.

128. Wilhelmsen KC, Forman MS, Rosen HJ, Alving LI, Goldman J, Feiger J, Lee JV, Segall SK, Kramer JH, Lomen-Hoerth C, Rankin KP, Johnson J, Feiler HS, Weiner MW, Lee VM, Trojanowski JQ, Miller BL. 17q-linked frontotemporal dementia-amyotrophic lateral sclerosis without tau mutations with tau and alpha-synuclein inclusions. Arch Neurol 2004; 61(3):398–406.

8

Objective Markers of Upper and Lower Motor Neuron Dysfunction: Electrophysiological Studies and Neuroimaging Technologies

Clifton L. Gooch, Petra Kaufmann, and Seth Pullman
Department of Neurology, The Neurological Institute, Columbia University College of Physicians and Surgeons, New York, New York, U.S.A.

INTRODUCTION

Since their inception, conventional electrodiagnostic techniques have played a critical role in the diagnosis and investigation of motor neuron disease. However, despite years of emphasis on electrodiagnosis in neurology training programs, patients continue to be misdiagnosed with amyotrophic lateral sclerosis (ALS) because of poorly performed and improperly interpreted electrodiagnostic studies. Consequently, an understanding of the proper role of electromyography and nerve conductions is essential for the clinical diagnosis of ALS.

Technological advances have provided a number of novel markers of motor neuron function in recent years, which have assumed increasing importance in the investigation of ALS. Prior to the mid-1990s, our ability to measure the integrity of the motor pathway was highly limited. However, significant advances in equipment and technology over the last decade have now made quantitative assessment of both upper and lower motor neuron (LMN) function not only possible but also feasible in the living human subject. As these methods are well tolerated, serial longitudinal measurements have become routine in many academic centers, enabling tracking of the effects of disease and therapy over time. Motor unit number estimation (MUNE) methods quantitatively track LMN deterioration, as well as providing an estimate of compensatory collateral reinnervation. Advanced neuroimaging techniques [e.g., magnetic resonance spectroscopy (MRS), single photon emission computed tomography (SPECT), and positron emission tomography (PET)] allow measurement of the metabolic health of the motor cortex and the upper motor neuron (UMN) pathway, while transcranial magnetic stimulation (TMS) enables the tracking of impulse transmission from the cortex to the muscle, assessing both the UMN and LMN.

ELECTROPHYSIOLOGIC TESTING IN THE DIAGNOSIS OF ALS

Introduction

Electromyographers have devoted considerable attention to ALS, not only because of the critical importance of insuring that this devastating diagnosis is properly made, but also because electrodiagnostic techniques provide unique physiologic information about the disease in the living human subject. The proper use of electrophysiologic techniques and the data they generate remains paramount, as a number of easily missed details can either obscure the recognition of ALS or prompt misdiagnosis in patients having other, less serious, disorders. Traditional electrodiagnostic investigations have also significantly contributed to our understanding of the effects of ALS on the LMN and the neuromuscular junction. Patients presenting to the electromyography laboratory with the diagnosis of possible ALS require a battery of investigations to rule out other causes of their symptoms and to provide further supportive evidence for the clinical diagnosis of motor neuron disease.

Nerve Conduction Studies

Nerve conduction studies (NCS) should be performed in a variety of sensory and motor nerves in at least one upper and one lower extremity; other nerves may need to be tested depending on the type and degree of abnormality observed. Standard sensory NCS involve transcutaneous stimulation of the sensory nerve, with transcutaneous recording from the same nerve either proximally or distally as the action potential spreads from the stimulation site. Nerve conduction velocity (NCV) and various parameters of the waveform [the sensory nerve action potential (SNAP)] are recorded and compared with normative data. Standard motor NCS involve transcutaneous stimulation of the nerve also, but with recording from an innervated muscle, rather than from the nerve itself. When adequate levels of stimulation are applied, complete depolarization of all motor axons within the nerve causes full depolarization and contraction of the muscle. The resultant electrical activity is recorded as the compound motor action potential (CMAP), a waveform representing the summated electrical activity of all the functional motor units and muscle fibers within the tested muscle. The amplitude of the CMAP is measured, and motor NCVs are also calculated. Late responses such as the F wave and H reflex measure depolarization up and down the entire peripheral nerve pathway and may also be performed.

In keeping with their lack of significant sensory loss, most ALS patients have normal sensory nerve conductions. Although subtle sensory abnormalities may be detected on somatosensory evoked potential testing, significant sensory abnormalities are rare and responses outside the limits of normal should prompt a more aggressive search for polyneuropathy (1–5). In early disease, motor NCS are also usually normal, but may demonstrate a range of abnormalities as the disease progresses. In most patients, CMAP amplitudes decline in a linear fashion with time, correlating with declines in the force of maximal isometric contraction as well as muscular atrophy (2–6). In motor nerves demonstrating significant loss of CMAP amplitude, mild slowing of conduction velocity may also be observed, although it rarely falls to less than 80% of the lower limits of normal (5–7). F wave and distal latency measures may also be abnormal under these conditions, but rarely exceed 1.25 times the upper limit of normal (7,8). Interestingly, another late response, the H reflex, appears with greater reliability in patients with ALS (perhaps because of increased excitability in the spinal motor neuron pool) and can be elicited from a wider range of muscles than in the normal patient (9,10).

Abnormalities in sensory or motor NCS exceeding the above parameters should suggest another disorder. Careful observation and testing for *conduction block* (a significant drop in the amplitude and/or area of a given motor nerve's CMAP when stimulation at a proximal site is compared with stimulation at a distal site) is also critical, as a number of eminently treatable demyelinative and ischemic neuropathies mimicking motor neuron disease may present with such findings (11,12). The precise degree of amplitude drop positively identifying a conduction block is a matter of some debate and probably varies somewhat from nerve to nerve, but strict research criteria (maximizing specificity rather than sensitivity) suggest a loss of at least 50% (13). If a discrete area of conduction block or an area of focal slowing is found in a motor nerve, extensive motor NCS of all extremities should be considered.

Standard Needle Electromyography

After completion of NCS, needle electromyography should be performed in at least three extremities, the paraspinous muscles, and at least one bulbar muscle (such as the genioglossus). This approach provides a thorough assessment of the extent and distribution of denervation in the cranial, cervical, thoracic, and lumbosacral myotomes, increasing sensitivity and allowing for the more accurate application of diagnostic criteria, such as the El Escorial system (see below). Although the needle electromyography (EMG) examination provides confirmatory evidence in areas where the clinical examination suggests denervation, it is most useful diagnostically for detecting denervation in areas where it is not clinically apparent, thereby demonstrating a wider distribution of LMN injury than the physical examination alone. Consequently, a thorough assessment of each major spinal and bulbar region, especially those without clear abnormalities by physical examination, is critical. As with other routine needle exams, five basic components should be assessed in different locations in each tested muscle: *insertional activity, spontaneous activity, motor unit configuration, recruitment, and the interference pattern.* As the needle is initially inserted, it transects the muscle and individual fibers causing a burst of insertional activity, which normally subsides in less than one second. Denervation renders the fiber membrane hyperexcitable, resulting in prolongation of this phenomenon (*increased insertional activity*). At rest, normal muscle (away from the end-plate zone) should be electrically silent but, with loss of innervation, lack of tonic neuronal influence will result in the spontaneous depolarizations of individual muscle fibers at rest, recorded as *spontaneous discharges* (fibrillations and positive sharp waves). Such spontaneous activity is widespread in ALS and is a hallmark of the disease, but is highly non-specific, requiring appropriate adjunctive NCS to rule out other denervating disorders. Spontaneous activity is most likely to be seen in weaker, atrophied muscles (6), and correlates with active, ongoing denervation. *Fasciculations* (the spontaneous and involuntary activation of individual motor units at the level of the anterior horn) are also commonly seen both at and during needle electromyography in ALS patients. They sometimes appear electrically when they cannot be observed by visual inspection of the overlying skin. Other discharges suggestive of muscular membrane irritability such as *simple* and *complex repetitive discharges* (prolonged trains of rapid and unusually regular discharges most probably resulting from ephaptic activation of groups of adjacent muscle fibers) may also appear following needle insertion or voluntary activation of the muscle (5,6,9,14).

The motor unit consists of a single anterior horn cell, its axon, and all of the muscle fibers it innervates. Analysis of the waveforms generated by voluntary activation of the motor units within a given muscle is an often overlooked, but critical step in the needle examination of the ALS patient. Assessment of motor unit action potential (MUAP) duration, complexity, and amplitude will help to identify normal, neuropathic, and myopathic abnormalities; at least 20 MUAPs should be analyzed in each sampled muscle. The normal MUAP should have a duration of 5 to 15 milliseconds, amplitude of several hundred microvolts to several millivolts, and have no more than four baseline crossings (phases) or five turns. Not more than 15% of the sampled MUAPs should exceed these parameters in a normal subject (9).

As motor axons die and deprive the muscle fibers they supplied of innervation, surviving axons branch to reinnervate these denervated muscle fibers, expanding and diversifying their territories. These modified motor units produce larger and more complex MUAPs due to their larger size and greater heterogeneity. This *neurogenic MUAP* therefore has a longer duration, greater amplitude, and increased complexity (greater numbers of turns and/or baseline crossings) and suggests a subacute or chronic denervation, as at least two to three months is required for reinnervation to become established. The most extreme examples of this process are the "giant units" exceeding 10 to 15 mV in amplitude, which sometimes appear in ALS patients. In contrast, the more random and global atrophy of myopathic diseases should characteristically produce MUAPs of shorter duration, lower complexity, and lower amplitude.

This process of collateral reinnervation is a very effective compensatory mechanism that enables patients to maintain normal strength despite loss of a considerable proportion of their motor units in ALS and other denervating diseases. Changes in the MUAP configuration provide a signature of the peripheral motor system's struggle to survive and enable the detection of chronic denervation in limbs, which appear normal symptomatically and by neurological examination.

In addition to measurements of motor unit configuration, the temporal patterns of motor unit firing should also be carefully assessed. This is typically studied in terms of the motor system's ability to properly activate or *recruit* appropriate numbers of motor units at different force levels during voluntary contraction. As initial voluntary contraction begins, a single motor unit (the first recruited) will appear. As voluntary effort increases, this motor unit increases its firing rate to generate greater force until it reaches a threshold (typically less than 15 Hz) known as the *recruitment frequency* at which point a second motor unit is also recruited and begins firing, adding its force to the first. As patient effort increases further, additional units join until maximal contraction appears. As motor units drop out with advancing disease, surviving units will increase their firing rates beyond the normal range in an attempt to generate enough force to compensate for the loss. A more global method of quantitating this phenomenon is the *recruitment ratio*, which is the ratio of the average firing rate to the total number of motor units firing (6,14–16).

As motor units die, the number of motor units available for recruitment decreases and the remaining motor units fire faster in an attempt to compensate for the lost force. Consequently, higher recruitment frequencies and ratios are characteristic of LMN lesions, particularly those affecting the anterior horn cell. Isolated UMN lesions result in a smaller number of recruited motor units, firing at slow rates despite maximal patient effort as coordination of firing rate fails at the central level. Although the UMN system is also affected in ALS, LMN degeneration often dominates the recruitment pattern, resulting in increased frequencies and ratios. Maximal voluntary effort by the patient is critical for the proper assessment of recruitment, as incomplete attempts due to pain or poor cooperation will not result in a full pattern. Typically, however, the recruitment ratio is normal under such circumstances and other clinical cues may also alert the examiner to this problem.

With normal maximal voluntary contraction, so many motor units are recruited that a nearly solid band of superimposed MUAPs is observed at slow sweep speeds (100 milliseconds per division or greater). This constitutes a *full interference pattern*. As motor units die and drop out, gaps appear in this band, getting wider and wider with increasing denervation until a "picket fence" pattern of MUAP activation appears, despite full efforts at voluntary contraction by the patient. Incomplete interference patterns can result from any process, which reduces motor unit activation (upper or LMN lesions; lack of full voluntary effort). Consequently, this test is much less specific and much less quantitatively reliable than the assessment of recruitment frequency and/or ratio. ALS patients manifest progressive reductions in the interference pattern over time, until they are left with only a few recruitable units and finally, one isolated survivor (a single firing motor unit) just prior to complete loss of all function in a given muscle.

As virtually all of these changes can be seen with a variety of lesions at every level of the peripheral nerve from root to motor nerve terminal, attention to the distribution of electrophysiologic abnormalities is essential. The widespread denervation characteristic of ALS is best confirmed when electrical changes are found in at least three separate and distinct areas (either three extremities or two extremities and the bulbar region). The most affected extremity should be tested initially in different proximal and distal myotomes, followed by other, more distant regions to confirm a diffuse process (14). In order to exclude regional polyradiculopathy and demonstrate diffuse involvement of the motor roots, testing of the paraspinal muscles is also crucial. This should include not only the cervical and lumbosacral but also the thoracic paraspinal muscles as the thoracic roots are rarely compressed by spondylosis or herniated discs, making denervation there a more reliable indicator of anterior horn cell disease. Similarly, denervation of the bulbar musculature can provide further supportive evidence for the diagnosis, though its absence by no means rules it out.

Diagnostic Criteria

In 1967, Lambert proposed a set of criteria for the electrodiagnosis of ALS that included: (i) fibrillations and fasciculations in the upper and lower extremities or in the extremities and the head, (ii) decreased numbers of MUAPs, (iii) increased MUAP amplitude and duration, (iv) normal motor NCS in the nerves of relatively unaffected muscles, (v) motor NCVs <30% below the normal range in affected muscles, and (vi) normal sensory NCS. Lambert's criteria were a starting point for further clarification and remain good basic guidelines, as evident from section "Standard Needle EMG".

The most ambitious and comprehensive criteria for the diagnosis of ALS were produced by the World Federation of Neurology Research Group on Neuromuscular Diseases in 1994 (17), and focused on clinical criteria (Table 1). These guidelines were created not only to insure standardized and reproducible diagnoses for international clinical trials, but also to provide a gold standard for the individual physician. The role of electrodiagnostic studies was summarized: "Patients with suspected, possible, probable, or definite ALS on clinical grounds should have electrophysiological studies to confirm LMN degeneration in clinically affected regions, to find electrophysiological evidence of LMN degeneration in clinically uninvolved regions and to exclude other pathophysiologic processes." These criteria were revised

Table 1 El Escorial Criteria for the Diagnosis of ALS (1994)

Definite ALS	UMN and LMN signs in bulbar and two spinal regions[a] or UMN and LMN signs in three spinal regions
Probable ALS	UMN and LMN signs in two regions (spinal or bulbar) and UMN signs in a region that is rostral to LMN signs
Possible ALS	UMN and LMN signs in one region (spinal or bulbar)
Suspected ALS	LMN signs in two or three regions (spinal or bulbar)

[a]Regions are bulbar/cranial, cervical, thoracic and lumbosacral.
Abbreviations: UMN, upper motor neuron; LMN, lower motor neuron; ALS, amyotrophic lateral sclerosis.

Table 2 Revised Criteria for the Diagnosis of ALS (1998)

Clinically Definite ALS is defined on clinical evidence alone by the presence of UMN, as well as LMN signs in three regions

Clinically Probable ALS is defined on clinical evidence alone by UMN and LMN signs in at least two regions with some UMN necessarily rostral to the LMN signs

Clinically Probable—Laboratory supported ALS is defined when clinical signs of UMN and LMN dysfunction are in only one region, or when UMN signs alone are present in one region, and LMN signs defined by EMG criteria are present in at least two limbs, with proper application of neuroimaging and clinical laboratory protocols to exclude other causes

Clinically Possible ALS is defined when clinical signs of UMN and LMN dysfunction are found together in only one region or UMN signs are found alone in two or more regions; or LMN signs are found rostral to UMN signs and the diagnosis of Clinically Probable—Laboratory supported ALS cannot be proven by evidence on clinical grounds in conjunction with electrodiagnostic, neurophysiologic, neuroimaging, or clinical laboratory studies

Other diagnoses must have been excluded to accept a diagnosis of Clinically Possible ALS

in 1998 (Table 2), with the addition of a new category of "Clinically Probable— Laboratory Supported" ALS (18).

Electrophysiologic Differential Diagnosis

Benign Fasciculations

Benign fasciculations are extremely common. Most patients pay little attention to these symptoms, but health care workers and others who learn of the association between diffuse fasciculations and ALS may be alarmed and seek medical evaluation. Benign fasciculations usually begin before 30 years and may persist for as little as a few weeks, or may last a lifetime. They are typically intermittent, and are often induced by stress, exercise, fatigue and sleep deprivation, alcohol, and caffeine. Cramps may also occur, as in the "cramp-fasciculation syndrome," but are generally less common than that in ALS. Prospective studies have clearly shown that benign fasciculations (defined as fasciculations without other symptoms or signs in a patient with an otherwise negative neurologic evaluation) are virtually never a prelude to ALS (19). As there are no distinctive electrophysiologic differences between "benign" and "malignant" fasciculations, their significance depends on associated electrophysiologic and clinical abnormalities (e.g., concurrent fibrillations, positive sharp waves, or neurogenic MUAPs in a clinically affected muscle). Fasciculations alone in an otherwise healthy patient with normal strength and a normal neurologic examination can be considered benign. Electrodiagnostic testing is useful to confirm the absence of any other denervation change and to reassure the patient.

Cervical Spondylitic Radiculomyelopathy

Cervical spondylitic radiculomyelopathy can cause weakness and wasting in the arms and hands due to spondylitic compression of the cervical nerve roots, with simultaneous spasticity due to spondylitic spinal cord compression, closely mimicking ALS. Although dermatomal sensory dysfunction and neck pain may also be seen, they are not invariably present and may not be a major component of the patient's presenting symptoms. In patients with diffuse spondylosis, lumbosacral polyradiculopathies may also be seen producing symptoms in the legs. NCS are unremarkable, with the exception of possible decreased motor amplitudes in areas in which muscle atrophy is present. EMG reveals denervation at several cervical and/or lumbosacral paraspinal levels and their corresponding myotomes. However, the thoracic paraspinal muscles are spared, as are the bulbar muscles. In patients with this electrophysiologic picture, further clinical evaluation, including imaging studies of the spine, is critically important.

Inclusion Body Myositis

Inclusion body myositis (IBM) is the most common myopathy in patients over 65 years of age. It typically presents with slowly progressive weakness and atrophy of the distal arm and hand muscles, with disproportionate involvement of the wrist and finger flexors, and later involvement of the proximal and distal legs. Early hand weakness can cause confusion with ALS. NCS are unremarkable, with the exception of possible decreased motor amplitudes in areas in which muscle atrophy is present. EMG typically demonstrates a predominately myopathic pattern with short duration motor unit potentials and early recruitment, most prominent in the forearm flexors. However, mild spontaneous activity including fibrillation potentials, positive sharp waves, and complex repetitive discharges, as well as neurogenic MUAPs, may also be seen, potentially causing diagnostic confusion. Careful motor unit analysis, however, usually distinguishes a dominant myopathic component in affected muscles. Muscle biopsy is definitive, demonstrating β-amyloid containing rimmed vacuoles within muscle fibers.

Polymyositis

Polymyositis is an inflammatory myopathy sometimes associated with other autoimmune diseases. Although weakness predominately affects the proximal leg and arm muscles (an unusual pattern for ALS), the absence of sensory symptoms in concert with some of the electrophysiologic features of this disorder can result in a misdiagnosis of ALS. NCS are typically normal. However, on needle EMG examination, widespread profuse spontaneous activity is seen, including the thoracic paraspinous muscles, presumably due to microdenervation and membrane irritation in inflamed muscle fibers. As spontaneous activity is usually a hallmark of denervation, these findings can be particularly misleading. Typically, complex repetitive discharges are somewhat more prominent in polymyositis than in ALS patients, but individual cases of each disease may vary in this respect. Consequently, MUAP configuration and the recruitment pattern become the critical elements on which the diagnosis rests, and should clearly demonstrate myopathic (not neuropathic) change. If these portions of the examination are not carefully performed, however, the chances of electrical misdiagnosis are significant.

Multifocal Motor Neuropathy with Conduction Block

This is rare and must be distinguished from true ALS, as it is potentially treatable. This disorder typically presents with weakness and wasting of one hand in an older man, with the progression to contralateral hand over months to years, followed by weakness of the proximal arms and legs. Multifocal motor neuropathy (MMN) is thought to be an autoimmune motor neuropathy, with focal demyelination affecting multiple nerves, especially in their proximal segments. However, these abnormalities may be detectable in only one or a few isolated areas on electrical testing, making extensive NCS critical for the diagnosis. Furthermore, proximal conduction block and focal slowing are often missed during NCS because most laboratories routinely test only the distal segments. When MMN is suspected, numerous motor NCS must be performed, often including all four extremities and any accessible proximal motor nerve segments. Mildly decreased sensory nerve amplitudes may sometimes also be seen, though sensory nerves are usually spared. EMG often demonstrates widespread acute and chronic denervation change (spontaneous activity, neurogenic MUAPs), although the paraspinal muscles are less frequently involved. In our experience and that of others, proximal conduction blocks of this type may occasionally be seen in patients with clear ALS by other criteria, whose clinical course is indistinguishable from patients with motor neuron disease. However, in the proper clinical setting, these findings should be considered diagnostic of MMN until proven otherwise.

Spinal Muscular Atrophies

Spinal muscular atrophies are a group of hereditary anterior horn cell diseases in both children and adults with progressive proximal and distal muscular weakness and atrophy over many years. In most forms, proximal weakness is most prominent. NCS are usually unremarkable, with the exception of possible decreased motor amplitudes in areas in which muscle atrophy is present. EMG findings may include fibrillations potentials, positive sharp waves, fasciculation potentials, and very large, complex motor units, with reduced recruitment patterns. Additionally, an unusual form of spontaneous activity consisting of an arrhythmic motor unit discharge at rest, having a frequency of 5 to 15 Hz, may also appear, thought to be due to the increased excitability of immature surviving motor neurons. Less prominent neurogenic features are usually seen in younger patients, which become more pronounced as age increases. Fibrillations, positive sharp waves, complex repetitive discharges, and fasciculations are less frequent in small infants and most common in patients older than four years of age. Motor unit size is usually the most useful parameter, and is usually most prominent in the proximal muscles of patients older than four years having more chronic disease.

Kennedy's Syndrome

Kennedy's syndrome is an X-linked motor neuron disorder affecting only males older than 30 to 40 years, causing progressive weakness of the bulbar and extremity muscles over many years. Motor NCS are frequently normal, although the sural and other

SNAPs may demonstrate reduced amplitudes or be absent. EMG demonstrates reduced motor unit recruitment patterns and complex motor unit potentials of long duration and increased amplitude in nearly all patients, with infrequent spontaneous activity. These changes typically affect arms, the legs, and the bulbar musculature. Heterozygous female carriers usually are not symptomatic, but 50% may demonstrate chronic reinnervation changes on EMG, including high amplitude long duration motor units, as well as fiber type grouping on muscle biopsy. Relatively specific grouped motor unit discharges occurring up to several times per second with mild voluntary activation of the mentalis muscle (with frequencies of 10–40 Hz within each group and durations of 0.1 to several seconds) may be found. Although these discharges are somewhat analogous to the syndrome of hereditary quivering of the chin, involuntary discharges are observed only with activation and not at rest.

Focal Motor Neuron Disease

Focal motor neuron disease is a form of motor neuron disease that remains restricted to one spinal segment and may be unilateral. *Monomelic amyotrophy* is a specific focal motor neuron syndrome affecting young males, restricted to one limb, usually the arm, with progressive weakness and wasting of the hand. In general, EMG of the focal motor neuron diseases demonstrates changes typical of ALS, but restricted to one region. This picture cannot be distinguished from early, focal onset ALS, and serial studies may be needed to document continued focality. In monomelic amyotrophy, spontaneous activity may be sometimes be sparse, though large, complex motor units are clearly seen.

Postpolio Syndrome

Postpolio syndrome begins about 30 years after an episode of poliomyelitis and is characterized by very slowly progressive muscle weakness and atrophy, usually in a previously affected area, without sensory changes. Progression of weakness is usually very slow. NCS are usually unremarkable, with the exception of possible decreased motor amplitudes in areas in which muscle atrophy is present. Electromyography reveals giant MUAPs, often more than 20 times the size of the average MUAP in affected muscles, with fasciculations but little other spontaneous activity.

Neuromuscular Junction Dysfunction

When an MUAP is isolated on needle examination and observed as it repetitively fires with voluntary contraction, its configuration should normally remain relatively stable. In patients with ALS (as in patients with disorders of the neuromuscular junction such as myasthenia gravis), however, the MUAP demonstrates instability by changing its configuration from discharge to discharge. The MUAP observed on EMG needle examination is the summated product of the simultaneous discharges of its component single muscle fibers and, as transmission fails at various different neuromuscular junctions (NMJs) from discharge to discharge, the shape of the waveform alters accordingly. This observation led Mulder, Lambert, and Eaton, in 1959, to further investigate this phenomenon with repetitive nerve stimulation (RNS). This test involves the supramaximal electrical stimulation of a motor nerve repeatedly at a given frequency (typically 2–3 Hz in low-frequency studies) with recording of the resulting train of CMAPs over an innervated muscle. As acetylcholine release from the nerve terminal declines with repeated depolarization, a reduced "safety factor" for neuromuscular transmission in diseases of the NMJ (such as myasthenia and the myasthenic syndromes) causes progressively more transmission failure at increasing numbers of NMJs, producing a decrement in CMAP amplitude. After a period of sustained exercise of the tested muscle, however, transiently increased acetylcholine pooling and release temporarily increase the CMAP and partially repair the decrement (postexercise facilitation). In 1959, Mulder et al. reported a CMAP amplitude decrement of 10% accompanied by postexercise facilitation in the distal musculature of an ALS patient and several other investigators subsequently reported similar results (20–23). The largest study of RNS in ALS (23) found that at least 50% of 190 ALS patients demonstrated some degree of decrementing, while 29% demonstrated decrement consistent with significant NMJ dysfunction. The higher incidence of decrement noted in this study was likely due to higher sensitivity resulting from examination of a more proximal muscle (the trapezius) than previous studies. No correlation with clinical severity or progression was noted and 25% of patients showing no decrement initially did not later develop it, despite the progression of their disease.

The most sensitive examination of NMJ function currently available, however, is single fiber electromyography (SFEMG), which provides an analysis of the variance in firing times between two muscle fibers correlating with NMJ function. This value, termed *jitter*, increases with increasing dysfunction of neuromuscular transmission and has been studied in ALS. SFEMG electrodes can also be used to calculate the density of fibers within a given motor unit [the *fiber density* (FD)] (24), which correlates with the degree of collateral reinnervation in a given muscle.

ALS patients demonstrate increased jitter, as well as complete failure of transmission (*blocking*), along with increased FD. Increased jitter in ALS has been attributed to the immaturity of new NMJs formed during collateral reinnervation. However, the degree of jitter abnormality in ALS often exceeds that expected on the basis of denervation/reinnervation alone (25,26). Symptomatically advanced cases with signs of denervation on routine EMG demonstrated higher jitter and more blocking, most prominent in the weakest muscles (25,26). In addition, abnormal jitter was noted in more than 30% of clinically normal muscles in ALS patients, leading some to suggest that increased jitter may be the earliest electrical abnormality in some patients (24,27). These higher jitter values and frequent blocking are consistent with a relatively rapidly progressive destruction of the motor neuron, possibly with a superimposed additional NMJ abnormality, and contrast with other disorders such as spinal muscular atrophy which have lower jitter and much less frequent blocking (25,28,29). There may be an additional (though likely subclinical) component of NMJ dysfunction in ALS, which might help explain these discrepancies, as animal models of motor neuron disease have demonstrated presynaptic NMJ abnormalities under a variety of circumstances (30–33).

FD measures in ALS are higher than normal subjects, but lower than those seen in polyneuropathy and spinal muscular atrophy. This may be the result of more rapid and aggressive denervation in ALS preventing the more extensive collateral reinnervation seen in more slowly progressive denervating diseases. FD values were generally higher in more clinically affected muscles, but remained abnormal even in clincally normal regions. FD increases also correlated with increases in mean MUAP amplitude measured during routine needle examination, though increased FD was seen in some muscles without increases in MUAP amplitude (25,27,29). In general, FD and MUAP appear to increase as strength in a given muscle remains normal (suggesting adequate compensatory reinnervation), then peak when moderate weakness appears and finally decline in the most severely affected muscles as reinnervation fails to keep up with the progression of the disease (24,25,27,29).

Selected Autonomic Studies

The autonomic nervous system may also be subtly affected in ALS, and electro-physiologic testing may best demonstrate these abnormalities. Decreased variability of the RR interval in the EKG with respiration has been reported in ALS patients compared with age-matched controls. This finding was consistent with parasympathetic dysfunction in at least one study and might possibly have some prognostic significance, although no correlation can be drawn between this abnormality and stage of disease at the time of measurement (34,35). The sympathetic skin response (SSR) is a measure of the change in electrical potential at the skin surface mediated by the autonomic pathway, involving a variety of central structures and efferent preganglionic myelinated and postganglionic non-myelinated axons and the neuro-glandular junction of the sweat gland. The SSR performed at the sole of the foot is absent in up to 40% of ALS patients and prolonged in onset in another significant number (36). Quantitative sudomotor axon reflex testing, a more specific test of postganglionic sympathetic axons, is also abnormal, failing in up to 31% of tested patients (34). Although these and other tests support some involvement of the autonomic nervous system in the disease, corresponding symptoms are extremely rare and these tests are not routinely recommended as part of a purely diagnostic investigation.

LOWER MOTOR NEURON DISEASE MARKERS: MOTOR UNIT NUMBER ESTIMATION

Basic Concepts of Motor Unit Number Estimation

The individual anterior horn cell and its motor axon, axonal branches and the muscle fibers it innervates are known as the *motor unit*. Most muscles contain hundreds of motor units and thousands of muscle fibers. Controlled external electrical stimulation can fully depolarize all of the functional motor axons within a peripheral nerve, sending action potentials down the terminal branches of every axon and across each NMJ into each muscle fiber within the innervated muscle. When an electrode is placed on the skin overlying the innervated muscle, the depolarization of these muscle fibers will generate an electrical potential, which can be recorded as a waveform (the CMAP). The CMAP is the traditional measure of motor nerve function used for many years in standard NCS (Fig. 1), and is the product of the total number of individual motor units the muscle contains and their sizes. The electrical signature of a single motor unit [*the single motor unit action potential* (SMUAP)] can also be derived using a variety of methods. A sample of SMUAPs recorded from the same muscle can be averaged to derive an average single motor unit size for the total motor unit population.

Since the CMAP represents the summated electrical signature of all the functional motor units within a given muscle firing together, the approximate number of motor units can be calculated by dividing the CMAP size (usually represented by amplitude or area) by the average S-MUAP waveform size (also in amplitude

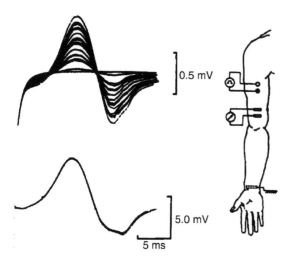

Figure 1 Incremental stimulation MUNE. Set up for recording from the biceps brachii with proximal stimulation of the musculocutaneous nerve (*right*). Superimposed waveforms, obtained following a series of progressively increasing stimuli (*top left*), are shown with the full CMAP (*bottom left*). The amplitude (or area) of each waveform increment is measured, and divided by the number of increments to obtain the average S-MUAP. The full CMAP amplitude (or area) is then divided by the average S-MUAP to derive the MUNE. *Abbreviations*: CMAP, compound motor action potential; MUNE, motor unit number estimation; MUAP, motor unit action potential. *Source*: From Ref. 37.

or area), yielding a MUNE. The formula for this calculation is:

$$\text{MUNE} = \frac{\text{CMAP Component}}{\text{Average S-MUAP Component}}$$

MUNE methods differ primarily in the techniques they use to derive the average S-MUAP size. Numerous methods for MUNE exist, but *incremental stimulation*, *multiple point stimulation* (MPS), and *the statistical method* are currently the most widely used.

Overview of MUNE Methods

As stimulation is applied to a peripheral nerve in small, progressively increasing increments, the size of the recorded waveform also increases in small incremental steps until the maximal CMAP appears. The *incremental stimulation method* assumes that each small incremental increase in waveform size corresponds with the activation and addition of another single motor unit to the growing waveform (Fig. 1). These waveform increments are averaged to derive an average S-MUAP size (37,38), which is then used to calculate the MUNE. The *multiple point stimulation method* (MPS) uses very low-intensity current to stimulate individual axons, producing a series of individual S-MUAP waveforms, which are then (Fig. 2) measured and averaged for MUNE calculation (39–43). The *statistical method* utilizes a proprietary software package to control repeated stimulation at several different stimulus levels. Variation of the CMAP at each of these levels is subjected to Poisson statistical analysis, producing values corresponding with single motor unit activation (Fig. 3) (44), which are then used to derive a MUNE. It is conceptually more

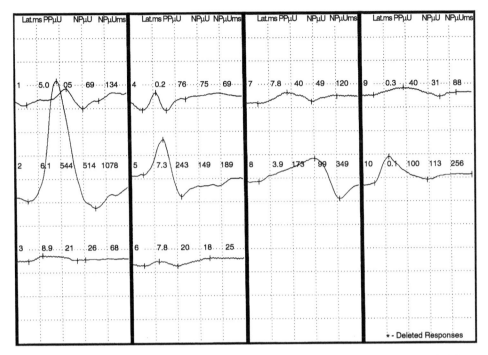

Figure 2 Multiple point stimulation MUNE. Individual motor unit waveforms recorded from the thenar muscles of an ALS patient via low intensity stimulation at multiple points along the median nerve (*above*) are averaged to obtain the representative S-MUAP for calculation of the MUNE. Note the high amplitude motor unit (*far left*) in this patient with motor neuron disease, a correlate of collateral reinnervation. *Abbreviations*: MUNE, motor unit number estimation; ALS, amyotrophic lateral sclerosis; MUAP, motor unit action potential.

complex than most other methods, but has been successfully applied to ALS patients and has been used in clinical trials of motor neuron disease.

Each of these methods has advantages and disadvantages that have been detailed elsewhere (45). The reproducibility of MPS and statistical MUNE, both in normal subjects and those with motor neuron disease, is very high and has been confirmed in numerous studies, with correlation coefficients for MPS ranging from 0.85 to 0.99 (39–43,46). Available data for the statistical method suggests reproducibility can reach 0.98 with particular technical modifications (47). As absolute MUNE values vary considerably from individual to individual, MUNE has its greatest utility in tracking motor unit loss over time through repeated studies in the same muscle. Rate and degree of change are especially useful in rapidly progressive conditions such as motor neuron disease, making reproducibility a critical issue.

All techniques are reasonably easy to teach to a trained electromyographer, but MPS, because of the low-stimulation intensities utilized, is more comfortable for the patients than the incremental and statistical methods. Both incremental stimulation and MPS can be performed on any standard EMG machine, while statistical MUNE requires special software currently available only on machines manufactured by one company. Incremental stimulation, MPS, and the statistical method each require approximately 15 to 20 minutes when performed by an experienced examiner.

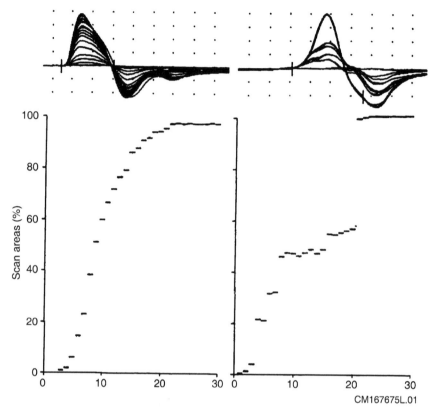

CM167675L.01

Figure 3 *The Statistical Method.* Recordings from a normal patient (*left*) and a patient with denervating disease (*right*). For each patient, a series of 30 progressively more intense stimuli (x-axis) are plotted against the size of the waveforms [expressed as a percentage of the full CMAP area (y-axis)]. The superimposed waveforms resulting from the 30 stimuli appear above each graph. The smooth progression of small incremental steps in the normal patient (*left*) contrasts markedly with the curve of the patient with denervating disease, which is interrupted by numerous large increments corresponding with larger, reinnervated S-MUAPs. *Source*: Adapted from Ref. 44.

MUNE and Amyotrophic Lateral Sclerosis

MUNE is the only technique providing a quantitative estimation of the number of functional motor units in the living human subject, and has been applied to ALS in numerous studies. Longitudinal rates of motor unit decline have been calculated for control patients, as well as for patients enrolled in clinical drug trials. As single motor unit size also provides a measure of collateral reinnervation, the data collected for MUNE calculations can also be used to measure the degree of compensatory response to motor axon injury.

In an early study using the incremental method, the average MUNE in ALS subjects was 62% lower and the average S-MUAP size was 145% higher than in control subjects (48). Incremental stimulation was also the first technique to study ALS patients longitudinally, providing a benchmark for future investigations (49). An average 50% loss of motor units was documented for every six months of disease progression (Figs. 4 and 5). This rate of loss has proven remarkably consistent over many subsequent studies using a variety of MUNE methods (42,44–46,49,50).

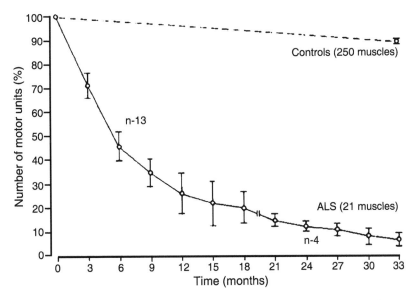

Figure 4 Motor unit loss in ALS. Motor unit decline in a group of ALS patients over 33 months by incremental MUNE. Motor unit loss averaged 50% for every six months of disease progression. The rate of decline in normal controls aged 60 and over for the same time period is also plotted as a dotted line (*above*), to serve as a reference for comparison. *Abbreviation*: ALS, amyotrophic lateral sclerosis. *Source*: From Ref. 49.

Another incremental study demonstrated strong correlations between MUNE and strength in the weak muscles of ALS patients (51) and a third used MUNE to calculate a linear estimate of rate of disease progression and survival, enabling accurate predictions of time to death or tracheostomy (52). Owing to technical concerns regarding its validity, the incremental method of MUNE is now less widely employed in humans. However, it remains the only technique practical thus far for the study of animal models of ALS, and has been used to calculate MUNE declines and to predict survival in SOD transgenic and knockout mice (53,54).

MPS MUNE has also been applied in numerous ALS studies. Early MPS studies demonstrated 80% reductions in average MUNE in the hand muscles of ALS patients and increases of greater than 600% in average S-MUAP size compared with controls (55). Because of this substantial compensatory reinnervation, CMAP amplitude remained normal until MUNE dropped to less than 10% of the average normal value, at which point clinical atrophy also appeared. MPS MUNE correlated strongly with other simultaneously acquired parameters [including the Medical Research Council (MRC) manual muscle testing score, the Appel ALS rating scale and forced vital capacity (FVC) measurements] in another study (46), and demonstrated a greater rate of change over time than MRC and FVC, especially in slowly progressive disease. MPS MUNE has also been employed as a secondary measure in clinical trials, demonstrating slowed rates of MUNE decline in patients treated with riluzole when compared with those treated with placebo alone (50). Most recently, MPS MUNE is being employed as one of several measures, including the ALS functional rating scale, quantitative strength measures, and transcortical magnetic stimulation (TMS) in a longitudinal natural history study of sporadic ALS (sALS), familial ALS (fALS), progressive muscular atrophy (PMA), and primary lateral

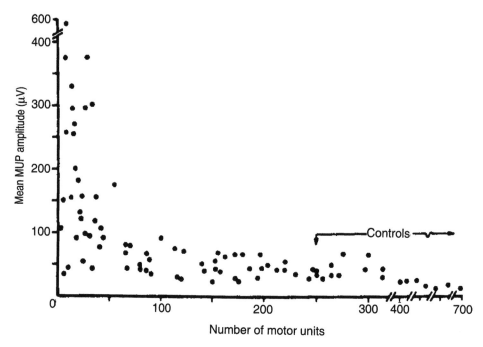

Figure 5 MUNE and single motor unit size in ALS. Average sizes of single motor units (amplitude) plotted against MUNE in the hypothenar muscles of patients with ALS. Note the asymptotic increase in motor unit size, consistent with aggressive reinnervation, as the MUNE falls below 50. *Abbreviations*: MUNE, motor unit number estimation; ALS, amyotrophic lateral sclerosis. *Source*: From Ref. 49.

sclerosis (PLS) (56). An interim analysis of the data generated by this study revealed that MUNE was clearly the most sensitive measure in detecting change over time (with average declines of 6% per month) and single MUNE measures at baseline enabled relative differentiation between the LMN disorders (sALS, fALS, and PMA) versus pure UMN disease (PLS). MUNE correlated significantly with the independent variables of pinch strength, grip strength, and manual muscle testing, as did CMAP. S-MUAP correlated significantly with pinch and grip, but not manual muscle testing. All MUNE measures were highly reproducible in all patient groups.

Statistical MUNE has also been applied extensively to the study of ALS (57). The statistical method demonstrated average motor unit decline of approximately 50% over several months in one study, with significant concurrent increases in FD measures (a correlate of collateral reinnervation) while CMAP and grip strength were maintained, supporting successful compensatory reinnervation. With further follow up, more rapid MUNE declines correlated with shorter survival. Statistical MUNE was the first method used in a multicenter clinical ALS trial. In the CNTF study, monthly measures over nine months demonstrated no statistically significant differences between rates of MUNE decline in the placebo and treatment groups, consistent with the overall negative results of the trial (58). This method was also employed in recent clinical trials of creatine (CR) in ALS with acceptable reproducibility and tolerability (59). However, the complexity of the statistical method and the assumptions on which it is based provide many potential sources of error, and those investigators most familiar with the method have proposed and tested a variety of modifications in attempts to improve both the technique and its accuracy (60–62). Recently, the issue of motor unit instability with extrinsic stimulation has been studied with greater precision, and has been cited as a possible cause of inherent error in the statistical method (63). Further studies are underway to see the magnitude of effect generated by this motor unit instability during statistical MUNE, and whether the technique or its algorithim can be sufficiently modified to adequately adjust for it.

Conclusions

Of the available MUNE methods, MPS and statistical MUNE are the most widely used, the most reproducible, and provide the greatest degree of patient comfort. Both can be performed relatively quickly. Of these methods, MPS MUNE has been most standardized. The statistical method (while more semiautomated and available on a widely used commercial EMG machine) is not yet fully standardized, as different investigators attempt different refinements to make it more likely to detect the increased number of large motor units present in ALS and other neurogenic disorders. Although it has been more commonly employed in recent multicenter clinical trials, some of those who championed the statistical MUNE have now cited a serious source of inherent error, which has the potential to render it unreliable for future application. The MPS method, in contrast, with accepted methods of performance and calculation among MUNE investigators routinely utilizing it, appears to be free of serious error and is ready for broad application. It requires no special software or proprietary EMG systems.

Motor unit loss is a hallmark of disease progression in ALS, and any measure which can detect early abnormalities in minimally affected or asymptomatic patients will be highly useful in the era of experimental therapeutics in motor neuron disease. MUNE appears to be the most sensitive quantitative measure of early disease progression in ALS, and can provide critical information about the efficacy of new drugs at an early stage when they are most likely to be effective. Early stratification of patients according to rate of progression and projected survival is another advantage of MUNE (52,64). In addition, changes in single motor unit size are also assessed by these techniques and can provide a gauge of collateral reinnervation, another important therapeutic target, as well as a potentially confounding variable (if not tracked) in clinical therapeutic trials.

UPPER MOTOR NEURON DISEASE MARKERS: MRI, MRS, AND OTHER IMAGING STUDIES

Introduction

Objective UMN markers are needed for clinical research and practice, and are often particularly important for helping to confirm the diagnosis of ALS. Currently, the diagnosis of ALS depends on detecting UMN signs by neurological examination (65–67). However, autopsy studies show corticospinal tract (CST) degeneration in more than half of cases having no clinical UMN signs (68–70). New imaging technology holds promise as a sensitive measure of UMN function, but needs further validation.

Magnetic Resonance Imaging

Magnetic resonance imaging (MRI) allows for the qualitative study of MR signal intensity within the brain and the quantitative study of brain volume.

CST hyperintensity extending from the precentral gyri into the subcortical white matter on T2-weighted images has been described in several ALS case series (71–73). Foci of abnormal intensity in the posterior limb of the internal capsule of ALS patients can be seen on T2-weighted images (74).

Newer MRI tools have been used to study ALS patients: proton density (PD)-weighted imaging can demonstrate signal abnormalities in the internal capsule of ALS patients (75). PD-weighted imaging may increase the specificity of MRI as CST signal changes in the internal capsule were presented in both ALS patients and controls on T2-weighted images, but in ALS patients only on PD-weighted images (76). Fluid attenuated inversion-recovery (FLAIR) may be more sensitive than T2-weighted images to visualize hyperintense changes in the subcortical white matter of the precentral gyrus (77–79). FLAIR and T2-weighted fast spin-echo imaging may be a more sensitive indicator of changes along the CST in ALS, but may also be abnormal in control subjects, decreasing specificity (77,79). Magnetization transfer imaging shows decreased ratios in ALS patients compared with healthy volunteers (80).

Diffusion tensor imaging (DTI) showed signal abnormalities in the CST, corpus callosum, and thalamus early in the course of the disease in 15 ALS patients, and 6 of these patients had such abnormalities prior to the development of clinical UMN signs (81). An association between DTI fractional anisotropy and central motor conduction time (CMCT) to the corresponding limb on TMS also supported these findings (82). High-angular resolution DTI may yield greater spatial resolution than six-direction DTI, but is less specific than other MRI methods (83).

In addition to imaging abnormalities in the CST, decreased T2 signal was seen in the *cortical motor strip* ALS patients (75,84,85). However, this finding is non-specific and can be seen in normal controls as well as in patients with neurological disease other than ALS (86). The size of the precentral gyrus and central sulcus may be decreased in ALS patients, but some case series report cortical volume changes on MRI only in a minority of ALS patients (87–89).

In the *spinal cord*, CST hyperintensity has been described in several case series using T2-weighted gradient echo axial images, and T1- and T2-weighted spin-echo axial images (90,91).

Evidence supporting the validity of MRI in ALS comes from two studies of five and nine ALS patients, respectively, correlating MRI with histopathological findings (74,76). Also, MR imaging changes in ALS are seen more frequently in patients with definite ALS compared with those in less definite diagnostic categories (89).

Magnetic Resonance Spectroscopy

Magnetic resonance spectroscopy (MRS) estimates the abundance of brain metabolites in a given volume of brain tissue (termed a "voxel" on neuroimaging studies). One of the metabolites studied, N-acetylaspartate (NAA), is thought to be a marker of neuronal integrity. Since it is technically difficult to measure absolute metabolite concentrations, the NAA results are usually given in relation to CR or choline (CHO).

Several studies of ALS patients have shown a decreased NAA/CR or NAA/CHO in a single voxel placed in the motor strip (89,92–97). NAA/CR seems lowest in ALS patients with definite clinical UMN signs (97), and one study suggests a threshold below which NAA/CR should be considered abnormal (89). Studies using multiple voxels have confirmed decreased NAA/CR or NAA/CHO in the motor cortex (98,99), and some case series also show MRS changes outside of the motor cortex, in areas such as the medulla, pons, or the internal capsule (100–103).

MRS may also have a role in the evaluation of treatment effects. One study found an increase in NAA/CR following three weeks of treatment with riluzole, the only FDA approved ALS medication (104–106), but this result was not reproduced in other studies (96,107). CR supplementation as a therapy for ALS poses particular problems in MRS, as CR is often used as a presumptively stable denominator for tracking NAA by ratio. In one study, CR administration for one month affected MRS parameters in normal controls in a different way than in ALS patients, where it was associated with stable NAA/CR and NAA/CHO ratios, but decreased glutamate/CR ratios (108). The NAA/CR change over about one month of gabapentin treatment did not differ between 8 treated and 10 untreated ALS patients (109). Neither CR nor gabapentine showed therapeutic efficacy in larger clinical trials (110,111).

More recent studies have suggested that both CR and CHO may be altered in ALS patients, even without CR supplementation, possibly artifactually influencing the accuracy of the NAA estimate as ratio to other metabolites (79,96,103,112,113). A longitudinal study found decreased absolute NAA levels after three months observation period in ALS patients, but unchanged NAA relative to CHO and CR (99). Several studies are under way addressing these problems through absolute metabolite quantitation. In addition to NAA, CR, and CHO, other metabolic changes have been described in ALS including excessive MRS glutamine and glutamate levels in ALS brainstem (100), and myo-inositol in the motor cortex (103).

Further studies are needed to clarify the role of MRI and MRS in the evaluation of UMN involvement in ALS, including comparative studies of different imaging techniques as well as comprehensive longitudinal observations correlating MRI and MRS with other biomarkers, clinical parameters, and, if available, histopathology (114) to confirm the validity of the technique.

Functional Imaging Studies

Functional Magnetic Resonance Imaging

Functional magnetic resonance imaging (fMRI) techniques use MR technology to track metabolic changes in brain tissue corresponding with brain activity, and these techniques have been applied to ALS patients in a few studies. fMRI performed during a motor task demonstrated a larger area of activation in the frontal cortex anterior to the motor strip in ALS patients than in controls (115). In 28 non-demented ALS patients, impaired frontal cortex activation was seen on fMRI using two sets of language and executive functions, letter fluency and confrontation naming (116).

Single Photon Emission Computed Tomography

Single photon emission computed tomography (SPECT) scanning tracks a radioactive isotope tracer introduced into the subject to study perfusion and other changes within various tissues. One SPECT study using ^{123}I-IMP showed decreased frontal lobe radionuclide uptake in ALS (117–119), though decreased radionuclide uptake restricted to the motor cortex was found in less than half of ALS patients studied (117,118). Two ^{99m}Tc-HMPAO SPECT studies found decreased blood flow in the frontal lobes of ALS patients (120,121).

Positron Emission Tomography

Positron emission tomography (PET) scans acquire physiologic images through the detection of positrons emitted from a radioactive substance administered to the subject, and also aids in the assessment of brain metabolism.[18]Fluro-deoxyglucose PET demonstrated decreased cerebral metabolic rates in ALS patients, mainly in the motor cortex and the putamen, but also in extramotor areas (119,122,123).[11]C-Flumazenil PET confirmed cortical involvement outside the motor strip (124).[11]C R-PK11195 PET demonstrated widespread cortical signal in ALS patients, suggesting cerebral microglial activation (125), while functional PET studies demonstrated abnormal activation on motor tasks, with recruitment of extramotor areas (126,127).

Conclusions

Functional imaging techniques offer great potential to the investigation of motor and extramotor systems of the brain in ALS. These methods, particularly MRS, remain the subject of ongoing investigation around the world. The published data are promising, but further work is needed to confirm their accuracy, validity, and reproducibility, as well as their specific role in clinical UMN assessment.

UPPER AND LOWER MOTOR NEURON DISEASE MARKERS: TRANSCRANIAL MAGNETIC STIMULATION

Introduction: Basic Concepts of Transcranial Magnetic Stimulation

Transcranial magnetic stimulation (TMS) is a method of evoking compound motor potentials through non-invasive stimulation of central motor systems. Developed for clinical application 20 years ago (128), TMS has become a useful tool for studying the conductivity, excitability, and abnormal circuitry of the corticospinal and corticobulbar systems in ALS (129–136). TMS is based on the principle that electromagnetic induction can stimulate neural tissue by generating high intensity (several kiloampere) current pulses from a series of capacitors and discharged through wire coils. The coils induce a magnetic flux of short duration (100–200 microseconds) and high intensity (1–3 T). The magnetic field, in turn, induces electrical current in the underlying cerebral cortex. Stimulus intensity is generally expressed as a percentage of maximal TMS machine output. TMS is relatively painless with compared with the clinically similar transcranial electrical stimulation (137,138) where uncomfortable shocks are sensed in the underlying skin and muscle tissues. Unlike transcranial electrical stimulation, which directly excites cortical long tracts, the induced electrical fields with TMS preferentially stimulate neural elements oriented parallel to the surface of the brain, primarily the interneurons and the apical dendrites of cortical motor neurons (139,140).

TMS measures two fundamental changes thought to occur in ALS: (1) cortical hyperexcitability or impaired inhibitory mechanisms and (2) the dropout of cortical motor neurons inducing subsequent degeneration of associated long tracts. TMS can be applied as a single pulse, in paired pulses, or in combination with peripheral stimulation and motor unit recordings. Single pulse, TMS provides information on the motor evoked potential (MEP) threshold, amplitude, and latency, and can be used to elicit the cortical silent period. TMS can also be used to map changes in cortical motor representation (141), which may correlate with the stages of ALS.

Such changes (attributed to loss of cortical cells) theoretically could serve as a sensitive measure for ALS progression.

TMS Techniques and Measures in ALS

Single Pulse TMS

Single pulse TMS provides MEP latency and amplitude data that can quantify the integrity of the UMN pathways. The latency from stimulation to recorded waveform represents the time required for a cortical impulse induced by TMS to travel from the motor cortex, through the brain, brainstem, spinal cord, and peripheral nerve to a hand or foot muscle, where it is recorded (through a surface electrodes placed over the muscle), as the MEP. This latency is the total TMS conduction time. The time for transit from the peripheral nerve root to the muscle can also be measured following stimulation of the cervical or lumbosacral roots, and is known as the peripheral motor conduction time. As the total TMS conduction time represents the time required for both central and peripheral conduction, the CMCT can be derived indirectly by subtracting the peripheral motor latency from the total TMS conduction time (142). CMCT prolongation may be due to the loss of large myelinated motor axons and correlates with UMN dysfunction. In ALS, CMCT is often prolonged with abnormally low-MEP amplitudes because the fast conducting, larger diameter Betz cells and axons are preferentially affected early in the course of disease (143), presumably due to increased metabolic requirements (144). CMCT prolongation, however, cannot clearly differentiate ALS from other conditions affecting the long motor tracts, but can assist in identifying UMN deterioration and thereby help clarify the diagnosis (e.g., PMA versus ALS, and PLS from normal controls) (Fig. 6), particularly as the disease progresses.

TMS stimulus intensity is expressed as a percent of the maximum stimulator output, or relative to the target muscle MEP threshold. MEP amplitude is usually measured peak-to-peak. It increases with stimulus intensity and plateaus at approximately 80% of amplitude of the peripherally stimulated M wave (145). In ALS, MEP amplitudes decrease due to drop out of both cortical and spinal motor neurons. The degree of central and/or peripheral deterioration can be distinguished to some extent by comparing TMS to the peripherally stimulated responses (see figure). Motor thresholds are defined as the lowest stimulus intensity that evokes MEPs (at least $50\,\mu V$ in amplitude) in just over 50% of stimulations (146,147). Cortical motor thresholds are low early in ALS and increase with disease progression. MEP threshold, latency, and amplitude are influenced by many factors, including configuration and placement of the TMS coil, stimulus intensity, conditioning pulses, muscle facilitation, synchrony of cortical discharges, temporal dispersion, and degree of MEP phase cancellation. In addition, the spinal motor neuron may fire repeatedly after a single TMS, adding to desynchronization and temporal dispersion.

The Cortical Silent Period

The cortical or central silent period is measured from an actively contracting muscle and represents the suppression of voluntary EMG activity for up to 300 milliseconds following a single TMS. The silent period typically follows the MEP induced by TMS, but the silent period may also be induced by stimuli beneath the threshold needed to produce an MEP (148). This latter characteristic provides strong support for the idea that this "negative effect" is mechanistically distinct from the positive effect seen during MEP induction. Although the origin of the initial segments of

		Normal (ms)	ALS (ms)	PMA (ms)	PLS (ms)
Total conduction time	A1: R ADM	19.5	22.8	28.3	73.8
	A2: L ADM	20.7	21.5	24.5	82.8
	A3: R TA	28.3	39.2	34.7	81.6
	A4: L TA	27.5	39.2	33.9	83.8
Peripheral conduction time	B5: R ADM	11.8	14.9	20.0	10.0
	B6: L ADM	12.4	15.9	18.8	12.5
	B7: R TA	13.1	17.9	20.0	14.0
	B8: L TA	12.7	15.5	19.7	15.8
Central conduction time	R ADM	7.7	7.9	8.3	63.8
	L ADM	8.3	5.6	5.7	70.2
	R TA	15.2	21.3	14.7	67.6
	L TA	14.8	23.7	14.2	68.0

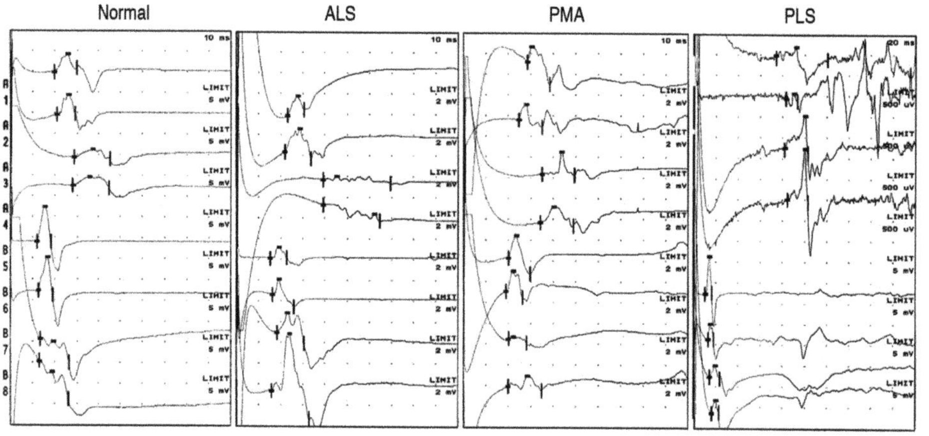

Figure 6 Single pulse TMS from normal example and ALS subtypes showing total conduction MEP responses from the cortex stimulating over the vertex (traces A1–A4). Peripheral responses are from the cervical spine (traces B5 and B6) and lumbosacral spine (B7 and B8) to bilateral ADM and bilateral TA. Onset latencies (in ms) are shown in the table and demarcated by the first vertical marker line in each trace in the figure. Central conductions, calculated by subtracting the peripheral conduction latencies from the total conduction latencies to each limb are listed at the bottom of the table. There are delayed onset MEP latencies in both central and peripheral responses in ALS, only in peripheral MEP latencies in PMA and only centrally in PLS. Note the increased time base for PLS (20 ms) illustrating the markedly prolonged CMCT and temporally dispersed MEPs with associated normal peripheral motor latencies. Also note the increased amplitude sensitivity compared to normal (5 mV) for all tracings apart from the peripheral recordings in PLS. *Abbreviations*: TMS, transcranial magnetic stimulation; ALS, amyotrophic lateral sclerosis; MEP, motor evoked potential; ADM, abductor digiti minimi; TA, tibialis anterior; PMA, progressive muscular atrophy; PLS, primary lateral sclerosis; CMCT, central motor conduction time.

the cortical silent period are controversial and may be caused by peripheral elements (e.g., transient neuronal hyperpolarization), the latter part of the TMS-induced silent period is likely determined by central mechanisms (149–151). The cortical silent period is shortened in ALS, correlating with hyperexcitability (132,135,136,152,153). It is shortest early in the disease, but becomes longer as the disease progresses.

Several lines of physiologic evidence (i.e., reduced MEP threshold, shortened cortical silent period, and reduced cortical inhibitory mechanisms) suggest that cortical motor neurons and their associated circuitry are hyperexcitable in ALS. It is hypothesized that the reduced inhibition early in the course of ALS reflects the effects of glutamate-induced neuronal excitotoxicity.

Paired Pulse TMS

Paired TMS pulses, time-locked at precise interstimulus intervals (ISIs), can demonstrate changes in cortical excitability, especially intracortical inhibition and facilitation. The first pulse, or the *conditioning stimulus*, is generally subthreshold compared with the second or *test pulse* in studies using short ISIs between 1 milliseconds and 15 milliseconds. At ISIs up to 6 milliseconds, inhibition of the MEP amplitude appears after the test pulse. In contrast, facilitation of MEP amplitudes may occur with ISIs between 6 milliseconds and 15 milliseconds (154). Paired pulse TMS at longer ISIs (100–250 milliseconds) using suprathreshold stimuli for both the conditioning and test pulses (155) has been used to investigate longer term effects. The cortical inhibitory mechanisms underlying MEP responses to short and long ISIs appear to be distinct (156). In ALS, both long and short interval paired pulse paradigms (154,157,158) have demonstrated decreased inhibition, again correlating with possible hyperexcitability, which again tends to diminish over time.

The Triple Stimulus Technique

The triple stimulus technique applies two collisions from a proximal (Erb's point) and distal (wrist) site to a single pulse TMS, and is used to reduce the effects of MEP desynchronization after TMS. In this manner, potentially subclinical UMN changes can be unmasked that would otherwise not be recordable, through an estimation of the proportion of motor units activated by the motor cortex (159–161). At the same time, it yields an estimate of LMN integrity. However, the technique is time consuming and painful due to the dual peripheral electrical stimuli at short intervals.

Peristimulus Time Histograms

Peristimulus time histograms (PSTHs) measure modulation of single fiber EMG recordings by TMS, and have been proposed as objective markers of disease progression in ALS (143,147,162–167). Changes in the discharge patterns of motor units appear as peaks and troughs in PSTHs. The first of these peaks (the D wave) represents direct activation through the UMN pathway. Subsequent peaks (I waves) result from indirect excitation of the UMNs via cortical interneurons. Inter-peak intervals corresponding to synaptic transmission support this interpretation (168–170). PSTHs peaks have been used to evaluate UMN dysfunction (e.g., the primary peak reflecting the initial rising phase of the excitatory postsynaptic potentials evoked in the anterior horn cell by converging UMNs is abnormal in form and desynchronized in ALS) (147).

PSTHs may be among the more sensitive UMN disease markers in ALS. Although there are normal age-dependent declines in PSTH responses (162), age-matched comparisons with ALS reveal changes reflective of cortical motor neuronal cell loss. In addition, PSTH may help discern subtypes of ALS, specifically PLS with its slower progression and predominant UMN features. PSTH primary peaks in PLS subjects are of higher threshold and longer duration than in those with ALS (143,144,171,172).

Repetitive TMS

Repetitive trains of stimulation (rTMS) are useful for studying the effects on brain function (173) and may have applications in ALS. High frequency rTMS (greater than

20 Hz) increase cerebral blood flow and neuronal "excitability" while low-frequency rTMS (1–2 Hz) have the opposite effect (174), suggesting some therapeutic potential for this technique (e.g., a painless and potentially safer alternative to direct electro-shock therapy of the brain for psyciatric treatment in depression and possible lasting motoric benefit in severe parkinsonism) (175). The potential of rTMS to enhance cortical excitability is supported by an increase in MEP amplitudes with rTMS (145) and by persistent focal metabolic activation on PET following rTMS (176). However, rTMS have also been shown to have negative effects on the motor system (177) in blinded studies, so its overall effects remain unclear.

In ALS, low frequency rTMS have the potential to limit or reverse cortical excitotoxicity. In a preliminary study, the rate of ALS progression appeared to slow in patients exposed to low frequency rTMS (178). However, no effects of rTMS were observed in transgenic rodent models, and all ALS patients studied eventually deteriorated, suggesting that rTMS effects may be limited and difficult to quantify (179).

Conclusions

TMS is the only tool capable of objectively quantifying impulse transmission through the UMN pathway and also provides a measure of excessive cortical excitability. TMS techniques and measures range from single pulse studies, paired pulse paradigms, cortical silent period analyses and peristimulus time histograms to potentially therapeutic rTMS regimens. The precise mechanisms by which TMS affect cortical excitability, the clinical significance of TMS measures, and the potential therapeutic value of this technique remain under investigation.

SUMMARY

In order to rule out the many clinical mimics of ALS and to confirm the presence and extent of denervation, a comprehensive electrodiagnostic study is critical. NCS should include both motor and sensory responses in a minimum of one arm and one leg. If the clinical picture or findings on NCS suggest a possible neuropathic component, a much broader screen may be required, with sampling of multiple motor nerves and specific testing of several proximal nerve segments. A thorough needle EMG examination is also mandatory and should include a minimum of three extremities and the cervical and lumbosacral paraspinal muscles, including the thoracic paraspinal muscles and, typically, at least one bulbar muscle. This study should be performed in a reputable electrodiagnostic laboratory having extensive experience in the evaluation of suspected motor neuron disease.

Over the last few years, technological advances have fostered the development of a number of new techniques for quantitative assessment of the upper and LMNs in the living human subject. The novel data generated by these methods is proving useful for the primary study of motor neuron and other diseases, and as a measure of therapeutic efficacy in clinical trials.

LMN assessment through MUNE has advanced considerably over the last decade, and has been increasingly applied to both natural history studies and clinical trials in ALS. MUNE appears to be the most sensitive measure of disease progression in ALS, and has the potential to detect the therapeutic effects of drugs during the earliest stages of the disease, when the possibility of altering the course of the disease is greater, but when other clinical measures are much less sensitive. MUNE may also facilitate early stratification of patients by rate of progression and projection of survival times, and corresponds with concurrent strength measures. It also has demonstrated greater sensitivity than other markers in several ALS studies. Single motor unit size data, a component of all MUNE measures, provides concurrent estimates of collateral reinnervation, another potential therapeutic target, which also may serve as a possible confounding variable (if not recognized) in clinical drug trials. Of the current MUNE methods, MPS and the statistical method have been the most extensively studied. Both have demonstrated good reproducibility, are well tolerated by patients, and can be performed relatively quickly. MPS is the simplest to perform and, unlike the statistical method, does not require specialized software. Consequently, MPS MUNE can be performed on any EMG machine. Statistical MUNE has been employed in a recent, negative, multicenter trial in ALS, and MPS is being incorporated into current multicenter therapeutic studies. A number of refinements have been proposed to improve the accuracy and reliability of the statistical method, but a recent study has suggested current methods of statistical MUNE may be inherently flawed. Further technical studies and refinements are needed to resolve the questions surrounding statistical MUNE, but MPS appears ready for wider use, and is now being incorporated into several multicenter trials of motor neuron disease.

Until recent years, the only objective markers of UMN function were clinical signs on physical examination and direct autopsy tissue analysis. Autopsy data confirms UMN deterioration occurs in the majority of patients having no clinical UMN signs, reinforcing the need for more sensitive UMN markers applicable to the living patient. However, with recent advances in neuroimaging technology, it has become possible to detect and quantitate UMN dysfunction well before structural imaging changes appear. As clear evidence of UMN disease is essential for making the diagnosis of ALS and differentiating it from the pure LMN syndromes, such markers, if valid, could play an important role in clinical diagnosis. MRS and other functional imaging technology show promise for both research and clinical application, but further confirmation of their accuracy, validity, and reproducibility in patients with motor neuron disease will help more clearly define their precise roles for the future.

TMS is the only tool with the capability to track and measure a motor impulse from its origin through both the upper and LMN pathways to an innervated muscle. In addition, TMS techniques enable quantitative measurement of UMN hyperexcitability. Although less sensitive to LMN deterioration than MUNE, TMS may provide relatively sensitive measures of UMN dysfunction. This important tool remains a subject of worldwide investigation in motor neuron and other neurologic diseases, and may also have a future therapeutic role for certain conditions. However, its accuracy, validity, and reproducibility and its precise value in the diagnosis of motor neuron disease and as a clinical trial marker remain under study.

REFERENCES

1. Lambert EH, Mulder DW. Electromyographic studies in ALS. Proc Mayo Clin 1957; 32:444–446.
2. Lambert EH. Diagnostic value of electrical stimulation of motor nerves. Electroenceph Clin Neurophys Suppl 1962; 22:9–16.
3. Ertekin C. Sensory and motor conduction in motor neurone disease. Acta Neurol Scand 1967; 43:499–512.

4.   Gregory R, Mills K, Donaghy M. Progressive sensory nerve dysfunction in ALS: a prospective clinical and neurophysiological study. J Neurol 1993; 240:309.
5.   Daube JR. EMG in motor neuron disease. American Association of Electrodiagnostic Medicine Minimonography #18. 1982:3–11.
6.   Lambert EH. Electromyographic studies in ALS. In: Norris FH, Kurland LT, eds. Motor Neuron Diseases: Research on ALS and Related Disorders. Contemporary Neurology Symposia. Vol. II. New York: Grune and Stratton, 1967:135–153.
7.   Cornblath DR, Kuncl RW, Mellits ED, Quaskey SA, Clawson L, Pestronk A, Drachman DB. Nerve conduction studies in amyotrophic lateral sclerosis. Muscle Nerve 1992; 15:1111–1115.
8.   Albizatti MG, Bassi S, Passerini D, Crespi V. F Wave velocity in motor neuron disease. Acta Neurol Scand 1976; 54:269–277.
9.   Kimura J. Electrodiagnosis in Diseases of Nerve and Muscle: Principles and Practice. Philadelphia: F.A. Davis, 1989.
10. Norris FH Jr. Adult spinal motor neuron disease. Progressive muscular atrophy (Aran's disease) in relation to ALS. In: Vinken PJ, Bruyn GW, eds. Handbook of Clinical Neurology. Vol. 22. System Disorders and Atrophies. Amsterdam: North-Holland, 1975:1–56.
11. Latov N. Neuropathy and anti-GM1 antibodies. Ann Neurol 1990; 27(s41–3):542–543.
12. Sumner AJ. Separating motor neuron disease from pure motor neuropathies. In: Rowland LP, ed. Advances in Neurology. Vol. 56. ALS and other motor neuron diseases. New York: Raven Press, 1991:399–410.
13. Lange DJ, Trojaborg W, Latov N, Hays AP, Younger DS, Uncini A, Blake DM, Hirano M, Burns SM, Lovelace RE. Multifocal motor neuropathy with conduction block: is it a distinct clinical entity?. Neurology 1992; 42:497–505.
14. Daube JR. Needle Examination in EMG. American Association of Electrodiagnostic Medicine Minimonograph #11. 1979:1–14.
15. Petajan JH. Clinical EMG studies of disease of the motor unit. EEG Clin Neurophys 1974; 36:395–401.
16. Milner-Brown H, Stein R, Lee R. Pattern of recruiting human motor units in neuropathies and motor neurone disease. J Neurol Neurosurg Psychiatry 1974; 37:665–669.
17. World Federation of Neurology Research Group on Neuromuscular Diseases. El Escorial World Federation of Neurology Criteria for the Diagnosis of Amyotrophic Lateral Sclerosis. J Neurologic Sci 1994; 124(suppl 96–107).
18. Brooks BR, Miller RG, Swash M, Munsat TL. The World Federation of Neurology Research Group on Motor Neuron Diseases. El Escorial revisited: revised criteria for the diagnosis of amyotrophic lateral sclerosis. Amyotroph Lateral Scler Other Motor Neuron Disord 2000; 1:293–299.
19. Blexrud MD, Windebank AJ, Daube JR. Long-term follow-up of 121 patients with benign fasciculations. Ann Neurol 1993; 34(4):622–625.
20. Mulder DW, Lambert EH, Eaton LM. Myasthenic syndrome in a patient with ALS. Neurology 1959; 9:627–631.
21. Denys EH, Norris FH. ALS: impairment of neurologic transmission. Arch Neurol 1957; 36:202–205.
22. Bernstein LP, Antel JP. Motor neuron disease: decremental responses to repetitive nerve stimulation. Neurology 1981; 31:204–205.
23. Killian JM, Wilfong AA, Burnett L, Appel SH, Boland D. Decremental motor responses to repetitive nerve stimulation in ALS. Muscle Nerve 1994; 17:747–754.
24. Sanders DB, Stalberg EV. Single fiber electromyography. Muscle Nerve 1996; 19: 1069–1083.
25. Stalberg E, Schwartz MS, Trontelj J. Single fiber EMG in various processes affecting the anterior horn cell. J Neurol Sci 1975; 24:403–425.
26. Schwartz MS, Swach M. Pattern of involvement in the cervical segments in the early stage of motor neuron diseases: a single fiber EMG study. Acta neurol Scand 1982; 65:424–431.

27. Stalberg E. Electrophysiological studies of reinnervation in ALS. In: Rowland LP, ed. Human Motor Neuron Diseases. New York: Raven Press, 1982:47–59.
28. Oh SJ. Electromyography: Neuromuscular Transmission Studies. Baltimore: Williams and Wilkins, 1988.
29. Schwatch M. Vulnerability of lower brachial myotomes in motor neuron disease. A clinical and single fiber EMG studies. J Neurol Sci 1980; 47:59–68.
30. Garcia J, Engelhardt J, Appel SH, Stefani E. Increased MEPP frequency as an early sign of experimental immune mediated motor neuron disease. Ann Neurol 1990; 28: 329–334.
31. Appel SH, Engelhardt J, Garcia J, Stefani E. Immunoglobulins from animal models of motor neuron disease and human ALS passively transfer physiological abnormalities of the neuromuscular junction. Proc Natl Acad Dis (USA) 1991; 88:647–651.
32. Smith RG, Hamilton S, Hofmann F, Schneider T, Nastainczyk W, Birnbaumer L, Stefani E, Appel SH. Serum antibodies to L-type calcium channels in patients with amyotrophic lateral sclerosis. N Engl J Med 1992; 327:1721–1728.
33. Llinas R, Sugimori M, Cherksey BD, Smith RG, Delbono O, Stefani E, Appel S. IgG from amyotrophic lateral sclerosis patients increases current through P-type calcium channels in mammalian cerebellar Purkinje cells and in isolated channel protein in lipid bilayer. Proc Natl Acad Sci U S A 1993; 90:11743–11747.
34. Daube JR, Litchy WJ, Low PA, Windebank AJ. Classificatioin of ALS by autonomic abnormalities. In: Tsubaki T, Yase Y, eds. Amyotrophic Lateral Sclerosis. Amsterdam: Elsevier Science Publishers B.V, 1989:189–191.
35. Pisano F, Miscio G, Mazzuero G, Lanfranchi P, Colombo R, Pinelli P. Decreased heart rate variability in amyotrophic lateral sclerosis. Muscle Nerve 1995; 18:1225–1231.
36. Dettmers C, Fatepour D, Faust H, Jerusalem F. Sympathetic skin response abnormalities in ALS. Muscle Nerve 1993; 16:930–934.
37. McComas AJ, Fawcett PRW, Campbell MJ, Sica REP. Electrophysiological estimation of the number of motor units within a human muscle. J Neurol Neurosurg Psychiatry 1971; 34:121–131.
38. De Bruin H, McComas A, Galea V. Automated motor unit counting in proximal limb muscles. Muscle Nerve 1989; 12:779.
39. Kadrie HA, Yates SK, Milner-Brown HS, Brown WF. Multiple point electrical stimulation of ulnar and median nerves. J Neurol Neurosurg Psychiatry 1976; 39:973–985.
40. Doherty TJ, Brown WF. The estimated numbers and relative sizes of thenar motor units as selected by multiple point stimulation in young and older adults. Muscle Nerve 1993; 16:355–366.
41. Felice KJ. Thenar motor unit number estimates using the multiple point stimulation technique: reproducibility studies in ALS patient and normal subjects. Muscle Nerve 1995; 18(12):1412–1416.
42. Gooch CL, Wagner T. Longitudinal S-MUAP tracking and MUNE: Validity of a combined method. Muscle Nerve 1998; 21:1601.
43. Doherty TJ, Brown WF. A method for the longitudinal study of human thenar motor units. Muscle Nerve 1994; 17:1029–1036.
44. Daube JR. Estimating the number of motor units in a muscle. J Clin Neurophysiol 1995; 12:585–594.
45. Gooch CL, Harati Y. Motor unit number estimation, ALS and clinical trials. Amyotroph Lateral Scler Other Motor Neuron Dis 2000; 1:71–82.
46. Felice K. A longitudinal study comparing thenar motor unit number estimates to other quantitative tests in patients with ALS. Muscle Nerve 1997; 20:179–185.
47. Lomen-Hoerth C, Olney R. A comparison of multipoint and statistical motor unit number estimation. Muscle Nerve 1999; 22:1304.
48. Hansen S, Ballantyne JP. A quantitative electrophysiological study of motor neurone disease. J Neurol Neurosurg Psychiatry 1978; 41:773–783.

49. Dantes A, McComas A. The extent and time course of motor neuron involvement in ALS. Muscle Nerve 1991; 14:416–421.

50. Gooch CL, Pleitez M, Harati Y. MUNE and single motor unit tracking: experience in a clinical ALS trial. EEG Clin Neurophys 1999:107.

51. Armon C, Brandstater ME, Peterson G. MUNE and quantitative strength measurements of distal muscles in patients with ALS. Muscle Nerve 1997; 20:499–501.

52. Armon C, Brandstater ME. Motor unit number estimate-based rates of progression of ALS predict patient survival. Muscle Nerve 1999; 22:1571–1575.

53. Azzouz M, Leclerc N, Gurney M, Warter JM, Poindron P, Borg J. Progressive motor neuron impairment in an animal model of familial amyotrophic lateral sclerosis. Muscle Nerve 1997; 20:45–51.

54. Shefner JM, Reaume AG, Flood DG, Scott RW, Kowall NW, Ferrante RJ, Siwek DF, Upton-Rice M, Brown RH. Mice lacking sytosolic Cu/ZN SOD display a distinctive motor axonopathy. Neurology 1999; 53:1239–1246.

55. Carleton SA, Brown WF. Changes in motor unit populations in motor neurone disease. J Neurol Neurosurg Psychiatry 1979; 42:42–51.

56. Gooch C, Tang M, Garcia J, Del Bene M, Battista V, Gad N, Montes J, Rowland L, Mitsumoto H. MUNE measures in ALS, fALS, PMA and PLS in a natural history biomarker study. Neurology 2004; 62:A278.

57. Yuen EC, Olney RK. Longitudinal study of fiber density and motor unit number estimate in patients with ALS. Neurology 1997; 49:573–578.

58. Smith B, Clarke J, Litchy W. Longitudinal electrodiagnostic studies in ALS patients treated with recombinant human ciliary neurotrophic factor. Neurology 1995; 45:A448.

59. Shefner JM, Cudkowicz ME, Schoenfeld D, Conrad T, Taft J, Chilton M, Urbinelli L, Qureshi M, Zhang H, Pestronk A, Caress J, Donofrio P, Sorenson E, Bradley W, Lomen-Hoerth C, Pioro E, Rezania K, Ross M, Pascuzzi R, Heiman-Patterson T, Tandan R, Mitsumoto H, Rothstein J, Smith-Palmer T, MacDonald D, Burke D. NEALS Consortium. A clinical trial of creatine in ALS. Neurology 2004; 63(9):1656–1661.

60. Olney RK, Yuen EC, Engstrom JW. Statistical motor unit number estimation: reproducibility and sources of error in patients with ALS. Muscle Nerve 2000; 23:193–197.

61. Shefner JM, Jillapalli D, Bradshaw DY. Reducing intersubject variability in motor unit number estimation. Muscle Nerve 1990; 22:1457–1460.

62. Slawnych M, Laszlo C, Hershler C. Motor unit number estimation: sample size considerations. Muscle Nerve 1997; 20:22–28.

63. Jillapalli D, Shefner JM. Single motor unit variability with threshold stimulation in patients with amyotrophic lateral sclerosis and normal subjects. Muscle Nerve 2004; 30(5):578–584.

64. Olney R, Yuen E, Engstrom J. The rate of change in motor unit number estimates predicts survival in patients with amyotrophic lateral sclerosis. Neurology 1999; 52 (suppl 2):A3.

65. Mitsumoto H, Chad DA, Pioro EP. Clinical features. In: Mitsumoto H, ed. Amyotrophic Lateral Sclerosis. New York: Oxford Press, 1998:47–64.

66. Brooks BR. El Escorial World Federation of Neurology criteria for the diagnosis of amyotrophic lateral sclerosis. J Neurol Sci 1994: 124(suppl 96–107). (www.wfnals.org).

67. World Federation of Neurology Research Group on Neuromuscular Diseases Subcommittee on Motor Neuron Disease: Airlie House Guidelines. Therapeutic trials in amyotrophic lateral sclerosis. J Neurol Sci 1995: 129(suppl 1–10).

68. Iwanaga K, Hayashi S, Oyake M, Horikawa Y, Hayashi T, Wakabayashi M, Kondo H, Tsuji S, Takahashi H. Neuropathology of sporadic amyotrophic lateral sclerosis of long duration. J Neurol Sci 1997; 146:139–143.

69. Brownell B, Oppenheimer D, Trevor-Hughes J. The central nervous system in motor neurone disease. J Neurol Neurosurg Psychiatry 1970; 33:338–357.

70. Lawyer T, Netsky MG. Amyotrophic lateral sclerosis: a clinicoanatomic study of fifty-three cases. Arch Neurol Psychiatry 1953; 69:171–192.

71. Goodin DS, Rowley HA, Olney RK. Magnetic resonance imaging in amyotrophic lateral sclerosis. Ann Neurol 1988; 23:418–420.

72. Mascalchi M, Salvi F, Valzania F, Marcacci G, Bartolozzi C, Tassinari CA. Corticospinal tract degeneration in motor neuron disease. AJNR Am J Neuroradiol 1995; 16(4 suppl):878–880.

73. Terao S, Sobue G, Yasuda T, Kachi T, Shimada N, Oguri C, Mitsuma T. Magnetic resonance imaging of spinal pyramidal tract degeneration in amyotrophic lateral sclerosis. J Neurol 1995; 242:178–180.

74. Yagishita A, Nakano I, Oda M, Hirano A. Location of the corticospinal tract in the internal capsule at MR imaging. Radiology 1994; 191:455–460.

75. Cheung G, Gawel MJ, Cooper PW, Farb RI, Ang LC, Gawal MJ. Amyotrophic lateral sclerosis: correlation of clinical and MR imaging findings. Radiology 1995; 194: 263–270.

76. Abe K, Fujimura H, Kobayashi Y, Fujita N, Yanagihara T. Degeneration of the pyramidal tracts in patients with amyotrophic lateral sclerosis. A premortem and postmortem magnetic resonance imaging study. J Neuroimaging 1997; 7:208–212.

77. Hecht MJ, Fellner F, Fellner C, Hilz MJ, Heuss D, Neundorfer B. MRI-FLAIR images of the head show corticospinal tract alterations in ALS patients more frequently than T2-, T1- and proton-density-weighted images. J Neurol Sci 2001; 186:37–44.

78. Zhang L, Ulug AM, Zimmerman RD, Lin MT, Rubin M, Beal MF. The diagnostic utility of FLAIR imaging in clinically verified amyotrophic lateral sclerosis. J Magn Reson Imaging 2003; 17:521–527.

79. Bowen BC, Pattany PM, Bradley WG, Murdoch JB, Rotta F, Younis AA, Duncan RC, Quencer RM. MR imaging and localized proton spectroscopy of the precentral gyrus in amyotrophic lateral sclerosis. AJNR Am J Neuroradiol 2000; 21:647–658.

80. Kato Y, Matsumura K, Kinosada Y, Narita Y, Kuzuhara S, Nakagawa T. Detection of pyramidal tract lesions in amyotrophic lateral sclerosis with magnetization-transfer measurements. AJNR Am J Neuroradiol 1997; 18:1541–1547.

81. Sach M, Winkler G, Glauche V, Liepert J, Heimbach B, Koch MA, Buchel C, Weiller C. Diffusion tensor MRI of early upper motor neuron involvement in amyotrophic lateral sclerosis. Brain 2004; 127:340–350.

82. Ellis CM, Suckling J, Amaro E Jr, Bullmore ET, Simmons A, Williams SC, Leigh PN. Volumetric analysis reveals corticospinal tract degeneration and extramotor involvement in ALS. Neurology 2001; 57:1571–1578.

83. Graham JM, Papadakis N, Evans J, Widjaja E, Romanowski CA, Paley MN, Wallis LI, Wilkinson ID, Shaw PJ, Griffiths PD. Diffusion tensor imaging for the assessment of upper motor neuron integrity in ALS. Neurology 2004; 63:2111–2119.

84. Oba H, Araki T, Ohtomo K, Monzawa S, Uchiyama G, Koizumi K, Nogata Y, Kachi K, Shiozawa Z, Kobayashi M. Amyotrophic lateral sclerosis: T2 shortening in motor cortex at MR imaging. Radiology 1993; 189:843–846.

85. Ishikawa K, Nagura H, Yokota T, Yamanouchi H. Signal loss in the motor cortex on magnetic resonance images in amyotrophic lateral sclerosis. Ann Neurol 1993; 33: 218–222.

86. Hirai T, Korogi Y, Sakamoto Y, Hamatake S, Ikushima I, Takahashi M. T2 shortening in the motor cortex: effect of aging and cerebrovascular diseases. Radiology 1996; 199:799–803.

87. Kiernan JA, Hudson AJ. Frontal lobe atrophy in motor neuron diseases. Brain 1994; 117:747–757.

88. Ellis CM, Suckling J, Amaro E Jr, Bullmore ET, Simmons A, Williams SC, Leigh PN. Volumetric analysis reveals corticospinal tract degeneration and extramotor involvement in ALS. Neurology. 2001; 57:1571–1578.

89. Chan S, Shungu DC, Douglas-Akinwande A, Lange DJ, Rowland LP. Motor neuron diseases: comparison of single-voxel proton MR spectroscopy of the motor cortex with MR imaging of the brain. Radiology 1999; 212:763–769.

90. Thorpe JW, Moseley IF, Hawkes CH, MacManus DG, McDonald WI, Miller DH. Brain and spinal cord MRI in motor neuron disease. J Neurol Neurosurg Psychiatry 1996; 61:314–317.

91. Waragai M, Shinotoh H, Hayashi M, Hattori T. High signal intensity on T1 weighted MRI of the anterolateral column of the spinal cord in amyotrophic lateral sclerosis. J Neurol Neurosurg Psychiatry 1997; 62:88–91.

92. Jones AP, Gunawardena WJ, Coutinho CM, Gatt JA, Shaw IC, Mitchell JD. Preliminary results of proton magnetic resonance spectroscopy in motor neurone disease (amytrophic lateral sclerosis). J Neurol Sci 1995; 129(Suppl 85–89).

93. Giroud M, Walker P, Bernard D, Lemesle M, Martin D, Baudouin N, Brunotte F, Dumas R. Reduced brain N-acetyl-aspartate in frontal lobes suggests neuronal loss in patients with amyotrophic lateral sclerosis. Neurol Res 1996; 18:241–243.

94. Block W, Karitzky J, Traber F, Pohl C, Keller E, Mundegar RR, Lamerichs R, Rink H, Ries F, Schild HH, Jerusalem F. Proton magnetic resonance spectroscopy of the primary motor cortex in patients with motor neuron disease: subgroup analysis and follow-up measurements. Arch Neurol 1998; 55:931–936.

95. Abe K, Takanashi M, Watanabe Y, Tanaka H, Fujita N, Hirabuki N, Yanagihara T. Decrease in N-acetylaspartate/creatine ratio in the motor area and the frontal lobe in amyotrophic lateral sclerosis. Neuroradiology 2001; 43:537–541.

96. Pohl C, Block W, Karitzky J, Traber F, Schmidt S, Grothe C, Lamerichs R, Schild H, Klockgether T. Proton magnetic resonance spectroscopy of the motor cortex in 70 patients with amyotrophic lateral sclerosis. Arch Neurol 2001; 58:729–735.

97. Kaufmann P, Mitsumoto H. Amyotrophic lateral sclerosis: objective upper motor neuron markers. Curr Neurol Neurosci Rep 2002; 2:55–60.

98. Pioro EP, Antel JP, Cashman NR, Arnold DL. Detection of cortical neuron loss in motor neuron disease by proton magnetic resonance spectroscopic imaging in vivo. Neurology 1994; 44:1933–1938.

99. Suhy J, Miller RG, Rule R, Schuff N, Licht J, Dronsky V, Gelinas D, Maudsley AA, Weiner MW. Early detection and longitudinal changes in amyotrophic lateral sclerosis by ^{1}H MRSI. Neurology 2002; 58:773–779.

100. Pioro EP, Majors AW, Mitsumoto H, Nelson DR, Ng TC. 1H-MRS evidence of neurodegeneration and excess glutamate + glutamine in ALS medulla. Neurology 1999; 53:71–79.

101. Cwik VA, Hanstock CC, Allen PS, Martin WR. Estimation of brainstem neuronal loss in amyotrophic lateral sclerosis with in vivo proton magnetic resonance spectroscopy. Neurology 1998; 50:72–77.

102. Rooney WD, Miller RG, Gelinas D, Schuff N, Maudsley AA, Weiner MW. Decreased N-acetylaspartate in motor cortex and corticospinal tract in ALS. Neurology 1998; 50:1800–1805.

103. Schuff N, Rooney WD, Miller R, Gelinas DF, Amend DL, Maudsley AA, Weiner MW. Reanalysis of multislice ^{1}H MRSI in amyotrophic lateral sclerosis. Magn Reson Med 2001; 45:513–516.

104. Kalra S, Cashman N, Arnold DL. Recovery of N-acetylaspartate in corticomotor neurons of patients with ALS after riluzole therapy. Neuroreport 1998; 9:1757–1761.

105. Bensimon G, Lacomblez L, Meininger V. A controlled trial of riluzole in amyotrophic lateral sclerosis. ALS/Riluzole Study Group. N Engl J Med 1994; 330:585–591.

106. Lacomblez L, Bensimon G, Leigh PN, Guillet P, Meininger V. Dose-ranging study of riluzole in amyotrophic lateral sclerosis. Amyotrophic Lateral Sclerosis/Riluzole Study Group II. Lancet 1996; 347:1425–1431.

107. Bradley WG, Bowen BC, Pattany PM, Rotta F. [1]H-magnetic resonance spectroscopy in amyotrophic lateral sclerosis. J Neurol Sci 1999; 169:84–86.

108. Vielhaber S, Kaufmann J, Kanowski M, Sailer M, Feistner H, Tempelmann C, Elger CE, Heinze HJ, Kunz WS. Effect of creatine supplementation on metabolite levels in ALS motor cortices. Exp Neurol 2001; 172:377–82.

109. Kalra S, Cashman NR, Caramanos Z, Genge A, Arnold DL. Gabapentin therapy for amyotrophic lateral sclerosis: lack of improvement in neuronal integrity shown by MR spectroscopy. AJNR Am J Neuroradiol 2003; 24:476–480.

110. Miller RG, Moore DH II, Gelinas DF, Dronsky V, Mendoza M, Barohn RJ, Bryan W, Ravits J, Yuen E, Neville H, Ringel S, Bromberg M, Petajan J, Amato AA, Jackson C, Johnson W, Mandler R, Bosch P, Smith B, Graves M, Ross M, Sorenson EJ, Kelkar P, Parry G, Olney R. Western ALS Study Group. Phase III randomized trial of gabapentin in patients with amyotrophic lateral sclerosis. Neurology 2001; 56:843–848.

111. Groeneveld GJ, Veldink JH, van der Tweel I, Kalmijn S, Beijer C, de Visser M, Wokke JH, Franssen H, van den Berg LH. A randomized sequential trial of creatine in amyotrophic lateral sclerosis. Ann Neurol 2003; 53:437–445.

112. Sarchielli P, Pelliccioli GP, Tarducci R, Chiarini P, Presciutti O, Gobbi G, Gallai V. Magnetic resonance imaging and ^{1}H-magnetic resonance spectroscopy in amyotrophic lateral sclerosis. Neuroradiology 2001; 43:189–197.

113. Gredal O, Rosenbaum S, Topp S, Karlsborg M, Strange P, Werdelin L. Quantification of brain metabolites in amyotrophic lateral sclerosis by localized proton magnetic resonance spectroscopy. Neurology 1997; 48:878–881.

114. Kaufmann P, Pullman SL, Shungu DC, Chan S, Hays AP, Del Bene ML, Dover MA, Vukic M, Rowland LP, Mitsumoto H. Objective tests for upper motor neuron involvement in amyotrophic lateral sclerosis (ALS). Neurology 2004; 62:1753–1757.

115. Konrad C, Henningsen H, Bremer J, Mock B, Deppe M, Buchinger C, Turski P, Knecht S, Brooks B. Pattern of cortical reorganization in amyotrophic lateral sclerosis: a functional magnetic resonance imaging study. Exp Brain Res 2002; 143:51–56.

116. Abrahams S, Goldstein LH, Simmons A, Brammer M, Williams SC, Giampietro V, Leigh PN. Word retrieval in amyotrophic lateral sclerosis: a functional magnetic resonance imaging study. Brain 2004; 127:1507–1517.

117. Udaka F, Sawada H, Seriu N, Shindou K, Nishitani N, Kameyama M. MRI and SPECT findings in amyotrophic lateral sclerosis. Demonstration of upper motor neurone involvement by clinical neuroimaging. Neuroradiology 1992; 34(5):389–393.

118. Abe K, Fujimura H, Toyooka K, Hazama T, Hirono N, Yorifuji S, Yanagihara T. Single-photon emission computed tomographic investigation of patients with motor neuron disease. Neurology 1993; 43:1569–1573.

119. Ludolph AC, Langen KJ, Regard M, Herzog H, Kemper B, Kuwert T, Bottger IG, Feinendegen L. Frontal lobe function in amyotrophic lateral sclerosis: a neuropsychologic and positron emission tomography study. Acta Neurol Scand 1992; 85:81–89.

120. Waldemar G, Vorstrup S, Jensen TS, Johnsen A, Boysen G. Focal reductions of cerebral blood flow in amyotrophic lateral sclerosis: a [^{99m}Tc]-d,l-HMPAO SPECT study. J Neurol Sci 1992; 107:19–28.

121. Caselli RJ, Smith BE, Osborne D. Primary lateral sclerosis: a neuropsychological study. Neurology 1995; 45:2005–2009.

122. Dalakas MC, Hatazawa J, Brooks RA, Di Chiro G. Lowered cerebral glucose utilization in amyotrophic lateral sclerosis. Ann Neurol 1987; 22:580–586.

123. Hatazawa J, Brooks RA, Dalakas MC, Mansi L, Di Chiro G. Cortical motor-sensory hypometabolism in amyotrophic lateral sclerosis: a PET study. J Comput Assist Tomogr 1988; 12:630–666.

124. Lloyd CM, Richardson MP, Brooks DJ, Al-Chalabi A, Leigh PN. Extramotor involvement in ALS: PET studies with the GABA$_A$ ligand [^{11}C]flumazenil. Brain 2000; 123:2289–2296.

125. Turner MR, Cagnin A, Turkheimer FE, Miller CC, Shaw CE, Brooks DJ, Leigh PN, Banati RB. Evidence of widespread cerebral microglial activation in amyotrophic lateral sclerosis: an [11C](R)-PK11195 positron emission tomography study. Neurobiol Dis 2004; 15:601–609.

126. Kew JJ, Brooks DJ, Passingham RE, Rothwell JC, Frackowiak RS, Leigh PN. Cortical function in progressive lower motor neuron disorders and amyotrophic lateral sclerosis: a comparative PET study.Neurology. 1994;44:1101–1110.

127. Abrahams S, Goldstein LH, Kew JJM. Frontal lobe dysfunction in amyotrophic lateral sclerosis: a PET study. Brain 1996; 119:2105–2120.

128. Barker AT, Jalinous R, Freeston IL. Non-invasive magnetic stimulation of human cortex. Lancet 1985; 1:1106–1107.

129. Schriefer TN, Hess CW, Mills KR, Murray NM. Central motor conduction studies in motor neurone disease using magnetic brain stimulation. Electroencephalogr Clin Neurophysiol 1989; 74(6):431–437.

130. Eisen A, Shytbel W, Murphy K, Hoirch M. Cortical magnetic stimulation in amyotrophic lateral sclerosis. Muscle Nerve 1990; 13(2):146–151.

131. Mills KR, Nithi KA. Peripheral and central motor conduction in amyotrophic lateral sclerosis. J Neurol Sci 1998; 159(1):82–87.

132. Siciliano G, Manca ML, Sagliocco L, Pastorini E, Pellegrinetti A, Sartucci F. Cortical silent period in patients with amyotrophic lateral sclerosis. J Neurol Sci 1999; 169(1–2): 93–97.

133. Kaufmann P, Pullman SL, Shungu DC, Chan S, Hays AP, Del Bene ML, Dover MA, Vukic M, Rowland LP, Mitsumoto H. Objective tests for upper motor neuron involvement in amyotrophic lateral sclerosis (ALS). Neurology 2004; 62:1753–1757.

134. Cruz MA, Trejo JM. Transcranial magnetic stimulation in amyotrophic and primary lateral sclerosis. Electromyogr Clin Neurophysiol 1999; 39(5):285–288.

135. Pouget J, Trefouret S, Attarian S. Transcranial magnetic stimulation (TMS): compared sensitivity of different motor response parameters in ALS. Amyotroph Lateral Scler Other Motor Neuron Disord 2000; 1(suppl 2):S45–S49.

136. Zanette G, Tamburin S, Manganotti P, Refatti N, Forgione A, Rizzuto N. Different mechanisms contribute to motor cortex hyperexcitability in amyotrophic lateral sclerosis. Clin Neurophysiol 2002; 113(11):1688–1697.

137. Fries W, Danek A, Witt TN. Motor responses after transcranial electrical stimulation of cerebral hemispheres with a degenerated pyramidal tract. Ann Neurol 1991; 29(6): 646–650.

138. Priori A, Bertolasi L, Dressler D, Rothwell JC, Day BL, Thompson PD. Transcranial electric and magnetic stimulation of the leg area of the human motor cortex: single motor unit and surface EMG responses in the tibialis anterior muscle. Electroencephalogr Clin Neurophysiol 1993; 89(2):131–137.

139. Day BL, Dressler D, Maertens de Noordhout A, Marsden CD, Nakashima K, Rothwell JC, Thompson PD. Electric and magnetic stimulation of human motor cortex: surface EMG and single motor unit responses. J Physiol 1989; 412; 449–473.

140. Amassian VE, Maccabee PJ, Cracco RQ, Cracco JB. Basic mechanisms of magnetic coil excitation of nervous system in humans and monkeys: application in focal stimulation of different cortical areas in humans. In: Chokroverty S, ed. Magnetic Stimulation in Clinical Neurophysiology. Stoneham, MA: Butterworth, 1990:73–111.

141. de Carvalho M, Miranda PC, Luis ML, Ducla-Soares E. Cortical muscle representation in amyotrophic lateral sclerosis patients: changes with disease evolution. Muscle Nerve 1999; 22(12):1684–1692.

142. Eisen AA, Shtybel W. Clinical experience with transcranial magnetic stimulation. Muscle Nerve 1990; 13:995–1011.

143. Kohara N, Kaji R, Kojima Y, Kimura J. An electrophysiological study of the corticospinal projections in amyotrophic lateral sclerosis. Clin Neurophysiol 1999; 110(6): 1123–1132.

144. Eisen A, Weber M. The motor cortex and amyotrophic lateral sclerosis. Muscle Nerve 2001; 24(4):564–573.

145. Pascual-Leone A, Valls-Sole J, Wassermann EM, Hallett M. Responses to rapid-rate transcranial magnetic stimulation of the human motor cortex. Brain 1994; 117(pt 4): 847–858.
146. Rothwell JC, Hallett M, Berardelli A, Eisen A, Rossini P, Paulus W. Magnetic stimulation: motor evoked potentials. The International Federation of Clinical Neurophysiology. Electroencephalogr Clin Neurophysiol Suppl 1999; 52:97–103.
147. Eisen A. Clinical electrophysiology of the upper and lower motor neuron in amyotrophic lateral sclerosis. Semin Neurol 2001; 21(2):141–154.
148. Rossini PM, Caramia MD, Iani C, Desiato MT, Sciarretta G, Bernardi G. Magnetic transcranial stimulation in healthy humans: influence on the behavior of upper limb motor units. Brain Res 1995; 676(2):314–324.
149. Uncini A, Treviso M, Di Muzio A, Simone P, Pullman S. Physiological basis of voluntary activity inhibition induced by transcranial cortical stimulation. Electroencephalogr Clin Neurophysiol 1993; 89(4):211–220.
150. Brasil-Neto JP, Cammarota A, Valls-Sole J, Pascual-Leone A, Hallett M, Cohen LG. Role of intracortical mechanisms in the late part of the silent period to transcranial stimulation of the human motor cortex. Acta Neurol Scand 1995; 92(5):383–386.
151. Chen R, Corwell B, Hallett M. Modulation of motor cortex excitability by median nerve and digit stimulation. Exp Brain Res 1999; 129(1):77–86.
152. Mills KR. The natural history of central motor abnormalities in amyotrophic lateral sclerosis. Brain 2003; 126(pt 11):2558–2566.
153. Triggs WJ, Menkes D, Onorato J, Yan RS, Young MS, Newell K, Sander HW, Soto O, Chiappa KH, Cros D. Transcranial magnetic stimulation identifies upper motor neuron involvement in motor neuron disease. Neurology 1999; 53:605–611.
154. Kujirai T, Caramia MD, Rothwell JC, Day BL, Thompson PD, Ferbert A, Wroe S, Asselman P, Marsden CD. Corticocortical inhibition in human motor cortex. J Physiol 1993; 471:501–519.
155. Berardelli A, Inghilleri M, Priori A, Marchetti P, Curra A, Rona S, Manfredi M. Inhibitory cortical phenomena studied with the technique of transcranial stimulation. Electroencephalogr Clin Neurophysiol Suppl 1996; 46:343–349.
156. Sanger TD, Garg RR, Chen R. Interactions between two different inhibitory systems in the human motor cortex. J Physiol 2001; 530(pt 2):307–317.
157. Yokota T, Yoshino A, Inaba A, Saito Y. Double cortical stimulation in amyotrophic lateral sclerosis. J Neurol Neurosurg Psychiatry 1996; 61(6):596–600.
158. Ziemann U, Winter M, Reimers CD, Reimers K, Tergau F, Paulus W. Impaired motor cortex inhibition in patients with amyotrophic lateral sclerosis. Evidence from paired transcranial magnetic stimulation. Neurology 1997; 49(5):1292–1298.
159. Rosler KM, Truffert A, Hess CW, Magistris MR. Quantification of upper motor neuron loss in amyotrophic lateral sclerosis. Clin Neurophysiol 2000; 111(12):2208–2218.
160. Komissarow L, Rollnik JD, Bogdanova D, Krampfl K, Khabirov FA, Kossev A, Dengler R, Bufler J. Triple stimulation technique (TST) in amyotrophic lateral sclerosis. Clin Neurophysiol 2004; 115:356–360.
161. Magistris MR, Rosler KM, Truffert A, Landis T, Hess CW. A clinical study of motor evoked potentials using a triple stimulation technique. Brain 1999; 122(pt 2):265–279.
162. Eisen A, Entezari-Taher M, Stewart H. Cortical projections to spinal motoneurons: changes with aging and amyotrophic lateral sclerosis. Neurology 1996; 46(5):1396–1404.
163. Kohara N, Kaji R, Kojima Y, Mills KR, Fujii H, Hamano T, Kimura J, Takamatsu N, Uchiyama T. Abnormal excitability of the corticospinal pathway in patients with amyotrophic lateral sclerosis: a single motor unit study using transcranial magnetic stimulation. Electroencephalogr Clin Neurophysiol 1996; 101:32–41.
164. Nakajima M, Eisen A, McCarthy R, Olney RK, Aminoff MJ. Reduced corticomotoneuronal excitatory postsynaptic potentials (EPSPs) with normal Ia afferent EPSPs in amyotrophic lateral sclerosis. Neurology 1996; 47(6):1555–1561.

165. Enterzari-Taher M, Eisen A, Stewart H, Nakajima M. Abnormalities of cortical inhibitory neurons in amyotrophic lateral sclerosis. Muscle Nerve 1997; 20(1):65–71.

166. Weber M, Eisen A. Assessment of upper and lower motor neurons in Kennedy's disease: implications for corticomotoneuronal PSTH studies [see comments]. Muscle Nerve 1999; 22(3):299–306.

167. Kleine BU, Praamstra P, Stegeman DF, Zwarts MJ. Impaired motor cortical inhibition in Parkinson's disease: motor unit responses to transcranial magnetic stimulation. Exp Brain Res 2001; 138(4):477–483.

168. Day BL, Dressler D, Maertens de Noordhout A, Marsden CD, Nakashima K, Rothwell JC, Thompson PD. Electric and magnetic stimulation of human motor cortex: surface EMG and single motor unit responses. J Physiol 1989; 412:449–473.

169. Berardelli A, Inghilleri M, Cruccu G, Manfredi M. Descending volley after electrical and magnetic transcranial stimulation in man. Neurosci Lett 1990; 112(1):54–58.

170. Boniface SJ, Mills KR, Schubert M. Responses of single spinal motoneurons to magnetic brain stimulation in healthy subjects and patients with multiple sclerosis. Brain 1991; 114(pt 1B):643–662.

171. Weber M, Stewart H, Hirota N, Eisen A. Corticomotoneuronal connections in primary lateral sclerosis (PLS). Amyotroph Lateral Scler Other Motor Neuron Disord 2002; 3(4):190–198.

172. Nakajima M, Eisen A, Stewart H. Diverse abnormalities of corticomotoneuronal projections in individual patients with amyotrophic lateral sclerosis. Electroencephalogr Clin Neurophysiol 1997; 105(6):451–457.

173. Hallett M. Transcranial magnetic stimulation and the human brain. Nature 2000; 406(6792):147–150.

174. Chen R, Classen J, Gerloff C, Celnik P, Wassermann EM, Hallett M, Cohen LG. Depression of motor cortex excitability by low-frequency transcranial magnetic stimulation. Neurology 1997; 48:1398–1403.

175. Friedman J, Gordon N. Electroconvulsive therapy in Parkinson's disease: a report on Five Cases. Convuls Ther 1992; 8(3):204–210.

176. Siebner HR, Mentschel C, Auer C, Lehner C, Conrad B. Repetitive transcranial magnetic stimulation causes a short-term increase in the duration of the cortical silent period in patients with Parkinson's disease. Neurosci Lett 2000; 284(3):147–150.

177. Boylan LS, Pullman SL, Lisanby SH, Spicknall KE, Sackeim HA. Repetitive transcranial magnetic stimulation to SMA worsens complex movements in Parkinson's disease. Clin Neurophysiol 2001; 112(2):259–264.

178. Di Lazzaro V, Oliviero A, Saturno E, Pilato F, Dileone M, Sabatelli M, Tonali PA. Motor cortex stimulation for amyotrophic lateral sclerosis? Clin Neurophysiol 2004; 115:1479–1485.

179. Ziemann U, Eisen A. TMS for ALS: why and why not. Clin Neurophysiol 2004; 115(6): 1237–1238.

9

Classification, Diagnosis, and Presentation of Diagnosis of ALS

David A. Chad
University of Massachusetts School of Medicine and UMass Memorial Health Care, Worcester, Massachusetts, U.S.A.

INTRODUCTION

In this chapter, our attention turns first to the classification of ALS, second to the diagnostic process—including criteria for diagnosis, differential diagnosis, and laboratory evaluation—and last, to the presentation of the diagnosis.

Patients referred to neurologists have generally been aware of the experience of weakness for some weeks or months. As we listen to their histories and make observations during their neurological examinations, we are determining if they have ALS or one of its subtypes (conditions classified as ALS or closely related to ALS that run a progressive course of increasing weakness, inexorably expanding in their distribution of clinical signs) or have one of the many neurological disorders that bear some resemblance to ALS, even mimic ALS but have a different character— the differential diagnostic considerations, more benign than ALS, often treatable, possibly curable. During the diagnostic process, we are helped in making this distinction—between establishing the diagnosis of ALS on the one hand, and excluding it with reassurance and diagnosing another differential diagnostic condition on the other—by well defined diagnostic criteria in concert with laboratory studies including electromyography (EMG) and other neurodiagnostic tests, neuroimaging, and clinical chemistry.

CLASSIFICATION OF ALS

ALS describes a progressive neurodegenerative disorder involving motor neurons in the cerebral cortex, brainstem, and spinal cord causing a clinical picture characterized by a combination of upper and lower motor neuron signs in a generalized distribution involving bulbar musculature and limb muscles. It is well recognized that, at onset, ALS may present with either upper motor neuron (UMN) or lower motor neuron (LMN) or exclusively bulbar signs (1). Thus, ALS may be designated UMN-onset, LMN-onset, or bulbar-onset disease. Although respiratory failure almost invariably occurs as a late manifestation of ALS, on rare occasions dyspnea is the

Table 1 Classification of ALS

Acquired
  ALS (classic Charcot type) with combined UMN and LMN signs bulbar-onset;
  LMN-onset; UMN-onset; dyspnea-onset
  Progressive bulbar palsy
  Progressive muscular atrophy
  Primary lateral sclerosis
  Guamanian ALS
  Inherited
Autosomal dominant
  ALS 1 [SOD1 mutation-associated (21q22.1)]
  ALS 3 adult-onset (18q21)
  ALS 4 juvenile-onset (9q34)
  ALS with FTD (9q21-q22)
  ALS 6 adult-onset (16q12)
  ALS 7 adult-onset (20ptel)
  ALS with dementia, disinhibition, parkinsonism, amyotrophy complex (17q21-q23)
Autosomal recessive
  ALS 2 juvenile-onset [alsin mutation-associated (2q33)]
  ALS 5 juvenile-onset (15q15.1-q21.1)

Abbreviations: ALS, amyotrophic lateral sclerosis; UMN, upper motor neuron; LMN, lower motor neuron; SOD, superoxide dismutase; FTD, frontotemporal dementia.

presenting clinical feature and hence ALS may also be designated dyspnea-onset disease (2). In a relatively small number of patients, the disease may remain exclusively in one of the first three categories (see below). Accordingly, the classification of ALS (Table 1) (3,4) comprises a set of acquired conditions: ALS per se with its four onset forms; progressive bulbar palsy (PBP), a disorder limited to the bulbar muscles; progressive muscular atrophy (PMA), a disease characterized by pure LMN involvement; and primary lateral sclerosis (PLS), a pure UMN disorder. The classification described in Table 1 also includes the inherited forms of ALS (described in chap. 6) and discussed briefly in this chapter (vide infra).

Acquired ALS

Sporadic ALS, described in detail (chaps. 4 and 5) is characterized by a combination of UMN signs that consist of loss of dexterity, spasticity, hyperreflexia, and pathological reflexes; and LMN signs including muscle weakness, atrophy, and fasciculations, in a widespread distribution. An ALS variant has been termed the "flail arm syndrome" with progressive muscle wasting and weakness of the arms that is symmetric and largely proximal, with little or no functional impairment of the bulbar muscles or the legs, but commonly with UMN signs in the legs (5). The age of onset is similar to ALS, while the male to female ratio is much greater than for ALS (9:1 vs. 1.5:1) and there is a trend toward a longer survival than ALS.

PBP per se is marked by increasing dysarthria and dysphagia with UMN and LMN findings in varying combination involving the bulbar musculature. In its pure form (affecting the bulbar musculature over the course of the illness), PBP is rare (6,7). The vast majority of affected individuals have either some evidence of UMN or LMN signs outside the bulbar muscles at the time of diagnosis, or will develop features of classic ALS with the passage of time.

PMA is characterized clinically as a disorder with signs of LMN involvement during its entire clinical course. Precise prevalence rates among all patients with ALS are difficult to ascertain because of the variability of diagnostic criteria among studies (8), but range from 1% to 19% (6,9) has been reported.

Patients with the PMA phenotype typically have a pattern of disease quite similar to classic ALS—with focal and asymmetrical onset followed by the gradual spread from initial involvement to contiguous muscles eventually involving both upper and lower extremities, bulbar and respiratory musculature. Like classic ALS, there are subsets of PMA patients whose clinical courses vary from rapidly progressive to very slowly evolving. In the rapidly progressive category (with a clinical course from onset to death or respiratory failure in <2 years) is a subset of patients who present with LMN signs and who are designated PMA by virtue of clinically unsuspected corticospinal tract degeneration during life (8). These patients and another subset of patients who develop ALS from an initial PMA presentation frequently have long tract pathology and most have ubiquinated inclusions typical of ALS. These findings led Ince et al. (8) to conclude that a patient presenting with PMA and rapid course has a disease with the character ("pathology and pathophysiology") of ALS whether or not UMN clinical signs develop and that "PMA represents one end of the spectrum of motor system disorders, spanning ALS." In the slowly evolving category, recently reviewed by Tsuchiya et al. (10), is a rare group of patients who have a very long course (>10 years) of progressive LMN weakness and qualify clinically for PMA, but are found to have neuropathological evidence of Betz cell loss and degeneration of the pyramidal tracts. These findings are in line with those of Ince et al. (8) and suggest that ALS is a single disease with a spectrum of clinical manifestations. Indeed, the occurrence of PMA, ALS, and PBP phenotypes in patients with familial ALS (see below) caused by various mutations in the gene for Cu/Zn superoxide dismutase-1 (SOD1) (11) indicate allelic heterogeneity (12) and suggest that these clinical presentations form a neurological spectrum reflecting diseased motor neurons within the central nervous system (3).

As already noted, a PLS phenotype is a well-known precursor to the onset of ALS (UMN-onset ALS). PLS per se (a pure and progressive UMN disorder over the course of many years) is a rare clinical syndrome, with some 50 reports in the world literature describing the insidious onset of a symmetrical spastic paraplegia of greater than 3 years duration in individuals more than 50 years old spreading over years to the arms and bulbar muscles; unlike ALS, there are no clinical or EMG features of LMN involvement; and bladder involvement (detrussor hyperreflexia) is common (4,13,14). Whether PLS represents a distinct entity or is part of the spectrum of ALS is unclear. There is consensus, however, that a predominance of UMN signs tends to characterize long survival in ALS (4,15) and that clinically diagnosed PLS has a more benign course than ALS (16). In his thoughtful review of the nosology of PLS, Rowland (17) suggests that there is evidence to view the disease from three distinct perspectives. In some cases of apparent PLS (exclusively UMN findings after three years) there is progression to typical features of ALS after five or more years (therefore, PLS may be a form of ALS). In other PLS cases, the disease is shown at autopsy to affect only the corticospinal tracts and spare the LMNs of the brainstem and spinal cord (therefore, PLS may be a separate disease). And finally in a third group, PLS may be caused by a biochemical or immune disturbance that has not yet been defined (therefore, PLS may be viewed as a syndrome). Recently, Zhai et al. (18) described what could be a distinct clinical subgroup of PLS patients with a relatively homogeneous pattern of smooth progression beginning in the legs and involving both legs before affecting the arms; quadriparesis was quickly followed by speech or swallowing difficulties. This pattern of involvement suggested a steady dying back of corticospinal axons. Physiological and biochemical correlates of these clinical findings were loss of the transcranial magnetic stimulation, motor-evoked responses, and a mean reduction in N-acetylaspartate/creatinine in the motor cortex by MRS, respectively.

Guamanian ALS

Like classic sporadic ALS, Guamanian ALS presents insidiously with a combination of UMN and LMN findings. Dysarthria and bulbar palsy occur in about one-third of Guamanian ALS patients. Parkinsonism or dementia occur in about 5% to 10% of patients with ALS (19). The neuropathology of Guamanian ALS is distinct from sporadic ALS, consisting of widespread neurofibrillary tangles identical to those found in Alzheimer's disease with minimal accompanying amyloid deposition (19). In the 1950s, the prevalence of the disease among Chamorros on Guam was >140 per 100,000, but the incidence has declined markedly to 7.5 per 100,000 [from an analysis of data available from 1980 through 1989 (20)]. During the period 1997–2000, ALS was diagnosed in five Chamarros who number about 50,000 on Guam. The dramatic decline in incidence of ALS over a period of some 50 years is compatible with the waning influence of an environmental factor with a genetic predisposition that has not been determined (19,21). Bearing a resemblance to some patients with Guamanian ALS (those with ALS plus cognitive and extrapyramidal disturbances) are rare reports of individuals in Western countries who develop a concurrence of dementia, Parkinsonism, and ALS (22) and family members with the dementia-Parkinsonism-amyotrophy complex linked to chromosome 17q21–23 (23).

Inherited ALS

The incidence of individuals with ALS who have another affected family member is thought to be around 8% to 10% (21). As shown in Table 1, both autosomal dominant and recessive forms of ALS have been described, the former making up the vast majority of the inherited cases. Approximately 20% of families with ALS have a mutation in the SOD1 gene [designated familial ALS 1 (FALS1)] and more than 100 different mutations of the gene have been described (24). Cudkowicz et al. (25) showed that the clinical features of FALS1 are broadly similar to sporadic ALS; that the mean age of onset of the FALS1 patients is 46.9 years (earlier than sporadic ALS by about 10 years); that bulbar-onset cases have a later age of onset than the limb-onset FALS1 patients; and that the alanine–valine substitution at codon 4 (A4V), the most commonly encountered SOD1 mutation in North America (50% of SOD1 patients), is associated with extremely short survival with a median disease duration of 1.4 (SD = 0.9) years. Although UMN findings are frequently combined with LMN signs in many patients with FALS1, for patients with the A4V mutation they are absent clinically and either absent or mild when studied pathologically (26). Indeed, prior to this observation, diagnostic criteria for ALS (vide infra) required a combination of LMN and UMN signs; currently the presence of widespread LMN signs in the presence of a demonstrable SOD1 mutation will suffice for the diagnosis of ALS even without evidence for UMN involvement.

   Other SOD1 mutations with a rapid course include A4T and H43R, in contrast to E100G with duration 5.1 ± 3.3 years and G37R and H46R, with average course of 17 to 18 years (27), highlighting how a specific type of SOD1 mutation determines disease duration and provides important prognostic information. There is also sometimes a striking variability of clinical phenotype among members of the same family with the identical SOD1 mutation that may relate to gene–gene or gene–environment interactions or both (3).

ALS2 is an autosomal recessive disorder with gene locus at 2q33, coding for the protein called alsin, reported in a large inbred Tunisian family with mean onset at age 12 (range from 3 to 23) and characterized by UMN signs, muscle atrophy, generalized fasciculations, bulbar signs, and normal sensation with slow progression over the course of decades (28). Approximately 80% of families with ALS do not have mutations in genes coding for either the SOD1 or alsin protein products. Linkage studies in families affected with ALS are beginning to elucidate the modes of inheritance and chromosomal locations for not yet identified genes whose mutated protein products lead to ALS (21,24).

THE DIAGNOSTIC PROCESS

The diagnosis of ALS per se may be challenging since there is no single diagnostic test for ALS (with the exception of finding a mutation in the SOD1 gene). ALS is a motor disorder without clinically significant sensory impairment, ocular palsy, or bladder and bowel dysfunction. Cognitive deficits once considered rare or uncommon occur in approximately 50% of sporadic ALS patients and are manifestations of frontotemporal lobar dementia (29).

The World Federation of Neurology (WFN) sought to develop workable, internationally acceptable diagnostic criteria that would enhance clinical and research studies in the field of ALS (Table 2) (30,31). To establish the diagnosis of ALS, a combination of LMN and UMN signs with evidence of spread within a region or to other regions of the body is required (Table 2). The four cardinal regions are defined as bulbar (including muscles of the jaw, face, palate, tongue, and larynx), cervical (including muscles of the neck, arm, hand, and diaphragm), thoracic (including muscles of the back and abdomen), and lumbosacral (including muscles of the back, abdomen, leg, and foot). Because progressive spread of signs from region to region is essential to the character of ALS, the WFN provided guidelines based on distribution of LMN and UMN findings so that the diagnosis could be established with varying levels of certainty (Table 3).

Table 2 Revised WFN Criteria for the Diagnosis of ALS

Features present	Features absent
Evidence of lower motor neuron degeneration by clinical, EMG, or neuropathological examination	EMG or pathological evidence of other disease processes that might explain signs of lower motor neuron or upper motor neuron degeneration or both
Evidence of upper motor neuron degeneration by clinical examination	Neuroimaging evidence of other disease processes that might explain the observed clinical and EMG signs
Progressive spread of signs within a region, or to other regions as determined by history or examination	

Abbreviations: WFN, World Federation of Neurology; ALS, amyotrophic lateral sclerosis; EMG, electromyography.
Source: From Ref. 31.

Table 3 Levels of Certainty in the Clinical Diagnosis of ALS

Level of certainty	Characteristic features
Definite ALS	UMN as well as LMN signs, in the bulbar region and at least two spinal regions; or UMN and LMN signs in three spinal regions
Definite familial ALS—Laboratory supported	UMN or LMN signs or both in at least a single region (in the absence of another cause for the abnormal signs) with an identified disease-causing mutation in the SOD1 gene in the proband or a positive family history of an individual with an identified disease-causing mutation in the SOD1 gene
Probable ALS	UMN and LMN signs in at least two regions with some UMN signs necessarily rostral to the LMN signs
Probable ALS—Laboratory Supported	Clinical signs of UMN and LMN dysfunction are in only one region; or UMN signs alone are present in one region; and LMN signs defined by EMG criteria are present in at least two limbs
Possible ALS	Clinical signs of UMN and LMN dysfunction are found together in only one region; or UMN signs are found in two or more regions; or LMN signs are found rostral to UMN signs

Abbreviations: ALS, amyotrophic lateral sclerosis; UMN, upper motor neuron; LMN, lower motor neuron; EMG, electromyography.
Source: From Ref. 31.

As shown in Table 3, clinically definite ALS is defined on clinical evidence alone by the presence of UMN as well as LMN signs in the bulbar region and at least two spinal regions, or the presence of UMN and LMN signs in three spinal regions. Definite familial ALS—laboratory supported is defined as UMN or LMN signs or both in at least a single region (in the absence of another cause for the abnormal signs) with an identified disease-causing mutation in the SOD1 gene in the proband or a positive family history of an individual with an identified disease-causing mutation in the SOD1 gene (24). Clinically probable ALS is defined on clinical evidence alone by UMN and LMN signs in at least two regions with some UMN signs necessarily rostral to the LMN signs. Clinically probable ALS—laboratory supported, is defined when clinical signs of UMN and LMN dysfunction are in only one region, or when UMN signs alone are present in one region and LMN signs defined by EMG criteria are present in at least two limbs. Additionally, there must be proper application of neuroimaging and clinical laboratory protocols to exclude other causes.

The addition of the category "clinically probable ALS—laboratory supported" marks a key difference from the first set of WFN El Escorial criteria because the combination of EMG and clinical findings is used in the diagnostic assessment. This new level of diagnostic certainty is derived from the experience of Ross et al. (32). They were motivated to relax the 1994 El Escorial criteria for establishing the diagnosis of ALS so that patients might have the opportunity to participate in clinical trials [in this instance, ciliary neurotrophic factor (CNTF)] in the early phases of their illness. The authors noted that early diagnosis might not be possible if it required widespread UMN and LMN disease since the clinical manifestations of ALS are often focal in the early stages. They cited the work of Chaudhuri et al. (33) who observed that when clinical features were correlated with postmortem neuropathologic findings, 25% of ALS patients died of the illness without meeting the initial El Escorial criteria for definite or probable ALS.

To facilitate early diagnosis, less restrictive criteria were created (32): UMN signs were required in at least one region, and EMG signs of LMN involvement (fibrillation potentials or positive sharp waves—evidence of acute denervation) were required in at least two limb muscles (innervated by different peripheral nerves and nerve roots) in each of two extremities for which there was no more likely cause than ALS. The criteria for the diagnosis of ALS used in this study incorporated neuroimaging, EMG, and laboratory investigations to exclude structural abnormalities, polyneuropathy and multifocal mononeuropathies, and a variety of immune-mediated, endocrine, metabolic, and toxic etiologies, respectively. All patients who met the criteria were given the diagnosis of ALS without further division into subcategories. Using these criteria, the diagnosis of ALS was made at a mean time of 9.7 months from onset of symptoms, which compared favorably with the 12-month period cited in the literature. At the end of the clinical trial, the authors believed that based on clinical grounds the diagnosis of ALS was accurate in every patient, but there was no pathological confirmation. Therefore, confidence in these criteria appeared to be justified and led to "probable ALS—laboratory supported" being added to the original WFN criteria.

Last, clinically possible ALS is defined when clinical signs of UMN and LMN dysfunction are found together in only one region or UMN signs are found in two or more regions or LMN signs are found rostral to UMN signs. The diagnosis of clinically possible ALS infers that EMG criteria for LMN involvement as established for clinically probable ALS—laboratory supported have not yet been met, but that other conditions that could mimic ALS have been excluded.

THE DIFFERENTIAL DIAGNOSIS OF ALS

Because ALS may disturb the structure and function of the upper and LMNs—elements crucial to motor control—its manifestations vary. Symptoms and signs of ALS are encountered in a large and varied group of disorders, both neurologic and systemic. Thus, in clinical practice, the differential diagnosis of ALS is extensive (34,35). In Table 4, the differential diagnosis of ALS is reviewed on the basis of the anatomy of the nervous system and, therefore, a heterogeneous group of disorders is considered: those characterized by pathological changes in anterior horn cells, corticospinal tracts, or both; and others in which the pathological alteration occurs outside of the central nervous system in a variety of areas including muscle, the neuromuscular junction, and peripheral nerve tissue. Another approach is to recall the three most common modes of clinical presentation of ALS: bulbar-onset, LMN- or PMA-onset, and UMN- or PLS-onset and to consider the differential diagnosis of each of these clinical patterns (Table 5) as we do in the following sections.

Differential Diagnosis of Bulbar-Onset ALS

Structural abnormalities of the brainstem and lower cranial nerves like brainstem infarction, glioma, and syrinx and tumors at the level of the foramen magnum bear consideration, but are usually easily diagnosed or excluded by the results of brain and spinal cord neuroimaging. The progressive dysphagia with onset in the fifth or sixth decade of life of oculopharyngeal dystrophy (OPD) might simulate bulbar-onset

Table 4 The Differential Diagnosis of ALS Classified Anatomically

Anatomic site	Possible disorder
Muscle	Inclusion body myositis, neck extensor myopathy, adult nemaline myopathy, distal myopathy, and oculopharyngeal dystrophy
Neuromuscular junction	Myasthenia gravis, Lambert-Eaton myasthenic syndrome
Roots, plexus, nerve	Spondylotic polyradiculopathy, multifocal motor neuropathy, diabetic polyradiculopathy, infectious polyradiculopathy, plexopathies, and mononeuropathies
Anterior horn cells	Monomelic amyotrophy, PMA (LMN syndrome) with benign course, paraneoplastic ALS (including lymphoproliferative disorders and ALS), paraproteinemia-associated ALS, postpolio muscular atrophy, bulbospinal neuronopathy, spinal muscular atrophy, and hexosaminidase deficiency
Spinal cord	Spondylotic radiculomyelopathy, syringomyelia, HTLV-1 myelopathy, hereditary spastic paraparesis (HSP), and adrenomyeloneuropathy
Central nervous system	Parkinson's disease, Creutzfeldt-Jacob disease, brainstem stroke, brainstem glioma, foramen magnum tumor, and Huntington's disease
Systemic disorder	Hyperthyroidism and hyperparathyroidism

Abbreviations: ALS, amyotrophic lateral sclerosis; LMN, lower motor neuron; PMA, progressive muscular atrophy; HTLV-1, human T-lymphotropic virus type 1.
Source: Modified from Ref. 34.

ALS, especially if the ocular features are minimal or mild and the familial nature of this ordinarily autosomal dominant disorder is not known. The dysphagia may become severe and lead to oropharyngeal or nasopharyngeal regurgitation, choking and aspiration; palatal and laryngeal weakness may lead to dysphonia (36). In the later stages of the illness, facial weakness and proximal muscle weakness become more pronounced. A clue to the presence of OPD, however, is its epidemiology with a high prevalence in the French-Canadian and the Bukhara-Jewish population and it is inherited in an autosomal dominant fashion—the mutation is a short (GCG) 8 to 13 expansion of a (GCG) six repeat encoding for a poly (A) binding protein (PABP 2) (37); genetic testing is available to confirm the diagnosis.

Myasthenia gravis and Lambert Eaton myasthenic syndrome (LEMS) are generally excluded by noting the absence of distinctive clinical attributes (fatigability and manifestations of dysautonomia, respectively) and lack of characteristic EMG findings that help make the distinction from ALS (38). In myasthenia gravis, there is typically a decremental motor response of >10% as well as an increase in jitter between two muscle fibers innervated by the same motor unit. Although these findings may be encountered in weakened muscles of patients with ALS, EMG evidence for LMN degeneration is lacking in myasthenia gravis. In LEMS, the diagnostic finding is very low-initial motor evoked responses that increase by more than 200% after a brief (15-second) period of exercise. Although initial motor evoked responses are also low in ALS, postactivation facilitation is generally not significant.

A more challenging differential diagnostic consideration is bulbospinal neuronopathy. Also known as Kennedy's disease, it is an X-linked disorder that results in slowly progressive, symmetric, bulbar and proximal limb muscle weakness, cramps, and atrophy (3,39). Fasciculations are prominent in perioral facial muscles and the tongue. Deep tendon reflexes are depressed or absent. Most cases lack UMN features although isolated patients have had UMN signs (40). In more than 50% of patients, there are signs of partial androgen deficiency like gynecomastia and infertility. The creatine kinase is typically elevated to a higher degree than would be seen in a purely denervating disorder. The EMG shows evidence of a LMN disorder (active and chronic denervation changes), but the sensory-evoked potentials are reduced or even absent suggesting involvement of sensory axons or dorsal root ganglia neurons (41), a finding that raises serious questions about the validity of the diagnosis of ALS. Nonetheless, at times Kennedy's disease may be mistaken for ALS (2% of cases of Kennedy's disease mistakenly diagnosed as ALS) for several reasons including lack of a family history, absence of gynecomastia, and absent or minimal sensory deficits (42). Accordingly, the diagnosis must be entertained in any male with predominantly LMN findings. Kennedy's disease may be established definitively by DNA testing, demonstrating an expansion of the cytosine-adenine-guanine (CAG) trinucleotide repeat within the translated portion (the first exon) of the androgen receptor gene. Normal individuals have a CAG repeat number ranging from 10 to 36, while in Kennedy's disease patients, the length range is 40 to 62. There is an inverse relationship between age of onset and repeat length.

Differential Diagnosis of PMA-Onset ALS

There is a wide range of disorders (listed in Table 5), both myopathic and neurogenic in nature, that present with weakness (and without definite UMN signs) and simulate PMA-onset ALS. The most important of the myopathic disorders to consider is inclusion body myositis (IBM). It is an inflammatory myopathy most often seen in older men. It tends to present in an asymmetric, patchy fashion with a predilection for weakness and atrophy of the forearm flexors, triceps, biceps and quadriceps; there are rare instances of primary respiratory failure (43). Accordingly, despite its myopathic nature, it may resemble a limb-onset LMN form of ALS. The creatine kinase is typically elevated to a modest degree and the muscle biopsy is diagnostic. The EMG findings usually suggest a necrotizing myopathy (evidence for active denervation with early recruited low-amplitude, short duration, and polyphasic

Table 5 The Differential Diagnosis of ALS Classified by Clinical Presentation

Clinical presentation	Differential diagnosis
Progressive bulbar palsy	Multiple sclerosis, foramen magnum tumor, cerebrovascular disease, syringobulbia, brainstem glioma myasthenia gravis, Lambert Eaton myasthenic syndrome, oculopharyngeal dystrophy, and bulbospinal neuronopathy
Progressive muscular atrophy	Inclusion body myositis, mononeuropathy, brachial or lumbar plexopathy, diabetic polyradiculoneuropathy, spinal muscular atrophy, bulbospinal neuronopathy, benign monomelic amyotrophy, motor neuronopathy with lymphoma, postpolio progressive muscular atrophy, and multifocal motor neuropathy
Progressive spastic paraparesis	Multiple sclerosis, cervical spondylotic myelopathy, syringomyelia, subacute combined degeneration, adrenoleukodystrophy, and hereditary spastic paraparesis

Abbreviation: ALS, amyotrophic lateral sclerosis.
Source: Modified from Ref. 34.

motor unit potentials) but when IBM is in its later phases, the EMG may show motor unit potentials and recruitment characteristics of chronic denervation, features seen in the context of ALS. Complicating the diagnostic process is the EMG finding of fasciculation potentials in some patients with IBM (44). Helping to make the distinction between ALS and IBM are specific clinical features in the latter disorder, especially early weakness of finger flexors, weakness of the quadriceps, slow progression, lack of UMN signs, and rarity of clinically visible fasciculations. Quantitative EMG may provide evidence for a myopathic disorder even when routine EMG does not show a myogenic disorder (44). A muscle biopsy should be obtained in circumstances that are diagnostically ambiguous, looking for evidence of an inflammatory myopathy with rimmed vacuoles, the morphological hallmark of IBM.

Disorders of individual named nerves (mononeuropathies) and plexopathies also bear consideration, but are usually differentiated from ALS by the presence of pain and numbness, and by the absence of progression or spread of clinical findings and by the limited distribution of EMG abnormalities. Diabetic polyradiculopathy may present with asymmetric lower extremity weakness and pain and over time a process of territorial spread may occur, simulating the progression of ALS but is usually distinguished from ALS by distinctive metabolic abnormalities and both clinical and electrophysiological evidence of sensory fiber involvement. A neoplastic polyradiculopathy might present with asymmetric weakness of the LMN type, but would probably be associated with sensory signs and one or more parameters of the cerebrospinal fluid analysis would almost certainly be abnormal. Certain neuronopathies, like adult-onset spinal muscular atrophy (SMA), postpolio progressive muscular atrophy (PPMA), and hexosaminidase deficiency (Hex-A deficiency), may be distinguished from ALS by slowly progressive, symmetrical limb-girdle weakness rarely affecting bulbar muscles and sparing respiratory muscles in the case of SMA (4), very slow progression (decades) and prior history of poliomyelitis for patients with PPMA, and young age of onset, tremor, cognitive impairment, and tremor with reduced Hex-A in serum and leukocytes in individuals with Hex-A deficiency (45).

Other differential diagnostic considerations include patients like those described by Van den Berg-Vos et al. (46). They reported three groups of patients with adult onset, sporadic LMN disease at least four years after onset (LMN syndrome) with benign course: Group 1 is designated slowly progressive spinal muscular atrophy, a severe generalized LMN disease with long duration (median duration, 11 years) and respiratory insufficiency in 2 of 13 patients; Group 2 is categorized as distal spinal muscular atrophy with slowly progressive symmetrical muscle weakness and atrophy involving the legs and arms (median duration, 14 years). Group 3 is subdivided into two subgroups—segmental distal LMN findings (3A), and segmental proximal LMN findings (3B). Katz et al. (47) described a group of patients similar to Group 3 of Van den Berg-Vos who presented with a pure LMN disorder at least 18 months after onset that they designated bibrachial amyotrophic diplegia; in follow-up periods ranging from 3 to 11 years these patients did not develop respiratory or bulbar dysfunction or lose the ability to walk.

Paraneoplastic disorders also find themselves in the category of differential diagnosis of a PMA-onset presentation of ALS (although for this group of diseases, UMN signs may be combined with LMN findings). In fact, there are three clinical situations in which a cause-and-effect relationship is regarded to exist between a PMA- or ALS-like syndrome and neoplasia (48). First, when patients with PMA or ALS substantially improve or stabilize with treatment of the underlying cancer, the PMA or ALS is considered paraneoplastic and there are rare reports of these syndromes behaving in this fashion (3,49). Casting doubt on the importance of this putative paraneoplastic relationship, however, is the much more common scenario described by Vigliani et al. (50) where none of the patients treated for cancer in a series of 14 patients with ALS and solid cancer improved after therapy.

Second, PMA or ALS may have a paraneoplastic origin when the neurological syndrome is tightly associated with the presence of a serum autoantibody—anti-Hu neuronal antibodies and lung cancer. With few exceptions, patients with small-cell lung carcinoma and paraneoplastic encephalomyelitis or a sensory neuronopathy have antineuronal antibodies (designated anti-Hu) in serum and cerebrospinal fluid (CSF) (51). Although PMA or ALS alone is typically not the sole manifestation of paraneoplastic encephalomyelitis (PEM), motor weakness occasionally is the first neurological symptom of PEM. No patient has developed a pure motor syndrome mimicking PMA or ALS, and all patients have had signs of dysfunction referable to other areas of the nervous system, but motor neuron dysfunction is a prominent symptom in about 20% of patients with the anti-Hu antibody (51). In general, symptoms begin with loss of strength proximally that affects the lower or upper extremities or both, sometimes in an asymmetric pattern mimicking PMA or ALS, but more rapidly progressive than usually seen in sporadic ALS. Weakness, atrophy, and fasciculations of the distal muscles are common findings; tendon reflexes may be decreased or increased in activity, and some patients have Hoffmann and Babinski signs. Rarely, patients may present with head drop. Thus, for some patients, prominent UMN and LMN signs that are seen in ALS or PMA occur in the context of cancer and a positive test for anti-Hu antibody.

A third situation in which there may be a paraneoplastic relationship between PMA or ALS and neoplasia is found in the special circumstance of these conditions in association with a lymphoproliferative disease (such as Hodgkin's or non-Hodgkin's lymphoma, multiple myeloma, Waldenstrom's macroglobulinemia, and chronic lymphatic leukemia) (52). Gordon et al. (53) found that more than half of their patients with lymphoproliferative disease and motor neuronopathies had typical ALS with a combination of UMN and LMN findings and that 5 of 42 patients treated for lymphoma improved or stabilized after treatment. Importantly, in the small group of responders, only one had classic ALS, the other had either motor neuropathy or a LMN syndrome. The nature of the association between PMA or ALS and lymphoproliferative disorders is not known, but in wild mice a spontaneous viral infection causes both leukemia and a motor neuron disease, suggesting the possibility that a persistent viral infection is involved in the pathogenesis of both conditions (54). Nobile-Orazio et al. (49) conclude that it is unlikely that patients with typical or classic ALS will benefit from therapy of concomitant lymphoma. Rowland (35) notes that less than 10% of patients with ALS (classic ALS and lower motor neuronopathy or PMA) and lymphoproliferative disease show improvement in their neurological disorder after treatment of the malignancy.

A related consideration is the PMA or ALS-like disorder found in association with a monoclonal gammopathy (MCG). In 1982, Rowland et al. (55) described a patient with a progressive LMN syndrome with clinical features resembling progressive spinal muscular atrophy. Laboratory features were unusual for PMA, however, in that nerve conduction velocities were less than 70% of normal, CSF protein was elevated (132 mg/dL), and the patient had a monoclonal IgM gammopathy. Postmortem examination revealed that the total number of motor neurons was essentially normal, although there was central chromatolysis of anterior cells. The brunt of the pathology was found in the ventral nerve roots. The condition resembled motor neuron disease clinically, but was best characterized as a predominantly proximal motor demyelinating radiculoneuropathy. This intriguing observation—that motor neuropathy associated with MCG could clinically simulate motor neuron disease or neuronopathy—spawned many studies that help to understand the relationship of paraproteins to motor neuron and motor nerve disorders (49,56). Younger et al. (57) found that almost 10% of patients with ALS have an associated MCG, while Willison et al. (58) found that the prevalence of MCG was identical in ALS patients and in controls. Reports show that some patients with ALS and MCG (sometimes reacting with glycoconjugate neural antigens, such as GM1 and asialo-GM1 ganglioside) improved with treatments that reduced the level of the circulating monoclonal proteins or antibodies or both (49) and led clinicians to search for serum protein abnormalities in patients suspected of having ALS with the view to treat individuals who proved to be seropositive. Treatment results have been disappointing, however, with only very rare reports of improvement in cases of typical ALS or PMA, leading most investigators to forego chemotherapy in the context of ALS associated with MCG, unless an underlying lymphoproliferative malignancy is found.

Another disorder to consider in the differential diagnosis of PMA-onset ALS is benign monomelic amyotrophy. It is a sporadic disorder that presents with focal weakness involving a single limb and affects men five times more frequently than women (59). The age of onset is between 15 and 30 years and although most of the patients described have been from Japan and India the condition has been encountered throughout the world (35). Most often, weakness begins in the hand intrinsic muscles and then spreads centripetally for 1 to 2 years to involve the forearm flexors and extensors. After this slow progression the condition usually stabilizes. Deep tendon reflexes are usually normal or reduced. UMN signs and bulbar involvement are not encountered. The EMG findings parallel the clinical signs in revealing evidence for a restricted LMN disorder. Routine nerve conduction studies are generally normal except for the presence of low motor amplitudes when recording from atrophic hand muscles. Modest reductions in sensory potentials are found in 30% of cases. The EMG reveals fibrillation potentials and positive sharp waves in less than half the patients, whereas recruitment is invariably reduced in a pattern corresponding to areas of weakness and atrophy (60). The EMG of muscles in the limb that appears to be uninvolved may reveal features of acute and chronic denervation, suggesting more widespread LMN disease than is apparent clinically (61). Magnetic resonance imaging (MRI) of the cervical spine may disclose focal atrophy of the spinal cord (62).

Arguably, the most important of the differential diagnostic conditions of a PMA-onset presentation of ALS is multifocal motor neuropathy with conduction block (35). This is because it can simulate ALS clinically but differs because it is responsive to immunotherapy (63). The disorder affects men primarily at a relatively young age (<45 years) and usually presents as slowly progressive, painless, remarkably focal weakness and amyotrophy involving the small hand muscles (64). Weakness begins typically unilaterally, progresses for a number of years, and then appears in the contralateral limb. Clinical deficits correspond to individual peripheral nerves and remain restricted in their anatomic distribution for years. After many years, the examination usually discloses marked atrophy of the intrinsic hand and forearm muscles, although in the initial phases the primary demyelinating character of the neuropathy leads to muscle weakness that is relatively less conspicuous than muscle atrophy. In general, compared to hand intrinsic muscles, the humeral and shoulder girdle muscles are relatively preserved. Lower extremity weakness is infrequent and cranial nerve involvement is rare. Fasciculations and cramps are common. Deep tendon reflexes may be attenuated, especially in weak limbs, but occasionally they are normally active or unexpectedly brisk for the degree of muscle atrophy and weakness. Most remarkable is the preservation of sensation, even in regions where muscles are markedly atrophic. Diagnosis rests on the findings from EMG studies that show evidence of a LMN disorder, but in contrast to ALS the defining abnormality is partial conduction block along focal segments of motor fibers in regions not usually susceptible to compression (65). Additional features of multifocal motor demyelination include temporal dispersion, segmentally reduced motor nerve conduction velocity, prolonged distal motor latency, and prolonged F-wave latency. In some series, conduction block per se is found only in 30% of patients, but virtually all patients have nerve conduction study evidence for demyelination (66). Fifty to sixty percent of patients with multifocal motor neuropathy have high titers of antibody reacting with the GM1 ganglioside, whereas the vast majority of patients with ALS are seronegative. As noted, the condition is responsive to immunotherapy including intravenous gamma globulin (as first line treatment) and cyclophosphamide (for refractory cases).

Differential Diagnosis of PLS-Onset ALS

A variety of acquired CNS disorders may present with UMN signs and suggest PLS-onset ALS, among them multiple sclerosis (MS), Vitamin B12 deficiency, and cervical spondylosis (Table 5). In a small subset of patients with MS, particularly in individuals more than 50 years old, the disorder presents and evolves as a slowly progressive spastic paraparesis. Because these patients may have few, if any, sensory symptoms or signs, the diagnosis of ALS may be considered. Similarly, occasional MS patients have pseudobulbar palsy that simulates bulbar ALS. In these patients, diagnostic uncertainity can usually be resolved with laboratory studies that are characteristically positive in MS and normal in ALS. In MS, MRI studies of the spinal cord and brain generally disclose areas of T2 brightening, and the CSF often has oligoclonal bands and an elevated gamma globulin fraction of the total protein. In Vitamin B12 deficiency, the first symptoms of spinal cord dysfunction are usually numbness and tingling in the feet and hands, which reflect abnormalities in the posterior columns. If the condition continues untreated, limb stiffness and weakness, particularly of the legs, develop as a result of corticospinal tract involvement. Ultimately, well-recognized UMN signs such as spasticity, hyperreflexia, clonus, and Babinski responses evolve and hence the disorder might resemble the PLS-onset form of ALS. One expects the serum B12 level, however, to be within normal limits in patients with ALS.

Perhaps the most important of the acquired diseases of the spinal cord in simulating ALS is spondylotic myelopathy. This disorder may lead to spinal cord compression and ischemia with or without nerve root compromise. Neck pain is a common but not invariable clinical feature. Some patients with myelopathy develop UMN signs in the legs and, if there is coexisting central gray matter or nerve root involvement or both, a subset of patients may have additional LMN signs in the arms, simulating ALS. In fact, in the experience of the Eleanor and Lou Gehrig Center at the New York Institute, Rowland reports that 5% of patients with ALS have had cervical (or lumbar) laminectomies early in their course (35). Unlike ALS, the clinical picture of spondylotic myelopathy often includes lower and upper extremity proprioceptive loss and sphincter abnormalities and the cervical MRI study typically discloses abnormal signal on FLAIR sequences intrinsic to the spinal cord. Importantly, although the EMG may disclose changes of active and chronic denervation in both arms in cervical spondylosis—and the legs if there is coexisting lumbosacral spondylotic disease—the EMG of bulbar and thoracic paraspinal muscles should be normal, in contrast to the frequent abnormal EMG findings in ALS.

Inherited disorders (adrenoleukodystrophy and familial spastic paraparesis) should also bear consideration in the differential diagnosis of PLS-onset ALS. The former is an X-linked peroxisomal disorder that may present as a relatively mild "spinal-neuropathic" form designated as "adrenomyeloneuropathy" (67). It is found in adult men and is characterized by progressive spastic paraparesis with a mild peripheral neuropathy. A chronic non-progressive spinal cord disorder has also been described in heterozygous women. Adrenomyeloneuropathy presents in the second to third decades of life with progressive spastic paraparesis, distal muscle weakness and sensory loss, impotence, and sphincter disturbances (67). Because the sensory, autonomic, and sphincter disturbances may be relatively mild, and the motor component of this syndrome (UMN signs of weakness and spasticity) may be striking, the disorder can resemble ALS. Most patients, however, do have some degree of peripheral neuropathy, and nerve conduction studies disclose reduced motor conduction velocities. Additional important diagnostic information may be obtained from a sural nerve biopsy specimen, which reveals loss of myelinated fibers, small onion bulbs, and characteristic lipid clefts in the Schwann cell cytoplasm, the so-called lamellar lipid inclusions (68). A laboratory chemistry clue is the presence of low sodium and elevated potassium concentrations reflecting atrophy of the adrenal gland. Diagnosis can be established by demonstrating increased levels of very long chain fatty acids in the plasma of patients and heterozygous carriers (69).

The hereditary spastic paraplegias (HSPs) represent a group of diverse disorders whose primary feature is insidiously progressive lower extremity weakness and spasticity (70). HSP may be inherited in an autosomal dominant, autosomal recessive, or X-linked recessive manner and the disorder is genetically heterogeneous, with 10 genes identified and at least 21 loci mapped (21). When neurologic impairment is largely restricted to progressive lower extremity spastic weakness, urinary urgency, and lower extremity paresthesias, HSP is designated "uncomplicated" (21,70). The examination of these patients typically discloses weakness and spasticity of the legs, lower limb hyperreflexia, Babinski signs, and mild diminution in vibratory sense with sparing of pain and temperature sensation. Some individuals have accompanying atrophy of the anterior tibial muscles that probably reflects mild LMN involvement (70). When these clinical features are accompanied by involvement of other systems (cutaneous abnormalities or cataracts) or additional neurological abnormalities such as seizures, dementia, amyotrophy, Parkinsonism, or peripheral neuropathy, the HSP is considered "complicated" (21,70). In recent years, however, the distinctions between the pure and complicated forms has become less clear as some patients in "pure" families have had features ordinarily associated with complicated phenotypes, such as cognitive impairment and cerebellar atrophy (21). The most common type of uncomplicated HSP accounting for 40% to 50% of autosomal dominant HSP families is caused by a mutation in the gene at chromosomal locus 2p21–24 coding for the chaperone protein, spastin (21). When family history is not available and onset is later in life, differentiating apparent sporadic HSP from classic ALS or UMN-onset ALS may pose a diagnostic challenge. The long clinical course, however, the absence of bulbar or respiratory muscle involvement, absence of prominent and diffuse LMN findings, presence of urinary symptoms, and mild but definite sensory findings help to separate HSP from ALS.

LABORATORY INVESTIGATIONS IN THE EVALUATION FOR ALS

After our initial histories and physical examinations in patients suspected of having ALS, we turn to various diagnostic studies. The framework for our work up is the classification scheme (Table 1) that includes classic ALS, PBP, PMA, and PLS. Before committing ourselves to the diagnosis of ALS, however, we view these subtypes generically, as clinical syndromes with the potential for a diverse set of causes or differential diagnostic considerations (Table 5) as we have discussed previously.

We employ four major categories of laboratory assessment when evaluating patients suspected to have ALS or an ALS subtype: the EMG, MRI of brain and spinal cord, clinical laboratory studies, and rarely muscle and nerve biopsy interpretation (70a). The rationale for each category of testing is outlined in Table 6.

EMG Studies

In virtually all patients presenting with motor neuron disease, we perform an EMG after completion of the history and physical examination. In ALS, we expect the EMG to reveal a characteristic pattern of normal sensory conduction studies, essentially normal motor conduction studies (although motor amplitudes are often reduced), and needle examination findings of fibrillation and fasciculation potential activity with evidence of motor unit potential remodeling in a wide distribution (38,71). We use the EMG to search for specific abnormalities that are recognizable neurophysiological signatures of disorders that may at times mimic ALS but in contrast to ALS are treatable, self-limited, or reversible, for example, the decremental motor response at slow rates of stimulation of myasthenia gravis, the postactivation facilitation of LEMS, the conduction block of multifocal motor neuropathy, and the attenuated or absent sensory potentials of bulbospinal neuronopathy.

Table 6 Steps in Diagnostic Evaluation When ALS Is Suspected

Investigation	Rationale/points to consider
Electromyography	Confirm lower motor neuron involvement Are there features of denervation and reinnervation? Is the process generalized or is it focal? Is there conduction block? Are sensory fibers involved? Is there a decremental motor response? Is there postactivation facilitation?
Neuroimaging of brain and spinal cord	Confirm normal anatomy and examine for motor pathway abnormalities seen in ALS on T-1 weighted MRI images Is there structural pathology of brain,brainstem, cervicomedullary junction, spinal cord, or nerve roots?
Clinical laboratory studies	Confirm normal results Is there evidence for treatable or reversible disorders of a metabolic, autoimmune, neoplastic, infectious, or vasculitic nature?
Muscle biopsy	Confirm denervation and reinnervation Is there evidence for inflammatory, metabolic, genetic, or toxic myopathy?

Abbreviations: ALS, amyotrophic lateral sclerosis; MRI, magnetic resonance imaging.
Source: Modified from Ref. 70a.

MRI Studies

Even when the EMG results strongly support a diagnosis of ALS, it is our practice to seek assurance that no structural abnormality exists that might even remotely explain a combination of UMN and LMN findings. Therefore, despite clinical features of ALS and confirmatory EMG evidence of involvement of the LMNs, we proceed with MRI studies of that portion of the CNS implicated by the physical examination and EMG evaluation to affirm the anatomical integrity of the brain stem and cervical spinal cord. Neuroimaging is especially important in patients presenting with features of a motor neuron disease subtype but without all the classic signs of ALS per se. For example, in patients presenting with PBP, the brain MRI scan is critical in identifying possible MS, brainstem glioma, or brainstem vascular disease. For patients with PMA, an MRI scan of the brain and spinal cord may provide a clue to pathology involving multiple nerve roots, such as neoplastic polyradiculopathy; and in a patient with features of PLS, the MRI may have an important role in supporting the diagnosis of myelopathies caused by MS or cervical spondylosis. In ALS or ALS subtypes, brain and spinal cord are expected to be normal or show only mild abnormalities (increased signal on T1-weighted MRI) without definite evidence of other brainstem, spinal cord, or nerve root pathology (72).

Clinical Laboratory Studies

We use laboratory studies for two major reasons. First, because ALS is not known to be mediated by conventional or well-established infectious, inflammatory, immunologic, toxic, or metabolic mechanisms, we expect clinical laboratory studies to be normal. Indeed, by definition, normal results from a variety of tests support the diagnosis of ALS. Second, in the few weeks after initially examining a patient we suspect may have ALS, we strive to find an alternate diagnosis, using our clinical judgment and experience to identify laboratory abnormalities that might explain UMN or LMN findings, or both. We have previously mentioned many of these alternate diagnoses in the section on differential diagnosis, but there are other important systemic disorders we did not list or discuss including endocrinopathy (hyperthyroidism and hyperparathyroidism) (73,74), connective tissue diseases, and chronic viral retroviral infections (75) whose pathogenesis may involve central or peripheral motor pathways and whose clinical findings may be reminiscent of ALS or an ALS subtype. This approach, therefore, forces us to cast a wide net and use various laboratory tests as we ascertain the overall health of our patients and search for treatable conditions.

In our clinical practice, therefore, virtually all patients evaluated for ALS are tested with the many and varied clinical laboratory studies listed in Table 7. The more closely the clinical features resemble classic ALS, the less likely we are to carry out additional or specialized laboratory evaluations (Table 8). In general, we reserve these tests for the patient whose ALS clinical presentation is atypical by virtue of age (less than 40 years, older than 80 years), with a positive family history of a central nervous system disorder, with features of an accompanying systemic disease (neoplastic, infectious, and endocrine), or with involvement of portions of the nervous system in addition to upper and LMNs.

In the setting of one or more of these atypical features, we may perform a lumbar puncture because this test is well tolerated, has virtually no serious morbidity, and may reveal evidence of treatable autoimmune, infectious, inflammatory, neoplastic, and paraneoplastic disorders. The CSF is usually normal in ALS, although 33% of patients

Table 7 Routine Clinical Laboratory Testing for Suspected ALS

Complete blood count, platelet count, Westergren sedimentation rate, prothrombin time, and
  urinalysis
Electrolytes (Na, K, Cl, CO_2, Ca, Mg, and PO_4), glucose, blood urea nitrogen, creatinine, and
  liver function tests
Serum VDRL
Chest roentenogram
Creatine kinase
Thyroid studies (T4, T3, Thyroid-stimulating hormone)
Assessment of stool for occult blood
Screening for connective-tissue diseases (antinuclear antibody, rheumatoid factor, complement)
Serum protein electrophoresis, serum immunoelectrophoresis with immunofixation
Anti-neural antigen testing (GM1, asialo-GM1)

Abbreviations: ALS, amyotrophic lateral sclerosis; VDRL, Venereal Disease Research Laboratory.
Source: Modified from Ref. 70a.

Table 8 Indications for Special Laboratory Testing for Suspected ALS

Test	Indication
Cerebrospinal fluid examination	Young age of onset (<40 years)
	Clinical evidence of infectious disease
	Clinical suspicion of meningeal metastases
	Clinical suspicion of multiple sclerosis
	Features of chronic neuropathy
Bone marrow examination	Clinical suspicion of lymphoma
	Monoclonal gammopathy
	Elevated CSF protein
	CSF oligoclonal bands
Anti-Hu antibody measurement	Multiple neural systems involved
	Suspicion of paraneoplastic syndrome
Leukocyte hexosaminadase-A assay	Young age of onset (<40 years)
	Mental changes
	Cramps
	Postural and action tremor
Test for cytosine-adenine-guanine	Young age of onset (<40years)
(CAG) repeat in androgen	Gynecomastia
receptor gene (X chromosome)	Sensory neuropathy
Anti-HIV antibody measurement	Risk factors for HIV
Anti-HTLV-1 antibody measurement	Risk factors for tropical spastic paraparesis
Serum very long chain fatty acids	Young age of onset (<40 years)
	Polyneuropathy (axon-loss)
	Adrenal insufficiency
Serum parathyroid hormone assay	Serum chemistry profile suggesting
	hyperparathyroidism
Muscle biopsy	Muscle weakness with few fasciculations
	No UMN signs
	Raised CK (>3–4-fold increased)
	Family history of a myopathic disorder
	Young age of onset (<40)

Abbreviations: CSF, cerebro spinal fluid; UMN, upper motor neuron; HIV, human immunodeficiency
virus; HTLV-1, human T-lymphotropic virus type I.
Source: Modified from Ref. 70a.

with pathologically confirmed ALS have elevated CSF protein (>45 mg/dL) (71); values in excess of 75 mg/dL are occasionally encountered (76,77). Rarely patients with ALS have mild pleocytosis or oligoclonal bands.

The possibility of lymphoma is strengthened by discovering an elevated CSF protein concentration and the presence of oligoclonal bands (78); in the setting of these abnormalities a bone marrow biopsy might be considered (79). We reserve anti-Hu antibody testing for those patients in whom the clinical presentation of a subacutely progressive LMN and UMN disorder is associated with an extra-muscular neurological abnormality (such as change in mentation, sensory signs, or cerebellar abnormalities) because the anti-Hu antibody is more accurately regarded as a marker for diffuse encephalomyelitis, rather than for a selective disorder of motor neurons (51). Serum parathyroid hormone is measured only if electrolyte concentrations suggest hyperparathyroidism (hypercalcemia and hypophosphatemia) (80). Leukocyte hexosaminadase A is measured in patients with earlier onset, slowly progressive ALS, or PMA (45). Genetic testing for bulbospinal neuronopathy is undertaken in younger men presenting with PBP or PMA phenotypes with slow progression (3). Evidence of HTLV-1 and HIV infection is sought in patients with a slowly progressive PLS syndrome (70). Last, evidence of adrenoleukodystrophy should be sought in younger men with a chronic PLS phenotype, especially if a mild peripheral neuropathy exists (67).

PRESENTATION OF THE DIAGNOSIS

The journey from good health to the latter stages of ALS presents a set of formidable challenges to the body, spirit, and psyche. Although this journey is often arduous and complicated, honesty and understanding from the neurologist help patients as they confront the hurdles of ALS. A tone of candor and hope should be set from the moment the neurologist meets with the patient to break the news of the diagnosis of ALS. Silani and Borasio (81) note that there are "few events that families and patients remember as vividly as the way the diagnosis was told to them." Smith (82) writes that in the process of breaking the news: "doctors are charged with a very delicate educational task." Miller et al. (83) alert us that: "Telling the patient the diagnosis is a daunting task for the physician. If not done appropriately, the effect can be devastating, leaving the patient with a sense of abandonment, and destroying the patient–physician relationship."

Before scheduling a meeting to disclose the diagnosis of ALS, the diagnosis must be established according to the criteria outlined earlier in this chapter. Using our experience and a review of recent literature as guidelines, we have found that 10 precepts serve as a solid foundation during the process of presenting the diagnosis, and we describe them in the following paragraphs.

1. *Adequate time.* First, there must be plenty of time set aside for the task. McCluskey et al. (84) found that greater time spent discussing the diagnosis was correlated with higher patient and caregiver satisfaction. They suggest that the process of breaking the news requires 45 minutes, at a minimum, and that a commitment be made to a near-term revisit for further discussion.
2. *Never alone.* Second, the patient should not hear the news alone. As the information to be revealed is profound and life altering in its implications, no patient should face it alone and if at all possible, a relative,

friend, or some representative of the patient's support network should be in attendance (83).

3. *Comfortable physical surroundings.* Third, the meeting room should be comfortable, quiet, and free of distractions, and the neurologist should sit at a desk next to the patient and make eye contact with the patient and companion (83).

4. *What does the patient know?* Fourth, the neurologist should ascertain what patients know before informing them of the diagnosis. Not uncommonly, before coming to the neurologist, many patients will already have the sense that their problem is a serious one and perhaps some may already know that ALS is a diagnostic possibility. We have encountered some individuals, however, who recognize their problem is serious and progressive but they have not yet become familiar with ALS, believing they may have some other neurological condition for which there are effective ameliorating treatments, such as MS or Parkinson's disease.

5. *Prepare the patient that bad news is imminent.* Fifth, the neurologist should provide a preliminary warning comment that bad news is coming with words to the effect: "I have been reviewing all the findings and I believe the problem is a serious one."

6. *Be caring and hopeful.* Sixth, it is probably best to reveal the diagnosis in a direct, empathetic, and caring manner with simple language free of medical jargon, calling the disease by its widely known name (ALS), noting that it is a progressive disorder with a variable prognosis (85). The neurologist should indicate that although there is no cure at present, research is very active around the world with scientists making progress in understanding the disease better. We repeat Dr. Lewis Rowland's "fifth level of hope," (86) which to paraphrase, is that one day, a very bright scientist/researcher is going to get lucky and unravel the mysterious biology of ALS so that we have more effective treatments.

7. *Strive to be empathetic, listen to the patient.* Seventh, it is best to attend to the patients' verbal and non-verbal responses to the revelations expressed during the encounter, and remain sensitive to how much information patients want to be conveyed about the disease, its course, and potential complications during this initial meeting. Miller et al. (83) suggest giving the news at the patients' pace, allowing the patients to dictate what they are told. In this spirit, Rose (87) observes that "a sudden blurting out of the nature of the disease can be shattering and there can be few patients who will face with equanimity being told that they have a progressive disease that may involve breathing muscles."

8. *Convey the concept of a multidisciplinary care team.* Eighth, the neurologist should provide reassurance that he or she views him or herself and health professional associates as an integral part of the patient's support system and will do whatever is possible to help maintain muscle functions and to manage any complications that arise during the course of the illness (88). The neurologist might indicate that the treatment team "is here" to ensure the patient's well being, that the patient's wishes will be respected at all times, and that the patient will never be abandoned (83).

9. *Provide a plan for management and revisits.* Ninth, the neurologist should consider summarizing the main points of the discussion verbally, in writing, or with an audiotape and propose at least a preliminary plan of care

for the patients before they leave the office. The neurologist might tell the patient how he proposes to ameliorate any symptoms the patient is now experiencing with medications or physical therapies, and that he would like the patient also to be seen and followed by colleagues in other disciplines. The neurologist should let the patient know his plans for a revisit [in the near term (1–3 weeks) for the patient to ask further questions about the illness after reflecting on today's discussion] and longer term for reassessment (range 1–3 months). It is important to inform patients about ALS resources, such as the Muscular Dystrophy Association (MDA) and the ALS Association, and to let patients know of therapeutic trials ongoing in your institution or nearby centers. Following the communication of bad news, McCluskey et al. (84) observe that the plan of care "fosters the physician–patient care bond while permitting patients and their caregivers to cope and to plan appropriately for the future."

10. *Suggest a second opinion.* Last, the neurologist should support the patient's desire to seek a second opinion and be open to facilitating the visit, providing a list of names of ALS specialists, making office notes and reports of all test results readily available. Bradley (89) points out that "the availability of the second opinion helps the patient and family members feel that the door is always left open, and that the initial physician's mind is not closed to other possibilities."

CONCLUSIONS

In this chapter, we have pointed out that ALS may be classified into acquired and inherited disorders. In the acquired category, we find ALS and the ALS subtypes of PBP, PMA, and PLS. The first two of these conditions, PBP and PMA, are probably part of the spectrum of ALS, with a comparable course and outcome. In contrast, PLS may in some cases be a pure UMN disorder distinct from ALS, and inherently much less severe in its manifestations.

During the evaluation of a patient suspected of having ALS, there are consensus diagnostic criteria that guide the neurologist in establishing one of several levels of certainty or confidence (definite, probable, suspected) in the diagnosis of ALS. Before accepting that ALS is the diagnosis that explains the patient's clinical features, however, a wide spectrum of neurological disorders that affect the UMN and the LMN must be considered in the differential diagnosis. It is helpful to categorize these disorders in the context of clinical presentations that manifest as one of three neurological syndromes: PBP, PMA, and PLS. The clinician is helped in ruling these conditions in or out by three categories of diagnostic studies— EMG, neuroimaging of the brain and spinal cord, and diverse clinical laboratory investigations.

Should ALS prove to be the most likely diagnosis that explains all aspects of the clinical presentation, then the diagnosis should be disclosed to the patient with honesty and compassion, emphasizing that there is now and will always be throughout the course of the illness specific plans for patient care and management. We feel it is important to point out to patients and family members that many ALS research projects and clinical studies are going on throughout the country and in many parts of the world, directed by scientists and clinicians whose work is imbued with imagination and passion.

REFERENCES

1. Mitsumoto H, Chad DA, Pioro EP. Clinical features: signs and symptoms. Amyotrophic Lateral Sclerosis. Philadelphia: FA Davis, 1998:47–64.
2. Scelsa SN, Yakubov B, Salzman SH. Dyspnea-fasciculation syndrome: early respiratory failure in ALS with minimal motor signs. Amyotroph Lateral Scler Other Motor Neuron Disord 2002; 3:239–243.
3. Swash M, Desai J. Motor neuron disease: classification and nomenclature. Amyotroph Lateral Scler Other Motor Neuron Disord 2000; 1:105–112.
4. Murray B, Mitsumoto HM. Disorders of upper and lower motor neurons. Neurology in Clinical Practice. Vol. 80. Boston: Butterworth-Heinemann, 2004; 2223–2266.
5. Hu MTM, Ellis CM, Al-Chalabi A, Leigh PN, Shaw CE. Flail arm syndrome: a distinctive variant of amyotrophic lateral sclerosis. J Neurol Neurosurg Psych 1998; 65:950–951.
6. Mortara P, Chio A, Rosso MG, Leone M, Schiffer D. Motor neuron disease in the province of Turin, Italy, 1966–1980. Survival analysis in an unselected population. J Neurol Sci 1984; 66:165–173.
7. Norris F, Shepherd R, Denys E, Mukai E, Elias L, Holden D, Norri H. Onset, natural history and outcome in idiopathic adult motor neuron disease. J Neurol Sci 1993; 118: 48–55.
8. Ince PG, Evans J, Knopp M, Forster G, Hamdalla HHM, Wharton SB, Shaw PJ. Corticospinal tract degeneration in the progressive muscular atrophy variant of ALS. Neurology 2003; 60:1252–1258.
9. Traynor B, Codd M, Corr B, Forde C, Frost E, Hardiman O. Incidence and prevalence of ALS in Ireland, 1995–1997: a population based study. Neurology 1999; 52:504–509.
10. Tsuchiya K, Sano M, Shiotsu H, Akiyama H, Watabiki S, Taki K, Kondo H, Nakano I, Ideda K. Sporadic amyotrophic lateral sclerosis of long duration mimicking spinal progressive muscular atrophy exists: additional autopsy case with a clinical course of 19 years. Neuropathology 2004; 24:228–235.
11. Andersen PM, Nilsson P, Keranen M-L, Forsgren L, Hagglund J, Karlsborg M, Ronnevi L-O, Gredal O, Marklund SL. Phenotypic heterogeneity in motor neuron disease patients with CuZn-superoxide dismutase mutations in Scandinavia. Brain 1997; 120:1723–1737.
12. Rowland LP. What's in a name? Amyotrophic lateral sclerosis, motor neuron disease, and allelic heterogeneity. Ann Neurol 1998; 43:691–694.
13. Pringle CE, Hudson AJ, Munoz DG, Kiernan JA, Brown WF, Ebers GC. Primary lateral sclerosis. Clinical features, neuropathology, and diagnostic criteria. Brain 1992; 115: 495–520.
14. Swash M, Desai J, Misra VP. What is primary lateral sclerosis. J Neurol Sci 1999; 170: 5–10.
15. Turner MR, Parton MJ, Shaw CE, Leigh PN, Al-Chalabi A. Prolonged survival in motor neuron disease: a descriptive study of the King's database 1990–2002. J Neurol Neurosurg Psychiatry 2003; 74:995–997.
16. Gordon PH, Pinto M, Mitsumoto H, Kaufmann P, Rowland LP. The clinical manifestations of primary lateral sclerosis. Amyotroph Lateral Scler Other Motor Neuron Disord 2004; 5(S2):112.
17. Rowland LP. Primary lateral sclerosis: disease, syndrome, both or neither? J Neurol Sci 1999; 170:1–4.
18. Zhai P, Pagan F, Statland J, Butman JA, Floeter MK. Primary lateral sclerosis. A heterogeneous disorder composed of different subtypes? Neurology 2003; 60:1258–1265.
19. Galasko D, Salmon DP, Craig UK, Thal LJ, Schellenberg G, Wiederholt W. Clinical features and changing patterns of neurodegenerative disorders on Guam, 1997–2000. Neurology 2002; 58:90–97.
20. Chen K-M, Kurland LT. Recent epidemiologic study of amyotrophic lateral sclerosis (ALS) and parkinsonism-dementia complex (PDC) in Guam island. Japanese J Clin Ecol 1995; 4:24–28.

21. Figlewicz DA, Orrell RW. The genetics of motor neuron diseases. Amyotroph Lateral Scler Other Motor Neuron Disord 2003; 4:225–231.

22. Hedera P, Lerner AJ, Castellani R, Friedland RP. Concurrence of Alzheimer's disease, Parkinson's disease, diffuse Lewy body disease, and amyotrophic lateral sclerosis. J Neurol Sci 1995; 128:219–224.

23. Lynch T, Sdano M, Marder KS, Bell KL, Foster NL, Defendini RF, Sima AA, Keohane C, Nygaard TG, Fahn S, et al. Clinical characteristics of a family with chromosome 17-linked disinhibition-dementia-parkinsonism-amyotrophy complex. Neurology 1994; 44: 1878–1884.

24. Gaudette M, Dellefave L, Siddique T. Amyotrophic lateral sclerosis overview. Gene Reviews www.genetests.org; 2004:1–25.

25. Cudkowicz ME, McKenna-Yasek D, Sapp PE, Chin W, Geller B, Layden DL, Schoenfeld DA, Hosler BA, Horvitz HR, Brown RH. Epidemiology of Mutations in Superoxide dismutase in amyotrophic lateral sclerosis. Ann Neurol 1997; 41:210–221.

26. Cudkowicz ME, McKenna-Yasek D, Chen C, Hedley-Whyte ET, Brown RH. Limited corticospinal tract involvement in amyotrophic lateral sclerosis subjects with the A4V mutation in the copper/zinc superoxide dismutase gene. Ann Neurol 1998; 43:703–710.

27. Mitsumoto H, Chad DA, Pioro EP. Familial ALS. Amyotrophic Lateral Sclerosis. Philadelphia: FA Davis, 1998:47–64.

28. Hentati A, Bejaoui K, Pericak-Vance MA, Hentati F, Speer MC, Hung WY, Figlewicz DA, Haines J, Rimmler J, Ben Hamida C, et al. Linkage of recessive familial amyotrophic lateral sclerosis to chromosome 2q33-q35. Nature Genet 1994; 7:425–428.

29. Lomen-Hoerth C, Murphy J, Langmore S, Kramer JH, Olney RK, Miller B. Are amyotrophic lateral sclerosis patients cognitively normal? Neurology 2003; 60:1094–1097.

30. Brooks BR. El Escorial World Federation of Neurology Criteria for the Diagnosis of Amyotrophic Lateral Sclerosis. J Neurol Sci 1994; 124(suppl):96–107.

31. Brooks BR, Miller RG, Swash M, Munsat TL, for the World Federation of Neurology Group on Motor Neuron Diseases. El Escorial revisited: Revised criteria for the diagnosis of amyotrophic lateral sclerosis. Amyotroph Lateral Scler Other Motor Neuron Disord 2000; 1:293–299.

32. Ross MA, Miller RG, Berchert L, Parry G, Barohn RJ, Armon C, Bryan WW, Petajan J, Stromatt S, Goodpasture J, McGuire D, The rhCNTF ALS study group. Toward earlier diagnosis of amyotrophic lateral sclerosis. Revised criteria. Neurology 1998; 50:768–772.

33. Chaudhuri KR, Crump SJ, Al-Sarraj S, et al. The validation of El Escorial criteria for the diagnosis of amyotrophic lateral sclerosis: a clinico-pathological study. J Neurol Sci 1995; 129(suppl):11–12.

34. Mitsumoto H, Chad DA, Pioro EP. The differential diagnosis of ALS. Amyotrophic Lateral Sclerosis. Philadelphia: FA Davis, 1998:87–121.

35. Rowland LP. Diagnosis of amyotrophic lateral sclerosis. J Neurol Sci 1998; 160:S6–S24.

36. Brais B, Rouleau GA, Bouchard J-P, Fardeau M, Tome FMS. Oculopharyngeal muscular dystrophy. Semin Neurol 1999; 19:59–66.

37. Blumen SC, Korczyn AD, Lavoie H, et al. Oculopharyngeal muscular dystrophy among Bukhara Jews is due to a founder (GCG) 9 mutation in the PABP2 gene. Neurology 2000; 55:1267–1270.

38. Chad DA. Electrodiagnostic approach to the patient with suspected motor neuron disease. Neurol Clin N Am 2002; 20:527–555.

39. Kennedy WB, Alter M, Sung JG. Report of an X-linked form of spinal muscular atrophy. Neurology 1968; 18:671–680.

40. Ferlini, et al. Androgen receptor gene (CAG)n repeat analysis in the differential diagnosis between Kennedy disease and other motor neuron disorders. Am J Med Genet 1995; 55: 105–111.

41. Olney RK, Aminoff MJ, So YT. Clinical and electrodiagnostic features of X-linked recessive bulbospinal neuronopathy. Neurology 1991; 41:823–828.

42. Parboosingh JS, Figlewicz DA, Krizus A, Meininger V, Azad NA, Newman DS, Rouleau GA. Spinobulbar muscular atrophy can mimic ALS: the importance of genetic testing in male patients with atypical ALS. Neurology 1997; 49:568–572.

43. Voermans NC, Vaneker M, Hengstman GJD, ter Laak HJ, Zimmerman C, Schelhaas HJ, Zwarets MJ. Primary respiratory failure in inclusion body myositis. Neurology 2004; 63:2191–2192.

44. Dabby R, Lange DJ, Trojaborg W, et al. Inclusion body myositis mimicking motor neuron disease. Arch Neurol 2001; 58:1253–1256.

45. Mitsumoto H, Sliman RJ, Schafer IA, et al. Motor neuron disease in adult hexosamini-dase A deficiency in two families: evidence for multisystem degeneration. Ann Neurol 1985; 17:378–385.

46. Van den Berg-Vos RM, Visser J, Franssen H, de Visser M, de Jong JMBV, Kalmijn S, Wokke JHJ, Van den Berg LH. Sporadic lower motor neuron disease with adult onset: classification of subtypes. Brain 2003; 126:1036–1047.

47. Katz JS, Wolfe GI, Andersson PB, Saperstein DS, Elliott JL, Nations SP, Bryan WW, Barohn RJBrachial amyotrophic diplegia. A slowly progressive motor neuron disease. Neurology 1999; 53:1071–1076.

48. Rosenfeld MR, Dalmau J. Paraneoplastic syndromes and progressive motor dysfunction. Semin Neurol 1993; 13:291–298.

49. Nobile-Orazio E, Carpo M, Meucci N. Are there immunologically treatable motor neuron diseases? Amyotroph Lateral Scler Other Motor Neuron Disord 2001; 2:S23–S30.

50. Vigliani MC, Polo P, Chio A, Giometto B, Mazzini L, Schiffer D. Patients with amyotrophic lateral sclerosis and cancer do not differ clinically from patients with sporadic amyotrophic lateral sclerosis. J Neurol 2000; 247:778–782.

51. Dalmau J, Graus F, Rosenblum MK, Posner JB. Anti-Hu-associated paraneoplastic encephalomyelitis/sensory neuronopathy. A clinical study of 71 patients. Medicine 1992; 71:59–72.

52. Chad DA, Harris NL. Case 16–1999. A 71-year-old man with progressive weakness and a gammopathy. N Engl J Med 1999; 340(21):1661–1669.

53. Gordon PH, Rowland LP, Younger DS, et al. Lymphoproliferative disorders and motor neuron disease: an update. Neurology 1997; 48:1671–1678.

54. Rowland LP, Schneider NA. Amyotrophic lateral sclerosis. N Engl J Med 2001; 344:1688–1700.

55. Rowland LP, Defendini R, ShermanWH, Hirano A, Olarte MR, Latov N, Lovelace RE, Inoue K, Osserman EF. Macroglobulinemia with peripheral neuropathy simulating motor neuron disease. Ann Neurol 1982; 11:532–536.

56. Rowland LP. Amyotrophic lateral sclerosis with paraproteins and antibodies. In: Serratrice G, Munsat TL, eds. Pathogenesis and Therapy of Amyotrophic Lateral Sclerosis. Philadelphia: Adv Neurol, Lippincott-Raven Press 1995:68:93–105.

57. Younger DS, Rowland LP, Latov N, et al. Motor neuron disease in amyotrophic lateral sclerosis: relation of high CSF protein content to paraproteinemia and clinical syndromes. Neurology 1990; 40:595–599.

58. Willison HJ, Chancellor AM, Patterson G, et al. Antiglycolipid antibodies, immunoglobulins, and paraproteins in motor neuron disease; a population-based case-control study. J Neurol Sci 1993; 114:209–215.

59. Hirayama K, Tomonaga M, Kitano K, Yamarta T, Korgema S, Arai K. Focal cervical poliopathy causing juvenile muscular atrophy of distal upper extremity: a pathological study. J Neurol Neurosurg Psychiatry 1987; 50:285–290.

60. Donofrio PD. Monomelic amyotrophy. Muscle Nerve 1994; 17:1129–1134.

61. Gourie-Devi M, Nalini A. Long term follow up of 44 patients with brachial monomelic amyotrophy. Acta Neurol Scand 2003; 107:215–220.

62. Tataroglu C, Bagdatoglu C, Apaydin FD, Celikbas H, Koksel T. Hirayama's disease: a case report. ALS 2003; 4:264–265.

63. Pestronk A. Invited review. Motor neuropathies, motor neuron disorders, and antiglyco-lipid antibodies. Muscle Nerve 1991; 14:927–936.

64. Parry GJ, Sumner AJ. Multifocal motor neuropathy. Neurologic Clinics 1992; 10:671–684.

65. Chaudhry V, Corse A, Cornblath DR, et al. Multifocal motor neuropathy: electrophysiological features. Muscle Nerve 1994; 17:198–205.

66. Katz JS, Wolfe GI, Bryan WW, Jackson CE, Amato AA, Barohn RJ. Electrophysiologic findings in multifocal motor neuropathy. Neurology 1997; 48:700–707.

67. Griffin JW, Goren E, Schaumberg H, Engel WK, Loriaux L. Adrenomyeloneuropathy: a probable variant of adrenoleukodystrophy. Neurology 1977; 27:1107–1113.

68. Bosch EP, Mitsumoto H. Neurology in Clinical Practice. Disorders of peripheral nerves. In: Bradley WG, Daroff RB, Fenichel GM, Marsden CD, eds. Neurology in Clinical Practice. Disorders of peripheral nerves. Boston: Butterworth-Heinemann, 2004:1881–1952.

69. Moser HW, Moser AB, Frayer KF, Chen W, Schulman JD, O'Neill BP, Kishimoto Y. Adrenoleukodystrophy: Increased plasma content of saturated very long chain fatty acids. Neurology 1981; 31:1241–1249.

70. Fink JK. Progressive spastic paraparesis: hereditary spastic paraplegia and its relation to primary and amyotrophic lateral sclerosis. Seminars in Neurology 2001; 21:199–207.

70a. Mitsumoto H, Chad DA, Pioro EP. Diagnostic investigation for ALS. In Amyotrophic Lateral Sclerosis. Philadelphia: FA Davis, 1998:122–133.

71. Mitsumoto H, Chad DA, Pioro EP. Electrodiagnosis. Amyotrophic Lateral Sclerosis. Philadelphia: FA Davis, 1998:65–86.

72. Mitsumoto H, Chad DA, Pioro EP. Neuroimaging. Amyotrophic Lateral Sclerosis. Philadelphia: FA Davis, 1998:134–150.

73. Fisher M, Mateer JE, Ullrich I, Gutrecht JA. Pyramidal tract deficits and polyneuropathy in hyperthyroidism. Combination clinically mimicking amyotrophic lateral sclerosis. Am J Med 1985; 78:1041–1044.

74. Ross MA, Bosch EP, Smith BE, Pingree MJ. Reversible endocrine disorders mimicking ALS. Amyotroph lat sclera and Other Motor Neuron Disorders 2004; 5(S2):118.

75. Gessain A, Gout O. Chronic myelopathy associated with human T-lymphotropic virus Type I (HTLV-I). Ann Intern Med 1992; 117:933–946.

76. Norris FH, Burns W, U KS, Mukai E, Norris H. Spinal fluid cells and protein in amyotrophic lateral sclerosis. Arch Neurol 1993; 50:489–491.

77. Guiloff RJ, McGregor B, Thompson E, Blackwood W, Paul E. Motor neurone disease with elevated cerebrospinal fluid protein. J Neurol Neurosurg Psychiatry 1980; 43:390–396.

78. Younger DS, Rowland LP, Latov N, et al. Lymphoma, motor neuron diseases, and amyotrophic lateral sclerosis. Ann Neurol 1991; 29:78–86.

79. Rowland LP, Sherman MD, Latov N, et al. Amyotrophic lateral sclerosis and lymphoma: bone marrow examination and other diagnostic tests. Neurology 1992; 42:1101–1102.

80. Tonner DR, Schlechte JA. Neurologic complications of thyroid and parathyroid disease. Med Clin North Am 1993; 77:251–263.

81. Silani V, Borasio GD. Honesty and hope: announcement of diagnosis of ALS. Neurology 1999; 53:S37–S39.

82. Smith RA. On behalf of the patient. Adv Exp Med Biol 1987; 209:319–322.

83. Miller RG, Rosenberg JA, Gelinas DF, Bradley WG, Bromberg MB, Brooks BR, Kasarskis EJ, Munsat TL, Oppenheimer EA. The ALS Practice Parameters Task Force. Practice parameter: the care of the patient with amyotrophic lateral sclerosis (an evidence-based review). Neurology 1999; 52:1311–1323.

84. McCluskey L, Casarett D, Siderowf A. Breaking the news: a survey of ALS patients and their caregivers. Amyotroph Lateral Scler Other Motor Neuron Disord 2004; 5:131–135.

85. Borasio GD, Sloan R, Pongratz DE. Breaking the news in amyotrophic lateral sclerosis. J Neurol Sci 1998; 160:S127–S133.

86. Rowland LP. Dr. Rowland's six levels of hope. ALSD33ALS-On-Line. ALS Interest Group. ALS Digest #332. May 27, 1997.

87. Rose FC. The management of motor neuron disease. Adv Exp Med Biol 1987; 209: 167–174.
88. Mitsumoto H, Del Bene M. Improving the quality of life for people with ALS: The challenge ahead. Amyotroph Lateral Scler Other Motor Neuron Disord 2000; 1:329–336.
89. Bradley WG. Amyotrophic Lateral Sclerosis. In: Mitsumoto H, Norris FH, eds. A comprehensive guide to management. New York: Demos Publications, 1994:2–28.

10

Natural History and Prognosis in Amyotrophic Lateral Sclerosis

Brian Murray
Department of Neurology, Mater Misericordiae University Hospital, Dublin, Ireland

INTRODUCTION

It is particularly difficult to discuss the prognosis with an individual who has just been diagnosed with amyotrophic lateral sclerosis (ALS). Indeed, this task has been made especially challenging in the light of current knowledge that ALS is not a homogeneous clinicopathological entity but rather encompasses a spectrum of related disorders each with different presentations and rates of progression. This chapter reviews the behavior of ALS in its "natural," untreated state, and not only compares clinical subtypes but also assesses various factors that significantly impact rates of progression, patterns of spread, and survival. The data so presented allow a greater degree of accuracy when discussing prognosis but it is important to realize that it is probably not possible to gain an absolutely accurate picture of the natural history of ALS for any one individual: many variables are difficult to assess either in clinics or in research trials including epigenetic influences, the environment, mental state, personality, cognitive function, diet, copathologies, and the use of medications. The mode of data collection has varied considerably across the many studies that have commented upon survival rates, rates of progression, and clinical progression patterns in ALS. Older studies were retrospective reviews of rather mixed patient populations containing sporadic and familial cases along with ALS variants such as progressive muscular atrophy (PMA), primary lateral sclerosis (PLS), and various other motor neuron disorders. One would think that the introduction of consensus criteria for the classification and diagnosis of ALS might have smoothed out such issues in modern studies but the accuracy of conclusions based upon post hoc analysis of even the most rigorously compiled modern ALS databases has also been the subject of debate (1–4). Furthermore, modern natural history studies must now account for the fact that some patients are receiving riluzole, which is itself an independent prognostic factor for survival. Moreover, many patients are treated with antioxidants such as vitamins C and E and/or receive interventions that may improve survival such as percutaneous gastrostomy and non-invasive positive pressure ventilation. As a consequence, it has become increasingly difficult, if not impossible, to perform true "natural" history studies (5–9).

THE ROLE OF NATURAL HISTORY CONTROL GROUPS
IN TREATMENT TRIALS

A number of ALS functional scales and neurophysiologic measurements have been designed to measure the progression of ALS both in terms of lower motor neuron (LMN) and non-motor function. Using various combinations of these measurements, clinical investigators have been afforded the opportunity to more accurately assess not only the natural history of disease over time but also the therapeutic benefit of research drugs in clinical trials (10). While placebo-controlled trials remain the gold standard, there is a place for using natural history control groups in exploratory treatment trials (11–13). For example, absence of benefit in a natural history phase would preclude the need to go to the considerable time and expense of a full-randomized placebo-controlled trial. Furthermore, relatively small patient numbers would be required and it would afford every study participant the chance to receive the therapeutic agent itself rather than placebo. On the other hand, the necessary time course of a natural history phase (likely to be several months) means that no study participant would be given any therapeutic agent for a defined period, which may not only dampen the enthusiasm of study participants but also generate a group of patients who are necessarily more advanced at the time of starting the treatment phase. Furthermore, there is evidence that a natural history phase in a drug trial of ALS is not identical to a placebo phase: the natural history study of gabapentin in ALS, e.g., showed significantly longer survival with treatment but this was not borne out in a subsequent randomized placebo-controlled trial (14,15). In the ciliary neurotrophic factor (CNTF) trial, no correlations were identified between natural history and placebo-control groups in the rate of decline of leg and pulmonary megascores. As the latter are particularly important measures of functional decline in ALS, it would appear that natural history control groups are not suitable to actually replace placebo-control groups in future trials (13).

PRECLINICAL PHASE

The pathological loss of motor neurons does not coincide with the onset of clinical symptoms in ALS. Rather, there is a preclinical phase of silent motor neuron attrition in both brain and spinal cord tissues during which patients may maintain normal muscle power in the face of up to 30% loss of motor units via collateral reinnervation (16,17). Aggarwal and Nicholson used motor unit number estimation (MUNE) to evaluate this preclinical phase in 84 family members of known SOD1 mutation-positive individuals of whom 19 were identified as asymptomatic carriers. Over a three-year period they identified significant drops in MUNE in two carriers of the val148gly mutation (51% and 37%, respectively) that clearly preceded clinical onset of disease by several months (Fig. 1) (18). Patients with the Leu144phe SOD1 and Asp90Ala mutations sometimes develop posterior lower limb pain and cramps many years prior to onset of muscle weakness that suggests the presence of a "preparetic" stage in some FALS syndromes (19,20). Swash and Ingram (16) also described one case of sporadic ALS whose illness was preceded by muscle fatigability for six years prior to onset of weakness, atrophy, cramps, and fasciculations. These findings indicate that there may be a dramatic loss of motor neurons that precedes clinical onset. The nature of this cellular loss remains to be determined but may represent large-scale programmed cell death or a breakdown in cellular protective mechanisms against

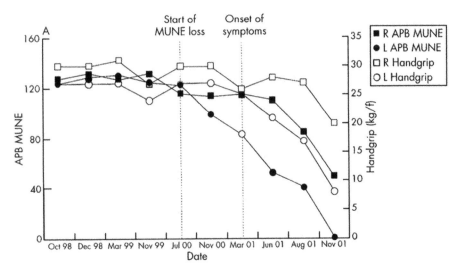

Figure 1 Preclinical loss of motor units from the left abductor pollicis brevis muscle of a human SOD1 mutation carrier as depicted by loss of number estimates (MUNE) prior to onset of symptoms. Note the steady decline in MUNE from the time of clinical onset. *Source*: From Ref. 18.

accumulating intracellular toxic substances (be they proteins, lipids, or other agents). This preclinical phase may be an important window of opportunity for the successful application of future therapeutic agents to at-risk carriers of ALS mutations.

CLINICAL SUBTYPES

Spinal ALS

"Spinal" ALS is clinically characterized by onset in limbs and trunk rather than bulbar musculature. Jean Martin Charcot recognized the progressive and inexorable nature of this disease; "One of the first distinctive features that in itself radically separates ALS from primary muscular atrophy is the comparative rapidity of its evolution, from the first symptoms to the fatal end. This does not usually extend more than three years" (21, p. 342). Charcot's observation has proven to be remarkably accurate; modern studies of ALS survival indicate that the mean duration from time of disease onset is indeed in the region of three years. Variations in this figure may be due to genuine differences in the characteristics of different populations or may be due to regional variations in case ascertainment, case characteristics, ALS classification, ALS care, or statistical analysis.

ALS survival is reported in different ways in different research papers: many prefer to express survival in terms of mean and median durations of disease expressed in months whereas others report survival in terms of probability of living beyond a 3-, 5-, or 10-year period from time of clinical onset. The duration of disease from the time of diagnosis rather than the time of onset is a particularly valuable figure to keep in mind not only when entering patients into research trials but also when discussing prognosis with patients and their families (8,9).

The mean duration of sporadic ALS from onset ranges from 23 to 43 months and the median duration (which excludes values from the extremes of a distribution) from 22 to 52 months (Table 1). However, within these studies there is a considerable

Table 1 ALS Disease Duration from Onset and Time of Diagnosis

Study (Reference); Method	Type of study	Location	Patient number	Mean duration from onset (months)	Mean duration from diagnosis (months)	Median duration from onset (months)	Median duration from diagnosis (months)
Mackay (22)	Retrospective, clinic based	USA	70	27			
Kristensen (23)	Retrospective, population-based Funen county	Denmark	118			31	
Juergens et al. (24)	Retrospective	USA	35			23	
Gubbay et al. (25)	Retrospective, population based	Israel	318			36	
Rosati et al. (26)	Retrospective, population-based Sardinia	Italy	64	30.5			
Li et al. (27)	Retrospective	UK	125	31			
Caroscio et al. (28)	Retrospective	USA	388				
Lopez-Vega (29)	Retrospective, population-based Cantabria	Spain	42	26.6		52	
Scarpa et al. (30)	Retrospective, population-based Modena	Italy	51	28.83		24.5	
Tysnes et al. (31)	Retrospective, population-based Hordaland county	Norway				28	

Reference	Study type	Country	N				
Tysnes et al. (32)	Retrospective, population-based Hordaland county	Norway	148				16.5
Jokelainen (33)	Retrospective	Finland	157	31		22 M, 31 F	
Alcaz et al. (34)	Retrospective, population-based Belgrade	Yugoslavia	58	27.7			
Louwerse et al. (35)	Retrospective, center based	Netherlands	307[c]				16[d]
Thijs et al. (36)	Retrospective, population based	Belgium	105			32	
Gamez et al. (37)	Retrospective	Spain	82 (Sporadic)	31.57			
Sorenson et al. (38)	Retrospective, population based Olmstead county	USA	77		36	28	
Turner et al. (5)	Retrospective, multivariate modeling, ALS center database	UK	802			43	
Magnus et al. (7)	Retrospective, ALS center database	Germany	155[b]	47			
Jablecki et al. (39)	Longitudinal, center based	USA	194			37	
Eisen et al. (40)	Longitudinal, center-based	Canada	138	43			
Ringel et al. (41)	Prospective, regional: Western USA	USA	165			48, 25.2 ND	
Haverkamp et al. (42)	Longitudinal, ALS center database	USA	506	33.6	36	29.1	

(Continued)

Table 1 ALS Disease Duration from Onset and Time of Diagnosis (*Continued*)

Study (Reference); Method	Type of study	Location	Patient number	Mean duration from onset (months)	Mean duration from diagnosis (months)	Median duration from onset (months)	Median duration from diagnosis (months)
Norris et al. (43)	Longitudinal, center based	USA	708	37		36.5	
Turner et al. (44)	Prospective, ALS center database	UK	769	43		39	
Chio et al. (8)	Prospective, population based	Italy	193[a]			30 Approximately 32	20 Approximately 19
del Aguila et al. (9)	Prospective, population-based, Western Washington	USA	174				

Abbreviation: ALS, amyotrophic lateral sclerosis.
[a]114 patients on Riluzole.
[b]All on riluzole and antioxidants. Some enrolled in Sanofi treatment trial EFC1923.
[c]Untreated.
[d]Sporadic ALS only.
ND = Newly diagnosed within one year of study.

degree of variability. Ringel et al. (41) point out (p. 1318) that inclusion of "long survivors" in a relatively short study period may have skewed their median survival figure upwards. On the other hand, many studies specifically excluded cases of PMA, PLS, and familial ALS in an effort to eliminate cases that would similarly skew the analysis of spinal and bulbar ALS (9,25,35,39,40,42,45). Crude estimation of average disease duration (derived from the referenced studies listed in Table 1) leaves us a with mean and median disease durations from onset of 33 and 32 months, respectively. Five-year survival rates from the time of disease onset range from 9% to 40% (rough average of studies listed in Table 2 = 22%), whereas 10-year survival rates range from 4% to 16% (rough average of studies listed in Table 3 = 9.4%) (Tables 1 and 2).

The pattern of deterioration in ALS is linear from the time of clinical onset to death, but there are three observations that must be borne in mind (1,7–9,11–13,35,39,42,54,55) (Fig. 2). First, the rate and pattern of decline in motor function varies (often considerably) from patient to patient. Second, the rate of progression at any one time varies between regions, but the overall rate of decline of different regions is similar in any one individual. Third, the rate of progression in any one region also varies over time. In Pradas' series, e.g., the rate of decline of arm function appeared to stabilize or even improve in rare cases whereas Swash and Ingram's Case 2 stabilized for two years after rapid upper limb onset before further progression in the lower limb (11,16,56). In other words, patients progress at their own rate in an overall linear fashion, the rate of deterioration varying within and between each region but the overall pattern being quite uniform.

The topographical spread of ALS was assessed in 702 patients attending the University of Wisconsin ALS Clinical Research Center over a seven-year period. For patients with lower limb-onset disease, symptom accrual began in the opposite lower limb followed by the ipsilateral upper limb, then by the contralateral upper limb, and finally the bulbar region (54, p. 525). In patients with upper limb onset, the rate of bulbar deterioration was faster than lower limb-onset disease. In bulbar-onset disease, initial dysarthria was followed by dysphagia more rapidly then by deficits in limb function (where there was no difference in the rate of accrual of upper versus lower limb symptoms). Patients who presented with bulbar-onset disease displayed a significantly faster rate of spread to the limbs than limb-onset patients did to the bulbar region. A previous study had also shown a "commonality of deterioration between motor units arising from similar regions of the CNS" (57). Together, these findings indicate that the spread of ALS within the CNS occurs in a segmental rather than multifocal pattern: onset in part of the cervical cord, e.g., is followed by spread throughout the rest of the cervical cord before there is spread to other regions of the CNS whereas onset in part of the bulbar region is followed by spread throughout the rest of the bulbar region before significant spread to other CNS regions. Furthermore, these studies show that the spread of symptoms in ALS is more rapid in the rostro-caudal then the caudo-rostral direction in ALS.

Clinical Variants

Several clinical variants are encompassed within the term ALS.

Mills' hemiplegic variant of ALS is a slowly progressive disorder that is largely upper motor neuron in type and, as the name suggests, presents as a progressive hemiplegia usually starting in one lower limb and spreading slowly to the ipsilateral upper limb (although both ascending and descending forms have been described). It

Table 2 Five-Year Survival in ALS

Study, Year	Country	Patient Number	5-Year Survival (%)
Mulder and Howard, 1976 (46)	USA	100	20
Rosen, 1978 (47)	USA	668	39.4
Juergens et al. 1980 (24)	USA	35	9
Kristensen et al. 1977 (23)	Denmark	118	18.7
Gubbay et al. 1985 (25)	Israel	318	29
Uebayashi, 1980 (48)	Japan/Guam	567	13
Granieri et al. 1988 (49)	Italy	61	40
Lopez-Vega et al. 1988 (29)	Spain	42	18
Scarpa et al. 1988 (30)	Italy	51	24.4
Tysnes et al. 1991 (31)	Norway	70	36.8 spinal, 8.8% bulbar
Chancellor et al. 1993 (50)	Scotland	229	28
Marti-Fabregas et al. 1996 (51)	Spain	71	25
Preux et al. 1996 (52)	France	158	14.7
Traynor et al. 2000 (53)	Ireland	388	17 (from diagnosis)
Alcaz et al. 1996 (34)	Yugoslavia	58	27
Lee et al. 1995 (45)	USA	439 referral, 97 incident	4 incident cohort, and 21 referral cohort
Louwerse et al. 1997 (35)	Netherlands	307	20
Thijs et al. 2000 (36)	Belgium	105	8.6
Chio et al. 2002 (8)	Italy	193	24.7 (onset); 20.2 (diagnosis)
del Aguila et al. 2003 (9)	USA	180	7 (diagnosis)

Mean value of all figures from onset is 22%.

Table 3 10-Year Survival in ALS

Study	Location	Total Patient Numbers	10-Year Survival (%)
Mulder and Howard (46)	USA	100	10
Kristensen et al. (23)	Denmark	118	7.6
Uebayashi (48)	Japan/Guam	552	14
Gubbay et al. (25)	Israel	318	16
Lopez-Vega (29)	Spain	42	6
Louwerse et al. (35)	Netherlands	307	8
Turner et al. (44)	UK	769	4[a]

[a]Eight cases received riluzole.
Mean value of all figures = 9.4%.

has been proposed that this may, in fact, represent a very asymmetric variant of PLS as supported by two cases with disease durations of 17 and 18 years at the time of the report (58).

The pseudoneuritic (or pseudopolyneuritic) variant refers to those cases of ALS that present with clinical deficits in the distribution of a major peripheral nerve but who have more widespread changes on electrodiagnostic examination and then progress to typical widespread of ALS. A few studies have identified a trend toward longer disease duration for this presentation but none have reached statistical

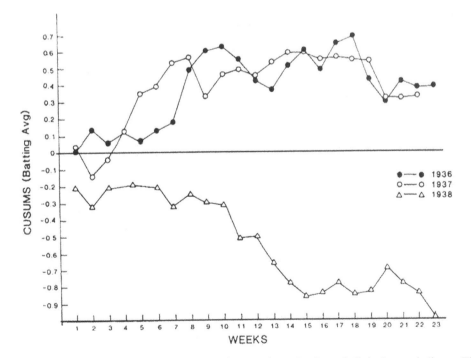

Figure 2 The overall pattern of decline in ALS from the time of clinical onset is linear. This graph illustrates the decline in Lou Gehrig's batting average (using CUSUM statistics) during the year 1938 and is compared to those of his previous two seasons. *Source*: From Ref. 55.

significance and the term itself may be misleading; in the French, Spanish, and Italian literature, the pseudopolyneuritic presentation actually refers to lower limb-onset disease (26,29,30,48,52).

The flail arm variant of ALS (also referred to as the bibrachial variant and Vulpian-Bernhardt's variant) is characterized by weakness and fatigue in the upper extremities often starting proximally and then progressing into the hands before there is spread to other regions (59–61). Couratier et al. (61) compared 20 such cases to 357 control ALS patients: the median survival of 49.5 months did not differ significantly from that of the ALS control group (32.8 months). In Hu et al. (60) retrospective analysis of 395 patients, 10% were classified as flail arm variants with a median survival of 57 months as compared to 39 months for the remaining members in the ALS group. Although intriguing, these results did not reach statistical significance (log rank test, $p = 0.204$). Chio et al. (62) also failed to identify any difference in survival when comparing shoulder girdle onset PMA (which they referred to as Vulpian Bernhardt's variety of PMA) to hand or lower limb-onset.

PLS has long been considered a pure upper motor neuron disorder throughout its course although in some cases there is evidence to support the involvement of LMNs (63,64). The rate of progression is significantly slower than spinal ALS. Bruyn et al. (65) reported three cases of PLS that subsequently developed the clinical features of ALS after intervals of 8,9, and 27 years, respectively. The interval between symptom onset and diagnosis was between 5 and 25 years in five cases reported by Gastaut et al. (43,66) (mean = 12.6 years) and in Norris's longitudinal study, the mean duration of 26 cases of PLS was 224 months (range 72–491) with 73% surviving on the last day of the study as compared to just 3% of patients with sporadic ALS. In Pringle's study of eight cases, the mean duration was 14.9 years with a median duration of 19 years (67). Although Mackay excluded surviving patients from his detailed analysis of 70 deceased patients with ALS, he did comment that three survivors had "purely spastic features whose disease has existed for 14, 21, and 8 years, respectively" (22). A recent five-year prospective study of 20 patients with PLS using the Pringle criteria described mean disease duration at the time of first examination of 8.5 years. The overall long-term pattern was that of slow steady progression but 10 cases had relatively stable periods lasting several months during which there was no clinical evidence of progression and three actually improved for a period. Ten patients required the use of a wheelchair within 48 months of starting the study and while half of the patients developed moderate muscle weakness (MRC grade 3 or greater, $n = 8$) during the five-year study period, a quarter of the patients experienced no weakness at all (63).

PMA, originally described by Francois Aran in 1850, is a pure LMN variant of ALS; there is no clinical evidence of upper motor neuron involvement during the first three years from clinical onset. Some cases continue as a pure lower neuron syndrome throughout the natural history of the disease whereas others evolve to ALS (PMA→ALS) (68). The usual clinical presentation is with distal weakness in the upper or lower (less common) extremities with gradual spread to proximal muscles. Bulbar and respiratory involvement is seen in the late stages. As for spinal ALS, men are slightly more often affected than women but the rate of disease progression is considerably slower. Furthermore, age of onset is younger than spinal ALS; mean age at onset in Norris' series (Ref. 43) was 47 years for PMA and 57.8 years for sporadic ALS; the mean age at diagnosis in Chio's series (Ref. 62) was 48.4 years. Norris et al. (43) reported mean disease duration of 159 months (range 43–407) in 17 cases longitudinally studied between the years 1970 and 1991. Seventy-one percent of PMA cases were surviving on the final day of study as compared to just 3% of sporadic ALS. The five-year survival rate for ALS was 36.8% and for PMA was 63.7% in a retrospective incidence study in Italy (49). Chio et al. (62) noted a significantly prolonged disease duration for 155 cases that they classified as PMA (from review of the records of 277 cases examined between 1955 and 1980): the rate of decline in the first three years steadied out and reached a stable rate by year 5 with little difference in survival at 5 and 10 years from disease onset. The three- and five-year survival figures for all cases were listed as 61.3% and 56.4 %, respectively, but for patients aged over 50 years, the five year survival was 40.1% as compared to 71.9% for those under the age of 50 years.

A subset of PMA may progress at a rapid rate; a recent report of 10 retrospectively assigned cases identified a mean disease duration of just 16.2 months (range 6–27). All 10 cases had ubiquitinated LMN inclusions in spinal cord tissue and five had evidence of corticospinal tract pathology. The authors proposed that such cases represent a more advanced point on the continuum from pure LMN disease (PMA) to an overlap with ALS (combined LMN and upper motor neuron disease) (68).

Although the muscles of ventilation may rarely be involved very early in the course of ALS, patients may not actually complain of dyspnea until there is severe loss of pulmonary function reserves (25,35,50,69–74). Those rare patients that do complain of dyspnea at onset may also complain of sleep disturbance, daytime sleepiness, have mild limb weakness with UMN signs at presentation and/or subtle evidence of bulbar dysfunction (70,74). Of 49 ALS cases evaluated by a pulmonary critical care team over a decade, 36 cases have objective evidence of ventilatory impairment but only seven complained of respiratory symptoms at presentation. Four cases were in a state of catastrophic respiratory failure at diagnosis and had to be ventilated prior to obtaining any formal pulmonary function tests. Seventeen of these patients were followed by serial pulmonary function tests from diagnosis to death or placement on mechanical ventilation; the mean survival was 15.9 months and the median 11.5 months (71). Similarly, in Bradley's review of 24 patients with respiratory failure, 17 were admitted to ICU prior to being diagnosed with ALS, 7 (29%) died between days 7 and 54 in the ICU, and 16 (67%) required long-term respiratory support (72). The median survival of patients with initial respiratory muscle weakness in the Netherlands ALS Consortium study of 1997 was only two months (35) whereas the two cases with early diaphragmatic paralysis of Parhad et al. (74) survived for 27 and 17 months, respectively. In Chio et al. (8) assessment, they noted that the presence of respiratory involvement at diagnosis led to a significantly reduced 3-year percent survivorship than for patients with no apparent respiratory compromise (34.5% vs. 75%, $p = 0.0001$).

The pattern of decline in respiratory function tends to be fairly linear (although non-linearity may be observed in individual patients) but the slope of deterioration may flatten out in the preterminal phase (71,75). Multiple studies have now confirmed that a reduction in percent predicted forced vital capacity (FVC) is a strong correlate of respiratory symptoms [although a less sensitive marker of respiratory muscle weakness than the maximal sniff nasal pressure (131)]. A low %FVC is also consistently associated with shorter survival (8,36,41,42,71,75,77) and in several studies has been the single best predictor of survival when compared to other variables such as age, gender, and site of onset (8,41,42).

It is important to distinguish between progressive bulbar palsy (PBP), an extremely rare disorder characterized by neurodegeneration that is limited to the bulbar region throughout the course of the disease, and bulbar-onset ALS, an altogether more common entity that presents with bulbar symptoms before spreading to other regions over time. Many of the studies referenced in this chapter do not make this distinction. PBP is so rare that it is difficult to state any true facts regarding its natural history and, in spite of personal experience with one such case with disease duration of 17 years, this author has been unable to unearth a single case in any of the studies listed in Table 1 of this chapter. The prognosis of bulbar-onset ALS is widely regarded as being unfavorable when compared to limb-onset ALS. The rate of symptom accrual in the limbs is faster in bulbar-onset disease than the rate of bulbar symptom accrual is in patients with limb-onset disease (54) and the median disease duration across all of the studies in Table 4 for bulbar-onset disease is 22 months and for spinal-onset is 38 months (4,5,7–9,23,25,31,32,34–36,39,41,43, 45,47,50,52,77). At first glance this would suggest that bulbar-onset disease uniformly portends a poorer prognosis, but some studies have not found any significant difference in prognosis between bulbar- and spinal-onset disease (28,30,44,51,78), while others have been unable to separate the apparently deleterious effect of bulbar-onset from an older age at onset and/or more advanced stage at presentation in the bulbar-onset group (5,39,40,42,79). It is also worthwhile to note that the presence of bulbar symptoms at onset does not guarantee a worse prognosis; in the recent analysis of long survivors (those living more than 10 years from disease onset) with definite ALS by El Escorial criteria, there were four cases with bulbar onset, one of whom remained alive after 20 years (44, p. 996).

Frank dementia is a rare initial presentation in the ALS population (circa 3%), but cognitive deficits, typically of the frontotemporal type (word generation deficits, fluency, executive control, personality change, etc.), may be detected in up to half of all patients with ALS/MND during the course of the illness (80). Hodges et al. (81) recently referred to ALS/FTD as a "malignant" disorder, in so far as the rate of progression is relatively rapid when compared with most other forms of FTD. In a subgroup of nine pathologically proven cases of FTD that later developed additional ALS/MND, the median duration from onset to death was two years and from diagnosis to death, just one year. This compared unfavorably to other FTD variants including frontal variant FTD, semantic dementia, corticobasal syndrome (with FTD pathology), and particularly, primary non-fluent progressive aphasia (median duration from onset of 6–8 years).

FAMILIAL ALS AND GENETIC RISK FACTORS

Mutations in the SOD1, alsin, and the p150 dynactin subunit genes are associated with familial forms of ALS. A detailed review for every available mutation is beyond the scope of this chapter (see Chap. 6) but from the selected data in Table 5, one can see that there is considerable variation in disease duration not only for the different mutations, but also both between and within different families bearing the same mutation. This marked genetic heterogeneity likely reflects the influence of additional genetic, epigenetic (e.g., gender), biochemical, and environmental influences that may render accurate prognostication difficult (94,95).

Apolipoprotein E may act as an injury response protein in sporadic ALS (96) but the results regarding its potential influence are somewhat conflicting. While the ApoE ε2 and ε3 proteins may be important in neuronal repair and maintenance, the ε4 protein might actually be toxic (97–100). In survival terms, Moulard et al. (98)

Table 4 Bulbar-Onset Versus Spinal Onset ALS: Mean Disease Duration and Percentage Interval (3, 5, and 10 Years) Survival

Study	Location	Bulbar-Onset mean or median duration	Bulbar-Onset percentage survival	Spinal-onset mean or median duration	Spinal-onset percentage survival
Mackay (23)	USA	Mean spastic 24.6 months, mean atrophic 17.3 months		Mean spastic 36.24 months, mean atrophic 33.05 months	
Kristensen et al. (23)	Denmark	Median two years		Median three years	
Rosen (47)	USA		Five years, 14.1% and 19.3% when age corrected		5-Year upper limb 41.6% and lower limb, 46.1%
Gubbay et al. (25)	Israel	Median 2.2 years		Median 3.3 years	
Chancellor et al. (50)	Scotland	Median 1.7 years approximately	8.8%, Five years	Median three years approximately	36.8%, five years
Tysnes et al. (31)	Norway	Median 24 months		Median 40 months	
Tysnes et al. (32)	Norway	Mean 12.1 months		Mean 26 months	
Lee et al. (45)	USA	Median 16.2 months incident and 15.4 months referral		Mean 22 months incident and 25 months referral approximately	
Louwerse et al. (35)	Netherlands	Median 1.3 years		Median 1.7 years	
Desport et al. (77)	France	Mean 30 months		Mean 37 months	
Thijs et al. (36)	Belgium	Median 20 months		Median 43 months	
Magnus et al. (7)	Germany	37 months		51 months	
Turner et al. (5) database analysis	UK	Median 30 months		Median 50 months	
Chio et al. (8)	Italy	Median 23.3 months	3-Year survival 24.6%	Median 45 months upper limbs and 35 months lower limbs	3-year survival 52.8% upper limbs and 46% lower limbs
del Aguila et al. (9)	USA	Median 12 months		Median 21 months	

Table 5 Familial ALS: Survival and Prognosis

Mutation	Clinical characteristic	Average duration from onset	References
A4V	LMN predominant. Rapid progression	1 ± 0.4 years	82
A4V	LMN predominant. Rapid progression	1.2 ± 0.8 years	133
A4T		0.75 years	84
A4T	Onset 32–60 years. LMN predominant	14 months (but one case > 76 months)	85
E100G		5.1 ± 3.3 years	82
G41D		11.6 ± 1.7 years	86
H46R		17.0 ± 11.0 years	87
H46R	Onset 39.7 ± 10.5 years. Distal lower limb onset. LMN predominant pathological evidence of UMN degeneration	18.1 ± 13.2 year. Longest duration 47 years	88
H46R	Onset ages 32–60; lower limb onset; LMN predominant. Peripheral dysesthesiae	12 ± 7.6 years (range 6–30 years). Suggest other influences	89
L84V		1.8 ± 5 years	90
V148I		1.5 years	91
D90A Homozygote	Preparetic myalgias, paresthesiae. Slowly ascending. Lower limb onset	14.2 years	20
D90A Heterozygote	Apparent sporadic inheritance. Unaffected (n = 1) or Bulbar-onset (n = 2)	2.5 years	20
L144F	Preparetic cramps. Slow progression. Lower limb onset. Onset age range 18–72 years	20.4 ± 14.6 years	19
V148G	Late onset if ≥1 copy of CNTF allele. Early onset and rapid progression to death if homozygous CNTF null mutation		92
N139H	Incomplete penetrance. Distal limb onset	4.0 years	93

study of 130 patients with sporadic ALS found that those patients with APOE ε2/ε3 alleles were more likely to have limb-onset rather than bulbar-onset disease and survive longer than those without the ε2 allele while Al-Chalabi et al. (99) reported a higher incidence of bulbar-onset ALS in those carrying at least one ε4 allele. High APOE plasma levels were associated with a significantly shorter survival time and more rapid rate of progression in 403 stringently categorized ALS patients when compared to controls, but there was no significant relationship between any APOE phenotype and any clinical ALS variable (e.g., age, body mass index, site of onset, and rate of deterioration) (101). Although Drory et al. (102) reported a survival disadvantage for those carrying at least a single APOE ε4 allele compared to those without (on average 39 months vs. 71 months, $p < 0.03$), four other separate research groups found no significant correlation between APOE ε4 and disease duration, site of onset, or age at onset (36,78,97,100,102).

The survival motor neuron genes, SMN1 and SMN2, underlie the pathogenesis and clinical presentation of spinal muscular atrophy but their respective roles in ALS are less certain. Although one study reported a shorter survival time in sporadic ALS patients with a homozygous SMN2 gene deletion, a further study was unable to identify any such pattern in 106 patients with sporadic and 18 with familial ALS (37,103).

Recent evidence suggests that the CNTF gene may act as a modifier in both familial and sporadic ALS. Approximately 2% of the population are homozygous for the CNTF null (−/−) mutation but this is not associated with any disease. Giess et al. (92) described FALS in a mother, sister, and brother with the SOD-1 V148G mutation. The brother, who also had a homozygous null mutation (−/−) in the CNTF gene, had a much more aggressive course than his sister and mother who lacked the CNTF mutation. In that same study, the presence of the CNTF −/− mutation in patients with sporadic ALS was associated with earlier age at onset but not with a change in disease duration. However, the CNTF −/− mutation was not associated with age at onset, rate of progression, or disease duration in a subsequent study of 400 cases of ALS and 236 controls (104).

VARIABLES OF PROGNOSTIC SIGNIFICANCE

Age

One of the most important prognostic indicators in sporadic ALS is the age of the patient at disease onset. This has been borne out repeatedly through both retrospective and prospective studies of a variety of ALS populations. In Norris' large series of 613 cases of sporadic ALS (excluding PMA and PLS), the mean disease duration was 72 months for those under 45 and 33 months for those over 55. Only one of their cases of sporadic ALS with onset under the age of 50 years died within the first 12 months, whereas 40 patients in the 50–74-year-old age group passed away in, the same period (26 of these were >60 years of age) (43). Eisen et al. (40) confirmed significantly longer survival in men with onset below the age of 40 years when compared with those with onset between the ages of 41 to 55, 56 to 65, and most significantly, those with onset over the age of 65 (Fig. 3). Over the past decade this relationship is still apparent in every study (5,7–9,35,36,44,51,52,77). In Chio's prospective population-based study, the median survival was 2000 days for patients with onset < 50 years of age, 1275 days for those between 51 and 60, 885 days for those between 61 and 70, and for the over 71 ages group it was 730 days ($p = 0.0003$) (8). Forbes et al. (79) recently described 135 cases of ALS that were aged

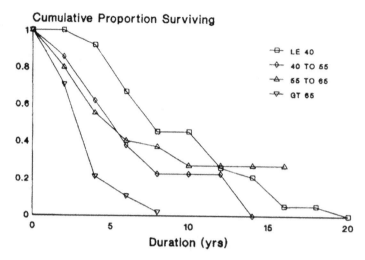

Figure 3 Age is an important prognostic indicator in ALS. The rate in decline of the Kaplan-Meier survival curve is worse for men greater than (GT) the age of 65 years when compared to men between the age of 55–65, 40–55, and, most strikingly, those less than or equal to (LE) 40 years old at the time of onset. *Source*: From Ref. 40.

80 years or older at the time of diagnosis (104 cases 80–84, 26 cases 85–90, and 5 cases > 90 years of age). Median time from onset to death in the patients > 80 years was 1.7 years (with a median time from onset to diagnosis of 0.79 years) whereas the median survival for the patients less than 80 was 2.09 years ($p = 0.0003$). It is interesting that bulbar-onset occurred in fully half of all of these late-onset cases and that only one had been prescribed riluzole.

Gender

Most, but not all, studies have not defined a true survival difference between males and females (not statistically significant in Refs. 5,7,31,32,35,39,41,43–45,47,77). Del Aguila et al. (9) reported that female sex was independently strongly associated with poor survival, although they were unable to tease out the relationship of female sex to other variables such as marital status, place of residence, and early progression rate. Other studies have ascribed the apparent worse outlook for women to either a higher frequency of bulbar palsy or more advanced age at the time of presentation (50,51).

Nonetheless, several studies have found significant differences between the sexes in terms of the regional pattern of progression. In Brooks et al. (54) series, females with leg-onset developed more spread of symptom than males after the third year ($p < 0.02$) whereas males with bulbar-onset had more rapid spread to the arms in the first three years ($p < 0.01$). Using serial Tufts Quantitative Neuromuscular Examinations, Munsat et al. (57) detected a slower rate of deterioration in arm strength in women than in men ($p < 0.01$). A gender difference was described in the Kii peninsula and Guam. Of those patients who survived more than 10 years from disease onset and who had an initial rapid progression with subsequent slowdown or stall, the ratio of male to female was 3:10. For those with continuous steady slow progression, the ratio was 1:1 and for those with an intermediate progression pattern the ratio was 9:2 (48). Ringel et al. (41) did not identify a survival disadvantage or difference in rate of decline based upon gender but did show that males were more likely to have four limb fasciculations than women ($p < 0.05$) whereas women were more likely to have dyspnea, dysphagia, and a positive family history ($p < 0.05$ for all three variables).

Nutrition

Malnutrition is an independent risk factor for a worse prognosis in ALS. Multivariate analysis of 55 patients (all classified as probable or definite ALS by El Escorial criteria) revealed that malnourishment, defined as a body mass index of $< 18.5 \, \text{kg/m}^2$, multiplied the risk of death by a factor of 7.4 and that the occurrence of malnutrition was equal in both spinal- and bulbar-onset disease (77). Malnourishment in ALS might reflect a hypermetabolic state that is independent of the mode of presentation (105). In support of these findings, a recent prospective study of 180 patients in western Washington revealed a trend towards longer survival in patients with a stable body mass index in the five years preceding the diagnosis of ALS (9).

Psychosocial Function

Two studies have identified a direct relationship between psychosocial function and survival in ALS. McDonald et al. (106) assessed a total of 138 subjects using seven different psychological assessment scales designed to probe life rating, purpose-in-life, disease control, anger expression, perceived stress, depression, and hopelessness. Those patients who fell into the low psychological score group had a mean survival time of 333 days as compared to those in the high scoring group whose mean survival was 1200 days ($p < 0.001$). After controlling for covariates of age, disease severity, and duration of illness, the relative risk of death per unit time was calculated to be 2.24 times greater for patients with psychological distress than that for patients with psychological well being. A subsequent longitudinal assessment of the impact of mood on survival involved an assessment at the time of initial diagnosis with follow-up assessments at six weeks and six months. From an original cohort of 38 study participants, 21 patients were available for interview at six months. Using a series of different measurement scales of mood and self-esteem, the investigators identified a pattern of greater disability (albeit as determined by an non-disease-specific measure, the Office of Population Census and Survey assessment), faster progression, and shorter survival in those individuals with lower mood. Yet again this finding appeared to be independent of other variables such as age and site of onset (126). Del Aguila et al. (9) were unable to make a significant association between measures of psychological well being and survival (as determined by the responses of patients to the Medical Outcome Short Form-36 questionnaire) but did determine that lack of a marital partner was an independent risk factor for worse prognosis (median survival from diagnosis of unmarried vs. married was 10 months vs. 21 months, $p < 0.05$). Overall, the authors concluded that unmarried older patients (70% of whom were women) with a shorter interval from onset to diagnosis had the shortest survival with a median duration of just nine months.

El Escorial Criteria

Diagnostic criteria for the diagnosis of ALS were devised in El Escorial, Spain, in 1990 and modified at Airlieo House, Virginia, in 1998. A longitudinal study of an Irish ALS population of 388 patients studied over a 6-year period concluded that these criteria were not reliable when used as prognostic indicators (53). However, a recent statistical analysis of a U.K. database involving 841 patients seen over a 10-year period concluded that El Escorial category at presentation was a highly significant independent prognostic variable ($p < 0.0001$) and was most marked when comparing clinically definite to suspected ALS (5). This association was confirmed in a further study of 769 patients that had been prospectively recorded in a database over a 12-year period although the authors were careful to highlight one case who remains alive after 20 years and who was clinically definite at the time of initial examination (44). Chio et al. (8) confirmed a poorer prognosis in patients with definite ALS at the time of diagnosis in their prospective study of 221 individuals listed in the Piemonte and Valle d'Aosta Register. Their patients with definite ALS had a mean survival of 23 months when compared with 34 months for those with probable ALS, 35 months for possible ALS, and 58 months for suspected ALS (definite vs. other categories, $p < 0.0001$).

Rate of Progression

Using a linear estimate of disease progression (measuring foot dorsiflexion and %FVC decline), Armon et al. (107) concluded that patients who progressed faster died sooner and that a faster estimated rate of decline prior to study entry (and thus prior to first evaluation) predicted shorter survival. In Magnus et al. (7) series of 155 patients (all of whom were on Riluzole $\pm$ antioxidants), shorter survival was associated with faster rates in decline of MRC compound score ($p < 0.003$), %FVC ($p < 0.002$), and ALS-Functional Rating Scale scores ($p < 0.0001$). Indeed administration of the latter scale (including a modified form that also addresses pulmonary symptoms) is a valuable and reliable tool that not only yields an estimate of survival at first assessment but also the slope of deterioration when sequentially tested (108). Studying 221 patients at six-month intervals, an Italian research group confirmed that the early course in ALS was predictive of the subsequent course until death. Patients with a more rapid rate of decline in lower limb muscle power (change in MRC scale, $p < 0.0011$), bulbar function (change in modified Appel Rating Scale subscore, $p < 0.009$), and pulmonary function (%FVC decline, $p < 0.0001$) had significantly shorter survival (8).

The Diagnostic Interval

A short interval between onset and diagnosis (or entry into a clinical trial) portends a worse prognosis (5,7,9,32,35,36,42,45,53,75,83). While this might simply reflect the fact that more aggressive disease is more easily diagnosed (9), Haverkamp et al. (42) also commented that "those with an initially slower course of disease delay longest in arriving at the clinic, and though their first examination totals may be high, their survival time will be somewhat greater" (p. 713). The more distressing initial symptoms of bulbar-onset ALS may precipitate earlier diagnosis: in the study of Iwasaki et al. (109), the time to diagnosis of disease for bulbar-onset was 10 months versus 14.25 months for limb-onset.

The Effect of Sub-Specialist Care

Lee et al. (45) noted that the favorable effect of a long diagnostic interval was more pronounced in those patients that were specifically referred to a specialist ALS center as opposed to those who were incident cases, the effect possibly reflecting, yet again, that faster progression prompts an individual to seek attention earlier before waiting for a referral to a specialist center. Indeed, the referral of patients to an Irish multidisciplinary ALS center was associated with prolonged survival: on average these patients lived 7.5 months longer than patients who were cared for in general neurology clinics. The two cohorts were not evenly matched in terms of size, age (the ALS Center group was five years younger on average), or use of riluzole (60.1% general vs. 98.8% ALS center). Nonetheless, using Cox model statistics, the authors concluded that these confounding variables were unlikely to have explained all of the difference in survival between the two groups (6). Forbes et al. (79) commented that patients older than 80 years of age with ALS were treated differently than their younger counterparts, with only one case out of 135 receiving riluzole and only 59% of cases managed by neurologists. However, they were unable to ascertain for certain if this "different process of care" was of actual prognostic significance. Further studies are certainly warranted to assess this apparent positive impact of specialist/multidisciplinary care on survival.

LONG DURATION ALS AND REVERSIBLE ALS

As seen in Table 3, about 9.4% of patients have "resistant" or "benign" ALS (22,23,43,46) and survive for more than 10 years. Indeed, some cases have been reported with disease durations lasting decades, the most striking example of which is a very thoroughly evaluated case with clinically definite sporadic ALS and a disease duration of more than 44 years (76). No clear blueprint for "long survival" emerges from these studies although certain features are suggestive, such as young age at onset (< 50 years), limb-onset (as apposed to bulbar-onset), male gender, and predominance of upper motor neuron features (32,35,43,44,48).

Reversible motor neuron disease is a distinctly rare entity that may be observed as a paraneoplastic phenomenon, in the setting of human immunodeficiency virus infection, and in cases of heavy metal poisoning. There have been sparse reports of otherwise unexplained cases that present with LMN predominant ALS-like symptoms and signs that progress for a period before making a recovery. Mulder and Howard commented that they had "several cases" in this category and then, to illustrate the point, described onset of typical asymmetrical weakness, wasting, fasciculations, atrophy, and some upper motor neuron features in a 49-year-old surgeon. The condition progressed but then the patient noted recovery of power and was not only back to normal at one year but remained so seven years later (46). Further case reports of a reversible motor neuron disease have been published but, as in the case of Tsai et al. (108) where the patient was not evaluated by MRI and in three of the four cases reported by Tucker et al. (111) where there were prominent sensory symptoms (albeit in the absence of objective sensory loss), atypical features or incomplete data are apparent (110). Overall, it is not possible to determine the true underlying cause for these unusual presentations in the absence of histopathological examination of brain and spinal cord tissue but it is unlikely that all of these cases represent true ALS.

CONCLUSION

Despite the considerable advances that have been made in our understanding of the natural history of ALS, it is still a difficult task to accurately predict the future for

Table 6 Summary of Good and Bad Prognostic Indicators in ALS

Factor	Good Prognosis	Bad Prognosis	Comment	References
Variable				
Age	Young age (<50 years)	Old age (>65 years)	Very strong association	See text
Gender	Inconsistent data	Inconsistent data	Inconsistent data	See text
mEECC		Worst for definite ALS	Not all studies agree	See text
Diagnostic delay	Long interval	Short interval	Strong association	See text
Rate of progression	Slow from onset	Rapid from onset	Strong association	See text
Nutrition	High/normal body mass index	Low BMI	Strong association	See text
Psychological/social well being/marital status	Good psychological status/ social support/married	Psychological distress/ isolation/single	Limited studies	See text
Pulmonary impairment	Slow rate of % FVC decline	Rapid rate of %FVC decline	Very strong association	See text
Clinical presentation				
Limb-onset	Overall, better	Overall worse	May be age related	See text
Bulbar-onset				See text
Pseudoneuritic	Trend only		Insufficient data, varied use of terminology	See text
Flail arm	Trend only		Insufficient data	See text
Mills hemiplegic variant	Possible: may be PLS		Insufficient data	See text
PMA	Long survival		Limited published data	See text
PLS	Long survival		Strong data	See text
FTD/ALS		Short survival	Strong data	See text
Genetic factors				
Familial ALS	Variable	Variable	Variable	Table 5
SMN 2 gene			Inconsistent data	See text
APOE gene status			Inconsistent data	See text
CNTF gene status			Inconsistent data	See text

(Continued)

				Table 5
Familial ALS	Variable	Variable	Variable	Table 5
SMN 2 gene			Inconsistent data	See text
APOE gene status			Inconsistent data	See text
CNTF gene status			Inconsistent data	See text
Lab tests				
CK	No relationship	No relationship	Small studies	112–114
Serum chloride	Normal	Low	Single study	75
Serum bilirubin		Low levels as patients progress	Small number. Single study. No clear correlation	115
Decremental response		Worse	Data conflicting	116–118, 127
Low motor-normal sensory pattern on EDX		Worse		119–122
NI	Slow rate of decline	Rapid rate of decline	Limited number of studies	123
MUNE		Rapid rate of decline	Good evidence	109,124,125, 128,129

Abbreviations: EDX, electrodiagnostic examination; UMN, upper motor neuron; CK, creatine kinase; PLS, primary lateral sclerosis; PMA, progressive muscular atrophy; mEECC, modified El Escorial Criteria classification; NI, Neurophysiological Index; SMN, survival motor neuron; APOE, apolipoprotein E; CNTF, ciliary neurotrophic factor.

any one person afflicted with the disease. However, certain factors should be apparent after the first bedside examination that may provide a reasonable guide to prognosis (Table 6). The most important of these are the age of the patient, the site of onset, the El Escorial classification, and the time to diagnosis from onset. The rate of disease progression is also critical and may be inferred from serial assessments of both muscle power and pulmonary function. The accuracy of these assessments relies upon reliable scoring systems to monitor disease progression, and, in particular, neurophysiological techniques to measure the evolution of LMN loss over time (10,130,132). Indeed, these techniques have enabled clinical investigators to carry out a natural history phase in treatment trials, which may be an effective means to study the likely benefit of a drug/intervention prior to embarking on an extensive (and expensive) randomized placebo-controlled trial. Additional information of prognostic value may be derived from ancillary investigations including blood testing and the electrodiagnostic examination (Table 6) but the search for reliable, disease-specific ALS biomarkers in blood, cerebrospinal fluid, and in the field of neuroimaging continues. There is a need to carry out further prospective natural history studies in carefully matched populations that not only include data on rates of change in cognitive function and psychological status but also serial measurement of the rate of loss of both lower and upper motor neurons.

ACKNOWLEDGMENT

This work was supported by a grant from the Programme for Research Training in Third Level Institutions and the Conway Institute of Biomolecular and Biomedical Research, Belfield, Dublin 4, Ireland.

REFERENCES

1. Armon C, Guiloff RJ, Bedlack R. Limitations of inferences from observational databases in amyotrophic lateral sclerosis: all that glitters is not gold. Amyotroph Lateral Scler Other Motor Neuron Disord 2002; 3(3):109–111.
2. Sufit RL. Issues in clinical trial design I: use of natural history controls. An antagonist view. Neurology 1996; 47(4 suppl 2):S98–S99.
3. Meinenger V. Database analyses: a reply. Amyotroph Lateral Scler Other Motor Neuron Disord 2002; 3:113.
4. Swash M. Controversies about databases. Amyotroph Lateral Scler Other Motor Neuron Disord 2002; 3:107.
5. Turner MR, Bakker M, Sham P, Shaw CE, Leigh PN, Al-Chalabi A. Prognostic modelling of therapeutic interventions in amyotrophic lateral sclerosis. Amyotroph Lateral Scler Other Motor Neuron Disord 2002; 3(1):15–21.
6. Traynor BJ, Alexander M, Corr B, Frost E, Hardiman O. Effect of a multidisciplinary amyotrophic lateral sclerosis (ALS) clinic on ALS survival: a population based study, 1996–2000. J Neurol Neurosurg Psychiatry 2003; 74(9):1258–1261.
7. Magnus T, Beck M, Giess R, Puls I, Naumann M, Toyka KV. Disease progression in amyotrophic lateral sclerosis: predictors of survival. Muscle Nerve 2002; 25(5):709–714.
8. Chio A, Mora G, Leone M, Mazzini L, Cocito D, Giordana MT, Bottacchi E, Mutani R. Piemonte and Valle d'Aosta Register for ALS (PARALS). Early symptom progression rate is related to ALS outcome: a prospective population-based study. Neurology 2002; 59(12):99–103.

9. del Aguila MA, Longstreth WT Jr, McGuire V, Koepsell TD, van Belle G. Prognosis in amyotrophic lateral sclerosis: a population based study. Neurology 2003; 60(5):813–819.

10. Bromberg MB. Diagnostic criteria and outcome measurement of amyotrophic lateral sclerosis. In: Pourmand R, Harati Y, eds. Neuromuscular Disorders. Adv Neurol (88) Philadelphia: Lippincott Williams & Wilkins publishers, 2002:53–62.

11. Pradas J, Finison L, Andres PL, Thornell B, Hollander D, Munsat TL. The natural history of amyotrophic lateral sclerosis and the use of natural history controls in therapeutic trials. Neurology 1993; 43:751–755.

12. Munsat TL. Issues in clinical trial design I: use of natural history controls. A Protagonist view. Neurology 1996; 47(suppl 2):S96–S97.

13. Bryan WW, Hoagland RJ, Murphy J, Armon C, Barohn RJ, Goodpasture JC, Miller RG, Parry GJ, Petajan JH, Ross MA, Stromatt SC, rhCNTF ALS Study Group. Amyotroph Lateral Scler Other Motor Neuron Disord 2003; 4(1):11–15.

14. Mazzini L, Mora G, Balzarini C, Brigatti M, Pirali I, Pastor E. The natural history and the effects of gabapentin in amyotrophic laterals sclerosis. J Neurol Sci 1998; 160(suppl 1): S57–S63.

15. Miller RG, Moore DH II, Gelinas DF, Dronsky V, Mendoza M, Barohn RJ, Ravits J, Yuen E, Neville H, Ringel S, et al. Western ALS Study Group. Phase III randomized trial of gabapentin in patients with amyotrophic lateral sclerosis. Neurology 2001; 56(7):843–848.

16. Swash M, Ingram D. Preclinical and subclinical events in motor neuron disease. J Neurol Neurosurg Psychiatry 1988; 51:165–168.

17. Wohlfart G. Collateral reinnervation in partially denervated muscle. Neurology 1958; 8:175–180.

18. Aggarwal A, Nicholson G. Detection of preclinical motor neurone loss in SOD1 mutation carriers using motor unit number estimation. J Neurol Neurosurg Psychiatry 2002; 73:199–201.

19. Ferrera L, Caponnetto C, Marini V, Rizzi D, Bordo D, Penco S, Amoroso A, Origone P, Garrè C. An Italian dominant FALS Leu144Phe SOD1 mutation; genotype–phenotype correlation. Amotroph Lateral Scler Other Motor Neuron Disord 2003; 4(3):167–170.

20. Andersen PM, Nilsson P, Keränen ML, Forsgren L, Hägglund J, Karlsborg M, Ronnevi L-O, Gredal O, Marklund SL. Phenotypic heterogeneity in motor neuron disease patients with CuZn-superoxide dismutase mutations in Scandinavia. Brain 1997; 120:1723–1737.

21. Goetz CG. Amyotrophic lateral sclerosis: early contributions of Jean-Martin Charcot. Muscle Nerve 2000; 23:336–343.

22. Mackay RP. Course and prognosis in amyotrophic lateral sclerosis. Arch Neurol 1963; 8:17–27.

23. Kristensen O, Melgaard B. Motor neuron disease prognosis and epidemiology. Acta Neur Scand 1977; 56:299–308.

24. Juergens SM, Kurland LT, Okazaki H, Mulder DW. ALS in Rochester, Minnesota. Neurology 1925–1977; 30:463–470.

25. Gubbay SS, Kahana E, Zilber N, Cooper G, Pintov S, Leibowitz Y. Amyotrophic lateral sclerosis. A study of its presentation and prognosis. J Neurol 1985; 232(5):295–300.

26. Rosati G, Pinna L, Granieri E, Aiello I, Tola R, Agnetti V, Pirisi A, de Bastiani P. Studies on epidemiological, clinical, and etiological aspects of ALS disease in Sardinia, Southern Italy. Acta Neurol Scand 1977; 55(3):231–244.

27. Li TM, Alberman E, Swash M. Clinical features and associations of 560 cases of motor neuron disease. J Neurol Neurosurg Psychiatry 1990; 53(12):1043–1045.

28. Caroscio JT, Mulvihill MN, Sterling R, Abrams B. Amyotrophic lateral sclerosis. Its natural history. Neurol Clin 1987; 5(1):1–8.

29. Lopez-Vega JM, Calleja J, Combarros O, Polo JM, Berciano J. Motor neuron disease in Cantabria. Acta Neurol Scand 1988; 77:1–5.

30. Scarpa M, Colombo A, Panzetti P, Sorgato P. Epidemiology of amyotrophic lateral sclerosis in the province of Modena, Italy. Influence of environmental exposure to lead. Acta Neurol Scand 1988; 77(6):456–460.

31. Tysnes O-B, Vollset SE, Aarli JA. Epidemiology of amyotrophic lateral sclerosis in Hordaland county, Western Norway. Acta Neurol Scand 1991; 83:280–285.

32. Tysnes O-B, Vollset SE, Larsen JP, Aarli JA. Prognostic factors and survival in amyotrophic lateral sclerosis. Neuroepidemiology 1994; 13(5):226–235.

33. Jokelainen M. Amyotrophic lateral sclerosis in Finland. II: Clinical characteristics. Acta Neurol Scand 1977; 56:194–204.

34. Alcaz S, Jarebinski M, Pekmezovic T, Stevic-Marinkovic Z, Pavlovic S, Apostolski S. Epidemiological and clinical characteristics of ALS in Belgrade, Yugoslavia. Acta Neurol Scand 1996; 94(4):264–268.

35. Louwerse ES, Visser CE, Bossuyt PMM, Weverling GJ. The Netherlands ALS Consortium. Amyotrophic lateral sclerosis: mortality risk during the course of the disease and prognostic factors. J Neurol Sci 1997; 152(suppl 1):S10–S17.

36. Thijs V, Peeters E, Theys P, Matthijs G, Robberecht W. Demographic characteristics and prognosis in a Flemish amyotrophic lateral sclerosis population. Acta Neurol Belg 2000; 100:84–90.

37. Gamez J, Barcelo MJ, Munoz X, Carmona F, Cusco I, Baiget M, Cervera C, Tizzano EF. Survival and respiratory decline are not related to homozygous SMN2 deletions in ALS patients. Neurology 2002; 59(9):1456–1460.

38. Sorenson EJ, Stalker AP, Kurland LT, Windebank AJ. Amyotrophic lateral sclerosis in Olmsted County, Minnesota, 1925–1998. Neurology 2002; 59(2):280–282.

39. Jablecki CK, Berry C, Leach J. Survival prediction in amyotrophic lateral sclerosis. Muscle Nerve 1989; 12:833–841.

40. Eisen A, Schulzer M, MacNeil M, Pant B, Mak E. Duration of amyotrophic lateral sclerosis is age dependent. Muscle Nerve 1993; 16:27–32.

41. Ringel SP, Murphy JR, Alderson MK, Bryan W, England JD, Miller RG, Petajan JH, Smith SA, Roelofs RI, Ziter F, et al. The natural history of amyotrophic lateral sclerosis. Neurology 1993; 43:1316–1322.

42. Haverkamp LJ, Appel V, Appel SH. Natural history of amyotrophic lateral sclerosis in a database population: validation of a scoring system and a model for survival prediction. Brain 1995; 118:707–719.

43. Norris F, Shepherd R, Denys E, Kwei U, Mukai E, Elias L, Holden D, Norris H. Onset, natural history and outcome in idiopathic adult motor neuron disease. J Neurol Sci 1993; 118:48–55.

44. Turner MR, Parton MJ, Shaw CE, Leigh PN, Al Chalabi A. Prolonged survival in motor neuron disease; a descriptive study of the King's database 1990–2002. J Neurol Neurosurg Psychiaty 2003; 74(7):995–997.

45. Lee JR-J, Annegers JF, Appel SH. Prognosis of amyotrophic lateral sclerosis and the effect of referral selection. J Neurol Sci 1995; 132:207–215.

46. Mulder DW, Howard FM Jr. Patient resistance and prognosis in amyotrophic lateral sclerosis. Mayo Clin Proc 1976; 51(9):537–541.

47. Rosen AD. Amyotrophic lateral sclerosis. Clinical features and prognosis. Arch Neurol 1978; 35(10):638–642.

48. Uebayashi Y. Epidemiological investigation of motor neuron disease in the Kii Peninsula, Japan, and on Guam—the significance of long survival cases. Wakayama Med Rep 1980; 23:13–27.

49. Granieri E, Carreras M, Tola R, Paolino E, Tralli G, Eleopra R, Serra G. Motor neuron disease in the province of Ferrara, Italy, in 1964–1982. Neurology 1988; 38:1604–1608.

50. Chancellor AM, Slattery JM, Fraser H, Swingler RJ, Holloway SM, Warlow CP. The prognosis of adult-onset motor neuron disease: a prospective study based on the Scottish Motor Neuron Disease Register. J Neurol 1993; 240(6):339–346.

51. Marti-Fabregas J, Pradas J, Illa I. Prognostic factors in amyotrophic lateral sclerosis. Neurologia 1996; 11(5):174–181.
52. Preux P-M, Couratier PH, Boutros-Toni F, Salle J-Y, Tabaraud F, Bernet-Bernady P, Vallat J-M, Dumas M. Survival prediction in sporadic amyotrophic lateral sclerosis. Age and clinical form at onset are independent risk factors. Neuroepidemiology 1996; 15:153–160.
53. Traynor BJ, Codd MB, Corr B, Forde C, Frost E, Hardiman OM. Clinical features of amyotrophic lateral sclerosis according to the El Escorial and Airlie House diagnostic criteria: a population-based study. Arch Neurol 2000; 57(8):1171–1176.
54. Brooks BR, Sufit RL, DePaul R, DeTan Y, Sanjak M, Robbins J. Design of clinical therapeutic trials in amyotrophic lateral sclerosis. In: Rowland LP, Ed. Amyotrophic Lateral Sclerosis and Other Motor Neuron Disorders. Adv Neurol 1991; 56:521–546.
55. Kasarskis EJ, Winslow M. When did Lou Gehrig's personal illness begin? Neurology 1989; 39(9):1243–1245.
56. Guiloff RJ, Goonetilleke A. Natural history of amyotrophic lateral sclerosis. Observations with the Charing Cross Amyotrophic Lateral Sclerosis Rating Scales. In: Serratrice G, Munsat TL, eds. Pathogenesis and Therapy of Amyotrophic Lateral Sclerosis. Adv Neurol (68) Philadelphia: Lippincott-Raven Press, 1995:185–198.
57. Munsat TH, Andres PL, Finison L, Conlon T, Thibodeau L. The natural history of motoneuron loss in amyotrophic lateral sclerosis. Neurology 1988; 38(3):409–413.
58. Gastaut JL, Bartolomei F. Mills' syndrome: ascending (or descending) progressive hemiplegia: a hemiplegic form of primary lateral sclerosis? J Neurol Neurosurg Psychiatry 1994; 57(10):1280–1281
59. Gamez J, Cervera C, Codina A. Flail arm variant or Vulpian-Bernhart's form of amyotrophic lateral sclerosis. J Neurol Neurosurg Psychiatry 1999; 67(2):258.
60. Hu MT, Ellis CM, Al-Chalabi A, Leigh PN, Shaw CE. Flail arm syndrome: a distinctive variant of amyotrophic lateral sclerosis. J Neurol Neurosurg Psychiatry 1998; 65(6):950–951.
61. Couratier P, Truong CT, Khalil M, Deviere F, Vallat JM. Clinical features of flail arm syndrome. Muscle Nerve 2000; 23(4):646–647.
62. Chio A, Brignolio F, Leone M, Mortara P, Rosso MG, Tribolo A, Schiffer D. A survival analysis of 155 cases of progressive muscular atrophy. Acta Neurol Scand 1985; 72:407–413.
63. Le Forestier N, Maisonabe T, Piquard A, Rivaud S, Crevier-Buchman L, Salachas F, Pradat PF, Lacomblez L, Meininger V. Does primary lateral sclerosis exist? A study of 20 patients and a review of the literature. Brain 2001; 124(10):1989–1999.
64. Younger DS, Chou S, Hays AP, Lange DJ, Emerson R, Brin M, Thompson H, Rowland LP. Primary lateral sclerosis. A clinical diagnosis reemerges. Arch Neurol 1988; 45:1304–1307.
65. Bruyn R, Koelman J, Troost D, de Jong J. Motor neuron disease (amyotrophic lateral sclerosis) arising from longstanding primary lateral sclerosis. J Neurol Neurosurg Psychiatry 1995; 58:742–744.
66. Gastaut JL, Michel B, Figarella-Branger D, Somma-Mauvais H. Chronic progressive spinobulbar spasticity. A rare form of primary lateral sclerosis. Arch Neurol 1988; 45:509–513.
67. Pringle CE, Hudson AJ, Munoz DG, Kiernan JA, Brown WF, Ebers GC. Primary lateral sclerosis. Clinical features, neuropathology and diagnostic criteria. Brain 1992; 115:495–520.
68. Ince PG, Evans J, Knopp M, Forster G, Hamdalla HHM, Wharton SB, Shaw PJ. Corticospinal tract degeneration in the progressive muscular atrophy variant of ALS. Neurology 2003; 60:1252–1258.
69. de Carvalho M, Matias T, Coelho F, Evangelista T, Pinto A, Luis ML. Motor neuron disease presenting with respiratory failure. J Neurol Sci 1996; 139(vi):117–122.

70. Scelsa SN, Yakubov B, Salzman SH. Dyspnea-fasciculation syndrome: early respiratory failure in ALS with minimal motor signs. Amyotroph Lateral Scler Other Motor Neuron Disord 2002; 3(4):239–243.

71. Schiffman PL, Belsh JM. Pulmonary function at diagnosis of amyotrophic lateral sclerosis. Chest 1993; 103(2):508–513.

72. Bradley MD, Orrell RW, Clarke J, Davidson AC, Williams AJ, Kullman DM, Hirsch N, Howard RS. Outcome of ventilatory support for acute respiratory failure in motor neurone disease. J Neurol Neurosurg Psychiatry 2002; 72(6):752–756.

73. Nightingale S, Bates D, Bateman DE, Hudgson P, Ellis DA, Gibson GJ. Enigmatic dyspnoea: an unusual presentation of motor neurone disease. Lancet 1982; 1(8278): 933–935.

74. Parhad IM, Clark AW, Barron KD, Staunton SB. Diaphragmatic paralysis in motor neuron disease. Report of two cases and a review of the literature. Neurology 1978; 28:18–22.

75. Stambler N, Charatan M, Cedarbaum JM. Prognostic indicators of survival in ALS. ALS CNTF Treatment Study Group. Neurology 1998; 50(1):66–72.

76. Grohme K, Maravic Mv, Gasser T, Borasio GD. A case of amyotrophic lateral sclerosis with a very slow progression over 44 years. Neuromusc Dis 2001; 11:414–416.

77. Desport JC, Preux PM, Truong TC, Vallat JM, Sautereau D, Couratier P. Nutritional status is a prognostic factor for survival in ALS patients. Neurology 1999; 53(5): 1059–1063.

78. Smith R, Haverkamp L, Case S, Appel V, Appel S. Apolipoprotein E E4 in bulbar-onset motor neuron disease. Lancet 1996; 348:334–335.

79. Forbes RB, Colville S, Swingler RJ. The epidemiology of amyotrophic lateral sclerosis (ALS/MND) in people aged 80 or over. Age Aging 2004; 33(2):131–134.

80. Strong MJ, Lomen-Hoerth C, Caselli RJ, Bigio EH, Yang W. Cognitive impairment, frontotemporal dementia, and the motor neuron diseases. Ann Neurol 2003; 54(suppl 5): S20–S23.

81. Hodges JR, Davies R, Xuareb J, Kril J, Halliday G. Survival in frontotemporal dementia. Neurology 2003; 61(3):349–354.

82. Juneja T, Pericak-Vance MA, Laing NG, Dave S, Siddique T. Prognosis in familial amyotrophic lateral sclerosis: progression and survival in patients with glu100gly and ala4val mutations in Cu, Zn superoxide dismutase. Neurology 1997; 48(1):55–57.

83. Turner M, Al-Chalabi A. Early symptom progression rate is related to ALS outcome: A prospective population-based study. Correspondence. Neurology 2002b; 59:2012–2013.

84. Takahashi H, Makifuchi T, Nakano R, Sato S, Inuzuka T, Sakimura K, Mishina M, Honma Y, Tsuji S, Ikuta F. Familial amyotrophic lateral sclerosis with a mutation in the Cu/Zn superoxide dismutase gene. Acta Neuropathol 1994; 88(2):185–188.

85. Aksoy H, Dean G, Elian M, Deng HX, Deng G, Juneja T, Storey E, McKinlay Gardner RJ, Jacob RL, Laing NG, et al. A4T mutation in the SOD1 gene causing familial amyotrophic lateral sclerosis. Neuroepidemiology 2003; 22:235–238.

86. Rainero I, Pinessi L, Tsuda T, Vignocchi MG, Vaula G, Calvi L, Carreto P, Rossi B, Bergamini L, McLachlan DR, et al. SOD1 missense mutation in an Italian family with ALS. Neurology 1994; 44:347–349.

87. Aoki M, Ogasawara M, Matsubara Y, Narisawa K, Nakamura S, Itoyama Y, Abe K. Familial amyotrophic lateral sclerosis (ALS) in Japan associated with H46R mutation in Cu/Zn superoxide dismutase gene: a possible new subtype of familial ALS. J Neurol Sci 1994; 126(1):77–83.

88. Ohi T, Saita K, Takechi S, Nabesima K, Tashiro H, Shiomi K, Sugimoto S, Akematsu T, Nakayama T, Iwaki T, et al. Clinical features and neuropathological findings of familial amyotrophic lateral sclerosis with a His46Arg mutation in Cu/Zn superoxide dismutase. J Neurol Sci 2002; 197(1–2):73–78.

89. Arisato T, Okubo R, Arata H, Abe K, Fukuda K, Sakoda S, Shimizu A, Qin XH, Izumo S, Osame M, et al. Clinical and pathological studies of familial amyotrophic lat-

eral sclerosis (FALS) with SOD1 H46R mutation in large Japanese families. Acta Neuropathol 2003; 106(6):561–568.

90. Aoki M, Abe K, Houi K, Ogasawara M, Matsubara Y, Kobayashi T, Mochio S, Narisawa K, Itoyama Y. Variance of age at onset in a Japanese family with amyotrophic lateral sclerosis associated with a novel Cu/Zn superoxide dismutase mutation. Ann Neurol 1995; 37(5):676–679.

91. Horton WA, Eldridge R, Brody JA. Familial motor neuron disease: evidence for at least three different types. Neurology 1976; 26:460–465.

92. Giess R, Holtmann B, Braga M, Grimm T, Muller-Myhsok B, Toyka KV, Sendtner M. Early onset of severe familial amyotrophic lateral sclerosis with SOD-1 mutation: potential impact of CNTF as a candidate modifier gene. Am J Hum Genet 2002; 70(5): 1277–1286.

93. Nogales-Gadea G, Carcia-Arumi E, Andreu AL, Cervera C, Gamez J. A novel exon 5 mutation (N139H) in the SOD1 gene in a Spanish family associated with incomplete penetrance. J Neurol Sci 2004; 219(1–2):1–6.

94. Radunovic A, Shaw CE, Akmen-Demir G, Idrisoglu H, Leigh PN. CuZnSOD-associated amyotrophic lateral sclerosis. Ann Neurol 1997; 42(2):273–274.

95. Cudkowicz ME, McKenna-Yasek D, Sapp PE, Chin W, Geller B, Hayden DL, Schoenfeld DA, Hosler BA, Horvitz HR, Brown RH. Epidemiology of mutations in superoxide dismutase in amyotrophic lateral sclerosis. Ann Neurol 1997; 41(2):210–221.

96. Haasdijk ED, Vlug A, Mulder MT, Jaarsma D. Increased apolipoprotein E expression correlates with the onset of neuronal degeneration in the spinal cord of G93A-SOD1 mice. Neurosci Lett 2002; 335(1):29–33.

97. Mui S, Rebeck GW, McKenna-Yasek D, Hyman BT, Brown RH Jr. Apolipoprotein E epsilon 4 allele is not associated with earlier age at onset in amyotrophic lateral sclerosis. Ann Neurol 1995; 38(3):460–463.

98. Moulard B, Sefiani A, Laamri A, Malafosse A, Camu W. Apolipoprotein E genotyping in sporadic amyotrophic lateral sclerosis: evidence for a major influence on the clinical presentation and prognosis. J Neurol Sci 1996; 139(vi):34–37.

99. Al-Chalabi A, Enayat ZE, Bakker MC, Sham PC, Ball DM, Shaw CE, Lloyd CM, Powell JF, Leigh PN. Association of apolipoprotein E epsilon 4 allele with bulbar-onset motor neuron disease. Association of apolipoprotein E E4 allele with bulbar-onset motor neuron disease. Lancet 1996; 347(8995):159–160.

100. Siddique T, Pericak-Vance MA, Caliendo J, Hong ST, Hung WY, Kaplan J, McKenna - Yasek D, Rimmler JB, Sapp P, Saunders AM, et al. Lack of association between apolipoprotein E genotype and sporadic amyotrophic lateral sclerosis. Neurogenetics 1998; 1(3):213–216.

101. Lacomblez L, Doppler V, Beucler I, Costes G, Salachas F, Raisonnier A, Le Forestier N, Pradat PF, Bruckert E, Meininger V. APOE: a potential marker of disease progression in ALS. Neurology 2002; 58(7):1112–1114.

102. Drory VE, Birnbaum M, Korczyn AD, Chapman J. Association of APOE ε4 allele with survival in amyotrophic lateral sclerosis. J Neurol Sci 2001; 190(1–2):17–20.

103. Veldink JH, van den Berg LH, Cobben JM, Stulp RP, De Jong JM, Vogels OJ, Baas F, Wokke JH, Scheffer H. Homozygous deletion of the survival motor neuron 2 gene is a prognostic factor in sporadic ALS. Neurology 2001; 56(6):749–753.

104. Al-Chalabi A, Scheffler A, Smith BN, Parton MJ, Cudkowicz ME, Andersen PM, Hayden DL, Hansen VK, Turner MR, Shaw CE, Leigh PN, Brown RH Jr. Ciliary neurotrophic factor genotype does not influence clinical phenotype in amyotrophic lateral sclerosis. Ann Neurol 2003; 54(1):130–134.

105. Desport JC, Preux PM, Magy L, Boirie Y, Vallat JM, Beaufrere B, Couratier P. Factors correlated with hypermetabolism in patients with amyotrophic lateral sclerosis. Am J Clin Nutr 2001; 74(3):328–334.

106. McDonald ER, Wiedenfeld SA, Hillel A, Carpenter C, Walter RA. Survival in amyotrophic lateral sclerosis. The role of psychological factors. Arch Neurol 1994; 51:17–23.

107. Armon C, Graves MC, Moses D, Forte DK, Sepulveda L, Darby SM, Smith RA. Linear estimates of disease progression predict survival in patients with amyotrophic lateral sclerosis. Muscle Nerve 2000; 23(6):874–888.

108. Tsai CP, Ho HH, Yen DJ, Wang V, Lin KP, Liao KK, Wu ZA. Reversible motor neuron disease. Eur Neurol 1993; 33(5):387–389.

109. Iwasaki Y, Ikeda K, Ichikawa Y, Igasashi O, Kinoshita M. The diagnostic interval in amyotrophic lateral sclerosis. Clin Neurol Neurosurg 2002; 104(2):87–89.

110. Miyoshi K, Ohyagi Y, Amano T, Inoue I, Miyoshi S, Tsuji S, Yamada T, Kira J. A patient with motor neuron syndrome clinically similar to amyotrophic lateral sclerosis, presenting spontaneous recovery. Rinsho Shinkeigaku 2000; 40(11):1090–1095.

111. Tucker T, Layzer RB, Miller RG, Chad D. Subacute reversible motor neuron disease. Neurology 1991; 41:1541–1544.

112. Sinaki M, Mulder DW. Amyotrophic lateral sclerosis: relationship between serum creatine kinase level and patient survival. Arch Phys Med Rehab 1986; 67(3):169–171.

113. Felice KJ, North WA. Creatine Kinase values in amyotrophic lateral sclerosis. J Neurol Sci 1998; 160(suppl 1):S30–S32.

114. Iłzecka J, Stelmasiak Z. Creatine kinase activity in amyotrophic lateral sclerosis. Neurol Sci 2003; 24(4):286–287.

115. Iłzecka J, Stelmasiak Z. Serum bilirubin in patients with amyotrophic lateral sclerosis. Clin Neurol Neurosurg 2003; 105:237–240.

116. Killian JM, Wilfong AA, Burnett L, Appel SH, Boland D. Decremental motor responses to repetitive nerve stimulation in ALS. Muscle Nerve 1994; 17(7):747–754.

117. Wang FC, De Pasqua V, Gerard P, Delwaide PJ. Prognostic value of decremental responses to repetitive nerve stimulation in ALS patients. Neurology 2001; 57(5):897–899.

118. Denys EH, Norris FH Jr. Amyotrophic lateral sclerosis. Impairment of neuromuscular transmission. Arch Neurol 1979; 36(4):202–205.

119. Daube JR. Electrophysiologic studies in the diagnosis and prognosis of motor neuron diseases. Neurol Clin 1985; 3:473–493.

120. Mitsumoto H, Schwartzman M, Levin KH, Shields RW, Wilbourn AJ. Electromyographic (EMG) changes and disease progression in ALS. Neurology 1990; 40(suppl 1):318.

121. Daube JR. Electrodiagnostic studies in amyotrophic lateral sclerosis and other motor neuron disorders. Muscle Nerve 2000; 23:1488–1502.

122. Wilbourn AJ. Generalized low motor-normal sensory conduction responses: the etiology in 55 patients (abstract). Muscle Nerve 1984; 7:564.

123. de Carvalho M, Scotto M, Lopes A, Swash M. Clinical and neurophysiological evaluation of progression in amyotrophic lateral sclerosis. Muscle Nerve 2003; 28:630–633.

124. Armon C, Brandstater ME. Motor unit number estimate-based rates of progression of ALS predict patient survival. Muscle Nerve 1999; 22:1571–1575.

125. Dantes M, McComas A. The extent and time course of motoneuron involvement in amyotrophic lateral sclerosis. Muscle Nerve 1991; 14:416–421.

126. Johnston M, Earll, Giles M, McClenahan R, Stevens D, Morrison V. Mood as a predictor of disability and survival in patients diagnosed with ALS/MND. Br J Health Psychol 1999; 4(2):127–136.

127. Bernstein LP, Antel JP. Motor neuron disease: decremental responses to repetitive nerve stimulation. Neurology 1981; 31:204–207.

128. Louwerse ES, Posthumus Meyjes FE, Sillevis Smitt JH, Redekop WK, Bossuyt PM, Vianney de Jong JM, Ongerboer de Visser BW. Prognostic values of electroneurographic and electromyographic features in amyotrophic lateral sclerosis. J Neurol Sci 1995; 129(suppl):29.

129. Kwon O, Lee K-W. Reproducibility of statistical motor unit estimates in amyotrophic lateral sclerosis: comparisons between size- and number-weighted modifications. Muscle Nerve 2004; 29:211–217.

130. Andres PL, Finison LJ, Conlon T, Thibodeau LM, Munsat TL. Use of composite scores (megascores) to measure deficit in amyotrophic lateral sclerosis. Neurology 1988; 38:405–408.
131. Lyall RA, Donaldson N, Polkey MI, Leigh PN, Moxham J. Respiratory muscle strength and ventilatory failure in amyotrophic lateral sclerosis. Brain 2001; 124:2000–2013.
132. Leigh NP, Swash M, Iwasaki Y, Ludolph A, Meininger V, Miller RG, Mitsumoto H, Shaw P, Tashiro K, van den Berg L. Amyotrophic lateral sclerosis: a consensus viewpoint on designing and implementing a clinical trial. Amyotroph Lateral Scler Other Motor Neuron Disord 2004; 5:84–98.
133. Rosen DR, Bowling AC, Patterson D, Usdin TB, Sapp P, Mezey F, McKenna Yasek D, O' Regan J, Rahmani Z, Ferrante RJ, et al. A frequent ala 4 to val superoxide dismutase-1 mutation is associated with a rapidly progressive familial amyotrophic lateral sclerosis. Hum Mol Genet 1994; 3:981–987.

11

Specifying Motor Neuron Identity in the Developing Spinal Cord

Thomas M. Jessell
Department of Biochemistry and Molecular Biophysics, Columbia University, New York, New York, U.S.A.

One of the most striking organizational features of the vertebrate central nervous system (CNS) is the extraordinary diversity of its component neuronal cell types. How this impressive feat of cellular diversification is achieved, and how molecular and morphological distinctions direct neuronal connectivity, physiology, and function remain enigmatic problems (1). Information on the mechanisms by which neurons acquire their specialized identities may also provide insights into the selectivity of neuronal loss that characterizes most neurodegenerative diseases.

Many advances in understanding the mechanisms of neuronal diversification in the CNS have emerged through the study of one of its major neural classes—the spinal motor neuron. Motor neurons share many core properties (2), but they also exhibit highly specialized features that are necessary for the precise coordination of motor output (3). Core features exhibited by all spinal motor neurons include the use of a common cholinergic-neurotransmitter system, and the extension of axons out of the CNS, a property that is exclusive to motor neurons (2). In almost every other respect, however, motor neurons exhibit divergent features—their location within the CNS, their connectivity with different peripheral target structures, their innervation by different classes of sensory neurons and interneurons, and their expression of ion channels that confer distinct firing properties (Fig. 1) (4–7).

This chapter outlines recent progress in defining the principles and mechanisms that are used to impose spinal motor neuron identity, and to link motor neuron identity with two later developmental stages of circuit formation—the establishment of precise axonal projection patterns and target connectivity. Progress in applying insights from the normal programs of motor neuron differentiation to the generation of functional motor neurons from stem cells are also discussed as a potential way in which basic motor neuron biology may have therapeutic relevance.

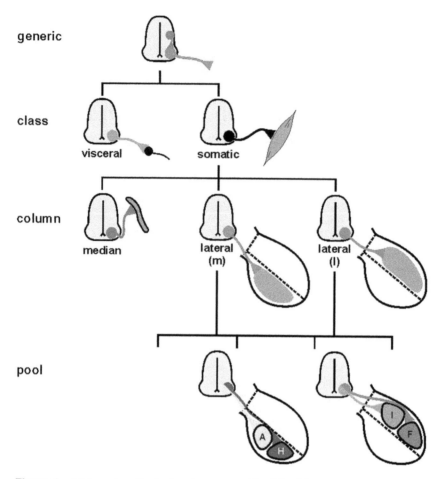

Figure 1 A hierarchy of spinal motor neuron identities. Motor neuron subtype organization in the developing spinal cord, defined on the basis of cell body position, axonal projections, and gene expression. *Generic*: features common to all motor neurons, such as the projection of axons out of the spinal cord, that distinguishes them from interneurons. *Class*: subdivision of motor neurons on the basis of the innervation of skeletal muscle targets (*somatic*) or neuronal or glandular targets (*visceral*). Visceral and somatic motor neurons are generated from the same ventral progenitor domain at spinal levels but from distinct progenitor domains at cranial levels. *Column*: sets of motor neurons arrayed in longitudinal columns and projecting to distinct regions in the periphery. LMC neurons are generated only at limb levels and send axons into the limb mesenchyme. Neurons in the medial (m) division of the LMC send axons into the ventral limb mesenchyme, and neurons in the lateral (l) division send axons into the dorsal limb mesenchyme. The MMC can be divided into a medial (m) group, which is found at all rostrocaudal levels and projects to axial muscles, and a lateral group (*not shown*), found only at thoracic levels and projecting to body wall muscles. *Pool*: clustered sets of motor neurons within the LMC that innervate a single muscle group in the limb. *Abbreviations*: LMC, lateral motor column, MMC, median motor column. (*See color insert.*)

SPECIFICATION OF GENERIC MOTOR NEURON IDENTITY

Within the neural tube, the differentiation of spinal motor neurons is triggered by the joint activation of two signaling pathways: a long-range gradient of Sonic hedgehog signaling (Shh) activity provided by the notochord and floor plate (8,9), and a more diffuse influence of retinoid signals provided by the paraxial mesoderm that flanks the neural tube (10–12). The major signaling activity of the notochord and floor plate was mediated by a secreted protein, Sonic hedgehog (Shh) (Fig. 2) (8,9). Ectopic expression of Shh in vivo and in vitro can induce the differentiation of motor neurons and ventral interneurons (13–17). Conversely, elimination of Shh signaling from the notochord by antibody blockade in vitro (13,15) or through gene targeting in mice (18) prevents the differentiation of motor neurons and most classes of ventral interneurons.

Studies of the actions of Shh on neural progenitor cells in vitro have shown that five molecularly distinct classes of ventral neurons can be generated in response to the progressive two-to-three fold changes in Shh concentration (Fig. 3) (9,15, 16,19,20). Moreover, the position of generation of each of these neuronal classes in vivo is predicted by the concentration of Shh required for their induction in vitro. Neurons generated in progressively more ventral regions of the neural tube require correspondingly higher concentrations of Shh for their induction (16,20). These findings have lent support to the proposal that the position of a progenitor cell within a ventral-to-dorsal gradient of Shh signaling activity directs its differentiation into specific neuronal subtypes (Fig. 3) (6,9).

There is now persuasive evidence that the secretion of Shh from the floor plate creates a long-range ventral-to-dorsal gradient of signaling activity, which exerts a direct influence on ventral cell fate and pattern. The secretion of Shh from notochord and floor plate cells depends on the function of a transmembrane protein dispatched (21). Once secreted, Shh protein and activity are detectable throughout the ventral neural tube, well away from the ventral sources of *Shh* synthesis (14,15,22), indicating that the active processed amino-terminal fragment of Shh, termed Shh-N, is transferred over many cell diameters through the ventral neural epithelium. Moreover, ectopic

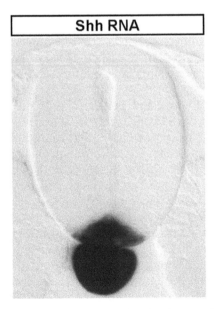
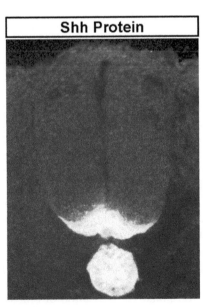

Shh RNA   **Shh Protein**

Figure 2   Shh expression by the notochord and floor plate. Cross-section through stage-18 chick spinal cord showing the expression of *Shh* RNA and protein by the notochord underlying the neural tube and floor plate at the ventral midline of the neural tube. *Abbreviation*: RNA, ribonucleic acid

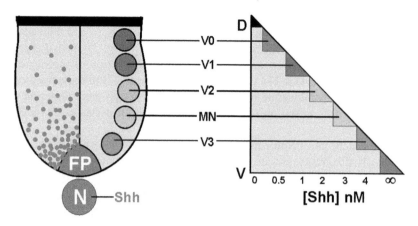

Figure 3 Graded Sonic hedgehog signaling and the positional specification of motor neuron identity. Left diagram shows the presumed gradient of Sonic hedgehog (Shh) activity in the ventral neural tube (*blue dots*), distributed in a ventral-high, dorsal-low profile within the ventral neural epithelium, and the position of five classes of neurons that are generated in response to graded Shh signaling. V0–V3 indicate four different classes of ventral interneurons. MN indicates motor neurons, and FP the floor plate. Right diagram shows the profile of neuronal generation in neural plate explants cultured in different concentrations of the recombinant amino-terminal fragment of Shh, termed Shh-N. D, dorsal neural tube; V, ventral neural tube. The more dorsal the position of neuronal subtype generation in vivo, the lower the concentration of Shh required to induce the same neuronal subpopulation in vitro. *Source*: From Refs. 9 and 16. (*See color insert.*)

expression of an activated form of *Smo*, the gene encoding the signal transducing subunit of the Shh receptor, appears to induce motor neurons in a cell-autonomous manner (23), indicating that Shh acts directly on target cells to specify motor neuron and interneuron fates. And in addition, the loss of Shh receptor function in neural progenitor cells blocks motor neuron and interneuron differentiation in a cell-autonomous manner (24,25). Thus, in the context of the neural tube, Shh appears to function as a gradient morphogen, assigning motor neuron and interneuron fates at distinct concentration thresholds (6).

These findings, in turn, pose the problem of how neural progenitor cells interpret graded Shh signals to generate motor neurons. Shh elicits responses in neural progenitor cells by interacting with a cell surface receptor complex that consists of two subunits: Patched, a multitransmembrane protein that serves as the Shh binding subunit, and Smoothened, a seven transmembrane protein that functions as the signal transducing subunit (26). The interaction of Shh with Patched relieves its tonic inhibition of Smoothened, leading in turn to the activation of an intracellular transduction pathway that is still poorly understood (27). However, it is clear that the key transcriptional mediators of Shh signaling in neural cells are a set of zinc finger transcription factors, the Gli proteins, which exist in both repressor and activator isoforms (28–30). Activation of Shh signaling in neural progenitor cells shifts the balance of Gli activities to the activator forms, and there is now persuasive evidence that the extracellular concentration of Shh sets the activator: repressor ratio of Gli protein activity, which in turn activates different target genes within neural precursor cells (30,31).

What are the targets of Gli transcriptional activity that specify different progenitor cell domains? A group of homeodomain transcription factors expressed by ventral progenitor cells act as a key intermediary factors in the interpretation of graded Shh and Gli signaling (16,19,20). These homeodomain proteins can be divided into two distinct classes based on their pattern of expression and mode of regulation by Shh (Fig. 4) (20). The expression of each class-I protein is repressed at a distinct Shh threshold concentration, and as a consequence the ventral boundaries of class-I homeodomain protein expression define ventral progenitor domains (20). In addition, the expression of class-I proteins is activated in a spatially unrestricted manner by retinoid signaling from the paraxial mesoderm, thus ensuring class-I protein expression despite the repressive actions of Shh signaling (11,12). The expression of class-II proteins, by contrast, requires Shh signaling, and with each protein activated at a distinct Shh threshold concentrations (20). Thus, the dorsal boundaries of class-II proteins delineate progenitor domains (Fig. 4). Together, the combinatorial profile of expression of these two classes of homeodomain proteins is sufficient to define five cardinal progenitor cell domains within the ventral neural tube (9,20).

These progenitor homeodomain proteins convert the gradient of extracellular Shh signaling and intracellular Gli activity into discrete progenitor domains through selective cross–repressive interactions between complementary pairs of class-I and class-II homeodomain proteins—those proteins that abut the same progenitor domain boundary (Fig. 5) (16,19,20,32,33). Such cross-repressive interactions serve three main roles (Fig. 5). First, they establish the initial dorsoventral domains of expression of class-I and -II proteins. Second, they ensure the existence of sharp boundaries between progenitor domains. Third, they help to relieve progenitor cells of a requirement for ongoing Shh signaling, thus consolidating progenitor domain identity (9,20).

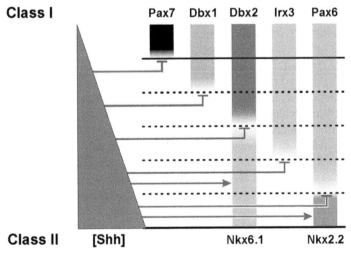

Figure 4 Graded Sonic hedgehog signaling patterns homeodomain protein expression. Shh signaling represses the expression of class-I homeodomain proteins (Pax7, Dbx1, Dbx2, Irx3, and Pax6) at different threshold concentrations and induces expression of class-II proteins (Nkx6.1 and Nkx2.2) at different threshold concentrations. Class-I and class-II proteins that abut a common progenitor domain boundary have similar Shh concentration thresholds for repression and activation of protein expression, respectively. The profile of homeodomain transcription factor expression established by graded Shh signaling defines five progenitor domains in the ventral neural tube. *Source*: From Refs. 9 and 20. (*See color insert.*)

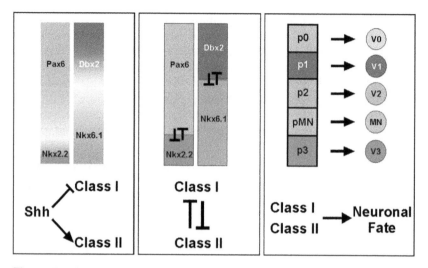

Figure 5 Three phases of ventral neural patterning. Phase 1: graded Shh signaling initiates dorsoventral restrictions in the domains of class-I and class-II protein expression within the ventral neural tube. Phase 2: cross-repressive interactions between class-I and class-II proteins that abut a common progenitor domain boundary refine and maintain progenitor domains. Phase 3: the profile of expression of class-I and class-II proteins within an individual progenitor domain controls neuronal fate. (*See color insert.*)

Strikingly, most of the homeodomain proteins involved in motor neuron generation possess a conserved motif—termed the eh1 domain—that mediates interaction with Gro/TLE class transcriptional corepressors (34). The progenitor homeodomain proteins that possess an eh1 domain can bind Gro/TLE proteins in vitro, and their neural patterning activity in vivo requires the presence of the eh1 domain, indicative of their function as Gro/TLE-dependent repressors (35). These findings have led to the idea that the pattern of motor neuron and interneuron generation in the ventral neural tube is achieved primarily through the spatially restricted repression of transcriptional repressors—a derepression strategy of neuronal specification. In this scheme, motor neuron specification depends on the selectivity of homeodomain repressor interactions with *cis*-acting DNA sequences present in the regulatory regions of other progenitor homeodomain proteins (35). Thus, the distinct activities of class-II and class-I repressor proteins in neural patterning appear to be encoded by the specificity of DNA recognition mediated solely by the homeodomain.

There is now extensive genetic evidence that the homeodomain proteins expressed by progenitor cells specify the identity of each of the classes of postmitotic neurons that derive from the individual progenitor domains (6,36). Evidence for their activity has come from ectopic expression studies in chick, and from gene targeting in mice. The misexpression of individual homeodomain proteins changes the fate and position at which individual classes of neurons are generated, as predicted by the normal profile of homeodomain protein expression (20). Conversely, there are predictable switches in progenitor domain identity and neuronal fate in mice in which individual class-I and class-II homeodomain proteins have been inactivated by gene targeting (16,32,33). Together, these studies provide an initial framework for defining Shh-regulated transcriptional cascades that direct neural progenitor cells into motor neurons.

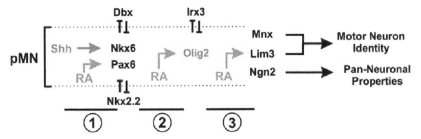

Figure 6 An interplay between inductive signals and transcription factors directs motor neuron identity. *Step 1*: within the motor neuron progenitor (pMN) domain, Shh and retinoic acid (RA) signaling direct the expression of Nkx6 and Pax6 proteins. The repressor activity of Nkx6 and Pax6 clear the pMN domain of transcriptional repressors, notably the Dbx proteins and Nkx2.2. *Step 2*: in this derepressed context, retinoid signaling is able to promote the expression of Olig2, a repressor that ensures the clearance of Irx3 from the pMN domain. Step 3: Olig2 repressor activity promotes the expression of pan-neuronal transcription factors such as Ngn2, and in addition promotes expression of motor neuron subtype transcription factors such as Lim3 (Lhx3) and Mnx class (Hb9 and Mnr2) homeodomain proteins. *Source*: From Refs. 9 and 11.

In particular, Shh-regulated homeodomain proteins can be ordered into a pathway that helps to explain how motor neurons acquire an identity distinct from that of adjacent interneurons (Fig. 4) (6). In this pathway, the combinatorial actions of three homeodomain proteins—Nkx6.1, Nkx2.2, and Irx3—restricts the generation of motor neurons to a single (pMN) progenitor domain (6). Within this domain, Nkx6.1 activity directs the domain-restricted expression of down-stream factors, most notably Olig2, a basic helix-loop-helix (bHLH) protein expressed selectively by motor neuron progenitors (37–40). Olig2 appears to specify the subtype identity of motor neurons (41–44) through cross-regulatory interactions with progenitor homeodomain transcription factors, and directs pan-neuronal properties by promoting Ngn2 expression, cell cycle exit, and neuronal marker expression (Fig. 6) (37,38,45,46). Moreover, Olig2 directs both branches of this neuronal differentiation program through its actions as a transcriptional repressor, providing further evidence that repressive interactions lie at the heart of generic motor neuron specification (37). Thus, an intricate interplay of inductive signals and repressor homeodomain and bHLH transcription factors directs naïve neural tube progenitors into postmitotic spinal motor neurons (Fig. 6).

SPECIFICATION OF MOTOR NEURON COLUMNAR IDENTITY

Although spinal motor neurons derive from a single ventral progenitor domain, they rapidly acquire distinct subtype identities. The classification of motor neuron subtypes has traditionally been based on cell body position in the spinal cord, and axonal projection pattern in the periphery. In higher vertebrates, one level of organization is evident in the alignment of motor neurons into longitudinally oriented columns, each with a distinct peripheral target (Fig. 1) (47–50). One motor column, the medial set of median motor column (MMC) neurons is found at all segmental levels of the spinal cord, but all other columns occupy distinct and discontinuous domains along the rostrocaudal axis (48–51). At limb levels of the spinal cord motor neurons of the lateral motor column (LMC) are generated in register with their limb target fields (48), whereas thoracic levels contain two distinct motor columns: the preganglionic autonomic motor column (termed Column of Terni in chick) (51), which innervates sympathetic neuronal targets, and a set of lateral MMC neurons that innervates intercostal and body wall musculature (48,49,52,53).

Recent studies have provided evidence that rostrocaudal differences in the columnar identity of spinal motor neurons are established in response to the sequential actions of two sets of extrinsic signals: an early gradient of FGF and GDF11 signaling activity derived from the node region, and a later influence of high-level retinoid signaling provided by cervical paraxial mesoderm (54–58). The rostrocaudal identity of neural progenitor cells and postmitotic motor neurons appears to be reflected in the position-specific expression of Hox class homeodomain proteins, notably members of the Hox-a and Hox-c clusters (Fig. 7) (55,57,59). Profiles of Hox expression characteristic of brachial, thoracic, and lumbar neural progenitor

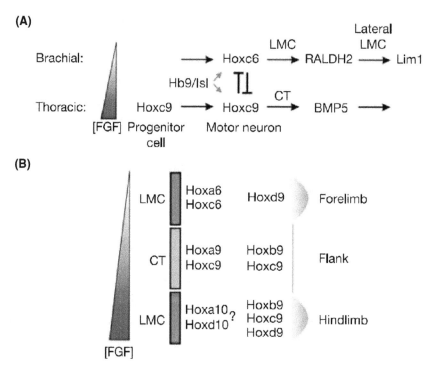

Figure 7 Hox protein activities control motor neuron columnar differentiation. (**A**) Model indicating the roles of FGF signaling and Hox6 and Hox9 protein expression in the specification of motor neuron columnar identity. Hoxc9 expression in progenitors and the cross-repressive interactions between Hox6 and Hox9 proteins in postmitotic Hb9+, Isl+ motor neurons consolidate the distinct Hox profiles of LMC and CT neurons. Hox6 activity in brachial motor neurons directs RALDH2 expression and late features of LMC identity, whereas Hox9 activity in thoracic motor neruons directs BMP5 expression and the dorsomedial migration of motor neruons. (**B**) Hox expression and the register between the rostrocaudal positions of LMC and limb formation. The diagram indicates how exposure of neural and lateral plate mesodermal cells to a common node-derived source of FGFs could establish distinct Hox expression profiles in these two tissues, directing LMC and limb formation in an aligned manner. *Abbreviations*: LMC, lateral motor column; RALDH2, retinaldehyde dehydrogenase-2. *Source*: From Ref. 55. (*See color insert.*)

cells are initially induced by exposure of neural progenitor cells to the increasing levels of FGF and GDF11 signaling (57), and consolidated by exposure to retinoids (58).

In response to these extrinsic pattering signals, an initial rostro-caudal pattern of Hox expression in neural progenitor cells is translated into a distinct postmitotic Hox pattern in LMC and CT neurons (Fig. 7) (55). Thus, Hox6 proteins are expressed by brachial level motor neurons and impose forelimb-level LMC identity, whereas Hox9 proteins are expressed at thoracic levels and impose CT identity, and Hox10 proteins are expressed at lumbar levels and impose hind-limb level LMC identity (55,59). The divergence of LMC and CT identities along the rostro-caudal axis of the spinal cord is reinforced by mutual transcriptional cross-repressive interactions between complementary Hox protein pairs (55). In addition, these Hox proteins also have intrinsic activator functions that are involved in the induction of differentiated markers of LMC and CT columnar identity (Fig. 7) (55). Together, these studies indicate that Hox proteins direct an early step in MN subtype diversification—the organization of columnar modules.

One unresolved issue in motor neuron columnar specification is the pathway used to assign the identity of medial MMC neurons—the sole motor column that is represented at all segmental levels of the spinal cord (60). The formation of this segmentally unrestricted column does not appear to involve Hox activities, since mis-expression of Hox proteins that determine LMC and CT identities has no impact on medial MMC fate (55). The immunity of medial MMC neurons to Hox activity appears to be linked to the activities of the LIM homeodomain transcription factors, Lhx3 (Lim3) and Lhx4 (Gsh4) (Fig. 8) (61–64). Lhx3 and Lhx4 are normally restricted to medial MMC neurons, and persistent ectopic expression of Lhx3 in other spinal motor neurons converts prospective LMC and preganglionic autonomic

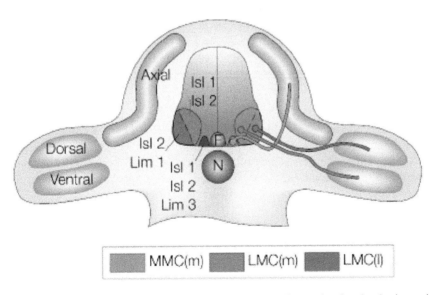

Figure 8 Spatial organizations of motor neuron columns in the developing spinal cord. Transverse section of the chick embryo at limb levels (similar at forelimb and hindlimb levels), showing the position of motor columns in relation to motor axonal projection pattern in the periphery and to LIM homeodomain protein expression. N, notochord; F, floor plate; LMC(m), medial division of the LMC; LMC(l), lateral division of the LMC. Brown regions indicate the positions of muscle targets. *Source*: From Refs. 60 and 69. (*See color insert.*)

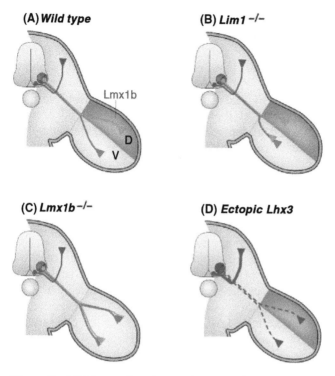

Figure 9 LIM homeodomain proteins control motor axon trajectory. (**A**) Wild type: projections of MMC(m) (*dark gray*), LMC(m) (*medium gray*) and LMC(l) (*light gray*) axons from the spinal cord at limb levels. (**B**) $Lim1^{-/-}$: $Lim1$ mutant LMC(l) neurons show aberrant ventral axonal projections. (**C**) $Lmx1b^{-/-}$: loss of $Lmx1b$ expression results in a ventral duplication of the limb mesenchyme. Consequently, motor axons from both divisions of the LMC randomly project axons into the dorsal (D) and ventral (V) limb mesenchyme. (**D**) Ectopic $Lhx3$: misexpression of $Lhx3$ in all motor neurons results in the conversion of most or all spinal LMC and visceral neurons to an MMC(m)-like identity. Many, but not all, motor axons now select a dorsal pathway to axial muscles. However, only a small increase in the net number of motor axons projecting into the axial pathway is permitted. *Source*: From Refs. 62 and 70. (*See color insert.*)

(CT) neurons to a medial MMC-like identity, as assessed by molecular markers, neuronal settling pattern, and the rerouting of motor axons to axial muscle targets (Fig. 9) (62,64). Thus, the persistence of expression of Lhx3 and Lhx4 by spinal motor neurons directs medial MMC identity and appears to render these neurons refractory to the columnar specification activities of Hox proteins.

ESTABLISHING THE DIVISIONAL IDENTITY AND AXONAL TRAJECTORY OF LMC NEURONS

How are motor neurons further diversified once their columnar fates have been established? Some insight into this issue has come from the study of LMC neurons and their connectivity with muscle targets in the limb. Within the LMC, motor neurons segregate into medial and lateral divisions, and send axons to ventral and dorsal limb muscles, respectively (48,49). Both sets of LMC neurons are generated from progenitor cells that occupy the same dorsoventral and rostrocaudal positions within the spinal cord, making it unlikely that signals from the axial or paraxial mesoderm impose this distinction. Strikingly, these two sets of LMC neurons differ most obviously in their birthdates: motor neurons destined to populate the medial LMC exit the cell cycle before those populating the lateral LMC (65). As a consequence, prospective lateral LMC neurons are required to migrate past their earlier born medial LMC counterparts to reach their final settling position (66).

Several observations indicate that a retinoid-mediated signal provided by early-born LMC neurons helps to specify the fate of later-born lateral LMC neurons. LMC neurons selectively express the retinoid synthetic enzyme retinaldehyde dehydrogenase-2 (RALDH2) (66,67) from the consequent synthesis of retinoids by early-born LMC neurons (68) acts in a cell non-autonomous manner to impose the LIM homeodomain profile that distinguishes medial (Isl1$^+$) and lateral (Lim1$^+$) LMC neurons (Fig. 8) (58,66). In turn, cross-repressive interactions between Isl1 and Lim1 consolidate the LMC divisional identities initiated by retinoid signaling (69). Thus, one strategy for generating diversity within motor columns involves local paracrine signaling between postmitotic motor neurons themselves.

The differential expression of LIM homeodomain proteins by LMC neurons, imposed in response to neuronal retinoid signaling, has a critical role in directing the dorsoventral trajectory of motor axons as they enter the limb (Fig. 8). In mice lacking *Lim1* function the axons of lateral LMC neurons project into the dorsal and ventral limb mesenchyme at equal incidence, apparently selecting their trajectories at random (Fig. 9) (70). Conversely, ectopic expression of Lim1 in prospective medial LMC neurons directs motor axons dorsally whereas expression of Isl1 directs axons ventrally (Fig. 9) (69). The ephrin-A:EphA-signaling system is a key effector of LIM homeodomain protein activity in the regulation of motor axon trajectory. EphA4 is preferentially expressed by the axons of lateral LMC neurons in response to the activities of Lim1 and Isl1 (Fig. 10) (69,71–73), and A-class Ephrins are concentrated in the ventral limb mesenchyme by the actions of the LIM homeodomain protein Lmx1b (69,70,72,74). Moreover, the ectopic expression of EphA4 in medial LMC neurons redirects their axons along a dorsal trajectory (69,73). Thus, the pattern of motor axon projections into the limb is established, in part, through the LIM homeodomain protein-dependent control of EphA receptors and ephrin-A ligands (Fig. 10).

Taken together, this analysis of motor neuron columnar differentiation has revealed a molecular cascade that links the specification of early progenitor cell identity to the selection of motor axon trajectories in the developing limb (55). Orthogonally acting gradients of Shh and FGF signaling establish a motor neuron homeodomain protein profile that activates RALDH2 expression and retinoid synthesis in postmitotic LMC neurons. In turn, retinoids induce Lim1 expression and high-level EphA4 expression in lateral LMC neurons, ensuring that motor axons select a dorsal axonal trajectory as they enter the limb mesenchyme.

THE EMERGENCE OF MOTOR NEURON POOL IDENTITY

From the perspective of locomotor function, the most critical aspect of motor neuron diversification is the assignment of motor neurons within the LMC to discrete motor pools (Fig. 1). Each muscle group in the limb is innervated by a specific pool of motor neurons (48,75,76). Thus the existence of about 50 distinct muscle groups in a typical amniote limb (53) implies the specification of an equivalent number of motor neuron pool identities. Each motor pool occupies a characteristic rostrocaudal and

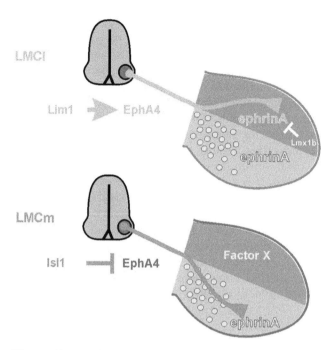

Figure 10 Ephrin-A signaling establishes the dorsoventral trajectory of motor axons in the developing limb. Top diagram shows the actions of LIM homeodomain transcription factors in LMC motor neurons and in the limb mesenchyme. Diagram also shows the distribution of EphA and ephrin-A proteins on LMC neurons and in the limb mesenchyme. The diagram also depicts a putative Ephrin-A: EphA independent repellent guidance signal (X) expressed by the dorsal limb mesenchyme, and the expression of a corresponding X receptor (Rx) on the axons of both medial and lateral LMC neurons. *Source*: From Ref. 69. (*See color insert.*)

mediolateral position within the LMC, and the axons of neurons in distinct pools pioneer stereotyped trajectories in the limb, and innervate individual target muscles, thus establishing specific patterns of connectivity (48,49).

Physiological and embryological studies have suggested that motor pool identity emerges soon after LMC neurons exit the cell cycle, with their distinct identities first revealed through their phasic firing patterns and the selection of specific nerve trajectories in the limb, en route to their muscle targets (50,77–79). Only somewhat later do motor neurons cluster into their characteristic intrasegmental pool positions, form stereotyped intramuscular nerve branching patterns, and receive selective proprioceptive sensory afferent input (80,81). Thus, motor pool specification appears to unfold in two main phases: an early phase linked to the assignment of muscle nerve trajectory (78) and a late phase linked to terminal branching, pool clustering, and sensory connectivity (Fig. 11) (81).

Recent studies have begun to identify molecular markers of LMC motor pool identity, and have provided a preliminary insight into the regulatory events that control the late phase of motor pool differentiation. Motor neuron pools can be defined by the expression of transcription factors of the ETS family, notably Pea3 and Er81 (80). The onset of expression of these genes by LMC neurons occurs well after cell cycle exit, coincides with axonal invasion of the limb mesenchyme, and depends on limb-derived signals that include GDNF and HGF (80–83). These and the other

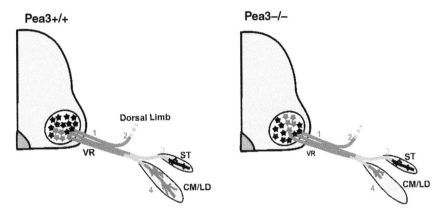

Figure 11 ETS protein Pea3 controls late aspects of the differentiation of specific motor neuron pools. The development of motor axonal projections into the limb mesenchyme can be subdivided into four phases, each controlled by the sequential expression of specific transcription factors. Phases of motor axon extension that appear to be preprogrammed at the time of axon outgrowth are indicated in blue, and phases that require a peripherally induced program of gene expression are indicated in purple. Pea3+/+: the establishment of ventral root projections (1) and axonal projections to distinct peripheral domains (e.g., dorsal limb, is regulated by Nkx6/Mnx, and LIM homeodomain proteins, respectively). The identity of transcription factors controlling the development of muscle-specific projections is not known, and it is uncertain whether this phase of axon extension requires peripherally induced gene expression. The invasion and branching of motor axons within target muscles is regulated by peripheral signals. Intramuscular nerve branches in a muscle not innervated by PEA3^{+} motor neurons (other muscles) are indicated in black. In *Pea3* mutant mice, the axons of specific motor pools (CM and LD, purple) fail to branch normally within their target muscles, and cell bodies are mispositioned within the spinal cord. *Abbreviations*: CM, cutaneous maximus; LD, latissimus dorsi; ETS, expression transcription factors. *Source*: From Ref. 81. (*See color insert.*)

observations have revealed that ETS protein expression marks the late, but not the early, phase of motor pool specification.

The induction of ETS protein expression has a critical role in directing late phases of motor pool differentiation. Thus in *Pea3* mutant mice, the axons of specific motor neuron pools fail to branch normally within their target muscles, and the cell bodies of these motor neurons fail to cluster and are mis-positioned within the spinal cord (Fig. 11) (81). The induction of a selective motor pool program of ETS gene expression by peripheral signals therefore coordinates cell body position within the LMC and axon terminal arborization in specific muscle targets. One target of ETS function in motor pool differentiation is a set of cell surface recognition proteins of the type-II cadherin family (84). The differential expression of type-II cadherins by chick motor neurons has been shown to regulate the segregation of motor neurons into characteristic pool patterns (84). Moreover, the expression of type-II cadherins is regulated by ETS gene activity: ectopic expression of Er81 results in the deregulation of type-II cadherin expression in the chick spinal cord, and the normal profile of expression of type-II cadherins in specific LMC pools is lost in *Pea3* mutant mice (81,84).

Together, these studies have therefore provided an initial insight into the late phase of the motor neuron pool specification. But how the early phase of motor pool specification that directs the trajectory of motor axons to specific limb muscles is achieved remains to be determined. The finding that Hox proteins have critical roles in the assignment of motor neuron columnar identity, together with fragmentary evidence that certain *Hox* genes are expressed by more restricted motor neuron subsets in the spinal cord and hindbrain (85–89), raises the possibility that Hox proteins have additional roles in the specification of motor neuron diversity.

APPLIED INSIGHTS FROM PATHWAYS OF MOTOR NEURON DIFFERENTIATION: TURNING EMBRYONIC STEM CELLS INTO MOTOR NEURONS

How can basic studies of motor neuron specification provide insights into clinically relevant aspects of motor neuron disease? The degeneration of specific classes of CNS neurons is the hallmark of many neurological disorders, a realization that has prompted interest in defining proliferative cell populations that could serve as replenishable sources of neurons for the treatment of neurodegenerative diseases. Recent studies by many different groups have begun to provide evidence that murine embryonic stem cells can be directed along specific pathways of neuronal differentiation in a systematic manner (90–94), raising the possibility that such stem cell-derived neurons could have clinical utility (95). The potential therapeutic efficacy of stem cell derived neurons, however, will depend critically on the fidelity with which in vitro generated neurons are able to recapitulate the functional properties of their embryo-derived counterparts. And even for the best characterized of ES cell derived neurons, this important issue remains far from resolved. Thus, one fundamental goal of ES cell research is to establish whether the neuronal progeny of ES cells possess functional properties that mimic those of highly differentiated neuronal subtypes generated in the context of the developing and embryo.

As discussed above, spinal motor neurons represent one class of CNS neuron that is reasonably well understood, both in their mature function and in their developmental origins. With such information about the normal pathway of motor neuron generation, it has become possible to ask whether ES cells can respond in vitro to the same extrinsic signals and generate postmitotic motor neurons through an authentic developmental pathway. Studies over the past few years have revealed that mouse ES cells can indeed generate spinal motor neurons at high efficiency, and that the pathway of motor neuron generation from ES cells recapitulates the steps of motor neuron generation in vivo (96–98).

ES cell-derived motor neurons that have been generated in vitro acquire electrophysiological properties that resemble their embryo-derived counterparts, they develop appropriate ionic currents in response to neurotransmitters, they can receive synaptic inputs and fire repetitively at rates sufficient for functional muscle contraction (98). In addition they can form functional synapses with cultured muscle cells (98). Moreover, ES cell-derived motor neurons can repopulate the embryonic and adult spinal cord in vivo (97). In an embryonic environment, ES cell motor neurons can extend axons into the periphery and form synapses with muscle targets (97). But in an adult environment, there is much more limited extension of motor axons out of the spinal cord, even under pharmacological conditions that promote axonal regeneration (99). Nevertheless, these initial studies have indicated that the feasibility of applying insights into normal developmental signaling cascades, in particular the development of extracellular inductive signals, to direct the differentiation of ES cells into spinal motor neurons. The potential for ES cell-derived motor neurons to innervate target muscle cells opens the way for a systematic evaluation of the use of such neurons to restore motor function, initially in animal models of spinal cord injury and motor neuron degenerative diseases.

There are, however, several major unanswered challenges in the analysis of ES cell differentiation into motor neurons. First, the studies performed to date on ES cell differentiation into motor neurons have only examined a set of generic motor neuron properties (97). Yet, as discussed in this review, the intact spinal cord harbors approximately 100 different classes of motor neurons, each acquiring subtype specializations that are critical for the effective innervation of their cognate muscle and neuronal targets. Despite the extensive evidence for motor neuron specialization in vivo, it remains unclear whether ES cell derived motor neurons are capable of acquiring these highly specialized motor neuron subtype characters. Defining pathways of motor neuron subtype diversity and applying this information to test the developmental potential of ES cell derived motor neurons will therefore be an important aim of ES cell research aimed at curing motor neuron diseases.

A second major challenge stems from the fact that almost all studies on ES cell differentiation into motor neurons have been performed on murine ES cells (98,100). Thus, a critical clinical issue—whether human ES cells can generate motor neurons in a manner similar to their murine counterparts—is only just beginning to be examined (101). Resolving this question will eventually be essential for the effective use of ES cell-derived motor neurons in a therapeutic context.

MOTOR NEURONS AND MOTOR CONTROL

This brief review has focused on the motor neuron as an exemplar of neuronal subtype identity. But motor neurons represent only a minor fraction of the neurons that populate the ventral spinal cord. Local circuit and projection interneurons predominate (3), and both serve critical roles in the coordination of motor output. Defining functional subsets of interneurons at early stages of spinal cord development is a more challenging task than is the recognition of motor neuron subtype, and consequently much less is known about the extent of spinal interneuron diversity or about their developmental of patterns of connectivity. Yet significant advances have been made recently towards this goal (102–105), and it is clear that any satisfying understanding of the development of motor circuits in the ventral spinal cord demands a detailed accounting of local interneurons and inputs from supraspinal neurons.

Finally, although there are still formidable challenges, it is encouraging that there is renewed interest in the use of the spinal cord as a model system for addressing the link between neuronal specification and motor circuit function, a trend that has begun to accelerate the rate of progress in tackling these issues. When combined with the recent methodological advances in the cellular and genetic analysis of neural development, some of the classical and once intractable questions about the physiology and pathology of spinal-motor systems may soon begin to yield informative and clinically relevant answers.

ACKNOWLEDGMENTS

I thank the many students and postdoctoral fellows who have contributed to the studies described in this review. I am grateful also to Kathy MacArthur and

Ira Schiren for their help in preparing the manuscript. Work on motor neurons in the Jessell lab is supported by grants from the NINDS, The Harold and Leila Mathers Foundation, The George Frederick Jewett Foundation, Wings Over Wall Street/ MDA, Project ALS, The Claire and Leonard Tow family, and by the Howard Hughes Medical Institute. TMJ is an Investigator of the Howard Hughes Medical Institute.

REFERENCES

1. Edlund T, Jessell TM. Progression from extrinsic to intrinsic signaling in cell fate specification: a view from the nervous system. Cell 1999; 96:211–224.
2. Tanabe Y, Jessell TM. Diversity and pattern in the developing spinal cord. Science 1996; 274:1115–1123.
3. Brown AG. Organization in the Spinal Cord. New York: Springer, 1981:154–214.
4. Goulding M. Specifying motor neurons and their connections. Neuron 1998; 21: 943–946.
5. Hultborn H, Brownstone RB, Toth TI, Gossard JP. Key mechanisms for setting the input–output gain across the motoneuron pool. Prog Brain Res 2002; 143:77–95.
6. Jessell TM. Neuronal specification in the spinal cord: inductive signals and transcriptional codes. Nat Rev Genet 2000; 1:20–29.
7. Shirasaki R, Pfaff SL. Transcriptional codes and the control of neuronal identity. Ann Rev Neurosci 2002; 25:251–281.
8. Patten I, Placzek M. The role of Sonic hedgehog in neural tube patterning. Cell Mol Life Sci 2000; 57:1695–1708.
9. Price SR, Briscoe J. The generation and diversification of spinal motor neurons: signals and responses. Mech Dev 2004; 121:1103–1115.
10. Pierani A, Brenner-Morton S, Chiang C, Jessell TM. A sonic hedgehog-independent, retinoid-activated pathway of neurogenesis in the ventral spinal cord. Cell 1999; 97: 903–915.
11. Novitch BG, Wichterle H, Jessell TM, Sockanathan S. A requirement for retinoic acid mediated transcriptional activation in ventral patterning and motor neuron specification. Neuron 2003; 40:81–95.
12. Diez del Corral R, Olivera-Martinez I, Goriely A, Gale E, Maden M, Storey K. Opposing FGF and retinoid pathways control ventral neural pattern, neuronal differentiation, and segmentation during body axis extension. Neuron 2003; 40:65–79.
13. Marti E, Bumcrot DA, Takada R, McMahon AP. Requirement of 19K form of Sonic hedgehog for induction of distinct ventral cell types in CNS explants. Nature 1995; 375:322–325.
14. Roelink H, Porter JA, Chiang C, Tanabe Y, Chang DT, Beachy PA, Jessell TM. Floor plate and motor neuron induction by different concentrations of the amino-terminal cleavage product of sonic hedgehog autoproteolysis. Cell 1995; 81:445–455.
15. Ericson J, Morton S, Kawakami A, Roelink H, Jessell TM. Two critical periods of Sonic Hedgehog signaling required for the specification of motor neuron identity. Cell 1996; 87:661–673.
16. Ericson J, Rashbass P, Schedl A, Brenner-Morton S, Kawakami A, van Heyningen V, Jessell TM, Briscoe J. Pax6 controls progenitor cell identity and neuronal fate in response to graded Shh signaling. Cell 1997; 90:169–180.
17. Tanabe Y, William C, Jessell TM. Specification of motor neuron identity by the MNR2 homeodomain protein. Cell 1998; 95:67–80.
18. Chiang C, Litingtung Y, Lee E, Young KE, Corden JT, Westphal H, Beachy PA. Cyclopia and defective axial patterning in mice lacking Sonic Hedgehog gene function. Nature 1996; 383:407–413.

19. Briscoe J, Sussel L, Serup P, Hartigan-O'Connor D, Jessell TM, Rubenstein JL, Ericson J. Homeobox gene Nkx2.2 and specification of neuronal identity by graded Sonic hedgehog signaling. Nature 1999; 398:622–625.

20. Briscoe J, Pierani A, Jessell TM, Ericson J. A homeodomain code specifies progenitor cell identity and neuronal fate in the ventral neural tube. Cell 2000; 101:435–445.

21. Tian H, Jeong J, Harfe BD, Tabin CJ, McMahon AP. Mouse Disp1 is required in sonic hedgehog-expressing cells for paracrine activity of the cholesterol-modified ligand. Development 2005; 132:133–142.

22. Gritli-Linde A, Lewis P, McMahon AP, Linde A. The whereabouts of a morphogen: direct evidence for short- and graded long-range activity of hedgehog signaling peptides. Dev Biol 2001; 236:364–386.

23. Hynes M, Weilan Y, Wang K, Stone D, Murone M, de Sauvage F, Rosenthal A. The seven-transmembrane receptor Smoothened cell-autonomously induces multiple ventral cell types. Nat Neurosci 2000; 3:41–46.

24. Briscoe J, Chen Y, Jessell TM, Struhl G. A hedgehog-insensitive form of patched provides evidence for direct long-range patterning activity of Sonic hedgehog in the neural tube. Mol Cell 2001; 7:1279–1291.

25. Wijgerde M, McMahon JA, Rule M, McMahon AP. A direct requirement for Hedgehog signaling for normal specification of all ventral progenitor domains in the presumptive mammalian spinal cord. Genes Dev 2002; 16:849–864.

26. Lum L, Beachy PA. The Hedgehog response network: sensors, switches, and routers. Science 2004; 304:1755–1759.

27. McMahon AP, Ingham PW, Tabin CJ. Developmental roles and clinical significance of hedgehog signaling. Curr Top Dev Biol 2003; 53:1–114.

28. Persson M, Stamataki D, te Welscher P, Andersson E, Bose J, Ruther U, Ericson J, Briscoe J. Dorsal-ventral patterning of the spinal cord requires Gli3 transcriptional repressor activity. Genes Dev 2002; 16:2865–2878.

29. Bai CB, Stephen D, Joyner AL. All mouse ventral spinal cord patterning by hedgehog is Gli dependent and involves an activator function of Gli3. Dev Cell 2004; 6:103–1015.

30. Briscoe J. Hedgehog signaling: measuring ligand concentrations with receptor ratios. Curr Biol 2004; 14:889–891.

31. Jacob J, Briscoe J. Gli proteins and the control of spinal-cord patterning. EMBO Rep 2003; 8:761–765.

32. Sander M, Paydar S, Ericson J, Briscoe J, Berber E, German M, Jessell TM, Rubenstein JL. Ventral neural patterning by Nkx homeobox genes: Nkx6.1 controls somatic motor neuron and ventral interneuron fates. Genes Dev 2000; 14:2134–2139.

33. Vallstedt A, Muhr J, Pattyn A, Pierani A, Mendelsohn M, Sander M, Jessell TM, Ericson J. Different levels of repressor activity assign redundant and specific roles to Nkx6 genes in motor neuron and interneuron specification. Neuron 2001; 31:743–970.

34. Smith ST, Jaynes JB. A conserved region of engrailed, shared among all en-, gsc-, Nk1-, Nk2- and msh-class homeoproteins, mediates active transcriptional repression in vivo. Development 1996; 122:3141–3150.

35. Muhr J, Andersson E, Persson M, Jessell TM, Ericson J. Groucho-mediated transcriptional repression establishes progenitor cell pattern and neuronal fate in the ventral neural tube. Cell 2001; 104:861–873.

36. Briscoe J, Price. 2004.

37. Novitch BG, Chen AI, Jessell TM. Coordinate regulation of motor neuron subtype identity and pan-neuronal properties by the bHLH repressor Olig 2. Neuron 2001; 31:773–789.

38. Mizuguchi R, Sugimori M, Takebayashi H, Kosako H, Nagao M, Yoshida S, Nabeshima Y, Shimamura K, Nakafuku M. Combinatorial roles of olig2 and neurogenin2 in the coordinated induction of pan-neuronal and subtype-specific properties of motoneurons. Neuron 2001; 31:757–771.

39. Lu QR, Sun T, Zhu Z, Ma N, Garcia M, Stiles CD. Common developmental requirement for Olig function indicates a motor neuron/oligodendrocyte connection. Cell 2002; 109: 75–86.

40. Zhou Q, Anderson DJ. The bHLH transcription factors OLIG2 and OLIG1 couple neuronal and glial subtype specification. Cell 2002; 109:61–73.

41. Arber S, Han B, Mendelsohn M, Smith M, Jessell TM, Sockanathan S. Requirement for the homeobox gene Hb9 in the consolidation of motor neuron identity. Neuron 1999; 23:659–674.

42. Pfaff SL, Mendelsohn M, Stewart CL, Edlund T, Jessell TM. Requirement for LIM homeobox gene Isl1 in motor neruon generation reveals a motor neuron-dependent step in interneuron differentiation. Cell 1996; 84:309–320.

43. Thaler J, Harrison K, Sharma K, Lettieri K, Kehrl J, Pfaff SL. Active suppression of interneuron programs within developing motor neurons revealed by analysis of homeo-domain factor HB9. Neuron 1999; 23:675–687.

44. Thaler JP, Koo SJ, Kania A, Lettieri K, Andrews S, Cox C, Jessell TM, Pfaff SL. A postmitotic role for Isl-class LIM homeodomain proteins in the assignment of visceral spinal motor neuron identity. Neuron 2004; 41:337–350.

45. Lee SK, Pfaff SL. Synchronization of neurogenesis and motor neuron specification by direct coupling of bHLH and homeodomain transcription factors. Neuron 2003; 38: 731–745.

46. Lee SK, Lee B, Ruiz EC, Pfaff SL. Olig2 and Ngn2 function in opposition to modulate gene expression in motor neuron progenitor cells. Genes Dev 2005; 19:282–294.

47. Hollyday M. Motoneuron histogenesis and the development of limb innervation. Curr Top Dev Biol 1980; 15:181–215.

48. Landmesser L. The distribution of motor neurons supplying the chick hind limb muscles. J Physiol 1978a; 284:371–389.

49. Landmesser L. The development of motor projection patterns in the chick hind limb. J Physiol 1978b; 284:391–414.

50. Tosney KW, Hotary KB, Lance-Jones C. Specifying the target identity of motoneurons. Bioessays 1995; 17:379–382.

51. Prasad A, Hollyday M. Development and migration of avian sympathetic preganglionic neurons. J Comp Neurol 1991; 307:237–258.

52. Gutman CR, Ajmera MK, Hollyday M. Organization of motor pools supplying axial muscles in the chicken. Brain Res 1993; 609:129–136.

53. Lance-Jones C. The morphogenesis of the thigh of the mouse with special reference to tetrapod muscle homologies. J Morphol 1979; 162:275–310.

54. Bel-Vialar S, Itasaki N, Krumlauf R. Initiating Hox gene expression: in the early chick neural tube differential sensitivity to FGF and RA signaling subdivides the HoxB genes in two distinct groups. Development 2002; 129:5103–5115.

55. Dasen JS, Liu JP, Jessell TM. Motor neuron columnar fate imposed by sequential phases of Hox-c activity. Nature 2003; 425:926–933.

56. Ensini M, Tsuchida TN, Belting HG, Jessell TM. The control of rostrocaudal pattern in the developing spinal cord: specification of motor neuron subtype identity is initiated by signals from paraxial mesoderm. Development 1998; 125:969–982.

57. Liu JP, Laufer E, Jessell TM. Assigning the positional identity of spinal motor neurons. Rostrocaudal patterning of Hox-c expression by FGFs, Gdf11, and retinoids. Neuron 2001; 32:997–1012.

58. Sockanathan S, Perlmann T, Jessell TM. Retinoid receptor signaling in postmitotic motor neurons regulates rostrocaudal positional identity and axonal projection pattern. Neuron 2003; 40:1–15.

59. Shah V, Drill E, Lance-Jones C. Ectopic expression of Hoxd10 in thoracic spinal segments induces motoneurons with a lumbosacral molecular profile and axon projections to the limb. Dev Dyn 2004; 231:43–56.

60. Tsuchida T, Ensini M, Morton SB, Baldassare M, Edlund T, Jessell TM, Pfaff SL. Topographic organization of embryonic motor neurons defined by expression of LIM homeobox genes. Cell 1994; 79:957–970.

61. Sharma K, Sheng HZ, Lettieri K, Li H, Karavanov A, Potter S, Westphal H, Pfaff SL. LIM homeodomain factors Lhx3 and Lhx4 assign subtype identities for motor neurons. Cell 1998; 95:817–828.

62. Sharma K, Leonard AE, Lettieri K, Pfaff SL. Genetic and epigenetic mechanisms contribute to motor neuron pathfinding. Nature 2000; 406:515–519.

63. Thaler JP, Lee SK, Jurata LW, Gill GN, Pfaff SL. LIM factor Lhx3 contributes to the specification of motor neuron and interneuron identity through cell-type-specific protein-protein interactions. Cell 2002; 110:237–249.

64. William CM, Tanabe Y, Jessell TM. Regulation of motor neuron subtype identity by repressor activity of Mnx homeodomain proteins. Development 2003; 130:1523–1536.

65. Hollyday M, Hamburger V. An autoradiographic study of the formation of the lateral motor column in the chick embryo. Brain Res 1977; 132:197–208.

66. Sockanathan S, Jessell TM. Motor neuron derived retinoid signals determine the number and subtype identity of motor neurons in the developing spinal cord. Cell 1998; 94:503–514.

67. Niederreither K, McCaffery P, Grager UC, Chambon P, Dolle P. Restricted expression and retinoic acid induced downregulation of the retinaldehyde dehydrogenase type 2 (RALDH-2) gene during mouse development. Mech Dev 1997; 62:67–78.

68. Solomin L, Johansson CB, Zetterstorm RH, Bissonette RP, Heyman RA, Olson L, Lendahl U, Frisen J, Perlmann T. Retinoid X receptor signaling in the developing spinal cord. Nature 1998; 395:398–402.

69. Kania A, Jessell TM. Topographic motor projections in the limb imposed by LIM homeodomain protein regulation of ephrin-A:EphA interactions. Neuron 2003; 38:581–596.

70. Kania A, Johnson RL, Jessell TM. Coordinate roles for LIM homeobox genes in directing the dorsoventral trajectory of motor axons in the vertebrate limb. Cell 2000; 102:161–173.

71. Helmbacher F, Schneider-Maunoury S, Topilko P, Tiret L, Charnay P. Targeting of the EphA4 tyrosine kinase receptor affects dorsal/ventral pathfinding of limb motor axons. Development 2000; 127:3313–3324.

72. Eberhart J, Swartz M, Koblar SA, Pasquale EB, Tanaka H, Krull CE. Expression of EphA4, ephrin-A2 and ephrin-A5 during axon outgrowth to the hindlimb indicates potential roles in pathfinding. Dev Neurosci 2000; 22:237–250.

73. Eberhart J, Swartz ME, Koblar SA, Pasquale EB, Krull CE. EphA4 constitutes a population-specific guidance cue for motor neurons. Dev Biol 2002; 247:89–101.

74. Riddle RD, Ensini M, Nelson C, Tsuchida T, Jessell TM, Tabin C. Induction of the LIM homeobox gene Lmx1 by WNT7a establishes dorsoventral pattern in the vertebrate limb. Cell 1995; 83:631–640.

75. Hollyday M, Jacobson RD. Location of motor pools innervating chick wing. J Comp Neurol 1990; 302:575–588.

76. McHanwell S, Biscoe TJ. The localization of motoneurons supplying the hindlimb muscles of the mouse. Philos. Trans R Soc Lond B Biol Sci 1981; 293:477–508.

77. Hanson MG, Landmesser LT. Normal patterns of spontaneous activity are required for correct motor axon guidance and the expression of specific guidance molecules. Neuron 2004; 43:687–701.

78. Milner LD, Landmesser LT. Cholinergic and GABAergic inputs drive patterned spontaneous motoneuron activity before target contact. J Neurosci 1999; 19:3007–3022.

79. Tosney KW, Landmesser LT. Development of the major pathways for neurite outgrowth in the chick hindlimb. Dev Biol 1985; 109:193–214.

80. Lin JH, Saito T, Anderson DJ, Lance-Jones C, Jessell TM, Arber S. Functionally related motor neuron pool and muscle sensory afferent subtypes defined by coordinate ETS gene expression. Cell 1998; 95:393–407.

81. Livet J, Sigrist M, Stroebel S, De Paola V, Price SR, Henderson CE, Jessell TM, Arber S. ETS gene Pea3 controls the central position and terminal arborization of specific motor neuron pools. Neuron 2002; 35:877–892.

82. Haase G, Dessaud E, Garces A, de Bovis B, Birling M, Filippi P, Schmalbruch H, Arber S, deLapeyriere O. GDNF acts through PEA3 to regulate cell body positioning and muscle innervation of specific motor neuron pools. Neuron 2002; 35:893–905.

83. Helmbacher F, Dessaud E, Arber S, deLapeyriere O, Henderson CE, Klein R, Maina F. Met signaling is required for recruitment of motor neurons to PEA3-positive motor pools. Neuron 2003; 39:767–777.

84. Price SR, De Marco Garcia NV, Ranscht B, Jessell TM. Regulation of motor neuron pool sorting by differential expression of type II cadherins. Cell 2002; 109:205–216.

85. Bell E, Wingate RJ, Lumsden A. Homeotic transformation of rhombomere identity after localized Hoxb1 misexpression. Science 1999; 284:2168–2171.

86. Studer M, Lumsden A, Ariza-McNaughton L, Bradley A, Krumlauf R. Altered segmental identity and abnormal migration of motor neurons in mice lacking Hoxb-1. Nature 1996; 384:630–634.

87. Carpenter EM, Goddard JM, Davis AP, Nguyen TP, Capecchi MR. Targeted disruption of Hoxd-10 affects mouse hindlimb development. Development 1997; 124:4505–4514.

88. Carpenter EM. Hox genes and spinal cord development. Dev Neurosci 2002; 24:24–34.

89. Tiret L, Le Mouellic H, Maury M, Brulet P. Increased apoptosis of motoneurons and altered somatotopic maps in the brachial spinal cord of Hoxc8-deficient mice. Development 1998; 125:279–291.

90. Bain G, Kitchens D, Yao M, Huettner JE, Gottlieb DI. Embryonic stem cells express neuronal properties in vitro. Dev Biol 1995; 168:342–357.

91. Kawasaki H, Mizuseki K, Nishikawa S, Kaneko S, Kuwana Y, Nakanishi S, Nishikawa SI, Sasai Y. Induction of midbrain dopaminergic neurons from ES cells by stromal cell-derived inducing activity. Neuron 2000; 28:31–40.

92. Munoz-Sanjuan I, Brivanlou AH. Neural induction, the default model and embryonic stem cells. Nat Rev Neurosci 2002; 3:271–280.

93. Tropepe V, Hitoshi S, Sirard C, Mak TW, Rossant J, van der Kooy D. Direct neural fate specification from embryonic stem cells: a primitive mammalian neural stem cell stage acquired through a default mechanism. Neuron 2001; 30:65–78.

94. Uchida N, Buck DW, He D, Reitsma MJ, Masek M, Phan TV, Tsukamoto AS, Gage FH, Weissman IL. Direct isolation of human central nervous system stem cells. Proc Natl Acad Sci USA 2000; 97:14,720–14,725.

95. Gage FH. Mammalian neural stem cells. Science 2000; 287:1433–1438.

96. Renoncourt Y, Carroll P, Filippi P, Arce V, Alonso S. Neurons derived in vitro from ES cells express homeoproteins characteristic of motoneurons and interneurons. Mech Dev 1998; 79:185–197.

97. Wichterle H, Lieberam I, Porter JA, Jessell TM. Directed differentiation of embryonic stem cells into motor neurons. Cell 2002; 110:385–397.

98. Miles GB, Yohn DC, Wichterle H, Jessell TM, Rafuse VF, Brownstone RM. Functional properties of motoneurons derived from mouse embryonic stem cells. J Neurosci 2004; 24:7848–7858.

99. Harper JM, Krishnan C, Darman JS, Deshpande DM, Peck S, Shats I, Backovic S, Rothstein JD, Kerr DA. Axonal growth of embryonic stem cell-derived motoneurons in vitro and in motoneuron-injured adult rats. Proc Natl Acad Sci USA 2004; 101:7123–71288.

100. Wichterle H, et al. 2000.

101. Li XJ, Du ZW, Zarnowska ED, Pankratz M, Hansen LO, Pearce RA, Zhang SC. Specification of motoneurons from human embryonic stem cells. Nat Biotechnol 2005; 23:215–221.

102. Butt SJ, Kiehn O. Functional identification of interneurons responsible for left-right coordination of hindlimbs in mammals. Neuron 2003; 38:953–963.

103. Lanuza GM, Gosgnach S, Pierani A, Jessell TM, Goulding M. Genetic identification of spinal interneurons that coordinate left-rightlocomotor activity necessary for walking movements. Neuron 2004; 42:375–386.

104. Kullander K, Butt SJ, Lebret JM, Lundfald L, Restrepo CE, Rydstrom A, Klein R, Kiehn O. Role of EphA4 and EphrinB3 in local neuronal circuits that control walking. Science 2003; 299:1889–1892.

105. Sapir T, Geiman EJ, Wang Z, Velasquez T, Mitsui S, Yoshihara Y, Frank E, Alvarez FJ, Goulding M. Pax6 and engrailed 1 regulate two distinct aspects of renshaw cell development. J Neurosci 2004; 24:1255–1264.

106. Briscoe J, Ericson J. Specification of neuronal fates in the ventral neural tube. Curr Opin Neurobiol 2001; 1:43–49.

12

Neurodegeneration in Amyotrophic Lateral Sclerosis

Gabriele Almer
Department of Neurology, Columbia University, New York, New York, U.S.A.

Wim Robberecht
Department of Neurology, School of Medicine, University Hospital Gasthuisberg, University of Leuven, Leuven, Belgium

INTRODUCTION

As discussed by Przedborski et al. (1), neurodegenerative diseases refer to a group of neurological disorders with heterogeneous clinical and pathological expressions affecting specific groups of neurons in specific functional anatomic systems. Most arise for unknown reasons and progress in a relentless manner. To date several approved drugs do, to some extent, alleviate symptoms of several neurodegenerative diseases, but their chronic use is often associated with serious side effects, and none seems to stop or even slow the inexorable clinical worsening. It is thus not surprising to note that neurodegenerative diseases represent a growing scientific and medical challenge with far-reaching social, ethical, and financial implications.

Among the most devastating neurodegenerative disorders is amyotrophic lateral sclerosis (ALS), which represents a prototype of fatal motor neuron degenerative conditions. Like for several other neurodegenerative disorders, our failure in developing effective preventive or protective therapies stems from our limited understanding of the etiology and the pathogenesis of ALS. Yet the intense research efforts in ALS, together with the explosion of new genetic and molecular discoveries in the field of motor neuron diseases, have considerably improved the odds of finding in near future, if not a cure, an effective means to alter the course of this fatal illness.

In this book, several chapters provide in-depth discussions about selected genetic and molecular advances relevant to the neurobiology of ALS such as apoptosis, oxidative stress, and mitochondrial dysfunction. These different chapters are expected to provide the readers with a comprehensive update on prominent aspects of ALS both from clinical and molecular viewpoints. As a preamble, we will discuss several more general issues related to neurodegeneration in ALS, which should help in setting the stage for the more focused chapters to follow.

ALS OR THE TALE OF THE LUMPERS AND THE SPLITTERS

One of the central issues that plagues ALS, which we believe goes to the heart of how one may have to study the molecular mechanisms responsible for the initiation and progression of the neurodegenerative process to develop effective neuroprotective strategies, is whether ALS is a *disease* or rather a *syndrome*. Usually, ALS is a diagnosis given to patients afflicted with an adult-onset paralytic condition due to the loss of upper motor neurons, lower motor neurons, or both (2). At the early stage of the disease, the clinical features of ALS can be confused with that of alternative neurological illnesses such as myopathy, spondylotic myelopathy, or radiculopathy (3). However, soon the combination of upper and lower motor neuron symptoms distinguishes ALS from any other neurological disease. Still, the question remains whether this diagnosis relates to nosological entity, or whether it covers a range of conditions with a variety of etiologies and pathogenic mechanisms.

Like many other prominent neurodegenerative disorders, ALS is essentially sporadic, and only in less than 5% to 10% of the cases it arises as a familial condition inherited as a simple Mendelien trait (Table 1). The clinical and pathological expressions of sporadic and familial cases of ALS are almost indistinguishable (2). As classification of neurodegenerative diseases still rely on the combination of clinical and neuropathological criteria, ALS might be looked at as a single entity. However, there is evidence that suggests that the common clinical picture (i.e., adult-onset progressive paralysis), as seen in ALS, could be provoked by many distinct etiological factors with completely different molecular bases. Although most experts in ALS recognize this issue, we still lack proper tools to either confirm or refute this view with confidence.

Table 1 ALS Phenotypes

Predominant motor neuron involvement	
Sporadic ALS	
FALS	
Autosomal-dominant FALS	
ALS1 (mutations in SOD1)	Chromosome 21
ALS3	Chromosome 18
ALS4 (mutations in senataxin)	Chromosome 9
ALS6	Chromosome 16
ALS7	Chromosome 20
ALS8 (mutations in VAPB)	Chromosome 20
ALSX	X Chromosome
Autosomal-recessive FALS	
Mutations in SOD1	Chromosome 21
ALS2 (mutations in alsin)	Chromosome 2
ALS5 (juvenile ALS)	Chromosome 15
Motor neuron involvement in other diseases	
Hereditary	
Frontotemporal dementia	Chromosome 9
Machado-Joseph disease	Chromosome 14
Hexosaminidase-A deficiency	Chromosome 15
Unknown origin	
ALS-PDC of Guam	

Abbreviations: FALS, Familial ALS; ALS, amyotrophic lateral sclerosis; SOD1, superoxide dismutase-1; ALS-PDC, ALS-Parkinsonism-Dementia-Complex.

A major change in the way clinicians and scientists now look at ALS results from the inclusion in the diagnostic criteria of information generated by other means than clinical- and neuropathological-based techniques. According to this new school of thought, one no longer favors classifying ALS solely upon clinical and neuropathological features, but also upon molecular characteristics. This view is particularly well illustrated by the discovery of mutations in the gene encoding for superoxide dismutase-1 (SOD1), which are linked to the occurrence of a familial form of adult-onset paralytic disorder that is unanimously named ALS (4). Yet, whether *mutant SOD1-linked* ALS (the best studied form of autosomal dominant ALS) is the same disease as *sporadic* ALS remains a question of fierce debate. This question is more than a simple point of semantics since the potential clinical heterogeneity of ALS may represent a critical hurdle in the successful design of neuroprotective therapies. Indeed, interventions geared toward suppressing the expression of mutant SOD1 to treat mutant SOD1-linked ALS may prove ineffective in improving sporadic ALS patients.

In light of this, it is our position that the conventional clinical- and neuropathological based lumping of all cases of ALS should be recast into a more molecular-based subclassification. This holds the promise of being more meaningful from a neurobiological point-of-view. On the other hand, common pathways may well be involved in several of the ALS subforms, allowing a strategy to be developed that will be applicable to all of these.

INITIATION OF MOTOR NEURON DEGENERATION

The cause of sporadic ALS is essentially unknown and even when, as in some rare familial cases, the etiology has been identified (i.e., SOD1 mutations), the mechanism by which the etiological factor initiates the demise of motor neuron remains, at best, speculative. In the following, we review the current knowledge about the etiology of the various forms of ALS.

SOD1 Mutations

In about 20% of families with autosomal dominant motor neuron diseases labeled as ALS, mutations in SOD1 are found (4). This gene on chromosome 21 encodes SOD1, an enzyme that acts as a homodimer and converts superoxide anions into hydrogen peroxide, which is then further inactivated, e.g., by catalase. More than 100 mutations have been identified in this 153 amino acid-long peptide (for an updated overview of these mutations please refer to www.alsod.org). Most of them are missense mutations, while a few deletions and insertions have been found affecting the *C*-terminal segment of the protein.

It remains unclear as to how mutations in this ubiquitous protein cause an adult-onset condition characterized by an almost selective death of motor neurons (5). Mice and rats overexpressing a mutated human SOD1 develop a motor neuron degeneration, which faithfully reflects human ALS (see below), while mice in which the SOD1 gene has been deleted do not develop a motor neuron degeneration. Therefore, and because of the dominant nature of its inheritance, it is generally accepted that the mutated SOD1 acquires a novel property apparently particularly toxic to motor neurons.

Two main hypotheses have been suggested to explain this newly gained effect (5,6). There is evidence that the mutations may subtly change the enzyme's conformation, so that "aberrant" substrates can interact with the copper in its active center, resulting in the generation of highly reactive oxidants. Hydrogen peroxide and peroxynitrite (formed by superoxide anions and NO) are two such possibilities through which the action of the mutant SOD1 may give rise to reactive species like hydroxyl radicals and nitronium ions. Alternatively, it has been suggested that the affinity of mutant SOD1 for zinc is reduced, resulting in reduction of the copper in its center. This would result in the formation of superoxide anions from oxygen through an inversed dismutation. These oxidative actions may explain the presence of oxidative damage to proteins, lipids, and nucleic acids observed in tissue of both human ALS and SOD1 mice (reviewed in Robberecht (7)). However, reducing the copper content of SOD1 [by deleting the gene for the copper chaperone for SOD (CCS), which is necessary for copper to be incorporated in SOD1] does not alter the disease course of mutant SOD1 mice (8), and mutation of the four copper binding histidine residues, which results in a copper-less enzyme, still causes motor neuron disease in mice (9).

Alternatively, the mutated SOD1 may have an abnormal tendency to form complexes with itself, wild type SOD1, and a variety of other cellular constituents (10). Structural studies have offered support for such action (11). These complexes may form fibrillary structures and cellular aggregates in a further stage. Such aggregates are indeed a characteristic feature in some mutant SOD1 models, and are also present in human ALS tissue (12). Some element in this process of multimerization and fibril and aggregate formation is thought to be toxic to the cell. Aggregates may strangulate the axonal transport system, sequester essential cellular constituents, or simply disturb cellular homeostasis by overwhelming the cellular protein chaperoning or proteasomal degrading system (5,13).

These two hypotheses are of course not mutually exclusive. Oxidative stress may induce conformational changes, making proteins prone to multimerization, and aggregates may be a source of reactive oxygen species, causing oxidative stress and damage.

The clinical phenotype associated with SOD1 mutations is quite variable. Some mutations (e.g., the A4V and the G93C mutations) are characterized by almost pure lower motor involvement (clinically and pathologically), while others are associated with prominent lower *and* upper motor neuron involvement. Some mutations (e.g., A4V) induce a fulminant disease being fatal within a year, while others (e.g., G93C) cause disease with a protracted course. Whether this phenotypic variation reflects a quantitative difference in the toxicity of the mutant SOD1 protein or is indicative of differences in the mechanism of toxicity of the different mutations is unknown, but is pivotal for our understanding of mutant SOD1-induced ALS. The recent finding that some SOD1 mutants may have different affinities to adhere to mitochondrial membranes and that mitochondrial membranes may show quantitative and qualitative differences among upper versus lower motor neurons, moves the field forward in that regard (14).

Other Genetic Causes for ALS

As shown in Table 1, other mutations that cause dominant ALS have been found in genes localized on chromosomes 16, 18, 20, and, surprisingly, on the X chromosome (15). A form associated with frontal dementia has been mapped to chromosome 9, and a juvenile form of dominant ALS (ALS4) has also been found. The latter is linked to mutations in senataxin, a protein possibly involved in RNA metabolism

(16). Of note, the phenotype of ALS4 is quite different from classical ALS and probably should be considered to be a distal hereditary motor neuropathy (HMN) with upper motor neuron signs. Apart from these dominant forms, two *recessive* forms of juvenile ALS have been mapped to chromosomes 2 and 15. Thus far, at least for the former, the actual gene harboring the ALS-like mutations has been identified (17,18). Its product, named alsin, of which a large and a small splice variant exist, contains guanosine exchange factor domains and appears as an endosomal protein (19,20). The clinical phenotype associated with alsin mutations is quite variable, but certainly seems to differ from classical ALS. How the absence of this protein gives rise to motor neuron degeneration is unclear. However, in light of its mode of inheritance, it is likely that alsin provokes motor neuron disease by a loss of function effect.

Mutations in other genes have also been identified in isolated cases, making their significance difficult to evaluate. In a handful of ALS patients, mostly sporadic cases, mutations in the heavy subunit of neurofilament have been identified (see below) (21–23). In addition, one patient was found to harbor a mutation in the gene encoding the glial glutamate transporter, EAAT2, possibly resulting in excitotoxic insult (see below) (24,25). One patient with a cytochrome oxidase (COX) subunit I mutation has been described (26).

Genetics and Sporadic ALS

Most investigators consider sporadic ALS to be the result of an interplay between genetic and environmental factors, interacting on the background of aging. Few environmental and genetic factors have been investigated thoroughly for their etiological significance. The important topic of the potential role of environmental factors in the etiology of ALS is reviewed by Dr. Shaw in chapter 18, whereas that of genetics is discussed by Dr. Vance in chapter 19.

In summary, it is thus fair to conclude that genetic forms have indeed provided some clues as to how motor neuron disease may be initiated in ALS. It is also clear that, at this time, little is known about the neurobiology of different mutations and that a plausible unifying scenario by which the different ALS-linked mutations initiate the degenerative process is yet to be formulated. Alternatively, it is also possible that the impression given by the different mutations of highly divergent mechanisms of neurodegeneration in ALS is accurate, a prospect that would be consistent with our position that ALS is a syndrome and not a disease.

NATURAL COURSE OF ALS

Typically, we follow the clinical expression of ALS in a patient to reach conclusions about the natural history of his/her disease. Again this is more than an academic preoccupation, as this information may help to link specific temporal events with the development of motor neuron disease as illustrated in the study from the Veterans Affairs Administration (27). It is also important to know with precision when ALS started and how it progresses in a patient for the purpose of neuroprotection clinical trials.

Once the neurodegenerative process in ALS is initiated under the effect of the etiological factor, the motor system becomes compromised, eventually leading to the emergence of a variety of specific symptoms, which, by the progressive nature of the disease, worsen over time. Most patients suffering from ALS can reasonably recall the onset of symptoms. However, it is quite important to remember that because of the neuronal redundancy in both the upper and lower motor neuronal pathways, the onset of symptoms does not equate with the onset of the disease. In reality, the beginning of symptoms corresponds to a situation in which either the number of residual motor neurons or their functionality falls below a threshold of what is required to maintain normal functioning of the neuromuscular system. This means the onset of the disease occurs at some earlier time, which can range from a few months to years. Unfortunately, in ALS, as in many other neurodegenerative diseases, the lack of presymptomatic markers and understanding of the kinetics of motor neuron death prevent determination of the disease onset per se.

It is also important to emphasize that in virtually all neurodegenerative disorders compromised neurons become dysfunctional well before succumbing to the disease. This means that a patient may grow weaker and more disabled over a short period of time because of a rapid functional deterioration of the compromised neurons, while the actual number of neurons remains essentially unchanged. Support for this scenario comes from the work of Kong and Xu (28) which clearly shows that transgenic mice expressing mutant SOD1 (used as a model of ALS) exhibited a rapid loss of their motor ability during a time frame in which obvious loss of lower motor neurons could not be demonstrated. A recent study confirmed that motor neurons remain present until mutant SOD1 mice have well advanced in their symptomatic stage (29). This may also be the case in human ALS, as suggested by the finding of normally appearing motor neurons in an ALS patient who accidentally happened to die early in the disease course (29).

It is difficult to determine the extent of contribution of decreased neuronal function and cell death to the overall disability of ALS patients. Yet, the contribution of both factors is important to recognize as therapeutic strategies aimed at boosting the function of sick motor neurons may be less challenging to develop than those aimed at preventing their death, and both could play a complementary and meaningful role for the optimal management of ALS patients.

In this context, it is also worth looking at the temporal distribution that the actual death of motor neurons in ALS follows during the course of disease. Notwithstanding the inherent limitations of applying in vitro data to in vivo situations, cell culture experiments have generated important insights into the temporal aspect of cell death within a given population of cells. Depending on the nature of the death stimulus, cells in vitro either die within a small time frame after the initial insult, more or less simultaneously or over an extended period of time with a small percentage of cells undergoing actual cell death at any point of time. The first, *synchronous demise*, is generally thought to be associated with neuronal death occurring in pathological situations such as trauma and stroke. The second, *asynchronous demise*, is often thought to be associated with less harsh and more chronic diseases of the brain such as neurodegenerative disorders. Indeed, the clinical course of neurodegenerative diseases with an insidious onset and a slow continuous progression of symptoms over a few years as in ALS is not consistent with a singular or even several distinct phases of simultaneous degeneration of a large number of neurons, but rather suggests a continuum of the degenerative process at a certain pace. The notion of an asynchronous form of cell death is in line with findings from neuropathology in ALS postmortem tissue and affected tissue in mutant SOD1 mice that invariably describe the coexistence of remaining healthy motor neurons next to motor neurons at different stages of degeneration (30,31). This view suggests that at any given time, motor neurons are at different stages of the pathogenic cascade and are subjected to the deleterious effects of different noxious molecular factors. Incidentally, if correct, this concept would argue that optimal treatment aimed at impeding ALS pathogenesis has to target multiple factors at once.

THE MECHANISM OF NEURONAL DEATH IN ALS

It is customarily considered that while etiology refers to the initiating factor of the disease, the mechanism by which the actual neuronal death occurs is called pathogenesis. It is true, however, that both etiology and pathogenesis are rather intermingled with no real beginning or end and that this popular division is somewhat artificial. Nevertheless, separating etiology from pathogenesis has many advantages, especially, as we will find below, for the purpose of discussing generic mechanisms of cell death recruited by the etiologic factor.

According to a popular scenario, once the disease is initiated by the etiologic factor, a cascade of deleterious events is set in motion, which ultimately leads to the cell's demise. Here, it is thus speculated that while the etiological factor may be different among all forms of ALS, the triggered pathogenic cascade would consistently be comprised of a similar set of noxious factors, such as impaired protein turnover, altered mitochondrial function, and apoptosis. The real challenges in terms of studying pathogenesis reside in cataloging all the molecular and cellular perturbations observed in postmortem tissues from ALS patients and experimental models of ALS, distinguishing between changes that reflect bystander alterations and true pathogenic changes, and finally defining in which sequence the different pathogenic events act within the neurodegenerative cascade of events.

NEUROPATHOLOGY OF ALS ILLUMINATES ITS PATHOGENESIS

Inspection of the sites of the neurodegenerative process in ALS may provide important information on the nature of cell death. In this regard, our interest in ALS neuropathology is two-fold: first, it is directed toward the morphology of the remaining motor neurons comprising both healthy and dying motor neurons at various stages of degeneration. Second, attention should be paid to the environment embedding motor neuron degeneration since numerous data suggest a contribution to motor neuron demise by phenomena originating in the surrounding of the motor neuron notably by inflammatory and glia-mediated processes.

Motor Neuron Pathology

As in other neurodegenerative diseases the target cells of the neurodegenerative process in ALS, i.e., motor neurons, display intracellular aggregates forming distinct inclusion bodies. They not only serve as neuropathological hallmarks of disease, but also represent intriguing phenomena that allow speculation on the nature of molecular mechanisms involved in the cell's demise. From a confusing plethora of nomenclatures, three types of inclusion bodies can be differentiated: ubiquitinated inclusions, Bunina bodies, and hyaline conglomerate inclusions (32).

Found abundantly in lower motor neurons of the brainstem and spinal cord, ubiquitinated inclusions can adapt a filamentous (skein-like) or a rounded and more compact shape (33). As implied by their name, these inclusions are invariably immuno-reactive for ubiquitin, a recognized cellular marker for proteins that are destined to be degraded in the cell's protein degradation machinery, ultimately leading to pro-teasomal digestion (ubiquitin/proteasome pathway). The main protein constituent of these inclusions, however, remains to be determined. In light of the physiologi-cal role of ubiquitin in the cellular protein degradation program, the abundance of this type of inclusion in ALS intrigues to speculate on a mechanism involving protein misfolding and accumulation and subsequent exhaustion of the protein degradation system. Along this line, identification of the mysterious ubiquitinated proteins that compose these inclusions becomes a crucially important issue that is likely to provide major insight into ALS pathobiology.

Bunina bodies are small eosinophilic inclusions detectable in the cell bodies of spinal motor neurons of ALS postmortem specimens. In contrast to ubiquitinated inclusions, Bunina bodies are not confined to motor neurons but have also been reported in other neurons (e.g., The subthalamic nucleus and the reticular formation of the brainstem) (34). Ultrastructural studies have revealed features suggestive of a lysosomal origin (35).

Less frequently, hyaline conglomerates are found in ALS motor neurons. This third type of intracellular inclusion is highly immunoreactive for neurofilament in both its phosphorylated and unphosphorylated forms. Notwithstanding the relative paucity of this type of intracellular inclusion in ALS postmortem tissue, the existence of inclusion bodies that are to a large extent composed of neurofilament subunits has prompted investigators to implicate a possible alteration of neurofilament assembly and transport in ALS pathophysiology. The potential implication of alterations in neurofilaments and other cytoskeletal elements in ALS pathophysiology will be addressed by Drs. Strong and Julien in Chapter 16.

Of special interest in our approach to revisit ALS pathology for potential clues for pathogenesis is the examination of motor neurons in familial cases of ALS (FALS) linked to mutations in the SOD1 gene. In line with the above mentioned hypotheses of pathological accumulation and aggregation of mutant SOD1, there is morphological evidence of SOD1 protein accumulation in at least a subset of SOD1-linked FALS cases (36). These formations display morphological features dis-tinct from inclusion bodies found in sporadic cases suggesting that different molecu-lar pathways underlie the formation of inclusions in familial and sporadic ALS cases. However, the presence of SOD1 containing inclusions in cases of FALS may repre-sent an important key to the puzzle of ALS pathophysiology.

Intracellular aggregation of mutant SOD1 is also well documented in transgenic mice expressing disease-linked human SOD1 mutations. Interestingly, SOD1 aggre-gates in these mice have been shown to contain ubiquitin, proteasome components, and molecular chaperones. Since all these molecules are known to be involved in the cellular protein degradation machinery, these findings provide yet another body of evidence that SOD1-mediated neurodegeneration involves an alteration of protein folding and degradation.

Non-Neuronal Pathology

Aside from the obvious selective neuronal loss and the above-described morphologi-cal changes of the remaining motor neurons affected, ALS tissue also invariably displays alterations of non-neuronal structures. Affected areas in both human ALS tissue and the mutant SOD1 mouse model have been shown to be the sites of a robust glial reaction composed of abundant activated microglia and astrocytes (37,38).

Increasing evidence has emerged suggesting an active role of glial cells in the process of neuronal death. Although this influence is not thought to be a primary event in ALS pathogenesis, there is reason to believe that glia-mediated secondary events significantly contribute to the propagation and progression of disease. The finding that expression of mutant SOD1 in neurons alone does not result in motor neuron degeneration in transgenic mice supports such a concept (39), but the interpretation of these results is hampered by the fact that the levels of expression in these mice may just have been too low. Deleting the mutant SOD1 gene from astrocytes in animals with ubiquitous overexpression of mutant SOD1 at a level sufficient for initiating disease is a currently pursued strategy to clarify this issue.

The marked microglial proliferation as part of an atypical inflammatory reaction seen in ALS, as in other neurodegenerative diseases, has attracted much attention recently. Activated microglia cells have been shown to release a variety of pro-inflammatory cytokines and enzymes including IL-6, TNF-alpha, and cyclooxygenase-2 (40,41). The local inflammatory reaction is enhanced by lymphocyte infiltrates releasing additional inflammatory mediators. It is tempting to speculate that these neurotoxic compounds contribute to the degeneration of motor neurons. The nature of the molecular pathways that are initiated by these events and their presumed influence on neuronal viability will be discussed in detail by Drs. Yen, Simpson, and Appel in Chapter 22.

NEURONAL DEATH PATHWAYS IN ALS

Programmed Cell Death (PCD)—Definition

Numerous data originating from transgenic mutant SOD1 mice suggest that motor neuron cell death is an active process in the sense that it is mediated by specific intracellular signaling pathways. Traditionally, the concept of an actively regulated cell death has been equated with apoptosis and was opposed to necrosis, which has been considered the passive mode of cell death. There is increasing evidence that this dichotomy that has dominated our view on neuronal death in both normal development and pathologic conditions for many years is obsolete as it fails to reflect the full spectrum of morphological and mechanistic diversity of cell death.

In essence, four different types of neuronal cell death can be differentiated on the basis of morphological criteria: apoptotic, autophagic, cytoplasmic, and necrotic cell death (42). The morphology of apoptotic cell death is characterized by nuclear and cytoplasmic condensation, chromatin clumping along the inside of the nuclear envelope, and preservation of cytoplasmic organelles. The dominant features of autophagic cell death are numerous cytoplasmic autophagic vacuoles. There has been debate about the distinctness of this type of cell death and apoptosis, but a number of data suggest a different mechanistic basis (43). Cytoplasmic cell death is associated with dilation of organelles and the perinuclear space. Little is known about the molecular pathways involved in this form of cell death. Finally, necrosis is characterized by dilation and fragmentation of organelles, scattering of nuclear chromatin, nuclear shrinkage, and loss of cell membrane integrity. While the first three forms of cell death are considered to be active in the sense of involving active intracellular signaling pathways, necrosis has generally been classified as a passive form of cell death. However, many of the doctrines regarding the paradigms and the classification of cell death have been subject to criticism and re-evaluation, as will be discussed later. Although little is known about the molecular mechanisms involved in these forms of cell death, there is evidence that they are distinct from the well-studied apoptotic pathways (44). Most noteworthy in this regard is the fact that there has been data suggestive of the presence of an inherent active signaling element also in necrotic cell death (45,46).

In light of the ongoing changes in the doctrine about apoptosis and necrosis, the use of the term PCD in the sense of a cell death that is actively mediated by specific signaling pathways has been advocated (47). As such, this term is defined by mechanistic instead of morphological criteria and therefore more useful and relevant in the context of studying mechanisms and pathways of cell death. By definition, apoptosis is a form of PCD and undoubtedly the most thoroughly studied form. However, since there are other forms of cell death that involve active intracellular programs, the use of the terms apoptosis and PCD as synonyms should be avoided.

Programmed Cell Death in ALS

Morphological Characteristics

When studying the nature of neuronal death in ALS in an attempt to elucidate the underlying pathobiological mechanisms, a key question relates to the morphological type of cell death. In ALS, ultrastructural analysis of the morphology of dying motor neurons in human postmortem samples has been performed in a detailed study, which proposed to categorize remaining motor neurons according to their appearance into three distinct groups supposedly corresponding to different stages of the neurodegenerative process (30). Along this line, the earliest changes detectable in the chromatolysis stage are an eccentrically placed nucleus and dispersion of the Nissl substance in an otherwise normally looking motor neuron. The second distinct morphological category, the attritional stage, shows a shrunken cell body of multipolar shape with nucleus and cytoplasm appearing homogenous and condensed. Finally, in the apoptotic stage the motor neuron substantially decreases in size and the cell body adopts a fusiform shape devoid of any process with cytoplasm and nucleus being extremely condensed. However, the morphological criteria of apoptosis consisting of cytoplasmic and nuclear condensation, formation of nuclear chromatin clumps along the inside of the nuclear membrane, and structural preservation of organelles are only partly met by some of these remaining neurons and therefore none of these cells can be identified as definitely apoptotic based on their structural morphology.

In light of the inconclusive data on the presence of apoptotic cells in human ALS tissue, it becomes an intriguing question whether morphological evidence for apoptosis can be found in mutant SOD1 mice. Morphological studies addressing this question have revealed a diversity of dying motor neurons (28,48). Most of the remaining motor neurons seen are atrophic with dilated cell organelles appearing as vacuoles in the cytoplasm. According to the above stated criteria for apoptosis, these cells cannot be categorized as apoptotic and are rather reminiscent of autophagic or cytoplasmic neuronal death. However, cells displaying all features of apoptosis have been encountered in rare cases in the spinal cords of mutant SOD1 mice, and these cells have been identified to be of both neuronal and glial origin (49,50).

In summary, the data on motor neuron pathology reviewed here yields inconclusive results on the morphological categorization of motor neuron cell death in ALS. Although certain findings are compatible with an apoptotic nature of the cell death process, a clear and confident statement about whether apoptosis plays a role in ALS cannot be made on the basis of morphological findings. Therefore, it seems more relevant to our research efforts to determine whether the neurodegenerative process involves known pathways of PCD.

Identification of PCD Pathways

PCD comprises a number of molecular pathways including survival and death pathways. The most thoroughly studied elements of the molecular death machinery include the regulatory members of the bcl-2 family and the death-promoting pathways effectuated by the sequential activation of caspases. The complex molecular events involving these elements of PCD will be discussed in detail by Dr. Friedlander in chapter 15.

Recent studies suggest that alternative pathways may be involved. These comprise activation of the p38 mitosis-activated protein kinase (MAPK) system as well as the binding of Fas ligand to its receptor, the recruitment and activation of Daxx, ASK1 and the transcriptional upregulation of neuronal nitric oxide synthase (nNOS) (51). Motor neurons cultured from mutant SOD1 mice were more sensitive to this pathway than wild-type motor neurons. Deleting the gene encoding the nNOS enzyme does not alter the clinical expression of the disease of mutant SOD1 mice, but the remaining NOS genes may be a sufficient source of NO to exert its deleterious effect (52). Treating mutant SOD1 animals with an inhibitor of nNOS paradoxically did affect the mouse life span (52). The effects of p38 activation are diverse, but an interesting aspect is the upregulation of the cyclin-dependent kinase (cdk)-4 system (53). A hypothetical mechanism to drive postmitotic neurons into cell death pathways may indeed be to activate a mitotic program. Whether these pathways are instrumental in motor neuron degeneration in ALS remains to be seen.

Other members of the cdk family have been studied in ALS as well. Cdk5 is known to be activated by two neuronally expressed proteins, p35 and p39. The p35 is well studied in ALS. It has been suggested that at least in the spinal cord of transgenic mice expressing SOD1^{G37R}, p35 is abnormally cleaved by calpain into p25 (53). This leads to abnormal cdk5 activation in the cytosol, which promotes hyperphosphorylation and cell death. Overexpression of p25 results in motor neuron loss in mice (54). Disappointingly, deletion of the p35 gene does not attenuate motor neuron disease in transgenic mice expressing SOD1^{G93A}, although the remaining p39 activator may be sufficient to maintain the abnormal cdk5 activity (55).

FACTORS CONTRIBUTING TO MOTOR NEURON DEATH IN ALS

Although not considered as primary etiological factors, numerous molecular events have been well established as potent contributors and/or modulators of the neurodegenerative process in ALS. In the following, we will review the most prominent scenarios and their presumed mode of influence on motor neuron cell death.

Excitotoxicity

Motor neurons appear to be prone to glutamate-induced excitotoxicity, both in vivo and in vitro. This is because they allow large amounts of calcium to enter their cytoplasm upon stimulation of the AMPA-type of glutamate receptors, due to the low abundance of the GluR2 subunit in the receptor in humans and some animal models. The involvement of excitotoxicity in the pathogenesis of ALS is suggested by a large set of experimental data, but the evidence remains indirect. Highly suggestive of such an involvement is the fact that compounds that interfere with glutamate transmission have been shown to provide a therapeutic effect in both human patients and SOD1 mice. The plethora of data documenting the relevance of glutamate-mediated cell death in ALS is reviewed in detail by Dr. Shaw in chapter 12.

Heat Shock Proteins and Motor Neurons

SOD1 mutations generate a stress response, characterized by the induction of heat shock proteins (HSP). This response is thought to represent a defense mechanism for the cell, although this has never been demonstrated. HSP27 and HSP70 are the most studied HSPs in ALS. HSP27 has known antiapoptotic activity in addition to its ATP-independent chaperoning activity. HSP70 is thought to be involved in ATP-dependent protein chaperoning.

In vivo, HSP27 and to a lesser degree αB-crystallin, but not HSP70, are up-regulated in the spinal cord of mutant SOD1 mice (56). This HSP27 is mainly present in proliferating glial cells, while it appears to disappear from the motor neurons' cytoplasm. This may contribute to the imbalance of pro- and antiapoptotic pathways in the mutant SOD1 motor neuron (57). This can only be speculated upon as the exact function of small HSPs in (motor) neurons remains far from being understood. However, the recent finding that mutations in HSP22 and HSP27 cause HMNs demonstrates, that these proteins are pivotal to the integrity of motor neurons and axons, an effect possibly mediated through an interaction with cytoskeletal elements (58,59).

HSP70 is not upregulated in the mutant SOD1 spinal cord, but it can be induced by treating animals with arimoclomol. This compound significantly prolongs the life span of mutant SOD1 mice (60). Whether this effect is mediated through the upregulation of HSP70, remains to be seen. In vitro, HSP70 can protect motor neurons from the toxic effect of overexpression of mutant SOD1 (61).

Finally, the ability to generate a HSP response has also been suggested to at least contribute to the selectivity of motor neuron death in ALS. Motor neurons seem to be poor inducers of HSPs, and this may be due to their lack of response to HSF-1 (62).

Hypoxia and Motor Neuron Vulnerability

The unexpected involvement of vascular endothelial growth factor (VEGF) in the pathogenesis of ALS is interesting, but needs further study. Mice, in which the hypoxia-responsive element of the VEGF promoter has been deleted, develop an adult-onset progressive motor neuron degeneration with progressive muscle atrophy and paresis (63). How low VEGF levels are in this model result in motor neuron loss is unclear, but it is known that VEGF can directly affect motor neuron biology, as a protective effect of this factor on motor neurons could be demonstrated in vitro (64). The relevance of this finding for human ALS comes from a collaborative study of Swedish, Belgian, and English investigators who found that sequence polymorphisms associated with low levels of VEGF were more frequent in ALS patients, albeit not in all populations (65). A recent study confirmed that ALS patients have lower VEGF levels in the cerebrospinal fluid than controls, but the number of individuals studied was low. The significance of VEGF for motor neuron survival, exerted through a vascular or neurotrophic mechanism of action, is also shown by the recent demonstration that viral vector-mediated delivery of VEGF to motor neurons in the mutant SOD1 mouse attenuates their disease progression (66). The finding that overexpression of the VEGF receptor equally protects motor neurons from mutant SOD1-induced degeneration suggests that a direct effect at least contributes to the observed protective effect of VEGF (67). The fact that intracerebroventricularly administrated VEGF appears to prolong survival of SOD1^{G93A} rats, even when the treatment is started at onset of clinical symptoms (67), suggests that exogenous administration of VEGF has a therapeutic potential for ALS patients.

Axonal Transport and Cytoskeleton

Motor neurons are heavily dependent upon transport along their long axons, the length of which can exceed up to one meter. Not surprisingly, therefore, abnormalities of cytoskeleton and the motor protein complexes of both anterograde and retrograde axonal transport can initiate or contribute to motor neuron degeneration.

Abnormalities of axonal transport are detected very early in the course of mutant SOD1-induced motor neuron degeneration (68,69). Dysfunction of the motor system for retrograde transport gives rise to motor neuron degeneration in both man and mouse. A dominant form of bulbar motor neuron involvement (distal HMN with vocal cord paralysis) is caused by a mutation in the dynactin gene (70). Dynactin is part of an enormous protein complex that is the motor of retrograde axonal transport. Likewise, mutations in two other components of this protein complex, dynein, and dynamitin, cause motor neuron degeneration in mice (71,72).

COMMON PATHOGENIC THEMES FOR MOTOR NEURON DEGENERATION

The study of the biology of motor neuron disorders including ALS, hereditary spastic paraparesis, spinomuscular atrophy, and HMN suggests common themes in their pathogenesis.

Some motor neuron disorders are caused by disturbances of the solubility of proteins, their turnover and degradation. Mutant SOD1-associated ALS may well be an example. X-linked bulbospinal muscular atrophy (Kennedy's disease), caused by a CAG repeat in the first exon of the androgen receptor protein leading to polyglutamin-mediated aggregate formation, is another (73).

Mutations in the molecular pathways of RNA metabolism can induce motor neuron degeneration. The best-studied example is spinomuscular atrophy caused by mutations in the survival motor neuron 1 (*SMN1*) gene (74). SMN1 is involved in the complex process of RNA transport and processing. Mutations in senataxin, which contains a helicase domain and is therefore likely to be involved in RNA processing, cause ALS4 (16). Mutations in immunoglobulin μ-binding protein 2 cause distal infantile spinal muscular atrophy with diaphragm paralysis (75); this protein has a DNA/RNA helicase domain and is known to play a role in RNA processing. In addition, glycyl-tRNA synthase mutations induce motor neuron disease with (Charcot-Marie-Tooth disease) or without (distal spinal muscular atrophy type V) sensory involvement (76).

Another common theme in the biology of motor neuron degeneration comprises abnormalities of axonal transport and/or the cytoskeleton. Mutations of dynein, dynactin, and dynamitin induce motor neuron degeneration, as described above. Of interest is the observation that mutations in one of the motor proteins of anterograde axonal transport, the kinesin proteins, also give rise to motor neuron disorders, such as CMT2A (77), congenital fibrosis of extra-ocular muscles (78), and spastic paraplegia (SPG10) (79).

As mentioned, alsin most likely plays a role in endosomal trafficking. Similarly, Rab7, mutated in CMT2B, is a regulator of vesicular transport and membrane trafficking, and is involved in recruitment of dynein/dynactin proteins and transport along microtubules through its effector protein RILF (80). In addition, spastin, a protein in which mutations cause SPG4, is a protein with microtubule severing properties (81).

Further examples for common mechanisms shared by different motor neuron diseases are abnormalities of chaperoning factors and the stress response. HSP22 and HSP27 mutations are found in CMT2F and HMN (58,59), possibly through their effect on the cytoskeleton. The role of HSPs in the pathogenesis of ALS has been mentioned above. HSP60, a mitochondrial protein with chaperoning activity is mutated in SPG13 (82). Paraplegin, mutations of which cause SPG7 (83), and sacsin, mutations of which cause the spastic ataxia of Charlevoix–Saguenay (84), are more examples of mutated chaperoning proteins causing motor neuron degeneration.

These examples further emphasize the importance of a classification of the motor neuron diseases on the basis of their molecular mechanism rather than on clinical grounds as a more relevant approach towards developing efficient therapeutic strategies.

CONCLUSION

While specific aspects of the biology of motor neuron degeneration in ALS will be discussed in depth in the respective chapters of this book, it has been our incentive for this chapter to address more general issues of neurodegeneration that underlie our views and approach towards this fatal disease. In this sense, we have challenged the conventional belief of ALS as a distinct clinical entity and have advocated a classification of motor neuron disease that is based on neurobiological rather than clinical or neuropathological criteria alone. In the light of increasing understanding and knowledge about the cellular and molecular events that are at the root of motor neuron disorders, we believe that such a strategy better captures the heterogeneity underlying ALS phenotypes. In our opinion, this is not only meaningful from a neurobiological point of view but may also have important implications for future therapeutic decisions. Along this line, the debates on the presence of apoptosis in ALS have prompted us to revisit data on this issue and to argue in favor of a categorization of cell death that avoids the narrow dichotomy of apoptosis-necrosis on the basis of morphological criteria, but instead relies upon mechanistic parameters.

We further addressed aspects of motor neuron disease that generally do not get a lot of attention, but may represent important determinants of success or failure of therapeutic strategies, such as the time course of ALS, notably the relationship between clinical disease and motor neuron cell death. In summary, it has been our goal in this chapter to broaden the reader's mind on a number of aspects of motor neuron disease as we believe that the plethora of new insights in the field requires adaptation of our way to look at ALS.

REFERENCES

1. Przedborski S, Vila M, Jackson-Lewis V. Series introduction: neurodegeneration: what is it and where are we? J Clin Invest 2003; 111:3–10.
2. Rowland LP, Shneider NA. Amyotrophic lateral sclerosis. N Engl J Med 2001; 344:1688–1700.
3. Mitsumoto H, Chad DA, Pioro EP. Amyotrophic Lateral Sclerosis. Philadelphia: F.A. Davis Company, 1998.
4. Rosen DR, Siddique T, Patterson D, Figlewicz DA, Sapp P, Hentati A, Donaldson D, Goto J, O'Regan JP, Deng H-X, et al. Mutations in Cu/Zn superoxide dismutase gene are associated with familial amyotrophic lateral sclerosis. Nature 1993; 362:59–62.
5. Bruijn LI, Miller TM, Cleveland DW. Unraveling the mechanisms involved in motor neuron degeneration in ALS. Annu Rev Neurosci 2004; 27:723–749.
6. Cleveland DW, Rothstein JD. From Charcot to Lou Gehrig: deciphering selective motor neuron death in ALS. Nat Rev Neurosci 2001; 2:806–819.
7. Robberecht W. Oxidative stress in amyotrophic lateral sclerosis. J Neurol 2000; 247(suppl 1):1–6.
8. Subramaniam JR, Lyons WE, Liu J, Bartnikas TB, Rothstein J, Price DL, Cleveland DW, Gitlin JD, Wong PC. Mutant SOD1 causes motor neuron disease independent of copper chaperone-mediated copper loading. Nat Neurosci 2002; 5:301–307.
9. Wang J, Slunt H, Gonzales V, Fromholt D, Coonfield M, Copeland NG, Jenkins NA, Borchelt DR. Copper-binding-site-null SOD1 causes ALS in transgenic mice: aggregates of non-native SOD1 delineate a common feature. Hum Mol Genet 2003; 12:2753–2764.
10. Wood JD, Beaujeux TP, Shaw PJ. Protein aggregation in motor neurone disorders. Neuropathol Appl Neurobiol 2003; 29:529–545.
11. Hough MA, Grossmann JG, Antonyuk SV, Strange RW, Doucette PA, Rodriguez JA, Whitson LJ, Hart PJ, Hayward LJ, Valentine JS, et al. Dimer destabilization in superoxide dismutase may result in disease-causing properties: structures of motor neuron disease mutants. Proc Natl Acad Sci USA 2004; 101:5976–5981.
12. Bruijn LI, Houseweart MK, Kato S, Anderson KL, Anderson SD, Ohama E, Reaume AG, Scott RW, Cleveland DW. Aggregation and motor neuron toxicity of an ALS-linked SOD1 mutant independent from wild-type SOD1. Science 1998; 281: 1851–1854.
13. Cleveland DW, Rothstein JD. From Charcot to Lou Gehrig: deciphering selective motor neuron death in ALS. Nat Rev Neurosci 2001; 2:806–819.
14. Liu J, Lillo C, Jonsson PA, Vande Velde C, Ward CM, Miller TM, Subramaniam JR, Rothstein JD, Marklund S, Andersen PM, et al. Toxicity of familial ALS-linked SOD1 mutants from selective recruitment to spinal mitochondria. Neuron 2004; 43:5–17.
15. Dewil M, Andersen PM, Van den Bosch L, Robberecht W. Genetics of motor neuron disease. In: Eisen A, ed. Clinical Neurophysiology of Motor Neuron Diseases. The Netherland: Elsevier Science, 2004.
16. Chen YZ, Bennett CL, Huynh HM, Blair IP, Puls I, Irobi J, Dierick I, Abel A, Kennerson ML, Rabin BA, et al. DNA/RNA helicase gene mutations in a form of juvenile amyotrophic lateral sclerosis (ALS4). Am J Hum Genet 2004; 74:1128–1135.
17. Yang Y, Hentati A, Deng HX, Dabbagh O, Sasaki T, Hirano M, Hung WY, Ouahchi K, Yan J, Azim AC, et al. The gene encoding alsin, a protein with three guanine-nucleotide exchange factor domains, is mutated in a form of recessive amyotrophic lateral sclerosis. Nat Genet 2001; 29:160–165.
18. Hadano S, Hand CK, Osuga H, Yanagisawa Y, Otomo A, Devon RS, Miyamoto N, Showguchi-Miyata J, Okada Y, Singaraja R, et al. A gene encoding a putative GTPase regulator is mutated in familial amyotrophic lateral sclerosis 2. Nat Genet 2001; 29: 166–173.
19. Topp JD, Gray NW, Gerard RD, Horazdovsky BF. Alsin is a Rab5 and Rac1 guanine nucleotide exchange factor. J Biol Chem 2004; 279:24612–24623.

20. Kanekura K, Hashimoto Y, Niikura T, Aiso S, Matsuoka M, Nishimoto I. Alsin, the product of ALS2 gene, suppresses SOD1 mutant neurotoxicity through RhoGEF domain by interacting with SOD1 mutants. J Biol Chem 2004; 279:19247–19256.

21. Al-Chalabi A, Andersen PM, Nilsson P, Chioza B, Andersson JL, Russ C, Shaw CE, Powell JF, Leigh PN. Deletions of the heavy neurofilament subunit tail in amyotrophic lateral sclerosis. Hum Mol Genet 1999; 8:157–164.

22. Figlewicz DA, Krizus A, Martinoli MG, Meininger V, Dib M, Rouleau GA, Julien JP. Variants of the heavy neurofilament subunit are associated with the development of amyotrophic lateral sclerosis. Hum Mol Genet 1994; 3:1757–1761.

23. Tomkins J, Usher P, Slade JY, Ince PG, Curtis A, Bushby K, Shaw PJ. Novel insertion in the KSP region of the neurofilament heavy gene in amyotrophic lateral sclerosis (ALS). Neuroreport 1998; 9:3967–3970.

24. Aoki M, Lin CL, Rothstein JD, Geller BA, Hosler BA, Munsat TL, Horvitz HR, Brown RH Jr. Mutations in the glutamate transporter EAAT2 gene do not cause abnormal EAAT2 transcripts in amyotrophic lateral sclerosis. Ann Neurol 1998; 43:645–653.

25. Trotti D, Aoki M, Pasinelli P, Berger UV, Danbolt NC, Brown RH Jr, Hediger MA. Amyotrophic lateral sclerosis-linked glutamate transporter mutant has impaired glutamate clearance capacity. J Biol Chem 2001; 276:576–582.

26. Comi GP, Bordoni A, Salani S, Franceschina L, Sciacco M, Prelle A, Fortunato F, Zeviani M, Napoli L, Bresolin N. Cytochrome c oxidase subunit I microdeletion in a patient with motor neuron disease. Ann Neurol 1998; 43:110–116.

27. Horner RD, Kamins KG, Feussner JR, Grambow SC, Hoff-Lindquist J, Harati Y, Mitsumoto H, Pascuzzi R, Spencer PS, Tim R, et al. Occurrence of amyotrophic lateral sclerosis among Gulf War veterans. Neurology 2003; 61:742–749.

28. Kong J, Xu Z. Massive mitochondrial degeneration in motor neurons triggers the onset of amyotrophic lateral sclerosis in mice expressing a mutant SOD1. J Neurosci 1998; 18:3241–3250.

29. Fischer LR, Culver DG, Tennant P, Davis AA, Wang M, Castellano-Sanchez A, Khan J, Polak MA, Glass JD. Amyotrophic lateral sclerosis is a distal axonopathy: evidence in mice and man. Exp Neurol 2004; 185:232–240.

30. Martin LJ. Neuronal death in amyotrophic lateral sclerosis is apoptosis: possible contribution of a programmed cell death mechanism. J Neuropathol Exp Neurol 1999; 58: 459–471.

31. Dal Canto MC, Gurney ME. Neuropathological changes in two lines of mice carrying a transgene for mutant human Cu,Zn SOD, and in mice overexpressing wild type human SOD: a model of familial amyotrophic lateral sclerosis (FALS). Brain Res 1995; 676: 25–40.

32. Wharton S, Ince PG. Pathology of motor neuron disorders. In: Shaw P, Strong MJ, eds. Motor neuron disorders. Philadelphia: Butterworth Heinemann, 2003.

33. Ince PG, Lowe J, Shaw PJ. Amyotrophic lateral sclerosis: current issues in classification, pathogenesis and molecular pathology. Neuropathol Appl Neurobiol 1998; 24:104–117.

34. Kusaka H. Neuropathology of the motor neuron disease—Bunina body. Rinsho Shinkeigaku 1999; 39:65–66.

35. Tomonaga M, Saito M, Yoshimura M, Shimada H, Tohgi H. Ultrastructure of the Bunina bodies in anterior horn cells of amyotrophic lateral sclerosis. Acta Neuropathol (Berl) 1978; 42:81–86.

36. Shibata N, Hirano A, Kobayashi M, Sasaki S, Kato T, Matsumoto S, Shiozawa Z, Komori T, Ikemoto A, Umahara T, et al. Cu/Zn superoxide dismutase-like immunoreactivity in Lewy body-like inclusions of sporadic amyotrophic lateral sclerosis. Neurosci Lett 1994; 179:149–152.

37. Kawamata T, Akiyama H, Yamada T, McGeer PL. Immunologic reactions in amyotrophic lateral sclerosis brain and spinal cord tissue. Am J Pathol 1992; 140:691–707.

38. Alexianu ME, Kozovska M, Appel SH. Immune reactivity in a mouse model of familial ALS correlates with disease progression. Neurology 2001; 57:1282–1289.

39. Gong YH, Parsadanian AS, Andreeva A, Snider WD, Elliott JL. Restricted expression of G86R Cu/Zn superoxide dismutase in astrocytes results in astrocytosis but does not cause motoneuron degeneration. J Neurosci 2000; 20:660–665.

40. Weydt P, Yuen EC, Ransom BR, Moller T. Increased cytotoxic potential of microglia from ALS-transgenic mice. Glia 2004; 48:179–182.

41. Almer G, Guégan C, Teismann P, Naini A, Rosoklija G, Hays AP, Chen C, Przedborski S. Increased expression of the pro-inflammatory enzyme cyclooxygenase-2 in amyotrophic lateral sclerosis. Ann Neurol 2001; 49:176–185.

42. Clarke PGH. Apoptosis versus necrosis. In: Koliatsos VE, Ratan RR, eds. Cell Death and Diseases of the Nervous System. New Jersey: Humana Press, 1999.

43. Kitanaka C, Kuchino Y. Caspase-independent programmed cell death with necrotic morphology. Cell Death Differ 1999; 6:508–515.

44. Sperandio S, de Belle I, Bredesen DE. An alternative, nonapoptotic form of programmed cell death. Proc Natl Acad Sci USA 2000; 97:14376–14381.

45. Moroni F, Meli E, Peruginelli F, Chiarugi A, Cozzi A, Picca R, Romagnoli P, Pellicciari R, Pellegrini-Giampietro DE. Poly(ADP-ribose) polymerase inhibitors attenuate necrotic but not apoptotic neuronal death in experimental models of cerebral ischemia. Cell Death Differ 2001; 8:921–932.

46. Borsello T, Bonny C, Riederer BM, Clarke PGH. Cell-permeable peptides inhibit JNK action, and completely protect neurons from NMDA-induced necrotic death. Soc Neurosci Abstr 2001; 27:267/15.

47. Guegan C, Przedborski S. Programmed cell death in amyotrophic lateral sclerosis. J Clin Invest 2003; 111:153–161.

48. Migheli A, Atzori C, Piva R, Tortarolo M, Girelli M, Schiffer D, Bendotti C. Lack of apoptosis in mice with ALS. Nat Med 1999; 5:966–967.

49. Pasinelli P, Houseweart MK, Brown RH Jr, Cleveland DW. Caspase-1 and -3 are sequentially activated in motor neuron death in Cu, Zn superoxide dismutase-mediated familial amyotrophic lateral sclerosis. Proc Natl Acad Sci USA 2000; 97:13901–13906.

50. Vukosavic S, Stefanis L, Jackson-Lewis V, Guégan C, Romero N, Chen C, Dubois-Dauphin M, Przedborski S. Delaying caspase activation by Bcl-2: a clue to disease retardation in a transgenic mouse model of amyotrophic lateral sclerosis. J Neurosci 2000; 20:9119–9125.

51. Raoul C, Estevez A, Nishimune H, Cleveland D, deLapeyriere O, Henderson C, Haase G, Pettmann B. Motoneuron death triggered by a specific pathway downstream of fas. potentiation by ALS-Linked SOD1 mutations. Neuron 2002; 35:1067–1083.

52. Facchinetti F, Sasaki M, Cutting FB, Zhai P, MacDonald JE, Reif D, Beal MF, Huang PL, Dawson TM, Gurney ME, Dawson VL. Lack of involvement of neuronal nitric oxide synthase in the pathogenesis of a transgenic mouse model of familial amyotrophic lateral sclerosis. Neuroscience 1999; 90:1483–1492.

53. Nguyen MD, Lariviere RC, Julien JP. Deregulation of Cdk5 in a mouse model of ALS: toxicity alleviated by perikaryal neurofilament inclusions. Neuron 2001; 30:135–147.

54. Bian F, Nath R, Sobocinski G, Booher RN, Lipinski WJ, Callahan MJ, Pack A, Wang KK, Walker LC. Axonopathy, tau abnormalities, and dyskinesia, but no neurofibrillary tangles in p25-transgenic mice. J Comp Neurol 2002; 446:257–266.

55. Takahashi S, Kulkarni AB. Mutant superoxide dismutase 1 causes motor neuron degeneration independent of cyclin-dependent kinase 5 activation by p35 or p25. J Neurochem 2004; 88:1295–1304.

56. Vleminckx V, Van Damme P, Goffin K, Delye H, Van den Bosch L, Robberecht W. Upregulation of HSP27 in a transgenic model of ALS. J Neuropathol Exp Neurol 2002; 61:968–974.

57. Okado-Matsumoto A, Fridovich I. Amyotrophic lateral sclerosis: a proposed mechanism. Proc Natl Acad Sci USA 2002; 99:9010–9014.

58. Evgrafov OV, Mersiyanova I, Irobi J, Van den Bosch L, Dierick I, Leung CL, Schagina O, Verpoorten N, Van Impe K, Fedotov V, et al. Mutant small heat-shock protein 27 causes

axonal Charcot-Marie-Tooth disease and distal hereditary motor neuropathy. Nat Genet 2004; 36:602–606.

59. Irobi J, Van Impe K, Seeman P, Jordanova A, Dierick I, Verpoorten N, Michalik A, De Vriendt E, Jacobs A, Van Gerwen V, et al. Hot-spot residue in small heat-shock protein 22 causes distal motor neuropathy. Nat Genet 2004; 36:597–601.

60. Kieran D, Kalmar B, Dick JR, Riddoch-Contreras J, Burnstock G, Greensmith L. Treatment with arimoclomol, a coinducer of heat shock proteins, delays disease progression in ALS mice. Nat Med 2004; 10:402–405.

61. Bruening W, Roy J, Giasson B, Figlewicz DA, Mushynski WE, Durham HD. Up-regulation of protein chaperones preserves viability of cells expressing toxic Cu/Zn-superoxide dismutase mutants associated with amyotrophic lateral sclerosis. J Neurochem 1999; 72:693–699.

62. Batulan Z, Shinder GA, Minotti S, He BP, Doroudchi MM, Nalbantoglu J, Strong MJ, Durham HD. High threshold for induction of the stress response in motor neurons is associated with failure to activate HSF1. J Neurosci 2003; 23:5789–5798.

63. Oosthuyse B, Moons L, Storkebaum E, Beck H, Nuyens D, Brusselmans K, Van Dorpe J, Hellings P, Gorselink M, Heymans S, et al. Deletion of the hypoxia-response element in the vascular endothelial growth factor promoter causes motor neuron degeneration. Nat Genet 2001; 28:131–138.

64. Van den Bosch L, Storkebaum E, Vleminckx V, Moons L, Vanopdenbosch L, Scheveneels W, Carmeliet P, Robberecht W. Effects of vascular endothelial growth factor (VEGF) on motor neuron degeneration. Neurobiol Dis 2004; 17:21–28.

65. Lambrechts D, Storkebaum E, Morimoto M, Del Favero J, Desmet F, Marklund SL, Wyns S, Thijs V, Andersson J, van M, et al. VEGF is a modifier of amyotrophic lateral sclerosis in mice and humans and protects motoneurons against ischemic death. Nat Genet 2003; 34:383–394.

66. Azzouz M, Ralph GS, Storkebaum E, Walmsley LE, Mitrophanous KA, Kingsman SM, Carmeliet P, Mazarakis ND. VEGF delivery with retrogradely transported lentivector prolongs survival in a mouse ALS model. Nature 2004; 429:413–417.

67. Storkebaum E, Carmeliet P. VEGF: a critical player in neurodegeneration. J Clin Invest 2004; 113:14–18.

68. Williamson TL, Bruijn LI, Zhu Q, Anderson KL, Anderson SD, Julien JP, Cleveland DW. Absence of neurofilaments reduces the selective vulnerability of motor neurons and slows disease caused by a familial amyotrophic lateral sclerosis-linked superoxide dismutase 1 mutant. Proc Natl Acad Sci USA 1998; 95:9631–9636.

69. Borchelt DR, Wong PC, Becher MW, Pardo CA, Lee MK, Xu ZS, Thinakaran G, Jenkins NA, Copeland NG, Sisodia SS, et al. Axonal transport of mutant superoxide dismutase 1 and focal axonal abnormalities in the proximal axons of transgenic mice. Neurobiol Dis 1998; 5:27–35.

70. Puls I, Jonnakuty C, LaMonte BH, Holzbaur EL, Tokito M, Mann E, Floeter MK, Bidus K, Drayna D, Oh SJ, et al. Mutant dynactin in motor neuron disease. Nat Genet 2003; 33:455–456.

71. LaMonte BH, Wallace KE, Holloway BA, Shelly SS, Ascano J, Tokito M, Van Winkle T, Howland DS, Holzbaur EL. Disruption of dynein/dynactin inhibits axonal transport in motor neurons causing late-onset progressive degeneration. Neuron 2002; 34:715–727.

72. Hafezparast M, Klocke R, Ruhrberg C, Marquardt A, Ahmad-Annuar A, Bowen S, Lalli G, Witherden AS, Hummerich H, Nicholson S, et al. Mutations in dynein link motor neuron degeneration to defects in retrograde transport. Science 2003; 300:808–812.

73. Lieberman AP, Fischbeck KH. Triplet repeat expansion in neuromuscular disease. Muscle Nerve 2000; 23:843–850.

74. Jablonka S, Sendtner M. Molecular and cellular basis of spinal muscular atrophy. Amyotroph Lateral Scler Other Motor Neuron Disord 2003; 4:144–149.

75. Grohmann K, Schuelke M, Diers A, Hoffmann K, Lucke B, Adams C, Bertini E, Leonhardt-Horti H, Muntoni F, Ouvrier R, et al. Mutations in the gene encoding

immunoglobulin mu-binding protein 2 cause spinal muscular atrophy with respiratory distress type 1. Nat Genet 2001; 29:75–77.

76. Antonellis A, Ellsworth RE, Sambuughin N, Puls I, Abel A, Lee-Lin SQ, Jordanova A, Kremensky I, Christodoulou K, Middleton LT, et al. Glycyl tRNA synthetase mutations in Charcot-Marie-Tooth disease type 2D and distal spinal muscular atrophy type V. Am J Hum Genet 2003; 72:1293–1299.

77. Zhao C, Takita J, Tanaka Y, Setou M, Nakagawa T, Takeda S, Yang HW, Terada S, Nakata T, Takei Y, et al. Charcot-Marie-Tooth disease type 2A caused by mutation in a microtubule motor KIF1Bbeta. Cell 2001; 105:587–597.

78. Yamada K, Andrews C, Chan WM, McKeown CA, Magli A, de Berardinis T, Loewenstein A, Lazar M, O'Keefe M, Letson R, et al. Heterozygous mutations of the kinesin KIF21A in congenital fibrosis of the extraocular muscles type 1 (CFEOM1). Nat Genet 2003; 35:318–321.

79. Fichera M, Lo Giudice M, Falco M, Sturnio M, Amata S, Calabrese O, Bigoni S, Calzolari E, Neri M. Evidence of kinesin heavy chain (KIF5A) involvement in pure hereditary spastic paraplegia. Neurology 2004; 63:1108–1110.

80. Verhoeven K, De Jonghe P, Coen K, Verpoorten N, Auer-Grumbach M, Kwon JM, FitzPatrick D, Schmedding E, De Vriendt E, Jacobs A, et al. Mutations in the small GTP-ase late endosomal protein RAB7 cause Charcot-Marie-Tooth type 2B neuropathy. Am J Hum Genet 2003; 72:722–727.

81. Hazan J, Fonknechten N, Mavel D, Paternotte C, Samson D, Artiguenave F, Davoine CS, Cruaud C, Durr A, Wincker P, et al. Spastin, a new AAA protein, is altered in the most frequent form of autosomal dominant spastic paraplegia. Nat Genet 1999; 23:296–303.

82. Hansen JJ, Durr A, Cournu-Rebeix I, Georgopoulos C, Ang D, Nielsen MN, Davoine CS, Brice A, Fontaine B, Gregersen N, et al. Hereditary spastic paraplegia SPG13 is associated with a mutation in the gene encoding the mitochondrial chaperonin Hsp60. Am J Hum Genet 2002; 70:1328–332.

83. Casari G, De Fusco M, Ciarmatori S, Zeviani M, Mora M, Fernandez P, De Michele G, Filla A, Cocozza S, Marconi R, et al. Spastic paraplegia and OXPHOS impairment caused by mutations in paraplegin, a nuclear-encoded mitochondrial metalloprotease. Cell 1998; 93:973–983.

84. Engert JC, Berube P, Mercier J, Dore C, Lepage P, Ge B, Bouchard JP, Mathieu J, Melancon SB, Schalling M, et al. ARSACS, a spastic ataxia common in northeastern Quebec, is caused by mutations in a new gene encoding an 11.5-kb ORF. Nat Genet 2000; 24:120–125.

13
Excitotoxicity

Paul R. Heath and Pamela J. Shaw
Academic Neurology Unit, Section of Neuroscience, University of Sheffield, Sheffield, U.K.

GLUTAMATERGIC NEUROTRANSMISSION

Glutamate is the major excitatory transmitter in the mammalian nervous system (1,2) and tremendous complexity has been uncovered, both in its mechanism of action and in the molecular structure of its receptors. This diversity means that specific types of neurons, such as motor neurons are likely to express a particular profile of glutamate receptors suited to cell specific physiological properties.

Glutamate is a non-essential dicarboxylic amino acid which exists in the nervous system in both metabolic and neurotransmitter pools. The neurotransmitter pool accounts for approximately 20% of stored glutamate, which is both synthesized and stored in synaptic nerve terminals and in perisynaptic glia. Glutamate is derived from α-ketoglutarate by reductive deamination catalyzed by glutamate dehydrogenase or from other amino acids through the action of aminotransferases (3).

During normal glutamatergic neurotransmission (Fig. 1), glutamate is released from presynaptic terminals in response to depolarization and crosses the synaptic cleft to activate postsynaptic receptors. The receptors are divided into two main types: those that form ion channels (ionotropic) and those that are linked to G-proteins (metabotropic). Each receptor type has been characterized according to its pharmacological agonist. There are three forms of ionotropic receptor, comprising *N*-methyl-D-aspartate (NMDA), α-amino-3-hydroxy-5-methyl-4-isoxazole propionic acid (AMPA), and kainate receptor subtypes, and three forms of metabotropic receptor. Each of the receptors is thought to exist as an oligomer, most likely a tetramer, of protein subunits. These may be homo-oligomeric or hetero-oligomeric.

The excitatory signal is terminated by active removal of glutamate from the synaptic cleft by glutamate reuptake transporter proteins. Currently there are five known subtypes of glutamate transporter proteins, which are located predominantly on perisynaptic astrocytes, though some subtypes are expressed by neurons (4). Synaptic glutamate that has been taken up by perisynaptic astroglial cells is converted to glutamine by the enzyme glutamine synthetase.

The glutamine is shuttled back to the neuronal terminal where glutaminase converts it back to glutamate (5,6). Some glutamate receptors are located on the

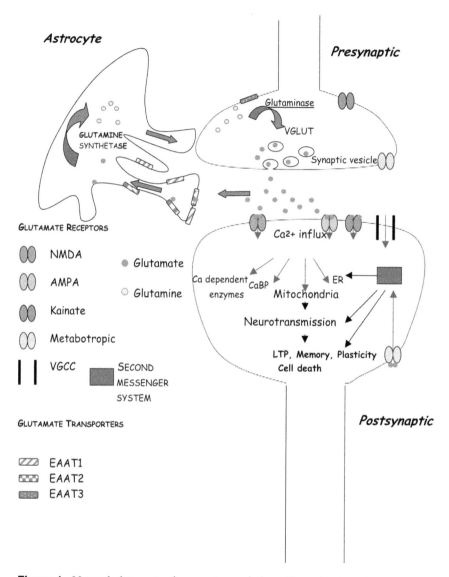

Figure 1 Normal glutamatergic neurotransmission. (*See color insert.*)

presynaptic neuronal terminal. Presynaptic metabotropic and kainate receptors may play a modulatory role in glutamate neurotransmission.

While the ionotropic glutamate receptors share the same overall topology (Fig. 2), they differ in their electrophysiological characteristics, permeabilities, developmental expression, and trafficking profiles (7). It has been shown that the cytosolic C-terminal domain of the constituent subunits of the receptors interacts with scaffolding, motor, and signaling proteins to promote proper receptor localization and regulation. For instance, the C-terminal domains of subunits of the NMDA receptor contain an endoplasmic reticulum retention motif (8), they can bind indirectly to the motor protein kinesin superfamily (9), and can interact with α-actinin and calcium calmodulin-activated protein kinase II (CAMKII) (10,11).

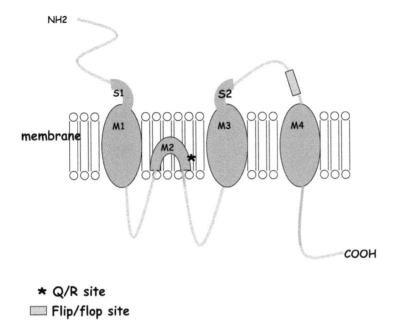

★ Q/R site
▨ Flip/flop site

Figure 2 Basic structure of ionotropic glutamate receptors.

Glutamate receptors are designed to invoke a variety of complex intracellular signal transduction processes (Fig. 1): including the activation or inhibition of enzymes, the release or inhibition of intracellular second messengers, the formation or release of transcellular messengers, and the regulation of calcium-dependent gene expression (7,12,13).

Classification of Glutamate Receptors

The first glutamate receptor subunit gene was identified in 1989 (14), and since then 26 further genes encoding glutamate receptor subunits have been discovered (15). An additional five proteins have been described whose function is less well defined but which may serve as receptor subunits or associated proteins (15). It is apparent that considerable molecular diversity of glutamate receptors can be generated from the existence of this plethora of genes encoding receptor subunits, with additional complexity made possible by alternative splicing and post-translational modifications (Fig. 3) (16).

This diversity means that the physiological properties of glutamate receptors can be finely tuned to the functional requirements of particular types of neurons.

NMDA Receptors

NMDA receptor activation produces excitatory currents characterized by a slow rise time and relatively slow decay (15). These properties confer integrative functions that are utilized in multiple physiological mechanisms including the generation of rhythmic motor activity (17) and as the first event in a complex biochemical cascade, long-term potentiation that underlies some forms of memory (18). NMDA receptors are sensitive to the coagonists glutamate and glycine, and the receptor channels demonstrate high permeability to calcium, are subject to voltage-dependent blockade by

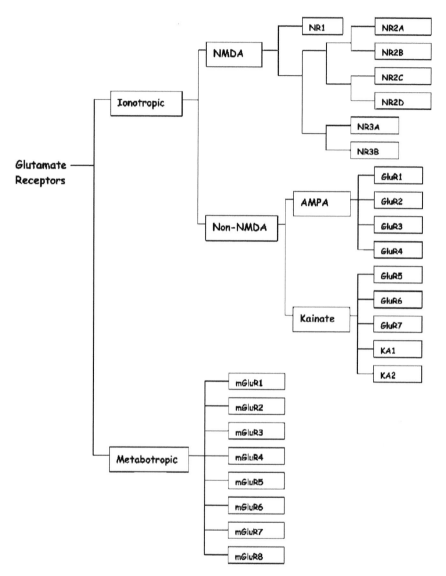

Figure 3 Classification of glutamate receptors.

Mg^{2+}, and the receptor sites are modulated by zinc, protons, polyamines, and redox agents (19). When the concept of excitotoxicity initially developed, the NMDA receptor incorporating an ion channel highly permeable to calcium, was considered to be the receptor subtype primary responsible for excitotoxic effects. However, it subsequently became apparent that other glutamate receptor subtypes could also be involved in excitotoxicity, especially with more prolonged glutamate exposure (20–22).

Seven genes encoding NMDA receptor subunits have been identified: NMDAR1, NMDAR2 (for which there are four subunits, A–D), and NMDAR3A/B (23). Of these, the NMDAR2D subunit appears to be the most abundantly expressed within the central nerous system (CNS). Each functional receptor complex requires the presence of two subunits, usually the NMDAR1 subunit combined with one of the NMDAR2 subunits. The NMDAR1 subunit can exist in one of eight forms generated by alternative splicing and appears to provide the essential part of the receptor complex with the NMDAR2 subunit providing functional variability (24). The NMDAR3 subunit appears to be developmentally regulated, but its precise function is as yet unknown (25).

There is evidence that the 3B subunit is preferentially expressed on somatic motor neurons where it may play a role in controlling the cell surface expression of NMDA receptors and the calcium permeability of the NMDA receptor complex (26–28).

Non-NMDA AMPA-Kainate Receptors

The kainate and AMPA receptors are often collectively referred to as non-NMDA receptors. These receptors possess functional similarities. They are both monovalent cation pores with fast excitation characteristics. Generally they are impermeable to calcium, which has major functional implications, but allow the rapid influx of the monovalent cations potassium and sodium and the associated monovalent anion chloride (16). Nine mammalian AMPA/kainate receptor subunits have been cloned and sequenced. The GluR1-4 are AMPA selective, whereas GluR5-7 and KA1-2 are kainate selective (Fig. 3).

AMPA Receptors

The AMPA glutamate receptor subunits GluR1-4 are each proteins of 95 to 163 kDa and the amino acid sequence and hydrophobicity plots suggest a structure in which there are three transmembrane domains and a fourth potential transmembrane domain which creates a loop into the cytoplasmic side of the membrane (16). The AMPA receptor complex appears to exist as a tetrameric structure in several potential arrangements determined by the cell type or the stage of development (12). There is evidence accumulating to demonstrate synaptic plasticity of AMPA receptors, which can be modulated by environmental conditions, including the activation status of the cell (29–32). The GluR2 subunit is of particular functional importance as it plays a key role in determining the calcium ion permeability of the assembled AMPA receptor (16). The presence of the GluR2 subunit in a heteromeric receptor confers the property of low permeability to Ca^{2+}, whereas AMPA receptors lacking GluR2 are permeable to calcium. Permeability of the receptor protein to calcium is governed by post-transcriptional editing of a site in the second transmembrane domain of GluR2 (Fig. 4) (14–16).

This occurs at amino acid 586 in the protein. In the other glutamate receptor subtypes this is a glutamine (Q) encoded by the triplet of bases CAG, but in the processing of the double stranded pre-mRNA for GluR2, the CAG triplet found at a point on the border between exon 11 and intron 11 is acted upon by the enzyme adenosine deaminase which converts the adenosine into an inosine, creating a novel triplet CIG. This triplet is recognized by the tRNA carrying an arginine (R) and hence the mature protein carries an altered sequence with replacement of the original glutamine by an arginine. This reaction is more than 90% efficient under normal conditions in vivo and therefore the majority of expressed GluR2 protein expressed in the CNS is edited in this way and confers on the GluR2 protein the property of calcium impermeability (Fig. 4). The adenosine deaminase enzyme has a further action on exon 13 of the GluR2,3 and 4 subtypes. An AGA triplet is modified to IGA, which causes a transition of arginine to glycine. The affected exon forms part of the extracellular loop between TM3 and TM4, and the alteration in

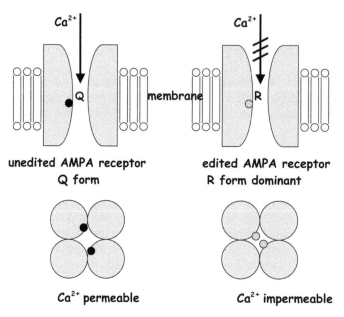

unedited AMPA receptor   edited AMPA receptor
        Q form   R form dominant

     Ca²⁺ permeable   Ca²⁺ impermeable

Figure 4 GluR2 subunit and calcium permeability of AMPA receptors.

the final protein improves the rate of recovery of the receptor protein following desensitization.

A further modification of the AMPA receptor subtypes occurs by alternative splicing of a region of the gene encoding 38 amino acids near the fourth transmembrane domain (Fig. 2). The different forms are denoted flip and flop, although they create no obvious alteration in the structure of the extracellular loop. The flip form includes exon 14 of the gene and it is the primary form of the protein produced in prenatal and early postnatal neurons. A postnatal developmental change results in increased expression of the flop isoforms of the AMPA receptor subunits. This change results in the replacement of exon 14 by exon 15 in the mature messenger RNA molecule. The resultant flop isoform shows more rapid glutamate-induced desensitization compared to the flip isoform.

It is likely that the flip/flop alternative splicing and R/G editing processes act cooperatively to control desensitization and recovery of the AMPA receptors.

Myers et al. (33) have investigated the transcriptional regulation of the *GluR2* gene. They have shown that initiation of transcription of GluR2 may occur at a number of sites. This allows for variations in the transcription, for example transcription initiation is different in adult cortex and cerebellar neurons. There is within the promoter of the *GluR2* gene a repressor-element-1 (RE-1) which acts as a negative regulatory element and also positive regulatory elements which use an Sp1 or a nuclear respiratory factor-1 (NRF-1) element. The RE1 element is found in the promoter of several neuron-specific genes and is controlled by interaction with the molecule REST (RE1 binding silencer protein) (34). The REST protein binds to the RE1 element in non-neuronal cells and is able to repress RNA transcription via an mSIN-3 feature at its N-terminal and/or a CoREST feature at its C-terminal. Both of these molecules bind to their corepressors, either mSIN-3 or CoREST, and the corepressor molecules both act through histone deacetylases to prevent gene transcription. The corepressors appear to be able to act either independently or synergistically. It is suggested that in normal neuronal tissue there is no activity of the REST protein but in instances of neuronal insult, such as excitotoxicity, the REST element might be invoked and GluR2 activity repressed in cells likely to die (33). However, the activity of the silencer in repressing GluR2 expression is quite weak, apparently acting to modulate rather than completely switch off expression. The same group (35) has recently extended this work in an investigation of the multiple initiation sites found in the 5' untranslated region of the *GluR2* gene. These sites may be of importance in the level of translation of the *GluR2* gene since some of the variants start sites appear to be more efficiently transcribed than others, leading to different levels of expression of GluR2 in different individuals.

Thus, there exists a subset of AMPA receptors, lacking the GluR2 subunit, which are permeable to Ca^{2+} and other divalent cations (36). The presence of these receptors could have a direct bearing upon the selective neurodegeneration of certain neuronal types. Cells, such as motor neurons, carrying AMPA receptors that are permeable to divalent cations may be more susceptible to oxidative damage and mitochondrial dysfunction resulting from the influx of calcium.

Some insights into the normal physiological function of calcium permeable AMPA receptors are beginning to emerge. For example, they are present on adult rat dorsal horn neurons, predominantly within inhibitory pathways where they play a distinct role in spinal nociceptive processing (37). Bergmann glia of the cerebellum of young rats also express calcium permeable AMPA receptors, where they appear to play an important role in regulating the innervation of Purkinje cells by climbing fibers (38).

Kainate Receptors

The first kainate receptor was cloned in the rat in 1990 and designated GluR5 (39), and since then four further kainate receptor subunits have been identified. These are designated GluR6, GluR7, KA1, and KA2 (40). The kainate receptor system is not as well characterized as the AMPA system. The exact functional role of the kainate receptors in the CNS beyond the mediation of fast excitatory neurotransmission is not known. However, it is recognized that the receptor complexes are present in both pre and postsynaptic neuronal membranes. Presynaptic kainate receptor complexes may have inhibitory effects on glutamatergic neurotransmission (41). Evidence is emerging that the kainate receptor subunit composition does influence physiological properties (41). There is also evidence that the kainate receptors display different kinetics compared to the AMPA receptors and may also have a substantial functional role in modulating interneuronal output (42).

As with the AMPA subunits, several mechanisms exist for the generation of molecular variants of kainate receptor subunits. GluR5 and GluR7 show significant variation generated by alternative splicing, with GluR5 having two N-terminal splice variants and four C-terminal splice variants and GluR7 having two N-terminal splice variants. The functional significance of this variation has not been fully investigated. The GluR6 subunit has two C-terminal splice variants and in addition, the GluR5 and GluR6 subunits undergo RNA editing similar to that undergone by the GluR2 subunit. They undergo incomplete Q/R (glutamine to arginine) editing in transmembrane domain 2 (39,43–45) which modulates the Ca^{2+} permeability of the receptors containing GluR5 or GluR6 receptors. The GluR6 has two further sites within its first transmembrane domain that undergo post-transcriptional RNA editing. These have been designated the I/V (isoleucine to valine) and Y/C (tyrosine to cysteine) sites but as yet the precise role of these editing patterns remains unknown (46).

The fully edited GluR6 predominates (V, C, and R), constituting approximately 65% of the GluR6 in the rat brain.

Functional kainate receptors are likely to be tetramers (12), with each subunit possessing a ligand binding site. Certain subunit arrangements are known to form functional receptors. For example, GluR5, GluR6, and GluR7 are able to form functional homomeric receptors and are also able to combine, to form functional heteromeric receptors (45,47–49). Each of the GluR kainate receptor subunits can also form heteromeric assemblies with KA1 and KA2.

For many years the understanding of kainate receptor function was hampered by a lack of specific agonists and antagonists that enabled a distinction to be made between actions at AMPA and kainate receptors. The discovery of the specific antagonistic action of compounds such as the 2,3-benzodiazepines, particularly GYK153655, at AMPA receptors has enabled a clearer analysis of the roles of both receptor types at synapses (46).

Some important insights into the functional properties of kainate receptors are emerging from the creation of knockout and transgenic mice (40).

Metabotropic Receptors

Metabotropic glutamate receptors were first characterized pharmacologically and electrophysiologically by Sladeczek et al. (50), and the first of these receptors was cloned in 1991 (51). The metabotropic receptors are membrane associated G-protein coupled receptors and operate by modulating intracellular second messenger systems. This receptor group appears to have roles in fast excitatory synaptic transmission and also in the regulation of neuronal excitability, presynaptic inhibition, and synaptic plasticity. Currently, eight types of metabotropic receptor are recognized and molecular diversity is again increased by the presence of splice variants (52). The mGluR subtypes are structurally related but highly heterogeneous in their agonist selectivity, signal transduction mechanisms, and distribution in the brain. The eight subtypes are classified into three groups based on their sequence homology, transduction mechanism, and pharmacology. The receptors of group I (mGluR1 and mGluR5) activate phospholipase C with production of inositol 1,4,5-triphosphate and diacylglycerol, which leads to the release of calcium from the endoplasmic reticulum and activation of protein kinase C. The group II (mGluR2 and mGluR3) and group III (mGluR4, mGluR6, mGluR7, and mGluR8) subtypes are negatively coupled to adenyl cyclase.

Metabotropic glutamate receptors are large proteins ranging from 854 to 1179 amino acids, with a large N-terminal region of about 550 amino acids, a core section of about 250 amino acids which is predicted to possess seven transmembrane domains, and a C-terminal region, the length of which varies with subtype (53). It has been proposed that the N-terminal domain is extracellular and contains the glutamate-binding site, while the C-terminal domain is intracellular (51).

The C-terminal domain may play a role in determining the potency of agonists as natural deletions of this domain in mGluR1, the splice variants mGluR1B and mGluR1C, result in a decrease of agonist potency. The sequences of the first and third intracellular loops are highly conserved among all the metabotropic glutamate receptors, suggesting that these domains are important for G-protein activation. The less conserved second intracellular loop and the intracellular portion adjacent to the seventh transmembrane domain may control the coupling of mGluR1 to phospholipase C (54).

Unravelling the physiological functions of metabotropic receptors has been impeded by the lack of potent subtype specific agonists and antagonists. However, some insights into their specific functions are emerging. They appear to be involved in induction of long-term changes in synaptic strength, and involvement in the control of movement and olfactory nociception has also been demonstrated (54,55). It is likely that presynaptic mGlu receptors will be active as autoreceptors regulating glutamate release from the nerve terminal, while postsynaptic receptors can modulate the activity of ionotropic AMPA or NMDA receptors and ion channels responsible for modulating postsynaptic responses.

Glutamate Reuptake Transporters

Five glutamate transporters have now been cloned and they show a high degree of homology between species (56). The human versions have been named excitatory amino acid transporters (EAAT) one to five. The role of these transporters is to regulate the concentration of extracellular glutamate by its reuptake, and hence maintain a concentration in the synaptic cleft of between 1 and 3 μM. To achieve this, they are able to concentrate glutamate several thousand fold across the cell membrane (57). The process of glutamate clearance is electrogenic, being coupled to the transport of two or three sodium ions and one proton from the extracellular space and the countertransport of a potassium ion.

EAAT1, EAAT2, and EAAT3 are found throughout the brain. EAAT1 is most abundant in the cerebellum and expressed by both glia and neurons (58). EAAT2 is the major glutamate transporter and is localized exclusively in glia. It is widely distributed in the human CNS, representing approximately one percent of brain protein (59). The expression of EAAT2 by glia makes this transporter of particular interest in terms of glutamate clearance at synapses and potential involvement in excitotoxicity. Reducing the expression of GLT1 (the rat homologue of EAAT2) using antisense oligonucleotides caused a dramatic elevation of extracellular glutamate and neuronal injury in specific regions of the CNS (60). GLT1 knockout mice undergo lethal spontaneous seizures, show increased susceptibility to acute brain injury, and rarely survive beyond three months of age (60). EAAT3 is highly expressed in neurons of the cortex, hippocampus, caudate, and putamen. EAAT4 is found in the Purkinje cells of the cerebellum and EAAT5 is located only in the retina (56).

Glutamate reuptake transporters appear to function as homomultimers and are regulated by soluble factors released from neurons, including glutamate itself (61). There is also evidence that these proteins are regulated by the redox environment in which they exist. Under oxidant conditions their activity is downregulated, and arachidonic acid has been shown to increase the affinity of EAAT2 for glutamate (62). In conditions where oxidative stress is severe, chronic, or associated with production of peroxynitrite, the transporters can become irreversibly oxidized, which impairs their function. This would increase neuronal vulnerability to glutamatergic toxicity and indicates that oxidative stress and excitotoxicity are interlinked mechanisms in the causation of neuronal injury.

Synaptic Vesicle Transporters

Neurotransmitter glutamate to be released at the synaptic cleft needs to be packaged into synaptic vesicles. Three molecules have now been described that are responsible for this process.

These are the vesicle glutamate transporters VGLUT1, VGLUT2, and VGLUT3, which are closely related proteins (63–67). VGLUT1 and VGLUT2 have complementary distributions in that they appear to be expressed by different groups of neurons (68). For example, many neurons in the cerebral cortex express VGLUT1, while most cells in the brainstem express VGLUT2. In the cerebellum, the neurons of the cortex express VGLUT1, but the deep cerebellar nuclei express VGLUT2. This suggests that different classes of glutamatergic excitatory synapses exist depending upon which vesicle transporter is involved. It has been suggested that VGLUT2 is located within neurons at synapses with a high chance of glutamate release, and VGLUT1 is localized at synapses with less glutamatergic activity (68). While VGLUT 1 and VGLUT 2 are overwhelmingly associated with excitatory neurons and appear presynaptically, VGLUT3 is found in other neuronal types and occasionally in cell bodies. Thus VGLUT3 might be involved in some novel glutamate signaling that is not necessarily excitatory and is often associated with other monoamine expression such as 5HT or dopamine (69). These vesicular transporters have not been demonstrated in glia, suggesting another mechanism is responsible for glial glutamate release.

The distribution of the vesicular glutamate transporters in rat spinal cord has recently been investigated (70). Using both immunohistochemistry and in situ hybridisation, the authors demonstrated that all three transporters are present to some degree in the spinal cord. However, VGLUT3 was only visible with immunohistochemistry and VGLUT1 and two proteins were only found in nerve fibers and not in cell bodies. VGLUT1 was observed at the mRNA level and as protein in dorsal root ganglia while VGLUT2 was only demonstrated in dorsal root ganglions (DRGs) as protein. As has shown previously, the two transporters VGLUT1 and VGLUT2 were found in different laminae of the spinal cord, but were mostly localized with interneurons and not motor neurons.

EXCITOTOXICITY

Lucas and Newhouse (71) initially demonstrated that glutamate can have lethal effects on neurons in the CNS. Olney (72) coined the term excitotoxicity and defined it as a phenomenon "whereby the excitatory action of glutamate and related excitatory amino acids becomes transformed into a neuropathological process that can rapidly kill CNS neurons." The phenomenon is largely described as a glutamate-mediated event, but other endogenous amino acids (e.g., aspartate, homocysteic acid, and quinolinic acid), synthetic glutamate analogues such as NMDA, and plant-derived glutamate receptor agonists (e.g., kainic acid, domoic acid, ibotenic acid, quisqualic acid, and acromelic acid) can also cause excitotoxicity (73).

Excessive activation of postsynaptic glutamate receptors could theoretically arise from several mechanisms including excessive presynaptic glutamate release, impaired glutamate reuptake transporter function, particular features of postsynaptic glutamate receptors (e.g., location and molecular properties), the activity of other ion channels, and downstream intracellular events following glutamate receptor activation.

Several cellular mechanisms have been elucidated, which may contribute to the toxic effects of excessive glutamatergic activation of neurons (Table 1). These include the activation of multiple, often calcium-dependent enzyme cascades such as calpain, protein kinase C, lipases, phospholipases, endonucleases, the arachidonic acid cascade, xanthine oxidase, and nitric oxide synthase (5). A key step in the excitotoxic process is the derangement of intracellular calcium homeostasis leading to increased levels of free intracellular calcium. Oxidative stress and the formation of reactive oxygen species (ROS) have also been identified as key components of excitotoxicity (74).

Table 1 Cellular Mechanisms Contributing to Excitotoxicity

Activation of Ca^{2+}-dependent pathways
Proteases (e.g., calpain and xanthine oxidase)
Protein kinases
Phosphatases
Phospholipases
Nitric oxide synthase
Endonucleases
Increased generation of intracellular free radicals
Arachidonic acid cascade
Xanthine oxidase
Nitric oxide synthase
Competitive interference with cystine uptake leading to glutathione depletion
Presence of mutant proteins, e.g., SOD1

Abbreviations: SOD, superoxide dismutase; Ca^{2+}, calcium ions.

The neurotoxic effects of glutamate might also occur indirectly through the toxic effects of depletion of intracellular glutathione, a major intracellular antioxidant (75).

Cystine is normally transported into cells via a cystine carrier which also counter-transports glutamate out of the cell. The action of this amino acid carrier is driven by the glutamate concentration gradient across the cell wall. An increase in extracellular glutamate concentration, as occurs in excitotoxicity, alters this gradient and decreases the intracellular transfer of cystine. Since cystine is a vital precursor of glutathione, the intracellular concentration of this important antioxidant and free radical scavenger will be compromised in conditions where the extracellular glutamate level is excessively high (76).

Other factors have also been implicated in mediating excitotoxic effects. It has been suggested that delayed cell death initiated by excitotoxic stress may be regulated through cell cycle components. Park et al. (77) reported that cell cycle pathways including the cyclin D1 associated kinase activity and ribosome (Rb) phosphorylation were activated in murine hippocampus following kainate administration. Additionally the CDK inhibitor flavopiridol, when coadministered with the glutamate receptor antagonist MK-801, protected cultured cells from death induced by the fungal toxin 3-NP. Dysregulation of cell cycle regulating proteins has been reported in ALS and models of this disease (78,79). Nguyen et al. (78) examined neuronal death in the G37R transgenic mouse model of ALS and found a dysregulation of Cdk5 leading to an increase in Cdk4 and its coactivator cyclin D1 and abnormal phosphorylation of the retinoblastoma protein. Ranganathan et al. (79) examined the levels of this group of proteins in postmortem tissue from both normal and ALS tissues. They demonstrated increased levels of cyclin D1 and Cdk4 and nuclear accumulation of hyperphosphorylated Rb, with an increase in cytoplasmic E2F-1. The increased levels of these proteins suggests aberrant induction of the cell cycle regulators moving the cell from post mitotic interphase into G1-S.

It was suggested that an abnormal stress such as excitotoxicity can cause the motor neuron to wrongly try and enter the G1 phase of cell division, and this leads to a premature cell death because postmitotic neurons are terminally differentiated and unable to proliferate (80).

There has also been recent work displaying an association between excitotoxicity and the pro-survival growth factor IGF-1 (81,82). IGF-1 has been shown to normally regulate lifespan and resistance to oxidative stress via its receptor (83). Garcia-Galloway et al. (81) examined the effect of glutamate excitotoxicity upon IGF-1 prosurvival factors. They found that the glutamate in excitotoxic doses caused attenuation of the IGF-1 signaling pathway by interfering with the P13K/Akt pathway. This attenuated the neuroprotective effect of IGF-1 signaling through its receptor. Interestingly, Chung et al. (82), examined the levels of expression of the IGF-1 receptor in the CNS of normal and G93A mutant transgenic mice and found the transgenic mice displayed increased levels of IGF-1 receptor in spinal cord reactive astrocytes. This may represent an attempt to overcome the loss of sensitivity to IGF-1 by increasing the level of expression of its receptor. Recently the protective effect of IGF-1 in blocking glutamate-mediated excitotoxicity was also demonstrated in an in vitro model of amyotrophic lateral sclerosis (ALS) using enriched cultures of embryonic rat spinal cord motor neurons (84).

Acute Excitotoxicity

Acute excitotoxicity has been implicated in pathogenesis of several neurological diseases including domoic acid poisoning, stroke, hypoxic-ischemic brain damage, hypoglycemic brain damage, status epilepticus, head injury, and some other toxic encephalopathies (14–16).

Acute excitotoxicity produces characteristic morphological changes in neurons. Initially there is swelling of the dendrites and perikaryon, which is followed by disruption of the cellular organelles, damage to the nucleus, and ultimately neuronal death (85).

There is evidence from in vitro studies that acute glutamatergic toxicity involves two distinct phases. First, depolarization-induced influx of sodium and chloride ions, together with water, causes acute neuronal swelling, which is reversible upon removal of the agonist (85). Second, there is an influx of calcium into the neuron through the ion channel of NMDA receptors, through calcium permeable AMPA receptors lacking the GluR2 subunit, or indirectly through the voltage-gated calcium channels (86). The intracellular calcium level is normally very tightly controlled and kept to a concentration below 0.1 μM by a complex system of compartmentalization and transportation that involves binding to calcium binding proteins, sequestration within organelles such as the endoplasmic reticulum and mitochondria, and return to the extracellular environment via ion exchangers (87,88). However, excessive activation of the glutamate receptors destabilizes intracellular calcium homeostasis, leading to a cascade of injurious biochemical events. These processes can cause both direct neuronal injury and indirect effects, through the generation of free radicals, but at least initially the damage is potentially reversible. Thus, glutamate receptor antagonists applied several hours after the excitotoxic insult show a neuroprotective effect. It is likely that the signals leading to cell death involve certain proapoptotic proteins and disorganization of the cytoskeleton (88).

Early evidence that excitotoxic neuronal death may occur by apoptosis was based upon characteristic morphological features (89). Several studies have indicated that activation of caspase 3 plays a key role in excitotoxic cell death (90,91). However, other studies have suggested that excitotoxic cell death can occur independently of caspase activation. Yu et al. (92) showed a direct relationship between glutamate excitotoxicity, PARP-1[Poly(ADP-ribose)polymerase] activation and cell death by a caspase independent pathway of programmed cell death.

Under homeostatic conditions PARP-1 participates in genome repair, DNA replication, and the regulation of transcription (93). However, should PARP-1 be massively upregulated there is depletion of the cell's energy resources and cell death. There has been some interesting recent work demonstrating an upregulation of PARP-1 in the CNS of transgenic mice bearing the G93A mutant *SOD1* gene (94).

Chronic Excitotoxicity

Evidence now exists indicating that excitotoxic effects can occur over a more chronic, as well as an acute time course. In several models including organotypic CNS tissue cultures (95) or following chronic intra-ventricular infusion of low concentrations of quinolinic acid (96), chronic excitotoxic effects have been observed. In spinal cord explants, motor neuron degeneration has been generated over a time course of several weeks by chronic pharmacological blockade of glutamate reuptake (97). It has been shown that activation of glutamate receptors can generate long-lasting changes both in neuronal gene expression and specific aspects of cellular biochemistry (98,99).

Secondary Excitotoxicity

Excitotoxicity can occur as a secondary process triggered by some other primary pathological event, if the initial insult compromises the neuronal energy status leading to a loss of normal resting membrane potential. In these circumstances the voltage-dependent magnesium block of NMDA receptor channels is lost, which results in excessive activation of the receptor in the presence of normal levels of extracellular glutamate.

This concept of secondary excitotoxicity may be a contributory mechanism that leads to cell death in certain chronic neurodegenerative disorders. In the context of neuronal energy compromise caused by some primary pathological process, activation of glutamate receptors may have toxic effects in the absence of an underlying abnormality in the expression of glutamate or its receptors.

Role of Specific Glutamate Receptor Subtypes in Mediating Excitotoxicity

It was initially thought that the NMDA subtype of glutamate receptor was primarily involved in the mediation of excitotoxic effects because it possesses an ion channel with high calcium permeability (22). However, it is now apparent that excitotoxicity can result from activation of non-NMDA receptors, particularly following more prolonged exposure to the agonist (21). As calcium is of great importance in mediating the toxic effects of glutamate, it could be predicted that neurons expressing calcium-permeable AMPA receptors are more susceptible to glutamate toxicity. Indeed it has been robustly demonstrated by several groups that populations of neurons such as spinal motor neurons, which have a high expression of calcium-permeable AMPA receptors and a low expression of the GluR2 AMPA receptor subunit, are more susceptible to excitotoxicity mediated by AMPA-kainate receptor activation compared to other neuronal populations (100–103).

The potential role of mGlu receptors in relation to excitotoxicity has also been explored. In certain experimental paradigms activation of mGlu receptors reduced the neurotoxic effect of NMDA receptor activation (104), whereas other reports support an opposing conclusion with the activation of mGlu receptors selectively potentiating NMDA toxicity (105). In mixed murine cortical cultures, group II metabotropic receptor agonists are neuroprotective against NMDA toxicity, and groups I and II receptor agonists have the same effect in cultures of cerebellar granule cells and in rat hippocampal slices (54,106). It has also been shown that activation of NMDA receptors can reverse the desensitization of the mGluR5 subtype (107). This suggests a reciprocal positive feedback mechanism between these two glutamate receptor subtypes. In addition, it has been demonstrated that the neuroprotective effect of group III metabotropic receptor activation against NMDA toxicity is primarily mediated by the mGluR4 subtype in both cell culture and in vivo models (108).

It has also been shown that in hippocampal slices from 14 to 19-day-old rats that activation of the kainate receptors causes downstream effects resembling metabotropic activity, which appear important in modulating the excitability of the pyramidal cells (109). Thus, metabotropic glutamate receptors may play an important role in regulating the sensitivity of neurons to excitotoxic stimuli.

THE GLUTAMATERGIC NEUROTRANSMITTER SYSTEM AND MOTOR NEURONS

Several glutamatergic pathways impinge on motor neurons, including corticospinal terminals, excitatory interneurons and collaterals from the Aα fibers innervating muscle spindles (110–112). Motor neurons are activated by stimulation of cell surface glutamate receptors, with other neurotransmitters, including thyrotropin releasing hormone (TRH) and serotonin, probably exerting modulatory effects (113). The AMPA glutamate receptor subtype is responsible for much of the routine fast excitatory neurotransmission and it appears that motor neurons are particularly susceptible to toxicity via activation of cell surface AMPA receptors (100).

NMDA Receptors

Autoradiographic studies have shown that NMDA receptors are present throughout the gray matter of the human spinal cord, with focal areas of high intensity binding in relation to motor neurons in the ventral horn (99,114). In the motor cortex, NMDA receptors are present in each layer, with the greatest density of receptors in layers I, II and the upper part of layer III (114). Brainstem motor neurons subserving eye movements, which tend to be spared in ALS, have significantly lower densities of NMDA receptors compared to other cranial nerve motor nuclei (V, VII, X, and XII), which tend to be affected (114).

Non-NMDA Receptors

Autoradiographic studies of the distribution of AMPA and kainate receptors in the human motor system have revealed the presence of these receptors through all layers of the motor cortex, with the highest receptor densities in the superficial layers (99,115).

In the spinal cord the receptors are present in all laminae of the gray matter, with the highest receptor density observed in the substantia gelatinosa (115). Brainstem motor nuclei subserving ocular movements expressed a higher density of AMPA and kainate receptor binding sites compared to bulbar motor nuclei vulnerable to the disease process in ALS (115).

Further studies examining the expression of the AMPA receptors by human motor neurons have focused on the GluR2 receptor subtype. As highlighted earlier, the fully Q/R edited GluR2 isoform has a profound effect upon the permeability of the neuron to calcium ions and thus may control susceptibility to excitotoxicity. Williams et al. (116) in an immunohistochemical study reported that human motor neurons express GluR2/3, GluR1, and GluR4 AMPA receptor subunits. The patterns of expression were similar in groups of motor neurons either typically affected or spared in ALS (117). Subsequently, using in situ hybridization with subunit specific riboprobes, it was found that the GluR2 subunit was expressed at a significantly lower level than the other three subunits in human motor neurons, compared to other neuronal groups. Petralia et al. (102) used a GluR2 specific antibody and demonstrated that motor neurons in the rat brainstem and spinal cord showed little or no GluR2 protein expression. Using this specific antibody for the GluR2 subunit, Shaw et al. (103) showed a low level of expression of GluR2 protein by normal human lower motor neurons in the spinal cord and upper motor neurons (Betz cells) in the motor cortex, in comparison with other neuronal groups. Tomiyama et al. (118) investigated the expression of the GluR subunits in the human spinal cord by in situ hybridization using oligonucleotide probes and demonstrated that motor neurons did appear to show some expression of the GluR2 flop isoform. Subsequently, two studies using laser capture microdissection of human motor neurons and quantitative PCR to measure expression levels of mRNA for GluR2 subunits have confirmed that motor neurons express relatively low levels of GluR2 compared to other neuronal groups (119,120).

In their studies of dissociated embryonic rat spinal cord neurons, Brorson et al. (121) and Vandenberghe et al. (122) have investigated the relative proportions of the different AMPA mediated receptor subtypes expressed by motor neurons and dorsal horn neurons in rats using a single cell RT–PCR approach allied to patch-clamp analysis. They reported that the GluR2 subunit forms up to 40% of the GluR isoforms found in both motor neurons and other cells, the GluR2 subunit was fully edited at the Q/R site, and the ratio of flip to flop forms was weighted towards the flop form. However, patch clamp analysis of AMPA receptor desensitization demonstrated that the motor neurons showed a two- to three-fold increased current density compared to the dorsal horn neurons. It was suggested that an important factor determining the selective vulnerability of motor neurons to excitotoxicity is the presence of a high number of AMPA receptors on the surface of motor neurons compared to dorsal horn neurons. In another study, cultured motor neurons were found to be selectively vulnerable to non-NMDA receptor toxicity via a calcium-dependent pathway (123). The susceptibility of the motor neurons was selective for calcium permeable AMPA receptors but some receptors on the motor neuron surface did possess the GluR2 subunit. It was suggested that the sensitivity of the motor neurons to excitotoxicity relies upon the presence of a proportion of AMPA receptors lacking the GluR2 subunit on the cell surface.

Laslo et al. (124) examined differential expression of GluR2 in selected normal rat motor nuclei. The selected nuclei were the oculomotor nucleus (III), which is resistant to degeneration in motor neuron disease, and the hypoglossal nucleus (XII), which is known to be vulnerable to degeneration in the disease. Using both in situ hybridization and immunocytochemistry, they found equivalent levels of GluR2 message and protein in both nuclei. Recently a GluR2 null mutant mouse line has been generated (125).

Using kainate to evoke AMPA receptor mediated excitotoxicity, it was possible to demonstrate that cells with reduced or absent GluR2 receptors were more calcium permeable and exhibited increased ionic currents in response to kainate. However, the dependence of excitotoxic vulnerability on GluR2 level corresponded with the evoked ionic current and not the predicted calcium permeability.

It is now apparent that the level of expression of the GluR2 subunit, and its editing at the Q/R site is a complex matter, dependent upon a number of variables. For example, it has recently been demonstrated that the level of expression of the GluR2 subunit by motor neurons varies in different strains of rat (126). Importantly, the differences observed appeared to reflect the background of the astrocyte feeder layer upon which the motor neurons were cultured. The relevance of this data might indicate some important translational control of GluR2 and could indicate the relevance of the polymorphic leader sequence in GluR2 reported by Myers et al. (35).

Thus motor neurons do appear to be differentially susceptible to toxicity mediated by activation of AMPA/kainate receptors. In some rodent models the intensity of the evoked ionic current appears to be an important factor underlying this vulnerability. The balance of evidence suggests that the molecular phenotype of AMPA receptors expressed by human motor neurons, in particular relating to the low relative expression of the GluR2 subunit, may be an important factor in selective vulnerability of these cells to the neurodegenerative process in ALS.

Metabotropic Receptors

Anneser et al. (127,128) have recently investigated the expression of group I metabotropic receptors mGluR1 and mGluR5 in human and rat spinal cord using in situ hybridization and immunohistochemistry. They demonstrated that mGluR5 was highly expressed by the autonomic neurons of Onuf's nucleus and thoracic sympathetic neurons, but not by the somatic motor neurons, which are vulnerable to the disease process in ALS.

In contrast, mRNA for the mGluR1 receptor was found only in the smaller somatic motor neurons that are spared in ALS. This suggested that the differential expression of the group I metabotropic receptors might have a role in the selective vulnerability of different populations of motor neurons. Tomiyama et al. (129) also examined mRNA expression of receptors mGluR 1–5 in the human spinal cord. They found mGluR1, 4, and 5 expression by spinal neurons. The mGluR4 was the most highly expressed in ventral horn motor neurons, which showed only weak expression of mGluR1. The mGluR5 showed most expression in dorsal horn neurons, with little expression by motor neurons. Thus, the group I receptors, mGluR5 and mGluR1, again were shown to be expressed in spinal cord neuronal groups which tend to be spared in ALS. In contrast, the group III receptor subtype mGluR4 appears to be enriched in the vicinity of motor neurons. The group III receptors have previously been thought to be predominantly presynaptic, where they may modulate glutamatergic transmission (130). However, the precise localization of the mGluR4 subunit in relation to motor neurons has not been determined. Valerio et al. (131) examined the expression of splice variants of mGluR1 in the human and rat spinal cord. They demonstrated that the mGluR1a splice variant was expressed at high levels by adult spinal motor neurons in both species, with increased levels of expression during development. This group also investigated the action of mGluR1 receptor agonists against kainate induced motor neuron toxicity. They applied toxic concentrations of kainate to adult rat lumbar spinal cord slices and showed that the group I metabotropic receptor agonist 3-hydroxyphenylglycine (3-HPG) was neuroprotective, suggesting a role for the group I receptor subtypes in protection of motor neurons from excitotoxicity.

Glutamate Transporter Expression in the Vicinity of Motor Neurons

Immunohistochemical approaches have been used to investigate the expression of specific glutamate transporter proteins in relation to the human motor system.

EAAT1 immunoreactivity in the normal human motor cortex was diffuse, with strongest staining in the outer molecular layer. In the spinal cord diffuse staining of astrocyte processes with EAAT1 was present as a felt-like neuropil across the whole spinal gray matter, with most intense staining in the substantia gelatinosa (132). EAAT2 immunoreactivity in the human motor cortex showed a laminated pattern, with a superficial intense band (corresponding to layers 1 and 2); a paler middle band (layer 3 and part of layer 5) and a more intense deep layer (layers 5 and 6) (133). In the spinal cord, the ventral horn showed strong immunoreactivity with dense perisomatic staining around motor neuron cell bodies, the substantia gelatinosa showed moderate diffuse staining and the intermediate spinal laminae showed weak staining (133). Motor neurons, which are vulnerable to pathology in ALS appear to have a much greater perisomatic expression of the EAAT2 protein compared to motor neuron groups such as the oculomotor nuclei which are normally spared in the disease (134). If the level of expression or functional capacity of EAAT2 is reduced, one could postulate that the consequences would be more damaging for cells that are normally reliant on high expression of this transporter in their vicinity.

POTENTIAL ROLE OF EXCITOTOXICITY IN ALS

ALS is a late-onset neurodegenerative disorder characterized by injury and cell death of motor neurons in the motor cortex, brainstem and spinal cord. This results in progressive failure of the neuromuscular system and death, usually from respiratory muscle weakness, within two to five years. Approximately 10% of ALS cases are familial and about 20% of cases with familial disease show mutations in the copper–zinc superoxide dismutase (*SOD1*) gene (135). The clinical phenotype and pathology of the sporadic and familial forms of ALS are very similar, suggesting common mechanisms of neurodegeneration.

Current evidence suggests that there may be a complex interplay between several pathogenetic mechanisms underlying motor neuron degeneration, as discussed elsewhere in this volume. There is a body of circumstantial evidence implicating a disturbance of glutamatergic neurotransmission and excitotoxicity as a contributory factor to motor neuron injury in ALS (Table 2), which is discussed below.

Levels of Glutamate and Glutamate Metabolism in ALS

Glutamate Levels in Blood, CSF, and CNS Tissue

Several studies have provided evidence of a possible underlying defect in glutamate metabolism in ALS patients. Thus, several reports have documented increased fasting levels of glutamate in the plasma or serum in ALS patients, and in one study, oral loading with glutamate resulted in significantly greater elevations in plasma glutamate and aspartate in ALS patients compared to controls (136–138). However, other studies have been unable to confirm any abnormality of blood levels of glutamate in ALS (139–142). A similar lack of consensus exists in the studies of levels of glutamate in the cerebrospinal fluid (CSF). The level of glutamate in CSF has been reported to be raised in at least a subgroup of ALS patients (142,143), although not all

Table 2 Evidence for Glutamate-Mediated Toxicity as a Contributory Factor to Motor
Neuron Injury in ALS

Levels of glutamate and glutamate metabolism in ALS
Toxicity of CSF from ALS patients
Alterations in the expression of glutamate receptor subtypes in ALS
Abnormalities of glutamate transporter mechanisms
Potentiation of excitotoxicity by mutant SOD1
Effect of antiglutamatergic therapy in ALS patients
Neurophysiological and imaging studies
Mitochondrial dysfunction
Inflammatory mediators and excitotoxicity
Cellular phenotype of motor neurons and vulnerability to excitotoxicity

Abbreviations: ALS, amyotrophic lateral sclerosis; SOD, superoxide dismutase; CSF, cerebrospinal fluid.

laboratories have been able to replicate this finding (141). It is apparent that there are
inherent difficulties in measuring glutamate levels in biological samples. Factors contributing to the lack of consensus in the literature on the levels of glutamate in blood
and CSF in ALS patients include the metabolic instability of glutamate in biological
samples, with the necessity for extremely rigorous sampling and processing protocols,
and the likely biochemical heterogeneity present in populations of ALS patients
(144–146). Spreux-Varoquaux et al. (147) also found two levels of glutamate in the
CSF of their ALS patients. One group had similar levels to normal but the second
group, with spinal onset disease, had much higher concentrations of glutamate. However, Tikka et al. (148) did not find any change in the levels of glutamate in the CSF
from ALS patients, although they did find the CSF to be toxic to cultured primary
motor neurons. Cid et al. (149) while demonstrating increased levels of glutamate
in the CSF of ALS patients, also demonstrated that concentrations of glutamate lower
than 10 μM can induce excitotoxic effects in cultured cortical neurons.

More consistently reported is a decrease in glutamate levels in various regions
of postmortem CNS tissue in ALS patients compared to controls (150,151). The
overall impression from these studies is that there may be some underlying disturbance in glutamate metabolism or transport in ALS. Failure to properly regulate
glutamate could potentially result in raised extracellular levels of glutamate and
reduced levels within CNS tissue.

Toxicity of CSF from ALS Patients

There is evidence that a component of CSF taken from ALS patients is toxic to
cultured neurons (152–154). This toxicity appears to be mediated by non-NMDA
glutamate receptors, suggesting that the toxic product is a non-NMDA receptor
agonist, though no direct evidence has emerged to implicate glutamate itself as the
toxic factor (155). This concept is supported by the evidence that the glutamate-
release inhibitor, riluzole, is neuroprotective in this paradigm. A further study (148)
examined the toxicity of CSF from five individuals homozygous for the D90A SOD1
mutation, five other familial ALS (fALS) cases, and 16 sporadic ALS cases compared
to 24 non-neurodegenerative controls. They demonstrated that the CSF from all the
ALS cases was toxic to rat embryo spinal cord cultures compared to the control
CSF. The toxicity was associated with a decline in neuronal numbers in the cultures
but a marked increase in microglia. Administration of NMDA (MK-801) or AMPA

(CNQX) antagonists prevented the toxicity of the CSF, but did not prevent the microglial proliferation. However, treatment with minocycline, an inhibitor of microglial proliferation, prevented both neuronal death and microglial expansion. These data suggest that the toxicity of CSF is mediated by factors other than the levels of excitatory amino acids in the CSF. This study is important because it highlights a possible role of microglia in excitotoxic cell death of motor neurons. Several mechanisms have been suggested for the role of glial cells in excitotoxic cell death: (i) astrocytes can release glutamate in the vicinity of neurons by a calcium dependent mechanism, (ii) activated microglia secrete TNFα which has been shown to mediate AMPA mediated excitotoxicity, and (iii) activated microglia release matrix metalloproteinases (MMP) which can exert neurotoxic effects (156). However, the toxicity of ALS CSF varies with the experimental paradigm used (156). At least one laboratory has not been able to confirm the neuronal toxicity of ALS CSF (157).

Glutamate Synthetic Enzymes

The enzyme responsible for synthesizing glutamate from α-ketoglutarate, glutamate dehydrogenase has been reported to show increased expression in both ventral horn and lateral spinal cord white matter in ALS (158). However, Gluck et al. (159) measured the activity levels of glutamate dehydrogenase and glutaminase in platelets from patients with sporadic ALS and uncovered no differences from controls. The enzyme glutamine synthetase (GS) within perisynaptic astrocytes is indirectly responsible for the synthesis of more than 50% of neurotransmitter glutamate (59). The levels of GS activity have been found to be normal in both ALS spinal cord tissue and in the SOD1 transgenic mouse model of familial ALS (59,160). These studies suggest that the abnormalities seen in levels of tissue or extracellular glutamate are not caused by derangement in the activity of the major biochemical synthetic pathways.

Alterations in the Expression of Glutamate Receptor Subtypes in ALS

Studies of NMDA glutamate receptors in relation to ALS have been limited. Autoradiographic studies have shown an increased density of binding sites in the deeper cortical laminae for the NMDA receptor ligand MK-801 in ALS cases (114). In the same study a decrease in binding was seen in the ventral horn of the spinal cord. This loss of signal may reflect a loss of spinal motor neurons as part of the disease process, since MK-801 binding was increased in intermediate gray matter. Krieger et al. (161) also reported a decrease of MK-801 binding in the ventral horn of spinal cord from ALS cases. In situ hybridization studies of the expression of the NMDA receptor subunits in ALS spinal cord have revealed decreased expression of both the NMDAR1 and NMDAR2A subunit compared to controls (162,163). The reduction in expression of the NMDAR1 subunit was localized to the ventral horn region, but the NMDAR2A reduction was found across all of the spinal cord gray matter.

Autoradiographic studies of non-NMDA receptors in ALS have demonstrated increased density of binding sites both in the intermediate gray matter of the spinal cord and in the deep layers of the motor cortex (115). Takuma et al. (164) demonstrated that the level of expression of GluR2 was reduced in the ventral horn of both ALS and other disease controls. They also demonstrated a reduction in the efficiency of editing of the GluR2 subunit in the ventral gray area of the spinal cord in the ALS cases, though the cell types expressing this change were not investigated. This was further investigated recently using individual motor neurons that were laser micro-dissected from the spinal cords of five ALS patients and five normal controls (165). Using a single cell RT–PCR followed by restriction enzyme digestion method, it was found that the editing efficiency of GluR2 was reduced in the motor neurons while remaining 100% efficient in similarly extracted and treated cerebellar Purkinje cells. Barbon et al. (166) examined the extent of editing of the AMPA receptor subunit GluR2 and the kainate receptor subunits GluR5 and GluR6 in the NT2 cell line using a quantified direct sequencing method.

It was found that editing efficiency of all these receptor subtypes increased during differentiation of the NT2 cells into neurons. The authors suggest a relationship between editing efficiency and the expression levels of the glutamate receptor genes, with higher levels of editing correlating with the higher levels of receptor subunit expression.

Aronica et al. (167) used immunohistochemistry to localise the groups I and II metabotropic receptors in spinal cords of both ALS patients and controls. They examined five familial ALS cases, 12 sporadic ALS cases, and eight normal (non-neurodegenerative) controls. They found expression of mGluR1a, mGluR2/3, and mGluR5 throughout the spinal cord with mGluR1a showing greatest expression in ventral horn neurons, but mGluR5 being more highly expressed in dorsal horn neurons. The mGluR2/3 receptors were expressed at a low level in neurons and confined to calbindin containing cells, which are thought to be spared in ALS. There were differences in expression between the ALS and control spinal cord, with the overall levels of mGluR1a and mGluR5 being comparable between control and ALS cases, but mGluR2/3 appeared to be reduced in neurons of ALS spinal cord. However, the reactive astrocytes in the ALS spinal cords showed markedly increased expression of mGluR proteins. This may have occurred as a direct result of up-regulation of the proteins in the glia, but might also be related to hyperplasia of mGluR expressing glia in the ALS cases. While mGluR1a showed the greatest increase in immunoreactivity, there was sufficient increase in mGluR5 expression to further suggest that these group I metabotropic receptor subtypes may play a role in the modulation of glial response and glial-neuronal communication in neurodegenerative diseases such as ALS.

Glutamate Transporters and Excitotoxicity in ALS

It has been suggested that the expression and function of the glutamate reuptake transporter system may be abnormal in ALS. Such a defect could potentially contribute to an elevation of extracellular glutamate levels, which could predispose to excitotoxic neuronal injury.

An initial study by Rothstein et al. (59) examined high-affinity Na^+-dependent glutamate transport in synaptosomes derived from postmortem brain and spinal cord tissue of ALS patients and controls. They reported that the synaptosomes from ALS patients showed a selective decrease in maximum transport velocity, but not affinity, for glutamate compared to those from controls. The transport defect appeared to be localized to areas of the brain and spinal cord pathologically damaged in ALS. A quantitative autoradiographic study revealed decreased binding of tritiated D-aspartate to glutamate transporter proteins in the spinal cord in ALS patients (168). A spinal cord explant model of chronic glutamatergic toxicity was developed by pharmacological inhibition of glutamate uptake using threohydroxy-aspartate (THA) (97). This experimental paradigm resulted in a slow, selective degeneration and loss of motor neurons over a period of weeks. The motor neuron toxicity was selectively prevented by non-NMDA antagonists and glutamate synthesis or release inhibitors, but not by NMDA antagonists.

Subsequent studies addressed the gene and protein expression levels of the glutamate transporters (60). Using antibodies generated against oligopeptides of rat proteins, which show 100% homology to the human proteins, reduction in expression of the EAAT2 protein by 30% to 90% in both spinal cord and motor cortex of ALS patients was demonstrated by Western blotting (60). A modest reduction was shown in EAAT3 expression in ALS motor cortex, but there was no change in EAAT1 expression. Immunohistochemical studies, using monoclonal antibodies to human glutamate transporter proteins, have also shown reduced expression of EAAT2, but increased expression of EAAT1 protein in the ALS spinal cord (133).

The hypothesis was put forward that abnormal RNA processing of EAAT2 could underlie the decreased expression and function of this protein in ALS (60).

Lin et al. (169) reported abnormal intron 7 retention and exon 9 skipping splice variants of EAAT2 as a disease specific finding in the CNS of ALS patients and this group also reported that abnormal EAAT2 transcripts could be detected in CSF. However, other groups have failed to replicate these findings, having demonstrated the presence of these EAAT2 splice variants in the CNS of normal controls as well as ALS cases (170,171). In the Flowers study, a real time RT–PCR assay was used to quantify to levels of intron 7 retaining and exon 9 skipping mRNAs in both affected and unaffected regions of tissue from both ALS and control cases. The two variants were present in the same proportions in control and ALS cases suggesting that these splice variant species are normal variants and not pathological. They were also unable to detect any expression of EAAT2 mRNA in CSF. Recently, Chen et al. (172) have described an alternative form of GLT1 (EAAT2) in neurons and astrocytes of rat brain although, as yet, they have not established a particular functional role for this splice variant. A study by Maragakis et al. (173) has examined the expression of an altered form of EAAT2, EAAT2b, in human motor cortex. The novel form of EAAT2, which has a truncated C-terminal domain, was found in increased levels in neurons from ALS tissue in addition to its expression in astrocytes. However, the increase in expression of the protein was not matched by an increase in glutamate transport. In a microarray study, Dangond et al. (174) analyzed expression changes of approximately 6800 human genes in ALS and normal human spinal cords. They investigated potential changes in the expression of the glutamate transporters and found no significant change in the gene expression level of EAAT2. However, there was some up-regulation of EAAT1 in ALS gray matter and downregulation of EAAT3 in the same areas.

Two studies have investigated the potential relationship between disruption of glial glutamate transport and the ROS produced by motor neurons (175,176).

These reports present an interesting model, wherein ROS released from motor neurons as a result of excessive glutamate receptor activation oxidatively damages glutamate transporter proteins present in glia in the vicinity of motor neurons, causing a disruption of glutamate transport and hence exacerbating motor neuron injury.

Several other studies have attempted to model glutamatergic toxic effects on motor neurons by experimental manipulation of glutamate transport. Reducing the expression of glutamate transporters using antisense oligonucleotides, both in organotypic rat spinal cord cultures and also by chronic intraventricular infusion

in vivo, produced elevated extracellular glutamate levels, neurodegeneration characteristic of excitotoxicity, and progressive paralysis in the *in vivo* experiments (97).
However, using an in vivo model involving microdialysis and chemical inhibitors
of glutamate transport, Massieu et al. (177) were unable to demonstrate neuronal
damage with increased extracellular glutamate alone.

A single patient has been described with a mutation in the *EAAT2* gene, an N
(Asparagine) to S (Serine) change at amino acid 206, which leads to impaired glutamate clearance capacity (178). This mutation appeared to have a dominant-negative
effect, since the mutant protein inhibited the capacity of the normal EAAT2 protein
to transport glutamate.

Based on current knowledge, it appears that alterations in the expression
and function of the glutamate transporter EAAT2 do accompany the ALS disease
state. However, it remains uncertain whether these changes represent a primary
defect, occur as part of an escalating cycle of motor neuron injury, or whether they
develop as secondary consequences of motor neuron depletion and an attempted
compensatory response in a failing motor system. At the present time the conclusion
must be that *EAAT2* gene regulation and its pathogenetic relevance for human diseases, including ALS, are incompletely understood and require further investigation.

Interaction Between SOD1 Mutations and the Glutamate Neurotransmitter System

Mutant SOD1 and Susceptibility of Motor Neurons to Excitotoxicity

Experiments using both transgenic animals and motor neuron cultures have demonstrated that the presence of the SOD1 mutation can have a marked effect on the
sensitivity of the motor neuron to excitotoxicity. This was first investigated in the
transgenic mouse model of the G93A SOD1 mutation by Gurney et al. (179) who
showed that the mutation was, at least in part, responsible for the increased susceptibility of the motor neurons to excitotoxicity. In a primary motor neuron culture
model, Durham et al. (180) showed that the presence of the mutant G93A SOD1
mutation caused aggregation of the SOD1 protein, and this was associated with
increased susceptibility of the cultured motor neurons to excitotoxicity (181).
Kruman et al. (182) using mixed spinal cord cultures derived from mutant SOD1
transgenic mice demonstrated an association between the SOD1 mutation and
increased susceptibility to excitotoxicity, both in vivo and in vitro. It was suggested
that the presence of the generated mutant SOD1 increased levels of cellular oxidative
stress and membrane lipid peroxidation, which in turn would disrupt calcium homeostasis and sensitize the motor neurons to excitotoxicity.

Following earlier work examining the altered expression of AMPA receptors in
mice expressing the human G93A mutant *SOD1* gene (183), Spalloni et al. (184)
demonstrated a direct link between the G93A SOD1 mutation and altered AMPA
receptor subunit expression within motor neurons in culture and hence susceptibility
to excitotoxicity induced by the non-NMDA receptor agonist kainate. They initially
demonstrated that cultured motor neurons from a G93A murine spinal cord were
more susceptible to kainate and AMPA induced neurotoxicity than those from mice
that are normal or carrying the wild type human SOD1.

Single cell RT–PCR analysis to quantify the levels of the different AMPA receptor subtypes showed that the levels of GluR3 and GluR4 were significantly higher in
G93A motor neurons than those of control or normal SOD1 motor neurons. There

was also a difference in the expression level of GluR1, with both control and G93A motor neurons expressing it at a higher level than normal SOD1 cells. There were also differences in the expression of splice variants of the AMPA receptors, with GluR3 and GluR4 flip isoforms being more prevalent in the G93A-bearing motor neurons, while the normal SOD1 bearing motor neurons expressed more GluR1 and GluR4 flop isoforms. Overall the data suggest that the presence of human SOD1 forms causes an alteration in the expression of AMPA receptor subunits. In particular, the G93A mutation causes an increased expression of the flip isoforms of the GluR3 and 4 sub-types, which would generate more slowly desensitizing AMPA receptors. Neurons bearing these receptors are more vulnerable to excess Ca^{2+} influx, which could be an important factor in the pathogenesis of motor neuron injury.

Effects of Mutant SOD1 on Glutamate Transporters

Bendotti et al. (185) showed in a G93A mutant SOD1 transgenic mouse that GLT1 (the mouse homolog of EAAT2) was expressed at a lower level in the ventral gray region of the spinal cord in aged transgenic mice than in the dorsal horn of the same mice. The decline in GLT1 seemed to develop after the clinical onset of disease and affected the protein, but not the mRNA level. Another study also examined the levels of GLT-1 in a G93A transgenic mouse model (186). Western blot analyses of protein derived from both transgenic and normal mice failed to show any significant differences in the level of GLT-1 in several CNS regions (cortex, brain stem, cervical, and lumbar cord). A similar result was obtained by direct immunohistochemistry. However, it was observed that the GLT-1 from end-stage G93A mice had altered mobility characteristics on Western blots, a proportion appearing as a higher molecular weight form, which might represent a dimer or a complex with another protein. It was suggested that this modification might cause some functional impairment of the transporter, but the fact that these changes were only strongly observed at end stage did not support a role in the early pathogenesis of motor neuron injury. Howland et al. (187) developed a G93A transgenic rat model and also showed loss of immunoreactive EAAT2 in the ventral gray region of the spinal cord, although in this model patchy loss of EAAT2 began at a presymptomatic stage of disease. Guo et al. (188) created a transgenic mouse over-expressing EAAT2 and crossed this with G93A mutant SOD1 transgenic animals. These animals developed an ALS-like phenotype as a result of the SOD1 mutation, but the onset of the disease was delayed. The authors suggested that the excitotoxic contribution to motor neuron injury was attenuated by the presence of increased expression levels of the EAAT2 glutamate reuptake transporter.

Tortarolo et al. (189) used primary murine astrocytes transiently transfected with either normal or G93A mutant SOD1 to demonstrate that when over-expressed in glial cells both normal and mutant human SOD1 caused downregulation of GLT1 (EAAT2) protein, though not the corresponding mRNA. The effect was greater in the presence of mutant SOD1. The downregulation appeared very rapid in this cellular model compared with that observed in transgenic mouse models where reduced expression of GLT1 is predominantly seen at the end stage of disease. In a *Xenopus* oocyte model, it has been shown that coexpression of the (Alanine) A4V (Valine) or (Isoleucine) I113T (Threonine) mutant forms of human SOD-1 protein with GLT1/EAAT2 caused inactivation of the glutamate transporter molecule (190). It has been demonstrated previously that the EAAT2 protein is vulnerable to oxidative modification by free radical species such as peroxynitrite, which could impair its clearance activity (57,191).

These experiments implicate a link between the reactive oxygen species produced as a result of the mutant SOD1 enzyme and damage to the glutamate transporter molecule GLT-1/EAAT2. This could lead to impaired glutamate clearance at the synaptic cleft and resultant exacerbation of motor neuron injury via excitotoxic mechanisms.

Efficacy of Antiglutamatergic Therapy in ALS

Several antiglutamate drugs (e.g., riluzole, gabapentin, and NBQX) have been shown to have neuroprotective effects on anterior horn cell degeneration in animal models of ALS (192–194). These compounds interfere with excitatory neurotransmission in the CNS, attenuate neuronal excitation, and have potent anticonvulsant activity in several model systems (195). Two large clinical trials have demonstrated that riluzole has a modest effect in prolonging survival in patients with ALS (196,197). Gabapentin, although showing a positive effect in animal models, does not appear to have a robust benefit in human ALS (198,199). Recently there have been clinical trials of two other potential antiexcitotoxic compounds, topiramate and lamotrigine (200,201). Topiramate had shown some promise in preventing excitotoxic neuron loss in an organotypic spinal cord model, although it was unable to increase survival in the G93A mutant SOD1 transgenic mouse model (202). Both the compounds were clinically tested in double blind placebo controlled crossover trials, but unfortunately neither demonstrated any patient benefit. Other compounds, which have been examined are reviewed elsewhere (203).

Neurophysiological and Imaging Studies in ALS

Transcranial magnetic stimulation of the motor cortex of patients with ALS has shown that a proportion of patients possess abnormalities related to hyperexcitable motor neurons (204,205). The hyperexcitable neurons appear to be largely cortical and not spinal with the increased excitation resulting from hyperexcitability of the corticomotoneurons accompanied by reduced inhibition owing to dysfunction of the cortical inhibitory interneurons (206).

Positron emission tomography (PET) studies have shown abnormalities in cerebral blood flow in ALS patients compared to controls in a paradigm involving upper limb movement (207). In the ALS group, there was abnormally widespread activation in several cortical areas outside the somatotropic representation of the upper limb, suggesting an imbalance between cortical excitatory and inhibitory neurotransmission in ALS. The altered excitability of motor neurons has also been examined in the G93A transgenic mouse model of ALS. It was found, by patch clamp analysis, that spinal motor neurons containing mutant SOD1 in culture displayed increased firing frequency of shorter duration than control motor neurons while having equivalent passive membrane properties (208,209). This further suggests a relationship between altered motor neuron excitability and the pathogenesis of ALS.

Mitochondrial Involvement and Excitotoxicity in ALS

The mitochondrial respiratory chain is one of the major sites for intracellular generation of free radicals, which might be expected to cause cell damage and increase cellular vulnerability to secondary excitotoxicity. The evidence that mitochondrial dysfunction may contribute to motor neuron injury in ALS has been reviewed (101,210,211). Morphological changes in mitochondria have been reported in the spinal motor neurons of ALS patients, and a decrease in cytochrome C oxidase activity in the ventral horn and in individual spinal motor neurons (212,213). In mutant SOD1 transgenic mice, swelling and vacuolar distortion of the mitochondria is seen as an early feature prior to signs of motor dysfunction.

It has been shown previously that glutamate receptor activation, free radical generation and mitochondrial energy metabolism are interconnected systems linked through the intracellular actions of calcium (211). The interaction of these pathways was investigated by Stout et al. (214), who showed that excessive activation of neuronal glutamate receptors caused excessive calcium influx.

It was demonstrated that blocking calcium uptake by mitochondria reduced glutamate toxicity. This indicated that the sequestration of intracellular calcium by mitochondria is an important factor in delayed neurotoxicity resulting from glutamate receptor activation.

Singh et al. (215) examined the effect of prolonged glutamate activation upon mitochondrial enzymes in a rat model. They found profound alteration of mitochondrial integrity leading to loss of enzymatic activity and functional impairment relating directly to the excessive glutamatergic activation. Kannurpati et al. (216) examined the effects of glutamatergic toxicity on mitochondrial function in cortical slices from young (21 days) and adult (80 days) rats. Particularly in the adult group the ATP/ADP ratios were reduced and the NAD/NADH ratio rose, suggesting a failing energy production by the mitochondria in the older rats. The addition of extra calcium in the culture medium caused increased glutamate induced ROS generation in both groups, but the rate of production was faster and markedly higher in the adult group. These data demonstrated that the adult rats were more susceptible to excitotoxic effects at the mitochondrial level.

Potentiation of Excitotoxicity by Inflammatory Mediators

The inducible enzyme cyclo-oxygenase-2 (COX-2) is an important component of the prostaglandin pathway, catalyzing the production of prostaglandins from arachidonic acid as a part of the inflammatory response. It is known that astrocytic glutamate release may be stimulated by prostaglandins via a calcium-dependent pathway (217). The levels of COX-2 are thus of importance in controlling the production of prostaglandins and, of relevance to ALS, is how this might interact with astrocytic glutamate release under stress conditions. Kelly et al. (218) examined the neuronal response to kainate-induced seizures and glutamate excitotoxicity using a murine transgenic model in which the human COX-2 (*hCOX-2*) gene was overexpressed under the control of a rat neuron-specific promoter. Overexpression of the *hCOX-2* caused upregulation of the immediate early genes c-fos and zif-268 in response to exposure to kainate, suggesting that COX-2 might regulate the sensitivity of the neurons to kainate by controlling the expression of these immediate early genes. The potential role of COX-2 in ALS was investigated by Drachman and Rothstein (217). They demonstrated a protective effect of a COX-2 inhibitor on motor neurons within spinal cord slices subjected to chronic glutamatergic toxicity and subsequently a neuroprotective effect was also observed in a mutant SOD1 mouse model (217). Almer et al. (219) demonstrated increased expression of COX-2 in the G93A SOD1 transgenic mouse model of ALS and in postmortem spinal cords from sporadic ALS patients.

Vulnerability Factors Predisposing Motor Neurons to Excitotoxicity

The molecular factors potentially underlying vulnerability of human motor neurons to excitotoxicity have been reviewed previously (220). Motor neurons are one of the largest cell groups in the nervous system. As well as a large somatic diameter, they possess axonal processes of up to 1m in length. These anatomical features would predict high metabolic demands, an accompanying high level of mitochondrial activity, and the requirement for a robust cytoskeletal organization. The possible role played by the particular profile of glutamate receptors expressed by motor neurons, and particularly the contribution of calcium permeable AMPA receptors generated by the low cellular expression of the GluR2 AMPA receptor subunit, has been discussed in the glutamatergic neurotransmitter system and motor neurons of this chapter. Motor neurons have a relatively high neurofilament content, and any disruption in the function and stoichiometric arrangement of the three neurofilament (NF) subunits, NF-light (NF-L), NF-medium (NF-M), and NF-heavy (NF-H), might have a profound effect on the viability of these neurons. It has been shown previously in ALS that motor neuron degeneration is associated with abnormal neurofilamentous accumulations (221,222).

Morrison et al. (223) examined a SOD1 transgenic mouse model of ALS by immunocytochemistry and demonstrated that motor neurons expressing phosphorylated neurofilaments were preferentially vulnerable to degeneration, except where calbindin was also expressed. In addition Williamson et al. (224) delayed the onset and progression of motor neuron degeneration in a SOD1 transgenic mouse by deleting the NF-L subunit gene. Bergeron et al. (43) demonstrated by in situ hybridization a decreased level of expression of the NF-L subunit (in association with an overall decrease in polyA mRNA production in these cells) in spinal cord motor neurons from ALS cases. Vartiainen et al. (225) examined the interaction between the expression of neurofilament subunits and glutamatergic receptors. They demonstrated in a rat spinal cord culture model that glutamate regulates the expression, distribution, and phosphorylation of the NF-M and NF-H subunits. Activation of the AMPA/kainate receptors caused an increase in the level of dephosphorylated NF-M and NF-H after 24 hours, even though the total amount of NF-M mRNA was decreased. These alterations might sensitize the cell to neurotoxic mechanisms such as calpain-mediated proteolysis. Under normal circumstances, neurofilaments are transported through axons by slow axonal transport, and it is believed that glutamatergic excitotoxicity can act to perturb this transport mechanism. By attaching green fluorescent protein to NF-M, it was shown that glutamate caused a slowing of axonal transport of neurofilaments (226). This was shown to be a result of increased phosphorylation of the NF-M side arm domains. The activity of the glutamate receptors also alters the expression of NF mRNAs and the subcellular location of their proteins, suggesting an interaction between glutamate receptor function, neurofilament expression, and the pathogenesis of ALS (225,227).

The maintenance of normal calcium homeostasis within neurons is of profound importance in preventing excitotoxicity.

This function is achieved by a complex system of compartmentalization, transportation involving binding to calcium-buffering proteins, sequestration within organelles, and transfer of excess calcium to the extracellular environment via ATP-dependent ion-exchangers (88). The level of expression of the calcium-binding proteins, calbindin, and calretinin, has been shown to correlate with resistance to excitotoxicity (228,229). Motor neuron groups vulnerable to the ALS disease-process have been shown to lack expression of the calcium-binding proteins calbindin D28K and parvalbumin, whereas, motor neuron groups less vulnerable to ALS, including the oculomotor nucleus and Onuf's nucleus, do show expression of these proteins.

It has been proposed that another factor directly involved in motor neuron injury is a low expression of molecular chaperones (230). In cell culture models, resistance to mutant SOD1 toxicity correlated with increased overall chaperone activity and up-regulation of individual chaperones/stress proteins. When the level of the stress inducible, chaperone, 70 kDa heat shock protein, was artificially raised by gene transfer into cultured primary motor neurons expressing the mutant human G93A SOD1 mutation, the production of SOD1-containing proteinaceous aggregates was reduced (230). In addition, in transgenic mice expressing the human G93A mutation, the level of protein chaperone activity was decreased in lumbar spinal cord, but in clinically unaffected tissues the level remained unchanged compared to control tissue.

EXCITOTOXICITY AND OTHER MOTOR SYSTEM DISORDERS

Several other types of neurodegenerative disease have been linked to excitotoxic neuronal injury. There are rare disorders in which a genetic defect disrupts normal excitatory amino acid metabolism. For example, sulfite oxidase deficiency, a metabolic disorder, which is normally fatal in childhood, leads to raised levels of the excitatory amino acid L-sulfo-cysteine (231).

A body of data exists in the literature reporting the association between chronic neurological disease and exogenous, environmentally encountered toxins. *Domoic acid poisoning* is a relatively acute disorder first described in 1987 in Canada. Ingestion of mussels contaminated with domoic acid led to an outbreak of neurological and gastrointestinal symptoms. Afflicted individuals developed headache, seizures, hemiparesis, ophthalmoplegia, and altered conscious level (232,233). Many victims of domoic acid poisoning had evidence of pure motor or sensorimotor neuropathy. Individuals who have ingested domoic acid develop gastrointestinal symptoms of poisoning within 24 hours and neurological signs within 48 hours (234). *Lathyrism*, a chronic progressive disorder that affects predominantly the upper motor neurons in the cerebral cortex and leads to anterograde amnesia and epileptic seizures, occurs as a result of ingestion of β-*N*-oxalyl-amino-L-alanine (BOAA) a glutamate analogue. BOAA is a naturally occurring excitotoxin present in chickling pea (*Lathyrus sativus*), which is a staple dietary component in areas, such as sub-Saharan Africa, where lathyrism is endemic (235). An investigation of the interaction of BOAA with non-NMDA receptors by autoradiography demonstrated that the compound inhibited both AMPA and kainate binding. This would suggest that the symptoms of lathyrism are caused by excitotoxic action on non-NMDA receptors (236). Another plant derived excitotoxin β-*N*-methylamino-L-alanine (BMAA), has been implicated in the *ALS and parkinsonism-dementia complex of Guam* (237). BMAA is present in the seed of the false sago palm (*Cycas circinalis*). The cycad seed is ground to make flour and also used as a poultice for skin wounds by the Chamorro Indian native population of Guam. BMAA in massive doses does appear to cause motor system injury in primates (237). However, evidence has emerged that the soaking and washing procedures used in the preparation of the cycad seeds are sufficient to remove most of the BMAA toxin (238).

Other compounds have been implicated in cycad toxicity, e.g., cycasin and several forms of the sterol β-D-glucoside (239,240). Recently, it has been suggested that the consumption of flying foxes by Guamanians may represent a way in which the dietary consumption of cycad toxins, including BMAA, is amplified in the human food chain (241). This hypothesis remains unproven. There is an acute form of a spastic paraparesis that occurs in Africa, which is caused by consumption of the toxic plant cassava. The leaves and tuber are eaten after attempts to remove the potentially harmful cyanogenic glucosides that are stored in the plant. The symptoms are similar to those of lathyrism, with early signs being difficulty in walking which develops into an asymmetrical spastic paraparesis (240). Victims of cassava poisoning may show clinical recovery, but there may be residual motor signs, optic atrophy, dysarthria, and hearing impairment. The precise cause of cassavism is unknown, but it may be related to insufficiently processed toxic cassava roots which are still loaded with cyanogenic glucosides. It has been suggested that the cyanide reacts with cysteine residues to form the excitotoxic compound 2-iminothiazolidine-4-carboxylic acid which is an agent proposed to have excitotoxic properties similar to those of BOAA (240).

ACKNOWLEDGMENTS

The authors are supported by the Wellcome Trust and the Motor Neuron Disease Association.

REFERENCES

1. Cotman CW, Monaghan DT, Ottersen OP, Storm-Mathisen J. Anatomical organization of excitatory amino acid receptors and their pathways. Trends Neurosci 1987; 10: 273–280.
2. Watkins JC, Evans RH. Excitatory amino acid transmitters. Annu Rev Pharmacol Toxicol 1981; 21:165–204.
3. Berg JM, Tymoczko JL, Stryer L. Biochemistry. New York: W.H. Freeman, 2002.
4. Maragakis NJ, Rothstein JD. Glutamate transporters: animal models to neurologic disease. Neurobiol Dis 2004; 15:461–473.
5. Ince PG, Eggett CJ, Shaw PJ. The role of excitotoxicity in neurological disease. Rev Contemp Pharmacother 1997; 8:195–212.
6. Broer S, Brookes N. Transfer of glutamine between astrocytes and neurons. J Neurochem 2001; 77:705–719.
7. McGee AW, Bredt DS. Assembly and plasticity of the glutamatergic postsynaptic specialization. Curr Opin Neurobiol 2003; 13:111–118.
8. Scott DB, Blanpied TA, Swanson GT, Zhang C, Ehlers MD. An NMDA receptor ER retention signal regulated by phosphorylation and alternative splicing. J Neurosci 2001; 21:3063–3072.
9. Setou M, Nakagawa T, Seog DH, Hirokawa N. Kinesin superfamily motor protein KIF17 and mLin-10 in NMDA receptor-containing vesicle transport. Science 2000; 288:1796–1802.
10. Wyszynski M, Kharazia V, Shanghvi R, Rao A, Beggs AH, Craig AM, Weinberg R, Sheng M. Differential regional expression AQ1 and ultrastructural localization of alpha-actinin-2, a putative NMDA receptor-anchoring protein, in rat brain. J Neurosci 1998; 18:1383–1392.
11. Leonard AS, Lim IA, Hemsworth DE, Horne MC, Hell JW. Calcium/calmodulin-dependent protein kinase II is associated with the N-methyl-D-aspartate receptor. Proc Natl Acad Sci USA 1999; 96:3239–3244.
12. Madden DR. The inner workings of the AMPA receptors. Curr Opin Drug Discov Devel 2002; 5:741–748.

13. Klauck TM, Scott JD. The postsynaptic density: a subcellular anchor for signal transduction enzymes. Cell Signal 1995; 7:747–757.
14. Hollmann M, O'Shea-Greenfield A, Rogers SW, Heinemann S. Cloning by functional expression of a member of the glutamate receptor family. Nature 1989; 342:643–648.
15. Michaelis EK. Molecular biology of glutamate receptors in the central nervous system and their role in excitotoxicity, oxidative stress and aging. Prog Neurobiol 1998; 54: 369–415.
16. Dingledine R, Borges K, Bowie D, Traynelis SF. The glutamate receptor ion channels. Pharmacol Rev 1999; 51:7–61.
17. Traven HG, Brodin L, Lansner A, Ekeberg O, Wallen P, Grillner S. Computer simulations of NMDA and non-NMDA receptor-mediated synaptic drive: sensory and supraspinal modulation of neurons and small networks. J Neurophysiol 1993; 70:695–709.
18. Bliss TV, Collingridge GL. A synaptic model of memory: long-term potentiation in the hippocampus. Nature 1993; 361:31–39.
19. Cull-Candy S, Brickley S, Farrant M. NMDA receptor subunits: diversity, development and disease. Curr Opin Neurobiol 2001; 11:327–335.
20. Van Den Bosch L, Schwaller B, Vleminckx V, Meijers B, Stork S, Ruehlicke T, Van Houtte E, Klaassen H, Celio MR, Missiaen L, Robberecht W, Berchtold MW. Protective effect of parvalbumin on excitotoxic motor neuron death. Exp Neurol 2002; 174:150–161.
21. Prehn JH, Lippert K, Krieglstein J. Are NMDA or AMPA/kainate receptor antagonists more efficacious in the delayed treatment of excitotoxic neuronal injury? Eur J Pharmacol 1995; 292:179–189.
22. Choi DW. Glutamate neurotoxicity and diseases of the nervous system. Neuron 1988; 1:623–634.
23. Prybylowski K, Wenthold RJ. N-Methyl-D-aspartate receptors: subunit assembly and trafficking to the synapse. J Biol Chem 2004; 279:9673–9676.
24. Zukin RS, Bennett MV. Alternatively spliced isoforms of the NMDARI receptor subunit. Trends Neurosci 1995; 18:306–313.
25. Takahashi T, Feldmeyer D, Suzuki N, Onodera K, Cull-Candy SG, Sakimura K, Mishina M. Functional correlation of NMDA receptor epsilon subunits expression with the properties of single-channel and synaptic currents in the developing cerebellum. J Neurosci 1996; 16:4376–4382.
26. Nishi M, Hinds H, Lu HP, Kawata M, Hayashi Y. Motoneuron-specific expression of NR3B, a novel NMDA-type glutamate receptor subunit that works in a dominant-negative manner. J Neurosci 2001; 21:RC185.
27. Matsuda K, Fletcher M, Kamiya Y, Yuzaki M. Specific assembly with the NMDA receptor 3B subunit controls surface expression and calcium permeability of NMDA receptors. J Neurosci 2003; 23:10064–10073.
28. Chatterton JE, Awobuluyi M, Premkumar LS, Takahashi H, Talantova M, Shin Y, Cui J, Tu S, Sevarino KA, Nakanishi N, Tong G, Lipton SA, Zhang D. Excitatory glycine receptors containing the NR3 family of NMDA receptor subunits. Nature 2002; 415:793–798.
29. Lissin DV, Carroll RC, Nicoll RA, Malenka RC, von Zastrow M. Rapid, activation-induced redistribution of ionotropic glutamate receptors in cultured hippocampal neurons. J Neurosci 1999; 19:1263–1272.
30. Lopez JC. AMPA receptors: now you see them, now you don't. Nat Rev Neurosci 2001; 2:5–7.
31. Luscher C, Nicoll RA, Malenka RC, Muller D. Synaptic plasticity and dynamic modulation of the postsynaptic membrane. Nat Neurosci 2000; 3:545–550.
32. Zhou Q, Xiao M, Nicoll RA. Contribution of cytoskeleton to the internalization of AMPA receptors. Proc Natl Acad Sci USA 2001; 98:1261–1266.
33. Myers SJ, Peters J, Huang Y, Comer MB, Barthel F, Dingledine R. Transcriptional regulation of the GluR2 gene: neural-specific expression, multiple promoters, and regulatory elements. J Neurosci 1998; 18:6723–6739.

34. Ballas N, Battaglioli E, Atouf F, Andres ME, Chenoweth J, Anderson ME, Burger C, Moniwa M, Davie JR, Bowers WJ, Federoff HJ, Rose DW, Rosenfeld MG, Brehm P, Mandel G. Regulation of neuronal traits by a novel transcriptional complex. Neuron 2001; 31:353–365.

35. Myers SJ, Huang Y, Genetta T, Dingledine R. Inhibition of glutamate receptor 2 translation by a polymorphic repeat sequence in the 5′-untranslated leaders. J Neurosci 2004; 24:3489–3499.

36. Weiss JH, Sensi SL. Ca^{2+}-Zn^{2+} permeable AMPA or kainate receptors: possible key factors in selective neurodegeneration. Trends Neurosci 2000; 23:365–371.

37. Stanfa LC, Hampton DW, Dickenson AH. Role of Ca^{2+}-permeable non-NMDA glutamate receptors in spinal nociceptive transmission. Neuroreport 2000; 11:3199–3202.

38. Iino M, Goto K, Kakegawa W, Okado H, Sudo M, Ishiuchi S, Miwa A, Takayasu Y, Saito I, Tsuzuki K, Ozawa S. Glia-synapse interaction through Ca2Þ–permeable AMPA receptors in Bergmannglia. Science 2001; 292:926–929.

39. Bettler B, Boulter J, Hermans-Borgmeyer I, O'Shea-Greenfield A, Deneris ES, Moll C, Borgmeyer U, Hollmann M, Heinemann S. Cloning of a novel glutamate receptor subunit, GluR5: expression in the nervous system during development. Neuron 1990; 5:583–595.

40. Lerma J. Roles and rules of kainate receptors in synaptic transmission. Nat Rev Neurosci 2003; 4:481–495.

41. Chittajallu R, Braithwaite SP, Clarke VR, Henley JM. Kainate receptors: subunits, synaptic localization and function. Trends Pharmacol Sci 1999; 20:26–35.

42. Frerking M, Ohliger-Frerking P. AMPA receptors and kainate receptors encode different features of afferent activity. J Neurosci 2002; 22:7434–7443.

43. Bergeron C, Beric-Maskarel K, Muntasser S, Weyer L, Somerville MJ, Percy ME. Neurofilament light and polyadenylated mRNA levels are decreased in amyotrophic lateral sclerosis motor neurons. J Neuropathol Exp Neurol 1994; 53:221–230.

44. Lomeli H, Wisden W, Kohler M, Keinanen K, Sommer B, Seeburg PH. High-affinity kainate and domoate receptors in rat brain. FEBS Lett 1992; 307:139–143.

45. Sommer B, Burnashev N, Verdoorn TA, Keinanen K, Sakmann B, Seeburg PH. A glutamate receptor channel with high affinity for domoate and kainate. EMBO J 1992; 11:1651–1656.

46. Kohler M, Burnashev N, Sakmann B, Seeburg PH. Determinants of Ca^{2+} permeability in both TM1 and TM2 of high affinity kainate receptor channels: diversity by RNA editing. Neuron 1993; 10:491–500.

47. Schiffer HH, Swanson GT, Heinemann SF. Rat GluR7 and a carboxy-terminal splice variant, GluR7b, are functional kainate receptor subunits with a low sensitivity to glutamate. Neuron 1997; 19:1141–1146.

48. Paternain AV, Herrera MT, Nieto MA, Lerma J. GluR5 and GluR6 kainate receptor subunits coexist in hippocampal neurons and coassemble to form functional receptors. J Neurosci 2000; 20:196–205.

49. Cui C, Mayer ML. Heteromeric kainate receptors formed by the coassembly of GluR5, GluR6, and GluR7. J Neurosci 1999; 19:8281–8291.

50. Sladeczek F, Pin JP, Recasens M, Bockaert J, Weiss S. Glutamate stimulates inositol phosphate formation in striatal neurones. Nature 1985; 317:717–719.

51. Masu M, Tanabe Y, Tsuchida K, Shigemoto R, Nakanishi S. Sequence and expression of a metabotropic glutamate receptor. Nature 1991; 349:760–765.

52. Nicoletti F, Bruno V, Copani A, Casabona G, Knopfel T. Metabotropic glutamate receptors: a new target for the therapy of neurodegenerative disorders? Trends Neurosci 1996; 19:267–271.

53. Hollmann M, Boulter J, Maron C, Heinemann S. Molecular biology of glutamate receptors. Potentiation of N-methyl-D-aspartate receptor splice variants by zinc. Ren Physiol Biochem 1994; 17:182–183.

54. Pin JP, Duvoisin R. The metabotropic glutamate receptors: structure and functions. Neuropharmacology 1995; 34:1–26.

55. Toms NJ, Roberts PJ, Salt TE, Staton PC. Latest eruptions in metabotropic glutamate receptors. Trends Pharmacol Sci 1996; 17:429–435.

56. O'Shea RD. Roles and regulation of glutamate transporters in the central nervous system. Clin Exp Pharmacol Physiol 2002; 29:1018–1023.

57. Trotti D, Danbolt NC, Volterra A. Glutamate transporters are oxidant-vulnerable: a molecular link between oxidative and excitotoxic neurodegeneration? Trends Pharmacol Sci 1998; 19:328–334.

58. Furuta A, Rothstein JD, Martin LJ. Glutamate transporter protein subtypes are expressed differentially during rat CNS development. J Neurosci 1997; 17:8363–8375.

59. Rothstein JD, Martin LJ, Kuncl RW. Decreased glutamate transport by the brain and spinal cord in amyotrophic lateral sclerosis. N Engl J Med 1992; 326:1464–1468.

60. Rothstein JD, Van Kammen M, Levey AI, Martin LJ, Kuncl RW. Selective loss of glial glutamate transporter GLT-1 in amyotrophic lateral sclerosis. Ann Neurol 1995; 38: 73–84.

61. Haugeto O, Ullensvang K, Levy LM, Chaudry FA, Honore T, Nielsen M, Lehre KP, Danbolt NC. Brain glutamate transporter proteins form homomultimers. J Biol Chem 1996; 271:27715–27722.

62. Fairman WA, Amara SG. Functional diversity of excitatory amino acid transporters: ion channel and transport modes. Am J Physiol 1999; 277:F481–F486.

63. Aihara Y, Mashima H, Onda H, Hisano S, Kasuya H, Hori T, Yamada S, Tomura H, Yamada Y, Inoue I, Kojima I, Takeda J. Molecular cloning of a novel brain-type Na(Þ)-dependent inorganic phosphate cotransporter. J Neurochem 2000; 74:2622–2625.

64. Bellocchio EE, Reimer RJ, Fremeau RT Jr., Edwards RH. Uptake of glutamate into synaptic vesicles by an inorganic phosphate transporter. Science 2000; 289:957–960.

65. Fremeau RT Jr, Burman J, Qureshi T, Tran CH, Proctor J, Johnson J, Zhang H, Sulzer D, Copenhagen DR, Storm-Mathisen J, Reimer RJ, Edwards RH. The identification of vesicular glutamate transporter 3 suggests novel modes of signaling by glutamate. Proc Natl Acad Sci USA 2002; 99:14488–14493.

66. Herzog E, Bellenchi GC, Gras C, Bernard V, Ravassard P, Bedet C, Gasnier B, Giros B, El Mestikawy S. The existence of a second vesicular glutamate transporter specifies subpopulations of glutamatergic neurons. J Neurosci 2001; 21:RC181.

67. Takamori S, Rhee JS, Rosenmund C, Jahn R. Identification of differentiation-associated brain-specific phosphate transporter as a second vesicular glutamate transporter (VGLUT2). J Neurosci 2001; 21:RC182.

68. Fremeau RT Jr, Troyer MD, Pahner I, Nygaard GO, Tran CH, Reimer RJ, Bellochio EE, Fortin D, Storm-Mathisen J, Edwards RH. The expression of vesicular glutamate transporters defines two classes of excitatory synapse. Neuron 2001; 31:247–260.

69. Fremeau RT Jr, Voglmaier S, Seal RP, Edwards RH. VGLUTs define subsets of excitatory neurons and suggest novel roles for glutamate. Trends Neurosci 2004; 27:98–103.

70. Oliveira AL, Hydling F, Olsson E, Shi T, Edwards RH, Fujiyama F, Kaneko T, Hokfelt T, Cullheim S, Meister B. Cellular localization of three vesicular glutamate transporter mRNAs and proteins in rat spinal cord and dorsal root ganglia. Synapse 2003; 50: 117–129.

71. Lucas DR, Newhouse JP. The toxic effect of sodium L-glutamate on the inner layers of the retina. Ama Arch Opthalmol 1957; 58:193–201.

72. Olney JW, Rhee V, Ho OL. Kainic acid: a powerful neurotoxic analogue of glutamate. Brain Res 1974; 77:507–512.

73. Whetsell WO Jr. Current concepts of excitotoxicity. J Neuropathol Exp Neurol 1996; 55:1–13.

74. Doble A. The role of excitotoxicity in neurodegenerative disease: implications for therapy. Pharmacol Ther 1999; 81:163–221.

75. Murphy TH, Miyamoto M, Sastre A, Schnaar RL, Coyle JT. Glutamate toxicity in a neuronal cell line involves inhibition of cystine transport leading to oxidative stress. Neuron 1989; 2:1547–1558.

76. Meister A, Anderson ME. Glutathione. Annu Rev Biochem 1983; 52:711–760.

77. Park DS, Obeidat A, Giovanni A, Greene LA. Cell cycle regulators in neuronal death evoked by excitotoxic stress: implications for neurodegeneration and its treatment. Neurobiol Aging 2000; 21:771–781.

78. Nguyen MD, Boudreau M, Kriz J, Couillard-Despres S, Kaplan DR, Julien JP. Cell cycle regulators in the neuronal death pathway of amyotrophic lateral sclerosis caused by mutant superoxide dismutase 1. J Neurosci 2003; 23:2131–2140.

79. Ranganathan S, Bowser R. Alterations in G(1) to S phase cell-cycle regulators during amyotrophic lateral sclerosis. Am J Pathol 2003; 162:823–835.

80. Klein JA, Ackerman SL. Oxidative stress, cell cycle, and neurodegeneration. J Clin Invest 2003; 111:785–793.

81. Garcia-Galloway E, Arango C, Pons S, Torres-Aleman I. Glutamate excitotoxicity attenuates insulin-like growth factor-I prosurvival signaling. Mol Cell Neurosci 2003; 24:1027–1037.

82. Chung YH, Joo KM, Shin CM, Lee YJ, Shin DH, Lee KH, Cha CI. Immunohistochemical study on the distribution of insulin-like growth factor I (IGF-I)receptor in the central nervous system of SOD1(G93A)mutant transgenic mice. Brain Res 2003; 994:253–259.

83. Holzenberger M, Dupont J, Ducos B, Leneuve P, Geloen A, Even PC, Cervera P, Le Bouc Y. IGF-1 receptor regulates lifespan and resistance to oxidative stress in mice. Nature 2003; 421:182–187.

84. Vincent AM, Mobley BC, Hiller A, Feldman EL. IGF-I prevents glutamate-induced motor neuron programmed cell death. Neurobiol Dis 2004; 16:407–416.

85. Choi DW. Ionic dependence of glutamate neurotoxicity. J Neurosci 1987; 7:369–379.

86. Miller RJ, Murphy SN, Glaum SR. Neuronal Ca^{2+} channels and their regulation by excitatory amino acids. Ann N Y Acad Sci 1989; 568:149–158.

87. Baimbridge KG, Celio MR, Rogers JH. Calcium-binding proteins in the nervous system. Trends Neurosci 1992; 15:303–308.

88. Orrenius S, McConkey DJ, Bellomo G, Nicotera P. Role of Ca^{2+} in toxic cell killing. Trends Pharmacol Sci 1989; 10:281–285.

89. Ankarcrona M, Dypbukt JM, Bonfoco E, Zhivotovsky B, Orrenius S, Lipton SA, Nicotera P. Glutamate-induced neuronal death:a succession of necrosis or apoptosis depending on mitochondrial function. Neuron 1995; 15:961–973.

90. Du Y, Dodel RC, Bales KR, Jemmerson R, Hamilton-Byrd E, Paul SM. Involvement of a caspase-3-like cysteine protease in 1-methyl-4-phenylpyridinium-mediated apoptosis of cultured cerebellar granule neurons. J Neurochem 1997; 69:1382–1388.

91. Mattson MP, Keller JN, Begley JG. Evidence for synaptic apoptosis. Exp Neurol 1998; 153:35–48.

92. Yu SW, Wang H, Poitras MF, Coombs C, Bowers WJ, Federoff HJ, Poirier GG, Dawson TM, Dawson VL. Mediation of poly(ADP-ribose)polymerase-1-dependent cell death by apoptosis-inducing factor. Science 2002; 297:259–263.

93. Chiarugi A, Moskowitz MA. Cell biology. PARP-1—a perpetrator of apoptotic cell death? Science 2002; 297:200–201.

94. Chung YH, Joo KM, Lee YJ, Shin DH, Cha CI. Reactive astrocytes express PARP in the central nervous system of SOD(G93A) transgenic mice. Brain Res 2004; 1003:199–204.

95. Whetsell WO Jr, Schwarcz R. Prolonged exposure to submicromolar concentrations of quinolinic acid causes excitotoxic damage in organotypic cultures of rat corticostriatal system. Neurosci Lett 1989; 97:271–275.

96. Susel Z, Engber TM, Kuo S, Chase TN. Prolonged infusion of quinolinic acid into rat striatum as an excitotoxic model of neurodegenerative disease. Neurosci Lett 1991; 121:234–238.

97. Rothstein JD, Jin L, Dykes-Hoberg M, Kuncl RW. Chronic inhibition of glutamate uptake produces a model of slow neurotoxicity. Proc Natl Acad Sci USA 1993; 90:6591–6595.

98. Jakoi ER, Sombati S, Gerwin C, DeLorenzo RJ. Excitatory amino acid receptor activation produces a selective and long-lasting modulation of gene expression in hippocampal neurons. Brain Res 1992; 582:282–290.

99. Monaghan DT, Bridges RJ, Cotman CW. The excitatory amino acid receptors: their classes, pharmacology, and distinct properties in the function of the central nervous system. Annu Rev Pharmacol Toxicol 1989; 29:365–402.

100. Carriedo SG, Yin HZ, Weiss JH. Motor neurons are selectively vulnerable to AMPA/kainate receptor-mediated injury in vitro. J Neurosci 1996; 16:4069–4079.

101. Heath PR, Shaw PJ. Update on the glutamatergic neurotransmitter system and the role of excitotoxicity in amyotrophic lateral sclerosis. Muscle Nerve 2002; 26:438–458.

102. Petralia RS, Wang YX, Mayat E, Wenthold RJ. Glutamate receptor subunit 2-selective antibody shows a differential distribution of calcium-impermeable AMPA receptors among populations of neurons. J Comp Neurol 1997; 385:456–476.

103. Shaw PJ, Williams TL, Slade JY, Eggett CJ, Ince PG. Low expression of GluR2 AMPA receptor subunit protein by human motor neurons. Neuroreport 1999; 10:261–265.

104. Siliprandi R, Lipartiti M, Fadda E, Sautter J, Manev H. Activation of the glutamate metabotropic receptor protects retina against N-methyl-D-aspartate toxicity. Eur J Pharmacol 1992; 219:173–174.

105. McDonald JW, Schoepp DD. The metabotropic excitatory amino acid receptor agonist 1S,3R-ACPD selectively potentiates N-methyl-D-aspartate-induced brain injury. Eur J Pharmacol 1992; 215:353–354.

106. Pizzi M, Consolandi O, Memo M, Spano PF. Activation of multiple metabotropic glutamate receptor subtypes prevents NMDA-induced excitotoxicity in rat hippocampal slices. Eur J Neurosci 1996; 8:1516–1521.

107. Alagarsamy S, Marino MJ, Rouse ST, Gereau RWt, Heinemann SF, Conn PJ. Activation of NMDA receptors reverses desensitization of mGluR5 in native and recombinant systems. Nat Neurosci 1999; 2:234–240.

108. Bruno V, Battaglia G, Ksiazek I, Van Der Putten H, Catania MV, Giuffrida R, Lukic S, Leonhardt T, Inderbitzin W, Gasparini F, Kuhn R, Hampson DR, Nicoletti F, Flor PJ. Selective activation of mGlu4 metabotropic glutamate receptors is protective against excitotoxic neuronal death. J Neurosci 2000; 20:6413–6420.

109. Melyan Z, Lancaster B, Wheal HV. Metabotropic regulation of intrinsic excitability by synaptic activation of kainate receptors. J Neurosci 2004; 24:4530–4534.

110. Burke RE. Spinal cord: ventral horn. In: Shepherd GM, ed. The Synaptic Organisation of the Brain. New York: Oxford University Press, 1990;88–132.

111. Molander C, Xu Q, Rivero-Melian C, Grant G. Cytoarchitectonic organization of the spinal cord in the rat: II. The cervical and upper thoracic cord. J Comp Neurol 1989; 289:375–385.

112. Young AB, Penney JB. Pharmacological aspects of motor dysfunction. In: Asbury AK, McKhann GM, McDonald WI, eds. Diseases of the Nervous System. Philadelphia: Saunders, 1992;1:342–352.

113. Shaw PJ, Ince PG, Falkous G, Mantle D. Cytoplasmic, lysosomal and matrix protease activities in spinal cord tissue from amyotrophic lateral sclerosis (ALS) and control patients. J Neurol Sci 1996; 139(suppl):71–75.

114. Shaw PJ, Ince PG, Matthews JN, Johnson M, Candy JM. N-methyl-D-aspartate (NMDA) receptors in the spinal cord and motor cortex in motor neuron disease: a quantitative autoradiographic study using [3H]MK-801. Brain Res 1994; 637: 297–302.

115. Shaw PJ, Chinnery RM, Ince PG. Non-NMDA receptors in motor neuron disease (MND): a quantitative autoradiographic study in spinal cord and motor cortex using [3H]CNQX and [3H]kainate. Brain Res 1994; 655:186–194.

116. Williams TL, Day NC, Ince PG, Kamboj RK, Shaw PJ. Calcium-permeable alpha-amino-3-hydroxy-5-methyl-4-isoxazole propionic acid receptors: a molecular determinant of selective vulnerability in amyotrophic lateral sclerosis. Ann Neurol 1997; 42:200–207.

117. Williams TL, Ince PG, Oakley AE, Shaw PJ. An immunocytochemical study of the distribution of AMPA selective glutamate receptor subunits in the normal human motor system. Neuroscience 1996; 74:185–198.

118. Tomiyama M, Rodriguez-Puertas R, Cortes R, Christnacher A, Sommer B, Pazos A, Palacios JM, Mengod G. Differential regional distribution of AMPA receptor subunit messenger RNAs in the human spinal cord as visualized by in situ hybridization. Neuroscience 1996; 75:901–915.

119. Heath PR, Tomkins J, Ince PG, Shaw PJ. Quantitative assessment of AMPA receptor mRNA in human spinal motor neurons isolated by laser capture microdissection. Neuroreport 2002; 13:1753–1757.

120. Kawahara Y, Kwak S, Sun H, Ito K, Hashida H, Aizawa H, Jeong SY, Kanazawa I. Human spinal motoneurons express low relative abundance of GluR2 mRNA: an implication for excitotoxicity in ALS. J Neurochem 2003; 85:680–689.

121. Brorson JR, Zhang Z, Vandenberghe W. Ca(2+) permeation of AMPA receptors in cerebellar neurons expressing glu receptor 2. J Neurosci 1999; 19:9149–9159.

122. Vandenberghe W, Ihle EC, Patneau DK, Robberecht W, Brorson JR. AMPA receptor current density, not desensitization, predicts selective motoneuron vulnerability. J Neurosci 2000; 20:7158–7166.

123. Van Den Bosch L, Vandenberghe W, Klaassen H, Van Houtte E, Robberecht W. Ca(2+)-permeable AMPA receptors and selective vulnerability of motor neurons. J Neurol Sci 2000; 180:29–34.

124. Laslo P, Lipski J, Nicholson LF, Miles GB, Funk GD. GluR2 AMPA receptor subunit expression in motoneurons at low and high risk for degeneration in amyotrophic lateral sclerosis. Exp Neurol 2001; 169:461–471.

125. Iihara K, Joo DT, Henderson J, Sattler R, Taverna FA, Lourensen S, Orser BA, Roder JC, Tymianski M. The influence of glutamate receptor 2 expression on excitotoxicity in Glur2 null mutant mice. J Neurosci 2001; 21:2224–2239.

126. Van Damme P. The AMPA receptor and ALS. Ph.D. Thesis, Neuroscience, Catholic University of Leuven, Leuven, 2004:107.

127. Anneser JM, Borasio GD, Berthele A, Zieglgansberger W, Tolle TR. Differential expression of group I metabotropic glutamate receptors in rat spinal cord somatic and autonomic motoneurons: possible implications for the pathogenesis of amyotrophic lateral sclerosis. Neurobiol Dis 1999; 6:140–147.

128. Anneser JM, Ince PG, Shaw PJ, Borasio GD. Differential expression of mGluR5 in human lumbosacral motoneurons. Neuroreport 2004; 15:271–273.

129. Tomiyama M, Kimura T, Maeda T, Tanaka H, Furusawa K, Kurahashi K, Matsunaga M. Expression of metabotropic glutamate receptor mRNAs in the human spinal cord: implications for selective vulnerability of spinal motor neurons in amyotrophic lateral sclerosis. J Neurol Sci 2001; 189:65–69.

130. Conn PJ, Pin JP. Pharmacology and functions of metabotropic glutamate receptors. Annu Rev Pharmacol Toxicol 1997; 37:205–237.

131. Valerio A, Ferrario M, Paterlini M, Liberini P, Moretto G, Cairns NJ, Pizzi M, Spano P. Spinal cord mGlu1a receptors:possible target for amyotrophic lateral sclerosis therapy. Pharmacol Biochem Behav 2002; 73:447–454.

132. Banner SJ, Fray AE, Ince PG, Steward M, Cookson MR, Shaw PJ. The expression of the glutamate re-uptake transporter excitatory amino acid transporter 1 (EAAT1) in the normal human CNS and in motor neurone disease: an immunohistochemical study. Neuroscience 2002; 109:27–44.

133. Fray AE, Ince PG, Banner SJ, Milton ID, Usher PA, Cookson MR, Shaw PJ. The expression of the glial glutamate transporter protein EAAT2 in motor neuron disease:an immunohistochemical study. Eur J Neurosci 1998; 10:2481–2489.

134. Milton ID, Banner SJ, Ince PG, Piggott NH, Fray AE, Thatcher N, Horne CH, Shaw PJ. Expression of the glial glutamate transporter EAAT2 in the human CNS: an immunohistochemical study. Brain Res Mol Brain Res 1997; 52:17–31.
135. Rosen DR. Mutations in Cu/Zn superoxide dismutase gene are associated with familial amyotrophic lateral sclerosis. Nature 1993; 364:362.
136. Plaitakis A, Caroscio JT. Abnormal glutamate metabolism in amyotrophic lateral sclerosis. Ann Neurol 1987; 22:575–579.
137. Plaitakis A, Constantakakis E, Smith J. The neuroexcitotoxic amino acids glutamate and aspartate are altered in the spinal cord and brain in amyotrophic lateral sclerosis. Ann Neurol 1988; 24:446–449.
138. Gredal O, Moller SE. Effect of branched-chain amino acids on glutamate metabolism in amyotrophic lateral sclerosis. J Neurol Sci 1995; 129:40–43.
139. Camu W, Billiard M, Baldy-Moulinier M. Fasting plasma and CSF amino acid levels in amyotrophic lateral sclerosis: a subtype analysis. Acta Neurol Scand 1993; 88:51–55.
140. Patten BM, Harati Y, Acosta L, Jung SS, Felmus MT. Free amino acid levels in amyotrophic lateral sclerosis. Ann Neurol 1978; 3:305–309.
141. Perry TL, Krieger C, Hansen S, Eisen A. Amyotrophic lateral sclerosis: amino acid levels in plasma and cerebrospinal fluid. Ann Neurol 1990; 28:12–17.
142. Shaw PJ, Forrest V, Ince PG, Richardson JP, Wastell HJ. CSF and plasma amino acid levels in motor neuron disease: elevation of CSF glutamate in a subset of patients. Neurodegeneration 1995; 4:209–216.
143. Rothstein JD, Tsai G, Kuncl RW, Clawson L, Cornblath DR, Drachman DB, Pestronk A, Stauch BL, Coyle JT. Abnormal excitatory amino acid metabolism in amyotrophic lateral sclerosis. Ann Neurol 1990; 28:18–25.
144. Ferrarese C, Pecora N, Frigo M, Appollonio I, Frattola L. Assessment of reliability and biological significance of glutamate levels in cerebrospinal fluid. Ann Neurol 1993; 33:316–319.
145. Iwasaki Y, Ikeda K, Kinoshita M. Plasma amino acid levels in patients with amyotrophic lateral sclerosis. J Neurol Sci 1992; 107:219–222.
146. Young AB. What's the excitement about excitatory amino acids in amyotrophic lateral sclerosis? Ann Neurol 1990; 28:9–11.
147. Spreux-Varoquaux O, Bensimon G, Lacomblez L, Salachas F, Pradat PF, Le Forestier N, Marouan A, Dib M, Meininger V. Glutamate levels in cerebrospinal fluid in amyotrophic lateral sclerosis: a reappraisal using a new HPLC method with coulometric detection in a large cohort of patients. J Neurol Sci 2002; 193.
148. Tikka TM, Vartiainen NE, Goldsteins G, Oja SS, Andersen PM, Marklund SL, Koistinaho J. Minocycline prevents neurotoxicity induced by cerebrospinal fluid from patients with motor neurone disease. Brain 2002; 125:722–731.
149. Cid C, Alvarez-Cermeno JC, Regidor I, Salinas M, Alcazar A. Low concentrations of glutamate induce apoptosis in cultured neurons: implications for amyotrophic lateral sclerosis. J Neurol Sci 2003; 206:91–95.
150. Perry TL, Hansen S, Jones K. Brain glutamate deficiency in amyotrophic lateral sclerosis. Neurology 1987; 37:1845–1848.
151. Tsai GC, Stauch-Slusher B, Sim L, Hedreen JC, Rothstein JD, Kuncl R, Coyle JT. Reductions in acidic amino acids and N-acetylaspartylglutamate in amyotrophic lateral sclerosis CNS. Brain Res 1991; 556:151–156.
152. Couratier P, Hugon J, Sindou P, Vallat JM, Dumas M. Cell culture evidence for neuronal degeneration in amyotrophic lateral sclerosis being linked to glutamate AMPA/kainate receptors. Lancet 1993; 341:265–268.
153. Roisen FJ, Bartfeld H, Donnenfeld H, Baxter J. Neuron specific in vitro cytotoxicity of sera from patients with amyotrophic lateral sclerosis. Muscle Nerve 1982; 5:48–53.
154. Wolfgram F, Myers L. Amyotrophic lateral sclerosis: effect of serum on anterior horn cells in tissue culture. Science 1973; 179:579–580.

155. Couratier P, Sindou P, Esclaire F, Louvel E, Hugon J. Neuroprotective effects of riluzole in ALS CSF toxicity. Neuroreport 1994; 5:1012–1014.

156. Shaw PJ. Toxicity of CSF in motor neurone disease: a potential route to neuroprotection. Brain 2002; 125:693–694.

157. Iwasaki Y, Ikeda K, Shiojima T, Tagaya M, Kinoshita M. Amyotrophic lateral sclerosis cerebrospinal fluid is not toxic to cultured spinal motor neurons. Neurol Res 1995; 17:393–395.

158. Malessa S, Leigh PN, Bertel O, Sluga E, Hornykiewicz O. Amyotrophic lateral sclerosis: glutamate dehydrogenase and transmitter amino acids in the spinal cord. J Neurol Neurosurg Psychiatry 1991; 54:984–988.

159. Gluck MR, Thomas RG, Sivak MA. Unaltered cytochrome oxidase, glutamate dehydrogenase and glutaminase activities in platelets from patients with sporadic amyotrophic lateral sclerosis—a study of potential pathogenetic mechanisms in neurodegenerative diseases. J Neural Transm 2000; 107:1437–1447.

160. Fray AE, Dempster S, Williams RE, Cookson MR, Shaw PJ. Glutamine synthetase activity and expression are not affected by the development of motor neuronopathy in the G93A SOD-1/ALS mouse. Brain Res Mol Brain Res 2001; 94:131–136.

161. Krieger C, Wagey R, Shaw C. Amyotrophic lateral sclerosis: quantitative autoradiography of [3H]MK-801/NMDA binding sites in spinal cord. Neurosci Lett 1993; 159: 191–194.

162. Samarasinghe S, Virgo L, de Belleroche J. Distribution of the N-methyl-D-aspartate glutamate receptor subunit NR2A in control and amyotrophic lateral sclerosis spinal cord. Brain Res 1996; 727:233–237.

163. Virgo L, de Belleroche J. Induction of the immediate early gene c-jun in human spinal cord in amyotrophic lateral sclerosis with concomitant loss of NMDA receptor NR-1 and glycine transporter mRNA. Brain Res 1995; 676:196–204.

164. Takuma H, Kwak S, Yoshizawa T, Kanazawa I. Reduction of GluR2 RNA editing, a molecular change that increases calcium influx through AMPA receptors, selective in the spinal ventral gray of patients with amyotrophic lateral sclerosis. Ann Neurol 1999; 46:806–815.

165. Kawahara Y, Ito K, Sun H, Aizawa H, Kanazawa I, Kwak S. Glutamate receptors: RNA editing and death of motor neurons. Nature 2004; 427:801.

166. Barbon A, Vallini I, La Via L, Marchina E, Barlati S. Glutamate receptor RNA editing: a molecular analysis of GluR2, GluR5 and GluR6 in human brain tissues and in NT2 cells following in vitro neural differentiation. Brain Res Mol Brain Res 2003; 117: 168–178.

167. Aronica E, Catania MV, Geurts J, Yankaya B, Troost D. Immunohistochemical localization of groups I and II metabotropic glutamate receptors in control and amyotrophic lateral sclerosis human spinal cord: upregulation in reactive astrocytes. Neuroscience 2001; 105:509–520.

168. Shaw PJ, Chinnery RM, Ince PG. [3H]D-aspartate binding sites in the normal human spinal cord changes in motor neuron disease: a quantitative autoradiographic study. Brain Res 1994; 655:195–201.

169. Lin CL, Bristol LA, Jin L, Dykes-Hoberg M, Crawford T, Clawson L, Rothstein JD. Aberrant RNA processing in a neurodegenerative disease: the cause for absent EAAT2, a glutamate transporter, in amyotrophic lateral sclerosis. Neuron 1998; 20:589–602.

170. Flowers JM, Powell JF, Leigh PN, Andersen P, Shaw CE. Intron 7 retention and exon 9 skipping EAAT2 mRNA variants are not associated with amyotrophic lateral sclerosis. Ann Neurol 2001; 49:643–649.

171. Meyer T, Fromm A, Munch C, Schwalenstocker B, Fray AE, Ince PG, Stamm S, Gron G, Ludolph AC, Shaw PJ. The RNA of the glutamate transporter EAAT2 is variably spliced in amyotrophic lateral sclerosis and normal individuals. J Neurol Sci 1999; 170:45–50.

172. Chen W, Aoki C, Mahadomrongkul V, Gruber CE, Wang GJ, Blitzblau R, Irwin N, Rosenberg PA. Expression of a variant form of the glutamate transporter GLT1 in

neuronal cultures and in neurons and astrocytes in the rat brain. J Neurosci 2002; 22:2142–2152.

173. Maragakis NJ, Dykes-Hoberg M, Rothstein JD. Altered expression of the glutamate transporter EAAT2b in neurological disease. Ann Neurol 2004; 55:469–477.

174. Dangond F, Hwang D, Camelo S, Pasinelli P, Frosch MP, Stephanopoulos G, Brown RH Jr, Gullans SR. Molecular signature of late-stage human ALS revealed by expression profiling of postmortem spinal cord gray matter. Physiol Genomics 2004; 16: 229–239.

175. Rao SD, Yin HZ, Weiss JH. Disruption of glial glutamate transport by reactive oxygen species produced in motor neurons. J Neurosci 2003; 23:2627–2633.

176. Rao SD, Weiss JH. Excitotoxic and oxidative cross-talk between motor neurons and glia in ALS pathogenesis. Trends Neurosci 2004; 27:17–23.

177. Massieu L, Morales-Villagran A, Tapia R. Accumulation of extracellular glutamate by inhibition of its uptake is not sufficient for inducing neuronal damage: an in vivo microdialysis study. J Neurochem 1995; 64:2262–2272.

178. Trotti D, Aoki M, Pasinelli P, Berger UV, Danbolt NC, Brown RH Jr, Heideger MA. Amyotrophic lateral sclerosis-linked glutamate transporter mutant has impaired glutamate clearance capacity. J Biol Chem 2001; 276:576–582.

179. Gurney ME, Cutting FB, Zhai P, Doble A, Taylor CP, Andrus PK, Hall ED. Benefit of vitamin E, riluzole, and gabapentin in a transgenic model of familial amyotrophic lateral sclerosis. Ann Neurol 1996; 39:147–157.

180. Durham HD, Roy J, Dong L, Figlewicz DA. Aggregation of mutant Cu/Zn superoxide dismutase proteins in a culture model of ALS. J Neuropathol Exp Neurol 1997; 56: 523–530.

181. Roy J, Minotti S, Dong L, Figlewicz DA, Durham HD. Glutamate potentiates the toxicity of mutant Cu/Zn-superoxide dismutase in motor neurons by postsynaptic calcium-dependent mechanisms. J Neurosci 1998; 18:9673–9684.

182. Kruman II, Pedersen WA, Springer JE, Mattson MP. ALS-linked Cu/Zn-SOD mutation increases vulnerability of motor neurons to excitotoxicity by a mechanism involving increased oxidative stress and perturbed calcium homeostasis. Exp Neurol 1999; 160: 28–39.

183. Pieri M, Gaetti C, Spalloni A, Cavalcanti S, Mercuri N, Bernardi G, Longone P, Zona C. alpha-Amino-3-hydroxy-5-methyl-isoxazole-4-propionate receptors in spinal cord motor neurons are altered in transgenic mice over-expressing human Cu Zn superoxide dismutase (Gly93 > Ala)mutation. Neuroscience 2003; 122:47–58.

184. Spalloni A, Albo F, Ferrari F, Mercuri N, Bernardi G, Zona C, Longone P. Cu/Zn-superoxide dismutase (GLY93 > ALA) mutation alters AMPA receptor subunit expression and function and potentiates kainate-mediated toxicity in motor neurons in culture. Neurobiol Dis 2004; 15:340–350.

185. Bendotti C, Tortarolo M, Suchak SK, Calvaresi N, Carvelli L, Bastone A, Rizzi M, Rattray M, Mennini T. Transgenic SOD1 G93A mice develop reduced GLT-1 in spinal cord without alterations in cerebrospinal fluid glutamate levels. J Neurochem 2001; 79:737–746.

186. Deitch JS, Alexander GM, Del Valle L, Heiman-Patterson TD. GLT-1 glutamate transporter levels are unchanged in mice expressing G93A human mutant SOD1. J Neurol Sci 2002; 193:117–126.

187. Howland DS, Liu J, She Y, Goad B, Maragakis NJ, Kim B, Erickson J, Kulik J, DeVito L, Psaltis G, DeGennaro LJ, Cleveland DW, Rothstein JD. Focal loss of the glutamate transporter EAAT2 in a transgenic rat model of SOD1 mutant-mediated amyotrophic lateral sclerosis (ALS). Proc Natl Acad Sci USA 2002; 99:1604–1609.

188. Guo H, Lai L, Butchbach ME, Stockinger MP, Shan X, Bishop GA, Lin CL. Increased expression of the glial glutamate transporter EAAT2 modulates excitotoxicity and delays the onset but not the outcome of ALS in mice. Hum Mol Genet 2003; 12:2519–2532.

189. Tortarolo M, Crossthwaite AJ, Conforti L, Spencer JP, Williams RJ, Bendotti C, Rattray M. Expression of SOD1 G93A or wild-type SOD1 in primary cultures of astrocytes down-regulates the glutamate transporter GLT-1: lack of involvement of oxidative stress. J Neurochem 2004; 88:481–493.

190. Trotti D, Rolfs A, Danbolt NC, Brown RH Jr, Hediger MA. SOD1 mutants linked to amyotrophic lateral sclerosis selectively inactivate a glial glutamate transporter. Nat Neurosci 1999; 2:848.

191. Trotti D, Rossi D, Gjesdal O, Levy LM, Racagni G, Danbolt NC, Volterra A. Peroxynitrite inhibits glutamate transporter sub-types. J Biol Chem 1996; 271:5976–5979.

192. Louvel E, Hugon J, Doble A. Therapeutic advances in amyotrophic lateral sclerosis. Trends Pharmacol Sci 1997; 18:196–203.

193. Ludolph AC. Treatment of amyotrophic lateral sclerosis—what is the next step? J Neurol 2000; 247:13–18.

194. Van Damme P, Leyssen M, Callewaert G, Robberecht W, Van Den Bosch L. The AMPA receptor antagonist NBQX prolongs survival in a transgenic mouse model of amyotrophic lateral sclerosis. Neurosci Lett 2003; 343:81–84.

195. Doble A. The pharmacology and mechanism of action of riluzole. Neurology 1996; 47:S233–S241.

196. Bensimon G, Lacomblez L, Meininger V. A controlled trial of riluzole in amyotrophic lateral sclerosis. ALS/Riluzole Study Group. N Engl J Med 1994; 330:585–591.

197. Lacomblez L, Bensimon G, Leigh PN, Guillet P, Meininger V. Dose-ranging study of riluzole in amyotrophic lateral sclerosis. Amyotrophic Lateral Sclerosis/Riluzole Study Group II. Lancet 1996; 347:1425–1431.

198. Miller RG, Moore D, Young LA, Armon C, Barohn RJ, Bromberg MB, Bryan WW, Gelinas DF, Mendoza MC, Neville HE, Parry GJ, Petajan JH, Ravits JM, Ringel SP, Ross MA. Placebo-controlled trial of gabapentin in patients with amyotrophic lateral sclerosis. WALS Study Group. Western Amyotrophic Lateral Sclerosis Study Group. Neurology 1996; 47:1383–1388.

199. Miller RG, Moore DH, Dronsky V, Bradley W, Barohn R, Bryan W, Prior TW, Gelinas DF, Iannaccone S, Kissel J, Leshner R, Mendell J, Mendoza M, Russman B, Samaha F, Smith S. A placebo-controlled trial of gabapentin in spinal muscular atrophy. J Neurol Sci 2001; 191:127–131.

200. Cudkowicz ME, Shefner JM, Schoenfeld DA, Brown RHJr, Johnson H, Qureshi M, Jacobs M, Rothstein JD, Appel SH, Pascuzzi RM, Heiman-Patterson TD, Donofrio PD, David WS, Russell JA, Tandan R, Pioro EP, Felice KJ, Rosenfeld J, Mandler RN, Sachs GM, Bradley WG, Raynor EM, Baquis GD, Belsh JM, Novella S, Goldstein J, Hulihan J. A randomized, placebo-controlled trial of topiramate in amyotrophic lateral sclerosis. Neurology 2003; 61:456–464.

201. Ryberg H, Askmark H, Persson LI. A double-blind randomized clinical trial in amyotrophic lateral sclerosis using lamotrigine: effects on CSF glutamate, aspartate, branched-chain amino acid levels and clinical parameters. Acta Neurol Scand 2003; 108:1–8.

202. Maragakis NJ, Jackson M, Ganel R, Rothstein JD. Topiramate protects against motor neuron degeneration in organotypic spinal cord cultures but not in G93A SOD1 transgenic mice. Neurosci Lett 2003; 338:107–110.

203. Brockington A, Shaw PJ. Developments in the treatment of Motor Neurone Disease. Adv Clin Neurosci Rehabil 2003; 3:13–19.

204. Eisen A, Pant B, Stewart H. Cortical excitability in amyotrophic lateral sclerosis: a clue to pathogenesis. Can J Neurol Sci 1993; 20:11–16.

205. Mills KR. Motor neuron disease. Studies of the corticospinal excitation of single motor neurons by magnetic brain stimulation. Brain 1995; 118 (Pt 4):971–982.

206. Eisen A, Weber M. Neurophysiological evaluation of cortical function in the early diagnosis of ALS. Amyotroph Lateral Scler Other Motor Neuron Disord 2001; 1: S47–S51.

207. Kew JJ, Leigh PN, Playford ED, Passingham RE, Goldstein LH, Frackowiak RS, Brooks DJ. Cortical function in amyotrophic lateral sclerosis. A positron emission tomography study. Brain 1993; 116(Pt 3):655–680.

208. Pieri M, Albo F, Gaetti C, Spalloni A, Bengtson CP, Longone P, Cavalcanti S, Zona C. Altered excitability of motor neurons in a transgenic mouse model of familial amyotrophic lateral sclerosis. Neurosci Lett 2003; 351:153–156.

209. Kuo JJ, Schonewille M, Siddique T, Schults AN, Fu R, Bar PR, Anelli R, Heckman CJ, Kroese AB. Hyperexcitability of cultured spinal motoneurons from presymptomatic ALS mice. J Neurophysiol 2004; 91:571–575.

210. Atlante A, Calissano P, Bobba A, Giannattasio S, Marra E, Passarella S. Glutamate neurotoxicity, oxidative stress and mitochondria. FEBS Lett 2001; 497:1–5.

211. Shaw PJ, Ince PG. Glutamate, excitotoxicity and amyotrophic lateral sclerosis. J Neurol 1997; 244(suppl 2):S3–S14.

212. Borthwick GM, Johnson MA, Ince PG, Shaw PJ, Turnbull DM. Mitochondrial enzyme activity in amyotrophic lateral sclerosis: implications for the role of mitochondria in neuronal cell death. Ann Neurol 1999; 46:787–790.

213. Menzies FM, Ince PG, Shaw PJ. Mitochondrial involvement in amyotrophic lateral sclerosis. Neurochem Int 2002; 40:543–551.

214. Stout AK, Raphael HM, Kanterewicz BI, Klann E, Reynolds IJ. Glutamate-induced neuron death requires mitochondrial calcium uptake. Nat Neurosci 1998; 1:366–373.

215. Singh P, Mann KA, Mangat HK, Kaur G. Prolonged glutamate excitotoxicity: effects on mitochondrial antioxidants and antioxidant enzymes. Mol Cell Biochem 2003; 243:139–145.

216. Kannurpatti SS, Sanganahalli BG, Mishra S, Joshi PG, Joshi NB. Glutamate-induced differential mitochondrial response in young and adult rats. Neurochem Int 2004; 44:361–369.

217. Drachman DB, Rothstein JD. Inhibition of cyclooxygenase-2 protects motor neurons in an organotypic model of amyotrophic lateral sclerosis. Ann Neurol 2000; 48:792–795.

218. Kelley KA, Ho L, Winger D, Freire-Moar J, Borelli CB, Aisen PS, Pasinetti GM. Potentiation of excitotoxicity in transgenic mice overexpressing neuronal cyclooxygenase-2. Am J Pathol 1999; 155:995–1004.

219. Almer G, Guegan C, Teismann P, Naini A, Rosoklija G, Hays AP, Chen C, Przedborski S. Increased expression of the pro-inflammatory enzyme cyclooxygenase-2 in amyotrophic lateral sclerosis. Ann Neurol 2001; 49:176–185.

220. Shaw PJ, Eggett CJ. Molecular factors underlying selective vulnerability of motor neurons to neurodegeneration in amyotrophic lateral sclerosis. J Neurol 2000; 247(suppl 1): I17–I27.

221. Figlewicz DA, Krizus A, Martinoli MG, Meininger V, Dib M, Rouleau GA, Julien JP. Variants of the heavy neurofilament subunit are associated with the development of amyotrophic lateral sclerosis. Hum Mol Genet 1994; 3:1757–1761.

222. Hirano A. Cytopathology of amyotrophic lateral sclerosis. Adv Neurol 1991; 56: 91–101.

223. Morrison BM, Gordon JW, Ripps ME, Morrison JH. Quantitative immunocytochemical analysis of the spinal cord in G86R superoxide dismutase transgenic mice: neurochemical correlates of selective vulnerability. J Comp Neurol 1996; 373:619–631.

224. Williamson TL, Bruijn LI, Zhu Q, Anderson KL, Anderson SD, Julien JP, Cleveland DW. Absence of neurofilaments reduces the selective vulnerability of motor neurons and slows disease caused by a familial amyotrophic lateral sclerosis-linked superoxide dismutase 1 mutant. Proc Natl Acad Sci USA 1998; 95:9631–9636.

225. Vartiainen N, Tikka T, Keinanen R, Chan PH, Koistinaho J. Glutamatergic receptors regulate expression, phosphorylation and accumulation of neurofilaments in spinal cord neurons. Neuroscience 1999; 93:1123–1133.

226. Ackerley S, Grierson AJ, Brownlees J, Thornhill P, Anderton BH, Leigh PN, Shaw CE, Miller C. Glutamate slows axonal transport of neurofilaments in transfected neurons. J Cell Biol 2000; 150:165–176.

227. Miller CC, Ackerley S, Brownlees J, Grierson AJ, Jacobsen NJ, Thornhill P. Axonal transport of neurofilaments in normal and disease states. Cell Mol Life Sci 2002; 59:323–330.

228. Ince P, Stout N, Shaw P, Slade J, Hunziker W, Heizmann CW, Baimbridge KG. Parvalbumin and calbindin D-28k in the human motor system and in motor neuron disease. Neuropathol Appl Neurobiol 1993; 19:291–299.

229. Alexianu ME, Ho BK, Mohamed AH, La Bella V, Smith RG, Appel SH. The role of calcium-binding proteins in selective motoneuron vulnerability in amyotrophic lateral sclerosis. Ann Neurol 1994; 36:846–858.

230. Bruening W, Roy J, Giasson B, Figlewicz DA, Mushynski WE, Durham HD. Up-regulation of protein chaperones preserves viability of cells expressing toxic Cu/Zn-super-oxide dismutase mutants associated with amyotrophic lateral sclerosis. J Neurochem 1999; 72:693–699.

231. Olney JW, Misra CH, de Gubareff T. Cysteine-S-sulfate: brain damaging metabolite in sulfite oxidase deficiency. J Neuropathol Exp Neurol 1975; 34:167–177.

232. Perl TM, Bedard L, Kosatsky T, Hockin JC, Todd EC, McNutt LA, Remis RS. Amnesic shellfish poisoning:a new clinical syndrome due to domoic acid. Can Dis Wkly Rep 1990; 16(suppl 1E):7–8.

233. Teitelbaum J, Zatorre RJ, Carpenter S, et al. Neurological sequelae of domoic acid intoxication. Due to ingestion of contaminated mussels. N Engl J Med 1990; 322:1781–1787.

234. Watters MR. Organic neurotoxins in seafoods. Clin Neurol Neurosurg 1995; 97:119–124.

235. Spencer PS, Schaumburg HH. Lathyrism: a neurotoxic disease. Neurobehav Toxicol Teratol 1983; 5:625–629.

236. Kunig G, Niedermeyer B, Krause F, Hartmann J, Deckert J, Ransmayr G, Heinsen H, Beckmann H, Riederer P. Interactions of neurotoxins with non-NMDA glutamate receptors:an autoradiographic study. J Neural Transm Suppl 1994; 43:59–62.

237. Spencer PS. Guam ALS/parkinsonism-dementia: a long-latency neurotoxic disorder caused by "slow toxin(s)" in food?. Can J Neurol Sci 1987; 14:347–357.

238. Duncan MW, Steele JC, Kopin IJ, Markey SP. 2-Amino-3-(methylamino)-propanoic acid (BMAA) in cycad flour: an unlikely cause of amyotrophic lateral sclerosis and parkinsonism-dementia of Guam. Neurology 1990; 40:767–772.

239. Khabazian I, Bains JS, Williams DE, Cheung J, Wilson JM, Pasqualotto BA, Pelech SL, Andersen RJ, Wang YT, Liu L, Nagai A, Kim SU, Craig UK, Shaw CA. Isolation of various forms of sterol beta-D-glucoside from the seed of Cycas circinalis:neurotoxicity implications for ALS-parkinsonism dementia complex. J Neurochem 2002; 82:516–528.

240. Spencer PS, Kisby GE, Ross SM, Roy DN, Hugon J, Ludolph AC, Nunn PB. Guam ALS-PDC:possible causes. Science 1993; 262:825–826.

241. Cox PA, Banack SA, Murch SJ. Biomagnification of cyanobacterial neurotoxins neurodegenerative disease among the Chamorro people of Guam. Proc Natl Acad Sci USA 2003; 100:13380–13383.

14

Superoxide Dismutase, Oxidative Stress, and ALS

Joseph S. Beckman
Linus Pauling Institute, Department of Biochemistry and Biophysics, Environmental Health Sciences Center, Oregon State University, Corvallis, Oregon, U.S.A.

Alvaro G. Estévez
Department of Physiology, The University of Alabama at Birmingham, Birmingham, Alabama, U.S.A.

INTRODUCTION

The discovery of mutations to the antioxidant enzyme copper, zinc superoxide dismutase (SOD) in 1993 led to still unfulfilled hopes that new treatments for amyotrophic lateral sclerosis (ALS) based on antioxidants might be forthcoming. While oxidative damage clearly occurs in degenerating tissues in ALS, a causal role of oxidation is difficult to prove (1) and in doubt by many (2,3). Several experiments from transgenic mice appear to argue strongly against copper being involved in the toxicity of mutant SOD (4,5). Many papers have now investigated the propensity of mutant SOD to aggregate when SOD is devoid of copper and zinc. Yet, there is precious little evidence that SOD aggregates are toxic and poor understanding of why they would be toxic. The available evidence is equally consistent for aggregation of SOD being protective by removing forms of SOD that are redox active. In the present review, we will re-examine the case that copper is involved in the toxicity of SOD in ALS in light of recent transgenic experiments. The hypothesis that the loss of zinc is what makes SOD initiate the death of motor neurons in both sporadic and familial ALS will be explored.

Recently, a remarkable finding just emerged from an observational cancer study involving 958,000 people followed since 1982. Those consuming vitamin E supplements regularly for more than 10 years had a 60% lower incidence of ALS and a 40% lower incidence when vitamin E was used regularly for 2 to 10 years (6). Similar observations have been made with reducing the incidence of Alzheimer's disease (7). Taking vitamin E after diagnosis of ALS at best gives only a mild improvement of symptoms and no effect on survival (8,9). However, it takes years to build tocopherol concentrations in human brain. The role of oxidative stress in ALS and in neurodegeneration in general needs to be explored in more depth.

SUPEROXIDE DISMUTASE

The discovery of the function of SOD dates to 1969 when McCord and Fridovich (10) published their findings that a copper, zinc-containing protein isolated from red blood cells efficiently scavenged superoxide radical. The protein had been first identified in the 1930s and was known as erythrocuprein or hemocuprein. Superoxide anion (O_2^-) is formed when molecular oxygen (O_2) picks up one electron, which is catalyzed by a number of enzymes such as NADPH oxidase (the NOX family), xanthine oxidase, and mitochondrial enzyme complexes. SOD reduces the intracellular concentration of superoxide by catalyzing a process called dismutation—converting two identical molecules into two different products. The copper in SOD is alternately reduced (Cu^+) and oxidized (Cu^{2+}) by superoxide in a two-step cyclic reaction producing oxygen and hydrogen peroxide (H_2O_2).

$$O_2^- + SOD - Cu^{2+} \rightarrow O_2 + SOD - Cu^+ \quad\quad\quad \text{(Step 1)}$$

$$O_2^- + SOD - Cu^+ \rightarrow H_2O_2 + SOD - Cu^{2+} \quad\quad\quad \text{(Step 2)}$$

Every reaction is reversible, so reduced copper produced in Step 1 can reoxidize and convert oxygen into superoxide. Similarly, oxidized copper in Step 2 can convert hydrogen peroxide back to superoxide. The reverse reactions are much slower than the forward reactions. However, these reverse reactions can have major consequences for the function of SOD, particularly when the zinc atom is missing from the molecule.

The structure of SOD is deceptively simple (Fig. 1). It is a small protein with 153 amino acids and remains associated tightly as a dimer of two identical subunits

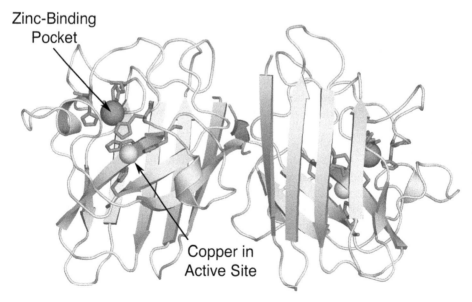

Figure 1 Dimeric structure of copper, zinc SOD. The copper represented by a lighter sphere sits in the middle of the left subunit and superoxide approaches from above the page to interact directly with the copper. Zinc represented by a darker sphere is completely inaccessible to solvent and held in place by a loop that also forms a substantial part of the dimer interface. Based upon the structure determined by Parge et al. (95).

with the active sites facing in opposite directions. Most of the protein is folded into an eight-strand β-barrel where the extensive hydrogen bonding along the peptide backbone produces one of the most stable proteins known. With copper and zinc bound, SOD retains its activity in 6 M urea and survives heating to 80°C. It denatures much more quickly in the apo state where copper and zinc are missing.

Two loops fold back onto the β-barrel to form the active site and one of these loops also forms a significant part of the dimer interface with the other subunit. One of the loops is critical in determining the propensity of mutated forms of the protein to aggregate (11). It extends from residues 49 to 83 in the sequence and is by far the largest part of the protein not involved in the β-barrel (Fig. 2). In addition to forming part of the dimer interface, this loop also forms the zinc-binding pocket. The loop is covalently held to the beta sheet by a disulfide bridge between cysteines 57 and 146 and further stabilized by histidines binding to both copper and zinc. The disulfide bridge is highly conserved among all eukaryotic Cu, Zn SODs and is extremely resistant to reduction (12). Disulfide bonds are uncommon in intracellular proteins because of the reducing potential by millimolar concentrations of glutathione and the actions of sulfhydryl-reducing enzymes such as thioredoxin. When SOD has lost copper and zinc, the zinc-binding loop becomes disordered and the disulfide bond becomes reducible by physiological concentrations of glutathione. Reduction of the disulfide bond in metal-deficient SOD destabilizes the dimer interface and leads to the dissociation of the subunits. Monomeric SOD subunits are far more prone to aggregation.

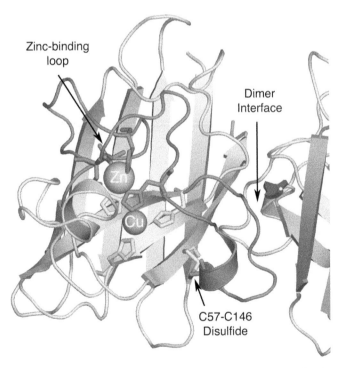

Figure 2 Copper and zinc bound to histidines are shown. The zinc-binding loop starts from His48 bound to the copper to make many contacts with the opposite subunit and is held in place by a disulfide bond between C57 and C146. It then loops back and twists to form the zinc-binding pocket.

SOD MUTATIONS AND ALS

The first 13 mutations to the antioxidant enzyme, copper, zinc SOD were discovered in 1993 (13). The list of mutations has expanded to over 105 known mutations (www.alsod.org), but still the occurrence is limited to only about 2% to 3% of ALS patients. The 97% to 98% of ALS cases without mutations in SOD have no other obvious deficiencies in their antioxidant defense systems. The mutations are widely distributed in the SOD protein, with the majority affecting structural stability (Fig. 3). Mutants expressed in cell culture often have near normal catalytic activity (14) and they do not necessarily decrease the activity of wild-type subunits (15). All but one familial ALS cases occur in heterozygotes and are dominant. The one exception is the mutation D90A, which was originally identified as a natural SOD polymorphism in Sweden and Finland long before a role of SOD in ALS was identified (16). After the discovery that other mutations in SOD were linked to ALS, it was established that homozygotes in Finland were susceptible to ALS. Further study revealed that in Belgium families with Finnish ancestors carrying the D90A mutation develop ALS as heterozygotes. Apparently, the inbred Finnish population has an adaptation that reduces the toxicity of an ALS mutant SOD, although the protein is still expressed in high levels in Finnish heterozygotes (17).

The majority of ALS SOD mutations are missense point mutations (Fig. 3). Mutations occur at over 65 of the 153 positions in the protein. The longest stretch without mutations is only 10 residues in length that forms the third beta strand on the back of the SOD protein. Mutation sites are scattered across all five exons of the protein and are generally located in positions that will structurally weaken the protein. Several truncation mutations have been found that delete up to 30 amino acids from the carboxy terminal. Two different mutations have been identified that mutate two histidines responsible for binding copper (His 46 and 48). Families with these mutants are reported to have an unusually slow progression of the disease (18–20). Only recently has a mutation affecting the zinc-binding site been found,

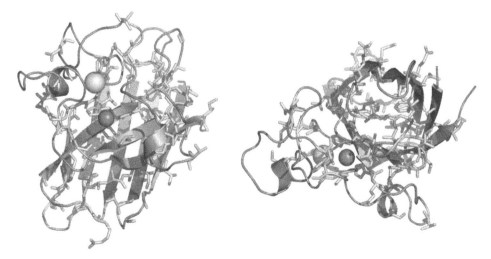

Figure 3 Amino acid side chains affected for 105 mutations so far identified are shown on one subunit of SOD viewed face on and from the top looking down the beta barrel. A majority of mutations occur in the beta barrel or in the short loops that interconnect the strands of the β-barrel.

which resulted in a rapid progressing form of the disease and appeared to be a spontaneous mutation in the afflicted individual (21).

Although afflicted individuals express SOD mutants from birth in all tissues assayed (22), symptoms of ALS typically develop after 40 years, whereupon the disease is largely restricted to motor neurons. Heterozygous SOD carriers have a greater than 85% chance of developing disease. There is no consistent correlation of any mutation with the age-of-onset, and individuals in the same family may develop the disease as early as 20 years of age and as late as age 85 (23). For most SOD mutations, the time to death is typically three to five years, which is similar to the death in sporadic ALS. Certain SOD mutations, such as A4V and A4T, cause a more rapid progression of the disease, with death occurring in a year after diagnosis. However, the A4V mutation in mice does not cause overt motor neuron disease when expressed at levels similar to G93A SOD, which develop disease at three to four months of age (24). The A4V mice might show some degenerative changes after two years at the end of a mouse's normal life. Yet, the A4V protein is still expressed and found in aggregates in motor neurons and associated with mitochondria.

Evidence for a Gain-of-Function

The loss of superoxide scavenging by SOD cannot solely be responsible for ALS. In Cu, Zn SOD-deficient "knock-out" mice, motor neurons develop normally, though they are more susceptible to cell death after axonal injury (25). The dominant nature of all the SOD mutations strongly suggests that the mutations enhance a previously unknown toxic function of SOD (26). Overwhelming experimental evidence supports the gain-of-function (24). Transgenic mice expressing the ALS-SOD mutants G93A, G37R, and G85R develop motor neuron degeneration, paralysis, and death even though they still express their endogenous wild-type SOD. More recently, two groups showed that expression of G93A SOD in transgenic rats also produces motor neuron disease with a profound astrogliosis (27). Disease onset in mice is proportional to the expression of ALS-SOD protein. Mice carrying a greater number of gene copies for the G93A mutation develop the disease at an earlier time. The highest expressing mouse line developed by Gurney et al. (24) is the most popular mouse line supplied by Jackson Laboratories because it develops disease at approximately 120 to 150 days. Lower expressing SOD mouse lines may take over a year to develop disease (24). In contrast, mice transgenic for wild-type SOD do not develop motor neuron disease. In general, wild-type SOD overexpressed in transgenic mice and rats is highly resistant to many forms of oxidative stress and is protective in models of neurodegeneration (28). However, subtle changes in neuromuscular junctions have been reported in one of the highest expressing lines of wild-type SOD (29,30) and aging wild-type mice can develop motor neuron disease and neuromuscular problems (31).

The Role of Copper in ALS

The copper chaperone protein for SOD (CCS), first identified in yeast (32), is important but not essential for delivering copper to SOD (33). In knockout mice lacking CCS, the activity of endogenous wild-type SOD is decreased by about 70% to 80% (34). Although these results indicate that CCS is the major source supplying copper to SOD in vivo, SOD can apparently acquire copper from other sources in cells since 20% to 30% of superoxide scavenging activity remained in the knock out mice. Copper is absolutely required for SOD to scavenge superoxide (10). A likely source for SOD to acquire copper is the mitochondria, where a separate copper transport and chaperone system provides substantial amounts of copper for cytochrome c oxidase.

The knockout of CCS has little effect on the development of motor neuron disease in three lines of ALS mutant SOD mice and might even accelerate the development of disease in some lines (35). Other studies have shown that CCS inserts copper into zinc-containing SOD (36), which will produce Cu, Zn SOD. However, the human SOD is also able to directly pick up copper from copper glutathione (33). When replete with zinc, even the ALS-SODs can be protective. In the absence of the CCS protein, the mutant SODs might acquire copper without zinc from other sources, contributing to the formation of zinc-deficient SOD. Because the mitochondria is the richest store of copper in the cell, this could also explain why mitochondrial pathology is one of the earliest markers of injury in the ALS-SOD mice (37,38).

Dual and Quad Copper Binding Site Mutants

By far the strongest evidence against copper having a role in the toxicity in the pathogenesis of ALS came from two papers from the Borchelt group (4,39). In the first study, they expressed SOD with the double mutation of H46R and H48Q, both of which are involved in copper binding (39). The double mutant SOD still caused motor neuron degeneration in transgenic mice. Then, they further mutated the two other histidines (H63 and H120) to glycine. The quad mutant SOD also caused motor neuron degeneration in transgenic mice, though apparently at a slower rate. Histidine 63 is also a ligand for zinc, so the zinc-binding site is also affected. Both the double and quad mutant SODs have no superoxide scavenging activity as evidenced in activity gels.

While several investigators have concluded that the role for copper in the toxicity of ALS mutant SOD is closed, the evidence is not air-tight and it is premature to reach a final conclusion. Since the early 1970s, copper has been known to bind in the zinc site of SOD (40,41). We have found that quad SOD can form a blue protein with copper bound tightly into the zinc-binding pocket and is much more redox reactive (unpublished observations). In the quad mutant protein, the remaining zinc binding site consists of a negatively charged aspartate (which strongly contributes to the binding of positively charged metals) and two histidines. The combination of these three ligands forms a classical binding motif for iron. Thus, the quad mutant may potentially bind with other transition metals. The extent to which metals are bound to SOD in ALS transgenic mice remains to be determined, but it is premature to conclude that copper cannot bind to the quad mutant or that copper is not causing oxidative stress in the transgenic mice.

AGGREGATION

A clear and common property of the ALS mutant SODs is their propensity to aggregate whether expressed in *Escherichia coli* (42), in transfected cells (43,44), or in transgenic animals (45,46). We found that the first 5% of SOD expressed in *E. coli* would fold into active and soluble protein, but once a threshold concentration was reached, subsequent protein was lost to inclusion bodies. If the growth temperature was reduced to slow the rate of SOD expression, then all of the mutant SOD would fold into soluble and active protein (47). Many reports have shown that SOD aggregates in transfected cells in culture, but the cells generally remain viable and cell death does not correlate with aggregation (48). It is not clear how aggregates would cause ALS, but some evidence suggests sequestration of chaperones might be involved (49).

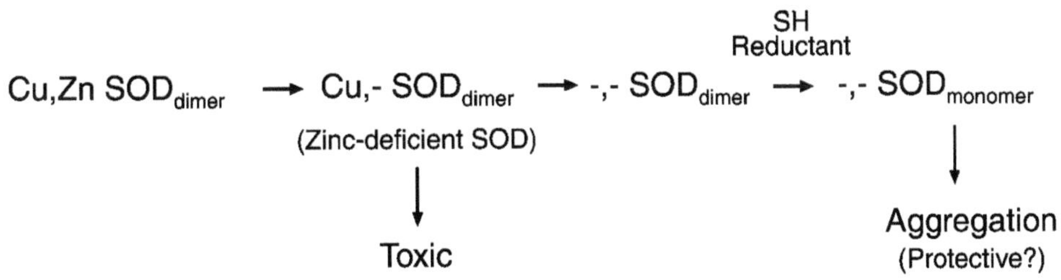

$$\text{Cu,Zn SOD}_{dimer} \longrightarrow \underset{\text{(Zinc-deficient SOD)}}{\text{Cu,- SOD}_{dimer}} \longrightarrow \text{-,- SOD}_{dimer} \overset{\underset{\text{Reductant}}{\text{SH}}}{\longrightarrow} \text{-,- SOD}_{monomer}$$

Toxic

Aggregation
(Protective?)

Figure 4 The aggregation of SOD appears to proceed by the loss of zinc followed by copper. A sulfhydryl reductant like glutathione is needed to reduce the C57-C146 disulfide bond to disrupt the dimer interface, which allows the SOD apoprotein to accumulate as monomers. The monomers are prone to aggregation through interactions of the beta sheets (96–98).

The processes leading to SOD aggregation have received considerable attention lately. A number of investigators have shown that oxidation of SOD can also cause aggregation of the enzyme. The sole tryptophan on SOD is particularly susceptible to oxidation by carbonate radical and can cause covalent dimerization of SOD monomers (50,51). However, mutant SODs do not need to be oxidatively damaged to aggregate (Fig. 4). The metal-deficient apoSOD protein is easily denatured and prone to aggregation when it becomes monomeric (52). Thus, Cu, Zn SOD would aggregate after losing its metals, with zinc being most likely lost first since it is not as tightly bound (42). An alternative explanation is that aggregation is protective by favoring the removal of zinc-deficient SOD, which is directly toxic to motor neurons. Some support for this radical interpretation can be found in the effects of crossing wild-type SOD overexpressing mice with G93A mice. Rather than providing protection, the mice die more quickly. Fukada et al. (53) showed that there was five-fold greater G93A SOD in the hydrid mice and concluded that heterodimers with wild-type SOD were stabilizing the mutant SOD.

In transgenic mice, SOD appears to accumulate in mitochondria of spinal cord and correlates with the disruption of mitochondrial structure and function. Several of the mutant SODs that are too unstable to accumulate in most tissues appear in the mitochondria of spinal cords in transgenic mice (54). SOD can be imported as an apoprotein into mitochondria where it can pick up copper and zinc (55). Although protein aggregation is a major hypothesis relative to oxidative stress (2), there is evidence that aggregation of SOD per se is not sufficient to cause motor neurons death. For example, the A4V SOD mutation causes the most rapidly progressing form of ALS in humans, but does not cause disease in mice. Yet, the A4V SOD is expressed at high levels similar to G93A in mice and principally accumulates in protein aggregates (24). This is further supported by growing evidence indicating that aggregation of SOD in motor neurons is not a sufficient explanation for the disease even in mice where mutant SOD is overexpressed to astonishing levels (48,56).

Zinc-Deficient SOD

One of the failings of the protein aggregation hypothesis is that it does not address how wild-type SOD might participate in ALS in 98% of patients without SOD mutations nor why the disease is selective for motor neurons. Rather than focusing on what makes mutant SOD different than wild-type SOD, one should examine what shared property between mutant and wild-type SOD results in toxicity to motor neurons. When expressing mutant SODs in *E. coli*, it was clear that all of the ALS mutants aggregated (42). However, bacterial expression of other mutations near the active site of SOD are still producing soluble proteins (57). A significant fraction formed soluble SOD that was capable of binding both copper and zinc and folded into fully functional and active SOD. In addition, many of the mutants have partial metal contents, which is due to a significant reduction in the affinity for zinc. The A4V mutation had the weakest affinity for zinc when compared with four other ALS mutants, consistent with it causing the most rapid progressing form of the disease (42). However, even in the mutant proteins the affinity for zinc is extremely high, which has been the cause of confusion (58). For SOD to become zinc deficient, there must either be something that strongly chelates zinc in the cell or the SOD expression must be so strongly induced, so that it exceeds the capacity of a cell to import zinc. In motor neurons, the huge abundance of neurofilaments presents a major binding site for zinc (42,59,60). A rapid induction of SOD expression may result in the formation of zinc-deficient SOD, as intracellular free zinc is normally kept at low levels due to its toxicity (61). It is relatively easy to make wild-type SOD zinc deficient in vitro (40). The simple dialysis of SOD at moderately acidic pH in phosphate buffer is sufficient to cause the preferential lose of zinc. Consequently, it is possible that zinc could be removed from wild-type SOD if strong zinc chelators are present in cells.

Zinc serves a structural role in SOD and is not directly involved in electron transfer reactions with superoxide. However, zinc substantially affects the coordination of copper through a shared histidine that binds to both copper and zinc (Fig. 2). In the reduced state, it is thought that the bridging histidine 63 detaches from the copper and binds a hydrogen ion (62). This hydrogen ion may be transferred to the superoxide anion entering the active site, thereby neutralizing the negative charge on superoxide (forming the powerful oxidant HO_2) and greatly enhancing the oxidation of the copper (63). Both wild-type and A4V SODs containing copper and zinc are visibly green. The green color is due to the shared ligand histidine 63 bridging copper and zinc, which creates an additional shoulder in the 450 nm region and adds a greenish hue. Simply removing the zinc from SOD turns the protein blue. Both Cu, Zn SOD and zinc-deficient SOD become colorless when the copper is reduced, which provides a simple assay to monitor the redox state of copper.

Valentine's group observed that some ALS mutant SODs expressed in yeast were readily reduced by ascorbate (becoming colorless) while others were not (64). We found that reduction depended on whether the SODs were zinc deficient and not on whether it was a mutant or wild-type Cu, Zn protein. Zinc-deficient SOD is reduced by ascorbate more than 3000 times faster than wild-type protein (65). The copper in zinc-deficient SOD is more accessible to intracellular reductants and could be kept entirely in a reduced state in motor neurons, where ascorbate concentrations are millimolar. The reduced SOD will favor the reverse reaction of the enzyme. As shown in Step 1 of the dismutation of superoxide, the back reaction of oxygen with superoxide is about a billion times slower than the forward reaction. Because motor neurons contain 10 to 40 µM SOD, superoxide concentrations are kept low so that paradoxically the oxygen concentration is about a hundred million times higher than the concentration of superoxide. If SOD was fully reduced, the rate of the back reaction is within an order of magnitude as the rate of the forward reaction. In transgenic mice, SOD concentrations can be 5 to 13 times higher than endogenous SOD. Because 10 µM zinc-deficient SOD would be kept fully reduced, it could potentially produce

1 to 2 nM superoxide per second. Although this is a significant flux of superoxide being produced inside the motor neuron, the intracellular steady state concentration of superoxide would still be kept low by the scavenging activity of SOD.

Only molecules that react quickly enough to compete with SOD will be able to react with this modest flux of superoxide. The one molecule that can do this is nitric oxide, which reacts at a diffusion-limited rate with superoxide to form peroxynitrite. This means that every time nitric oxide collides with superoxide, peroxynitrite is formed. In addition, nitric oxide is one of the smallest possible molecules and can diffuse much faster than a protein the size of SOD. Consequently, nitric oxide reacts at least 10 times faster with superoxide than SOD can scavenge it. In these conditions, zinc-deficient SOD can effectively produce peroxynitrite from oxygen and nitric oxide. Using physiologically relevant concentrations of SOD and nitric oxide, we showed that 10 µM zinc-deficient SOD could make 1 to 2 µM peroxynitrite per hour (65). Curiously, this rate of production was not significantly slowed by adding 10 µM wild-type Cu, Zn SOD. It only takes a few hours at this rate of production to kill a motor neuron.

Endogenous production of peroxynitrite by motor neurons is able to activate apoptotic cascades. When grown in the presence of any of the several different neurotrophic factors, motor neurons isolated from spinal cords of embryonic rats develop the phenotype of a mature motor neuron over a period of about a week (66). If these trophic factors are withdrawn at any point, the motor neurons undergo apoptosis (67). Motor neuron death requires the simultaneous production of both nitric oxide and superoxide, implicating peroxynitrite as an early intermediate for activating apoptosis after trophic factor-deprivation (66). Before motor neurons undergo apoptosis, they induce neuronal nitric oxide synthase and become immunoreactive for nitrotyrosine, a marker for peroxynitrite. Inhibiting nitric oxide synthesis prevented apoptosis and the protection is lost when a low concentration of less than 100 nM nitric oxide is generated extracellularly. These concentrations of nitric oxide production have previously been directly measured in intact brain under physiological rather than pathological conditions (68–70).

To specifically scavenge superoxide, wild-type Cu, Zn SOD was delivered intracellularly to motor neurons using liposomes (67). Intracellular SOD was as protective as inhibiting nitric oxide synthesis, while adding extracellular SOD was not protective. Any of eight different ALS mutant SODs containing their full complement of copper and zinc also fully protected motor neurons in culture from trophic factor withdrawal (65). The ability to deliver SOD entrapped in liposomes to motor neurons enabled us to directly test whether zinc-deficient SOD is toxic to motor neurons (67). Delivery of wild-type Cu, Zn SOD or any of the eight different ALS mutant SODs replete with Cu and Zn protected motor neurons equally well from trophic factor deprivation. However, the zinc-deficient forms of ALS mutant and wild-type SOD induced tyrosine nitration and motor neuron apoptosis even in the presence of trophic factors. Inhibition of nitric oxide synthesis prevented death and blocked accumulation of nitrotyrosine in the motor neurons. In these in vitro experiments, copper was essential for the toxicity of zinc-deficient SOD and apoSOD itself was not toxic to the motor neurons (65). Adding equivalent amounts of copper either in free form or complexed to bovine serum albumin was not toxic to motor neurons in culture. Zinc-deficient wild-type SOD was just as toxic as the mutant SODs. On the basis of these results, we proposed that the mutations to SOD do not directly confer the gain-of-function but rather increase the susceptibility to lose zinc with zinc-deficient SOD being responsible for the death of motor neurons. Thus, wild-type SOD can participate in sporadic ALS if it becomes zinc deficient (71).

This work was supported by studies from the Henderson group, who showed that FAS ligand-stimulated motor neuron death by increasing endogenous peroxynitrite formation (72). In the same paper, motor neurons from G93A, G37R, or G85R SOD transgenic mice were isolated and shown to be viable. However, if a nitric oxide donor was added to maintain a steady state concentration of nitric oxide as low as 40 nM, the motor neurons underwent apoptosis. With non-transgenic mice, the same concentration of nitric oxide had no effect on viability. These data provide indirect evidence that the overexpression of G93A SOD in motor neurons was partially zinc deficient, based upon our previous results of supplying zinc-deficient SOD to motor neurons.

Tyrosine Nitration

A marker left by peroxynitrite is the nitration of proteins. One line of evidence supporting a role of peroxynitrite in the pathogenesis of ALS is the finding by multiple laboratories of increased nitrotyrosine in lower motor neurons of transgenic mice and ALS patients (73–84). Although observed by many laboratories in both transgenic mice and rats, the findings are controversial. Bruijn et al. (85) reported increased free nitrotyrosine but could not demonstrate a difference in protein bound nitrotyrosine between control versus transgenic SOD mice. Strong et al. (86) isolated neurofilaments from ALS patients and found that neurofilaments were nitrated. A difficulty is that motor neurons constitute only a miniscule fraction of spinal cord, contributing less than about 1% of total protein. Recently, 20 nitrated proteins have been identified in G93A SOD mice with active disease (87).

ZINC-DEFICIENT DIETS

If zinc-deficient SOD is responsible for motor neuron death in ALS, a zinc-deficient diet fed to transgenic animals should accelerate disease and zinc supplements might be protective. Some evidence supporting this premise exists. Metallothioneins are major intracellular zinc-binding proteins that are important for protecting cells when zinc is low (88). Genetic deletion of the three major isoforms of metallothionein in brain accelerates the development of ALS in G93A transgenic mice (89,90). Importantly, the two astrocytic isozymes for metallothionein were found to be as important as the neuronal isozyme for delaying the disease. We found that zinc deficiency accelerated the progression of ALS in G93A SOD mice by seven days (91).

Conversely, zinc supplementation should be protective if dietary zinc is limiting in the SOD transgenic mice. In apparent opposition of this premise, high dosages of zinc given in the drinking water were reported to paradoxically accelerate the death of ALS-SOD transgenic mice (92). However, the dosages were 75 and 375 mg/kg/day of zinc, which were 15 to 75 times greater than current recommendations established for rodents (93). Excessive zinc blocks copper absorption and zinc is used to treat copper overload in Wilson's disease. However, copper is also crucial for ceruloplasmin to insert iron into heme and its deficiency can lead to a fatal anemia (94). We found using modest levels of zinc (12 mg/kg/day) extended life by 11 days compared to the zinc-deficient group. Raising the dosage to 18 mg/kg/day resulted in more rapid death, but the early mortality was prevented by the addition of a low dosage of copper to the drinking water. These results indicate that zinc is a limiting nutrient for the SOD transgenic mice and moderate supplements with zinc could reduce the variability in transgenic SOD ALS models.

SUMMARY

Twelve years have passed since the discovery of mutations to SOD, the major sentiment in the literature is that the SODs are causing ALS by protein aggregation. Yet, apoSOD appears to be non-toxic to motor neurons compared with wild-type SOD. Although several studies suggest copper may not have a role in the toxicity of mutant SODs, the case against copper mediating the toxicity of SOD is not closed. The zinc-deficient hypothesis explains many of the perplexing questions about the role of SOD in ALS. How can wild-type SOD participate in 98% of ALS cases without SOD mutations? Why do so many different mutations to SOD cause the same phenotype? Why the dominant gain of function is not prevented by wild-type Cu, Zn SOD? The striking epidemiological studies just published on the 60% reduction of ALS among people regularly taking vitamin E further supports a role for oxidative stress as a major role in the pathogenesis of ALS.

REFERENCES

1. Ischiropoulos H, Beckman JS. Oxidative stress and nitration in neurodegeneration: cause, effect, or association? J Clin Invest 2003; 111:163–169.
2. Cleveland DW, Liu J. Oxidation versus aggregation: how do SOD1 mutants cause ALS? Nature Med 2000; 6:1320–1321.
3. Bruijn LI, Miller TM, Cleveland DW. Unraveling the mechanisms involved in motor neuron degeneration in als. Annu Rev Neurosci 2004; 27:723–749.
4. Wang J, Slunt H, Gonzales V, Fromholt D, Coonfield M, Copeland NG, Jenkins NA, Borchelt DR. Copper-binding-site-null SOD1 causes ALS in transgenic mice: aggregates of non-native SOD1 delineate a common feature. Hum Mol Genet 2003; 12:2753–2764.
5. Orr HT. A proposed mechanism of ALS fails the test in vivo. Nat Neurosci 2002; 5: 287–288.
6. Ascherio A, Weisskopf MG, O'Reilly EJ, Jacobs EJ, McCullough ML, Calle EE, Cudkowicz M, Thun MJ. Vitamin E intake and risk of amyotrophic lateral sclerosis. Ann Neurol 2005; 57:104–10.
7. Zandi PP, Anthony JC, Khachaturian AS, Stone SV, Gustafson D, Tschanz JT, Norton MC, Welsh-Bohmer KA, Breitner JC. Reduced risk of Alzheimer disease in users of antioxidant vitamin supplements: the Cache County Study. Arch Neurol 2004; 61:82–88.
8. Desnuelle C, Dib M, Garrel C, Favier A. A double-blind, placebo-controlled randomized clinical trial of alpha-tocopherol (vitamin E) in the treatment of amyotrophic lateral sclerosis. ALS riluzole-tocopherol Study Group. Amyotroph Lateral Scler Other Motor Neuron Disord 2001; 2:9–18.
9. Graf M, Ecker D, Horowski R, Kramer B, Riederer P, Gerlach M, Hager C, Ludolph AC, Becker G, Osterhage J, Jost WH, Schrank B, Stein C, Kostopulos P, Lubik S, Wekwerth K, Dengler R, Troeger M, Wuerz A, Hoge A, Schrader C, Schimke N, Krampfl K, Petri S, Zierz S, Eger K, Neudecker S, Traufeller K, Sievert M, Neundorfer B, Hecht M. High dose vitamin E therapy in amyotrophic lateral sclerosis as add-on therapy to riluzole: results of a placebo-controlled double-blind study. J Neural Transm 2005; 5:649–660.
10. McCord JM, Fridovich I. Superoxide dismutase: an enzymic function for erythrocuprein (hemocuprein). J Biol Chem 1969; 244:6049–6055.
11. Furukawa Y, O'Halloran TV. ALS mutations have the greatest destabilizing effect on the apo, reduced form of SOD1, leading to unfolding and oxidative aggregation. J Biol Chem 2005; 280:17266–17274.
12. Arnesano F, Banci L, Bertini I, Martinelli M, Furukawa Y, O'Halloran TV. The unusually stable quaternary structure of human Cu,Zn-superoxide dismutase 1 is controlled by both metal occupancy and disulfide status. J Biol Chem 2004; 279:47998–48003.

13. Rosen DR, Siddique T, Patterson D, Figlewicz DA, Sapp P, Hentati A, Donaldson D, Goto J, O'Regan JP, Deng HX, et al. Mutations in Cu/Zn superoxide dismutase gene are associated with familial amyotrophic lateral sclerosis. Nature 1993; 362:59–62.
14. Borchelt DR, Lee MK, Slunt HS, Guarnieri M, Xu ZS, Wong PC, Brown RH, Jr. Price DL, Sisodia SS, Cleveland DW. Superoxide dismutase 1 with mutations linked to familial amyotrophic lateral sclerosis possesses significant activity. Proc Natl Acad Sci USA 1994; 91:8292–8296.
15. Borchelt DR, Guarnieri M, Wong PC, Lee MK, Slunt HS, Xu Z-S, Sisodia SS, Price DL, Cleveland DW. Superoxide dismutase 1 subunits with mutations linked to familial amyotrophic lateral sclerosis do not affect wild-type subunit function. J Biol Chem 1995; 270:3234–3238.
16. Parton MJ, Broom W, Andersen PM, Al-Chalabi A, Nigel Leigh P, Powell JF, Shaw CE. D90A-SOD1 mediated amyotrophic lateral sclerosis: a single founder for all cases with evidence for a Cis-acting disease modifier in the recessive haplotype. Hum Mutat 2002; 20:473.
17. Jonsson PA, Backstrand A, Andersen PM, Jacobsson J, Parton M, Shaw C, Swingler R, Shaw PJ, Robberecht W, Ludolph AC, Siddique T, Skvortsova VI, Marklund SL. CuZn-superoxide dismutase in D90A heterozygotes from recessive and dominant ALS pedigrees. Neurobiol Dis 2002; 10:327–333.
18. Abe K, Aoki M, Ikeda M, Watanabe M, Hirai S, Itoyama Y. Clinical characteristics of familial amyotrophic lateral sclerosis with Cu/Zn superoxide dismutase gene mutations. J Neurol Sci 1996; 136:108–116.
19. Aoki M, Ogasawara M, Matsubara Y, Narisawa K, Nakamura S, Itoyama Y, Abe K. Familial amyotrophic lateral sclerosis (ALS) in Japan associated with H46R mutation in Cu/Zn superoxide dismutase gene: a possible new subtype of familial ALS. J Neurol Sci 1994; 126:77–83.
20. Arisato T, Okubo R, Arata H, Abe K, Fukada K, Sakoda S, Shimizu A, Qin XH, Izumo S, Osame M, Nakagawa M. Clinical and pathological studies of familial amyotrophic lateral sclerosis (FALS) with SOD1 H46R mutation in large Japanese families. Acta Neuropathol (Berl) 2003; 106:561–568.
21. Alexander MD, Traynor BJ, Miller N, Corr B, Frost E, McQuaid S, Brett FM, Green A, Hardiman O. "True" sporadic ALS associated with a novel SOD-1 mutation. Ann Neurol 2002; 52:680–683.
22. Bowling AC, Schulz JB, Brown Jr. RH, Beal MF. Superoxide dismutase activity, oxidative damage, and mitochondiral energy metabolism in familial and sporadic amyotrophic lateral sclerosis. J. Neurochem 1993; 61:2322–2325.
23. Brown RH. Amyotrophic lateral sclerosis: recent insights from genetics and transgenic mice. Cell 1995; 80:687–692.
24. Gurney ME, Pu H, Chiu AY, Dal Corto MC, Polchow CY, Alexander DD, Caliendo J, Hentati A, Kwon YW, Deng H-X, Chen W, Zhai P, Sufit RL, Siddique T. Motor neuron degeneration in mice that express a human Cu,Zn superoxide dismutase mutation. Science 1994; 264:1772–1775.
25. Reaume AG, Elliott JL, Hoffman EK, Kowall NW, Ferrante RJ, Siwek DF, Wilcox HM, Flood DG, Beal MF, Brown RH, Jr Scott RW, Snider WD. Motor neurons in Cu/Zn superoxide dismutase-deficient mice develop normally but exhibit enhanced cell death after axonal injury. Nature Genetics 1996; 13:43–47.
26. Rosen DR, Siddique T, Patterson D, Figlewicz DA, Sapp P, Hentati A, Donaldson D, Goto J, O'Regan JP, Deng H-X, Rahmani Z, Krizus A, McKenna-Yasek D, Cayabyab A, Gaston SM, Berger R, Tanszi RE, Halperin JJ, Herzfeldt B, Van den Bergh R, Hung W-Y, Bird T, Deng G, Mulder DW, Smyth C, Lang NG, Soriana E, Pericak-Vance MA, Haines J, Rouleau GA, Gusella JS, Horvitz HR, Brown RH, Jr Mutations in Cu/Zn superoxide dismutase gene are associated with familial amyotrophic lateral sclerosis. Nature 1993; 362:59–62.
27. Howland DS, Liu J, She Y, Goad B, Maragakis NJ, Kim B, Erickson J, Kulik J, DeVito L, Psaltis G, DeGennaro LJ, Cleveland DW, Rothstein JD. Focal loss of the glutamate transporter EAAT2 in a transgenic rat model of SOD1 mutant-mediated amyotrophic lateral sclerosis (ALS). Proc Natl Acad Sci USA 2002; 99:1604–1609.

28. Chan PH, Kawase M, Murakami K, Chen SF, Li Y, Calagui B, Reola L, Carlson E, Epstein CJ. Overexpression of SOD1 in transgenic rats protects vulnerable neurons against ischemic damage after global cerebral ischemia and reperfusion. J Neurosci 1998; 18:8292–8299.

29. Avraham K, Schickler M, Sapoznoikov D, Yarom R, Groner Y. Down's syndrome: abnormal neuromuscular junction in tongue of transgenic mice with elevated levels of human Cu/Zn-superoxide dismutase. Cell 1988; 54:823–829.

30. Groner Y, Elroy-Stein O, Avraham KB, Schickler M, Knobler H, Minc-Golomb D, Bar-Peled O, Yarom R, Rotshenker S. Cell damage by excess CuZnSOD and Down's syndrome. Biomed Pharmacother 1994; 48:231–240.

31. Rando TA, Crowley RS, Carlson EJ, Epstein CJ, Mohapatra PK. Overexpression of copper/zinc superoxide dismutase: a novel cause of murine muscular dystrophy. Ann Neurol 1998; 44:381–386.

32. Culotta VC, Klomp LWJ, Strain J, Casareno RLB, Krems B, Gitlin JD. The copper chaperone for superoxide dismutase. J Biol Chem 1997; 272:23469–23472.

33. Carroll MC, Girouard JB, Ulloa JL, Subramaniam JR, Wong PC, Valentine JS, Culotta VC. Mechanisms for activating Cu- and Zn-containing superoxide dismutase in the absence of the CCS Cu chaperone. Proc Natl Acad Sci USA 2004; 101:5964–5969.

34. Wong PC, Waggoner D, Subramaniam JR, Tessarollo L, Bartnikas TB, Culotta VC, Price DL, Rothstein J, Gitlin JD. Copper chaperone for superoxide dismutase is essential to activate mammalian Cu/Zn superoxide dismutase. Proc Natl Acad Sci 2000; 10:1073.

35. Subramaniam JR, Lyons WE, Liu J, Bartnikas TB, Rothstein J, Price DL, Cleveland DW, Gitlin JD, Wong PC. Mutant SOD1 causes motor neuron disease independent of copper chaperone-mediated copper loading. Nat Neurosci 2002; 5:301–307.

36. Rae TD, Schmidt PJ, Pufahl RA, Culotta VC, O'Halloran TV. Undetectable intracellular free copper: the requirement of a copper chaperone for superoxide dismutase. Science 1999; 284:805–808.

37. Wong PC, Pardo CA, Borchelt DR, Lee MK, Copeland NG, Jenkins NA, Sisodia SS, Cleveland DW, Price DL. An adverse property of a familial ALS-linked SOD1 mutation causes motor neuron disease characterized by vacuolar degeneration of mitochondria. Neuron 1995; 14:1105–1116.

38. Kong J, Xu Z. Massive mitochondrial degeneration in motor neurons triggers the onset of amyotrophic lateral sclerosis in mice expressing a mutant SOD1. J Neurosci 1998; 18:3241–3250.

39. Wang J, Xu G, Gonzales V, Coonfield M, Fromholt D, Copeland NG, Jenkins NA, Borchelt DR. Fibrillar inclusions and motor neuron degeneration in transgenic mice expressing superoxide dismutase 1 with a disrupted copper-binding site. Neurobiol Dis 2002; 10:128–138.

40. Forman JH, Fridovich I. On the stability of bovine superoxide dismutase. J Biol Chem 1973; 248:2645–2649.

41. Pantoliano MW, McDonnell PJ, Valentine JS. Reversible loss of metal ions from the zinc binding site of copper-zinc superoxide dismutase. The low pH transition. J Am Chem Soc 1979; 101:6454–6456.

42. Crow JP, Sampson JB, Zhuang Y, Thompson JA, Beckman JS. Decreased zinc affinity of amyotrophic lateral sclerosis-associated superoxide dismutase mutants leads to enhanced catalysis of tyrosine nitration by peroxynitrite. J Neurochem 1997; 69:1936–1944.

43. Ghadge GD, Lee JP, Bindokas VP, Jordan J, Ma L, Miller RJ, Roos RP. Mutant superoxide dismutase-1-linked familial amyotrophic lateral sclerosis: molecular mechanisms of neuronal death and protection. J Neurosci 1997; 17:8756–8766.

44. Stathopulos PB, Rumfeldt JA, Scholz GA, Irani RA, Frey HE, Hallewell RA, Lepock JR, Meiering EM. Cu/Zn superoxide dismutase mutants associated with amyotrophic lateral sclerosis show enhanced formation of aggregates in vitro. Proc Natl Acad Sci USA 2003; 100:7021–7026.

45. Bruijn LI, Cleveland DW. Mechanisms of selective motor neuron death in ALS: insights from transgenic mouse models of motor neuron disease. Neuropathol Appl Neurobiol 1996; 22:373–387.
46. Watanabe M, Dykes-Hoberg M, Culotta VC, Price DL, Wong PC, Rothstein JD. Histological evidence of protein aggregation in mutant SOD1 transgenic mice and in amyotrophic lateral sclerosis neural tissues. Neurobiol Dis 2001; 8:933–941.
47. Leinweber B, Barofsky E, Barofsky DF, Ermilov V, Nylin K, Beckman JS. Aggregation of ALS mutant superoxide dismutase expressed in Escherichia coli. Free Radic Biol Med 2004; 36:911–918.
48. Lee JP, Gerin C, Bindokas VP, Miller R, Ghadge G, Roos RP. No correlation between aggregates of Cu/Zn superoxide dismutase and cell death in familial amyotrophic lateral sclerosis. J Neurochem 2002; 82:1229–1238.
49. Okado-Matsumoto A, Fridovich I. Amyotrophic lateral sclerosis: A proposed mechanism. Proc Natl Acad Sci USA 2002; 99:9010–9014.
50. Zhang H, Andrekopoulos C, Joseph J, Crow J, Kalyanaraman B. The carbonate radical anion-induced covalent aggregation of human copper, zinc superoxide dismutase, and alpha-synuclein: intermediacy of tryptophan- and tyrosine-derived oxidation products. Free Radic Biol Med 2004; 36:1355–1365.
51. Zhang H, Joseph J, Gurney M, Becker D, Kalyanaraman B. Bicarbonate enhances peroxidase activity of Cu,Zn-superoxide dismutase. Role of carbonate anion radical and scavenging of carbonate anion radical by metalloporphyrin antioxidant enzyme mimetics. J Biol Chem 2002; 277:1013–1020.
52. Lynch SM, Boswell SA, Colon W. Kinetic stability of Cu/Zn superoxide dismutase is dependent on its metal ligands: implications for ALS. Biochemistry 2004; 43:16,525–16,531.
53. Fukada K, Nagano S, Satoh M, Tohyama C, Nakanishi T, Shimizu A, Yanagihara T, Sakoda S. Stabilization of mutant Cu/Zn superoxide dismutase (SOD1) protein by coexpressed wild SOD1 protein accelerates the disease progression in familial amyotrophic lateral sclerosis mice. Eur J Neurosci 2001; 14:2032–2036.
54. Jonsson PA, Ernhill K, Andersen PM, Bergemalm D, Brannstrom T, Gredal O, Nilsson P, Marklund SL. Minute quantities of misfolded mutant superoxide dismutase-1 cause amyotrophic lateral sclerosis. Brain 2004; 127:73–88.
55. Field LS, Furukawa Y, O'Halloran TV, Culotta VC. Factors controlling the uptake of yeast copper/zinc superoxide dismutase into mitochondria. J Biol Chem 2003; 278:28052–28059.
56. Lino MM, Schneider C, Caroni P. Accumulation of SOD1 mutants in postnatal motoneurons does not cause motoneuron pathology or motoneuron disease. J Neurosci 2002; 22:4825–4832.
57. Macfadyen AJ, Reiter C, Zhuang YX, Beckman JS. A novel superoxide dismutase-based trap for peroxynitrite used to detect entry of peroxynitrite into erythrocyte ghosts. Chem Res Toxicol 1999; 12:223–229.
58. Hayward LJ, Rodriguez JA, Kim JW, Tiwari A, Goto JJ, Cabelli DE, Valentine JS, Brown RH, Jr. Decreased metallation and activity in subsets of mutant superoxide dismutases associated with familial amyotrophic lateral sclerosis. J Biol Chem 2002; 277:15,923–15,931.
59. Crow JP, Strong MJ, Zhuang Y, Ye Y, Beckman JS. Superoxide dismutase catalyzes nitration of tyrosines by peroxynitrite in the rod and head domains of neurofilament L. J Neurochem 1997; 69:1945–1953.
60. Pierson KB, Evenson MA. 200 KD neurofilament protein binds Al, Cu and Zn. Biochem Biophys Res Commun 1988; 152:598–604.
61. Outten CE, O'Halloran TV. Femtomolar sensitivity of metalloregulatory proteins controlling zinc homeostasis. Science 2001; 292:2488–2492.
62. Ogihara NL, Parge HE, Hart PJ, Weiss MS, Goto JJ, Crane BR, Tsang J, Slater K, Roe JA, Valentine JS, Eisenberg D, Tainer JA. Unusual trigonal-planar copper configuration

revealed in the atomic structure of yeast copper-zinc superoxide dismutase. Biochemistry 1996; 35:2316–2321.

63. Ellerby LM, Cabelli DE, Graden JA, Valentine JS. Copper-zinc superoxide dismutase: why not pH-dependent?. J Am Chem Soc 1996; 118:6556–6561.

64. Wiedau-Pazos M, Goto JJ, Rabizadeh S, Gralla EB, Roe JA, Lee MK, Valentine JS, Bredesen DE. Altered reactivity of superoxide dismutase in familial amyotrophic lateral sclerosis. Science 1996; 271:515–518.

65. Estevez AG, Crow JP, Sampson JB, Reiter C, Zhuang Y, Richardson GJ, Tarpey MM, Barbeito L, Beckman JS. Induction of nitric oxide-dependent apoptosis in motor neurons by zinc-deficient superoxide dismutase. Science 1999; 286:2498–2500.

66. Estevez AG, Spear N, Manuel SM, Radi R, Henderson C, E, Barbeito L, Beckman JS. Nitric oxide and superoxide contribute to motor neuron apoptosis induced by trophic factor deprivation. J Neurosci 1998; 18:923–931.

67. Estévez AG, Sampson JB, Zhuang Y-X, Spear N, Richardson GJ, Crow JP, Tarpey MM, Barbeito L, Beckman JS. Liposome-delivered superoxide dismutase prevents nitric oxide-dependent motor neuron death induced by trophic factor withdrawal. Free Radic Biol Med 2000; 28:437–446.

68. Shibuki K, Okada D. Endogenous nitric oxide release required for long-term synaptic depression in the cerebellum. Nature (Lond) 1991; 349:326–329.

69. Malinski T, Taha Z. Nitric oxide release from a single cell measured in situ by a porphyrinic-based microsensor. Nature 1992; 358:676–678.

70. Malinski T, Bailey F, Zhang ZG, Chopp M. Nitric oxide measured by a porphyrinic microsensor in rat brain after transient middle cerebral artery occlusion. J Cereb Blood Flow Metab 1993; 13:355–358.

71. Beckman JS, Estevez AG, Crow JP, Barbeito L. Superoxide dismutase and the death of motoneurons in ALS. Trends Neurosci 2001; 24:S15–20.

72. Raoul C, Estevez AG, Nishimune H, Cleveland DW, deLapeyriere O, Henderson CE, Haase G, Pettmann B. Motoneuron death triggered by a specific pathway downstream of Fas. potentiation by ALS-linked SOD1 mutations. Neuron 2002; 35:1067–1083.

73. Abe K, Pan L-H, Watanabe M, Kato T, Itoyama Y. Induction of nitrotyrosine-like immunoreactivity in the lower motor neuron of amyotrophic lateral sclerosis. Neurosci Lett 1995; 199:152–154.

74. Abe K, Pan L-H, Watanabe M, Konno H, Kato T, Itoyama Y. Upregulation of protein-tyrosine nitration in the anterior horn cells of amyotrophic lateral sclerosis. Neurol Res 1997; 19:124–128.

75. Tohgi H, Abe T, Yamazaki K, Murata T, Ishizaki E, Isobe C. Remarkable increase in cerebrospinal fluid 3-nitrotyrosine in patients with sporadic amotrophic lateral sclerosis. Ann Neurol 1999; 46:129–131.

76. Tohgi H, Abe T, Yamazaki K, Murata T, Ishizaki E, Isobe C. Increase in oxidized NO products and reduction in oxidized glutathione in cerebrospinal fluid from patients with sporadic form of amyotrophic lateral sclerosis. Neurosci Lett 1999; 260:204–206.

77. Sasaki S, Shibata N, Komori T, Iwata M. iNOS and nitrotyrosine immunoreactivity in amyotrophic lateral sclerosis. Neurosci Lett 2000; 291:44–48.

78. Sasaki S, Warita H, Abe K, Iwata M. Inducible nitric oxide synthase (iNOS) and nitro-tyrosine immunoreactivity in the spinal cords of transgenic mice with a G93A mutant SOD1 gene. J Neuropathol Exp Neurol 2001; 60:839–846.

79. Sasaki S, Warita H, Abe K, Iwata M. Neuronal nitric oxide synthase (nNOS) immunoreactivity in the spinal cord of transgenic mice with G93A mutant SOD1 gene. Acta Neuropathol (Berl) 2002; 103:421–427.

80. Chou SM, Wang HS, Taniguchi A. Role of SOD-1 and nitric oxide/cyclic GMP cascade on neurofilament aggregation in ALS/MND. J Neurol Sci 1996; 139(suppl):16–26.

81. Chou SM, Wang HS, Komai K. Colocalization of NOS and SOD1 in neurofilament accumulation within motor neurons of amyotrophic lateral sclerosis: an immunohisto-chemical study. J Chem Neuroanat 1996; 10:249–258.

82. Ferrante RJ, Browne SE, Shinobu LA, Bowling AC, Baik MJ, MacGarvey U, Kowall NW, Brown RH, Jr, Beal MF. Evidence of increased oxidative damage in both sporadic and familial amyotrophic lateral sclerosis. J Neurochem 1997; 69:2064–2074.

83. Ferrante RJ, Shinobu LA, Schulz JB, Matthews RT, Thomas CE, Kowall NW, Gurney ME, Beal MF. Increased 3-nitrotyrosine and oxidative damage in mice with a human copper/zinc superoxide dismutase mutation. Ann Neurol 1997; 42:326–334.

84. Beal MF, Ferrante RJ, Browne SE, Matthews RT, Kowall NW, Brown RH, Jr, Increased 3-nitrotyrosine in both sporadic and familial amyotrophic lateral sclerosis. Ann Neurol 1997; 42:646–654.

85. Bruijn LI, Beal MF, Becher MW, Schulz JB, Wong PC, Price DL, Cleveland DW. Elevated free nitrotyrosine levels, but not protein-bound nitrotyrosine or hydroxyl radicals, throughout amyotrophic lateral sclerosis (ALS)-like disease implicate tyrosine nitration as an aberrant in vivo property of one familial ALS-linked superoxide dismutase 1 mutant. Proc Natl Acad Sci USA 1997; 94:7606–7611.

86. Strong MJ, Sopper MM, Crow JP, Strong WL, Beckman JS. Nitration of the low molecular weight neurofilament is equivalent in sporadic amyotrophic lateral sclerosis and control cervical spinal cord. Biochem Biophys Res Commun 1998; 248:157–164.

87. Casoni F, Basso M, Massignan T, Gianazza E, Cheroni C, Salmona M, Bendotti C, Bonetto V. Protein nitration in a mouse model of familial amyotrophic lateral sclerosis: Possible multifunctional role in the pathogenesis. J Biol Chem 2005; 280:16295–16304.

88. Suhy DA, Simon KD, Linzer DI, O'Halloran TV. Metallothionein is part of a zinc-scavenging mechanism for cell survival under conditions of extreme zinc deprivation. J Biol Chem 1999; 274:9183–9192.

89. Nagano S, Satoh M, Sumi H, Fujimura H, Tohyama C, Yanagihara T, Sakoda S. Reduction of metallothioneins promotes the disease expression of familial amyotrophic lateral sclerosis mice in a dose-dependent manner. Eur J Neurosci 2001; 13:1363–1370.

90. Puttaparthi K, Gitomer WL, Krishnan U, Son M, Rajendran B, Elliott JL. Disease progression in a transgenic model of familial amyotrophic lateral sclerosis is dependent on both neuronal and non-neuronal zinc binding proteins. J Neurosci 2002; 22:8790–8796.

91. Ermilova I, Ermilov V, Levy M, Ho E, Pereira C, Beckman J. Protection by dietary zinc in ALS mutant G93A SOD transgenic mice. Neurosci Lett 2005; 379:42–46.

92. Groeneveld GJ, de Leeuw van Weenen J, van Muiswinkel FL, Veldman H, Veldink JH, Wokke JH, Bar PR, van den Berg LH. Zinc amplifies mSOD1-mediated toxicity in a transgenic mouse model of amyotrophic lateral sclerosis. Neurosci Lett 2003; 352:175–178.

93. Reeves PG, Nielsen FH, Fahey GC Jr. AIN-93 purified diets for laboratory rodents: final report of the American Institute of Nutrition ad hoc writing committee on the reformulation of the AIN-76A rodent diet. J Nutr 1993; 123:1939–1951.

94. Fox PL. The copper-iron chronicles: the story of an intimate relationship. Biometals 2003; 16:9–40.

95. Parge HE, Getzoff ED, Scandella CS, Hallewell RA, Tainer JA. Crystallographic characterization of recombinant human CuZn superoxide dismutase. J Biol Chem 1986; 261:16215–16218.

96. Hough MA, Grossmann JG, Antonyuk SV, Strange RW, Doucette PA, Rodriguez JA, Whitson LJ, Hart PJ, Hayward LJ, Valentine JS, Hasnain SS. Dimer destabilization in superoxide dismutase may result in disease-causing properties: structures of motor neuron disease mutants. Proc Natl Acad Sci USA 2004; 101:5976–5981.

97. Strange RW, Antonyuk S, Hough MA, Doucette PA, Rodriguez JA, Hart PJ, Hayward LJ, Valentine JS, Hasnain SS. The structure of holo and metal-deficient wild-type human Cu, Zn superoxide dismutase and its relevance to familial amyotrophic lateral sclerosis. J Mol Biol 2003; 328:877–891.

98. DiDonato M, Craig L, Huff ME, Thayer MM, Cardoso RM, Kassmann CJ, Lo TP, Bruns CK, Powers ET, Kelly JW, Getzoff ED, Tainer JA. ALS mutants of human superoxide dismutase form fibrous aggregates via framework destabilization. J Mol Biol 2003; 332:601–615.

15

Neuronal and Non-neuronal Cell Interactions in ALS

Jeffrey L. Elliott
University of Texas, Southwestern Medical Center, Dallas, Texas, U.S.A.

Although neurons, particularly motor neurons, are susceptible to the pathophysiologic process in amyotrophic lateral selerosis (ALS) and eventually undergo degeneration, there is increasing experimental evidence to suggest an important role for nonneuronal cell populations in contributing to neuronal dysfunction and the disease phenotype. Within the central nervous system (CNS), neurons exist in close contact with a variety of other cell types including astrocytes, oligodendrocytes, and microglia, while motor neuron axons projecting into the periphery are in proximity with Schwann cells and, of course, muscle. These differing nonneuronal cell types can be affected directly by the disease process in ALS, thereby contributing directly to the overall phenotype, or nonneuronal cells might indirectly impact neuron survival and function. Evidence for non-neuronal cell involvement in ALS has arisen directly from studies using autopsied human tissue from patients with sporadic and familial forms of ALS. However, more definitive insights have come from experiments using mutant Cu,Zn superoxide dismutase (SOD1) transgenic mice that serve as an excellent model of one inherited form of ALS. This animal model has allowed novel genetic approaches to be used in evaluating the role of nonneuronal cells to the ALS disease process, which has potential treatment implications for human ALS.

PATHOLOGIC EVIDENCE FOR NON-NEURONAL CELL INVOLVEMENT IN HUMAN ALS

Early evidence supporting a role for nonneuronal cells in ALS had its basis in careful pathologic studies of postmortem CNS tissue from patients with ALS. Although much attention was focused primarily on neuronal changes in disease, by the late 1980s and early 1990s neuropathologists had recognized that nonneuronal cells also underwent substantial pathologic alterations in tissues from patients with classic ALS. Initial studies observed significant "reactive" changes in astrocytes occurring in the gray matter of primary motor cortex as defined by GFAP immmuno-reactivity and cellular hypertrophy (1,2). Subsequent investigations extended these results, finding reactive astrocytosis to be a more diffuse process involving areas distant from degenerating motor pools. Reactive astrocytes were found widely distributed throughout subcortical white matter and cortical gray matter extending well into parietal, temporal, and, to a lesser extent, occipital areas in patients dying from ALS but not in control subjects (3–5). The distribution of these GFAP reactive astrocytes differed slightly in the various brain regions with superficial laminae being more positive in motor cortex and deeper laminae more positive in frontal (non-motor) and temporal cortex.

Reactive astrocytes have also been well documented in the ventral horn of ALS spinal cord sections in close proximity to degenerating anterior horn cells (6,7). However, as in cortex, astrogliosis is also evident in areas of spinal cord distant from motor neuron pools including white matter tracts of the ventral and lateral columns and dorsal areas of gray matter. These widespread changes observed in ALS patient brain and spinal cord clearly indicate astrocytic involvement in disease and suggest three possible interpretations: (i) astrocytes are reacting to diffuse neuronal injury in ALS not limited to motor populations, (ii) that the disease itself has some overall primary influence on astrocytes in general, and (iii) astrocytic changes can both be reactive and primary. Several experiments to be discussed later have tried to address this important question of whether astrocytic involvement is primary or secondary, and whether that involvement influences disease phenotype.

Although alterations in GFAP immunoreactivity clearly are pathologic markers of the "reactive" changes occurring within ALS tissue astrocytes, these indicators by themselves are not specific and unlikely related to the disease process. Indeed, part of the difficulty in trying to define ALS specific and disease related pathology in astrocytes is due to an incomplete understanding of sporadic ALS itself. In contrast, the recognition that mutations in SOD1 cause familial ALS has led to the identification of a disease-related astrocytic pathology that is shared with neuronal populations. One pathologic hallmark of familial ALS is the presence of ubiquitin and SOD1 positive cytosolic inclusions within many remaining neurons in the spinal cord, brainstem, and cortex (8–11). Similar cytoplasmic inclusions have been observed in astrocytes within the spinal cord, brainstem, and telencephalon in patients dying from SOD1 related familial ALS (8,10,12,13). Like their neuronal counterparts, these astrocytic inclusions are strongly SOD1 and ubiquitin positive. Ultratructurally, astrocytic inclusions are composed of 15 to 25 nm granule coated fibrils and closely resemble the neuronal dense Lewy-like body inclusion. Both neuronal and astrocytic SOD1 inclusions colocalize with markers for end glycation products (n-carboxymethyl lysine), and assorted other proteins like tubulin and tau. Neuronal and astrocytic inclusions do differ with regard to certain cell type specific proteins that are detected by immunocolocalization. For instance, S-100 protein is associated with astrocytic inclusions, while neurofilament, neuron-specific enolase (NSE), and synaptophysin reactivity are linked with neuronal inclusions. The observation that astrocytes and neurons share a characteristic and specific pathologic feature of ALS is highly significant because it suggests both cell types are directly affected by the production of the aberrant protein and respond in an overall similar biological manner with aggregate formation.

Microglial cells also undergo substantial pathologic change in tissue from ALS patients suggesting potential involvement in the disease process. Within control human non-diseased spinal cord, only scattered resting microglia are observed in gray and white matter, based on a characteristic dendritic morphologic appearance and immunoreactivity with major histocompatability complex (MHC) II glycoproteins (14). In contrast, ALS spinal cord exhibits a substantial increase in the number of total and activated microglia cells present. The increased number of spinal cord microglia can be found primarily as foamy macrophages within white matter tracts (anterior and lateral columns), presumably digesting myelin and other cellular debris, or maintaining a more ramified morphology within gray matter (15). Microgliosis is not limited to spinal cord regions but also occurs within motor cortex of ALS patients, extending beyond the vicinity of motor neuron pools (14,16). The source for this increased number of microglia is not entirely clear. Microglia are frequently observed in close proximity to blood vessel walls within both white and gray matter regions of ALS spinal cord suggesting that migration of peripherally derived macrophages may be a principle contributor for the increase in microglia number. However, proliferation of resident CNS microglia may also be occurring and contribute substantially to the exuberant microglial reaction. There is little experimental evidence available to distinguish between these two possibilities.

There have been no detailed studies of oligodendroglial, ependymal, or leptomeningeal cell changes in the CNS of ALS patients. However, the absence of such reports does not preclude either primary or secondary involvement of these cell types in disease.

Lymphocytic cell infiltrates have been reported in the spinal cord tissue of many but not all ALS patients (17–19). These infiltrating lymphocytes are almost exclusively composed of T-cells, with little if any positive B-cell identification, and are found in white matter tracts, ventral horn gray matter and scattered through the leptomeninges. CD4 positive T-cells predominate in white matter, while both CD4 and CD8 positive T-cells equally populate ventral horn gray matter. In contrast to ALS spinal cord, lymphocytes are not generally observed in spinal cords from control patients. Engelhardt et al. found no correlation between the degree of lymphocytic infiltration in ALS spinal cord and the rate of disease progression premortem. Interestingly, several of their patients had been given immunosuppressive agents, including steroids or cyclosporin, but the investigators noted no significant effect of such treatments in the presence or distribution of lymphocytes within spinal cord.

These studies, dating largely from the early- and mid-1990s, clearly identified pathologic changes in multiple nonneuronal cell types found within the CNS of patients dying from ALS. Although these findings demonstrate the involvement of nonneuronal cells in the end stage of disease, their relevance to the disease process itself could not be addressed. Were these changes in nonneuronal cells artifacts of terminal disease stage, merely responses triggered by significant neuronal injury and death, or were they indicative of a more smoldering and chronic participation in the disease course, more consistent with an integral role? Because human pathologic studies can be performed only on autopsied tissue, no temporal information detailing the course of nonneuronal cell pathology can be obtained. However, the advent of a mutant SOD1 transgenic mouse model for FALS has allowed better definition of the temporal changes pertaining to nonneuronal cells and clearly demonstrates that such pathology is not an end-stage disease artifact (20).

NON-NEURONAL INVOLVEMENT IN A MURINE MODEL OF FALS

Many studies have investigated the time course of astroglial involvement in mutant SOD1 expressing transgenic mice that go on to develop a progressive motor phenotype. Transgenic mice expressing G85R human SOD1 (line 148) develop motor symptoms at 7 to 7.5 months and reach end-stage by eight months of age (21). However, the earliest recognized pathology in these mice occurs at six months of age, significantly earlier than onset of motor symptoms and consists of both astroglial and neuronal cytoplasmic inclusions. These inclusions are both SOD1 and ubiquitin positive, closely resembling what is found in human 21q linked FALS tissue. Astrocytosis, characterized by increased GFAP reactivity in the spinal cord of these G85R SOD1 mice, begins somewhat later at 6.5 months, although even this change occurs prior to the onset of disease symptoms and significant motor neuron loss. Because astroglial pathology is an early phenomenon in these mice, occurring roughly contemporaneously to early neuronal changes, this finding suggests that astrocytic involvement in disease is neither just a reaction to neuronal degeneration nor only a marker of terminal cellular events. These results imply parallel rather than sequential cellular dysfunction in astrocytes and neurons induced by mutant SOD1 protein expression.

Within transgenic mouse lines expressing a G93A SOD1 mutation, an overall similar temporal pattern of astroglial involvement emerges. In high-expressing G93A SOD1 mouse lines with a survival of 140 days, significant astrogliosis is noted within the spinal cord by 100 days of age, which correlates well with disease onset but is well after the initiation of neuronal pathology (22). In the low-expressing G93A SOD1 lines, spinal cord astrocytosis, as manifested by increased GFAP reactivity and cell hypertrophy, is well established by 150 days, significantly earlier than end-stage disease, which is about 240 days (Fig. 1). Interestingly, this astrocytosis does not begin diffusely but clearly originates within the ventral horn of spinal cord in the vicinity of motor pools, and only later appears to spread and involve ventral portions of spinal cord and beyond (Fig. 2) (23).

The onset of astrocytosis in these mice also correlates with the onset of motor weakness (150 days), but occurs after the initiation of neuronal pathology. Although these results suggest that significant astrocytosis in G93A SOD1 mice occurs as a reaction to neuronal pathology, no systematic temporal examination of astroglial inclusion formation has been done in G93A SOD1 mice to better document the onset of astroglial changes. If astroglial inclusion formation precedes "astrocytosis" as it does in G85R SOD1 mice, then the onset of astroglial reaction has been underestimated in G93A SOD1 lines.

Although subtle differences in overall astrocytic pathology have been observed in mouse lines harboring various SOD1 mutations, certain key features appear to be constant. Astroglial pathology is not a terminal disease event but occurs near the onset or even before the development of motor symptoms. Astrocytic changes correlate with motor symptom progression but not necessarily with neuronal pathology. The difficulty in correlating astrocytic changes with neuronal pathology or disease phenotype arises from the ambiguity of establishing initial astrocytic abnormalities. Astrocytic SOD1 inclusions appear to form before increased GFAP immunoreactivity and thus may represent an earlier marker of astrocytic involvement in disease. However, earlier markers of disease may yet be identified that push back the onset of non-neuronal cell involvement even farther.

There has been remarkably little study of non-astrocytic glial cell pathology in mutant SOD1 transgenic mice. One study did find filamentous SOD1 positive aggregates in the periaxonal process of oligodendrocytes from G93A high-expressing mice (24). These aggregates were found to form early in the disease time course (two months) and preceded neuronal and astroglial SOD1 perikaryal aggregation. Whether these oligodendroglial aggregates are also ubiquitin positive is unclear.

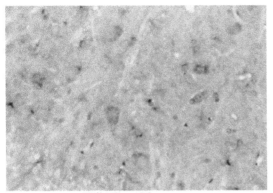

Wild Type Mouse

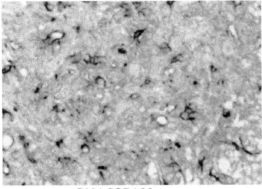

G93A SOD1 Mouse

Figure 1   GFAP immunoreactivity in the lumbar spinal cord of 7.5-month-old wild-type and G93A SOD1 mice. There is marked astroglial reaction in the G93A SOD1 spinal cord.

The temporal and spatial course of inflammatory cell involvement has been well studied in G93A SOD1 transgenic mice. In high-expressing G93A SOD1 trans-genic lines, microglial activation manifested by MHC II or by CD11b immunoreac-tivity is observed by about 80 days of age (22,25). This time period again precedes onset of motor symptoms but is after initiation of neuronal pathology (Fig. 3). Spatially, microgliosis begins in the ventral horn and proximal ventral roots. Only later by 100–120 days does microglial activation involve dorsal spinal cord and spinal cord white matter tracts (Fig. 4). In contrast to the relatively early appearance of microglial changes, T-lymphocyte infiltration occurs only at terminal stages of dis-ease at 120 days or later (25). These results suggest that comparable T-cell lympho-cytic infiltrates found in human ALS tissue on autopsy may also represent terminal cellular reactions with little contribution to the overall disease process.

Overall, these studies using mutant SOD1 transgenic mice provide some impor-tant insights into the potential involvement of nonneuronal cells in ALS. Clearly, the pathology observed in astrocytes, oligodendrocytes, and microglia does not repre-sent reactive change to end-stage neuronal degeneration, since nonneuronal changes precede substantial neuronal losses. Rather, the temporal and spatial patterns of astrocytic, oligodendroglial, and microglial pathology are consistent with the hypothesis that these cells contribute, directly or indirectly, to the ALS disease pro-cess. Such nonneuronal cells may be direct targets of the underlying pathogenesis.

Wild Type Mouse

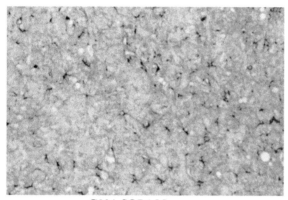

G93A SOD1 Mouse

Figure 2   GFAP immunoreactivity in the pons of 7.5-month-old wild-type and G93A SOD1 mice. There is marked astroglial reaction in the G93A SOD1 tissue.

For instance, in 21q linked FALS, mutant SOD1 expression within astrocytes or oligodendrocytes might directly perturb important cellular pathways required for normal motor function or trigger biochemical cascades harmful for cell survival. Nonneuronal cells may be important indirect targets. For instance, astroglial or microglial function may be unaffected by mutant SOD1 expression, but may be altered in response to cues derived from injured neurons. It is also possible that rather than accelerating disease progression, non-neuronal cell involvement may be important in retarding disease manifestation. Several groups have recently used novel genetic manipulations of the mutant SOD1 mouse in attempts to address these complex questions.

TRANSGENIC, KNOCKOUT, AND CHIMERA MICE: GENETIC EVIDENCE FOR NON-NEURONAL CELL INVOLVEMENT IN ALS

Given the pathologic evidence implicating astrocytic involvement in ALS, initial research was directed towards understanding whether mutant SOD1 related FALS was a primary disorder of astrocytes with only secondary neuronal injury. Although the original mutant SOD1 transgenic mouse lines are excellent models of the human disease, they are not ideally suited for sorting out the contributory role of specific cell

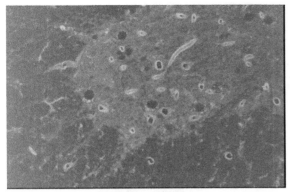

Wild Type Mouse

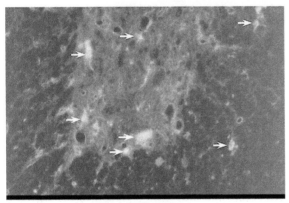

G93A SOD1 Mouse

Figure 3 Microgliosis in G93A SOD1 spinal cord. Tomato lectin staining in ventral horn of 7.5 months wild-type and G93A SOD1 lumbar spinal cord. Arrows indicate positive microglia.

types to the disease process. Traditional mutant SOD1 mouse lines were generated using the endogenous SOD1 promoter (human or mouse) to recapitulate the normal expression patterns found in vivo (20,21,26,27). However, SOD1 is a ubiquitously expressed protein in eukaryotic cells, and the SOD1 promoter drives transgene expression in virtually all cell types making it difficult to isolate effects in particular cell types. Cell type specific expression of mutant SOD1 in vivo was needed to evaluate cell type specific contributions to disease.

The first cell type specific mutant SOD1 transgenic mouse line was generated using the human GFAP promoter to drive expression of murine G86R SOD1 (28). The GFAP promoter is highly specific to astrocytes within the CNS, but does drive some expression in extra CNS cell types including Schwann cells. Still, this promoter does not drive expression in neurons and is appropriate to distinguish effects from mutant SOD1 expression in astrocytes from neurons. These GFAP driven G86R SOD1 mice are viable, grow normally, and do not develop any progressive motor phenotype. Interesting, these mice do develop a progressive astrocytosis as manifested by hypertrophy and increased GFAP staining, but without concomitant neuronal pathology. Two important conclusions can be reached from this experiment. First, mutant SOD1-induced ALS is not a primary disorder of astrocytes, nor is

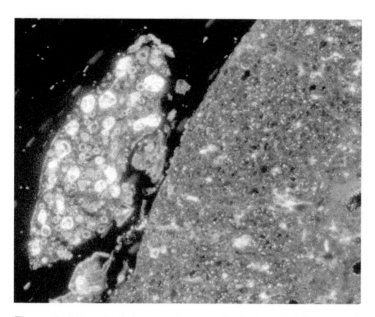

Figure 4 Microgliosis in ventral root and spinal cord white matter from G93A SOD1 mice. Numerous lectin positive cells are evident in the degenerating ventral root and white matter tracts.

expression of mutant protein in astrocytes sufficient to yield a disease phenotype. Expression of mutant SOD1 in another cell type is required for motor dysfunction, and this familial form of ALS is clearly distinguished from disorders like Alexander's disease where primary astroglial dysfunction is sufficient to produce neurological disease (29,30). Second, this work indicates that mutant SOD1 expression has direct and primary effects on astrocytes causing pathology that cannot be viewed as merely reactive to neuronal dysfunction. What effects mutant SOD1 expression may have directly on astrocytic function are unclear, and although insufficient to produce ALS alone, these primary induced changes still may contribute substantially to disease. For instance, astrocytic dysfunction induced by mutant SOD1 expression may not be capable of initiating the disease process but may play important roles in allowing its propagation. However, an important caveat to consider for experiments using transgenic mice is whether expression of the transgene is sufficiently high to produce the expected biological effect. Thus is it possible that with higher GFAP driven mutant SOD1 expression, a different phenotype may have been observed.

Because restricted expression of mutant SOD1 in astrocytes did not cause weakness in transgenic mice, other cell types must be involved in the disease process. Perhaps ALS is a primary neuronal disorder and does not require the participation of other cell types for the disease phenotype. In this case, one would predict that mutant SOD1 expression limited to neurons would be sufficient to produce disease. In order to test this hypothesis, three lines of neuronal specific mutant SOD1 expressing mice have been generated. Expression of human G37R SOD1 under the control of the neurofilament light chain promoter did not yield a motor phenotype in transgenic mice (31). No significant neuronal or overall pathology was observed in these mice. In the following year, transgenic mice expressing human G85R or G93A SOD1 under the control of the mouse Thy-1 promoter were generated (32). These mice did not develop motor weakness and did not manifest any pathologic features, either neuronal or astrocytic. Neither neurons nor astrocytes in these mice formed ubiquitin positive inclusions that are a hallmark of conventional mutant SOD1 transgenic mice.

These results would seem to indicate that expression of mutant SOD1 limited to neurons is insufficient to cause disease, however, some caution is warranted in interpreting these experiments because transgene expression of mutant SOD1 was low in both studies. In NFL-G37R SOD1 mice, transgene expression level was significantly lower than that of native murine SOD1. G37R SOD1 is a relatively non-toxic mutant requiring high-protein levels to give disease in traditional transgenic mouse lines expressing the protein in multiple cell types (26). Even traditional G37R SOD1 lines expressing transgene at levels lower than a threshold value develop neither disease nor pathologic features such as neuronal ubiquitin inclusion bodies. Similarly, levels of transgene expression were low in the Thy-1 driven mutant SOD1 mice and may also be below the critical threshold level required to develop disease or pathology (33). If transgene levels were sufficiently high and above threshold, then one might expect limited cell specific pathology even without a motor phenotype, as one observes in the astrocytes of GFAP driven G86R SOD1 mice. The fact that no neuronal pathology is observed in these NFL-SOD1 or Thy-1 SOD1 lines favors the interpretation that threshold levels of transgene protein expression were not attained.

However, an alternative interpretation might hold that threshold levels of neuronal protein expression were indeed achieved in these mice, and the lack of a phenotype signifies the critical importance of nonneuronal cells to disease initiation. Perhaps expression of mutant SOD1 in oligodendrocytes, microglia or another cell type (neither neuronal nor astroglial) would be sufficient to produce disease. There is no strong evidence available to prove or disprove this possibility, although for microglia, the pathologic evidence presented earlier strongly argues against primary microglial contribution to disease (rather than secondary). Perhaps ALS pathogenesis is a more complex process that requires multiple hits for generating a "successful" disease phenotype. Direct neuronal involvement by mutant SOD1 may be absolutely necessary for the disease phenotype but not sufficient in itself to initiate or propagate disease. Similarly, astrocytic involvement may be necessary but not sufficient in itself to produce disease. The possibility that dual neuronal and astrocytic involvement is necessary for the disease phenotype could easily be tested by breeding GFAP mutant SOD1 mice with the neuronal mutant SOD1 restricted lines to determine whether this cross could recapitulate the disease process. To date, there are no published results concerning the results of this experiment. There is, however, additional evidence from in vivo studies supporting the hypothesis that both neuronal and nonneuronal cells both contribute to the mutant SOD1-induced disease phenotype.

Genetic knockout experiments targeting molecules potentially important in disease but with restricted cellular expression patterns have been used to address neuronal and nonneuronal contributions to disease in G93A SOD1 transgenic mice. The metallothioneins (MTs) represent a family of zinc binding proteins important in the regulation of zinc bioavailability by acting as chaperones within cells.

Within the CNS, MT-I, and MT-II proteins are not expressed within neurons, but are primarily restricted to astrocytes and ependymal cells. The expression of these molecules is significantly upregulated in G93A SOD1 transgenic mice as they age and develop motor deficits (23). Two groups have reported that crossing G93A SOD1 transgenic mice with MT-I/MT-II double knockout mice results in a substantially earlier onset of motor deficits and a significant decrease in the survival of the G93A SOD1 mice (34,35). There are enhanced pathologic changes observed in G93A SOD1 lacking MT-I and MT-II that appeared limited to nonneuronal populations. These mice have more extensive astrocytosis than what is observed in comparable G93A SOD1 mice with normal MT levels but do not exhibit a change in the degree of neuronal loss. These results indicate that primary changes restricted to nonneuronal cells in G93A SOD1 mice can influence disease course and motor function independent of any direct neuronal effect.

In contrast, MT-III, another member of the metallothionein family of metal chaperones, is normally expressed only within neurons. MT-III expression also increases in G93A SOD1 spinal cord as the mice mature and develop motor symptoms (23). Crossing G93A SOD1 transgenic mice with MT-III knockout mice produces an even more significant impact on survival and motor function (35). Survival is reduced by over 20% in G93A SOD1 mice lacking MT-III. While the onset of motor deficits is comparable in G93A SOD1 mice with or without MT-III, the rate of motor decline is significantly more rapid in G93A SOD1 mice lacking MT-III. Pathologic examination demonstrates more marked spinal cord motor neuron loss in the G93A SOD1 mice lacking MT-III compared with G93A SOD1 mice with normal MT-III levels. These results indicate that primary events occurring within neurons can alter disease parameters without requiring any concomitant non-neuronal cell involvement.

Taken together these complimentary studies suggest that both neuronal and nonneuronal dysfunction can impact disease in G93A SOD1 mice, and do so in differing ways. Altering MT expression levels within nonneuronal cell populations influences the onset of motor deficits without affecting neuronal number suggesting that the extent of motor dysfunction and motor loss is discordant. In contrast, removal of neuronal MT-III produces changes in survival and function that are concordant with motor neuron loss. This effect might not be unexpected since the neuronal compartment was specifically targeted. If contributions from both neuronal and nonneuronal cells can impact the disease, understanding the nature of that interaction is an important issue. Are there interactions between the cell types or is cell dysfunction autonomous?

In order to address this issue, wild-type and mutant SOD1 chimeric mice were generated either by morula aggregation (G37R or G93A with wild-type) or by blastocyst injection (G37R or G85R with wild-type) (36). Because individual cells in such a chimeric mouse arising either from mutant SOD1 transgenic or wild-type progenitors can be labeled, this procedure allows investigation of interactions between differing cell types as well as differing genotypes that are in close proximity. This study found not surprisingly that the survival of wild-type/mutant SOD1 chimera correlated well with the number of wild-type cells present within spinal cord. For instance, chimeric mice with 40% of their cells derived from wild-type mice lived longer than those having only 20% of cells derived from wild-type mice. This makes sense, as there are a larger number of normal cells present, including neurons that can preserve strength and maintain motor function longer. However, in one G37R chimera, no motor neuron pathology was observed at the L5 level even though 30% of the cells were mutant. No astroglial or microglial changes were noted in this animal as well. The authors conclude that this point argues for non-cell autonomous neuronal injury, because one would expect mutant neurons to show a certain degree of pathology based on their intrinsic expression of mutant SOD1. The observation that these neurons did not exhibit pathology suggests that the presence of neighboring wild-type healthy cells was sufficient to retard or prevent pathology. This conclusion is supported by findings in two additional chimeras. In these mice, all lumbar spinal motor neurons were derived from mutant SOD1 progenitors, but yet had asymmetric proportions of wild-type nonneuronal cells, which differentially affected motor neuron survival. Interactions between wild-type and mutant SOD1 expressing cells also appeared to influence wild-type cells. Remarkably, the authors found that even some wild-type neurons in G37R and G85R chimera would form ubiquitin positive (? SOD1 positive) inclusions when surrounded by mutant nonneuronal cells suggesting that neuronal deficits in ubiquitin dependent protein degradation can be acquired from nonneuronal cells.

Results from this complicated study involving chimera provide some additional support for important nonneuronal cell contributions to disease but are not definitive for several reasons. Part of the difficulty arises from the fact that each chimeric mouse represents an experimental N of one, which cannot be duplicated in another mouse. Each chimeric mouse is unique in terms of the percentage of wild-type to transgenic cells present (ranging 5–90% wild-type), the distribution of those cells (cervical vs. thoracic; left vs. right), and even the type of cells (motor neuron vs. glia). Moreover, chimerization in these mice extends beyond the CNS. Thus each mouse is also unique in the degree of mutant to wild-type cells comprising muscle, Schwann cell, macorph-age, etc. Because each mouse is unique, it cannot readily be compared with another mouse nor can studies of temporal progression be performed in an animal once the pathologic and chimeric character is known. Because neurons and their processes are three-dimensional structures extending over long distances, it is difficult in serial sections to determine the exact genotype of nonneuronal cells that envelop or border neuronal cell bodies, dendrites, and axons across the many microns which these structures traverse. The authors had little choice but to simplify this important point in analyzing their chimeric mice, but such assumptions diminish the impact of their findings.

The conclusions reached from experiments using genetic approaches to understand the contributions of nonneuronal cells have been less than satisfying. These experiments have failed to show which cell type (neuronal or nonneuronal) is primarily targeted by mutant SOD1 and responsible for the large share of the phenotype. Although such failure may result from the complexity of the question, methodologic difficulties (i.e., insufficient transgene expression, etc.) likely play some role in making the experimental results challenging to interpret. However, the conclusions from these experiments in total are most consistent with the idea that neurons and nonneuronal cells are altered in the disease and contribute to the motor phenotype.

MECHANISMS OF NEURONAL AND NON-NEURONAL CELL INTERACTION

Several differing mechanisms can account for neuronal and nonneuronal cell interactions that contribute to the ALS disease phenotype, although none has yet been proved to be absolutely critical in vivo. Moreover, there is no reason to suppose that the differing mechanisms for that interaction are exclusionary, and some combination of very differing pathways may in fact be quite possible.

The production and release of potent cytokines within the spinal cord of mutant SOD1 transgenic mice is one potential mechanism for paracrine or autocrine signaling that might impact motor function and cell survival. Several groups have longitudinally assayed the expression levels of various cytokines, either at the mRNA or protein level, within G37R or G93A SOD1 transgenic mice, and have reported significant increases over time (37–41). A compilation of these findings is given in Tables 1 and 2, but results for several key cytokines will be discussed. Expression of the pro-inflammatory cytokine, TNF-α, is observed beginning at around 75 to 80 days of age in high-expressing G93A SOD1 mice and by 120 days in low-expressing G93A SOD1 mice. This time period correlates well with the initiation of microglial and astroglial activation observed in those lines and clearly precedes the development of actual motor deficits. Over time as the mice develop weakness, levels of TNF-α mRNA substantially rise, by over sevenfold at 120 days in the high-expressing G93A SOD1 line while protein increases by 55%. These increasing values of TNF-α production also correlate with the progressive microgliosis and astrocytosis that are occurring in the G93A SOD1 mouse spinal cord. However, since both astrocytes and microglia are capable of synthesizing TNF-α, it has been difficult to determine which particular cell type is primarily responsible for synthesis or whether multiple cell types contribute significantly (42–45). Importantly, there is clear expression of receptors, TNFR1 and TNFR2, within the spinal cord of G93A SOD1 mice that are necessary for transducing the biological effects of TNF-α. These TNF receptors can be expressed in multiple cell types including astrocytes, microglia, oligodendrocytes, and neurons (46–48) indicating that these cells are potentially responsive to TNF-α via paracrine and autocrine loops. Given that TNF-α may transduce very different cellular responses depending on whether effects are mediated via TNFR1 or TNFR2 receptors and that both receptors may be present in any given cell type, the level of biologic complexity is quite great. Thus, understanding the precise role of TNF-α in disease is daunting. Similar challenges exist for other cytokines that are altered in mutant G93A SOD1 spinal cord including TGF-β family, γ-interferon, etc.

One approach that can be used to assess the overall importance of a particular cytokine, such as TNF-α, on a complex disease phenotype is with genetic cytokine or cytokine receptor knockouts. For example, TNF-α, TNFR1, or TNFR2 knockout mice can be used crossed with mutant SOD1 mice in order to assess what overall

Table 1 Cytokine Expression in Mutant SOD1 Transgenic Mice

Cytokine	mRNA	Protein
IL-1a	+	++
IL-1b	+	+
IL-2	+	++
IL-3	+	+
IL-4	+	+
IL-5		+
IL-6	+	++
IL-10		+
IL-12	+	+
TNF-α	+	++
IFN-γ	+	+
MIP-1a	+	
M-CSF	+	
TGFβ1	+	
TGFβ2	+	
TGFβ3	+	
RANTES		++

For protein levels (+) = 20–50% increase; (++) = 50% or greater increase.

Table 2 Cytokine with Little Change in ALS

IL-15
IL-17
GM-CSF
G-CSF

influence, if any, TNF-α may have on disease. However, this approach will not be able to determine important biologic differences in specific cell–cell type interactions that TNF-α may afford such as the biological importance of astroglial versus microglial production, or of astrocytic versus neuronal response to TNF-α. Surprisingly, results for this important experiment have yet to be published.

Nguyen et al. have crossed G37R SOD1 mice with mice deficient of IL-1β, a pro-inflammatory cytokine produced by microglia as well as other cell types within the CNS that is upregulated in both G37R and G93A SOD1 transgenic mouse spinal cord by nearly twofold in mRNA and by 37% in protein levels (38,40,41). However, crossing IL-1β deficient mice to G37R SOD1 mice had little effect on the survival or course of G37R SOD1 mediated disease in the mice indicating that the loss of this upregulated pro-imflammatory cytokine, IL-1β did not impact disease.

Despite the marked induction of many inflammatory cytokines that correlate with disease progression in mutant SOD1 mice, there is actually little data presently available to prove that changes in expression of individual cytokines in fact do contribute to the disease process. There has been relatively little published regarding the effect of knocking out or inducing specific cytokines expression in G93A SOD1 mice (see above), but one interesting study has recently addressed whether induction of a chronic inflammatory state would affect mutant SOD1-induced disease (49). In this work, administration of bacterial lipopolysaccharide endotoxin significantly shortens survival in G37R SOD1 mice by three weeks (49 vs. 46 weeks) and worsens axonal loss. This change in motor phenotype is accompanied by an increased induction of TNF-α and IL-12 mRNA, even beyond the already increased levels observed in the untreated G37R SOD1 mouse. Moreover, this treatment resulted in an induction of the Toll-like receptor-2 within microglia suggesting (but not proving) that microglia are primarily responding to the inflammatory challenge. No infiltration of T-cells was observed in the treated mice to suggest that input from these cells was in any way contributing to the change in phenotype. These results demonstrate that general stimulation of the immune response, even peripherally, can influence disease progression, although the overall impact is modest. Changes in cytokine production correlated with worsening phenotype, but whether enhanced cytokine expression was truly responsible for the effects of LPS administration, or whether other microglial-derived factors contributed preferentially remains unclear.

To date much of the research on cytokines in ALS as it relates to microglia or astrocytes has focused on characterizing any changes in cytokine expression patterns and understanding the biologic relevance of those altered expression profiles on disease. However, the primary disease process might also fundamentally alter how microglial or astrocytic cells respond to conditions that would usually induce cytokine production. One recent study has found evidence to support the concept that microglial function may be altered by the disease process but not necessarily by mutant SOD1 protein expression (50). Weydt et al. found that microglial cells cultured from adult G93A SOD1 mice responded to LPS stimulation with enhanced

TNF-α production (twofold increase in protein level) compared with stimulated microglia isolated from adult non-transgenics, while baseline unstimulated TNF-α levels were comparable in the two groups. In contrast, microglia isolated from neonatal mutant SOD1 mice and non-transgenics demonstrated no difference in baseline or stimulated TNF-α expression levels. These results suggest that microglia may be in some way primed for mounting an abnormal immunologic response with altered cytokine expression patterns by cues stemming from the disease state. However, the precise nature of those signals and whether their interruption would improve clinical outcome remain unclear.

The changing expression patterns demonstrated by multiple cytokines during the progression of disease in mutant G93A SOD1 mice correlate well with the progression of motor dysfunction in mutant SOD1 mice. However, correlation does not prove effect, and to date there has been little in vivo data to definitively establish clear roles for cytokines, beneficial or harmful, in the disease process itself. More cytokine or cytokine receptor knockouts crossed with SOD1 mutant mice would certainly provide some answer to the importance of cytokine function in disease, particularly if a limited number of cytokines significantly influenced survival or motor function. However, negative results from such a crossing experiment might not completely rule out a functional role for a particular cytokine, given possible redundancy in cytokine function. Even if deleting a specific cytokine would profoundly alter the disease course, it would be extremely difficult to ascertain upon which cell type(s) that effect was manifested. Because cytokines can act via paracrine or autocrine pathways, it becomes extremely difficult to sort out which cell is responsible for secreting or reacting to a particular cytokine. Virtually every cytokine that is altered in ALS can be synthesized by multiple cell types within the CNS and can then induce effects in multiple cell types as well. This complexity is well demonstrated in Table 3.

GROWTH FACTORS: BENEFICIAL NEURONAL–NON-NEURONAL INTERACTIONS

Although much research has focused on the possible deleterious interactions between neuronal and nonneuronal cells in ALS, there is also evidence that this relationship may be beneficial, providing some protection against the disease process. For example neuronal growth factors such as GDNF secreted by astrocytes can provide neuronal protection and enhance motor neuron survival during programmed cell death and after neonatal axotomy (51). Indeed, several other growth factors (CNTF, BDNF, and IGF-1), which had been shown to similarly support motor neuron survival and function postaxotomy, have been unsuccessful in human ALS trials (52–54). These failures may have derived in part because of the route of administration selected for testing as well as from a lack of actual medical benefit. However, the interest in using growth factors in ALS has increased due to the identification of potentially more efficacious growth factors in several recent studies.

Vascular endothelial growth factor-A (VEGF) is perhaps one of the more promising growth factors recently identified that may play an important role in ALS via cell–cell signaling. VEGF is one member of an enlarging family of growth factors (VEGF, VEGF-B, VEGF-C, and VEGF-D in mammals) that were originally recognized as critical factors in promoting angiogenesis (for extensive reviews, see Ref. 55). The biologic actions of VEGF are mediated by binding to high-affinity tyrosine kinase receptors, VEGFR-1, VEGFR-2, and VEGFR-3, on the cell surface. Certain

Table 3 Expression Pattern of ALS Related Cytokines and Receptors in the CNS

Cytokine	Synthesis[a]	Receptors[b]
IL-1a	N, A, M	A, M
IL-1b	N, A, M, O	N, A, M, O
IL-2	A, M	N, M, O (?)[c]
IL-3	N, A, M	N, M
IL-4	A, M	A, M, O
IL-5	A, M	A, M (?)
IL-6	N, A, M	N, A, M, O (?)
IL-10	A, M	A, M, O
IL-12	N, M, A	N, M
TNF-α	N, A, M, O	N, A, M, O
IFN-γ	N, A, M,	N, A, M, O
MIP-1a	A, M	A, M
M-CSF	N, A, M	N, A, M, O
TGFβ1	N, A, M, O	N, A, M
TGFβ2	A, O	N, A, M
TGFβ3	A, O	N, A, M
RANTES	N, A, M	N, A, M

[a]Synthesis, cells known to express the cytokine. [b]Receptors, cells with known specific cytokine receptor. [c]?, possible. *Abbreviations*: N, neuron; A, astrocyte; M, microglia; O, oligodendrocyte.

VEGF isoforms may also interact with neuropilin-1 or -2 coreceptors, which serve to increase VEGF binding affinity to the tyrosine kinase receptors. Control of VEGF expression is in part achieved via the binding of several transcription factors, including hypoxia-inducible factor 1 (HIF-1), to different response elements in the VEGF promoter. A deletion in the HIF-1 response element within the VEGF promoter results in a neurologic phenotype where 60% of mice die at birth, but the remaining 40% developed a slowly progressive, non-lethal motor phenotype beginning at five months of age (56). Pathologic examination revealed moderate motor neuron loss with a prominent astroglial reaction. Biochemical analysis confirmed that HIF-1 element knockouts had a 33% reduction in spinal cord levels of VEGF suggesting that a loss of growth factor synthesis might account for the motor phenotype. Further analysis in human populations found that certain homozygous polymorphisms in the HIF-1 element of the human VEGF promoter conveyed a 1.8 times greater risk of having sporadic ALS (57). Because these experiments suggested a relationship between lower VEGF levels and impaired motor neuron survival, VEGF has been tested as disease modifying agent in mutant SOD1 transgenic mice (58,59). Intramuscular injection of a lentiviral vector-based VEGF delivery system prior to onset of motor deficits resulted in a significant prolongation of survival (146 vs. 127 days). If the injections were given in young mice (21 days), survival improved by an additional 17 days. Another group reported improved survival in G93A SOD1 mice receiving intraperitoneal injections of VEGF beginning at 74 days of age. In both paradigms, administration of VEGF also served to delay onset and retard the decline in motor function.

Although precise mechanisms underlying the relationship between VEGF levels and ALS remain unclear, there is evidence to suggest such effects may involve neuronal and non-neuronal cell interactions. VEGF can be synthesized by multiple cell types within the CNS, including neurons and astrocytes implying both multiple paracrine and autocrine signaling possibilities (56,60–63). High-affinity receptors for VEGF (VEGFR-1, VEGFR-2, and VEGFR-3) are expressed on neurons, endothelial cells, astrocytes, and microglia indicating potential responsiveness of multiple cell types to VEGF (56,63–66). VEGF is a potent angiogeneisis factor and may promote neuronal survival indirectly via this mechanism, but VEGF also has direct effects on neurons, astrocytes, and microglia. VEGF can promote neurite outgrowth and improve survival in primary motor neuron cultures via either direct actions on neurons or via effects on astrocytes (56,67). VEGF also has direct effects on microglia including enhanced chemotaxis and proliferation primarily mediated via the VGEFR-2 receptor (65). Although VEGF is constitutively expressed, its expression can be significantly altered by a host of factors including reactive nitrogen species, reactive oxygen species, and numerous cytokines, including those elevated in ALS spinal cord (55,68).

At a systems level, there are interesting questions about the nature of growth factor responsiveness in ALS raised by the VEGF experience. The VEGF promoter HIF element knockout mice suggest that diminished VEGF levels contribute to motor dysfunction while increased VEGF levels improve motor phenotypes. But are VEGF levels altered in ALS? In the original paper, Lambrechts et al. found low plasma VEGF levels in SALS patients, even those without the promoter polymorphism (57). However, this result was not seen in a smaller Swedish study that found elevated VEGF levels in ALS patients compared with controls (69). This group also found no difference in spinal cord VEGF levels obtained postmortem from ALS patients and controls. Similarly within G93A SOD1 mice, there is no difference in VEGF levels compared with controls when measured in plasma, CSF fluid, or spinal cord homogenates from 60-, 80-, 120-, and 140-day-old mice (67). Moreover, reducing VEGF levels in G93A SOD1 mice by crossing them with the HIF-1 element knockout mice has only minimal impact on survival. These results would indicate that reductions in VEGF levels within spinal cord are not a significant event in either mutant SOD1 mice or in human ALS patients, and suggest that some error in intrinsic VEGF production by cell populations within the CNS, such as neurons or astrocytes, is not a major factor in the disease. However, this data does not exclude the possibility of decreased responsiveness to VEGF in ALS by other mechanisms such as alterations in VEGF receptor expression.

Although VEGF has survival promoting effects directly on neurons/glia in vitro, it is possible that VEGF may exert some of its benefits in ALS via more peripheral actions. The success of the viral lentiviral vector injections in mutant SOD1 mice does not prove that the effects are mediated within the CNS. By definition, this experiment involved intramuscular injections, which would allow for local and even some systemic spread of virus and therefore potential effects on peripheral tissues. This is certainly possible given that direct administration of VEGF by intraperitoneal injection has somewhat comparable survival promoting effect in G93A SOD1 mice (59). Whether VEGF prolongs survival or motor function in mutant G93A SOD1 mice partially via its influence on peripheral targets such as muscle is unclear.

There are several growth factors besides VEGF which have also been shown to improve motor function and survival in G93A SOD1 mice after peripheral administration using viral vectors. Both glial cell line derived neurotrophic factor (GDNF) and insulin-like growth factor-1 (IGF-1) have been administered with adeno-associated virus bearing vectors injected into muscle and modestly improve survival of mutant SOD1 transgenic mice (70,71). Like VEGF, these factors can exert autocrine and paracrine functions on multiple cell types and the precise mechanisms of action are unknown. Hepatocyte growth factor (HGF) is another growth factor with previously shown neurotrophic properties that can ameliorate the phenotype of mutant G93A SOD1 mice. Crossing G93A SOD1 mice with a transgenic line expressing HGF under the control of the NSE promoter results in 27 days improvement in survival (175 vs. 148 days) (72). HGF can be expressed and secreted from several differing cell types within the CNS including neurons, astrocytes microglia, and oligodendrocytes allowing for many potential interactions between differing cell types (73–76). The high-affinity receptor for HGF, c-met, is also expressed by virtually all cell types within the CNS including neurons, astrocytes, microglia, and oligodendrocytes implicating both autocrine and paracrine signaling pathways in HGF actions (72,76–78).

Although several neuronal growth factors have been shown to improve motor function and survival in mutant SOD1 transgenic mice, it has been difficult to understand the mechanisms underlying those benefits. This issue is particularly complex considering neuronal–non-neuronal cell interactions with growth factors. Growth factor expression can be modulated by expression of cytokines or other growth factors. For example, VEGF expression can be stimulated by interleukin-1, IL-3, IL-6, IL-12, interferon-γ, TGF β, and TNF-α, while VEGF expression can be down regulated by the actions of IL-4 or IL-10 (55,79–82). Because IGF-1 and HGF administration can induce VEGF synthesis in certain tissues, the beneficial effects of these growth factors in ALS might in part be mediated via the actions of VEGF (83–86). These complex interactions make it even more difficult to define precise relationships between neuronal and nonneuronal cells in disease.

NON-PROTEIN MEDIATED CELL–CELL INTERACTIONS IN ALS

Important disease-related interactions between neurons and nonneuronal cells might also occur via non-protein associated signaling mechanisms. Glutamate mediated excitoxicity has been implicated as a potential contributor to motor neuron dysfunction in both sporadic and familial ALS, and such a hypothesis includes a prominent role for astrocytes. Studies from the early 1990s found elevated levels of glutamate, the primary CNS excitatory neurotransmitter, in the spinal fluid of ALS patients coupled with abnormalities in synaptosome glutamate transport function (87,88).

Rothstein et al. (89) addressed the possible biologic consequences of these biochemical changes by using an in vitro spinal cord slice model, and showing that chronic pharmacologic blockade of glutamate transport results in selective motor neuron degeneration. Subsequent work in the mid-1990s established the likely molecular basis for abnormal glutamate transport function in ALS patients by documenting a selective reduction in protein expression for the principal glutamate transport protein, EAAT2 (90). Furthermore, abnormal splicing of EAAT2 transcripts that caused reductions in functional EAAT2 protein levels appeared specific to ALS to patients (91). Because EAAT2 is primarily expressed in astrocytes, the glutamate hypothesis placed astrocytic cell dysfunction as the primary candidate responsible for elevating extracellular glutamate levels, increasing glutamate receptor activation, and ultimately causing motor neuron degeneration (92).

Findings of abnormal glutamate homeostasis were not limited to sporadic ALS patients but also were found in mutant SOD1-induced FALS suggesting some commonality in pathogenesis. Elevated CSF glutamate levels, diminished glutamate transport function, and reduced murine EAAT2 protein levels were all reported in mutant SOD1 transgenic mice, mirroring results from sporadic ALS patients (21,93,94). Moreover, expression of mutant SOD1 in culture seemed to promote inactivation of murine EAAT2 resulting in diminished glutamate transport function (95). These studies compellingly suggest a shared pathologic process between sporadic and familial ALS centered on abnormal astrocytic uptake of glutamate leading to eventual motor neuron degeneration.

Although the glutamate hypothesis in ALS is certainly an attractive theory that clearly emphasizes astrocytic–neuronal interaction, experiments designed to test its validity in vivo have yielded little evidence to support the hypothesis predictions. GLT-1 knockout mice do have elevated glutamate levels and diminished glutamate transport function as would be predicted (96). However, these mice develop epilepsy and not motor neuron disease, indicating that loss of this protein function is not by itself sufficient to cause motor neuron disease. In addition, over-expression of the EAAT2 transporter, while clearly improving astrocytic glutamate uptake, had no impact on the survival of G93A SOD1 mice and only minimal effect on disease onset and pathology (97). This result would be unexpected if reductions in astrocytic glutamate transport proteins really were a central part of disease pathogenesis. Furthermore, additional studies did not confirm the specificity of aberrant EAAT2 mRNA transcripts in ALS patients, but rather found such mRNA species also occur in normal and other neurologic disease control subjects (98,99). Taken together, these experiments indicate that abnormalities in glutamate homeostasis and changes in glutamate transport function are not primary causes of motor neuron dysfunction in ALS. Glutamate excess can harm motor neurons in certain experimental paradigms, so it may be reasonable to still consider that glutamate mediated toxicity as one of many pathways that in total contribute to declines in motor function (100).

Nitric oxide (NO) represents another non-proteinacious diffusible factor hypothesized to mediate neuronal–non-neuronal interactions in ALS. NO is produced by any of the three distinct nitric oxide synthases (NOS), endothelial (eNOS), neuronal (nNOS), or inducible (iNOS), which catalyze the reaction of molecular oxygen with arginine to form NO and citrulline (101). NO can freely diffuse between cells and through cell membranes, directly contributing to the formation of potentially toxic reactive nitrogen species. NO can also combine with superoxide anions to form highly reactive intermediates such as peroxynitrite, that may produce lipid peroxidation or protein nitration (102–104). The presence of such species has been reported in spinal cords of both human ALS (sporadic and familial) and SOD1 transgenic mice suggesting possible contributions to disease pathophysiology (105–108). NO can be synthesized by microglia, astrocytes, and neurons within the CNS via the actions of the differing NOS enzymes, but does not appear to made by oligodendrocytes (109–111). Expression patterns of NOS can be modulated by inflammatory molecules, such as TNF-α and interferon-γ, by growth factors including VEGF and IGF-1 or by free radicals (112–115). Such triggers may be responsible for the increased expression of neuronal NOS within motor neurons and inducible NOS within astrocytes and microglia, which characterizes ALS spinal cord (116–118).

The potential in vivo role of NO in ALS has been examined by several groups. Upton-Rice et al. (119) administered highly selective inhibitors of nNOS to mutant SOD1 transgenic mice. These compounds reduced nNOS activity in the brain and plasma by 95%, but did not affect survival or motor function testing in G93A SOD1 mice. Similarly, Dawson et al. (120) found that treating G93A SOD1 with either a non-selective NOS or an nNOS specific inhibitor did not significantly alter survival or disease course in G93A SOD1 mice. This group also crossed nNOS knockout mice with G93A SOD1 mice to insure ablation of nNOS enzymatic activity. G93A SOD1 lacking nNOS showed no significant difference in survival or motor function loss compared with G93A SOD1 mice expressing normal nNOS levels. The role of inducible NOS in ALS was examined by crossing iNOS knockout mice with G93A SOD1 mice (121). G93A SOD1 transgenic mice lacking iNOS demonstrated no change in survival or motor function decline compared with G93A SOD1 mice with normal iNOS expression levels. These experiments, using both pharmacological and genetic manipulation of NOS, strongly suggest that NO does not play a significant role in ALS pathogenesis either via cell signaling or via direct toxicity.

CONCLUSION

There is compelling evidence that nonneuronal cells play an important role in ALS. Nonneuronal cells, including asytrocytes, oligodendrocytes, and microglia, undergo significant pathologic change during the disease process and produce multiple factors capable of altering both their own and neuronal function. Despite many experiments, it is still not entirely clear which of these cell types influence disease or which precise mechanisms are involved. To determine specific roles of distinct nonneuronal populations will require complex experiments using cell type restricted expression or knockouts. However, even such difficult experiments may not provide satisfactory answers. It is possible that a functional motor system requires neuronal fitness in the context of a beneficial environment provided by nonneuronal neighbors. Abnormal responses in nonneuronal cells resulting from either primary or secondary disease related insults might serve to further undermine already precarious neuronal function. Because nonneuronal cells may provide beneficial as well as harmful factors, their interactions with neurons in total are likely a balance between these opposing drives. Understanding these relationships in the setting of disease is complex, but might allow for better insights into treatment strategies.

REFERENCES

1. Kamo H, Haebara H, Akiguchi I, Kameyama M, Kimura H, McGeer PL. A distinctive distribution of reactive astroglia in the precentral cortex in amyotrophic lateral sclerosis. Acta Neuropathol (Berl) 1987; 74(1):33–38.
2. Murayama S, Inoue K, Kawakami H, Bouldin TW, Suzuki K. A unique pattern of astrocytosis in the primary motor area in amyotrophic lateral sclerosis. Acta Neuropathol (Berl) 1991; 82(6):456–461.
3. Nagy D, Kato T, Kushner PD. Reactive astrocytes are widespread in the cortical gray matter of amyotrophic lateral sclerosis. J Neurosci Res 1994; 38(3):336–347.
4. Kushner PD, Stephenson DT, Wright S. Reactive astrogliosis is widespread in the subcortical white matter of amyotrophic lateral sclerosis brain. J Neuropathol Exp Neurol 1991; 50(3):263–277.
5. Feigin I. Astrocytic changes in white matter of ALS brain. J Neuropathol Exp Neurol 1991; 50(5):678–679.
6. O'Reilly SA, Roedica J, Nagy D, et al. Motor neuron-astrocyte interactions and levels of Cu, Zn superoxide dismutase in sporadic amyotrophic lateral sclerosis. Exp Neurol 1995; 131(2):203–210.

7. Schiffer D, Cordera S, Cavalla P, Migheli A. Reactive astrogliosis of the spinal cord in amyotrophic lateral sclerosis. J Neurol Sci 1996; 139(suppl)27–33.

8. Kato S, Shimoda M, Watanabe Y, Nakashima K, Takahashi K, Ohama E. Familial amyotrophic lateral sclerosis with a two base pair deletion in superoxide dismutase 1: gene multisystem degeneration with intracytoplasmic hyaline inclusions in astrocytes. J Neuropathol Exp Neurol 1996; 55(10):1089–1101.

9. Shibata N, Hirano A, Kobayashi M, et al. Intense superoxide dismutase-1 immunoreactivity in intracytoplasmic hyaline inclusions of familial amyotrophic lateral sclerosis with posterior column involvement. J Neuropathol Exp Neurol 1996; 55(4):481–490.

10. Kato S, Hayashi H, Nakashima K, et al. Pathological characterization of astrocytic hyaline inclusions in familial amyotrophic lateral sclerosis. Am J Pathol 1997; 151(2):611–620.

11. Watanabe M, Dykes-Hoberg M, Culotta VC, Price DL, Wong PC, Rothstein JD. Histological evidence of protein aggregation in mutant SOD1 transgenic mice and in amyotrophic lateral sclerosis neural tissues. Neurobiol Dis 2001; 8(6):933–941.

12. Kato S, Horiuchi S, Nakashima K, et al. Astrocytic hyaline inclusions contain advanced glycation endproducts in familial amyotrophic lateral sclerosis with superoxide dismutase 1 gene mutation: immunohistochemical and immunoelectron microscopical analyses. Acta Neuropathol (Berl) 1999; 97(3):260–266.

13. Kato S, Takikawa M, Nakashima K, et al. New consensus research on neuropathological aspects of familial amyotrophic lateral sclerosis with superoxide dismutase 1 (SOD1) gene mutations: inclusions containing SOD1 in neurons and astrocytes. Amyotroph Lateral Scler Other Motor Neuron Disord 2000; 1(3):163–184.

14. McGeer PL, McGeer EG. Inflammatory processes in amyotrophic lateral sclerosis. Muscle Nerve 2002; 26(4):459–470.

15. Lampson LA, Kushner PD, Sobel RA. Major histocompatibility complex antigen expression in the affected tissues in amyotrophic lateral sclerosis. Ann Neurol 1990; 28(3): 365–372.

16. Troost D, Claessen N, van den Oord JJ, Swaab DF, de Jong JM. Neuronophagia in the motor cortex in amyotrophic lateral sclerosis. Neuropathol Appl Neurobiol 1993; 19(5): 390–397.

17. Troost D, van den Oord JJ, de Jong JM, Swaab DF. Lymphocytic infiltration in the spinal cord of patients with amyotrophic lateral sclerosis. Clin Neuropathol 1989; 8(6): 289–294.

18. Troost D, Van den Oord JJ, Vianney de Jong JM. Immunohistochemical characterization of the inflammatory infiltrate in amyotrophic lateral sclerosis. Neuropathol Appl Neurobiol 1990; 16(5):401–410.

19. Engelhardt JI, Tajti J, Appel SH. Lymphocytic infiltrates in the spinal cord in amyotrophic lateral sclerosis. Arch Neurol 1993; 50(1):30–36.

20. Gurney ME, Pu H, Chiu AY, et al. Motor neuron degeneration in mice that express a human Cu,Zn superoxide dismutase mutation. Science 1994; 264(5166):1772–1775.

21. Bruijn LI, Becher MW, Lee MK, et al. ALS-linked SOD1 mutant G85R mediates damage to astrocytes and promotes rapidly progressive disease with SOD1-containing inclusions. Neuron 1997; 18(2):327–338.

22. Hall ED, Oostveen JA, Gurney ME. Relationship of microglial and astrocytic activation to disease onset and progression in a transgenic model of familial ALS. Glia 1998; 23(3):249–256.

23. Gong YH, Elliott JL. Metallothionein expression is altered in a transgenic murine model of familial amyotrophic lateral sclerosis. Exp Neurol 2000; 162(1):27–36.

24. Stieber A, Gonatas JO, Gonatas NK. Aggregates of mutant protein appear progressively in dendrites, in periaxonal processes of oligodendrocytes, and in neuronal and astrocytic perikarya of mice expressing the SOD1 (G93A) mutation of familial amyotrophic lateral sclerosis. J Neurol Sci 2000; 177(2):114–123.

25. Alexianu ME, Kozovska M, Appel SH. Immune reactivity in a mouse model of familial ALS correlates with disease progression. Neurology 2001; 57(7):1282–1289.
26. Wong PC, Pardo CA, Borchelt DR, et al. An adverse property of a familial ALS-linked SOD1 mutation causes motor neuron disease characterized by vacuolar degeneration of mitochondria. Neuron 1995; 14(6):1105–1116.
27. Ripps ME, Huntley GW, Hof PR, Morrison JH, Gordon JW. Transgenic mice expressing an altered murine superoxide dismutase gene provide an animal model of amyotrophic lateral sclerosis. Proc Natl Acad Sci USA 1995; 92(3):689–693.
28. Gong YH, Parsadanian AS, Andreeva A, Snider WD, Elliott JL. Restricted expression of G86R Cu/Zn superoxide dismutase in astrocytes results in astrocytosis but does not cause motoneuron degeneration. J Neurosci 2000; 20(2):660–665.
29. Brenner M, Johnson AB, Boespflug-Tanguy O, Rodriguez D, Goldman JE, Messing A. Mutations in GFAP, encoding glial fibrillary acidic protein, are associated with Alexander disease. Nat Genet 2001; 27(1):117–120.
30. Namekawa M, Takiyama Y, Aoki Y, et al. Identification of GFAP gene mutation in hereditary adult-onset Alexander's disease. Ann Neurol 2002; 52(6):779–785.
31. Pramatarova A, Laganiere J, Roussel J, Brisebois K, Rouleau GA. Neuron-specific expression of mutant superoxide dismutase 1 in transgenic mice does not lead to motor impairment. J Neurosci 2001; 21(10):3369–3374.
32. Lino MM, Schneider C, Caroni P. Accumulation of SOD1 mutants in postnatal motoneurons does not cause motoneuron pathology or motoneuron disease. J Neurosci 2002; 22(12):4825–4832.
33. Liu J, Lillo C, Jonsson PA, et al. Toxicity of familial ALS-linked SOD1 mutants from selective recruitment to spinal mitochondria. Neuron 2004; 43(1):5–17.
34. Nagano S, Satoh M, Sumi H, et al. Reduction of metallothioneins promotes the disease expression of familial amyotrophic lateral sclerosis mice in a dose-dependent manner. Eur J Neurosci 2001; 13(7):1363–1370.
35. Puttaparthi K, Gitomer WL, Krishnan U, Son M, Rajendran B, Elliott JL. Disease progression in a transgenic model of familial amyotrophic lateral sclerosis is dependent on both neuronal and nonneuronal zinc binding proteins. J Neurosci 2002; 22(20):8790–8796.
36. Clement AM, Nguyen MD, Roberts EA, et al. Wild-type nonneuronal cells extend survival of SOD1 mutant motor neurons in ALS mice. Science 2003; 302(5642):113–117.
37. Elliott JL. Cytokine upregulation in a murine model of familial amyotrophic lateral sclerosis. Brain Res Mol Brain Res 2001; 95(1–2):172–178.
38. Nguyen MD, Julien JP, Rivest S. Induction of proinflammatory molecules in mice with amyotrophic lateral sclerosis: no requirement for proapoptotic interleukin-1beta in neurodegeneration. Ann Neurol 2001; 50(5):630–639.
39. Yoshihara T, Ishigaki S, Yamamoto M, et al. Differential expression of inflammation- and apoptosis-related genes in spinal cords of a mutant SOD1 transgenic mouse model of familial amyotrophic lateral sclerosis. J Neurochem 2002; 80(1):158–167.
40. Hensley K, Floyd RA, Gordon B, et al. Temporal patterns of cytokine and apoptosis-related gene expression in spinal cords of the G93A-SOD1 mouse model of amyotrophic lateral sclerosis. J Neurochem 2002; 82(2):365–374.
41. Hensley K, Fedynyshyn J, Ferrell S, et al. Message and protein-level elevation of tumor necrosis factor alpha (TNF alpha) and TNF alpha-modulating cytokines in spinal cords of the G93A-SOD1 mouse model for amyotrophic lateral sclerosis. Neurobiol Dis 2003; 14(1):74–80.
42. Katsuse O, Iseki E, Kosaka K. Immunohistochemical study of the expression of cytokines and nitric oxide synthases in brains of patients with dementia with Lewy bodies. Neuropathology 2003; 23(1):9–15.
43. Ohtori S, Takahashi K, Moriya H, Myers RR. TNF-alpha and TNF-alpha receptor type 1 upregulation in glia and neurons after peripheral nerve injury: studies in murine DRG and spinal cord. Spine 2004; 29(10):1082–1088.

44. Fernandes A, Silva RF, Falcao AS, Brito MA, Brites D. Cytokine production, glutamate release and cell death in rat cultured astrocytes treated with unconjugated bilirubin and LPS. J Neuroimmunol 2004; 153(1–2):64–75.

45. Jana M, Dasgupta S, Saha RN, Liu X, Pahan K. Induction of tumor necrosis factor-alpha (TNF-alpha) by interleukin-12 p40 monomer and homodimer in microglia and macrophages. J Neurochem 2003; 86(2):519–528.

46. Arnett HA, Mason J, Marino M, Suzuki K, Matsushima GK, Ting JP. TNF alpha promotes proliferation of oligodendrocyte progenitors and remyelination. Nat Neurosci 2001; 4(11):1116–1122.

47. Yan P, Liu N, Kim GM, et al. Expression of the type 1 and type 2 receptors for tumor necrosis factor after traumatic spinal cord injury in adult rats. Exp Neurol 2003; 183(2):286–297.

48. Dopp JM, Mackenzie-Graham A, Otero GC, Merrill JE. Differential expression, cytokine modulation, and specific functions of type-1 and type-2 tumor necrosis factor receptors in rat glia. J Neuroimmunol 1997; 75(1–2):104–112.

49. Nguyen MD, D'Aigle T, Gowing G, Julien JP, Rivest S. Exacerbation of motor neuron disease by chronic stimulation of innate immunity in a mouse model of amyotrophic lateral sclerosis. J Neurosci 2004; 24(6):1340–1349.

50. Weydt P, Yuen EC, Ransom BR, Moller T. Increased cytotoxic potential of microglia from ALS-transgenic mice. Glia 2004; 48(2):179.

51. Zhao Z, Alam S, Oppenheim RW, Prevette DM, Evenson A, Parsadanian A. Overexpression of glial cell line-derived neurotrophic factor in the CNS rescues motoneurons from programmed cell death and promotes their long-term survival following axotomy. Exp Neurol 2004; 190(2):356–372.

52. Borasio GD, Robberecht W, Leigh PN, et al. A placebo-controlled trial of insulin-like growth factor-I in amyotrophic lateral sclerosis. European ALS/IGF-I Study Group. Neurology 1998; 51(2):583–586.

53. A controlled trial of recombinant methionyl human BDNF in ALS: the BDNF Study Group (Phase III). Neurology 1999; 52(7):1427–1433.

54. Miller RG, Petajan JH, Bryan WW, et al. A placebo-controlled trial of recombinant human ciliary neurotrophic (rhCNTF) factor in amyotrophic lateral sclerosis. rhCNTF ALS Study Group. Ann Neurol 1996; 39(2):256–260.

55. Xie K, Wei D, Shi Q, Huang S. Constitutive and inducible expression and regulation of vascular endothelial growth factor. Cytokine Growth Factor Rev 2004; 15(5):297–324.

56. Oosthuyse B, Moons L, Storkebaum E, et al. Deletion of the hypoxia-response element in the vascular endothelial growth factor promoter causes motor neuron degeneration. Nat Genet 2001; 28(2):131–138.

57. Lambrechts D, Storkebaum E, Morimoto M, et al. VEGF is a modifier of amyotrophic lateral sclerosis in mice and humans and protects motoneurons against ischemic death. Nat Genet 2003; 34(4):383–394.

58. Azzouz M, Ralph GS, Storkebaum E, et al. VEGF delivery with retrogradely transported lentivector prolongs survival in a mouse ALS model. Nature 2004; 429(6990):413–417.

59. Zheng C, Nennesmo I, Fadeel B, Henter JI. Vascular endothelial growth factor prolongs survival in a transgenic mouse model of ALS. Ann Neurol 2004; 56(4):564–567.

60. Chow J, Ogunshola O, Fan SY, Li Y, Ment LR, Madri JA. Astrocyte-derived VEGF mediates survival and tube stabilization of hypoxic brain microvascular endothelial cells in vitro. Brain Res Dev Brain Res 2001; 130(1):123–132.

61. Salhia B, Angelov L, Roncari L, Wu X, Shannon P, Guha A. Expression of vascular endothelial growth factor by reactive astrocytes and associated neoangiogenesis. Brain Res 2000; 883(1):87–97.

62. Hossain MA, Bouton CM, Pevsner J, Laterra J. Induction of vascular endothelial growth factor in human astrocytes by lead. Involvement of a protein kinase C/activator

protein-1 complex-dependent and hypoxia-inducible factor 1-independent signaling pathway. J Biol Chem 2000; 275(36):27874–27882.

63. Islamov RR, Chintalgattu V, Pak ES, Katwa LC, Murashov AK. Induction of VEGF and its Flt-1 receptor after sciatic nerve crush injury. Neuroreport 2004; 15(13): 2117–2121.

64. Krum JM, Rosenstein JM. VEGF mRNA and its receptor flt-1 are expressed in reactive astrocytes following neural grafting and tumor cell implantation in the adult CNS. Exp Neurol 1998; 154(1):57–65.

65. Forstreuter F, Lucius R, Mentlein R. Vascular endothelial growth factor induces chemotaxis and proliferation of microglial cells. J Neuroimmunol 2002; 132(1–2):93–98.

66. Spliet WG, Aronica E, Ramkema M, et al. Immunohistochemical localization of vascular endothelial growth factor receptors-1, -2 and -3 in human spinal cord: altered expression in amyotrophic lateral sclerosis. Neuropathol Appl Neurobiol 2004; 30(4):351–359.

67. Van Den Bosch L, Storkebaum E, Vleminckx V, et al. Effects of vascular endothelial growth factor (VEGF) on motor neuron degeneration. Neurobiol Dis 2004; 17(1):21–28.

68. Rosenstein JM, Krum JM. New roles for VEGF in nervous tissue—beyond blood vessels. Exp Neurol 2004; 187(2):246–253.

69. Nygren I, Larsson A, Johansson A, Askmark H. VEGF is increased in serum but not in spinal cord from patients with amyotrophic lateral sclerosis. Neuroreport 2002; 13(17):2199–2201.

70. Kaspar BK, Llado J, Sherkat N, Rothstein JD, Gage FH. Retrograde viral delivery of IGF-1 prolongs survival in a mouse ALS model. Science 2003; 301(5634):839–842.

71. Wang LJ, Lu YY, Muramatsu S, et al. Neuroprotective effects of glial cell line-derived neurotrophic factor mediated by an adeno-associated virus vector in a transgenic animal model of amyotrophic lateral sclerosis. J Neurosci 2002; 22(16):6920–6928.

72. Sun W, Funakoshi H, Nakamura T. Overexpression of HGF retards disease progression and prolongs life span in a transgenic mouse model of ALS. J Neurosci 2002; 22(15):6537–6548.

73. Nagayama T, Nagayama M, Kohara S, et al. Post-ischemic delayed expression of hepatocyte growth factor and c-Met in mouse brain following focal cerebral ischemia. Brain Res 2004; 999(2):155–166.

74. Kato S, Funakoshi H, Nakamura T, et al. Expression of hepatocyte growth factor and c-Met in the anterior horn cells of the spinal cord in the patients with amyotrophic lateral sclerosis (ALS): immunohistochemical studies on sporadic ALS and familial ALS with superoxide dismutase 1 gene mutation. Acta Neuropathol (Berl) 2003; 106(2): 112–120.

75. Zhang L, Himi T, Murota S. Induction of hepatocyte growth factor (HGF) in rat microglial cells by prostaglandin E(2). J Neurosci Res 2000; 62(3):389–395.

76. Yan H, Rivkees SA. Hepatocyte growth factor stimulates the proliferation and migration of oligodendrocyte precursor cells. J Neurosci Res 2002; 69(5):597–606.

77. Yang XM, Toma JG, Bamji SX, et al. Autocrine hepatocyte growth factor provides a local mechanism for promoting axonal growth. J Neurosci 1998; 18(20):8369–8381.

78. Yamada T, Tsubouchi H, Daikuhara Y, et al. Immunohistochemistry with antibodies to hepatocyte growth factor and its receptor protein (c-MET) in human brain tissues. Brain Res 1994; 637(1–2):308–312.

79. Brizzi MF, Formato L, Dentelli P, et al. Interleukin-3 stimulates migration and proliferation of vascular smooth muscle cells: a potential role in atherogenesis. Circulation 2001; 103(4):549–554.

80. Nagineni CN, Samuel W, Nagineni S, et al. Transforming growth factor-beta induces expression of vascular endothelial growth factor in human retinal pigment epithelial cells: involvement of mitogen-activated protein kinases. J Cell Physiol 2003; 197(3):453–462.

81. Nabors LB, Suswam E, Huang Y, Yang X, Johnson MJ, King PH. Tumor necrosis factor alpha induces angiogenic factor up-regulation in malignant glioma cells: a role for RNA stabilization and HuR. Cancer Res 2003; 63(14):4181–4187.

82. Silvestre JS, Mallat Z, Duriez M, et al. Antiangiogenic effect of interleukin-10 in ischemia-induced angiogenesis in mice hindlimb. Circ Res 2000; 87(6):448–452.

83. Zhang YW, Su Y, Volpert OV, Vande Woude GF. Hepatocyte growth factor/scatter factor mediates angiogenesis through positive VEGF and negative thrombospondin 1 regulation. Proc Natl Acad Sci USA 2003; 100(22):12718–12723.

84. Poulaki V, Mitsiades CS, McMullan C, et al. Regulation of vascular endothelial growth factor expression by insulin-like growth factor I in thyroid carcinomas. J Clin Endocrinol Metab 2003; 88(11):5392–5398.

85. Burroughs KD, Oh J, Barrett JC, DiAugustine RP. Phosphatidylinositol 3-kinase and mek 1/2 are necessary for insulin-like growth factor-I-induced vascular endothelial growth factor synthesis in prostate epithelial cells: a role for hypoxia-inducible factor-1? Mol Cancer Res 2003; 1(4):312–322.

86. Wojta J, Kaun C, Breuss JM, et al. Hepatocyte growth factor increases expression of vascular endothelial growth factor and plasminogen activator inhibitor-1 in human keratinocytes and the vascular endothelial growth factor receptor flk-1 in human endothelial cells. Lab Invest 1999; 79(4):427–438.

87. Rothstein JD, Tsai G, Kuncl RW, et al. Abnormal excitatory amino acid metabolism in amyotrophic lateral sclerosis. Ann Neurol 1990; 28(1):18–25.

88. Rothstein JD, Martin LJ, Kuncl RW. Decreased glutamate transport by the brain and spinal cord in amyotrophic lateral sclerosis. N Engl J Med 1992; 326(22):1464–1468.

89. Rothstein JD, Jin L, Dykes-Hoberg M, Kuncl RW. Chronic inhibition of glutamate uptake produces a model of slow neurotoxicity. Proc Natl Acad Sci USA 1993; 90(14):6591–6595.

90. Rothstein JD, Van KM, Levey AI, Martin LJ, Kuncl RW. Selective loss of glial glutamate transporter GLT-1 in amyotrophic lateral sclerosis. Ann Neurol 1995; 38(1):73–84.

91. Lin CL, Bristol LA, Jin L, et al. Aberrant RNA processing in a neurodegenerative disease: the cause for absent EAAT2, a glutamate transporter, in amyotrophic lateral sclerosis. Neuron 1998; 20(3):589–602.

92. Rothstein JD, Martin L, Levcy AI, et al. Localization of neuronal and glial glutamate transporters. Neuron 1994; 13(3):713–725.

93. Alexander GM, Deitch JS, Seeburger JL, Del VL, Heiman-Patterson TD. Elevated cortical extracellular fluid glutamate in transgenic mice expressing human mutant (G93A) Cu/Zn superoxide dismutase. J Neurochem 2000; 74(4):1666–1673.

94. Canton T, Pratt J, Stutzmann JM, Imperato A, Boireau A. Glutamate uptake is decreased tardively in the spinal cord of FALS mice. Neuroreport 1998; 9(5):775–778.

95. Trotti D, Rolfs A, Danbolt NC, Brown RH, Jr, Hediger MA. SOD1 mutants linked to amyotrophic lateral sclerosis selectively inactivate a glial glutamate transporter. Nat Neurosci 1999; 2(5):427–433.

96. Tanaka K, Watase K, Manabe T, et al. Epilepsy and exacerbation of brain injury in mice lacking the glutamate transporter GLT-1. Science 1997; 276(5319):1699–1702.

97. Guo H, Lai L, Butchbach ME, et al. Increased expression of the glial glutamate transporter EAAT2 modulates excitotoxicity and delays the onset but not the outcome of ALS in mice. Hum Mol Genet 2003; 12(19):2519–2532.

98. Honig LS, Chambliss DD, Bigio EH, Carroll SL, Elliott JL. Glutamate transporter EAAT2 splice variants occur not only in ALS, but also in AD and controls. Neurology 2000; 55(8):1082–1088.

99. Flowers JM, Powell JF, Leigh PN, Andersen P, Shaw CE. Intron 7 retention and exon 9 skipping EAAT2 mRNA variants are not associated with amyotrophic lateral sclerosis. Ann Neurol 2001; 49(5):643–649.

100. Hermann GE, Rogers RC, Bresnahan JC, Beattie MS. Tumor necrosis factor-alpha induces cFOS and strongly potentiates glutamate-mediated cell death in the rat spinal cord. Neurobiol Dis 2001; 8(4):590–599.
101. Liu B, Gao HM, Wang JY, Jeohn GH, Cooper CL, Hong JS. Role of nitric oxide in inflammation-mediated neurodegeneration. Ann NY Acad Sci 2002; 962:318–331.
102. Crow JP, Sampson JB, Zhuang Y, Thompson JA, Beckman JS. Decreased zinc affinity of amyotrophic lateral sclerosis-associated superoxide dismutase mutants leads to enhanced catalysis of tyrosine nitration by peroxynitrite. J Neurochem 1997; 69(5):1936–1944.
103. Crow JP, Ye YZ, Strong M, Kirk M, Barnes S, Beckman JS. Superoxide dismutase catalyzes nitration of tyrosines by peroxynitrite in the rod and head domains of neurofilament-L. J Neurochem 1997; 69(5):1945–1953.
104. Trotti D, Rossi D, Gjesdal O, et al. Peroxynitrite inhibits glutamate transporter subtypes. J Biol Chem 1996; 271(11):5976–5979.
105. Ferrante RJ, Browne SE, Shinobu LA, et al. Evidence of increased oxidative damage in both sporadic and familial amyotrophic lateral sclerosis. J Neurochem 1997; 69(5):2064–2074.
106. Abe K, Pan LH, Watanabe M, Konno H, Kato T, Itoyama Y. Upregulation of protein-tyrosine nitration in the anterior horn cells of amyotrophic lateral sclerosis. Neurol Res 1997; 19(2):124–128.
107. Sasaki S, Shibata N, Komori T, Iwata M. iNOS and nitrotyrosine immunoreactivity in amyotrophic lateral sclerosis. Neurosci Lett 2000; 291(1):44–48.
108. Beal MF, Ferrante RJ, Browne SE, Matthews RT, Kowall NW, Brown RH, Jr. Increased 3-nitrotyrosine in both sporadic and familial amyotrophic lateral sclerosis. Ann Neurol 1997; 42(4):644–654.
109. Hewett JA, Hewett SJ, Winkler S, Pfeiffer SE. Inducible nitric oxide synthase expression in cultures enriched for mature oligodendrocytes is due to microglia. J Neurosci Res 1999; 56(2):189–198.
110. Keilhoff G, Seidel B, Wolf G. Absence of nitric oxide synthase in rat oligodendrocytes: a light and electron microscopic study. Acta Histochem 1998; 100(4):409–417.
111. Zhao W, Xie W, Le W, et al. Activated microglia initiate motor neuron injury by a nitric oxide and glutamate-mediated mechanism. J Neuropathol Exp Neurol 2004; 63(9):964–977.
112. Cassina P, Peluffo H, Pehar M, et al. Peroxynitrite triggers a phenotypic transformation in spinal cord astrocytes that induces motor neuron apoptosis. J Neurosci Res 2002; 67(1):21–29.
113. Wang Y, Nagase S, Koyama A. Stimulatory effect of IGF-I and VEGF on eNOS message, protein expression, eNOS phosphorylation and nitric oxide production in rat glomeruli, and the involvement of PI3-K signaling pathway. Nitric Oxide 2004; 10(1):25–35.
114. Shin HH, Lee HW, Choi HS. Induction of nitric oxide synthase (NOS) by soluble glucocorticoid induced tumor necrosis factor receptor (sGITR) is modulated by IFN-gamma in murine macrophage. Exp Mol Med 2003; 35(3):175–180.
115. Wu W, Li L, Yiek LW, et al. GDNF and BDNF alter the expression of neuronal NOS, c-Jun, and p75 and prevent motoneuron death following spinal root avulsion in adult rats. J Neurotrauma 2003; 20(6):603–612.
116. Phul RK, Shaw PJ, Ince PG, Smith ME. Expression of nitric oxide synthase isoforms in spinal cord in amyotrophic lateral sclerosis. Amyotroph Lateral Scler Other Motor Neuron Disord 2000; 1(4):259–267.
117. Almer G, Vukosavic S, Romero N, Przedborski S. Inducible nitric oxide synthase up-regulation in a transgenic mouse model of familial amyotrophic lateral sclerosis. J Neurochem 1999; 72(6):2415–2425.
118. Kashiwado K, Yoshiyama Y, Arai K, Hattori T. Expression of nitric oxide synthases in the anterior horn cells of amyotrophic lateral sclerosis. Prog Neuropsychopharmacol Biol Psychiatry 2002; 26(1):163–167.

119. Upton-Rice MN, Cudkowicz ME, Mathew RK, Reif D, Brown RH, Jr. Administration of nitric oxide synthase inhibitors does not alter disease course of amyotrophic lateral sclerosis SOD1 mutant transgenic mice. Ann Neurol 1999; 45(3):413–414.
120. Facchinetti F, Sasaki M, Cutting FB, et al. Lack of involvement of neuronal nitric oxide synthase in the pathogenesis of a transgenic mouse model of familial amyotrophic lateral sclerosis. Neuroscience 1999; 90(4):1483–1492.
121. Son M, Fathallah-Shaykh HM, Elliott JL. Survival in a transgenic model of FALS is independent of iNOS expression. Ann Neurol 2001; 50(2):273.

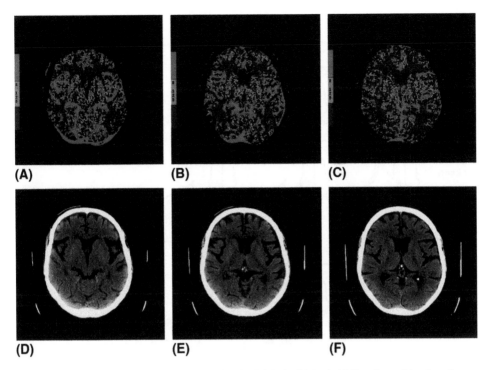

Figure 6-1 Cerebral blood flow studies of an individual with both ALS and cognitive impairment consistent with FTD. (*See p. 121.*)

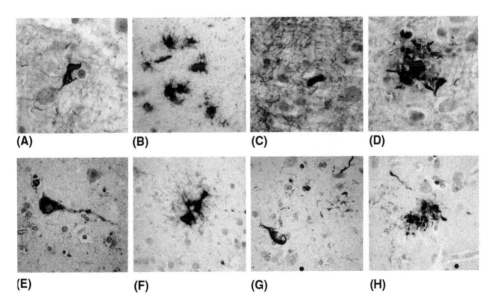

Figure 6-3 Tau protein aggregation characteristic of frontotemporal lobar degeneration in ALSci. (*See p. 128.*)

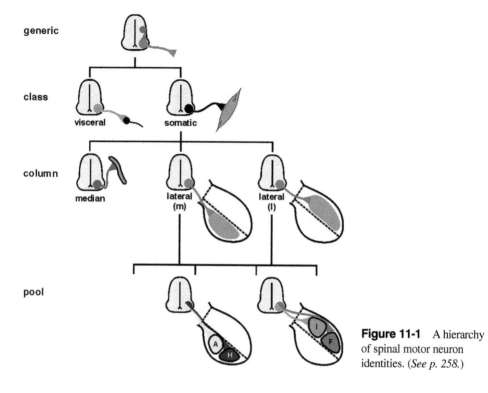

generic

class

visceral   somatic

column

median   lateral (m)   lateral (l)

pool

Figure 11-1 A hierarchy of spinal motor neuron identities. (*See p. 258.*)

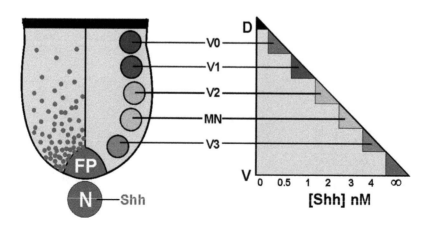

Figure 11-3 Graded Sonic hedgehog signaling and the positional specification of motor neuron identity. (*See p. 260.*)

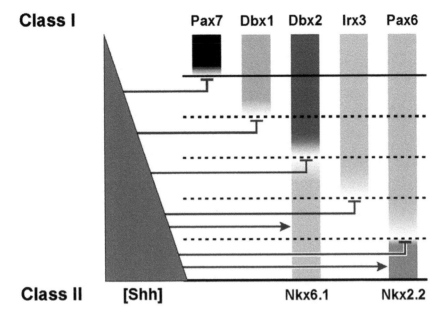

Figure 11-4 Graded Sonic hedgehog signaling patterns homeodomain protein expression. (*See p. 261.*)

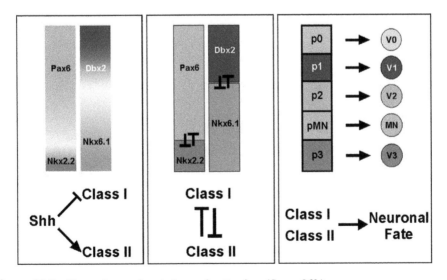

Figure 11-5 Three phases of ventral neural patterning. (*See p. 262.*)

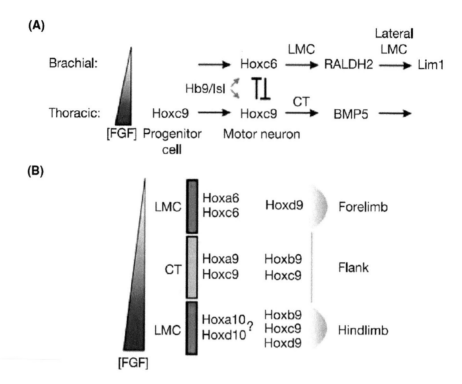

Figure 11-7 Hox protein activities control motor neuron columnar differentiation. (*See p. 264.*)

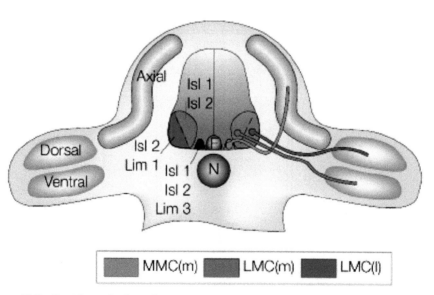

Figure 11-8 Spatial organizations of motor neuron columns in the developing spinal cord. (*See p. 265.*)

(A) Wild type

(B) *Lim1* ⁻/⁻

(C) *Lmx1b* ⁻/⁻

(D) Ectopic *Lhx3*

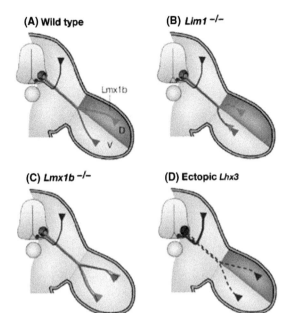

Figure 11-9 LIM homeodomain proteins control motor axon trajectory. (*See p. 266.*)

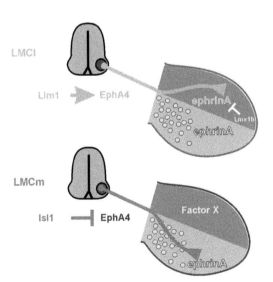

Figure 11-10 Ephrin-A signaling establishes the dorsoventral trajectory of motor axons in the developing limb. (*See p. 268.*)

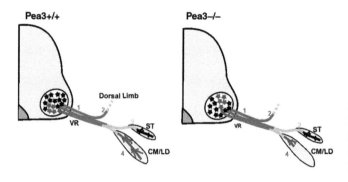

Figure 11-11 ETS protein Pea3 controls late aspects of the differentiation of specific motor neuron pools. (*See p. 269.*)

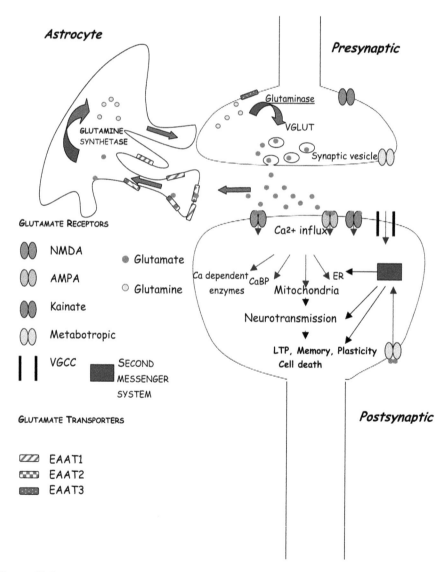

Figure 13-1 Normal glutamatergic neurotransmission. (*See p. 300.*)

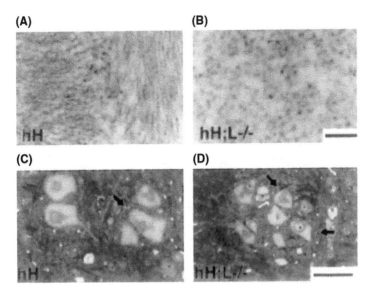

Figure 17-3 Perikaryl accumulation in the absence of NF-L. (*See p. 404.*)

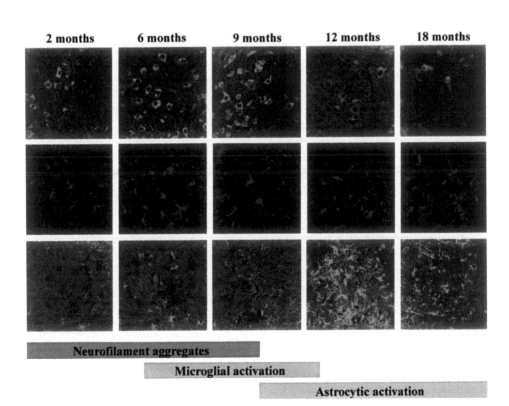

Figure 17-4 The temporal pattern of neurofilamentous aggregate formation in a transgenic NF-L knockout. (*See p. 406.*)

7

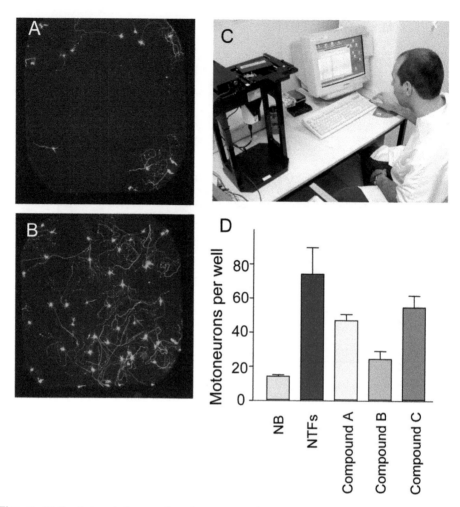

Figure 25-3 Automated screening for compounds that enhance motor neuron survival. (*See p. 567.*)

16

Apoptosis in Amyotrophic Lateral Sclerosis

Ian F. Dunn and Robert M. Friedlander
Department of Neurosurgery, Brigham and Women's Hospital, Harvard Medical School, Boston, Massachusetts, U.S.A.

INTRODUCTION

Amyotrophic lateral sclerosis (ALS) remains a fatal disorder characterized by progressive paralysis terminating in an inevitable loss of respiratory function and death within five years of diagnosis. The most common motor neuron disease in adults, ALS—known through history as Charcot's sclerosis and Lou Gehrig's disease—has as its signature neuropathologic effect the selective and progressive loss of motor neurons in the brain, brainstem, and spinal cord (1). The clinical hallmarks are muscle atrophy, weakness, and fasciculations—or lower motor neuron syndrome—along with attendant long tract signs of hyperactive tendon reflexes, clonus, and Hoffman's and Babinski's signs reflecting the clinical manifestations of the lateral sclerosis observed at autopsy. Disease specificity is highlighted by the complete absence of cognitive impairment in the disease despite the near-complete paralysis of extremities and muscles of speech and eventually of respiration.

The prevalence of ALS is 2 to 3/100,000 (2). The mean age of onset is in the fourth and fifth decades of life, but risk increases by an order of magnitude after 60 years of age. In rare cases, onset occurs in adolescence. Death ensues within one to five years after onset in the most common forms of the disease, with denervation of respiratory muscles and diaphragm usually the terminal event. The only available therapy is riluzole, shown to extend survival by only three months.

Pathologically, ALS is characterized by a loss of upper motor neurons in the cerebral cortex and of α-motor neurons and up to 30% of interneurons in the spinal cord. Microscopic hallmarks include a variety of neuronal inclusions; among these are small eosinophilic aggregates termed Bunina bodies, hyaline inclusions, and gliosis in the lateral columns (3). Nearly 90% to 95% of cases of ALS show no specific genetic linkage and are sporadic, 5% to 10% are inherited; nearly 20% of inherited forms carry a dominant mutation in the gene superoxide dismutase 1 (SOD1) encoding the cytoplasmic Cu/Zn SOD (1). More recently, mutations in the ALS2 gene encoding the guanine nucleotide exchange factor *Alsin* have been linked to juvenile type-3 ALS (4,5).

While investigators are beginning to shed light on the genetic underpinnings of familial forms of ALS, the molecular events set into motion by mutant gene products culminating in motor neuron death and the disease phenotype are poorly understood. Proposed hypotheses include oxidative damage from SOD1 mutation (6); pathologic accumulation of abnormal intracellular inclusions; and excitotoxic death from glutamate toxicity (2). More recently, mounting evidence from cellular morphologic analyses, postmortem studies, and molecular studies in mice and humans has suggested the critical involvement of programmed cell death pathways in the etiopathogenesis of ALS, which may be the final common pathway for current disease hypotheses. In this chapter, we review current understanding of the putative contributions of programmed cell death pathways to the molecular pathogenesis of ALS by drawing on animal and human data. We first review briefly the genetic basis of the disease and mouse models. Second, we review the general apoptotic cascade and take an in-depth look at its relevance in ALS. Lastly, we discuss current and future prospects in the pharmacologic targeting of the apoptotic cascade and their therapeutic applications to combat ALS.

THE GENETICS OF ALS

SOD1

The identification of mutations in SOD1 as the primary cause of 15% to 20% of cases of familial ALS comprising 1% to 2% of all cases was a landmark discovery in the current understanding of the molecular details of the disease (6). Linked to chromosome 21q22.2, its gene product, SOD, is a ubiquitous 153-amino-acid cytoplasmic free-radical scavenger (7,8). To date, over 100 mutations in the gene have been identified; all but one is dominant, and mutations have been found throughout the primary and three-dimensional structure of the protein and produce a nearly full-length polypeptide (9–11) and similar disease phenotypes.

Existing data suggest that mutations in SOD1 are gain-of-function mutations. Mice with deficient levels of SOD1 fail to develop motor neuron disease (12), while transgenic mice bearing the SOD1^{G93A} mutation develop an ALS-like disorder with varying levels of SOD1 activity (13–15). The pathologic effects of the gain-of-function mutant SOD are unclear. Some have hypothesized that an abnormal protein product could generate undue oxidative stress (16–18) through overly permissive catalytic activity while others contend that intracellular protein aggregates of mutant SOD1 could soak up important chaperone proteins and disrupt cellular transport as well as the policing machinery of the cell, the proteasome, thereby preventing normal protein unfolding, disrupting vital axonal transport, and perpetuating nefarious proteins which would otherwise be degraded (19,20). A role for SOD1 in the initiation of the apoptotic cascade is discussed later in this chapter.

SOD1-mutant-mediated ALS and its transgenic mouse model have served as models for the study of ALS despite subtle differences in disease characteristics and pathology when compared with the more common, sporadic form of the disease. There appears to be an increased sensitivity of sensory neurons in the dorsal columns and spinocerebellar tract in the familial form of the disease (21). Moreover, while corticospinal tract sclerosis and neurofilament aggregates are pathologic hallmarks of the human disease, these findings are conspicuously absent in the transgenic mouse (22,23). These differences notwithstanding, studies of familial ALS and its SOD1 transgenic murine model in the absence of appropriate models of sporadic ALS have been invaluable to date.

ALS2

A second gene called *ALS2* mapped to chromosome 2q33 has been convincingly linked to juvenile ALS type 3, a slowly progressive form of the disease characterized by recessive inheritance and age of onset in adolescence (4,5). The *ALS2* gene product is *Alsin*, a large protein recently identified as a Rab5/Rac1 guanine nucleotide exchange factor (GEF) (24). Rab5 and Rac1 are GTPases linked with functions linked to receptor-mediated endocytosis/pineocytosis and cytoskeletal organization, respectively (25). Alterations in the *ALS2* gene appear to confer loss-of-function mutations. The mechanisms by which deficient or dysfunctional Alsin leads to motor neuron disease—as in the SOD1-mediated form—are also poorly understood. Alsin has recently been localized to membrane ruffles and lamellipodia (24) which when taken together with its association with Rab5 and Rac1 suggests a role in membrane transport events, potentially linking endocytic processes, and cytoskeleton remodeling. Whether or not dysfunctional membrane transport plays a role in the pathogenesis of *ALS2*-mutant-mediated ALS is unknown, and there are currently no transgenic models of this particular form of ALS. A role for the *ALS2* gene product in the initiation of the apoptotic cascade is unknown.

GENERAL OVERVIEW OF APOPTOSIS

Apoptosis is to be distinguished from necrotic cell death. In necrosis, cell death ensues at the epicenter of injury as a direct result of an ischemic or traumatic insult and is characterized by mitochondrial and nuclear swelling, organelle dissolution, and condensation of chromatin around the nucleus. Nuclear and cytoplasmic membrane rupture follow, and DNA is thereafter randomly degraded (26,27). In contrast, apoptosis is characterized by a biochemical cascade that activates molecules mediating a program of cell suicide. Cells are fragmented into "apoptotic bodies" and chromosomal DNA is enzymatically cleaved to 180 bp internucleosomal fragments. Other features of apoptosis are a reduction in the membrane potential of the mitochondria, intracellular acidification, generation of free radicals, and externalization of phosphatidylserine residues (27–31).

While the morphologic sequelae of apoptosis are well recognized, its molecular mediators were largely unknown until 1993 when several genes controlling cell death were identified in studies of the nematode *Caenorhabditis elegans* (*C. elegans*). In *C. elegans*, four genes are required for the orderly implementation of the developmental apoptotic program. The ced-3, ced-4, and egl-1 genes mediate cell death; worms bereft of these genes harbor additional cells (32,33). The fourth gene, ced-9, functions as an inhibitor of apoptosis and, accordingly, ced-9 −/− worms are characterized by diffuse apoptotic cell death. Metazoan homologs of ced-3 (caspases), ced-4 (Apaf-1), ced-9 (Bcl-2), and egl-1 (BH3-only proteins) have been identified (32–37).

Caspases

The principal executioners in the vertebrate apoptotic program are cysteine dependent, aspartate-specific proteases called caspases, which are homolgous to the *C. elegans* gene product ced-3 and are highly conserved through evolution. The interleukin-1β-converting enzyme, known as caspase-1 or ICE, was the first vertebrate caspase identified by virtue of its homology with ced-3 (32,34). Fourteen caspases have been identified to date, eleven of which are present in humans (32).

Caspases exist as latent precursors or zymogens which when activated initiate the death program by destroying key components of the cellular infrastructure and activating factors that mediate cellular damage. Procaspases are composed of p10 and p20 subunits and an N-terminal recruitment domain; caspases in their active forms are heterotetramers of two p10 and two p20 subunits from two procaspase molecules. Caspases are further subdivided into either upstream initiators or downstream executioners. Upstream caspases are activated by the cell death signal from molecules such as tumor necrosis factor-α (TNF-α) and have a long N-terminal prodomain which regulates their activation (28,38). Upstream caspases in turn activate downstream caspases that directly mediate the events leading to cellular demise.

The specific activation of upstream initiator caspases is an important event in caspase-mediated cell death. Upstream caspases may be subclassified into two groups depending on the molecules that modulate their activation. Procaspases 1, 2, 4, 15, 9, 11, 12, and 13 have a long N-terminal prodomain called the caspase-recruiting domain (CARD), while caspases 8 and 10 have a long N-terminal prodomain called the death-effector domain (DED). A regulating molecule is then required for specific binding to the CARD/DED ddomain, which results in caspase activation. These molecules are caspase and trigger specific. For example, after the binding of TNF-α to its receptor, TNF-receptor binds the DED domain to mediate caspase-8 activation. Of this class of caspases with long prodomains, caspases 2, 8, 9, and 10 are initiators of apoptosis and caspases 1, 4, 5, 11, 12, and 13 are involved with cytokine activation. As a general rule, protein–protein interactions are instrumental in the activation of initiator caspases, while downstream executioner caspases are usually proteolytically cleaved by an upstream caspase. Caspase-1 also has an important role as an upstream initiator in addition to its role in inflammation (39,40), with a pivotal role in ischemic neuronal cell death only recently demonstrated (41). Caspase-1, the founding member of the caspase family, is responsible for cleavage of pro-IL-1β to the mature and active form of the cytokine (42). Evidence indicates that following caspase-1 activation, binding of mature IL-β to its type-1 receptor plays an important role mediating neuronal cell death (43,44).

Among the targets of upstream initiator caspases are their downstream executioner counterparts, caspases 3, 6, and 7. Cell death then occurs in one of two ways: destruction and activation. Key cellular substrates are destroyed systematically, and DNA degradation machinery is activated to herald the terminal phase of the death process. Downstream targets are many and include infrastructural proteins as well as DNA. One of the targets of caspase-3 is the nuclease responsible for cleaving DNA into 180-bp fragments. This DNA ladder nuclease (caspase-active DNase, or CAD) exists as an inactive complex with an inhibitory subunit (ICAD). Caspase-3 cleaves ICAD, thus releasing CAD to degrade DNA (45).

The manner by which the downstream executioner caspases are activated has clarified at least two caspase-dependent apoptotic pathways to date. The "death-receptor" pathway, as mentioned above, is triggered by members of the death-receptor superfamily such as TNFR or CD95 which when activated by their respective extracellular ligands lead to formation of a death-inducing protein assembly. Caspase-8 is summoned to the complex and may then activate the downstream effector caspase-3. Another way by which the apoptotic cascade is set into motion is by releasing mitochondrial apoptogenic proteins that activate downstream caspases, a process in which the Bcl-2 family members play important roles.

Bcl-2 Family Members and Their Regulation of Release of Mitochondrial Cytochrome c

Cytochrome c is a member of the mitochondrial electron-transport chain required for the generation of ATP. In addition to its role in bioenergetics, cytochrome c is an important trigger of the caspase cascade and a key member of the mitochondrial apoptotic cascade. Cytochrome c-mediated activation of cell death occurs if cytochrome c is released from the mitochondria into the cytoplasm. There, it binds to Apaf-1 to form the apoptosome—a molecular complex comprising cytochrome c, Apaf-1, ATP, and procaspase-9. The apoptosome then activates caspase 9, which is an upstream initiator of apoptosis. Cytochrome c release is now recognized as a key step in the initiation of apoptosis (28).

Members of the Bcl-2 family—so named for its founding member, isolated in B-cell lymphoma—are proapoptotic or antiapoptotic, and the balance between these activating and inhibitory signals form the Bcl-2 family has a critical role in the release of cytochrome c. Moreover, members of the caspase family can influence the balance of pro- and antiapoptotic signals from the Bcl-2 family. For instance, caspases 1 and 8 cleave Bid—a Bcl-2 family member—to a truncated pro-apoptotic form, which translocates to the mitochondria and induces the release of cytochrome c. The particular mechanism by which tBid leads to cytochrome c translocation to the cytosol is unclear, but may involve stabilization of other Bcl-2 family members such as Bax in the mitochondrial membrane to enhance membrane permeability (46,47). Bcl-2 family members implicated in apoptosis include cell-death suppressors Bcl-2 and Bcl-XL as well as pro-apoptotic members Bad, Bak, Bid, Bax, Bcl-xS, and Hrk (48).

Other Mitochondrial Pro-apoptotic Proteins

Other pro-apoptotic proteins released from the mitochondria in addition to cytochrome c are Smac/Diablo, HtrA2/Omi, AIF (apoptosis-inducing factor), and endonuclease G. Smac/Diablo and HtrA2/Omi may facilitate caspase activation by inactivating a class of proteins known as inhibitors of apoptosis proteins (IAPs) including the X chromosome-linked inhibitor of apoptosis (XIAP) (49–51). While these proteins are involved in caspase-dependent pathways, endonuclease-G and AIF are pro-apoptotic mitochondrial proteins that play roles in caspase-independent cell death. AIF, like cytochrome c, has dual functions—it participates in physiologic oxidative phosphorylation but upon cytosolic translocation participates in the activation of apoptosis by inducing large-scale DNA fragmentation and chromatin condensation (52). Endonuclease-G, like AIF, cleaves DNA upon cytosolic relocation. Neither AIF nor endonuclease-G is impaired by pharmacologic caspase inhibitors (53,54), suggesting that both proteins participate in a caspase-independent apoptotic cascade.

IAPs: Inhibitors of Apoptosis

The apoptosis pathway also includes its endogenous inhibitors. The IAPs are an additional group of antiapoptotic proteins in addition to select Bcl-2 family members. Human IAPs include the neuronal apoptosis inhibitory protein (NAIP), c-IAP1, c-IAP2, XIAP. Interestingly, genetic inactivation of the *NAIP* gene, the deletion of which is associated with spinal muscular atrophy, is associated with neuronal cell death (55,56). XIAP, c-IAP1, and c-IAP2 block cytochrome-c activation of caspase-9 as well as directly inhibiting activated caspase-3 (28).

THE ABCs OF ALS: APOPTOSIS, BCL-2, AND CASPASES

A putative role for apoptosis in the onset and progression of ALS was suggested by early in vitro and in vivo experiments aimed at delineating a pathogenic role of the mutant SOD1 gene product. Neurons or PC12 cells harboring mutant SOD1 cDNA died with features of apoptotic cell death, shaping the hypothesis that mutant SOD1 in some way deleteriously activates apoptosis in alpha motor neurons. In morphologic studies, Troost et al. (57) detected the presence of apoptotic bodies within macrophages in the motor cortex, brain stem, and spinal cord in post-mortem studies of ALS patients. Intense TUNEL staining has been detected in the motor cortex, brain stem, and spinal cord in patients with ALS (58), as has internucleosomal DNA cleavage (26), though other reports have been more equivocal. Other apoptotic markers including fractin, the Le^Y antigen and prostate apoptosis respone-4 are highly expressed in spinal cords of ALS cases and transgenic SOD1 mice as compared to controls (59–63).

Family Feud: Bcl-2 Members in ALS

The morphologic data suggesting a prominent role for apoptosis in ALS have been followed by a wealth of convincing molecular and genetic data, much of it drawn from studies in the SOD1 mouse. The Bcl-2 family—containing both pro- and anti-apoptotic members—has been studied in particular depth. Overexpression of Bcl-2 in transgenic SOD1 mice has been shown to not only lengthen survival in SOD1 mice, but also to attenuate the magnitude of spinal cord degeneration (64); in vitro work has similarly shown an increased survival of mutant SOD1-transfected PD12 cells overexpressing Bcl-2 (65). Correlative studies in both humans and SOD1 mice have shown that Bcl-2 mRNA is markedly decreased in ALS patients and SOD1 mice, but that Bax mRNA is present at high levels when compared with controls (66,67). The expression of their corresponding protein products follow these trends (63). Przedborski's group have also shown that the pro-apoptotic protein Bax is not only upregulated in the SOD1 mouse, but that it translocates from the cytosol to the mitochondria, and that cytochrome c conversely moves from mitochondria to cytosol (63). These events occur in the early symptomatic stage of disease progression. Messenger levels of Hrk, a prop-apoptotic Bcl-2 family member, are also elevated in the spinal cords of ALS patients (68).

The Bcl-2 family member Bid deserves particular mention. Bid, a pro-apoptotic protein, is thought to be activated early in the mitochondrial apoptotic cascade by truncation to tBid and subsequent translocation to the mitochondria, where it is thought to be instrumental in the release of cytochrome c and hence downstream activation of caspases 3 and 9. Bid mRNA is expressed in the spinal cord of transgenic SOD1 mice, with levels corresponding to the severity of disease (69). Interestingly, the full-length Bid translation product is expressed at similar levels in transgenic and non-transgenic SOD1 mice, but the truncated activated form (tBid) was observed unequivocally in disease mice and not in unaffected mice (69)—this study was, in fact, the first demonstration of Bid cleavage in neurodegenerative disease.

The same authors also detected continued translocation of Bax from cytosol to mitochondria throughout the disease and suggested that Bid cleavage may be a more critical event than Bax translocation in activating apoptosis in this particular model. What is emerging, then, is a cellular balance between pro- and antiapoptotic members of the Bcl-2 family in ALS that appears to be tipped in favor of apoptosis induction. Two central issues requiring elucidation include the mechanisms by which the mutant *SOD1* gene product leads to Bid truncation and translocation and how tBid and Bax function to facilitate the translocation of cytochrome c to the cytosol.

Caspases

Recent data from transgenic mice and from humans also suggest a prominent role for caspase family members in the pathogenesis of ALS. The first definitive evidence suggesting that caspases may be involved in the pathogenesis of ALS came from experiments in which the mutant SOD1 transgenic mouse was crossbred with a mouse expressing a dominant negative caspase 1 (ICE) that inhibited caspase 1 in neurons. Compared with mice expressing only the mutant *SOD1* transgene, mice expressing both the mutant *SOD1* transgene and mutant caspase-1 transgene had duration of survival that was greater by 9%; moreover, disease progression was slowed by more than 50% (70). Further studies showed caspases 1 and 3 activities are present in neurons of SOD1 mice (71). In this same study, intraventricular administration of the broad caspase inhibitor *N*-benzyloxycarbonyl-Val-Asp-fluoromethylketone (zVAD-fmk) was neuroprotective and extended survival in the ALS mice by 22%; this activity was dose dependent, as lower doses of inhibitor resulted in shorter survival benefit. Furthermore, motor neurons in the cervical cord were preserved. As the mice aged, there was progressive transcriptional up-regulation of caspase 1 messenger RNA (mRNA), followed by upregulation of capsase-3 mRNA. These sequential events are also detected at the level of enzymatic activity (59,70,72).

The discovery of caspases 1 and 3 activation in spinal cord samples from patients with ALS indicates the clinical relevance of these animal models of ALS (70,72).

More recent data support a prominent role of caspase 1 in the apoptotic pathway in ALS. Earlier data demonstrated that caspase-8-mediated Bid cleavage in the death-receptor pathway (73). However, caspase-8 activation has been shown to occur in the late symptomatic stage of ALS progression in the SOD1 mouse (69), while Bid cleavage occurs earlier. These data, together with the finding that caspase-1 inhibition attenuates Bid cleavage, suggest that caspase 1, and not caspase 8, is responsible for Bid truncation and hence activation of the mitochondrial apoptotic pathway. This is consistent with findings that caspase-1 activation occurs early in the disease process. A definitive role for caspase 1 in neuronal cell death and the mechanism by which caspase 1 may function as an apical caspase in the apoptotic cascade was recently demonstrated in a murine ischemia model. Under ischemic conditions, the CARD-containing molecule Rip2/Cardiac/Rick was activated, in turn activating caspase 1, which mediated Bid truncation. This resulted in release of the mitochondrial apoptogenic factors cytochrome-c, AIF, and Smac/Diablo, and in the subsequent activation of caspases 9 and 3. This study clarifies the role of caspase 1 as an apical caspase whose functions include Bid activation and hence initiation of the mitochondrial apoptosis pathway (41). A putative mechanism by which the mutant *SOD1* gene product activates caspase 1 early in the course of ALS has not been proposed.

The time course of caspase activation is also becoming clearer. In the presymptomatic stage, caspase 1 is activated but no neuronal cell death is detected. In the early symptomatic stage, neuronal cell death is detected; caspases 1 and 3 are detected and proapoptotic changes in Bcl-2 family expression are detected with early muscle atrophy and axonal loss (74).

Caspase 9 is activated in the spinal cords of ALS patients (75) in SOD1 mice (22) and is also active in the early presymptomatic stage. In the late symptomatic stage, progressive neuronal cell death is detected and severe muscle atrophy and axonal loss are observed.

A critical question remains in the field. How neurons survive for weeks or even months harboring such apoptotic signals. Two hypotheses have surfaced. First, it may be that the apoptotic signals do not reach such magnitude to trigger the full-blown apoptotic machinery. Second, given the gradual increase in apoptotic signals, neurons build up protective mechanisms resulting the prevention of cell death. These important questions are the subject of intense investigation.

Therapeutic Options: Minocycline, Creatine, and Celebrex

Further demonstration that apoptosis plays a role in the progression of ALS is provided by the survival benefit conferred by pharmacologic caspase inhibitors in SOD1 mice. The broad-spectrum caspase inhibitor zVAD-fmk has been shown to extend survival and delay disease progression in mutant SOD1 transgenic mice (76). Work from our laboratory has also shown the therapeutic potential of the antibiotic min-ocylcine. Minocycline, a second-generation tetracycline, crosses the blood–brain barrier and has remarkable neuroprotective properties in models of cerebral ischemia, traumatic brain injury, and Huntington's and Parkinson's disease (77–81). In SOD1 transgenic mice, minocycline delays disease onset and extends survival; in these studies, minocycline administration was shown to inhibit caspase-1 activity as well permeability-transition-mediated mitochondrial cytochrome-c release, both pivotal steps in the mitochondrial apoptotic cascade (76). Importantly, this finding has been independently confirmed by two additional laboratories (82,83). The therapeutic implications of a non-toxic inhibitor of apoptosis for use in patients with ALS—for which no therapies with significant benefit are available—are clear. Phase III trials are currently underway (84).

A related approach is the combination of minocycline with the amino acid creatine, also non-toxic and shown to be neuroprotective in the SOD1 mouse (85). In animal studies, creatine potentiated the neuroprotective effect conferred by min-ocycline administration (86). Both drugs' lack of toxicity and demonstrated efficacy in animal models may make them suitable for clinical trials in patients with ALS.

A third class of commonly used compounds, the cyclooxygenase-2 (COX-2) inhibitors, have also shown promise as therapeutic agents in animal models of ALS. COX-2, induced in response to inflammatory stimuli, cytokines, and mitogens, produces prostaglandins (87). In vivo and in vitro data have shown that prostaglandins may contribute to motor neuron degeneration, and that prostaglandin-mediated neuronal degeneration may be mediated by caspase-dependent apoptosis (88,89). Inhibiting COX-2 with celecoxib in transgenic SOD1 mice delayed onset of weakness and weight loss and prolonged survival in these mice by 25% (90).

Contagious Apoptosis: "The Kindergarten Effect"

The process of cell death in one cell can affect the dynamics of cell death in neighboring cells (72). Factors generated by cells as they die and after they die are also detrimental to bordering cells; they are exposed to triggering factors that are similar to those affecting a dying cell. For example, in stroke a neuron is exposed to an ischemic environment triggering the apoptotic cascade producing IL-1-β, TNF-α, and fee radicals (91). These diffusible factors affect neighboring neurons that have been similarly exposed to ischemia. Since there is a gradient of ischemia, neurons that might not behave died as the result of the ischemic insult from a combination of exposure to a sublethal ischemic environment and the diffusible toxic factors generated by their dying neighbors. This phenomenon also occurs in chronic neurodegenerative disease. For example, in ALS mediated by mutant SOD1, the mutant SOD1 protein initiates the cell-death cascade in one neuron. As the neuron progresses through the cascade and dies, it releases proapoptotic factors affecting neighboring cells in a paracrine fashion. Since these cells have the same genetic predisposition as their dying neighbors, such factors might induce them, too, to initiate the cascade. From a therapeutic standpoint, this concept is important as an inhibitor of apoptosis not only will slow the process of cell death in one cell but will also inhibit the production of the diffusible toxic factors that might initiate the cell-death cascade in a neighboring cell.

CONCLUSION

We have herein reviewed the available data on the role of apoptosis in the ALS. Particular emphasis has been placed on the roles of the Bcl-2 family members and caspases, with convincing data showing definitive roles of each family of proteins in disease progression. The emerging model of apoptosis in ALS appears to involve, to some degree, a balance between pro- and antiapoptotic Bcl-2 proteins, one which may be tipped towards programmed cell death initiation by an as-yet unknown pathway involving the mutant *SOD1* gene product. Recent data suggest that an early event may be caspase-1 activation, which in turn cleaves Bid to its activated truncated form leading to mitochondrial translocation. The next critical sequence of events is the release of apoptogenic proteins such as cytochrome c from the mitochondria, leading in turn to formation of the apoptosome and activation of caspase 9. The downstream caspases 3 and 7 are then activated, and cellular demise ensues. Caspase-1 activation also cleaves pro-IL-1β to its active form, and this diffusible factor may act in paracrine fashion to initiate apoptosis in neighboring cells.

Further research will clarify the specific roles played by mutant *SOD1* and *ALS2* gene products in the initiation of the apoptotic cascade. While these pathways are unclear, a large body of evidence has nevertheless implicated apoptosis as a central process in the death of motor neurons in ALS. In this cascade, caspases are emerging as specific molecular targets whose inhibition has resulted in meaningful survival benefit in transgenic SOD1 mice. These encouraging animal data suggest that large-scale human clinical trials of non-toxic compounds such as minocycline are warranted.

REFERENCES

1. Rowland LP, Shneider NA. Amyotrophic lateral sclerosis. N Engl J Med 2001; 344(22): 1688–1700.
2. Cleveland DW, Rothstein JD. From Charcot to Lou Gehrig: Deciphering selective motor neuron death in ALS.. Vat Rev Neurosci 2001; 2(11):802–819.

3. Graham DI, Lantos PL, eds. Greenfield's Neuropathology. 7th ed. New York: Arnold, 2002.
4. Yang Y, Hentati A, Deng HX, Dabbagh O, Sasaki T, Hirano M, Hung WY, Ouahchi K, Yan J, Azim AC, et al. The gene encoding alsin, a protein with three guanine-nucleotide exchange factor domains, is mutated in a form of recessive amyotrophic lateral sclerosis. Nat Genet 2001; 29(2):160–165.
5. Hadano S, Hand CK, Osuga H, Yanagisawa Y, Otomo A, Devon RS, Miyamoto N, Showguchi-Miyata J, Okada Y, Singaraja R, et al. A gene encoding a putative GTPase regulator is mutated in familial amyotrophic lateral sclerosis 2. Nat Genet 2001; 29(2): 166–173.
6. Rosen DR, Siddique T, Patterson D, Figlewicz DA, Sapp P, Hentati A, Donaldson D, Goto J, O'Regan JP, Deng HX, Rahaman B, Krieus A, Mukenra-Yasek D, Gayabyab A, Gasin SM, Baqer R, Tausi RE, Halperin TJ, Hefrfeldt B, Van Den Bingle R, Hung WY, Bird T, Ding G, Mulden Dut, Sugle C, Laving NE, Sorian E, Perricak-Vance MA, Haine J, Roulean GA, Gusella JS, Hong HR, Brown Jr.R. Mutations in Cu/Zn superoxide dismutase gene are associated with familial amyotrophic lateral sclerosis. Nature 1993; 362(6415):59–62.
7. Longo VD, Gralla EB, Valentine JS. Superoxide dismutase activity is essential for stationary phase survival in Saccharomyces cerevisiae. Mitochondrial production of toxic oxygen species in vivo. J Biol Chem 1996; 271(21):12,275–12,280.
8. Deng HX, Hentati A, Tainer JA, Iqbal Z, Cayabyab A, Hung WY, Getzoff ED, Hu P, Amyotrophic lateral sclerosis and structural defects in Cu, Zn superoxide dismutase. Science 1993; 261(5124):1047–1051.
9. Cudkowicz ME, McKenna-Yasek D, Sapp PE, Chin W, Geller B, Hayden DL, Schoenfeld DA, Hosler BA, Horvitz HR, Brown RH. Epidemiology of mutations in superoxide dismutase in amyotrophic lateral sclerosis. Ann Neurol 1997; 41(2):210–221.
10. Gaudette M, Hirano M, Siddique T. Current status of SOD1 mutations in familial amyotrophic lateral sclerosis. Amyotroph Lateral Scler Other Motor Neuron Disord 2000; 1(2):83–89.
11. Andersen PM. Genetic factors in the early diagnosis of ALS. Amyotroph Lateral Scler Other Motor Neuron Disord 2000; 1(suppl 1):S31–S42.
12. Reaume AG, Elliott JL, Hoffman EK, Kowall NW, Ferrante RJ, Siwek DF, Wilcox HM, Flood DG, Beal MF, Brown RH Jr, et al. Motor neurons in Cu/Zn superoxide dismutase-deficient mice develop normally but exhibit enhanced cell death after axonal injury. Nat Genet 1996; 13(1):43–47.
13. Wong PC, Pardo CA, Borchelt DR, Lee MK, Copeland NG, Jenkins NA, Sisodia SS, Cleveland DW, Price DL. An adverse property of a familial ALS-linked SOD1 mutation causes motor neuron disease characterized by vacuolar degeneration of mitochondria. Neuron 1995; 14(6):1105–1116.
14. Bruijn LI, Becher MW, Lee MK, Anderson KL, Jenkins NA, Copeland NG, Sisodia SS, Rothstein JD, Borchelt DR, Price DL, et al. ALS-linked SOD1 mutant G85R mediates damage to astrocytes and promotes rapidly progressive disease with SOD1-containing inclusions. Neuron 1997; 18(2):327–338.
15. Gurney ME, Pu H, Chiu AY, Dal Canto MC, Polchow CY, Alexander DD, Caliendo J, Hentati A, Kwon YW, Deng HX, et al. Motor neuron degeneration in mice that express a human Cu, Zn superoxide dismutase mutation. Science 1994; 264(5166):1772–1775.
16. Crow JP, Sampson JB, Zhuang Y, Thompson JA, Beckman JS. Decreased zinc affinity of amyotrophic lateral sclerosis-associated superoxide dismutase mutants leads to enhanced catalysis of tyrosine nitration by peroxynitrite. J Neurochem 1997; 69(5):1936–1944.
17. Wiedau-Pazos M, Goto JJ, Rabizadeh S, Gralla EB, Roe JA, Lee MK, Valentine JS, sclerosis. Science 1996; 271(5248):515–518.
18. Beckman JS, Carson M, Smith CD, Koppenol WH. ALS, SOD and peroxynitrite. Nature 1993; 364(6438):584.

19. Bruening W, Roy J, Giasson B, Figlewicz DA, Mushynski WE, Durham HD. Up-regulation of protein chaperones preserves viability of cells expressing toxic Cu/Zn-superoxide dismutase mutants associated with amyotrophic lateral sclerosis. J Neurochem 1999; 72(2):693–699.

20. Bruijn LI, Houseweart MK, Kato S, Anderson KL, Anderson SD, Ohama E, Reaume AG, Scott RW, Cleveland DW. Aggregation and motor neuron toxicity of an ALS-linked SOD1 mutant independent from wild-type SOD1. Science 1998; 281(5384):1851–1854.

21. Hirano A, Donnenfeld H, Sasaki S, Nakano I. Fine structural observations of neurofilamentous changes in amyotrophic lateral sclerosis. J Neuropathol Exp Neurol 1984; 43(5):461–470.

22. Guegan C, Przedborski S. Programmed cell death in amyotrophic lateral sclerosis. J Clin Invest 2003; 111(2):153–161.

23. Mulder DW, Kurland LT, Offord KP, Beard CM. Familial adult motor neuron disease: amyotrophic lateral sclerosis. Neurology 1986; 36(4):511–517.

24. Topp JD, Gray NW, Gerard RD, Horazdovsky BF. Alsin is a Rab5 and Rac1 guanine nucleotide exchange factor. J Biol Chem 2004; 279(22):29612–29623.

25. Spaargaren M, Bos JL. Rab5 induces Rac-independent lamellipodia formation and cell migration. Mol Biol Cell 1999; 10(10):3239–3250.

26. Martin LJ, Price AC, Kaiser A, Shaikh AY, Liu Z. Mechanisms for neuronal degeneration in amyotrophic lateral sclerosis and in models of motor neuron death (Review). Int J Mol Med 2000; 5(1):3–13.

27. Kerr JF, Wyllie AH, Currie AR. Apoptosis: a basic biological phenomenon with wide-ranging implications in tissue kinetics. Br J Cancer 1972; 26(4):239–257.

28. Hengartner MO. The biochemistry of apoptosis. Nature 2000; 407(6805):770–776.

29. Wyllie AH, Kerr JF, Currie AR. Cell death: the significance of apoptosis. Int Rev Cytol 1980; 68:251–306.

30. Wyllie AH. Glucocorticoid-induced thymocyte apoptosis is associated with endogenous endonuclease activation. Nature 1980; 284(5756):555–556.

31. Liu X, Zou H, Slaughter C, Wang X. DFF, a heterodimeric protein that functions downstream of caspase-3 to trigger DNA fragmentation during apoptosis. Cell 1997; 89(2): 175–184.

32. Yuan J, Shaham S, Ledoux S, Ellis HM, Horvitz HR. The C. elegans cell death gene ced-3 encodes a protein similar to mammalian interleukin-1 beta-converting enzyme. Cell 1993; 75(4):641–652.

33. Yuan JY, Horvitz HR. The Caenorhabditis elegans genes ced-3 and ced-4 act cell autonomously to cause programmed cell death. Dev Biol 1990; 138(1):33–41.

34. Miura M, Zhu H, Rotello R, Hartwieg EA, Yuan J. Induction of apoptosis in fibroblasts by IL-1 beta-converting enzyme, a mammalian homolog of the C. elegans cell death gene ced-3. Cell 1993; 75(4):653–660.

35. Li P, Nijhawan D, Budihardjo I, Srinivasula SM, Ahmad M, Alnemri ES, Wang X. Cytochrome c and dATP-dependent formation of Apaf-1/caspase-9 complex initiates an apoptotic protease cascade. Cell 1997; 91(4):479–489.

36. Hengartner MO, Horvitz HR. C. elegans cell survival gene ced-9 encodes a functional homolog of the mammalian proto-oncogene bcl-2. Cell 1994; 76(4):665–676.

37. Conradt B, Horvitz HR. The C. elegans protein EGL-1 is required for programmed cell death and interacts with the Bcl-2-like protein CED-9. Cell 1998; 93(4):519–529.

38. Shi Y. Mechanisms of caspase activation and inhibition during apoptosis. Mol Cell 2002; 9(3):459–470.

39. Friedlander RM. Role of caspase 1 in neurologic disease. Arch Neurol 2000; 57(9): 1273–1276.

40. Friedlander RM, Yuan J. ICE, neuronal apoptosis and neurodegeneration. Cell Death Differ 1998; 5(10):823–831.

41. Zhang WH, Wang X, Narayanan M, Zhang Y, Huo C, Reed JC, Friedlander RM. Fundamental role of the Rip2/caspase-1 pathway in hypoxia and ischemia-induced neuronal cell death. Proc Natl Acad Sci USA 2003; 100(26):16,012–16,017.

42. Thornberry NA, Molineaux SM. Interleukin-1 beta converting enzyme: a novel cysteine protease required for IL-1 beta production and implicated in programmed cell death. Protein Sci 1995; 4(1):3–12.

43. Friedlander RM, Gagliardini V, Rotello RJ, Yuan J. Functional role of interleukin 1 beta (IL-1 beta) in IL-1 beta-converting enzyme-mediated apoptosis. J Exp Med 1996; 184(2):717–724.

44. Troy CM, Stefanis L, Prochiantz A, Greene LA, Shelanski ML. The contrasting roles of ICE family proteases and interleukin-1β in apoptosis induced by trophic factor withdrawal and by copper/zinc superoxide dismutase down-regulation. Proc Natl Acad Sci USA 1996; 93:5635–5640.

45. Nagata S. Apoptotic DNA fragmentation. Exp Cell Res 2000; 256:12–18.

46. Crompton M. Bax, Bid and the permeabilization of the mitochondrial outer membrane in apoptosis. Curr Opin Cell Biol 2000; 12(4):414–419.

47. Desagher S, Osen-Sand A, Nichols A, Eskes R, Montessuit S, Lauper S, Maundrell K, Antonsson B, Martinou JC. Bid-induced conformational change of Bax is responsible for mitochondrial cytochrome c release during apoptosis. J Cell Biol 1999; 144(5):891–901.

48. Chao DT, Korsmeyer SJ. BCL-2 family: regulators of cell death. Annu Rev Immunol 1998; 16:395–419.

49. Verhagen AM, Ekert PG, Pakusch M, Silke J, Connolly LM, Reid GE, Moritz RL, Simpson RJ, Vaux DL. Identification of DIABLO, a mammalian protein that promotes apoptosis by binding to and antagonizing IAP proteins. Cell 2000; 102(1):43–53.

50. Du C, Fang M, Li Y, Li L, Wang X. Smac, a mitochondrial protein that promotes cytochrome c-dependent caspase activation by eliminating IAP inhibition. Cell 2000; 102(1): 33–42.

51. Suzuki Y, Imai Y, Nakayama H, Takahashi K, Takio K, Takahashi R. A serine protease, HtrA2, is released from the mitochondria and interacts with XIAP, inducing cell death. Mol Cell 2001; 8(3):613–621.

52. Susin SA, Daugas E, Ravagnan L, Samejima K, Zamzami N, Loeffler M, Costantini P, Ferri KF, Irinopoulou T, Prevost MC, et al. Two distinct pathways leading to nuclear apoptosis. J Exp Med 2000; 192(4):571–580.

53. Leist M, Jaattela M. Four deaths and a funeral: from caspases to alternative mechanisms. Nat Rev Mol Cell Biol 2001; 2(8):589–598.

54. Li LY, Luo X, Wang X. Endonuclease G is an apoptotic DNase when released from mitochondria. Nature 2001; 412(6842):95–99.

55. Liston P, Roy N, Tamai K, Lefebvre C, Baird S, Cherton-Horvat G, Farahani R, McLean M, Ikeda JE, MacKenzie A, et al. Suppression of apoptosis in mammalian cells by NAIP and a related family of IAP genes. Nature 1996; 379(6563):349–353.

56. Roy N, Mahadevan MS, McLean M, Shutler G, Yaraghi Z, Farahani R, Baird SBesner-Johnston A, Lefebvre C, Kang X, Salih M, Avlery H, Tamai K, Gvan X, Ioannou P, Craniford TD, da Joug PJ, Surh L, Ikeda JE, Morneluk RE, Mademaie PC. The gene for neuronal apoptosis inhibitory protein is partially deleted in individuals with spinal muscular atrophy. Cell 1995; 80(1):167–178.

57. Troost D, Aten J, Morsink F, de Jong JM. Apoptosis in amyotrophic lateral sclerosis is not restricted to motor neurons. Bcl-2 expression is increased in unaffected post-central gyrus. Neuropathol Appl Neurobiol 1995; 21(6):498–504.

58. Ekegren T, Grundstrom E, Lindholm D, Aquilonius SM. Upregulation of Bax protein and increased DNA degradation in ALS spinal cord motor neurons. Acta Neurol Scand 1999; 100(5):317–321.

59. Vukosavic S, Stefanis L, Jackson-Lewis V, Guegan C, Romero N, Chen C, Dubois-Dauphin M, Przedborski S. Delaying caspase activation by Bcl-2: A clue to disease

retardation in a transgenic mouse model of amyotrophic lateral sclerosis. J Neurosci 2000; 20(24):9119–9125.

60. Yoshiyama Y, Yamada T, Asanuma K, Asahi T. Apoptosis related antigen, Le(Y) and nick-end labeling are positive in spinal motor neurons in amyotrophic lateral sclerosis. Acta Neuropathol (Berl) 1994; 88(3):207–211.

61. Rangnekar VM. Apoptosis mediated by a novel leucine zipper protein Par-4. Apoptosis 1998; 3(2):61–66.

62. Pedersen WA, Luo H, Kruman I, Kasarskis E, Mattson MP. The prostate apoptosis response-4 protein participates in motor neuron degeneration in amyotrophic lateral sclerosis. FASEB J 2000; 14(7):913–924.

63. Guegan C, Vila M, Rosoklija G, Hays AP, Przedborski S. Recruitment of the mitochondrial-dependent apoptotic pathway in amyotrophic lateral sclerosis. J Neurosci 2001; 21(17):6569–6576.

64. Kostic V, Jackson-Lewis V, de Bilbao F, Dubois-Dauphin M, Przedborski S. Bcl-2: prolonging life in a transgenic mouse model of familial amyotrophic lateral sclerosis. Science 1997; 277(5325):559–562.

65. Ghadge GD, Lee JP, Bindokas VP, Jordan J, Ma L, Miller RJ, Roos RP. Mutant superoxide dismutase-1-linked familial amyotrophic lateral sclerosis: molecular mechanisms of neuronal death and protection. J Neurosci 1997; 17(22):8756–8766.

66. Mu X, He J, Anderson DW, Trojanowski JQ, Springer JE. Altered expression of bcl-2 and bax mRNA in amyotrophic lateral sclerosis spinal cord motor neurons. Ann Neurol 1996; 40(3):379–386.

67. Vukosavic S, Dubois-Dauphin M, Romero N, Przedborski S. Bax and Bcl-2 interaction in a transgenic mouse model of familial amyotrophic lateral sclerosis. J Neurochem 1999; 73(6):2460–2468.

68. Shinoe T, Wanaka A, Nikaido T, Kanazawa K, Shimizu J, Imaizumi K, Kanazawa I. Upregulation of the pro-apoptotic BH3-only peptide harakiri in spinal neurons of amyotrophic lateral sclerosis patients. Neurosci Lett 2001; 313(3):153–157.

69. Guegan C, Vila M, Teismann P, Chen C, Onteniente B, Li M, Friedlander RM, Przedborski S, Teissman P. Instrumental activation of bid by caspase-1 in a transgenic mouse model of ALS. Mol Cell Neurosci 2002; 20(4):553–562.

70. Friedlander RM, Brown RH, Gagliardini V, Wang J, Yuan J. Inhibition of ICE slows ALS in mice. Nature 1997; 388(6637):31.

71. Pasinelli P, Houseweart MK, Brown RH Jr, Cleveland DW. Caspase-1 and -3 are sequentially activated in motor neuron death in Cu, Zn superoxide dismutase-mediated familial amyotrophic lateral sclerosis. Proc Natl Acad Sci USA 2000; 97(25): 13,901–13,906.

72. Li M, Ona VO, Guegan C, Chen M, Jackson-Lewis V, Andrews LJ, Olszewski AJ, Stieg PE, Lee JP, Przedborski S, et al. Functional role of caspase-1 and caspase-3 in an ALS transgenic mouse model. Science 2000; 288(5464):335–339.

73. Li H, Zhu H, Xu CJ, Yuan J. Cleavage of BID by caspase 8 mediates the mitochondrial damage in the Fas pathway of apoptosis. Cell 1998; 94(4):491–501.

74. Friedlander RM. Apoptosis and caspases in neurodegenerative diseases. N Engl J Med 2003; 348(14):1365–1375.

75. Inoue H, Tsukita K, Iwasato T, Suzuki Y, Tomioka M, Tateno M, Nagao M, Kawata A, Saido TC, Miura M, et al. The crucial role of caspase-9 in the disease progression of a transgenic ALS mouse model. EMBO J 2003; 22(24):6665–6674.

76. Zhu S, Stavrovskaya IG, Drozda M, Kim BY, Ona V, Li M, Sarang S, Liu AS, Hartley DM, Wu du C, et al. Minocycline inhibits cytochrome c release and delays progression of amyotrophic lateral sclerosis in mice. Nature 2002; 417(6884):74–78.

77. Yrjanheikki J, Keinanen R, Pellikka M, Hokfelt T, Koistinaho J. Tetracyclines inhibit microglial activation and are neuroprotective in global brain ischemia. Proc Natl Acad Sci USA 1998; 95(26):15,769–15,774.

78. Sanchez Mejia RO, Ona VO, Li M, Friedlander RM. Minocycline reduces traumatic brain injury-mediated caspase-1 activation, tissue damage, and neurological dysfunction. Neurosurgery 2001; 48(6):1393–1399; discussion 1399–1401.
79. Chen M, Ona VO, Li M, Ferrante RJ, Fink KB, Zhu S, Bian J, Guo L, Farrell LA, Hersch SM, et al. Minocycline inhibits caspase-1 and caspase-3 expression and delays mortality in a transgenic mouse model of Huntington disease. Nat Med 2000; 6(7): 797–801.
80. Wu DC, Jackson-Lewis V, Vila M, Tieu K, Teismann P, Vadseth C, Choi DK, Ischiropoulos H, Przedborski S. Blockade of microglial activation is neuroprotective in the 1-methyl-4-phenyl-1,2,3,6-tetrahydropyridine mouse model of Parkinson disease. J Neurosci 2002; 22(5):1763–1771.
81. Du Y, Ma Z, Lin S, Dodel RC, Gao F, Bales KR, Triarhou LC, Chernet E, Perry KW, Nelson DL, et al. Minocycline prevents nigrostriatal dopaminergic neurodegeneration in the MPTP model of Parkinson's disease. Proc Natl Acad Sci USA 2001; 98(25): 14,669–14,674. Epub November 27, 2001.
82. Kriz J, Nguyen MD, Julien JP. Minocycline slows disease progression in a mouse model of amyotrophic lateral sclerosis. Neurobiol Dis 2002; 10(3):268–278.
83. Van Den Bosch L, Tilkin P, Lemmens G, Robberecht W. Minocycline delays disease onset and mortality in a transgenic model of ALS. Neuroreport 2002; 13(8):1067–1070.
84. Gordon PH, Moore DH, Gelinas DF, Qualls C, Meister ME, Werner J, Mendoza M, Mass J, Kushner G, Miller RG. Placebo-controlled phase I/II studies of minocycline in amyotrophic lateral sclerosis. Neurology 2004; 62(10):1845–1847.
85. Klivenyi P, Ferrante RJ, Matthews RT, Bogdanov MB, Klein AM, Andreassen OA, Mueller G, Wermer M, Kaddurah-Daouk R, Beal MF. Neuroprotective effects of creatine in a transgenic animal model of amyotrophic lateral sclerosis. Nat Med 1999; 5(3):347–350.
86. Zhang W, Narayanan M, Friedlander RM. Additive neuroprotective effects of minocycline with creatine in a mouse model of ALS. Ann Neurol 2003; 53(2):267–270.
87. O'Banion MK. Cyclooxygenase-2: molecular biology, pharmacology, and neurobiology. Crit Rev Neurobiol 1999; 13(1):45–82.
88. Takadera T, Yumoto H, Tozuka Y, Ohyashiki T. Prostaglandin E(2) induces caspase-dependent apoptosis in rat cortical cells. Neurosci Lett 2002; 317(2):61–64.
89. Almer G, Teismann P, Stevic Z, Halaschek-Wiener J, Deecke L, Kostic V, Przedborski S. Increased levels of the pro-inflammatory prostaglandin PGE2 in CSF from ALS patients. Neurology 2002; 58(8):1277–1279.
90. Drachman DB, Frank K, Dykes-Hoberg M, Teismann P, Almer G, Przedborski S, Rothstein JD. Cyclooxygenase 2 inhibition protects motor neurons and prolongs survival in a transgenic mouse model of ALS. Ann Neurol 2002; 52(6):771–778.
91. Yuan J, Yankner BA. Apoptosis in the nervous system. Nature 2000; 407(6805):802–809.

17

Cytoskeletal Proteins in the Pathogenesis of ALS

Michael J. Strong
Department of Clinical Neurological Sciences, The University of Western Ontario, and Robarts Research Institute, London, Ontario, Canada

Jesse McLean
Department of Cell Biology, Robarts Research Institute, London, Ontario, Canada

Jean-Pierre Julien
Department of Anatomy and Physiology, Research Centre of CHUQ, Quebec City, Quebec, Canada

INTRODUCTION

Protein aggregation is increasingly recognized as a common pathological hallmark of a number of neurodegenerative diseases. Amyotrophic lateral sclerosis (ALS) is no exception. The motor neuron degeneration that is typical of ALS is accompanied by a range of intraneuronal protein aggregates that take the form of inclusions, the most common of which are Bunina bodies, ubiquitinated inclusions and neurofilament-rich "hyaline conglomerate inclusions" (1). Increasingly, however, protein aggregation in non-neuronal cells is observed in both experimental models of ALS and in postmortem ALS tissue. Understanding the genesis of these proteinaceous aggregates and their role in the pathogenesis of motor neuron degeneration in ALS is the primary focus of this chapter.

INTERMEDIATE FILAMENT METABOLISM

Developmental Expression Patterns

Intermediate filaments (IFs) are a highly conserved family of proteins that share a great deal of homology and which exhibit tissue-specific patterns of expression (Table 1). Within the central nervous system, there is a developmentally specific pattern of IF expression. Nestin is expressed early and is followed by vimentin, thus laying down the initial cytoskeletal network. Thereafter, there is a coordinated pattern of expression of peripherin, α-internexin, and the neurofilament (NF) subunit proteins, giving rise to the mature neuronal cytoskeletal network (2–11). This initial cytoskeletal

Table 1 Intermediate Filament Classification

Class	Identity	Molecular Weight (kDa)	Cell Expression
Type I	Acidic Keratins	40–64	Epithelial
Type II	Basic Keratins	52–68	Epithelial
Type III	Desmin	53	Muscle
	GFAP	51	Astrocytes
	Peripherin	54	Neuronal
	Vimentin	55	Mesenchymal
	α-internexin	66	Neuronal
	β-internexin	70	Neuronal
Type IV	NF-L	68	Neuronal
	NF-M[a]	110	Neuronal
	NF-H[a]	130	Neuronal
Type V	Lamin A	70	Most
	Lamin B	64	Most
	Lamin C	58	Most
Type VI	Nestin	240	CNS stem cells
Misc	Septins A–C		Nucleated cells
	Filensin	100	Lens
	Phakinin	Variable	Lens

[a]Post-translational modification (hyperphosphorylation) yields molecular weights of 160 kDa (NF-M) and 200 kDa (NF-H).

network is either completely or partially replaced, presumably through heteropolymer formation, with the more stable NF network (12). Layered onto this process is a somatotopically specific pattern of expression, such that α-internexin is expressed primarily within neurons residing in the central nervous system and peripherin is expressed in externally projecting neurons (e.g., motor neurons). Mature neurons thus possess the ability to express a number of related IFs, many of which relate to their initial phylogenetically determined pattern of expression.

Within the adult neuron, the NF proteins are the primary IFs (13). The individual NF proteins can be defined on the basis of molecular mass as determined by SDS.PAGE and include a 200 kDa (NF-H—high molecular weight NF), a 160 kDa (NF-M—intermediate molecular weight NF), and a 68 kDa (NF-L—low molecular weight NF) protein. Each one of them is composed of a highly conserved α-helical core region of approximately 310 amino acids that forms double stranded coils flanked by head-(amino) and tail-(carboxy) domains (Fig. 1) (14). The individual NF subunit proteins form obligate heteropolymers and assemble in the neuronal perikaryon into a single NF triplet protein prior to the initiation of their transport into the neuronal processes (15,16). The dimerization of NF-L is key to the initiation of this process, although heteropolymerization with related IFs in which the central rod domains of the two IF proteins wind around each other can also trigger this process. These dimers then assemble in a staggered, antiparallel array in which NF-M and NF-H subunits associate to form the intact NF triplet protein and in which the C-terminal tail domains project laterally from the filament core allowing for interaction among neighboring NF and microtubules (10,17). Elongation of the protein occurs by head to tail assembly of NF-L in a complex process involving

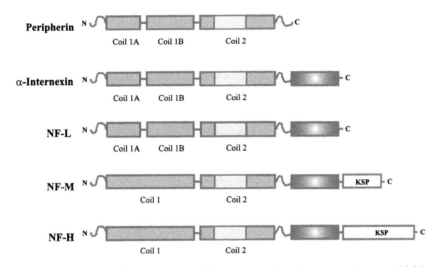

Figure 1 Intermediate filaments. The intermediate filaments share a highly common conserved α-helical core region that forms double stranded coiled-coils flanked by head-(amino) and tail-(carboxy) domains.

antagonistic effects of the C-terminus and N-terminus domains (18). The N-terminus domain is involved in the regulation of this assembly (19,20).

Both NF-M and NF-H are highly phosphorylated proteins, with the majority (but not all) phosphorylation sites located at multiphosphorylation repeats within the C-terminus domain. Neurofilament can be directly phosphorylated by a number of kinases, including cyclin-dependant kinase 5, glycogen synthase kinase-3, casein kinases I and II, members of the mitogen-activated protein kinase family, and stress-activated kinases. Phosphorylation appears to be a key determinant of the interaction between NF proteins and neighboring structures, but in also determining their rate of axonal transport, with the more highly phosphorylated NF residing within a less dynamic, slowly moving phase than those that are less phosphorylated.

Not surprisingly given this intricate pattern of NF assembly and post-translational modification, disruption of NF metabolism can have significant consequences on neuronal function and lead to the formation of proteinaceous aggregates. For example, N-terminal deletions of the NF-L gene yields assembly-incompetent NF-L polypeptides (21); cleavage of the NF-L N-terminus inhibits assembly of NF-L into 10 nm filaments (22); and a single missense mutation in the rod domain (Leu394Pro) of NF-L leads to a profound accumulation of NF within motor neurons resulting in motor neuron death and atrophy of muscle fibers (23). In this latter transgenic mouse, the mutation disrupts the binding of a ribonucleoprotein complex to the 3′ UTR of NF-L mRNA and thereby alters mRNA stability (24,25).

Although their exact relationships to the induction of ALS are not known, multiple mutations in NF-H have now been identified in approximately 1% of sporadic ALS patients (Fig. 2) (26–30). Virtually all of these mutations (small in-frame deletions or insertions) occur in the multiphosphorylation repeats of the carboxy terminus, where they would be predicted to interfere not with the primary structure of the neurofilament triplet protein, but with the interaction of the triplet with adjacent cytoskeletal proteins.

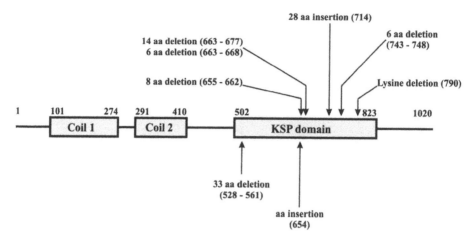

Figure 2 Schematic illustration of the human NF-H protein and the sites of mutations identified in sALS. All mutations to date have been isolated within the multiphosphorylation repeat domain (lys-ser-pro) in the C-terminus domain. Extensive post-translational modification of this domain, predominantly through phosphorylation, is key to the interactions of the NF triplet protein in determining axonal caliber and to regulating NF proteolysis.

Of additional interest to a discussion of the pathobiology of ALS is the potential role of peripherin, a type-III IF. Although encoded by a single gene located on chromosome 12, three alternative splice variants have been identified with molecular weights of 56, 58, and 61 kDa (31). The 58 kDa variant is the most common, while the 61 kDa variant carries an addition 96-base pair insertion within the α-helical rod domain. Peripherin can coassemble with the NF subunits in vitro and has been observed to coaggregate with NF aggregates in ALS. Of importance to understanding the pathogenesis of ALS, the expression of the 61 kDa isoform is associated with an enhanced rate of motor neuron death (32). Moreover, the screening for sequence variants of the peripherin gene in a cohort of ALS patients led to the discovery of one variant consisting of a nucleotide deletion within exon 1 that predicts a truncated peripherin species of 85 amino acids (33). Expression of this frameshift peripherin mutant in SW13 cells caused disruption of neurofilament network assembly. These results suggest that peripherin mutations may be the cause of a small percentage of ALS cases and they further support the view of NF disorganization as a contributor of ALS pathogenesis.

Molecular Motors

The cytoskeletal proteins are synthesized in the neuronal cell body and transported down the axon toward the nerve ending. Recently, many studies showed that defects in the microtubule-based transport machinery could provoke motor neuron disease. The over-expression in mice of dynamitin disrupts dynein/dynactin function and induces motor neuron disease with neurofilamentous swellings in motor axons (34). Mutations in dynein were shown to cause motor neuron disease in mice (35), whereas mutant dynactin gene was discovered in human cases of motor neuron disease (36). Further proof that defects in axonal transport can provoke neurodegeneration came from the characterization of a mouse knockout for the kinesin KIF1B gene (37) and from the identification of mutations in the motor domain of the KIF1B gene in some cases of Charcot-Marie-Tooth disease type 2A (37). The disruption of KIF5A gene in the mouse led to abnormal NF transport (38). Moreover, two laboratories recently identified that the progressive motor neuronopathy (PMN) mutation in the mouse is due to a mutation in the tubulin-specific chaperone (Tbce) protein (39,40). Tbce is essential for proper tubulin assembly and for the maintenance of microtubules in motor axons. Mutations in the gigaxonin gene can also cause neuropathy (41,42). The over-expression of tau, a stabilizer of microtubules, can also provoke motor neuron disease in mice (43). This suggests that altered function of tubulin cofactors might be implicated in human motor neuron disease.

MOLECULAR NEUROPATHOLOGY OF ALS RELEVANT TO THE CYTOSKELETON

The pathology of ALS has been reviewed elsewhere (Chapter 3). Of specific relevance to this discussion of the cytoskeleton in ALS are the numerous intracellular inclusions that have been described in degenerating motor neurons in ALS, involving both the cell body and neuritic processes (44–46). Of the intraneuronal aggregates traditionally associated with ALS, Bunina bodies appear to be unique. These are dense, refractile eosinophilic inclusions of lysosomal origin that are immunoreactive for the lysosomal cystein proteinase inhibitor cystatin C (47). Typically, the degenerating motor neurons of ALS also contain ubiquitin-immunoreactive structures that take the form of either skeins or aggregates (48,49). Both can be seen within the same cell. While the underlying substrate giving rise to skein formation remains unknown, the more dense, discrete ubiquitinated aggregates share immunoreactivity with the neuronal IF (NF, peripherin, α-internexin) (44–46,48–52). Although these latter aggregates may be surrounded by a peripheral halo, giving rise to an appearance of "Lewy body like inclusions," the absence of α-synuclein within these aggregates indicates that these are not Lewy bodies, typical of Parkinson's disease, and hence this term should not be applied. The final major class of inclusions to affect degenerating motor neurons in ALS is neurofilamentous in origin.

While many of the inclusions described above can be immunostained with antibodies recognizing phosphorylated NF-H, both peripherin and α-internexin immunoreactivity may also be observed (50,51). Coimmunostaining with antibodies recognizing SOD1, dorfin, and nitric oxide (53–56), suggests a potential role for the oxidative modification of NF in the induction of aggregates. The observation of serpin–serine protease complexes within NF aggregates further suggests an inhibition of the degradation of oxidatively modified NF (57). The presence of galectin-1 immunoreactivity colocalizing to neurofilamentous aggregates suggests that this protein, involved in axonal regeneration, cell growth, and differentiation, has also been mislocalized within the neuron or entrapped in the process giving rise to the NF aggregate (58).

In the subsequent sections, we will examine the role of altered IF metabolism inducing the formation of these aggregates in ALS.

Alterations in IF Expression in ALS

There is considerable evidence that supports an alteration in the stoichiometry of steady-state levels of NF mRNA in ALS in a manner it is experimentally associated with the induction of NF aggregate formation (reviewed in next section). This has included the finding of reduced NF-L steady-state mRNA levels in degenerating spinal motor neurons in which inclusions were also observed (59). This observation was subsequently shown using in situ hybridization to reflect a selective suppression of NF-L mRNA in ALS in which the motor neuron-specific steady-state level of both NF-M and NF-H mRNA was unchanged from that observed in controls (51). In the latter study, both peripherin and α-internexin mRNA levels were reduced, while β-actin mRNA levels were elevated in the absence of an increase in Tα1-tubulin. The former implied a lack of compensatory increased expression of either of the two intermediate filaments that would be expected to participate in the formation of the NF triplet protein in the absence of NF-L, while the latter observation regarding Tα1-tubulin implies that the alterations in IF expression were not reflective of a regenerative response (60,61). In a subsequent study using single cell PCR from microdissected spinal motor neurons, the observation of selective loss of NF-L mRNA was further validated (62).

Interestingly, these observations are the converse of the elevated NF-L, NF-M, and NF-H steady-state mRNA levels observed when crude homogenates of ALS spinal cord are examined and which appear to be due to an enhanced stability of the mRNA species (63). In support of the latter, when heterogeneously expressed NF-L mRNA is incubated with crude protein extracts from age-matched neurologically normal control spinal cord, NF-L mRNA decay rates are significantly more rapid than when incubated in the presence of ALS-derived crude spinal cord protein extracts (64). By heat denaturing the control extracts, or by the use of proteinase K digestion of the extract, or by adjusting the ratio of ALS to control tissue protein homogenates (in admixture studies), the rate of degradation of NF-L mRNA can be made to approximate that of NF-L mRNA exposed to ALS protein extract alone. This effect is mediated through the binding of novel *trans*-acting destabilizing proteins interacting with *cis*-acting elements of the NF-L mRNA 3′ UTR.

One such *trans*-acting binding protein, capable of destabilizing NF-L mRNA, is mutant copper/zinc superoxide dismutase (SOD1) (65). The latter, a novel gain of function for the SOD1 protein, not evident in wild-type SOD1, was first suggested when a significant suppression of the NF-L mRNA steady-state levels was observed in a motor neuron hybridoma cell line (NSC-34) that had been stably transfected with SOD1^{G93A} (62). We have subsequently observed that mutant, but not wild-type, SOD1 binds directly to the NF-L mRNA 3′ UTR, destabilizing the mRNA and leading to an enhanced rate of NF-L mRNA degradation. This provides a potential linkage between the expression of a familial ALS-associated mutation and the genesis of an alteration in NF stoichiometry.

Transgenic Mouse Models of Altered IF Metabolism

Many factors can potentially lead to formation of abnormal IF accumulations including deregulation of IF expression, defective axonal transport, IF gene mutations, or post-translational protein modifications, and proteolysis. Initial evidence for a deleterious effect of NF disorganization came from transgenic mice overexpressing human NF-H (66,67) or mouse NF-L (68). In both cases, there was abnormal perikaryal accumulation of NFs in spinal motor neurons that was accompanied by axonal atrophy and motor dysfunction, but without massive neuronal death. Subsequently, the concept that an alteration in IF expression patterns can lead to a motor neuronal degeneration has been established through a number of transgenic and gene knockout mouse models (Table 2) (Fig. 3). These models have helped us to establish the concept that altering the expression NF-L, either by altering the stoichiometry of NF expression through targeted deletions or in altering

Table 2 Murine Transgenic Models of Targeted Disruption of Neuronal IF Gene Expression

	Age[a] (months)	Mouse strain	Neuropathological effect	Axonal loss	Effects on IF content	Phenotype	Reference
NF-L							
Murine NF-L (−/−); (+/−)	2–3	C57BL/6	≥50% reduction in ventral root axonal caliber	∼20% loss	Reduction in both NF-M and NF-H protein levels in sciatic nerves and brain homogenates; significant loss of NF in myelinated axons	Normal development, no overt phenotype; reduced rate of regeneration post-axotomy	69
Murine NF-L (+/+)	6	B6AF₁J (108)	Massive perikaryal aggregates of neurofilament; axonal NF aggregates	None	Increased NF density, no alteration in NF-L or NF-H expression levels	No overt motor phenotype in Monterio et al; motor dysfunction observed in Xu et al; cataract formation	68,108
Murine NF-L (−/−), α-internexin (−/−)			≥50% reduction in ventral root axonal caliber	∼20%	Scarcity	Normal development, no overt phenotype	109
Human NF-L (+/+)		C57BL/6	None	None	None	No overt phenotype	70
Human NF-L (+/+)	P70 (adult)	C57BL/6	Prominent perikaryal NF-L immunostaining	None stated	None stated	None stated	110
NF-M							
Murine NF-M (−/−)	4	129 Sv/J bred to C57BL/6	≥50% reduction in ventral root axonal caliber; loss of large diameter myelinated axons	∼10% loss	Significant reduction in NF-L protein levels in NF-M (−/−) mice; concomitant increase in NF-H protein levels in brain but not spinal cord	Normal development; no overt phenotype	111,112

(Continued)

Table 2 Murine Transgenic Models of Targeted Disruption of Neuronal IF Gene Expression (*Continued*)

	Age[a] (months)	Mouse strain	Neuropathological effect	Axonal loss	Effects on IF content	Phenotype	Reference
Human NF-M (+/+)	3–12	C57BL6/ DBA2J	Age-dependent prominent NF aggregate formation		Increased levels of NF-L expression; reduced phosphorylation of NF-H; increased axonal NF density	Age-dependent deficits on reference and memory tasks	113–116
Murine NF-M/ NF-H double (−/−) mutants	3	C57BL/6 or 129 Sv/J bred to C57BL/6	≥50% reduction in ventral root axonal caliber; enhanced NF-L immunoreactivity in motor neuron perikarya	25%	Significant loss of intermediate filaments within axonal processes; most axons devoid of NFs; loss of NF-L	No overt phenotype	117,118
NF-H							
Murine NF-H (−/−)	4	129 Sv/J bred to C57BL/6	Significant reduction in the development of large diameter myelinated axons with concomitant increase in smaller diameter fibres	No	Approximately 10–25% reduction in NF-L protein level; no effect on NF-M protein levels	Normal development; no overt phenotype; reduced axonal conductivity	119–121
Murine NF-H (+/+)	4 weeks, 9 weeks, and 1 year	C57BL6/ C3	NF-H dose-dependent induction of severe axonal and perikaryal NF aggregate fomation in spinal cord, reduction in axonal calibre	Reduced large diameter axons if peri- karyal aggre- gates formed	Reduced NF-L and NF-M molar ratios	Normal phenotype; no evidence of neurogenic atrophy (even at 2 years)	122
Human NF-H (+/+)	4	C57BL6/ C3H	Prominent perikaryal NF aggregate formation; dying back axonopathy	Severe axono- pathy	Elevated level of NF-H expression, no alteration in NF-L or NF-H levels	Progressive motor neuronopathy; reduced axonal conductivity	66,123

	Age[a]	Strain					Ref
Amino terminal deletion, NF-H	9 weeks	C57BL/6J	~20% reduction in both large and small motor neuron axonal area	No	No alteration in NF-L; approximately 2-fold increase in NF-M levels	No phenotype	124
Peripherin Knockout Murine			Normal	30% loss of small sensory fibers	Normal		125
Murine peripherin (+/+)	6–10	C57BL/ C3H	Diffuse, increased peripherin immunoreactivity in perikaryal and neurites; peripherin immunoreactive aggregates in aged mice	~35% motor axonal loss, age-dependant	Normal	Late onset (> 2 years) motor dysfunction	71
Murine peripherin (+/+); NF-L (−/−)	6–8	C57BL/ C3H	Significant (~64%) loss of large motor neurons, increasing with age; increased peripherin staining in motor neurons with peripherin aggregates	~46% loss of ventral root motor axons	Not stated	Progressive loss of hindlimb mobility beginning at 6–8 months	71
α-Internexin Murine (−/−)	3	C57BL6/ 129 Sv	Normal	No	Normal	No developmental delay; no overt phenotype	109
Murine (+/+)	12–18	B6CBA F₁/J	Enhanced α-internexin immunostaining in cerebellum, neocortex and thalamus	None	Normal	Reduced motor coordination and balance on rotorod	126

[a]Age at which neuropathological analysis undertaken.

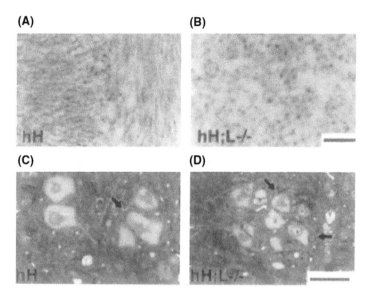

Figure 3 Perikaryal accumulations in absence of NF-L. Spinal cord section stained with
Toluidine blue show the presence of hyaline inclusions in the cell body of motor neurons from
a transgenic mouse over-expressing human NF-H in NF-L normal background (**A**) and in
context of NF-L knockout (**B**). Perikaryal accumulations are observed (*arrow*) in each.
Electron microscopic examination revealed IF structures in the perikaryon of hNF-H over-
expressor (**C**) and their absence in protein inclusions of hNF-H over-expressor in absence
of NF-L (**D**). *Scale bars*: **A, B**, 50 μm; **C, D**, 2 μm. (*See color insert.*)

the interactions between NF-L and either NF-M or NF-H, provokes an aggregation
of NF proteins, reduced axonal IF density, and motor neuron degeneration. However, this concept cannot be applied indiscriminately. For example, knockout mice
individually for the NF proteins or α-internexin do not develop an overt phenotype,
or exhibit developmental delay. Given the proceeding discussion on the key role of
NF-H phosphorylation, the failure of NF-H knockout mice, or mice lacking the
C-terminus domain, to develop an overt phenotype was also of concern in spite of
the reduction in axonal caliber. However, many of the models do demonstrate a
reduction in the number of motor neurons, impairments in conduction velocity,
impaired axonal regeneration, or concomitant reductions in the expression of other
NF proteins. For instance, the NF-L knockout mice show a significant reduction in
both NF-M and NF-H protein levels.

In part, some of these results can be attributed to genetic strain backgrounds,
increasingly recognized as a key determinant of the phenotypic expression of a number
of transgenic mice. A more critical observation is, however, that a specific temporal
profile exists with regards to the neuropathological process of motor neuron degeneration in these models, an observation lacking from the literature. Quite simply, the
analysis may have been too early and too restricted to the effect on neuronal cell
populations alone. This is exemplified by an analysis of the natural history of NF aggregate formation in two murine transgenic models of motor neuron degeneration: NF-L
(−/−) in which the NF-L is not expressed, or hNF-L (+/+) in which the human NF-L
protein is over-expressed (69,70). The formation of NF aggregates is clearly time-
dependent in both transgenics being maximal by 4 to 6 months of age (127). In the case
of NF-L (−/−), the majority (>90%) of motor neurons contained NF aggregates,

whereas 40% to 50% of the hNF-L (+/+) motor neurons are aggregate bearing. Thereafter, there is a relentless decline in the number of NF-aggregate bearing neurons such that in mice that are 12 months of age; few NF aggregate bearing neurons remain. By 18 months, motor neuron numbers are reduced, with the majority of remaining aggregate-bearing neurons being large motor neurons in the lateral fasciculus. In both instances, but most profoundly in the NF-L (−/−) mice, the formation of NF aggregates is accompanied by a robust microglial inflammatory response in the adjacent neuropil. This too, however, is self-limited, being maximal by 4 to 12 months, declining thereafter until only minimal microglial proliferation is observed by 15 to 18 months. Only the NF-L (−/−) mice demonstrate significant astrogliosis, beginning at month six, becoming maximal by 12 months, and declining thereafter.

This temporal relationship among the appearance and subsequent loss of motor neuron NF aggregates, and the microglial and astrocytic responses, suggests that stage-specific neuropathological phenotypes exist, including (i) an early NF aggregate predominant variant with preserved motor neuron numbers with profound microglial activation, (ii) an intermediate phase of prominent NF-aggregate bearing neurons with reduced motor neuron numbers accompanied by a robust microglial proliferative response with early astrogliosis, and (iii) a late (>12 months) response with few NF-aggregate bearing neurons, minimal microglial proliferation, and prominent astrogliosis (Fig. 4).

The utility for such models in understanding the pathogenesis of ALS thus lie in their ability to not only recapitulate specific aspects of the motor neuron degeneration of ALS, but in providing a window to view the complex inter-relationship between motor neuron degeneration and adjacent non-neuronal cells. In contrast to transgenic models in which the timing of disease onset at the individual motor neuron level is relatively homogeneous, ALS motor neuron degeneration is non-homogeneous and thus one should not be surprised to see varying levels of NF aggregate formation, motor neuron loss, microglial proliferation, and astrogliosis—even among differing regions of the same individual spinal cord.

Neurofilamentous aggregates also intensely colocalize peripherin, a related intermediate filament protein. The over-expression of the most abundant isoforms of peripherin (per58) induces motor neuron degeneration in vivo (71). In addition, the expression of a more neurotoxic splice variant (per61) that induces motor neuron death in vitro has been observed in ALS lumbar spinal motor neurons (32). It is of interest that the regulation of peripherin expression may be driven by microglial factors, in particular TNF-α, again stressing the close inter-relationship between neuronal and non-neuronal cells in ALS (72).

A difficult observation to reconcile is the impact that alterations in NF expression have on transgenic mice that also express mutant copper/zinc superoxide dismutase (SOD1). In these latter mice, reductions in the expression of axonal NF, in association with an increased level of either NF-M or NF-H expression within the perikaryon, result in a slowing of disease progression. The most impressive prolongation of survival in the SOD1^{G93A} mutant is associated with increased expression of NF-H, resulting in five months improved survivorship (73). To date, there has not been a satisfactory explanation for such a phenomenon, although it is tantalizing to suggest that the formation of intraneuronal aggregates associated with alterations in NF expression results in the sequestration, or buffering, of key cellular proteins or oxidative species, thus reducing their impact on neuronal function. One such example is the presence of cyclin-dependant kinase 5 (cdk5) colocalizing to NF aggregates in SOD1^{G37R} mice (74). An alternate hypothesis would hold that

2 months   6 months   9 months   12 months   18 months

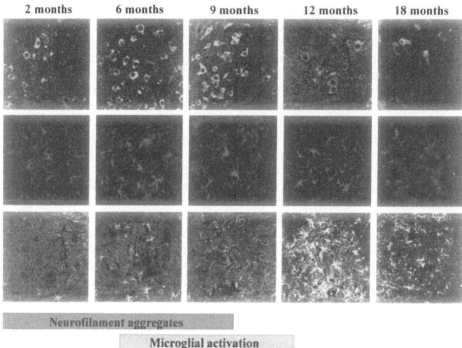

Neurofilament aggregates

Microglial activation

Astrocytic activation

Figure 4 The temporal pattern of neurofilamentous aggregate formation in a transgenic
NF-L knockout. Transgenic mice will be autopsied at time points of 2, 6, 9, 12, and 18 months
of age and paraffin embedded lumbar sections immunostained and viewed by confocal microscopy for either NF-H (SMI-31 monoclonal antibody; row 1), microglia (Iba-1 monoclonal
antibody, row 2), or astrocytes (antiGFAP polyclonal antibody; row 3). A schematic representation of the time course of neurofilament aggregate predominance (0–9 months), microglial
proliferation (6–12 months), and astrocytic proliferation (10–18 months) suggests that the
up-regulation of both microglial and astrocytes in response to motor neuron injury precipitated by the presence of neurofilamentous inclusions follows a specific hierarchical pattern.
(*See color insert.*)

reduced levels of axonal NF expression results in reduced axonal transport of mutant
SOD1, thereby modulating its extent of damage (75).

Post-Translational Modifications of NF Expression in ALS

Based on the observation of highly phosphorylated NF aggregation in ALS, it has
been tempting to suggest that NF aggregate formation in ALS is due to alterations
in the phosphorylation state of the NF subunit proteins, particularly NF-H. To date,
however, there has been no evidence to support such a process, and indeed NF-H
isolated from patients with ALS shows no alteration in phosphorylation state
beyond that observed in age-matched control cases (76).

The observation of mutant SOD1 in familial ALS raised the intriguing possibility
of an alteration in the extent of reactive nitrating species formation in ALS. In immunohistochemical studies, it had been proposed that through the SOD1-mediated catalysis
of peroxynitrite, an enhanced level of reactive nitrating species formation would be

evident in ALS (53,77). In support of this, concentrations of free 3-nitrotyrosine (a specific marker of reactive nitrating species formation) and its metabolite, 3-nitro-4-hydroxyphenol acetic acid as measured by HPLC chromatography, are elevated in spinal cord homogenates of ALS patients compared to controls and are reminiscent of those observed in transgenic mice expressing the human $SOD1^{G93A}$ mutation (78,79). When bovine brain homogenates were incubated with peroxynitrite and SOD1 in vitro, NF-L was observed to be the primary intraneuronal protein targeted for nitration, suggesting a potential role for NF-L in mediating oxidative injury through buffering reactive nitrating species, a postulate supported by the finding of equivalent levels of NF-L nitration in both ALS and control derived NF-L (80,81). Using dissociated monolayer cultures of murine spinal motor neurons from either NF-L (–/–) or hNF-L (+/+) mice in which NF aggregates occur within 14 days post-plating, NF-L deficient neurons were shown to be distinctly more sensitive to oxidative injury (82). This observation lends support to the hypothesis that NF-L can be served to protect against toxicity mediated by reactive nitrating species. A deficiency of NF-L protein might thus be predicted to increase the susceptibility of motor neurons to an oxidative stress beyond its role in leading to the formation of NF aggregates.

Intraneuronal Neurofilamentous Aggregate Formation—Impact on Cellular Metabolism

The formation of neurofilamentous aggregates will also have a significant effect on neuronal metabolism. We have already addressed the observation of nNOS sequestration to the aggregate and failure of NMDA down-regulation (83), but in addition, NF-L deficient neurons are at a heightened risk for oxidatively mediated cell death (82). The formation of perikaryal aggregates is also associated with the sequestration and deregulation of cdk5 in transgenic mice expressing a mutant SOD1 (74). This may not be deleterious, however, in that the formation of neurofilamentous aggregates in mutant SOD1 transgenic mice improves survival, perhaps by buffering cdk5 activity.

This does not, however, explain the colocalization of NF-L, nitrotyrosine, and nNOS immunoreactivity within neurofilamentous aggregates of ALS. To examine this, we first demonstrated in NGF-differentiated PC12 cells that, in the absence of neurofilamentous aggregates, the application of a NMDA agonist would lead to an up-regulation of the expression of nNOS (84). While unexpected, the studies also demonstrated that synchronously with the up-regulation of nNOS expression and the generation of NO, there was a translocation of nNOS from a predominantly cytosolic localization to a membrane-bound localization. We hypothesized that the effect of a neurofilamentous aggregate would be to shunt the nNOS into the neurofilamentous aggregate and thus prevent its translocation to the cell surface membrane, where it would normally down-regulate the NMDA receptor and inhibit calcium influx. Using primary cultures of dissociated motor neurons from either C57Bl/6 or hNF-L(+/+) mice, we have confirmed that this is in fact the case, and that there is a complete disruption of the regulation of calcium influx in response to a NMDA administration (83). This is accompanied by an enhanced rate of motor neuron apoptosis.

NON-IF PROTEIN AGGREGATION

Although the topic of protein aggregation will be further examined in detail elsewhere (Chapter 21), two specific intraneuronal or astrocytic protein aggregates are relevant to this discussion of alterations in cytoskeletal protein metabolism in ALS. The first, aggregation of tau protein, relates specifically to the occurrence of cognitive dysfunction in ALS. The second, aggregation of mutant SOD1 protein, is of direct relevance to understanding the complex inter-relationship between the cytoskeleton, especially NF, and the mechanisms of mutant SOD1-mediated neuro-degeneration.

Tau Protein

As discussed in a previous chapter (Chapter 6), the occurrence of a frontotemporal lobar degeneration (FTLD) is increasingly recognized in ALS with estimates ranging from 30% to 70% of the ALS population having some component of a frontotemporal lobar degenerative syndrome (85–87). Thus, in addition to the core features of ALS described above, one must include the neuropathological characteristics of FTLD in ALS, among which are tau immunoreactive intraneuronal aggregates. Tau immunoreactive thread-like structures have been described in the neuropil and in glial cells (as coiled bodies) in the hippocampus, parahippocampal gyrus, and amygdala of ALS patients (88). Suggesting that tau aggregate formation may be a more ubiquitous process in ALS, neuronal, extraneuronal, and glial tau aggregates have been observed in both cognitively impaired and cognitively intact ALS subjects (89). Both cognitively intact and cognitively impaired ALS patients demonstrated astrocytic tau immunoreactive inclusions in cortical layer I, deeper cortical layers, and subcortical white matter. Unique to cognitively impaired ALS patients has been the observation of extraneuronal tau aggregates that appear as curvilinear neuropil threads, argyrophilic granules, or as dense rounded aggregates with irregular fibrillary margins. We have subsequently reported that tau isolated from ALS patients, particularly within the frontal cortex and subcortical white matter, is more highly detergent insoluble than that isolated from neurologically normal control patients, and that this correlated with tau hyperphosphorylation (90).

This observation is reminiscent of that of the ALS/parkinsonism–dementia complex of Guam in which ALS and parkinsonism/dementia can coexist in the same individual (91–93). Tau-immunoreactive neuronal inclusions have been observed throughout frontal cortical layers II and III, reminiscent of the distribution of neurofibrillary tangles (NFT) in Guamanian ALS/parkinsonism–dementia patients (94). Severe cortical atrophy and widespread NFT formation are among the neuropathological hallmarks of this disorder with the NFTs bearing the immunohistochemical and ultrastructural characteristics of Alzheimer disease NFTs (95–99). In this entity, highly insoluble, hyperphosphorylated tau (the fundamental constituent of the NFT) is evident (100).

The association of ALS with disturbances in tau metabolism is also apparent from studies of dementia with parkinsonism due to mutations in the tau gene on chromosome 17 (FTDP-17) (101,102). At the core of the FTDP-17 syndrome are behavioral changes, psychosis, loss of executive functioning, and for the majority of variants, a lack of motor phenomenon with the exception of a progressive loss of speech output. However, among more than 30 kindreds with FTD having linkage to chromosome 17, corticospinal disturbances, muscle wasting, and fasciculations typical of ALS have been found in 4. Tau immunoreactive neuropil threads are prominent as are glial tangles and dense intracellular deposits of tau.

Thus, among the cytoskeletal protein alterations known to be associated with ALS, we must now include alterations of tau protein metabolism and the formation of intracellular protein aggregates thought to be the consequence of these processes.

Copper/Zinc Superoxide Dismutase

The expression of mutant forms of copper/zinc SOD1 is associated with formation of ubiquitin-immunoreactive intraneuronal and astrocytic SOD1 protein aggregates. This is consistent in both transgenic mice expressing mutant SOD1 protein and in type I familial ALS patients (103,104). In addition, mutant SOD1 induced aggregates colocalize dorfin, a RING finger-type E3 ubiquitin ligase, important for targeting for proteosomal degradation. The origin of these SOD1 aggregates is not yet entirely clear, although mutant SOD1 and not wild-type form detergent insoluble aggregates that associate with Hsp70 and Hsp 40 (105). The critical role of Hsp 70 in preventing protein folding and aggregation has been demonstrated by the observation that increased Hsp 70 expression in cultured primary motor neurons harboring mutant SOD1 (G93A) reduces the extent of SOD1 aggregate formation and prolongs survival (106). The failure to express HSF1 in motor neurons, required for upregulation of Hsp 70 expression, may place motor neurons at a heightened risk for SOD1 aggregate formation (107).

CONCLUSIONS

Among the competing theories for the pathogenesis of ALS, none has gained supremacy as being clearly linked to the triggering of the disease process. In part, this is almost certainly due to the tight integration among the many disturbances in neuronal metabolism in ALS. The exact role that alterations in IF metabolism can play in the disease process remains to be fully defined, but if ALS is viewed as a disorder of protein aggregation, then IFs must be considered a primary target. There is little doubt that altering the stoichiometry of expression of IF, and specifically of NF, induces motor neuron degeneration in those neurons in which NF are the most abundant protein. The pathology observed in transgenic mice in which NF stoichiometry is altered is variable in terms of severity and in clinical phenotype, but in two such transgenics in which the human disease state is most closely recapitulated [NF-L (–/–) with or without peripherin over-expression], it is parallel to ALS. Moreover, the former shows a clear age dependency in the development of a phenotype, and the temporal correlation between NF aggregate formation and motor neuron death with astrocytic and microglial activation is striking.

Once established, intraneuronal proteinaceous aggregates are not insoluble rocks with no dynamic impact. They serve as sinks for the mislocalization of a variety of proteins, including SOD1, nNOS, dorfin, and cdk5. In doing so, fundamental alterations in cellular metabolism are induced, including alterations in NMDA-mediated calcium influx.

Understanding the genesis of these alterations in neuronal cytoskeletal protein has been the domain of few labs in the recent decade. However, just as NF aggregates serve to recruit a number of metabolic players to become integrated within them, perhaps these advances will serve to recruit others into understanding their biology as it applies to ALS.

ACKNOWLEDGMENTS

Research support Canadian Institutes of Health Research (CIHR NRP) (MJS and JPJ), The American ALS Association (ALSA) (MJS), the NIH (JPJ), and the Robert Packard Centre for ALS Research at Johns Hopkins (JPJ).

REFERENCES

1. Wharton S, Ince PG. Pathology of motor neuron disorders. In: Shaw PJ, Strong MJ, eds. Motor Neuron Disorders. Philadelphia: Butterworth Heinemann, 2003:17–50.
2. Bignami A, Raju T, Dahl D. Localization of vimentin, the nonspecific intermediate filament protein, in embryonal glia and in early differentiating neurons. In vivo and in vitro immunofluorescence study of the rat embryo with vimentin and neurofilament antisera. Dev Biol 1982; 91:286–295.
3. Shaw G, Weber K. Differential expression of neurofilament triplet proteins during brain development. Nature 1982; 298:277–279.
4. Cochard P, Paulin D. Initial expression of neurofilaments and vimentin in the central and peripheral nervous system of the mouse embryo in vivo. J Neurosci 1984; 4:2080–2094.
5. Hoffman PN, Cleveland DW, Griffin JW, Landes PW, Cowan NJ, Price DL. Neurofilament gene expression: a major determinant of axonal caliber. Proc Natl Acad Sci USA 1987; 84:3472–3476.
6. Fliegner KH, Ching GY, Liem RKH. The predicted amino acid sequence of α-internexin is that of a novel neuronal intermediate filament protein. EMBO 1990; 9:749–755.
7. Kaplan MP, Chin SSM, Fliegner KH, Liem RKH. α-Internexin, a novel neuronal intermediate filament protein, precedes the low molecular weight neurofilament protein (NF-L) in the developing rat brain. J Neurosci 1990; 10:2735–2748.
8. Schlaepfer WW, Bruce J. Simultaneous up-regulation of neurofilament proteins during the postnatal development of the rat nervous system. J Neurosci Res 1990; 25:39–49.
9. Kost SA, Chacko K, Oblinger MM. Developmental patterns of intermediate filament gene expression in the normal hamster brain. Brain Res 1992; 95:270–280.
10. Nixon RA, Shea TB. Dynamics of neuronal intermediate filaments: a developmental perspective. Cell Motil Cytoskel 1992; 22:81–91.
11. Athlan ES, Sacher MG, Mushynski WE. Associations between intermediate filament proteins expressed in cultured dorsal root ganglion neurons. J Neurosci Res 1997; 47:300–310.
12. Giasson BI, Mushynski WE. Developmentally regulated stabilization of neuronal intermediate filaments in rat cerebral cortex. Neurosci Lett 1997; 229:77–80.
13. Trojanowski JQ, Walkenstein N, Lee VMY. Expression of neurofilament subunits in neurons of the central and peripheral nervous system: an immunohistochemical study with monoclonal antibodies. J Neurosci 1986; 6:650–660.
14. Geisler N, Fischer S, Vandekerckhove J, Van Damme J, Plessmann U, Weber K. Protein-chemical characterization of NF-H, the largest mammalian neurofilament component; intermediate filament-type sequences followed by a unique carboxy-terminal extension. EMBO 1985; 4:57–63.
15. Ching GY, Liem RKH. Assembly of type IV neuronal intermediate filaments in non-neuronal cells in the absence of preexisting cytoplasmic intermediate filaments. J Cell Biol 1993; 122:1323–1335.
16. Lee MK, Xu Z, Wong PC, Cleveland DW. Neurofilaments are obligate heteropolymers in vivo. J Cell Biol 1993; 122:1337–1350.
17. Sihag RK, Nixon RA. Identification of Ser-55 as a major protein kinase A phosphorylation site on the 70-kDa subunit of neurofilaments. J Biol Chem 1991; 266:18861–18867.

18. Heins S, Wong PC, Muller S, Goldie K, Cleveland DW, Aebi U. The rod domain of NF-L determines neurofilament architecture, whereas the end domains specifiy filament assembly and network formation. J Cell Biol 1993; 123:1517–1533.

19. Hisanaga S, Gonda Y, Inagaki M, Ikai A, Hirokawa N. Effects of phosphorylation on neurofilament L protein on neurofilamentous structures. Cell Regul 1990; 1:237–248.

20. Nakamura Y, Takeda M, Angelides KJ, Tanaka T, Tada K, Nishimura T. Effect of phosphorylation on 68 kDa neurofilament subunit protein assembly by the cyclic AMP dependant protein kinase in vitro. Biochem Biophys Res Comm 1990; 169:744–750.

21. Gill SR, Wong PC, Monteiro MJ, Cleveland DW. Assembly properties of dominant and recessive mutations in the small mouse neurofilament (NF-L) subunit. J Cell Biol 1990; 111:2005–2019.

22. Schmalbruch H, Jensen H-JS, Bjaerg M, Kamieniecka Z, Kurland L. A new mouse mutant with progressive motor neuronopathy. J Neuropathol Exp Neurol 1991; 50:192–204.

23. Lee MK, Marszalek JR, Cleveland DW. A mutant neurofilament subunit causes massive, selective motor neuron death: implications for the pathogenesis of human motor neuron disease. Neuron 1994; 13:975–988.

24. Schwartz ML, Bruce J, Shneidman PS, Schlaepfer WW. Deletion of 3′-untranslated region alters the level of mRNA expression of a neurofilament light subunit transgene. J Biol Chem 1995; 270:26,364–26,369.

25. Cañete-Soler R, Silberg DG, Gershon MD, Schlaepfer WW. Mutation in neurofilament transgene implicates RNA processing in the pathogenesis of neurodegenerative disease. J Neurosci 1999; 19:1272–1283.

26. Figlewicz DA, Krizus A, Martinoli MG, Meininger V, Dib M, Rouleau GA, Julien JP. Variants of the heavy neurofilament subunit are associated with the development of amyotrophic lateral sclerosis. Hum Mol Genet 1994; 3:1757–1761.

27. Al-Chalabi A, Andersen PM, Nilsson D, Chioza B, Andersson JL, Russ C, et al. Deletions of the heavy neurofilament subunit tail in amyotrophic lateral sclerosis. Hum Mol Genet 1999; 8:157–164.

28. Rooke K, Figlewicz DA, Han FY, Rouleau GA. Analysis of the KSP repeat of the neurofilament heavy subunit in familial amyotrophic lateral sclerosis. Neurology 1996; 46:789–790.

29. Tomkins J, Usher P, Slade JY, Ince PG, Curtis A, Bushby K, et al. Novel insertion in the KSP region of the neurofilament heavy gene in amyotrophic lateral sclerosis (ALS). NeuroReport 1998; 9:3697–3670.

30. Meyer MA, Potter NT. Sporadic ALS and chromosome 22: evidence for a possible neurofilament gene defect. Muscle Nerve 1995; 18:536–539.

31. Landon F, Lemonnier M, Benarous R, Huc C, Fiszman M, Gros F, et al. Multiple mRNAs encode peripherin, a neuronal intermediate filament protein. EMBO 1989; 8: 1719–1726.

32. Robertson J, Doroudchi MM, Nguyen MD, Durham HD, Strong MJ, Shaw G, et al. A neurotoxic peripherin splice variant in a mouse model of ALS. J Cell Biol 2003; 160:939–949.

33. Gros-Louis F, Larivière RC, Gowing G, Laurent S, Camu W, Bouchard J-P, et al. A frameshift deletion in peripherin gene associated with amyotrophic lateral sclerosis. J Biol Chem 2004; 279(44):45,951–45,956.

34. LaMonte BH, Wallace KE, Holloway BA, Shelly SS, Ascano J, Tokito M, et al. Disruption of dynein/dynactin inhibits axonal transport in motor neurons causing late-onset progressive degeneration. Neuron 2002; 34:715–727.

35. Hafezparast M, Klocke R, Ruhrberg C, Marquardt A, Ahmad-Annuar A, Bowen S, et al. Mutations in dynein link motor neuron degeneration to defects in retrograde transport. Science 2003; 300:808–812.

36. Puls I, Jonnakuty C, LaMonte BH, Holzbaur EL, Tokito M, Mann E, et al. Mutant dynactin in motor neuron disease. Nat Genet 2003; 33:455–456.

37. Zhao C, Takita J, Tanaka Y, Setou M, Nakagawa T, Takeda S, et al. Charcot-Marie-Tooth disease type 2A caused by mutation in a microtubule motor KIF1Bbeta. Cell 2001; 105:587–597.

38. Xia CH, Roberts EA, Her LS, Liu X, Williams DS, Cleveland DW, et al. Abnormal neurofilament transport caused by targeted disruption of neuronal kinesin heavy chain KIF5A. J Cell Biol 2003; 161:55–66.

39. Bommel H, Xie G, Rossol W, Wiese S, Jablonka S, Boehm T, et al. Missense mutation in the tubulin-spedific chaperone E (Tbce) gene in the mouse mutnt progressive motor neuronopathy, a model of human motoneuron disease. J Cell Biol 2002; 159:563–569.

40. Martin N, Jaubert J, Gounon P, Salido E, Haase G, Szatanik M, et al. A missense mutation in Tbce causes progressive motor neuronopathy in mice. Nat Genet 2002; 32:455–456.

41. Bomont P, Cavalier L, Blondeau F, Ben Hamida C, Belal S, Tazir M, et al. The gene encoding gigaxonin, a new member of the cytoskeletal BTB/kelch repeat family, is mutated in giant axonal neuropathy. Nat Genet 2000; 26:370–374.

42. Ding J, Liu JJ, Kowal AS, Nardine T, Bhattacharya P, Lee A, et al. Microtubule-associated protein 1B: a neuronal binding partner for gigaxonin. J Cell Biol 2002; 158: 427–433.

43. Ishihara T, Hong M, Zhang B, Nakagawa Y, Lee MK, Trojanowski JQ, et al. Age-dependant emergence and progression of a tauopathy in transgenic mice overexpressing the shortest human tau isoform. Neuron 1999; 24:751–762.

44. Carpenter S. Proximal axonal enlargement in motor neuron disease. Neurology 1968; 18:841–851.

45. Delisle MB, Carpenter S. Neurofibrillary axonal swellings and amyotrophic lateral sclerosis. J Neurol Sci 1984; 63:241–250.

46. Averback P. Unusual particles in motor neuron disease. Arch Pathol Lab Med 1981; 105:490–493.

47. Wada M, Uchihara T, Nakamura A, Oyanagi K. Bunina bodies in amyotrophic lateral sclerosis on Guam: a histochemical, immunohistochemical and ultrastructural investigation. Acta Neuropathol 1999; 98:150–156.

48. Murayama S, Mori H, Ihara Y, Bouldin W, Suzuki K, Tomonaga M. Immunocytochemical and ultrastructural studies of lower motor neurons in amyotrophic lateral sclerosis. Ann Neurol 1990; 27:137–148.

49. Leigh PN, Dodson A, Swash M, Brion J-P, Anderton BH. Cytoskeletal abnormalities in motor neuron disease. An immunohistochemical study. Brain 1989; 112:521–535.

50. Migheli A, Pezzulo T, Attanasio A, Schiffer D. Peripherin immunoreactive structures in amyotrophic lateral sclerosis. Lab Invest 1993; 68:185–191.

51. Wong N, He BP, Strong MJ. Characterization of neuronal intermediate filament protein expression in cervical spinal motor neurons in sporadic amyotrophic lateral sclerosis (ALS). J Neuropathol Exp Neurol 2000; 59:972–982.

52. Strong MJ. Neurofilament metabolism in sporadic amyotrophic lateral sclerosis. J Neurol Sci 1999; 169:170–177.

53. Chou SM, Wang HS, Komai K. Colocalization of NOS and SOD1 in neurofilament accumulation within motor neurons of amyotrophic lateral sclerosis: an immunohistochemical study. J Chem Neuroanat 1996; 10:249–258.

54. Chou SM, Wang HS, Taniguchi A. Role of SOD-1 and nitric oxide/cyclic GMP cascade on neurofilament aggregation in ALS/MND. J Neurol Sci 1996; 139:16–26.

55. Shibata N, Hirano A, Klapporth K. Immunohistochemical demonstration of Cu/Zn superoxide dismutase in the spinal cord of patients with familial amyotrophic lateral sclerosis. Acta Histochem Cytochem 1993; 26:619–621.

56. Shibata N, Hirano A, Kobayashi M, Siddique T, Deng H-X, Hung W-Y, et al. Intense superoxide dismutase-1 immunoreactivity in intracytoplasmic hyaline inclusions of familial amyotrophic lateral sclerosis with posterior column involvement. J Neuropathol Exp Neurol 1996; 55:481–490.

57. Chou SM, Taniguchi A, Wang HS, Festoff BW. Serine = serine protease-like complexes within neurofilament conglomerates of motoneurons in amyotrophic lateral sclerosis. J Neurol Sci 1998; 160:S73–S79.

58. Kato T, Kurita K, Seino T, Kadoya T, Horie H, Wada M, et al. Gelatin-1 is a component of neurofilamentous lesions in sporadic and familial amyotrophic lateral sclerosis. Biochem Biophys Res Comm 2001; 282:166–172.

59. Bergeron C, Beric-Maskarel K, Muntasser S, Weyer L, Somerville M, Percy ME. Neurofilament light and polyadenylated mRNA levels are decreased in amyotrophic lateral sclerosis motor neurons. J Neuropathol Exp Neurol 1994; 53:221–230.

60. Miller FD, Tetzlaff W, Bisby MA, Fawcett JW, Milner RJ. Rapid induction of the major embryonic α-tubulin mRNA, Tα1, during nerve regeneration in adult rats. J Neurosci 1989; 9:1452–1463.

61. Tetzlaff W, Alexander SW, Miller FD, Bisby MA. Response of facial and rubrospinal neurons to axotomy: changes in mRNA expression for cytoskeletal proteins and GAP-43. J Neurosci 1991; 11:2528–2544.

62. Menzies FM, Grierson AJ, Cookson MR, Heath PR, Tomkins J, Figlewicz DA, et al. Selective loss of neurofilament expression in Cu/Zn superoxide dismutase (SOD1) linked amyotrophic lateral sclerosis. J Neurochem 2002; 82:1118–1128.

63. Strong MJ, Leystra-Lantz C, Ge W. Intermediate filament steady state mRNA levels in amyotrophic lateral sclerosis (ALS). Biochem Biophys Res Comm 2004; 316:317–322.

64. Ge W, Leystra-Lantz C, Wen W, Strong MJ. Selective loss of trans-acting instability determinants of neurofilament mRNA in amyotrophic lateral sclerosis spinal cord. J Biol Chem 2003; 278:26558–26563.

65. Ge WW, Wen W, Strong WL, Leystra-Lantz C, Strong MJ. Mutant copper/zinc superoxide dismutase binds to and destabilizes human low molecular weight neurofilament mRNA. J Biol Chem 2005; 280(1):118–124.

66. Côte F, Collard J-F, Julien J-P. Progressive neuronopathy in transgenic mice expressing the human neurofilament heavy gene: a mouse model of amyotrophic lateral sclerosis. Cell 1993; 73:35–46.

67. Collard J-F, Côté F, Julien J-P. Defective axonal transport in a transgenic mouse model of amyotrophic lateral sclerosis. Nature 1995; 375:61–64.

68. Xu Z, Cork LC, Griffin JW, Cleveland DW. Increased expression of neurofilament subunit NF-L produces morphological alterations that resemble the pathology of human motor neuron disease. Cell 1993; 73:23–33.

69. Zhu Q, Couillard-Després S, Julien J-P. Delayed maturation of regenerating myelinated axons in mice lacking neurofilaments. Exp Neurol 1997; 148:299–316.

70. Julien J-P, Tretjakoff I, Beaudet L, Peterson A. Expression and assembly of a human neurofilament protein in transgenic mice provide a novel neuronal marking system. Genes Dev 1987; 1:1085–1095.

71. Beaulieu J-M, Nguyen MD, Julien J-P. Late-onset death of motor neurons in mice overexpressing wild-type peripherin. J Cell Biol 1999; 147:531–544.

72. Robertson J, Beaulieu J-M, Doroudchi MM, Durham HD, Julien J-P, Mushynski WE. Apoptotic death of neurons exhibiting peripherin aggregates is mediated by the proinflammatory cytokine tumor necrosis factor-α. J Cell Biol 2001; 155:217–226.

73. Couillard-Després S, Zhu Q, Wong PC, Price DL, Cleveland DW, Julien J-P. Protective effect of neurofilament heavy gene overexpression in motor neuron disease induced by mutant superoxide dismutase. Proc Natl Acad Sci USA 1998; 95: 9626–9630.

74. Nguyen MD, Larivière RC, Julien J-P. Deregulation of Cdk5 in a mouse model of ALS: toxicity alleviated by perikaryal neurofilament inclusions. Neuron 2001; 30:135–147.

75. Williamson TL, Bruijn LI, Zhu Q, Anderson KL, Anderson SD, Julien J-P, et al. Absence of neurofilaments reduces the selective vulnerability of motor neurons and slows disease caused by a familial amyotrophic lateral sclerosis-linked superoxide dismutase 1 mutant. Proc Natl Acad Sci USA 1998; 95:9631–9636.

76. Strong MJ, Strong WL, Jaffe H, Traggert B, Sopper MM, Pant HC. Phosphorylation state of the native high molecular weight neurofilament subunit protein (NFH) from cervical spinal cord in sporadic amyotrophic lateral sclerosis. J Neurochem 2001; 76:1315–1325.

77. Abe K, Pan L-H, Watanabe M, Kato T, Itoyama Y. Induction of nitrotyrosine-like immunoreactivity in the lower motor neuron of amyotrophic lateral sclerosis. Neurosci Lett 1996; 199:152–154.

78. Ferrante RJ, Shinobu LA, Schulz JB, Matthews RT, Thomas CE, Kowall NW, et al. Increased 3-nitrotyrosine and oxidative damage in mice with a human copper/zinc superoxide dismutase mutation. Ann Neurol 1997; 42:326–334.

79. Beal FM, Ferrante RJ, Browne SE, Matthews RT, Kowall NW, Brown RH Jr. Increased 3-nitrotyrosine in both sporadic and familial amyotrophic lateral sclerosis. Ann Neurol 1997; 42:646–654.

80. Crow JP, Ye YZ, Strong MJ, Kirk M, Barnes S, Beckman JS. Superoxide dismutase catalyzes nitration of tyrosines by peroxynitrite in the rod and head domains of neuro-filament-L. J Neurochem 1997; 69:1945–1953.

81. Strong MJ, Sopper MM, Crow JP, Strong WL, Beckman JS. Nitration of the low mole-cular weight neurofilament (NFL) is equivalent in sporadic amyotrophic lateral sclerosis and control cervical spinal cord. Biochem Biophys Res Comm 1998; 248:157–164.

82. Strong MJ, Sopper MM, He BP. In vitro reactive nitrating species toxicity in dissociated spinal motor neurons from NFL (−/−) and hNFL (+/+) transgenic mice. ALS Other Motor Neuron Disord 2003; 11:81–89.

83. Sanelli T, Sopper MM, Strong MJ. Sequestration of nNOS in neurofilamentous aggre-gate bearing neurons leads to enhanced glutamate-mediated calcium influx. Brain Res 2004; 1004:8–17.

84. Arundine M, Sanelli T, He BP, Strong MJ. NMDA induces NOS 1 translocation to the cell membrane in NGF-differentiated PC12 cells. Brain Res 2003; 976:149–158.

85. Wilson CM, Grace GM, Munoz DG, He BP, Strong MJ. Cognitive impairment in sporadic ALS. A pathological continuum underlying a multisystem disorder. Neurology 2001; 57:651–657.

86. Strong MJ, Grace GM, Orange JB, Leeper HA, Menon R, Aere C. A prospective study of cognitive impairment in ALS. Neurology 1999; 53:1665–1670.

87. Lomen-Hoerth C, Murphy J, Langmore S, Kramer JH, Olney RK, Miller B. Are amyo-trophic lateral sclerosis patients cognitively normal? Neurology 2003; 60:1094–1097.

88. Noda K, Katayama S, Watanabe C, Yamamura Y, Nakamura S. Gallyas- and tau-positive glial strucutres in motor neuron disease with dementia. Clin Neuropath 1999; 18:218–225.

89. Yang W, Sopper MM, Leystra-Lantz C, Strong MJ. Microtubule-associated tau protein positive neuronal and glial inclusions in amyotrophic lateral sclerosis. Neurology 2003; 61:1766–1773.

90. Strong MJ, Yang W, Strong WL, Pant H. Insoluble tau protein isoforms in amyotrophic lateral sclerosis with cognitive impairment (ALSci). Neurology 2004; 62(suppl 5):A185.

91. Garruto RM. Amyotrophic lateral sclerosis and Parkinsonism-dementia of Guam: Clin-ical, Epidemiological and Genetic Patterns. Am J Hum Biol 1989; 1:367–382.

92. Garruto RM. Cellular and Molecular mechanisms of neuronal degeneration: Amyo-trophic lateral sclerosis, parkinsonism-dementia, and Alzheimer disease. Am J Hum Biol 1989; 1:529–543.

93. Trojanowski JQ, Ishihara T, Higuchi M, Yoshiyama Y, Hong M, Zhang B, et al. Amyotrophic lateral sclerosis/parkinsonism dementia complex: transgenic mice provide insights into mechanisms underlying a common tauopathy in an ethnic minority on Guam. Exp Neurol 2002; 176:1–11.

94. Buée-Scherrer V, Buée L, Hof PR, Leveugle B, Gilles C, Loerzel AJ, et al. Neurofibril-lary degeneration in amyotrophic lateral sclerosis/parkinsonism-dementia complex of Guam. Immunochemical characterization of tau proteins. Am J Pathol 1995; 146: 924–932.

95. Rodgers-Johnson P, Garruto RM, Yanigahara R, Chen KM, Gajdusek DC, Gibbs CJ Jr. Amyotrophic lateral sclerosis and parkinsonism-dementia on Guam: A 30-year evaluation of clinical and neuropathological trends. Neurology 1986; 36:7–13.
96. Shankar SK, Yanagihara R, Garruto RM, Grundke-Iqbal I, Kosik KS, Gajdusek DC. Immunocytochemical characterization of neurofibrillary tangles in amyotrophic lateral sclerosis and Parkinsonism-Dementia of Guam. Ann Neurol 1989; 25:146–151.
97. Hirano A. Neuropathology of amyotrophic lateral sclerosis and parkinsonism-dementia complex on Guam. In: Luthy L, Bischoff A, eds. Proceedings of the fifth international congress of neuropathology. Amsterdam: Excerpta Medica, 1966:190–194.
98. Hirano A, Dembitzer HM, Kurland LT, Zimmerman HM. The fine structure of some intraganglionic alterations: neurofibrillary tangles, granulovacuolar bodies, and "rod-like" structures in Guam amyotrophic lateral sclerosis and parkinsonism-dementia complex. J Neuropathol Exp Neurol 1968; 27:167–182.
99. Hirano A, Arumugasamy N, Zimmerman HM. Amyotrophic lateral sclerosis. A comparison of Guam and classical cases. Arch Neurol 1967; 16:357–363.
100. Buée-Scherrer V, Buée L, Hof PR, Leveugle B, Gilles C, Loerzel AJ, et al. Neurofibrillary degeneration in amyotrophic lateral sclerosis/parkinosnism-dementia complex of Guam. Am J Pathol 1995; 68:924–932.
101. Lee VMY, Goedert M, Trojanowski JQ. Neurodegenerative tauopathies. Ann Rev Neurosci 2001; 24:1121–1159.
102. Foster NL, Wilhelmsen K, Sima AAF, Jones MZ, D'Amato CJ, Gilman S, et al. Frontotemporal dementia and parkinsonism linked to chromosome 17: A consensus conference. Ann Neurol 1997; 41:706–715.
103. Bruijn LI, Houseweart MK, Kato S, Anderson KL, Anderson SD, Ohama E, et al. Aggregation and motor neuron toxicity of an ALS-linked SOD1 mutant independent from wild-type SOD1. Science 1998; 281:1851–1854.
104. Kato S, Horiuchi S, Liu J, Cleveland DW, Shibata N, Nakashima K, et al. Advanced gylcation endproduct-modified superoxide dismutase-1 (SOD-1)-positive inclusions are common to familial amyotrophic lateral sclerosis patients with SOD1 gene mutations and transgenic mice expressing human SOD1 with a G85R mutation. Acta Neuropathol 2000; 100:490–505.
105. Steiber A, Gonatas JO, Gonatas NK. Aggregates of mutant protein appar progressively in dendrites, in periaxonal processes of oligodendrocytes, and in neuronal and astrocytic perikarya of mice expressing the SOD1^{G93A} mutation of familial amyotrophic lateral sclerosis. J Neurol Sci 2000; 177:114–123.
106. Bruening W, Roy J, Giasson B, Figlewicz DA, Mushynski WE, Durham HD. Upregulation of protein chaperones preserves viability of cells expressing toxic Cu/Zn superoxide dismutase mutants associated with amyotrophic lateral sclerosis. J Neurochem 1999; 72:693–699.
107. Batulan Z, Shinder GA, Minotti S, He BP, Doroudchi MM, Strong MJ, et al. The stress response of spinal motor neurons: high threshold for induction of heat shock proteins in primary culture and transgenic mouse models and in patients with amyotrophic lateral sclerosis. J Neurosci 2003; 23:5789–5798.
108. Monteiro MJ, Hoffman PN, Gearhart JD, Cleveland DW. Expression of NF-L in both neuronal and nonneuronal cells of transgenic mice: increased neurofilament density in axons without affecting caliber. J Cell Biol 1990; 11:1543–1557.
109. Levavasseur F, Zhu Q, Julien JP. No requirement of alpha-internexin for nervous system development and for radial growth of axons. Brain Res Mol Brain Res 1999; 69:104–112.
110. Ma D, Descarries L, Julien J-P, Doucet G. Abnormal perikaryal accumulation of neurofilament light protein in the brain of mice transgenic for the human protein: sequence of postnatal development. Neuroscience 1995; 63:135–149.
111. Elder GA, Friedrich VL Jr, Bosco P, Kang C, Gourov A, Tu PH, et al. Absence of the mid-sized neurofilament subunit decreases axonal calibre, levels of light neurofilament (NF-L), and neurofilament content. J Cell Biol 1998; 141:727–739.

112. Elder GA, Friedrich VL Jr, Margita A, Lazzarini RA. Age-related atrophy of motor axons in mice deficient in the mid-sized neurofilament subunit. J Cell Biol 1999; 146:181–192.

113. Lee VM, Elder GA, Chen LC, Liang Z, Snyder SE, Friedrich VL Jr, et al. Expression of human mid-sized neurofilament subunit in transgenic mice. Brain Res Mol Brain Res 1992; 15:76–84.

114. Tu P-H, Elder G, Lazzarini RA, Nelson D, Trojanowski JQ, Lee VMY. Overexpression of the human NFM subunit in transgenic mice modifies the level of endogenous NFL and the phosphorylation state of NFH subunits. J Cell Biol 1995; 129:1629–1640.

115. Vickers JC, Morrison JH, Friedrich VL Jr, Elder GA, Perl DP, Katz RN, et al. Age-associated and cell-type-specific neurofibrillary pathology in transgenic mice expressing the human midsized neurofilament subunit. J Neurosci 1994; 14:5603–5612.

116. Haroutunian V, Zhou Y, Elder G, Li C, Lazzarini RA. Age-dependant spatial memory deficits in transgenic mice expressing the human mid-sized neurofilament gene: I. Mol Brain Res 1996; 42:62–70.

117. Elder GA, Friedrich VL Jr, Pereira D, Tu PH, Zhang B, Lee VM, et al. Mice with disrupted midsized and heavy neurofilament genes lack axonal neurofilaments but have unaltered numbers of axonal microtubules. J Neurosci Res 1999; 57:23–32.

118. Jacomy H, Zhu Q, Couillard-Després S, Beaulieu JM, Julien JP. Disruption of type IV intermediate filament network in mice lacking the neurofilament medium and heavy subunits. J Neurochem 1999; 81:525–532.

119. Elder GA, Friedrich VL Jr, Kang C, Bosco P, Gourov A, Tu PH, et al. Requirement of heavy neurofilament subunit in the development of axons with large calibers. J Cell Biol 1998; 143:195–205.

120. Zhu Q, Lindenbaum M, Levavasseur F, Jacomy H, Julien J-P. Disruption of the NF-H gene increases axonal microtubule content and velocity of neurofilament transport: relief of axonopathy resulting from the toxin beta, beta'-iminodiproprionitrile. J Cell Biol 1998; 143:183–193.

121. Kriz J, Zhu Q, Julien J-P, Padjen AL. Electrophysiological properties of axons in mice knock-out for neurofilament genes: Disparity between conduction velocity and axon diameter in absence of NF-H. Brain Res 2000; 885:32–44.

122. Marszalek JR, Williamson TL, Lee MK, Xu Z, Hoffman PN, Becher MW, et al. Neurofilament subunit NF-H modulates axonal diameter by selectively slowing neurofilament transport. J Cell Biol 1996; 135:711–724.

123. Kriz J, Meier J, Julien J-P, Padjen AL. Altered ionic conductances in axons of transgenic mouse expressing the human neurofilament heavy gene: A mouse model of amyotrophic lateral sclerosis. Exp Neurol 2000 Jun; 163(2):414–421.

124. Rao MV, Houseweart MK, Williamson TL, Crawford TO, Folmer J, Cleveland DW. Neurofilament-dependant radial growth of motor axons and axonal organization of neurofilaments does not requrie the neurofilament heavy subunit (NF-H) or its phosphorylation. J Cell Biol 1998; 143:171–181.

125. Larivière RC, Nguyen MD, Ribeiro-da-Silva A, Julien JP. Reduced number of unmyelinated sensory axons in peripherin null mice. J Neurochem 2002; 81:525–532.

126. Ching GY, Chien C-L, Plores R, Liem RKH. Overexpression of α-internexin causes abnormal neurofilamentous accumulations and motor coordination deficits in transgenic mice. J Neurosci 1999; 19:2974–2986.

127. McLean Jr, Leystra-Lantz C, He B-P, Strong MJ. Temporal profiles of neuronal degeneration, glial proliferation, and cell death in hNFL +/+ and NFL −/− mice. Glia 2005; May 26; [Epub ahead of print].

18

Role of Mitochondria in Motor Neuron Degeneration in ALS

Zuoshang Xu
Department of Biochemistry and Molecular Pharmacology, University of Massachusetts Medical School, Worcester, Massachusetts, U.S.A.

Jiming Kong
Department of Human Anatomy and Cell Science, University of Manitoba, Winnipeg, Manitoba, Canada

INTRODUCTION

Mitochondrial involvement in amyotrophic lateral sclerosis (ALS) was initially suggested by circumstantial evidence from ultrastructural studies in human autopsies. Afifi et al. (1) first reported abnormal mitochondrial morphology in atrophic muscles of ALS patients in 1966. They observed aggregates of mitochondria in subsarcolemmal regions of muscle fibers. The mitochondria were dense and large, and distributed in a pattern of "sentinel mitochondria" along the Z line, perpendicular to the myofibrils. Other studies have supplied a continuous stream of evidence suggesting the involvement of mitochondrial abnormality in the pathogenesis of ALS. Mitochondrial abnormalities and dysfunction have been reported in liver biopsies and peripheral blood lymphocytes from individuals with sporadic ALS (2–4). Atsumi (5) found a reduction in the number of mitochondria in intramuscular nerves. Siklos et al. (6) found increased mitochondrial volume and elevated calcium levels within the mitochondria from muscle biopsy of ALS patients. Although early studies in the central nervous system (CNS) focused on neurofilament accumulation in proximal axons because of their conspicuous presence, careful examination of the published EM micrographs reveals numerous vacuolated mitochondria among swirls of disorganized neurofilaments in both sporadic and familial cases (7). Other studies found numerous abnormal mitochondria in upper and lower motor neurons in human ALS cases (8–10).

Although human studies provided the initial suggestion that mitochondrial degeneration was involved in motor neuron death in ALS, they were limited in two ways. First, in almost all cases, only the end stage pathology could be observed since it was not possible to study pathological changes before disease onset. Second, there was always the issue of postmortem tissue preservation. Poor preservation might result in artifactual changes that did not reflect the true pathology. These limitations have been compensated in recent years because excellent animal models for ALS became available.

HOW MITOCHONDRIAL DEGENERATION DEVELOPS: OBSERVATIONS IN TRANSGENIC MICE EXPRESSING MUTANT CU, ZN SUPEROXIDE DISMUTASE (SOD1)

In 1993, the first genetic cause for ALS was identified as mutations in Cu, Zn superoxide dismutase (SOD1) (see chap. 5). Shortly after this breakthrough, several lines of transgenic mice expressing various SOD1 mutants were generated. These mice develop age-dependent motor neuron degeneration similar to human ALS (11–13), and thus are excellent ALS models. The first studies on mutant SOD1 transgenic mice reported mitochondrial vacuolation as well as neurofilament accumulation in motor neurons (13,14). The neurofilament pathology was expected but the severe mitochondrial abnormalities were a surprise. Nevertheless, an in vitro study suggested that mutant SOD1 could indeed cause mitochondrial damage; when mutant SOD1 was introduced into cultured neuroblastoma cells, mitochondrial damage and dysfunction were observed (15). These early studies raised this question: Was mitochondrial degeneration a crucial step in motor neuron degeneration pathway, or was it merely a byproduct of degenerative process—a consequence of cellular degeneration?

Mitochondrial Degeneration Is an Early Event in Motor Neuron Degeneration Pathway

To answer this question, Kong and Xu (16) took an approach that defines the sequence of the pathological events in a transgenic mouse model that expresses SOD1G93A mutant. The rationale for this approach was that early pathological changes would be more likely to associate with causes than consequences of neuronal degeneration. In contrast, late pathological changes, those that occur at a time when substantial neuronal death had already been underway, were more likely to be consequences of early degenerative processes. Identifying early pathological events would also facilitate the development of therapeutic interventions, as stopping disease progression early in its track enhances the probability of motor neuron rescue. This kind of study would have been impossible in humans, and thus took the full advantage of this robust animal model for ALS.

Because the onset and progression of the disease in the mutant SOD1 transgenic animals were heterogeneous, Kong and Xu first used a muscle strength assay to determine the process of clinical disease progression. By this assay the disease progression was divided into four stages according to the relative muscle strength: a pre-muscle weakness (PMW) stage during which the muscle strength remained steady in mutant mice and was indistinguishable from wild-type mice; a rapid declining (RD) stage during which the muscle strength declined suddenly and precipitously; a slow declining (SD) stage during which the muscle strength declined further but gradually in a prolonged period; and finally the paralysis stage during which one or multiple limbs became totally immobile. Interestingly, similar patterns of clinical progression, particularly the RD of muscle strength at the onset of ALS, have been reported in human longitudinal observations (17,18).

Studies of the animals synchronized for their disease stage revealed several surprises. First, at the RD stage when the disease began (60–90 days before paralysis), the loss of motor neurons was minor (less than 10%). The largest loss of motor neurons occurred at the paralysis stage. This pattern inversely correlated with the changes in the number of active motor neuron degeneration profiles and astrogliosis, which sharply rose at the paralysis stage (16,19). This suggested that early and effective therapeutic intervention after onset of ALS could rescue the majority of motor neurons and prevent further degeneration. Second, deliberate searching for prominent neurofilament abnormalities revealed few sites of neurofilament accumulation, which occurred mostly in late SD and paralysis stages. In contrast, widespread vacuoles in the spinal cord were conspicuous. Importantly, the largest number of these vacuoles was at the RD stage, indicating that vacuoles are a prominent early pathology (16).

Detailed microscopic observations confirmed that these vacuoles were derived from vacuolated mitochondria (16,20,21). The vacuoles developed mostly in neuronal processes, including dendrites and axons. Early stages of mitochondrial vacuolation were observed during the PMW stage, before the onset of the disease (16,22). These observations demonstrate that mitochondrial degeneration is a prominent early event in mutant SOD1-induced motor neuron degeneration.

Mitochondrial Vacuolation by Intermembrane Space Expansion (MVISE)

How do mitochondria become vacuolated in the SOD1G93A mutant mice? Two known mechanisms might provide the answer. The first is mitochondrial permeability transition (MPT), which is classically induced by exposing mitochondria to high concentrations of Ca^{2+}. MPT involves matrix swelling and can be inhibited by cyclosporine A (23). The second is autophagy, which is a cellular mechanism to digest and recycle damaged, old organelles, and cytoplasmic proteins. One step in autophagy is the formation of autophagic vacuoles, which are membrane-bound intracellular vesicles containing proteins and organelles. These vacuoles deliver their contents to lysosomes to be digested and recycled. Increased autophagy has been observed in neurodegenerative diseases including Alzheimer's disease, Huntington's disease, Parkinson's disease, and Friedreich ataxia (24–27). The mitochondrial vacuoles might be developed through either of these two mechanisms. Some evidence suggested that MTP occurs in mutant SOD1-induced motor neuron degeneration (28,29). The involvement of autophagy was a speculation.

Early electron microscopic (EM) observations raised the possibility that mitochondrial vacuoles were developed from the expansion of intermembrane space (20,21). Higgins et al. (22) investigated this issue in detail. On the basis of their EM observations, they proposed a pattern of progression in mitochondrial vacuolation. Initially, mitochondria were swollen and their cristae were disorganized, but they maintained their general structure. The outer membrane then folded at a focal point, forming a small protrusion on the mitochondrial surface and creating a small space between the outer and inner membranes. This might be caused by damage to the attachment structure between the inner and outer mitochondrial membranes. Following the formation of this small protrusion was a further detachment between the inner and outer membranes and expansion of the intermembrane space. As the space became increasingly large, the inner membrane components disintegrated, forming the inner membrane remnants inside the mitochondrial vacuoles (22,30).

This model for mitochondrial vacuolation was plausible because several other studies had shown that both wild-type and mutant SOD1 existed in mitochondrial intermembrane space (31–34). To further verify this model, Higgins et al. (22) localized various markers for different mitochondrial compartments on the vacuoles. They found that the inner mitochondrial membrane marker cytochrome c oxidase was located with the inner membrane remnants inside the vacuoles, while the outer mitochondrial membrane markers were located on the outer vacuolar membrane. Cytochrome c, an intermembrane space marker, colocalized with SOD1 in mitochondria at the beginning stage of vacuolation, but disappeared when the vacuoles enlarged. The disappearance of cytochrome c in large vacuoles could be due to either a dilution of cytochrome c as the intermembrane space expanded, and/or to cytochrome c leaking out of mitochondrial intermembrane space. Further observation that the outer membranes of the large vacuoles were often porous supported the latter possibility. The expansion of the intermembrane space rather than mitochondrial matrix, combined with the evidence showing the involvement of peroxisomes but not lysosomes, suggests that the mutant SOD1-induced mitochondrial vacuolation is neither the classical MPT (which involves expansion of the mitochondrial matrix) nor the autophagic vacuolation (which involves lysosomes), but rather the vacuolation by intermembrane space expansion or MVISE (30,35).

How Mutant SOD1 Damages Mitochondria: The Mechanistic Models

The studies on transgenic mice expressing mutant SOD1G93A or SOD1G37R have provided unequivocal evidence that mitochondrial degeneration is involved in motor neuron degeneration in ALS. However, mitochondrial vacuolation is not observed in all mutant SOD1 transgenic lines. Some SOD1 mutants such as G85R and H46R/H48Q cause motor neuron degeneration without mitochondrial vacuolation (12,36,37). These facts raise the following questions: how does mutant SOD1 damage mitochondria? Is mitochondrial damage involved in all motor neuron degeneration induced by all SOD1 mutants? And more broadly, how could mitochondria be damaged in all ALS cases including the sporadic cases? Definitive answers to these questions are not yet available but we will discuss several alternative, but not necessarily mutually exclusive models.

The first model is based on the hypothesis that aberrant redox chemistry mediated by the SOD1 mutants damage mitochondria. Beckman, Crow, Estevez, and their colleagues (38–40) proposed that the mutated SOD1 had an enhanced activity to catalyze nitration of tyrosine by producing peroxynitrite ($ONOO^-$), which was generated by the reaction of superoxide with nitric oxide. This enhanced activity might be brought about by a reduced Zn^{2+} affinity as a consequence of the mutations. Loss of Zn^{2+} from SOD1 resulted in a structural change so that the Cu^{2+} could be readily reduced to Cu^+ by cellular reductants. This increased the readiness for SOD1 to generate peroxynitrate, a potent oxidative free radical that ultimately produces cellular damage.

Two other groups, Wiedau-Pazos et al. (41) and Yim et al. (42,43), proposed a different mechanism. Their data suggested that the mutant SOD1 had an enhanced peroxidase activity. Yim et al. (44,45) first demonstrated that wild-type SOD1 possessed the peroxidase activity. These two groups produced evidence that this peroxidase activity was elevated in some SOD1 mutants in vitro. This proposal, however, is not universally supported. Singh et al. (46) carried out similar experiments and found no enhancement of the peroxidase activity in several SOD1 mutants.

The mechanism by aberrant redox chemistry could produce direct mitochondrial damage because SOD1 mutants are localized to mitochondria besides the cytoplasm and other organelles (31–34). However, this model has been contradicted by several other experiments. Because both of these two aberrant redox mechanisms required the Cu^{2+} in SOD1, Subramaniam (47) tested these hypotheses by crossing multiple lines of mutant SOD1 transgenic mice with a transgenic line in which the copper chaperone for SOD1 (CCS) expression was eliminated. CCS delivers copper to SOD1 (48,49). In the absence of CCS, the copper content in SOD1 was reduced and the SOD1 activity was reduced by ~85% in mice (49). If the aberrant redox theories were correct, the anticipation was that the motor neuron degeneration should be alleviated because these aberrant redox reactions would be reduced due to a reduction of copper in SOD1. Contrary to this expectation, however, a lack of CCS did not modify the course of ALS (47). Recently, SOD1 mutants that lack copper binding at their active center have been proved to cause motor neuron degeneration in mice (37,50). These experiments suggest that the redox chemistry derived directly from the SOD1 mutants is unlikely to play a prominent role in causing motor neuron degeneration in vivo, although a debate is underway regarding whether copper bound at aberrant sites on SOD1 can still mediate oxidative damage (51–53).

The second model has been proposed by Okado-Matsumoto and Fridovich (31). These investigators and Shinder et al. (54) found that SOD1 mutants interact with several chaperones and chaperone activity was inhibited in SOD1 mutant-expressing cells as well as in the spinal cord of mutant SOD1 transgenic mice (55,56). On the basis of these observations, they proposed that SOD1 mutants inhibit chaperone functions by this interaction and sequestration (31). Because mitochondrial protein import, proper refolding of the imported proteins, and assembly of mitochondrial protein complexes all depend on chaperone functions (57), it is conceivable that mutant SOD1 might damage mitochondrial function by diminishing chaperone functions.

The third model is that mutant SOD1 might damage mitochondria by forming aggregates on mitochondrial membranes. Mutant SOD1 aggregates were first observed on the outer mitochondrial membrane in mitochondrial vacuoles in SOD1G93A transgenic mice (22). Recent biochemical analyses suggest that SOD1 mutants and their aggregates, including G93A, G85R, G37R, and H46R/H48Q and G127X, concentrate in mitochondrial fractions, and the mutant proteins appear to be attached to the outside of mitochondria (58). This association might be mediated by interaction between mutant SOD1 and Bcl-2 (59). Evidence for protein aggregates damaging biomembranes has been reported in studies on Parkinson's disease, where mutant α-synuclein forms aggregates and annular rings on membranes (60), causing permeabilization of membranes (61). Similar annular structures formed by mutant SOD1 have been shown recently (62).

CONSEQUENCES OF MITOCHONDRIAL DYSFUNCTION AND DEGENERATION

Vulnerability of Motor Neuron Mitochondria and the Role of Excitotoxicity

Strong experimental evidence suggests that excitotoxicity plays a role in motor neuron cell death in ALS (see chap. 12). Adult motor neurons express glutamate receptors (63–65) and are susceptible to injury by high concentrations of glutamate receptor agonists (66–69). Glutamate levels are elevated in ALS patients' plasma and cerebrospinal fluid (CSF) (70–72). These abnormalities are likely caused by deficient glutamate transport capacity (73) as confirmed by the observations that inhibitors of glutamate uptake cause selective motor neuron degeneration in organotypic slices (66) and in dissociated spinal cord cultures (74). Although excitotoxicity was initially thought to be associated only with sporadic ALS (75), several experiments suggest that it also plays a role in familial ALS. Expression of mutant SOD1 in cultured motor neurons enhances their sensitivity to excitatory amino acids (76,77). Mutant SOD1 is capable of impairing the function of glial glutamate transporter GLT-1 (78–80), which could increase the extracellular concentration of glutamate. In a transgenic mutant SOD1 rat model, a region-specific reduction in glutamate transporter is correlated with motor neuron degeneration (81). The only drug proven to slow the course of human as well as mouse ALS, riluzole, acts at least in part by antiexcitotoxic mechanisms (82,83).

Mutant SOD1 could enhance the sensitivity to excitotoxicity by damaging mitochondria. Excitotoxicity, in turn, could induce further mitochondrial damage, forming a vicious degenerative cycle. Mitochondrial dysfunction sensitizes neurons to glutamate toxicity (84,85). Conversely, mitochondria in motor neurons are particularly susceptible to mitochondrial calcium overload when exposed to AMPA (86). Importantly, mitochondrial calcium overload appears to be required for neuronal excitotoxicity (86,87). Chronic partial disruption of mitochondrial function causes motor neuron death, which can be inhibited by applying excitatory amino acid blockers, suggesting the involvement of excitotoxicity in mitochondrial dysfunction-induced motor neuron death (88,89). These factors, compounded by a decrease in glutamate clearance by astrocytes, might induce the final motor neuron death by excitotoxicity.

This combined effect of mitochondrial dysfunction and excitotoxicity might explain the selective vulnerability of motor neurons in ALS. Motor neurons are more vulnerable to AMPA induced excitotoxicity than other neurons (86). This could be the result of several characteristics of motor neurons, including their high AMPA receptor density (90), the propensity of their mitochondria to overload calcium during cell excitation (86), and the tendency of their mitochondria to generate high levels of reactive oxygen species (ROS) upon excitatory stimuli (91,92). The unique properties of mitochondria in the spinal cord might be the basis for the susceptibility of motor neurons to mutant SOD1 or other noxious assaults, combined with excitotoxicity (92).

Dysfunction of Oxidative Phosphorylation and Elevation of ROS

One manifestation of mitochondrial damage in ALS is impairment in the mitochondrial energy production system. Electron transport chain (ETC) activities are decreased in muscle biopsies from patients with sporadic ALS (93,94). In the CNS, complexes I, II, and III activities are increased in the cortex of human ALS cases and in mutant SOD1 transgenic mice, suggesting a compensatory reaction in unaffected regions (95,96). In the spinal cord, decreases in the ETC activities have been consistently observed in human ALS and transgenic mice expressing mutant SOD1, particularly in the activities of complexes I and IV (10,34,96–99). Of note, a systematic analysis at different disease stages in mutant SOD1 transgenic mice detected dysfunction of complex I several months before the disease onset and the widespread mitochondrial vacuolation (99).

How the ETC dysfunction is initiated is not clear, but in ALS caused by mutant SOD1, localization and aggregation of mutant SOD1 in mitochondria and compromised chaperone functions might play a role (see section "How Mutant SOD1 Damages Mitochondria: The Mechanistic Models"). The consequence of ETC dysfunction could, perhaps, be predicted. Mitochondrial oxidative phosphorylation produces the proton gradient across the inner mitochondrial membrane (which is used to produce ATP) by transferring electrons through the ETC and finally to oxygen. During this process, some electrons escape the ETC and are captured by oxygen to produce superoxide, which can be converted to other chemically unstable and highly ROS (100). Cells maintain low levels of ROS via its antioxidant defense system, which includes the antioxidant enzymes SOD, glutathione peroxidase, glutathione reductase, and catalase, and small molecular weight compounds such as vitamin E and glutathione (101). Dysfunction of ETC can elevate ROS levels by increasing the escape of electrons from the ETC (101).

Indeed, production of ROS is increased in ALS and this increase appears to associate with the disease onset and progression (102,103). In addition, protein carbonyls and protein nitration, and other oxidative damage indicators in DNA and lipids, are elevated in both ALS patients and mutant SOD1 transgenic mice (104–109). The increased ROS levels could contribute to motor neuron degeneration in two ways. First, ROS can react with cellular macromolecules and disrupt the functions of these molecules as well as the cell. This may be particularly detrimental to mitochondria themselves because of their proximity to ROS. For example, ROS can damage mitochondrial DNA and induce mutations in mitochondrial genes. These mutations can further weaken mitochondrial function including ETC activities, further increasing in ROS production. This establishes a vicious cycle, which could lead to the ultimate mitochondrial destruction. Not surprisingly, increasing mitochondrial antioxidative capacity by overexpression of antioxidative genes such as Mn^{2+} SOD2 and glutathione peroxidase isotype-4 (GPX4) significantly reduces mutant SOD1-mediated motor neuron death (110,111). Likewise, treatment of mutant SOD1G93A transgenic mice with antioxidants modestly slowed the disease progression (83,112–115) (see chap. 13).

The second way ROS may contribute to motor neuron degeneration is that ROS can act as small signaling molecules to stimulate the expression of genes that are associated with inflammation. ROS can activate various transcription factors associated with inflammation, including NF-κB, TNF-α, c-Jun, AP-1, and HIF-1 (116–121). Some of these molecules are increased and activated in ALS (122–125). The consequence of these changes is complex (see chap. 14). Some have roles that might be beneficial, such as up-regulating protective proteins including the heat shock proteins and the antioxidant enzymes. Others may be detrimental because they activate death-inducing proteins such as BNIP3 and Bax to cause further mitochondrial dysfunction and cell death (126–130).

Mitochondrial DNA Mutations and Their Dysfunction

Mitochondrial DNA mutates at a higher rate than nuclear DNA (131,132). This is probably due to its proximity to the source of ROS, which are thought to be responsible for the high mutation rate of mitochondrial DNA (133). Another contributing factor could be its lack of histone coat, as the histone coat might have protective effects against damage by ROS (134). As a consequence, the steady-state level of oxidized bases in mitochondrial DNA appears at least 10-fold higher than the level of nuclear DNA (135). The further increased levels of oxidative stress observed in ALS naturally aroused suspicion that mitochondrial DNA damage might be increased.

Comi, Swerdlow, and their colleagues (136,137) produced first pieces of evidence suggesting mitochondrial DNA damage in ALS. Comi et al. (136) found a case of motor neuron disease with severe complex IV deficiency in the muscle fibers. They found a 5 bp deletion in the mitochondrial DNA coding for subunit I of complex IV, leading to premature termination of translation. Swerdlow et al. (137) created hybrid neuroblastoma cells using mitochondria that were derived from platelets of sporadic ALS patients. They observed reduced ETC activity, increased ROS production, and decreased calcium-buffering capacity in mitochondria from ALS patients. This result, however, was not replicated in a recent study (138).

Several studies confirmed the increased mitochondrial DNA mutations in ALS. Vielhaber et al. (139) found a reduced mitochondrial DNA content and increase in the frequency of mitochondrial DNA mutations. Dhaliwal and Grewal (140) examined a mitochondrial DNA mutation mtDNA^{4977} that was commonly associated with aging and found that, in the ALS patients, the frequency of this mutation was much higher in the motor cortex than in the temporal cortex. This difference was not found in control cases. Similar increases in this mutation were found in skeletal muscle samples from ALS patients (141). Wiedemann et al. (10) analyzed mitochondrial DNA isolated from spinal cords of ALS patients and found that mitochondrial mutations were increased. These data are consistent with the conclusion that mitochondrial DNA mutations are probably not the primary cause for ALS but occur during the pathogenic process because tissues not involved in degeneration did not show an increased mutation rate (140). Further support for this conclusion is the finding by Warita et al. (142). They found increased immunoreactivity to 8-hydroxy-2-deoxyguanosine in the cytoplasm, but not in the nuclei, of spinal cord motor neurons in transgenic mice expressing mutant SOD1G93A, suggesting the presence of oxidative damage in mitochondrial DNA caused by the expression of mutant SOD1. These mutations are likely to further exacerbate mitochondrial dysfunction and degeneration.

Mitochondrial Dysfunction and Cell Death

Detailed mechanism of cell death is discussed in chapter 15. Here we touch upon a few specific points related to the role of mitochondrial dysfunction and degeneration in motor neuron death. The exact mechanism whereby motor neurons die is unclear. What is clear is that this mechanism shares molecular pathways with apoptosis (143). For example, several pro-apoptotic molecules are increased in the spinal cord of ALS patients and in transgenic mice expressing mutant SOD1 (144–146). Caspases 1 and 3, two cysteine proteases key to the apoptosis pathway, are activated in a sequential manner in transgenic mice expressing mutant SOD1 (147,148). Furthermore, therapeutic intervention designed to block apoptosis showed efficacy in mutant SOD1 transgenic mice (144,146,149). Yet the motor neuron death mechanism is unlikely to be the typical apoptosis. Morphological hallmarks of apoptosis, such as chromatin condensation and nuclear shrinkage, have not been observed in mutant SOD1 transgenic mice (Xu, unpublished observations; also see Refs. 21 and 150). Genetic ablation of caspase 11, which is an upstream regulator of caspases 1 and 3, caused significant decrease in caspases 1 and 3 levels in mice, but had no effect on the onset and progression of motor neuron degeneration in mutant SOD1 transgenic mice (151).

Regardless of the exact pathway of motor neuron death in ALS, mitochondria seem involved. In addition to their function in energy production for cells, mitochondria also serve as a pivotal point in controlling cell death programs. Mitochondria participate in both typical and atypical cell death programs (152–157). Damage to mitochondria, either by MVISE or other mechanisms, could release pro-apoptotic proteins that reside in the mitochondrial intermembrane space, such as cytochrome c, AIF, SMAC/DIABLO, endo G, and Htra/Omi. The absence of cytochrome c in the porous large vacuoles and the presence of cytochrome c in the small vacuoles are consistent with this possibility. Because the majority of vacuoles develop in distal small dendrites (19), the release of these pro-apoptotic molecules may not cause typical apoptotic changes in cell bodies including chromatin condensation and cytoplasmic blebbing, but may induce a neuritic death program (158).

CONCLUSIONS AND PROSPECTS

Compelling evidence suggests that mitochondria play a crucial role in the pathogenesis of motor neuron death in ALS. Dramatic morphological abnormalities in mitochondria are found in human ALS cases and in mutant SOD1 transgenic mice. In the transgenic mice, these abnormalities peak at the early stage of the disease. Deficiencies in mitochondrial function have also been detected in humans and mutant SOD1 transgenic mice. In the transgenic mice, these deficiencies occur early, before the onset of the disease and probably exacerbated further by mitochondrial DNA damage and mutations. Mitochondrial abnormalities may cause motor neurons, to die by sensitizing motor neurons to excitotoxicity, by increasing generation of ROS, and by releasing mitochondrial death factors. The mechanism whereby mitochondria are damaged in ALS is not clear. But because mutant SOD1 is localized to mitochondria, we may be able to understand how SOD1 mutants damage mitochondria. Our future challenge is to establish an in vitro system where the effects of mutant SOD1 on mitochondria can be measured in a controlled environment.

REFERENCES

1. Afifi AK, Aleu FP, Goodgold J, MacKay B. Ultrastructure of atrophic muscle in amyotrophic lateral sclerosis. Neurology 1966; 16:475–481.
2. Masui Y, Mozai T, Kakehi K. Functional and morphometric study of the liver in motor neuron disease. J Neurol 1985; 232:15–19.
3. Nakano Y, Hirayama K, Terao K. Hepatic ultrastructural changes and liver dysfunction in amyotrophic lateral sclerosis. Arch Neurol 1987; 44:103–106.
4. Curti D, Malaspina A, Facchetti G, Camana C, Mazzini L, Tosca P, Zerbi F, Ceroni M. Amyotrophic lateral sclerosis: oxidative energy metabolism and calcium homeostasis in peripheral blood lymphocytes. Neurology 1996; 47:1060–1064.
5. Atsumi T. The ultrastructure of intramuscular nerves in amyotrophic lateral sclerosis. 1980; 55:193–198.
6. Siklos L, Engelhardt J, Harati Y, Smith RG, Joo F, Appel SH. Ultrastructural evidence for altered calcium in motor nerve terminals in amyotropic lateral sclerosis. Ann Neurol 1996; 39:203–216.
7. Hirano A, Donnenfeld H, Sasaki S, Nakano I. Fine structural observations of neurofilamentous changes in amyotrophic lateral sclerosis. J Neuropathol Exp Neurol 1984; 43:461–470.

8. Sasaki S, Iwata M. Ultrastructural change of synapses of Betz cells in patients with amyotrophic lateral sclerosis. Neurosci Lett 1999; 268:29–32.

9. Sasaki S, Iwata M. Ultrastructural study of synapses in the anterior horn neurons of patients with amyotrophic lateral sclerosis. Neurosci Lett 1996; 204:53–56.

10. Wiedemann FR, Manfredi G, Mawrin C, Beal MF, Schon EA. Mitochondrial DNA and respiratory chain function in spinal cords of ALS patients. J Neurochem 2002; 80:616–625.

11. Gurney ME, Pu H, Chiu AY, Dal_Canto MC, Polchow CY, Alexander DD, Caliendo J, Hentati A, Kwon YW, Deng HX. Motor neuron degeneration in mice that express a human Cu, Zn superoxide dismutase mutation. Science 1994; 264:1772–1775.

12. Ripps ME, Huntley GW, Hof PR, Morrison JH, Gordon JW. Transgenic mice expressing an altered murine superoxide dismutase gene provide an animal model of amyotrophic lateral sclerosis. Proc Natl Acad Sci USA 1995; 92:689–693.

13. Wong PC, Pardo CA, Borchelt DR, Lee MK, Copeland NG, Jenkins NA, Sisodia SS, Cleveland DW, Price DL. An adverse property of a familial ALS-linked SOD1 mutation causes motor neuron disease characterized by vacuolar degeneration of mitochondria. Neuron 1995; 14:1105–1116.

14. Dal_Canto MC, Gurney ME. Neuropathological changes in two lines of mice carrying a transgene for mutant human Cu, Zn SOD, and in mice overexpressing wild-type human SOD: a model of familial amyotrophic lateral sclerosis (FALS). Brain Res 1995; 676:25–40.

15. Carri MT, Ferri A, Battistoni A, Famhy L, Gabbianelli R, Poccia F, Rotilio G. Expression of a Cu, Zn superoxide dismutase typical of familial amyotrophic lateral sclerosis induces mitochondrial alteration and increase of cytosolic Ca^{2+} concentration in transfected neuroblastoma SH-SY5Y cells. FEBS Lett 1997; 414:365–368.

16. Kong J, Xu Z. Massive mitochondrial degeneration in motor neurons triggers the onset of amyotrophic lateral sclerosis in mice expressing a mutant SOD1. J Neurosci 1998; 18:3241–3250.

17. Aggarwal A, Nicholson G. Detection of preclinical motor neurone loss in SOD1 mutation carriers using motor unit number estimation. J Neurol Neurosurg Psychiatry 2002; 73:199–201.

18. Kasarskis EJ, Winslow M. When did Lou Gehrig's personal illness begin? Neurology 1989; 39:1243–1245.

19. Levine JB, Kong J, Nadler M, Xu Z. Astrocytes interact intimately with degenerating motor neurons in mouse amyotrophic lateral sclerosis (ALS). Glia 1999; 28:215–224.

20. Jaarsma D, Rognoni F, van Duijn W, Verspaget HW, Haasdijk ED, Holstege JC. Cu, Zn superoxide dismutase (SOD1) accumulates in vacuolated mitochondria in transgenic mice expressing amyotrophic lateral sclerosis-linked SOD1 mutations. Acta Neuropathol (Berl) 2001; 102:293–305.

21. Bendotti C, Calvaresi N, Chiveri L, Prelle A, Moggio M, Braga M, Silani V, De_Biasi S. Early vacuolization and mitochondrial damage in motor neurons of FALS mice are not associated with apoptosis or with changes in cytochrome oxidase histochemical reactivity. J Neurol Sci 2001; 191:25–33.

22. Higgins C, Jung C, Xu Z. ALS-associated mutant SODIG93A causes mitochondrial vacuolation by expansion of the intermembrane space and involvement of peroxisomes. BMC Neurosci 2003; 4:1–14.

23. Petronilli V, Cola C, Massari S, Colonna R, Bernardi P. Physiological effectors modify voltage sensing by the cyclosporin A-sensitive permeability transition pore of mitochondria. J Biol Chem 1993; 268:21939–21945.

24. Anglade P, Vyas S, Javoy-Agid F, Herrero MT, Michel PP, Marquez J, Mouatt-Prigent A, Ruberg M, Hirsch EC, Agid Y. Apoptosis and autophagy in nigral neurons of patients with Parkinson's disease. Histol Histopathol 1997; 12:25–31.

25. Nixon RA, Cataldo AM, Mathews PM. The endosomal-lysosomal system of neurons in Alzheimer's disease pathogenesis: a review. Neurochem Res 2000; 25:1161–1172.

26. Ravikumar B, Vacher C, Berger Z, Davies JE, Luo S, Oroz LG, Scaravilli F, Easton DF, Duden R, O'Kane CJ, et al. Inhibition of mTOR induces autophagy and reduces toxicity of polyglutamine expansions in fly and mouse models of Huntingin disease. Nat Genet 2004; 36:585–595.

27. Simon D, Seznec H, Gansmuller A, Carelle N, Weber P, Metzger D, Rustin P, Koenig M, Puccio H. Friedreich ataxia mouse models with progressive cerebeller and sensory ataxia reveal autophagic neurodegenaration in dorsal root ganglia. J Neurosci 2004; 24:1987–1995.

28. Zhu S, Stavrovskaya IG, Drozda M, Kim BY, Ona V, Li M, Sarang S, Liu AS, Hartley DM, Wu DUC, et al. Minocycline inhibits cytochrome c release and delays progression of amyotrophic lateral sclerosis in mice. Nature 2002; 417:74–78.

29. Kirkinezos IG, Hemandez D, Bradley WG, Moraes CT. An ALS mouse model with a permeable blood-brain barrier benefits from systemic cyclosporine & nbsp; a treatment. J Neurochem 2004; 88:821–826.

30. Xu ZS, Jung C, Higgins CM, Levine JB, Kong J. Mitochondrial degeneration in amyotrophic lateral sclerosis. J Bioenerg Biomembranes 2004; 36:395–399.

31. Okado_Matsumoto A, Fridovich I. Amyotrophic lateral sclerosis: a proposed mechanism. Proc Natl Acad Sci USA 2002; 99:9010–9014.

32. Sturtz LA, Diekert K, Jensen LT, Lill R, Culotta VC. A fraction of yeast Cu, Zn-superoxide dismutase and its metallochaperone, CCS, localize to the intermembrane space of mitochondria. A physiological role for SOD1 in guarding against mitochondrial oxidative damage. J Biol Chem 2001; 276:38084–38089.

33. Higgins CM, Jung C, Ding H, Xu Z. Mutant Cu, Zn superoxide dismutase that causes motoneuron degeneration is present in mitochondria in the CNS. J Neurosci 2002; 22:RC215.

34. Mattiazzi M, D'_Aurelio M, Gajewski CD, Martushova K, Kiaei M, Beal MF, Manfredi G. Mutated human SOD1 causes dysfunction of oxidative phosphorylation in mitochondria of transgenic mice. J Biol Chem 2002; 277:29626–29633.

35. Higgins CM, Jung C, Xu Z. ALS-associated mutant SOD1G93A causes mitochondrial vacuolation by expansion of the intermembrane space and by involvement of SOD1 aggregation and peroxisomes. BMC Neurosci 2003; 4:16.

36. Bruijn LI, Houseweart MK, Kato S, Anderson KL, Anderson SD, Ohama E, Reaume AG, Scott RW, Cleveland DW. Aggregation and motor neuron toxicity of an ALS-linked SOD1 mutant independent from wild-type SOD1. Science 1998; 281:1851–1854.

37. Wang J, Slunt H, Gonzales V, Fromholt D, Coonfield M, Copeland NG, Jenkins NA, Borchelt DR. Copper-binding-site-null SOD1 causes ALS in transgenic mice: aggregates of non-native SOD1 delineate a common feature. Hum Mol Genet 2003; 12:2753–2764.

38. Beckman JS, Carson M, Smith CD, Koppenol WH. ALS, SOD and peroxinitrate. Nature 1993; 364:584.

39. Crow JP, Sampson JB, Zhuang Y-X, Thompson JA, Beckman JS. Decreased zinc affinity of amyotrophic lateral sclerosis-associated superoxide dismutase mutants leads to enhanced catalysis of tyrosine nitration by peroxynitrite. J Neurochem 1997; 69:1936–1944.

40. Estevez AG, Crow JP, Sampson JB, Reiter C, Zhuang YX, Richardson GJ, Tarpey MM, Barbeito L, Beckman JS. Induction of nitric oxide-dependent apoptosis in motor neurons by zinc-deficient superoxide dismutase. Science 1999; 286:2498–2500.

41. Wiedau-Pazos M, Goto JJ, Rabizadeh S, Gralla EB, Roe JA, Lee MK, Valentine JS, Bredesen DE. Altered reactivity of superoxide dismutase in familial amyotrophic lateral sclerosis. Science 1996; 271:515–518.

42. Yim MB, Kang J-H, Yim H-S, Kwak H-S, Chock PB, Stadtman ER. A gain-of-function of an amyotrophic lateral sclerosis-associated Cu, Zn-superoxide dismutase mutant: an enhancement of free radical formation due to a decrease in Km for hydrogen peroxide. Proc Natl Acad Sci USA 1996; 93:5709–5714.

43. Yim HS, Kang JH, Chock PB, Stadtman ER, Yim MB. A familial amyotrophic lateral sclerosis-associated A4V Cu, Zn-superoxide dismutase mutant has a lower Km for

hydrogen peroxide. Correlation between clinical severity and the Km value. J Biol Chem 1997; 272:8861–8863.

44. Yim MB, Chock PB, Stadtman ER. Copper, zinc superoxide dismutase catalyzes hydroxyl radical production from hydrogen peroxide. Proc Natl Acad Sci USA 1990; 87:394–398.

45. Yim MB, Chock PB, Stadtman ER. Enzyme function of copper, zinc superoxide dismutase as a free radical generator. J Biol Chem 1993; 268:4099–4105.

46. Singh RJ, Karoui H, Gunther MR, Beckman JS, Mason RP, Kalyanaraman B. Reexamination of the mechanism of hydroxyl radical adducts formed from the reaction between familial amyotrophic lateral sclerosis-associated Cu, Zn superoxide dismutase mutants and H_2O_2. Proc Natl Acad Sci USA 1998; 95:6675–6680.

47. Subramaniam JR, Lyons WE, Liu J, Bartnikas TB, Rothstein J, Price DL, Cleveland DW, Gitlin JD, Wong PC. Mutant SOD1 causes motor neuron disease independent of copper chaperone-mediated copper loading. Nat Neurosci 2002; 5:301–307.

48. Culotta VC, Klomp LWJ, Strain J, Casareno RLB, Krems B, Gitlin JD. The copper chaperone for superoxide dismutase. J Biol Chem 1997; 272:23469–23472.

49. Wong PC, Waggoner D, Subramaniam JR, Tessarollo L, Bartnikas TB, Culotta VC, Price DL, Rothstein J, Gitlin JD. Copper chaperone for superoxide dismutase is essential to activate mammalian Cu/Zn superoxide dismutase. Proc Natl Acad Sci USA 2000; 97:2886–2891.

50. Wang J, Xu G, Gonzales V, Coonfield M, Fromholt D, Copeland NG, Jenkins NA, Borchelt DR. Fibrillar inclusions and motor neuron degeneration in transgenic mice expressing superoxide dismutase 1 with a disrupted copper-binding site. Neurobiol Dis 2002; 10:128–138.

51. Beckman JS, Estvez AG, Barbeito L, Crow JP. CCS knockout mice establish an alternative source of copper for SOD in ALS. Free Radic Biol Med 2002; 33:1433–1435.

52. Bush AI. Is ALS caused by an altered oxidative activity of mutant superoxide dismutase? Nat Neurosci 2002; 5:919; author reply 919–920.

53. Wong PC. Is ALS caused by an altered oxidative activity of mutant superoxide dismutase–reply. Nat Neurosci 2002; 5:919–920.

54. Shinder GA, Lacourse MC, Minotti S, Durham HD. Mutant Cu/Zn-superoxide dismutase proteins have altered solubility and interact with heat shock/stress proteins in models of amyotrophic lateral sclerosis. J Biol Chem 2001; 276:12791–12796.

55. Bruening W, Roy J, Giasson B, Figlewicz DA, Mushynski WE, Durham HD. Upregulation of protein chaperones preserves viability of cells expressing toxic Cu/Zn-superoxide dismutase mutants associated with amyotrophic lateral sclerosis. J Neurochem 1999; 72:693–699.

56. Batulan Z, Shinder GA, Minotti S, He BP, Doroudchi MM, Nalbantoglu J, Strong MJ, Durham HD. High threshold for induction of the stress response in motor neurons is associated with failure to activate HSF1. J Neurosci 2003; 23:5789–5798.

57. Neupert W, Brunner M. The protein import motor of mitochondria. 2002; 3:555–565.

58. Liu J, Lillo C, Jonsson PA, Velde CV, Ward CM, Miller TM, Subramaniam JR, Rothstein JD, Marklund S, Andersen PM. Toxicity of familial ALS-linked SOD1 mutants from selective recruitment to spinal mitochondria. Neuron 2004; 43:5–17.

59. Pasinelli P, Belford ME, Lennon N, Bacskai BJ, Hyman BT, Trotti D, Brown J, Robert H. Amyotrophic lateral sclerosis-associated SOD1 mutant proteins bind and aggregate with Bcl-2 in spinal cord mitochondria. Neuron 2004; 43:19–30.

60. Lashuel HA, Petre BM, Wall J, Simon M, Nowak RJ, Walz T, Lansbury PT. Alphasynuclein, especially the Parkinson's disease-associated mutants, forms pore-like annular and tubular protofibrils. J Mol Biol 2002; 322:1089–1102.

61. Volles MJ, Lee SJ, Rochet JC, Shtilerman MD, Ding TT, Kessler JC, Lansbury PT. Vesicle permeabilization by protofibrillar alpha-synuclein: implications for the pathogenesis and treatment of Parkinson's disease. Biochemistry 2001; 40:7812–7819.

62. Ray SS, Nowak RJ, Strokovich K, Brown RH Jr, Walz T, Lansbury PT Jr. An inter-subunit disulfide bond prevents in vitro aggregation of a superoxide dismutase-1 mutant linked to familial amytrophic lateral sclerosis. Biochemistry 2004; 43:4899–4905.

63. Bonnot A, Corio M, Tramu G, Viala D. Immunocytochemical distribution of ionotro-pic glutamate receptor subunits in the spinal cord of the rabbit. J Chem Neuroanat 1996; 11:267–278.

64. Robinson D, Ellenberger H. Distribution of N-methyl-D-aspartate and non-N-methyl-D-aspartate glutamate receptor subunits on respiratory motor and premotor neurons in the rat. J Comp Neurol 1997; 389:94–116.

65. Williams TL, Ince PG, Oakley AE, Shaw PJ. An immunocytochemical study of the dis-tribution of AMPA selective glutamate receptor subunits in the normal human motor system. Neuroscience 1996; 74:185–198.

66. Rothstein JD, Jin L, Dykes-Hoberg M, Kuncl, RW. Chronic inhibition of glutamate uptake produces a model of slow neurotoxicity. Proc Natl Acad Sci USA 1993; 90:6591–6595.

67. Carriedo SG, Yin HZ, Weiss JH. Motor neurons are selectively vulnerable to AMPA/kainate receptor-mediated injury in vitro. J Neurosci 1996; 16:4069–4079.

68. Ikonomidou, C, Qin Qin Y, Labruyere J, Olney JW. Motor neuron degeneration induced by excitotoxin agonists has features in common with those seen in the SOD-1 transgenic mouse model of amyotrophic lateral sclerosis. J Neuropathol Exp Neurol 1996; 55:211–224.

69. Rothstein JD. Excitotoxicity hypothesis. Neurology 1996; 47:S19–S25.

70. Plaitakis A, Caroscio JT. Abnormal glutamate metabolism in amyotrophic lateral sclerosis. Ann Neurol 1987; 22:575–579.

71. Rothstein JD, Tsai G, Kuncl RW, Clawson L, Cornblath DR, Drachman DB, Pestronk A, Stauch BL, Coyle JT. Abnormal excitatory amino acid metabolism in amyotrophic lateral sclerosis. Ann Neurol 1990; 28:18–25.

72. Spreux-Varoquaux O, Bensimon G, Lacomblez L, Salachas F, Pradat PF, Le Forestier N, Marouan A, Dib M, Meininger V. Glutamate levels in cerebrospinal fluid in amyotrophic lateral sclerosis: a reappraisal using a new HPLC method with coulometric detection in a large cohort of patients. J Neurol Sci 2002; 193:73–78.

73. Rothstein JD, Martin LJ, Kuncl RW. Decreased glutamate transport by the brain and spinal cord in amyotrophic lateral sclerosis. New Engl J Med 1992; 326:1464–1468.

74. Carriedo SG, Yin HZ, Weiss JH. Motor neurons are selectively vulnerable to AMPA/kainate receptor-mediated injury in vitro. J Neurosci 1996; 16:4069–4079.

75. Rothstein JD, Kuncl R, Chaudhry V, Clawson L, Cornblath DR, Coyle JT, Drachman DB. Excitatory amino acids in amyotrophic lateral sclerosis: an update. Ann Neurol 1991; 30:224–225.

76. Roy J, Minotti S, Dong L, Figlewicz DA, Durham HD. Glutamate potentiates the toxi-city of mutant Cu/Zn-superoxide dismutase in motor neurons by postsynaptic calcium-dependent mechanisms. J Neurosci 1998; 18:9673–9684.

77. Kruman II, Pedersen WA, Springer JE, Mattson MP. ALS-linked Cu/Zn-SOD mutation increases vulnerability of motor neurons to excitotoxicity by a mechanism involving increased oxidative stress and perturbed calcium homeostasis. Exp Neurol 1999; 160:28–39.

78. Canton T, Pratt J, Stutzmann JM, Imperato A, Boireau A. Glutamate uptake is decreased tardively in the spinal cord of FALS mice. Neuroreport 1998; 9:775–778.

79. Pedersen WA, Fu W, Keller JN, Markesbery WR, Appel S, Smith RG, Kasarskis E, Mattson MP. Protein modification by the lipid peroxidation product 4-hydroxynonenal in the spinal cords of amyotrophic lateral sclerosis patients. Ann Neurol 1998; 44: 819–824.

80. Trotti D, Rolfs, A, Danbolt NC, Brown RH Jr, Hediger MA. SOD1 mutants linked to amyotrophic lateral sclerosis selectively inactivate a glial glutamate transporter [pub-lished erratum appears in Nat Neurosci 1999; 2(9):848]. Nat Neurosci 1999; 2:427–433.

81. Howland DS, Liu J, She Y, Goad B, Maragakis NJ, Kim B, Erickson J, Kulik J, DeVito L, Psaltis G, et al. Focal loss of the glutamate transporter EAAT2 in a transgenic rat model of SOD1 mutant-mediated amyotrophic lateral sclerosis (ALS). Proc Natl Acad Sci USA 2002; 99:1604–1609.

82. Dib M. Amyotrophic lateral sclerosis: progress and prospects for treatment. Drugs 2003; 63:289–310.

83. Gurney ME, Cutting FB, Zhai P, Doble A, Taylor CP, Andrus PK, Hall ED. Benefit of vitamin E, riluzole, and gabapentin in a transgenic model of familial amyotrophic lateral sclerosis [see comments]. Ann Neurol 1996; 39:147–157.

84. Ikonomidou C, Turski L. Neurodegenerative disorders: clues from glutamate and energy metabolism. Crit Rev Neurobiol 1996; 10:239–263.

85. Bittigau P, Ikonomidou C. Glutamate in neurologic diseases. J Child Neurol 1997; 12:471–485.

86. Carriedo SG, Sensi SL, Yin HZ, Weiss JH. AMPA exposures induce mitochondrial Ca(2+) overload and ROS generation in spinal motor neurons in vitro. J Neurosci 2000; 20:240–250.

87. Stout AK, Raphael HM, Kanterewicz BI, Klann E, Reynolds IJ. Glutamate-induced neuron death requires mitochondrial calcium uptake. Nat Neurosci 1998; 1:366–373.

88. Kanki R, Nakamizo T, Yamashita H, Kihara T, Sawada H, Uemura K, Kawamata J, Shibasaki H, Akaike A, Shimohama S. Effects of mitochondrial dysfunction on glutamate receptor-mediated neurotoxicity in cultured rat spinal motor neurons. Brain Res 2004; 1015:73–81.

89. Kaal EC, Vlug AS, Versleijen MW, Kuilman M, Joosten EA, Bar PR. Chronic mitochondrial inhibition induces selective motoneuron death in vitro: a new model for amyotrophic lateral sclerosis. J Neurochem 2000; 74:1158–1165.

90. Vandenberghe W, Ihle EC, Patneau DK, Robberecht W, Brorson JR. AMPA receptor current density, not desensitization, predicts selective motoneuron vulnerability. J Neurosci 2000; 20:7158–7166.

91. Rao SD, Yin HZ, Weiss JH. Disruption of glial glutamate transport by reactive oxygen species produced in motor neurons. J Neurosci 2003; 23:2627–2633.

92. Sullivan PG, Rabchevsky AG, Keller JN, Lovell M, Sodhi A, Hart RP, Scheff SW. Intrinsic differences in brain and spinal cord mitochondria: implication for therapeutic interventions. J Comp Neurol 2004; 474:524–534.

93. Vielhaber S, Kunz D, Winkler K, Wiedemann FR, Kirches E, Feistner H, Heinze HJ, Elger CE, Schubert W, Kunz WS. Mitochondrial DNA abnormalities in skeletal muscle of patients with sporadic amyotrophic lateral sclerosis. Brain 2000; 123(Pt 7):1339–1348.

94. Wiedemann FR, Winkler K, Kuznetsov AV, Bartels C, Vielhaber S, Feistner H, Kunz WS. Impairment of mitochondrial function in skeletal muscle of patients with amyotrophic lateral sclerosis. J Neurol Sci 1998; 156:65–72.

95. Bowling AC, Schulz JB, Brown RH, Beal MF. Superoxide dismutase activity, oxidative damage, and mitochondrial energy metabolism in familial and sporadic amyotrophic lateral sclerosis. J Neurochem 1993; 61:2322–2325.

96. Browne SE, Bowling AC, Baik MJ, Gurney M, Brown RH, Beal MF. Metabolic dysfunction in familial, but not sporadic, amyotrophic lateral sclerosis. J Neurochem 1998; 71:281–287.

97. Borthwick GM, Johnson MA, Ince PG, Shaw PJ, Turnbull DM. Mitochondrial enzyme activity in amyotrophic lateral sclerosis: implications for the role of mitochondria in neuronal cell death. Ann Neurol 1999; 46:787–790.

98. Fujita K, Yamauchi M, Shibayama K, Ando M, Honda M, Nagata Y. Decreased cytochrome c oxidase activity but unchanged superoxide dismutase and glutathione peroxidase activities in the spinal cords of patients with amyotrophic lateral sclerosis. J Neurosci Res 1996; 45:276–281.

99. Jung C, Higgins CM, Xu Z. Mitochondrial electron transport chain complex dysfunction in a transgenic mouse model for amyotrophic lateral sclerosis. J Neurochem 2002; 83:535–545.
100. Scheffler IE. Mitochondria. New York: Wiley-Liss, 1999.
101. Cassarino DS, Bennett JPJ. An evaluation of the role of mitochondria in neurodegenerative diseases: mitochondrial mutations and oxidative pathology, protective nuclear responses, and cell death in neurodegeneration. Brain Res Reviews 1999; 29:1–25.
102. Said Ahmed M, Hung W-Y, Zu JS, Hockberger P, Siddique T. Increased reactive oxygen species in familial amyotrophic lateral sclerosis with mutations in SOD1. J Neurol Sci 2000; 176:88–94.
103. Liu D, Wen J, Liu J, Li L. The roles of free radicals in amyotrophic lateral sclerosis: reactive oxygen species and elevated oxidation of protein, DNA, and membrane phospholipids. FASEB J 1999; 13:2318–2328.
104. Bruijn LI, Beal MF, Becher MW, Schulz JB, Wong PC, Price DL, Cleveland DW. Elevated free nitrotyrosine levels, but not protein-bound nitrotyrosine or hydroxyl radicals, throughout amyotrophic lateral sclerosis (ALS)-like disease implicate tyrosine nitration as an aberrant in vivo property of one familial ALS-linked superoxide dismutase 1 mutant. Proc Natl Acad Sci USA 1997; 94:7606–7611.
105. Ferrante RJ, Browne SE, Shinobu LA, Bowling AC, Baik MJ, MacGarvey U, Kowall NW, Brown JRH, Beal MF. Evidence of increased oxidative damage in both sporadic and familial amyotrophic lateral sclerosis. J Neurochem 1997; 69:2064–2074.
106. Ferrante RJ, Shinobu LA, Schulz JB, Matthews RT, Thomas CE, Kowall NW, Gurney ME, Beal MF. Increased 3-nitrotyrosine and oxidative damage in mice with a human copper/zinc superoxide dismutase mutation. Ann Neurol 1997; 42:326–334.
107. Andrus PK, Fleck TJ, Gurney ME, Hall ED. Protein oxidative damage in a transgenic mouse model of familial amyotrophic lateral sclerosis. J Neurochem 1998; 71:2041–2048.
108. Hall ED, Andrus PK, Oostveen JA, Fleck TJ, Gurney ME. Relationship of oxygen radical-induced lipid peroxidative damage to disease onset and progression in a transgenic model of familial ALS. J Neurosci Res 1998; 53:66–77.
109. Oteiza PI, Uchitel OD, Carrasquedo F, Dubrovski AL, Roma JC, Fraga CG. Evaluation of antioxidants, protein, and lipid oxidation products in blood from sporadic amyotrophic lateral sclerosis patients. Neurochem Res 1997; 22:535–539.
110. Liu R, Li B, Flanagan SW, Oberley LW, Gozal D, Qiu M. Increased mitochondrial antioxidative activity or decreased oxygen free radical propagation prevent mutant SOD1-mediated motor neuron cell death and increase amyotrophic lateral sclerosis-like transgenic mouse survival. J Neurochem 2002; 80:488–500.
111. Flanagan SW, Anderson RD, Ross MA, Oberley LW. Overexpression of manganese superoxide dismutase attenuates neuronal death in human cells expressing mutant (G37R) Cu/Zn-superoxide dismutase. J Neurochem 2002; 81:170–177.
112. Jung C, Rong Y, Doctrow S, Baudry M, Malfroy B, Xu Z. Synthetic superoxide dismutase/catalase mimetics reduce oxidative stress and prolong survival in a mouse amyotrophic lateral sclerosis model. Neurosci Lett 2001; 304:157–160.
113. Dugan LL, Turetsky DM, Du C, Lobner D, Wheeler M, Almli CR, Shen CK-F, Luh T-Y, Choi DW, Lin T-S. Carboxyfullerenes as neuroprotective agents. Proc Natl Acad Sci USA 1997; 94:9434–9439.
114. Reinholz MM, Merkle CM, Poduslo JF. Therapeutic benefits of putrescine-modified catalase in a transgenic mouse model of familial amyotrophic lateral sclerosis. Exp Neurol 1999; 159:204–216.
115. Nagano S, Ogawa Y, Yanagihara T, Sakoda S. Benefit of a combined treatment with trientine and ascorbate in familial amyotrophic lateral sclerosis model mice. Neurosci Lett 1999; 265:159–162.
116. Rahman I, Gilmour PS, Jimenez LA, MacNee W. Oxidative stress and TNF-alpha induce histone acetylation and NF-kappaB/AP-1 activation in alveolar epithelial cells:

potential mechanism in gene transcription in lung inflammation. Mol Cellular Biochem 2002; 234–235, 239–248.

117. Rokutan K, Teshima S, Miyoshi M, Kawai T, Nikawa T, Kishi K. Glutathione depletion inhibits oxidant-induced activation of nuclear factor-kappa B, AP-1, and c-Jun/ATF-2 in cultured guinea-pig gastric epithelial cells. J Gastroenterol 1998; 33:646–655.

118. Chandel NS, Trzyna WC, McClintock DS, Schumacker PT. Role of oxidants in NF-kappa B activation and TNF-alpha gene transcription induced by hypoxia and endotoxin. J Immunol 2000; 165:1013–1021.

119. Chandel NS, McClintock DS, Feliciano CE, Wood TM, Melendez JA, Rodriguez AM, Schumacker PT. Reactive oxygen species generated at mitochondrial complex III stabilize hypoxia-inducible factor-1alpha during hypoxia: a mechanism of O_2 sensing. J Biol Chem 2000; 275:25130–25138.

120. Duyndam MC, Hulscher TM, Fontijn D, Pinedo HM, Boven E. Induction of vascular endothelial growth factor expression and hypoxia-inducible factor 1alpha protein by the oxidative stressor arsenite. J Biol Chem 2001; 276:48066–48076.

121. Chandel NS, Maltepe E, Goldwasser E, Mathieu CE, Simon MC, Schumacker PT. Mitochondrial reactive oxygen species trigger hypoxia-induced transcription. Proc Natl Acad Sci USA 1998; 95:11715–11720.

122. Hensley K, Fedynyshyn J, Ferrell S, Floyd RA, Gordon B, Grammas P, Hamdheydari L, Mhatre M, Mou S, Pye QN. Message and protein-level elevation of tumor necrosis factor [alpha] [TNF(alpha)] and TNF[alpha]-modulating cytokines in spinal cords of the G93A-SOD1 mouse model for amyotrophic lateral sclerosis. Neurobiol Dis 2003; 14: 74–80.

123. Yoshihara T, Ishigaki S, Yamamoto M, Liang Y, Niwa J, Takeuchi H, Doyu M, Sobue G. Differential expression of inflammation- and apoptosis-related genes in spinal cords of a mutant SOD1 transgenic mouse model of familial amyotrophic lateral sclerosis. J Neurochem 2002; 80:158–167.

124. Casciati A, Ferri A, Cozzolino M, Celsi F, Nencini M, Rotilio G, Carri MT. Oxidative modulation of nuclear factor-kappa B in human cells expressing mutant fALS-typical superoxide dismutases. J Neurochem 2002; 83:1019–1029.

125. Migheli A, Piva R, Atzori C, Troost D, Schiffer D. c-Jun, JNK/SAPK kinases and transcription factor NF-kappa B are selectively activated in astrocytes, but not motor neurons, in amyotrophic lateral sclerosis. J Neuropathol Exp Neurol 56:1314–1322.

126. Sowter H, Ratcliffe P, Watson P, Greenberg A, Harris A. HIF-1-dependent regulation of hypoxic induction of the cell death factors BNIP3 and NIX in human tumors. Cancer Res 2001; 61:6669–6673.

127. Guo K, Searfoss G, Krolikowski D, Pagnoni M, Franks C, Clark K, Yu KT, Jaye M, Ivashchenko Y. Hypoxia induces the expression of the pro-apoptotic gene BNIP3. Cell Death Differ 2001; 8:367–376.

128. Bruick RK. Expression of the gene encoding the proapoptotic Nip3 protein is induced by hypoxia. Proc Natl Acad Sci USA 2000; 97:9082–9087.

129. Naderi J, Hung M, Pandey S. Oxidative stress-induced apoptosis in dividing fibroblasts involves activation of p38 MAP kinase and over-expression of Bax: resistance of quiescent cells to oxidative stress. Apoptosis 2003; 8(1):91–100.

130. Jungas T, Motta I, Duffieux F, Fanen P, Stoven V, Ojcius DM. Glutathione levels and BAX activation during apoptosis due to oxidative stress in cells expressing wild-type and mutant cystic fibrosis transmembrane conductance regulator. J Biol Chem 2002; 277:27912–27918.

131. Bandy B, Davison AJ. Mitochondrial mutations may increase oxidative stress: implications for carcinogenesis and aging? Free Radic Biol Med 1990; 8:523–539.

132. Wallace DC. Mitochondrial genetics: a paradigm for aging and degenerative diseases? Science 1992; 256:628–632.

133. Shenkar R, Navidi W, Tavare S, Dang MH, Chomyn A, Attardi G, Cortopassi G, Arnheim N. The mutation rate of the human mtDNA deletion mtDNA4977. Am J Hum Genet 1996; 59:772–780.

134. Madigan JP, Chotkowski HL, Glaser RL. DNA double-strand break-induced phosphorylation of Drosophila histone variant H2Av helps prevent radiation-induced apoptosis. Nucl Acids Res 2002; 30:3698–3705.

135. Richter C, Park JW, Ames BN. Normal oxidative damage to mitochondrial and nuclear DNA is extensive. Proc Natl Acad Sci USA 1988; 85:6465–6467.

136. Comi GP, Bordoni A, Salani S, Franceschina L, Sciacco M, Prelle A, Fortunato F, Zeviani M, Napoli L, Bresolin N, et al. Cytochrome c oxidase subunit I microdeletion in a patient with motor neuron disease. Ann Neurol 1998; 43:110–116.

137. Swerdlow RH, Parks JK, Cassarino DS, Trimmer PA, Miller SW, Maguire DJ, Sheehan JP, Maguire RS, Pattee G, Juel VC, et al. Mitochondria in sporadic amyotrophic lateral sclerosis. Exp Neurol 1998; 153:135–142.

138. Gajewski CD, Lin MT, Cudkowicz ME, Beal MF, Manfredi G. Mitochondrial DNA from platelets of sporadic ALS patients restores normal respiratory functions in [rho]0 cells. Exp Neurol 2003; 179:229–235.

139. Vielhaber S, Kunz D, Winkler K, Wiedemann FR, Kirches E, Feistner H, Heinze HJ, Elger CE, Schubert W, Kunz WS, et al. Mitochondrial DNA abnormalities in skeletal muscle of patients with sporadic amyotrophic lateral sclerosis impairment of mitochondrial function in skeletal muscle of patients with amyotrophic lateral sclerosis. Brain 2000; 123:1339–1348.

140. Dhaliwal GK, Grewal RP. Mitochondrial DNA deletion mutation levels are elevated in ALS brains. Neuroreport 2000; 11:2507–2509.

141. Ro LS, Lai SL, Chen CM, Chen ST. Deleted 4977-bp mitochondrial DNA mutation is associated with sporadic amyotrophic lateral sclerosis: a hospital-based case-control study. Muscle Nerve 2003; 28:737–743.

142. Warita H, Hayashi T, Murakami T, Manabe Y, Abe K. Oxidative damage to mitochondrial DNA in spinal motoneurons of transgenic ALS mice. Mol Brain Res 2001; 89:147–152.

143. Guegan C, Przedborski S. Programmed cell death in amyotrophic lateral sclerosis. J Clin Invest 2003; 111:153–161.

144. Kostic V, Jackson-Lewis V, de Bilbao F, Dubois-Dauphin M, Przedborski S. Bcl-2: prolonging life in a transgenic mouse model of familial amyotrophic lateral sclerosis. Science 1997; 277:559–562.

145. Martin LJ. Neuronal death in amyotrophic lateral sclerosis is apoptosis: possible contribution of a programmed cell death mechanism. J Neuropathol Exp Neurol 1999; 58:459–471.

146. Li M, Ona VO, Gueacutegan C, Chen M, Jackson-Lewis V, Andrews LJ, Olszewski AJ, Stieg PE, Lee J-P, Przedborski S, et al. Functional role of Caspase-1 and Caspase-3 in an ALS transgenic mouse model. Science 2000; 288:335–339.

147. Pasinelli P, Houseweart MK, Brown RH Jr, Cleveland DW. Caspase-1 and Caspase-3 are sequentially activated in motor neuron death in Cu, Zn superoxide dismutase-mediated familial amyotrophic lateral sclerosis. Proc Natl Acad Sci USA 2000; 97:13901–13906.

148. Vukosavic S, Stefanis L, Jackson-Lewis V, Guegan C, Romero N, Chen C, Dubois-Dauphin M, Przedborski S. Delaying caspase activation by Bcl-2: a clue to disease retardation in a transgenic mouse model of amyotrophic lateral sclerosis. J Neurosci 2000; 20:9119–9125.

149. Friedlander RM, Brown RH, Gagliardini V, Wang J, Yuan J. Inhibition of ICE slows ALS in mice [letter] [published erratum appears in Nature 1998; 392(6676):560]. Nature 1997; 388:31.

150. Migheli A, Atzori C, Piva R, Tortarolo M, Girelli M, Schiffer D, Bendotti C. Lack of apoptosis in mice with ALS. Nat Med 1999; 5:966–967.

151. Kang SJ, Sanchez I, Jing N, Yuan J. Dissociation between neurodegeneration and Caspase-11-mediated activation of Caspase-1 and Caspase-3 in a mouse model of amyotrophic lateral sclerosis. J Neurosci 2003; 23:5455–5460.
152. Danial NN, Korsmeyer SJ. Cell death: critical control points. Cell 2004; 116:205–219.
153. Sperandio S, de Belle I, Bredesen DE. An alternative, nonapoptotic form of programmed cell death. Proc Natl Acad Sci USA 2000; 97:14376–14381.
154. Hegde R, Srinivasula SM, Zhang Z, Wassell R, Mukattash R, Cilenti L, DuBois G, Lazebnik Y, Zervos AS, Fernandes-Alnemri T, et al. Identification of Omi/HtrA2 as a mitochondrial apoptotic serine protease that disrupts inhibitor of apoptosis protein-caspase interaction. J Biol Chem 2002; 277:432–438.
155. Vande Velde C, Cizeau J, Dubik D, Alimonti J, Brown T, Israels S, Hakem R, Greenberg AH. BNIP3 and genetic control of necrosis-like cell death through the mitochondrial permeability transition pore. Mol Cell Biol 2000; 20:5454–5468.
156. Yu S-W, Wang H, Poitras MF, Coombs C, Bowers WJ, Federoff HJ, Poirier GG, Dawson TM, Dawson VL. Mediation of poly(ADP-Ribose) polymerase-1-dependent cell death by apoptosis-inducing factor. Science 2002; 297:259–263.
157. Guegan C, Vila M, Rosoklija G, Hays AP, Przedborski S. Recruitment of the mitochondrial-dependent apoptotic pathway in amyotrophic lateral sclerosis. J Neurosci 2001; 21:6569–6576.
158. Mattson MP, Duan W. "Apoptotic" biochemical cascades in synaptic compartments: roles in adaptive plasticity and neurodegenerative disorders. J Neurosci Res 1999; 58:152–166.

19

Environmental Toxicity and ALS: Novel Insights from an Animal Model of ALS-PDC

C. A. Shaw
Departments of Ophthalmology, Neuroscience, and Experimental Medicine, University of British Columbia, Vancouver, British Columbia, Canada

J. M. B. Wilson
Department of Neuroscience, University of British Columbia, Vancouver, British Columbia, Canada

INTRODUCTION

Amyotrophic lateral sclerosis (ALS) is a rapidly progressive and incurable neurological disorder which typically kills its victims within three to five years of clinical diagnosis. ALS is characterized pathologically by the loss of upper and lower motor neurons in the CNS accompanied by muscle wasting and the loss of motor function. Over 90% of cases are sporadic ALS (SALS) with no clear etiology (1,2). Of the familial cases of ALS, approximately 20% appear to arise due to a toxic gain of function mutation in genes coding for the antioxidant enzyme superoxide dismutase (SOD) (1). Five percent of people with SALS also have Cu/Zn superoxide dismutase (SOD1) mutations (3). A second mutation in a gene coding for a protein of unknown function, "alsin," produces a rare juvenile variant form of the disease (ALS2) (4).

The various notions concerning the etiology of ALS (and other neurological diseases) can be reduced to three basic hypotheses. The first, largely driven by enthusiasm for mutant forms of SOD, favors a genetic etiology. In this view, inherited genes produce abnormal gene products whose action on neurons or other CNS cells is direct and toxic. Implicit in this hypothesis is the notion that most cases of ALS now termed "sporadic" will be found to contain one or more still unknown genetic abnormalities. This hypothesis retains much support in the field and remains hard to refute, not because this view has amassed any particularly compelling experimental evidence besides that provided for the SOD mutation, but rather due to the fact that some future study might indeed still show novel genes or synergies between genes as key causal factors for most sporadic forms of the disease. The second hypothesis postulates that environmental substances and/or specific molecules are the key etiological factor in SALS. While a variety of neurotoxins are well known and while various neurological disorders can be attributed to some of these, evidence for specific molecules giving rise to ALS is not particularly compelling (2) and there are few good animal models currently available. We will summarize some of the existing data below, including our own for an animal model of a variant form of ALS, ALS-parkinsonism dementia complex (ALS-PDC). A third hypothesis links genetic and epigenetic events, suggesting that potential neurotoxins are able to exert their fatal actions due to unique interactions with some genetic susceptibility factors. For example, a particular environmental neurotoxin might cause the death of motor neurons, but only in individuals deficient in genes coding for a specific detoxifying enzyme. This hypothesis of gene–environment interactions in ALS (and other neurological diseases) has only recently attracted significant attention in the field, and to date few studies have addressed it in any detail. Figure 1 provides a schematic view of the various factors that may be involved in ALS, including the one that is well known but often neglected, age.

In this chapter, we will focus on environmental toxicity in relation to ALS-PDC of the Western Pacific and describe a novel animal model of the disease. We will also suggest that the creation of a detailed time-line of disease progression provides the best hope of developing early strategic and targeted therapy designed to either prevent disease onset or to halt disease progression before irreparable harm has occurred in the nervous system.

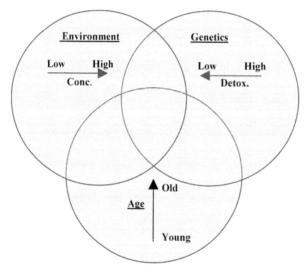

Figure 1 Synergistic interactions of presumed risk factors in SALS. Motor neuron death in ALS may occur following exposure to a neurotoxin(s) in the environment or one arising from internal biochemical processes. The toxins may be naturally occurring or synthetic. A toxic factor component is represented in the Venn diagram by the set on the left side of the schematic. The potential range of toxic effects runs from left to right and is labeled as "low to high." Intersecting the first set is another representing some undefined genetic susceptibility factor. Such genetic susceptibilities might reflect the polymorphic expression patterns of various alleles, such as those for ApoE. More generally, such variants could reflect gene products involved in detoxification mechanisms. For this schematic, we have shown an arbitrary range from "high to low," with "low" corresponding to higher risk of a deleterious interaction with the toxic factor. The intersection of these two sets represents the subset of individuals who may be at risk for developing ALS. Note that the intersecting region can increase or decrease depending on strength of either variable. Intersecting these sets is a set representing the variable of age, with the level of risk increasing from young to old. *Abbreviations*: SALS, sporadic amyotrophic lateral sclerosis; Conc., toxin concentration; Detox., detoxification ability dependant on genetics.

ENVIRONMENTAL FACTORS AND ALS CLUSTERS

A major avenue in ALS research has sought to recreate SALS as a result of exposure to some environmental factor(s). Candidate factors have included various natural or synthetic molecules, including mitochondrial inhibitors or other molecules acting to increase oxidative stress, specific excitotoxins [glutamate or agonists (5)], heavy metal and transition metal ions, infectious agents, skeletal trauma, and electrical shock (for review, see Mitchell (2); Nelson et al. in preparation). Of these, glutamate consumption, smoking, and heavy metal exposure are significantly associated risk factors.

Accepting the notion of an environmental etiology thus introduces myriad possible candidates, and while no one factor seems likely to account for most cases of ALS, two general molecular categories have emerged as the most likely. They are molecules that increase oxidative stress or those that mimic the excitatory action of the neurotransmitter glutamate. Those that impact oxidative stress can do so either by increasing free radical production or by decreasing antioxidant defense mechanisms. Molecules that increase excitotoxicity are those that directly activate any of the glutamate receptor subtypes or those that act indirectly to cause glutamate release.

The major evidence for oxidative stress in neurological disease or in animal models arises from studies showing mitochondrial degeneration, notably in Parkinsonism (6,7). A variant form of Parkinsonism on Guadeloupe is attributed to chronic ingestion of tea made from varieties of soursop (*Annona muricata*) containing annonacin (8). In addition, the natural herbicide rotenone has also been linked to Parkinsonism (9). Notably, both compounds inhibit mitochondrial enzyme-I activity in a manner similar to that shown for the well-known parkinsonism-inducing toxins 1-methyl-4-phenyl-1,2,3,6-tetrahydropyridine and 6-hydroxydopamine (10). Evidence for oxidative damage to mitochondrial DNA leading to the accumulation of mutations, as well as other mitochondrial damage, could be an important mechanism contributing to the selective loss of motor neurons in ALS as well, and mitochondrial pathology has been documented in central nervous system tissue from ALS victims. A selective decrease in the activity of the mitochondrial DNA-encoded cytochrome c oxidase has been detected in human spinal cord motor neurons in ALS (11). In transgenic mice expressing a mutation in SOD1, morphological changes indicative of mitochondrial damage are seen early in the disorder (12). Enzyme activities of the mitochondrial electron transport chain are decreased in the spinal cords of mutant SOD transgenic mice, beginning at early stages and persisting throughout the progression of the disorder. A partial deficiency of another mitochondrial enzyme, manganese superoxide dismutase (SOD2), exacerbates motor neuron death in transgenic SOD1 mice (13). Another antioxidant molecule, glutathione, is significantly altered both in ALS and in other neurodegenerative disorders (14).

Evidence for excitotoxicity mediated by glutamate or glutamate agonists in neurological disease is now well established such as in ischemic conditions following stroke (15). A classic example of excitotoxicity in a neurodegenerative disorder is lathyrism, a disease of upper motor neurons caused by excessive consumption of the chickling pea (*Lathyrus sativus*), which contains the amino acid β-*N*-oxalylamino-L-alanine (BOAA) (16,17), an agonist at the AMPA subtype of the glutamate receptor. The disease expresses as disturbed motor function and muscle wasting. A related glutamate agonist found in the seed of the cycad palm (β-*N*-methylamino-L-alanine, BMAA) is an NMDA receptor agonist and has been reported to induce upper and lower motor neuron death in macaques. This finding is controversial (5), and the reported neural deficits were not reproducible in mice [(18); Cruz-Aguado et al. in preparation]. Cognitive dysfunction is associated with hippocampal damage combined with limb weakness suggestive of motor neuron dysfunction followed by injection of phytoplankton-contaminated mussels containing domoic acid, an agonist of the kainate subytpe of the glutamate receptor (19).

Other neurological disorders have been attributed to environmental excitotoxins including globus pallidus degeneration in horses following ingestion of yellow star thistle (*Centaurea solstitialis*), which may contain high levels of glutamate and aspartate (20) and consumption of cassava root which contains a cyanogenic glucosides leading to the muscle wasting disease konzo (21). Monosodium glutamate also causes hypothalamic and other CNS lesions in young mice (22).

The above will have made clear that a key source for human exposure to glutamate and glutamate agonists may be through diet or other forms of environmental exposure and that such exposure can lead to neurodegeneration of motor and other neurons. In regard to the overall action of such molecules, it is important to keep in mind that toxins impacting neuronal survival via excitotoxic mechanisms do not have to do so directly by activating the various glutamate receptor subtypes, but can equally induce excitotoxic events by either causing the uncontrolled release of glutamate from intracellular stores or by diminishing the uptake capacity of glutamate transporters whose role is to maintain glutamate homeostasis (23).

While oxidative stress and excitotoxicity are sometimes considered to be mutually exclusive as mechanisms inducing neurodegeneration, this is not necessarily the case. In fact, excitotoxicity and oxidative stress are intimately interlinked. Excitotoxic over-stimulation of neurons, for example, has as one consequence an increase in cellular activity leading to greater oxidative phosphorylation. The latter, in turn, increases free radical production with free radicals able to oxidatively damage proteins, lipids, and DNA. In addition, toxins that increase oxidative stress by inhibiting mitochondrial complex-I activity also impact the mitochondrial transmembrane potential. Alterations in this potential affect the resting potential across the neuronal cell membrane, leading to increased resting and active ionic influxes through NMDA and other glutamate receptor subtypes. For these reasons, it is not possible to view the long-term consequences of an excitotoxicity or increased oxidative stress in isolation. In addition, some molecules, methionine sulfoximine (MSO), for example, may have dual actions with direct impacts on both glutamate release and glutathione synthesis (24), thus immediately providing both excitotoxic actions while diminishing antioxidant defense mechanisms. The capacity for such molecules to have an immediate negative effect on neural function will be obvious (25). In addition, the notion of a synergistic interaction of separate excitotoxins and oxidative stressors contained in the same dietary item is not only plausible but in some circumstances likely.

In spite of the literature cited above, there is still no clear and definitive demonstration of an environmental factor that is universally causal for ALS. This fact can be contrasted with the acute neurotoxicity arising from domoic acid exposure cited above (19). One possibility raised by this comparison is that the molecules inducing SALS are discretely distributed or only present in subacute concentrations too low to impact motor neuron function or survival except following prolonged exposure. Alternatively, subthreshold levels of toxins may require synergistic interaction with other molecules or with susceptibility genes (26). The number of permutations for environmental synergies or gene–environmental factors is thus exceedingly large. Tracking down such factors remains a daunting task, especially when one adds on the clear evidence for the influence of aging in disease pathogenesis, not to mention the likelihood that there may be a considerable incubation period of years to decades during which the causal factors interact and in which abnormal biochemical and cellular processes accumulate. As clinical diagnosis for ALS only occurs once motor behavior has been significantly impacted, retrospective epidemiological searches for identifiable causal factors are difficult and often inconclusive.

One solution to identifying promising candidate molecules or genes lies in studying ALS disease clusters in which sufficient numbers of individuals are afflicted to generate statistical significance. Currently, the field recognizes one definitive ALS cluster, the Guamanian disorder ALS-PDC (for review, see Ref. 27). Recently, another potential cluster has been considered: the form of ALS that may be associated with Gulf War Syndrome (28), although this remains controversial.

ALS-PDC was recognized as such in the early 1950s (27,29). Found on Guam and Rota in the Marianas Islands chain and at other sites in the Western Pacific (e.g., New Guinea, Kii Peninsula of Japan) the disease can present as a relatively classical ALS ("lytico" or "paralytico"), as an Alzheimer's-like disorder with strong parkinsonism features ("bodig"), or, less frequently, as a combination of the separate disorders. For those cases exhibiting a combination of features, these commonly occur sequentially, with ALS preceding dementia (Steele, personal communication). The disease has been documented for hundreds of years from early in the period of the Spanish occupation of Guam, but was only the subject of intense neurological study after World War II (WWII). Kurland and others noted the unusual combination of features in some individuals, the extremely high-incidence rates, and the early onset of symptoms compared to North American neurological diseases. Chamorros who moved away from Guam were equally likely to get ALS-PDC, provided that they had lived on Guam early in life (30). The latter observation suggested some slow toxic factor, perhaps a virus, which could remain dormant for many years. Overall, however, most of the early epidemiological data supported a cultural/dietary link between the incidence of the disease and the consumption of flour made from the seed of a local variety of cycad palm (*Cycas micronesia K.D. Hill,* formerly incorrectly termed *C. circinalis,* T. Marler, personal communication) long used as traditional and/or famine food and as a medicine (27), both on Guam and elsewhere in the Western Pacific. Cycad seed was found to contain various toxins and early studies focused on potential links between these compounds and the disease. The amino sugar, cycasin, was found to exert cytotoxic actions, acutely affecting the liver via its aglycone, methylazoxymethanol (MAM). While both cycasin and MAM induced developmental abnormalities of the nervous system in rodents and could produce an acute loss of motor function in cattle, they did not otherwise mimic ALS-PDC in either behavioral or neuropathological outcomes [see Wilson et al. (31), for further citations]. Other toxins found in cycad, e.g., BOAA and BMAA, evoked differing forms of neurodegeneration through activation of either AMPA or NMDA glutamate receptor subtypes (32), as cited above. Renewed interest in BMAA neurotoxicity in ALS-PDC via biomagnification has been actively promoted recently by one group (33), but the latter has provided no experimental evidence to date to support neurological deficits associated with BMAA exposure. We have recently revisited the issue, feeding adult male CD-1 mice BMAA at 1 mg/kg [equivalent to the dose proposed to cause the disorder in humans by Cox et al. (33)] but have not seen any evidence for alterations in motor or cognitive behaviors or neural damage in the CNS (Cruz-Aguado et al. in preparation). These results mirror those of Perry et al. (18). Studies showing that water soluble toxins like BMAA and cycasin were removed from cycad flour by the extensive washing that was part of traditional Chamorro preparation (31,34) did not bolster the original "cycad hypothesis" for environmental toxicity associated with ALS-PDC.

While the ALS cluster on Guam remains the definite cluster for the disease, results such as the above suggested to many researchers that environmental toxicity would prove difficult or impossible. In addition, ALS-PDC incidence had been in decline for years, with rates falling to near North American levels (35). Although enthusiasm for the "cycad hypothesis" has declined, epidemiological studies continue to show strong links between ALS-PDC and cycad consumption. Kurland et al. (36) noted that cycad consumption on Guam was not uniform and that regions of Guam with the highest levels of consumption were ALS-PDC "hotspots". In addition, Kurland, Steele, and others noted that while the Chamorro peoples of Guam and Saipan are of similar ethnic/genetic stock, the rates of ALS-PDC were dissimilar, correlated with the fact that Guamanian Chamorros consumed cycad, especially during WWII, while their fellow Chamorros on Saipan did not. Another reason to abandon the cycad hypothesis was that, until recently, few studies have provided detailed behavioral and histological analyses of neural function and morphology following prolonged exposure to *washed* cycad as part of diet, i.e., in experiments designed to mimic typical patterns of Chamorro cycad preparation and consumption. An exception to this was a preliminary study by Dastur (37,38). In this experiment, several rhesus monkeys that were fed washed cycad seed showed motor deficits and motor neuron loss that resembled ALS, a promising outcome, which was not followed up with more detailed studies. After a 20-year lapse, the next experiments were those of Spencer and colleagues using pure BMAA. We will present in detail our studies of cycad toxicity in which we have attempted to model the disease by feeding washed cycad to mice (31) and which we believe validates Dastur's work and the general notion that cycad toxicity is intimately associated with ALS-PDC.

A MURINE MODEL OF ALS-PDC

In Vivo Cycad Toxicity: Motor, Cognitive, and Sensory Phenotypes

We have attempted to reproduce ALS-PDC in the simplest possible way by feeding adult male CD-1 mice washed cycad seed flour as approximately 25% of their total diet. The reasons for this included the following: (i) an intent to mimic dietary exposure to putative cycad neurotoxins; (ii) to provide evidence that any such neurotoxins could be absorbed through the gastrointestinal tract; (iii) to demonstrate that such toxins or metabolites could enter the CNS to inflict neural damage. In our experimental paradigm, we used cycad seeds obtained from Guam that had been subjected to a multiple and prolonged washing. The washed seeds were ground into flour and formed into pellets with water. The overall procedure was designed to mimic as far as possible the preparations of cycad by the Chamorros (34). To assess possible neural deficits over time, cycad-fed and control mice were subjected to a weekly battery of motor, cognitive, and olfactory function tests over a period of months, then sacrificed and processed for various histological and/or biochemical indices of neuronal death/dysfunction (31,39–41). Behavioral motor tests included leg extension, gait length, wire hang, and rotarod. Cognitive function was assessed using the Morris water maze or radial arm maze. Olfactory discrimination as well as behavior in an open field test was also measured.

Figure 2 summarizes some of these behavioral outcomes which have been described in detail elsewhere (26,31,41). Briefly, cycad feeding led to a significant

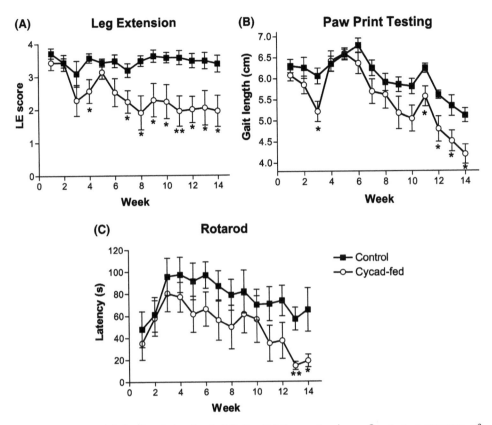

Figure 2 Cycad-fed mice: behavioral deficits. (**A**) Leg extension reflex test, a measure of motor neuron integrity. (**B**) Paw-print testing for walking gait length. (**C**) Rotarod test of balance and motor coordination. Cycad-fed mice show significant deficits on these tests begin-ning at weeks 3 and 4 and consistently thereafter for at least 10 to 12 of cycad feeding.

progressive decrease in the leg extension reflex, diminished gait length, loss of muscle strength, and diminished latency to fall on the rotarod. In regard to the latter, cycad-fed mice appeared to adapt their behavior on the rotarod to eventually achieve comparable durations to control mice (31). Cognitive tests revealed a trend toward diminished spatial learning and a highly significant decrease in reference memory. Olfactory function test showed a significant loss of odor detection, although we were not able to distinguish olfactory discrimination versus memory in our preliminary results. The altered behavior for the different functions did not emerge simultaneously, but generally showed a tendency for the earlier appearance of motor versus cognitive behavioral phenotypes. Although the level of effect varied between cycad-fed mice, cycad seed batches demonstrated to be toxic in vitro studies (42) showed that approxi-mately 85% of mice in such groups had motor deficits. Overall, the spectrum of behavioral outcomes remarkably resembled the human distribution of ALS-PDC, with some mice having dominant motor outcomes, some mice showing more pronounced cognitive effects, and some mice showing the full range of behavioral deficits (31).

Recently, we have observed a behavioral deficit that mimics yet another feature of the human disease. As cited above, early exposure to some factor on Guam led to high disease incidence rates in Chamorros outside of Guam. As part of a study of the age-dependence of cycad toxicity, we had fed cycad flour to animals of various ages.

Some of these mice showed no initial behavioral deficits, an outcome we attributed to low levels of the putative cycad neurotoxins and for these animals the cycad-feeding paradigm was halted after a month. Some of these mice (5 of 20 cycad fed; 1 of 20 controls), now over 18 months of age, have begun to show profound motor deficits characterized by ataxia, head tremor, and an inability to stay on the rotarod (Schulz et al. in preparation). We continue to monitor the responses of the remaining mice of this group and histological studies are underway to see the nature of the pathology generating this motor outcome.

Morphological and histological analyses of CNS tissue from cycad-fed animals have revealed pathological correlates to the altered behavioral functions. These included a significant volume decrease in ventral lumbar cord and internal capsule measured by magnetic resonance microscopy (MRM), correlating with a significant net loss of motor neurons in spinal cord (41). In cord, terminal deoxytransferase-mediated dUTP nick-end labeling (TUNEL) and caspase-3 positive cells were found. In addition, there was diminished cortical thickness in the motor and somatosensory cortices. Corresponding to the parkinsonism and dementia behavioral features, we found decreased MRM volume in the substantia nigra pars compacta (SNpc), hippocampus, and olfactory bulb along with TUNEL and caspase-3 positive cells in these areas. The olfactory bulb showed a disruption of glomerulus morphology. The striatum showed significant decreases in tyrosine hydroxylase and dopamine transporter (DAT) levels and increased D_2 dopamine receptor levels in cycad-fed mice; increased astrogliosis was seen in the SNpc of cycad-fed mice [(39); Schulz et al. in preparation]. Tau protein expression was also increased (cortex, SNpc, and hippocampus) (31). Some of these data are illustrated in Figures 2 and 3 (31,39–41). Oxidative stress markers were seen in various areas, including the hippocampus and motor cortex (43). The spinal cord, striatum, hippocampus, and some regions of cortex showed decreased GLT-1 (EAAT2) glutamate transporter levels and a coincident decline in AMPA and NMDA receptors (44).

Cycasin/MAM and BMAA concentrations were not present in our washed cycad flour (42) except in trace amounts. As cited above, BMAA alone did not mimic the behavioral or histological impacts of washed cycad (Cruz-Aguado et al. in preparation). Overall, we saw no evidence for liver or other system damage outside the CNS (31).

Preliminary age-dependent studies showed greater impacts of weight-adjusted cycad feeding with increasing age. Young (30–60 days old) mice that were fed with cycad flour showed initial motor deficits that recovered to normal values after the end of cycad feeding, in contrast to older mice in which the deficits were pronounced and progressive (45). These studies are ongoing. In human ALS and ALS-PDC, male victims predominate. We examined gender in relation to cycad toxicity using three-month-old female mice fed washed cycad flour compared to male mice of the same age. Female mice had disturbed gait length, as well as deficits in grip strength and balance, but these effects did not match the loss of function in male mice. Ovariectomized (OVR) mice and OVR mice in which physiological levels of β-estradiol 3-benzoate and/or progesterone were applied via implanted silastic capsules were also tested. OVR mice resembled male mice when fed cycad. Replacement of physiological levels of estradiol and progesterone provided some protection against cycad-induced motor deficits in grip strength and gait (46). These studies are also ongoing.

Cycad feeding in C57/Bl6 mice initiated the same behavioral and neuropathological outcomes as previously seen in CD-1 mice. C57/Bl6 mice were used in experiments to show the interaction of cycad feeding and a known genetic risk factor for

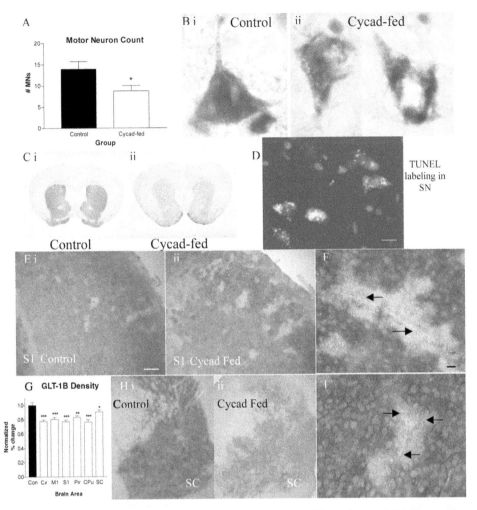

Figure 3 Cycad-fed mice: morphological and histological indices of neuronal degeneration. **(A)** In cervical spinal cord (SC) ventral horn motor neurons counts, cycad-fed mice show a significant decrease in motor neurons compared to control mice. **(B)** Photomicrographs of ventral motor neurons from control (i) and cycad-fed mice (ii). **(C)** Tyrosine hydroxylase (TH) labeling in the striatum of control (i) and cycad-fed (ii) mice as a measure of intrinsic dopamine levels. Cycad-fed mice show decreased TH labeling (−50% of control see Ref. 39). **(D)** Fluorescent TUNEL (terminal deoxytransferase-mediated dUTP nick-end labeling) labeling in the SNpc of a cycad-fed mouse. (*Gray*): Nucleus of cell body (DAPI). (*White*): TUNEL labeling of fragmented DNA as a measure of apoptosis. **(E–I)** Immunolabeling of Glutamate transporter 1B (GLT-1B) in cortex **(E)** and spinal cord **(H)** of control (E i, H i) and cycad-fed (E i, H ii) mice. **(F, I)** High-magnification photos of apparent blood vessels in areas lacking GLT-1B labeling. (*Arrows*): Indicate blood vessels. **(G)** Density of GLT-1B labeling in several CNS areas. The data represent standardized and averaged results of antibody-labeled sections measured using computerized densitometry (NIH Scion Image) (mean ± SEM) from three cycad-fed mice and three control mice. Multiple sections (2–4) were used from each animal. Dashed line represent control values for each area. Cycad fed mice show significantly decreased GLT-1B labeling. D: scale bar = 50 μm. **(E, H)** scale bar = 80 μm. **(F, I)** scale bar = 20 μm. $^*p < 0.05$, $^{**}p < 0.01$, $^{***}p < 0.001$. *Abbreviations*: Cx, total cortex; M1, primary motor cortex; S1, primary somatosensory cortex; pir, piriform cortex; CPu, caudate putamen; SC, spinal cord. *Source*: From Ref. 44.

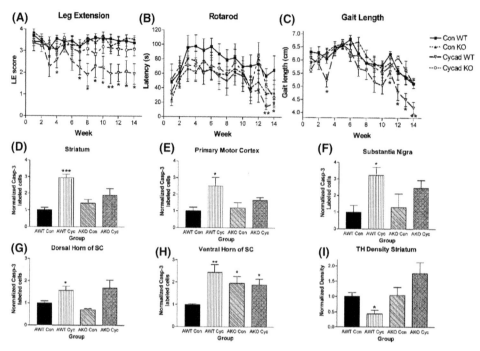

Figure 4 ApoE and cycad: motor function and quantitative apoptosis results. (A–C) Motor tests. (A) Leg extension, lower score indicated altered motor reflex. (B) Rotarod, latency to fall recorded as test of muscle strength and balance. (C) Gait Length, hind limb gait length was measured to see progressive changes. All three motor tests reveal progressive deficits of cycad-fed WT mice only. (D–I) active caspase-3 cell counts. Active caspase-3 labeling is significantly increased in AWT Cyc mice, but not in AKO Cyc mice in most areas. (L) TH labeling in striatum. TH density is significantly decreased in AWT Cyc mice only. $^{*}p < 0.05$, $^{**}p < 0.01$, $^{***}p < 0.001$. *Abbreviations*: (A–C) Con WT, Control Wild type; Con KO, Control ApoE Knockout; Cycad-fed WT, Cycad Wild-type; Cycad-fed KO, Cycad ApoE Knockout. (D–I) AWT Con, ApoE wild-type control; AWT Cyc, ApoE wild type cycad-fed; AKO Con, ApoE knockout control; AKO Cyc, ApoE knockout cycad-fed; TH, tyrosine hydroxylase.

neurodegenerative disease, apolipoprotein E (ApoE). ApoE wild-type (WT) mice fed with cycad showed behavioral and histological results similar to previous experiments. However, cycad-fed ApoE knockout mice appeared to be significantly protected from the neurotoxic impact of cycad feeding (40), although the amount of protection was dependent on the level of analysis. For example, behavioral motor tests showed near control values on leg extension, pawprint, and rotarod while motor neuron counts, apoptosis, tyrosine hydroxylase, and GLT-1 labeling revealed deficits following cycad feeding, but not to the level seen in the cycad-fed WT mice. Some of these data are shown in Figure 4 (40). More selective studies employing cycad-fed transgenic mice dominantly expressing ApoE2, E3, or E4 alleles are ongoing.

In Vitro Studies of Cycad-Induced Neurotoxicity

To isolate the principal toxin in washed cycad, we performed a series of studies using compounds isolated from washed cycad flour as described in detail in Khabazian et al. (42). In brief, serial isolation using HPLC/column chromatography methods were used to provide different fractions which were tested in an in vitro rat or mouse cortical wedge preparation for neural activity and neurotoxicity by measurements of cell death (lactate dehydrogenase, LDH, release assay). The most active fraction was found to contain a water insoluble mixture of phytosterol β-D-glucosides (abbreviated as SG), including β-sitosterol β-D-glucoside (the largest fraction, BSSG), campesterol/dihydro-brassicasterol β-D-glucoside, and stigmasterol β-D-glucoside (42). In vitro studies showed that the isolated SGs, as well as synthetic steryl glucosides made by us including BSSG and a cholesterol glucoside, were highly toxic with at least part of their action due to glutamate release *prior* to cell death. Exposure to these molecules gave a significant up-regulation of protein kinases, including PKC and CDKs 2 and 5 in cortical slices in vitro.

Recently, we have expanded our studies of SG neurotoxicity in neural cell cultures (Singh et al. in preparation). Astrocytes, neurons, or mixed neuron-glia culture preparations of human fetal cells showed that cholesterol glucoside was toxic in the low-micromolar range (tested at $50\,\mu M$). Exposure to this SG induced increased expression of hyperphosphorylated tau in neurons, decreased GLT-1 expression in astrocytes, increased HSP 70 in both cell types, and is followed by increased caspase-3 labeling. A higher percentage of neurons than astrocytes showed apoptosis.

DISCUSSION

Our modeling of ALS-PDC in mice replicates the presumed etiology and neural-systems outcomes of the human disorder. The results from the model are robust, reproducible, and, crucially, quantifiable. Variances within groups of animals in the level and site of impact on neurological function closely match the outcomes for ALS-PDC. The most pronounced effects of cycad toxicity were from batches of seeds containing the highest concentrations of phytosterol glucosides [Wilson et al. (31), Wilson et al. in preparation] and vice versa. There was a clear age-dependence with older animals more susceptible to cycad toxicity [Schulz et al. (39) and in preparation]; additionally, there was a greater impact of cycad toxins on male than female mice [Wong et al. (46), and in preparation], both features of ALS-PDC. The level of neurodegeneration induced by cycad toxins were clearly linked to specific genetic susceptibility factors, i.e., ApoE (40).

Cycad toxins previously associated with ALS-PDC are not present in our washed cycad flour and hence not in the source of the observed neurodegeneration and loss of behavioral function. Our in vitro data show acute toxicity of SGs in the low to medium μM range [compared to BMAA that acts in the mM range; Weiss et al. (32)]. Our in vivo data show a range of SG concentrations of 21 to $155\,\mu g/g$ dry cycad seed weight with an average concentration of approximately $88\,\mu g/g$. Adjusting for mouse weight ($40\,g$ being an approximate value), the total dose/animal was calculated to be $1.1\,mg/kg$; an equivalent human toxic dosage based on a $70\,kg$ human of $77.7\,mg$, or the amount provided by approximately $0.88\,kg/d$ cycad flour. In times of food shortage as proposed by Kurland (27), this amount of flour consumed per day may be a realistic estimate. [Note that not all SGs have equivalent toxicity as shown in Khabazian et al. (42); some may not be toxic at all, others much more so.]

The results to date, while still preliminary and speculative, support the notion that the causal neurotoxin in cycad is a steryl glucoside. Experiments in progress are attempting to reproduce the full cycad toxicity paradigm in mice fed steryl glucosides alone. A successful outcome to this experiment would suggest that such molecules are indeed the cause of the ALS-PDC outcomes in our mice and, by extension, in

ALS-PDC. The implications for ALS and other neurological diseases outside of Guam are obvious.

However, if we are unable to reproduce the cycad effect with SGs alone, we will be forced to reisolate the neurotoxin(s) responsible. In either case, the successful isolation of causal neurotoxins would lead to the following crucial questions: can the presence of molecules deemed causal to ALS serve as biomarkers for early stage disease processes? If we can identify such toxins and their origins, as well as understand their mechanisms of action, will we be able to design pharmaceutical strategies to prevent the initiation and progression of neural cell death in ALS? A key part of this goal is that we must also understand the temporal events from initial toxin exposure to motor neuron degeneration. The creation of an ALS "time-line" is thus crucial. Such a time-line would describe the process in four "dimensions," providing a full description of behavioral, structural, cellular, and biochemical events for different neural subsets as a function of time from initial toxin exposure [see Shaw and Wilson (26) for a more detailed discussion].

The identification of potential neurotoxins, a better understanding of the interactions of such toxins with genetic susceptibility factors, and the provision of a detailed time-line remain some of the most pressing experimental problems in current ALS research. The solution to these problems, however, will ultimately be accomplished through the use of appropriate animal models such as the one we have described in this chapter. Remaining, however, will be the far greater theoretical and practical challenge of how to apply the knowledge so gained to a successful search for the early behavioral and biochemical indices of ALS in the hope of preventing irreversible damage to the CNS *before* it has occurred.

ACKNOWLEDGMENTS

This work was supported by Grants from US Army Medical Research and Materiel Command (#DAMD17-02-1-0678), the Scottish Rite Charitable Fdn. of Canada, ALSA, NSERC. The authors thank Cheryl Melder, Jeff Schulz, Erin Hawkes, and Swaraj Singh for valuable comments. We thank Drs. Ulla Craig, Tom Marler, and John Steele for providing cycad seeds.

REFERENCES

1. Majoor-Krakauer D, Willems PJ, Hofman A. Genetic epidemiology of amyotrophic lateral sclerosis. Clin Genet 2003; 63:83–101.
2. Mitchell JD. Amyotrophic lateral sclerosis: toxins and environment. Amyotroph Lateral Scler Other Motor Neuron Disord 2000; 1:235–250.
3. Rowland LP, Shneider NA. Amyotrophic lateral sclerosis. N Engl J Med 2001; 344: 1688–1700.
4. Yang Y, Hentati A, Deng HX, Dabbagh O, Sasaki T, Hirano M, Hung WY, Ouahchi K, Yan J, Azim AC, et al. The gene encoding alsin, a protein with three guanine-nucleotide exchange factor domains, is mutated in a form of recessive amyotrophic lateral sclerosis. Nat Genet 2001; 29:160–165.
5. Spencer PS, Nunn PB, Hugon J, Ludolph AC, Ross SM, Roy DN, Robertson RC. Guam amyotrophic lateral sclerosis-parkinsonism-dementia linked to a plant excitant neurotoxin. Science 1987; 237:517–522.
6. Greenamyre JT, MacKenzie G, Peng TI, Stephans SE. Mitochondrial dysfunction in Parkinson's disease. Biochem Soc Symp 1999; 66:85–97.

7. Betarbet R, Sherer TB, Di Monte DA, Greenamyre JT. Mechanistic approaches to Parkinson's disease pathogenesis. Brain Pathol 2002; 12:499–510.

8. Lannuzel A, Michel PP, Hoglinger GU, Champy P, Jousset A, Medja F, Lombes A, Darios F, Gleye C, Laurens A, et al. The mitochondrial complex I inhibitor annonacin is toxic to mesencephalic dopaminergic neurons by impairment of energy metabolism. Neuroscience 2003; 121:287–296.

9. Betarbet R, Sherer TB, MacKenzie G, Garcia-Osuna M, Panov AV, Greenamyre JT. Chronic systemic pesticide exposure reproduces features of Parkinson's disease. Nat Neurosci 2000; 3:1301–1306.

10. Orth M, Tabrizi SJ. Models of Parkinson's disease. Mov Disord 2003; 18:729–737.

11. Borthwick GM, Johnson MA, Ince PG, Shaw PJ, Turnbull DM. Mitochondrial enzyme activity in amyotrophic lateral sclerosis: implications for the role of mitochondria in neuronal cell death. Ann Neurol 1999; 46:787–790.

12. Jung C, Higgins CM, Xu Z. Mitochondrial electron transport chain complex dysfunction in a transgenic mouse model for amyotrophic lateral sclerosis. J Neurochem 2002; 83:535–545.

13. Andreassen OA, Ferrante RJ, Klivenyi P, Klein AM, Shinobu LA, Epstein CJ, Beal MF. Partial deficiency of manganese superoxide dismutase exacerbates a transgenic mouse model of amyotrophic lateral sclerosis. Ann Neurol 2000; 47:447–455.

14. Bains JS, Shaw CA. Neurodegenerative disorders in humans: the role of glutathione in oxidative stress-mediated neuronal death. Brain Res Brain Res Rev 1997; 25:335–358.

15. Arundine M, Tymianski M. Molecular mechanisms of glutamate-dependent neurodegeneration in ischemia and traumatic brain injury. Cell Mol Life Sci 2004; 61:657–668.

16. Ravindranath V. Neurolathyrism: mitochondrial dysfunction in excitotoxicity mediated by L-beta-oxalyl aminoalanine. Neurochem Int 2002; 40:505–509.

17. Spencer PS, Schaumburg HH. Lathyrism: a neurotoxic disease. Neurobehav Toxicol Teratol 1983; 5:625–629.

18. Perry TL, Bergeron C, Biro AJ, Hansen S. Beta-N-methylamino-L-alanine. Chronic oral administration is not neurotoxic to mice. J Neurol Sci 1989; 94:173–180.

19. Teitelbaum JS, Zatorre RJ, Carpenter S, Gendron D, Evans AC, Gjedde A, Cashman NR. Neurologic sequelae of domoic acid intoxication due to the ingestion of contaminated mussels. N Engl J Med 1990; 322:1781–1787.

20. Roy DN, Peyton DH, Spencer PS. Isolation and identification of two potent neurotoxins, aspartic acid and glutamic acid, from yellow star thistle (Centaurea solstitialis). Nat Toxins 1995; 3:174–180.

21. Howlett WP, Brubaker GR, Mlingi N, Rosling H. Konzo, an epidemic upper motor neuron disease studied in Tanzania. Brain 1990; 113(pt 1):223–235.

22. Perez VJ, Olney JW, Martin JF, Cannon WO. Minimal tissue concentrations of glutamate required to produce necrosis of hypothalamic neurons in newborn mice. Biol Neonate 1979; 35:17–22.

23. Danbolt NC. Glutamate uptake. Prog Neurobiol 2001; 65:1–105.

24. Shaw CA, Bains JS, Pasqualotto BA, Curry K. Methionine sulfoximine shows excitotoxic actions in rat cortical slices. Can J Physiol Pharmacol 1999; 77:871–877.

25. Shaw CA, Bains JS. Synergistic versus antagonistic actions of glutamate and glutathione: the role of excitotoxicity and oxidative stress in neuronal disease. Cell Mol Biol (Noisylegrand) 2002; 48:127–136.

26. Shaw CA, Wilson JM. Analysis of neurological disease in four dimensions: insight from ALS-PDC epidemiology and animal models. Neurosci Biobehav Rev 2003; 27:493–505.

27. Kurland LT. Amyotrophic lateral sclerosis and Parkinson's disease complex on Guam linked to an environmental neurotoxin. Trends Neurosci 1988; 11:51–54.

28. Horner RD, Kamins KG, Feussner JR, Grambow SC, Hoff-Lindquist J, Harati Y, Mitsumoto H, Pascuzzi R, Spencer PS, Tim R, et al. Occurrence of amyotrophic lateral sclerosis among Gulf War veterans. Neurology 2003; 61:742–749.

29. Whiting MG. Toxicity of cycads. Econ Botany 1963; 17:271–302.

30. Garruto RM, Gajdusek C, Chen KM. Amyotrophic lateral sclerosis among Chamorro migrants from Guam. Ann Neurol 1980; 8:612–619.

31. Wilson JM, Khabazian I, Wong MC, Seyedalikhani A, Bains JS, Pasqualotto BA, Williams DE, Andersen RJ, Simpson RJ, Smith R, et al. Behavioral and neurological correlates of ALS-parkinsonism dementia complex in adult mice fed washed cycad flour. Neuromolecular Med 2002; 1:207–221.

32. Weiss JH, Koh JY, Choi DW. Neurotoxicity of beta-N-methylamino-L-alanine (BMAA) and beta-N-oxalylamino-L-alanine (BOAA) on cultured cortical neurons. Brain Res 1989; 497:64–71.

33. Cox PA, Banack SA, Murch SJ. Biomagnification of cyanobacterial neurotoxins and neurodegenerative disease among the Chamorro people of Guam. Proc Natl Acad Sci USA 2003; 100:13,380–13,383.

34. Duncan MW, Steele JC, Kopin IJ, Markey SP. 2-Amino-3-(methylamino)-propanoic acid (BMAA) in cycad flour: an unlikely cause of amyotrophic lateral sclerosis and parkinsonism-dementia of Guam. Neurology 1990; 40:767–772.

35. Plato CC, Garruto RM, Galasko D, Craig UK, Plato M, Gamst A, Torres JM, Wiederholt W. Amyotrophic lateral sclerosis and parkinsonism-dementia complex of Guam: changing incidence rates during the past 60 years. Am J Epidemiol 2003; 157:149–157.

36. Lessell S, Hirano A, Torres J, Kurland LT. Parkinsonism-dementia complex. Epidemiological considerations in the Chamorros of the Mariana Islands and California. Arch Neurol 1962; 7:377–385.

37. Dastur DK. Cycad toxicity in monkeys: clinical, pathological, and biochemical aspects. Fed Proc 1964; 23:1368–1369.

38. Dastur DK, Palekar RS, Manghani DK. Toxicity of various forms of cycas circinalis in rhesus monkeys: pathology of brain, spinal cord and liver. In: Rose FC, Norris FH, eds. Amyotrophic Lateral Sclerosis: New Advances in Toxicology and Epidemiology. New York, NY: Smith-Gordon/Nishimura press, 1990:129–141.

39. Schulz JD, Khabazian I, Wilson JM, Shaw CA. A muring model of als-pdc with behavioural and neuropathological features of parkinsonism. Ann N Y Acad Sci 2003; 991:326–329.

40. Wilson JM, Petrik MS, Moghadasian MH, Shaw CA. Examining the role of apoe in neurodegenerative disorders using an environmentally-induced murine model of ALS-PDC. Canadian Jorn & Physiology an Pharmacology 2005; 83(2):131–14.

41. Wilson JM, Petrik MS, Grant SC, Blackband SJ, Lai J, Shaw CA. Quantitative measurement of neurodegeneration in an ALS-PDC model using MR microscopy. NeuroImage 2004; 23(1):336–343.

42. Khabazian I, Bains JS, Williams DE, Cheung J, Wilson JM, Pasqualotto BA, Pelech SL, Andersen RJ, Wang YT, Liu L, et al. Isolation of various forms of sterol beta-d-glucoside from the seed of Cycas circinalis: neurotoxicity and implications for ALS-parkinsonism dementia complex. J Neu rochem 822002516–528.

43. Cruz-Aguado R, Schulz JD, Hawkes EL, Shaw CA. Oxidative damage and differential neuronal vulnerability in a mouse model of amyotrophic lateral sclerosis-parkinsonism-dementia complex. Sixth Biennial Advanced School of Neurochemistry of the ISN, Abstracts book 2004 [abst.].

44. Wilson JM, Khabazian I, Pow DV, Craig UK, Shaw CA. Decrease in glial glutamate transporter variants and excitatory amino acid receptor down-regulation in a murine model of ALS-PDC. Neuromolecular Med 2003; 3:105–118.

45. Hawkes EL, Schulz JD, Shaw CA. Recovery of Motor Function In Mice Fed Cycad Toxin: Implication For ALS? Program No. 630.11. 2003 Abstract Viewer/Itinerary Planner. Washington, DC: Society for Neuroscience, 2003. Online. 2003 [abst.].

46. Wong MC, Lukic V, Shaw CA. Cycad Toxicity in a Female Mouse Model of ALS-PDC. Abstract Viewer/Itinerary Planner. Washington, DC: Society for Neuroscience 2003; Online Abstract.

20
Genetic Causes and Predisposition

Silke Schmidt and Jeffery M. Vance
Department of Medicine, Center for Human Genetics, Duke University Medical Center, Durham, North Carolina, U.S.A.

INTRODUCTION

This chapter will focus on the genetic dissection of complex traits, specifically the non-Mendelian forms of amyotrophic lateral sclerosis (ALS). In contrast to the methods that have successfully been applied to discover the genes responsible for Mendelian (monogenic) ALS (chap. 6), the analysis of the more common form of the disorder is complicated by several factors. For example, instead of a single *causal* gene such as SOD1, the more common forms of ALS are likely due to one or more *susceptibility* genes, each conferring a relatively small risk increase ("predisposition"), as well as to interactions between these genes and between genes and environmental exposures. Even patients with non-Mendelian forms of ALS may present with a family history (e.g., they may have an affected first-degree relative), but no specific inheritance pattern is apparent in their families. Different individuals within the same family do not necessarily share the same genetic factors. For example, in one individual, gene A could contribute more to the disease than gene B, while in another individual, due to different allelic variations in interacting genes or different environmental challenges, gene B could be the major determinant of disease. Because of these complexities, the probability (penetrance) of expressing a particular phenotype given genotypes at one or more disease-associated loci will depend on many factors typically unknown to the investigator. Many statistical analysis methods for mapping complex disease genes have been specifically developed to accommodate this greater uncertainty in genotype–phenotype relationships.

BACKGROUND

Linkage Analysis

The goal of linkage analysis is to identify regions in the human genome likely to harbor causal or susceptibility genes for the phenotype of interest, which we will assume to be qualitative in nature (i.e., affected with ALS, unaffected, or unknown). In order to detect such regions, the investigator has to collect families in which at least two biologically related individuals (e.g., siblings) are affected with ALS and

449

are able to provide a DNA sample. The DNA samples are then analyzed for certain types of genetic variation (polymorphisms) distributed at known positions all across the human genome (*markers*). The most common types of polymorphisms used today are (i) *microsatellite* markers, which vary in the number of times certain nucleotide sequences are repeated, e.g., $(CA)_n$, or $(GATA)_n$ and (ii) single-nucleotide polymorphisms (SNPs), which vary by the nucleotide (A, C, G, or T) at a single base-pair position and typically exist in only two versions (alleles). In contrast, microsatellite markers typically have many (up to 20 or more) different alleles.

Regardless of the type of marker used, the biological process that allows us to perform linkage analysis on human pedigrees is *meiosis*, the cell division that leads to the formation of gametes (ova and sperm). During meiosis, homologous chromosomes pair up and exchange genetic material by the crossing-over of an individual's maternal and paternal chromosome strand, thus creating a mosaic of "recombinant" segments with different parental origin. The key observation for linkage analysis is the fact that recombination between any two loci on the same chromosome is more likely to occur the further apart the loci are, since greater distance provides more physical opportunity for recombination to occur. Therefore, the distance between two loci can be measured by the frequency with which new combinations of grandparental alleles are observed in the offspring resulting from the fusion of two parental gametes (*recombination frequency*).

Genotypes at a large number of marker loci with known position in the human genome are easily measured in the laboratory using a variety of techniques (1). *Linkage analysis* on the collected pedigrees then evaluates whether the disease phenotype and marker genotype travel together (cosegregate) more often than expected by chance. If so, this suggests that the disease locus we want to map and the marker locus whose position is known are physically located close to one another ("linked") on the same chromosome. The presence of linkage is relatively easy to evaluate in clearly Mendelian pedigrees in which multiple generations are affected with the phenotype of interest, since much information about the recombination frequency between disease and marker loci can be obtained from even one large pedigree. However, in complex disorders like ALS or Alzheimer disease, each pedigree typically provides limited information about cosegregation of disease phenotype and marker genotype. It is common that only one generation of affected individuals is available for DNA sampling. In this situation, the extent of linkage can be measured by examining marker allele sharing among affected relative pairs (e.g., affected sibling pairs). This approach is based on the intuitive idea that pairs of relatives who share the same phenotype (e.g., both are affected with ALS) are expected to show above-average sharing of alleles at marker loci that are physically close to the disease locus causing the shared phenotype (2). However, because much less information is gained from each of these small pedigrees, the total number of patient samples needed for complex disease studies is much greater than that needed for Mendelian diseases.

Statistically, linkage analysis of complex disorders can be performed with model-based ("parametric") and model-free ("non-parametric") methods (3). Parametric analysis is similar to the traditional method used for mapping Mendelian disease genes, with modifications allowing for the greater uncertainty in genotype–phenotype relationships, including unknown inheritance patterns. Non-parametric analysis simply scores the evidence for excess marker allele sharing in pairs of sampled affected relatives, without making any assumptions about genotype–phenotype relationships. With both approaches, the evidence for linkage is summarized by a measure known as the LOD score. Originally used as an abbreviation for "log of the odds," the LOD score is more appropriately referred to as the log-likelihood ratio for linkage (4). For Mendelian diseases with known inheritance patterns, a parametric LOD score > 3.0 is generally accepted as the minimum level of significance suggesting linkage. Because of the $\log_{10}$ scale of LOD scores, pedigree data giving a score above 3.0 can be interpreted to be more than $10^3 = 1000$ times more likely to have arisen under linkage of marker and disease locus than under no linkage. For complex diseases and in the context of a genome-wide linkage screen, any LOD score over 2.0 is typically considered "interesting" by most investigators (5). Statistical significance levels for LOD scores are more formally discussed elsewhere (6).

It should be pointed out that an identical clinical phenotype for a complex disorder might be due to one of several rare Mendelian disease genes, usually with autosomal-recessive inheritance, or one of several susceptibility genes. In ALS, mutations in SOD1 or ALS2 yield the same phenotype as observed in the sporadic form of the disorder. Similarly, idiopathic Parkinson disease (PD) may be due to known mutations in several rare autosomal recessive genes, including Parkin, PINK1, and DJ1 (7–9). While these genes often produce a form of PD with earlier age at onset, the clinical phenotype is otherwise identical to sporadic PD. To complicate matters further, it now appears that heterozygous carriers of at least Parkin and glucocerebrosidase mutations are also at increased risk of late-onset PD (10,11).

Association Analysis

The difference between association and linkage analysis is often confusing to the non-geneticist. The goal of *linkage* analysis is to detect a relatively large chromosomal region that travels with the disease in multiple *pedigrees* and is thus likely to harbor a disease susceptibility gene. The goal of *association* analysis is to identify a particular DNA sequence variant in that region that is found more commonly in people affected with the disease than in people without it when the entire *population* of interest, or a representative subset of it, is evaluated. The following analogy may be useful.

A policeman determines, after investigating all the blocks of a large city, that prank telephone calls (the disorder) affecting a community are coming from a specific block of houses (genes) on a street (chromosome) in the city (genome). This would be the equivalent of successfully detecting linkage (location) of the disorder. His linkage method, however, cannot tell him which of the houses and which of the residents inside them is the culprit; it can only identify the location of the block. Thus, he must determine which of the houses on this linked block and then which of the residents in the houses (which specific polymorphism) is the cause of the phone calls. After watching cars coming to the houses, he determines that resident A drives home and is present in the house during most of the times the calls are made, more often than the policeman would expect to observe this simply by chance. He thus suspects resident A. This is the equivalent of establishing association of the polymorphic allele (resident A) with the disorder (phone calls). However, further research reveals that resident B rides to work each day with resident A and thus is very closely linked to him in time and space [linkage disequilibrium of two polymorphisms (haplotype) on the same chromosome]. This confuses the policeman, as he realizes that either could be the caller. But deeper investigation leads the policeman to find out that on the weekends, resident B is not with resident A (linkage disequilibrium is broken up), and that in fact, resident B is present in the house at the time the prank phone calls are made, while resident A is not. Thus the officer determines that resident B is most closely associated with the phone calls and is thus the most likely culprit, based on circumstantial evidence.

In the human genome, allelic association may be created by various mechanisms, but the only one that is of interest for mapping disease genes is association due to tight physical linkage of two loci, i.e., *linkage disequilibrium* (LD). LD is generated when a susceptibility allele first arises by mutation and at that particular point of time only exists on the single ancestral combination of alleles (haplotype) at polymorphic loci surrounding it. This originally very tight association due to physical linkage is gradually broken up over time and the primary factor determining the rate of LD decay in a randomly mating population is the recombination frequency between the disease locus and the adjacent polymorphic loci. However, LD is also strongly influenced by stochastic factors, which makes it difficult to predict the amount of LD as a function of physical distance alone. Commonly used statistical measures of LD in present-day chromosomes include D' and r^2, both of which are reviewed and comprehensively compared elsewhere (12). In a genetically homogeneous population, strong LD will only persist over many generations of chromosomes when marker and disease loci are so tightly linked that their alleles almost never recombine. Thus, the detection of LD between a putative disease allele and a measured marker allele provides a much greater resolution of the most likely location of the susceptibility gene than the detection of linkage, which is a measure of very recent recombination events within families. This is an intuitive explanation for the greater statistical power to detect disease susceptibility genes provided by association analysis, relative to linkage analysis (13).

For LD mapping of complex disease genes, different types of data sets may be used. A *family-based test of allelic association* can be applied to pedigrees with at least two sampled first-degree relatives, of which at least one is affected with the disease of interest. The second sampled relative has to be either a parent (or ideally both parents) or a sibling. Parental affection status is not used in the analysis (14,15). Some methods require phenotypically unaffected siblings, while others only use sibling genotypes to infer the most likely parental transmissions of marker alleles (16). An alternative to family-based association analysis is to collect a data set of unrelated patients (cases) and unrelated individuals without the disease of interest (controls) to perform a *case–control test of allelic association*. The controls need to be matched to the cases in terms of their genetic background and should represent the source population that gave rise to the cases. They should be sampled from an age group that is at risk of being affected with the disease of interest. General control selection strategies for epidemiologic studies are extensively reviewed elsewhere (17).

There has been much discussion about the relative merits of family-based versus case–control association designs. The main advantage of family-based designs is that "controls" (alleles *not* transmitted from parents to affected offspring) are by definition genetically perfectly matched to "cases" (alleles transmitted to affected offspring). Thus, the investigator is protected from detecting spurious (false-positive) allelic association due to reasons other than close physical proximity of marker and disease locus, such as population stratification or admixture (3). However, the protection against spurious results comes at the cost of a loss of statistical power of the family-based design when population structure is indeed absent (18). Family-based designs have additional advantages when the investigator is interested in estimating gene–gene and gene–environment interactions (19–21), or maternal genotype and parent-of-origin (imprinting) effects (22).

Genomic Convergence

A tremendous and unprecedented resource of DNA polymorphisms has been provided by the Human Genome Project and the more recently initiated HapMap Project (23). There are currently over five million validated SNPs in the public database (dbSNP, http://www.ncbi.nlm.nih.gov/SNP) and the number continues to grow rapidly. It is estimated that SNPs occur on average every 300 to 500 base pairs and that the number of SNPs within the human genome, defined as having a minor allele frequency of $\geq 1\%$ in at least one population, is likely to be at least 10 million (23). The much greater density and lower mutation rate of SNPs, compared to microsatellite polymorphisms, and the fact that assays for affordable high-throughput genotyping are much more easily developed, have made SNPs the marker of choice for modern association analysis.

In parallel with this development, gene expression data for various human tissues have become available through sophisticated microarray and Serial Analysis of Gene Expression (SAGE) techniques. Thus, a key concept in complex disease gene mapping is the combination of evidence from multiple experiments or study types to narrow down the list of plausible candidate genes for a given disorder or phenotype. This paradigm has been coined the "genomic convergence" approach to complex trait analysis (24). To illustrate with an example from PD research (24), SAGE was used to identify sequence tags expressed in normal substantia nigra (SN) and adjacent midbrain tissue. Bioinformatics methods were then used to map the genes corresponding to the SAGE tags to the human genome and thus determine the subset of genes located in genomic regions identified in a previous linkage screen of PD (25). In this example, the number of candidate genes to investigate was reduced from almost 5000, which mapped to one of five large linkage intervals identified in the genome screen, to 402, fewer than 10%, which were actually expressed in normal SN. A further refinement to achieve even greater "convergence" might include genetic studies on experimental animals, or the evaluation of expression changes in PD patients compared with controls using SAGE or microarray techniques.

ASSOCIATION STUDIES FOR SPORADIC ALS

The majority of association studies in non-Mendelian ALS have been performed on case–control data sets, but of highly variable sample size. This is a problem, as small sample sizes often lead to difficulty in replicating initial results. To provide some indication of the required sample size to detect plausible effect sizes for complex disorders with reasonably high probability (statistical power), we performed some example calculations with the program QUANTO (19,20). Effect sizes are measured as the relative risk (RR) for carriers of a susceptible genotype to develop ALS relative to non-carriers. Assuming a 5% significance level for a two-sided test, a sample of 100 cases and 100 controls (unmatched design) has 81% power to detect an RR of 2.3 if the susceptibility SNP allele frequency is 0.3 and the mode of inheritance is dominant, but only 29% power to detect an RR of 1.5 with the same allele frequency. Lower allele frequency and a recessive mode of inheritance greatly decrease statistical power, e.g., for an allele frequency of 0.1, the same sample size of 100 cases and 100 controls has only 11% power to detect an RR of 2.3 and 6% power to detect an RR of 1.5.

Mendelian Genes in Sporadic ALS

SOD1 screening has been performed on samples of sporadic ALS patients and has generally indicated that the gene does not appear to play a major role in the non-Mendelian forms of the disorder, although mutations have been detected in up to 2% of apparently sporadic cases (26–28). Mixed results have been reported for the survival motor neuron gene (SMN1), which causes spinal muscular atrophy (MIM 253300). The gene exists in two closely flanking, nearly identical copies, the telomeric *SMN1* and the centromeric *SMN2* genes, which are distinguished by sequence differences in exons seven and eight. A homozygous deletion in SMN2 was proposed to be predictive of survival and respiratory decline in sporadic ALS (110 cases, 100 controls) (29), but this result was not confirmed in another study (124 cases, 200 controls) (30).

An abnormal SMN1 copy number was reported to be a susceptibility factor for ALS based on comparing 167 cases and their unaffected spouses (31). No difference in SMN2 copy number between the two groups was observed. Thus, the roles of the *SMN1* and *SMN2* genes in ALS remain unclear. Other candidate genes selected for association studies with non-SOD1 mediated ALS have primarily been derived from the major etiologic hypotheses for ALS pathogenesis. Example studies are listed below.

Neurotrophic Growth Factor Malfunction

Neurotrophic growth factors (NGFs) are a group of neuropeptides that play an important role in regulating the growth, differentiation, and survival of neurons in the peripheral (PNS) and central nervous systems (CNS). If they are absent or not readily available to repair injured motor neurons or maintain healthy neurons, cell death will occur. This is consistent with the observed loss of motor neurons in upper and lower body extremities in ALS and suggests NGF-regulating genes as plausible candidates. There are only few published association studies of NGF-regulating genes for ALS. A study of 400 cases and 236 controls failed to support an effect of genotypes at the ciliary neurotrophic factor (CNTF) locus on ALS risk or clinical phenotype (32).

Neurofilament Accumulation

Abnormal accumulation of intermediate filaments in the perikarya and proximal axons of motor neurons is a common pathological hallmark of ALS (33). This observation, along with our general understanding of the functions of intermediate filaments in neuronal development (34), suggests that abnormalities in neurofilament (NF) organization may be involved in ALS pathogenesis. NFs are the principal intermediate filament type expressed by motor neurons and are formed by the coassembly of three subunits: NF-L (light), NF-M (medium), and NF-H (heavy subunit). A potentially important, although likely very small, role of polymorphisms in the NF genes in ALS etiology was supported by the presence of codon deletions and insertions in the KSP repeat region of the NF-H gene in a total of about 1% of the combined set of patients ($n > 1000$) from three independent studies (35–37). Interestingly, the codon deletions in affected individuals almost always occurred in combination with the long (L) allele of NF-H (45 motif repeats), while most individuals harboring a deletion along with the short (S) allele were unaffected. On the other hand, when genotype frequencies were compared between sporadic ALS patients and controls from a Russian population, the S/S genotype was more frequent in patients than controls (38). The reason for the difference between these results is not clear. More recently, a frameshift deletion in the peripherin gene, another type of intermediate filament protein, was detected in one out of 190 ALS patients and none out of 190 controls (39). Should this polymorphism contribute to ALS at all, it would clearly explain only a small fraction of the disease.

Excitotoxicity

Glutamate is a by-product of glutamic acid metabolism in the cells and is the major excitatory transmitter in the motor neuron system. The over-activation of excitatory amino acid receptors is known as excitotoxicity and results in damage and ultimately death of the affected cells. Thus, a malfunction in the glutamate uptake system may lead to toxic effects on motor neurons. The glial glutamate transporter EAAT2 is responsible for approximately 90% of glutamate removal from motor neurons (40) and suppressed expression of EAAT2 was observed in 60% of patients with sporadic ALS (41). Abnormal splice variants of EAAT2 have been detected in human CNS, however, they may not be due to polymorphisms in the *EAAT2* gene (42). A recent study of the glutamate AMPA receptor in patients with sporadic ALS and controls suggested that defective RNA editing of the GluR2 subunit of the AMPA receptor may contribute to motor neuron death (43). This report, as well as experimental data on mice and in vitro studies of motor neurons, continue to support a role of impaired glutamic acid metabolism in ALS (44). Excitotoxicity actually appears to be a mechanistic link to SOD1-mediated ALS (45) and is also the basis of the only FDA-approved ALS therapy, Riluzole, which decreases glutamate toxicity. Thus, studies of ALS candidate genes involved in glutamic acid metabolizing pathways appear to be well justified.

Oxidative Stress and Mitochondria

Oxidative stress arises from an imbalance between the intracellular production of potentially toxic reactive oxygen species (ROS) and reactive nitrogen species (RNS) and the elimination of ROS and RNS by the scavenging activities of various antioxidant molecules. The CNS is known to be particularly susceptible to oxidative stress, which has strongly been implicated in many neurodegenerative disorders, including Alzheimer, Parkinson, and Huntington disease (46). A role of ROS-mediated oxidative stress in ALS has been supported by increased levels of typical oxidation products found in both familial and sporadic ALS patients (47) as well as mouse models of ALS (48). The number of candidate genes contributing to oxidative stress pathways is quite large. However, only a few such genes have been examined in ALS association studies so far.

For example, the RNS nitric oxide (NO) is an important biological messenger that plays a prominent role in the physiology of the CNS. Thus, the three isoforms responsible for NO production, the neuronal, inducible, and endothelial NO synthase genes [nNOS (NOS1), iNOS (NOS2A), and eNOS (NOS3), respectively], are an excellent group of candidate genes for association studies of ALS (49). It has also been proposed that membrane-associated oxidative stress (e.g., lipid peroxidation and oxidative modification of membrane proteins) in neurodegenerative disorders is promoted by redox-active metals, such as iron and copper (50). Metal-catalyzed oxidative stress may contribute to the elevated ALS risk observed in several Western

Pacific island populations, such as the native Chamorros of Guam (reviewed in more detail later in this chapter). This theory was supported by significantly increased iron levels in the brains of Chamorro patients affected with a combination of ALS and Parkinson—dementia complex (ALS/PDC), compared with neurologically normal controls from the same region (51).

Since mitochondria are capable of antioxidant activity, but are also known to produce ROS, both nuclear and mitochondrial genes may be involved in oxidative stress pathways leading to ALS. Mitochondria are organelles with unique genetic properties. They have their own genome which codes for 13 polypeptides, 22 tRNAs and two rRNAs and consists of a single circular chromosome, meaning that mitochondrial alleles do not recombine. They also have poor DNA repair capabilities and are inherited exclusively through the maternal lineage. Thus, they are like molecular "passports" tracing the travels of our female ancestral mitochondria, and have been very useful in studies of population migrations and evolutionary relationships. These molecular "passports" are known as "haplogroups," similar to haplotypes in the nuclear genome, except that haplogroups are much more specific to the continental origin of different ethnic groups. For example, northern Europeans tend to have specific haplogroups, which distinguish them from individuals originating from Asia, Africa, etc. Interestingly, recent studies suggested a protective effect of certain haplogroups on the risk of Parkinson disease. Relative to the most common European haplogroup H, haplogroups K and J were found to be protective in females (52). This result was specifically due to the 10398 polymorphism found in the ND3 subunit of complex I, whose G allele is part of both protective haplogroups. A subsequent study with relatively small sample size examined the role of haplogroups in ALS (53) and found that haplogroup I may be protective for ALS, but with no sex effect. Haplogroup I is the only other group that shares the 10398 G allele with the K and J haplogroups in Europeans.

A small study conducted in Taiwan suggested that the 4977 bp deletion mitochondrial polymorphism, located between the D loop and CO1 gene, might also be significantly associated with ALS risk (54). These findings provide support for additional studies of the role of mitochondrial polymorphisms in ALS.

Apolipoprotein E

Apolipoprotein E (APOE) is a ubiquitous cholesterol transport protein, which plays an important role in promoting the general health and survival of neurons, and clearly has a role in how neuronal tissue responds to cellular stress. It is a major apolipoprotein in the CNS and is also found in the PNS. The human APOE protein exists in three functionally distinct isoforms, E2, E3, and E4. The three isoforms are coded by three alleles (haplotypes) composed of combinations of two SNPs in exon four of the gene and vary at amino acid positions 112 and 158. Frequencies of the three alleles vary widely across different human populations (55), but APOE-3 is always more common than APOE-2 and APOE-4. Strong associations between APOE and human diseases of the CNS exist. The APOE-4 allele has long been known to confer an approximately threefold increased risk of Alzheimer disease (AD) to heterozygous carriers and a much greater risk increase to homozygous carriers, and is also associated with an earlier age of onset (56). In contrast, each APOE-2 allele decreases AD risk and increases the age of onset (57). The APOE-4 allele was also shown to increase the risk and decrease the age-at-onset of Parkinson disease, with this association apparently not being dependent upon cognitive impairment (58).

The role of APOE in sporadic ALS has been examined in multiple case–control and one family-based study (59–63). Conflicting results were obtained, although most studies did not support an association between ALS risk or age at onset and APOE genotypes. However, several studies did support a tendency of APOE-4 carriers to experience more rapid disease progression and shorter survival (59–61). Interestingly, APOE was found to be significantly up regulated in the spinal cord of SOD1-mutant mice at the time of onset of paralysis, providing some biological support for these reports (64). Two studies of the ALS/PDC phenotype observed in the Chamorro population of Guam examined disease associations with APOE genotypes. Both of them had very small sample sizes of 12 and 29 patients, respectively, who were compared with the same 12 Chamorro controls (65,66). The Chamorro population has one of the highest APOE-2 frequencies in the world (33.3%) and the frequency of this allele was found to be substantially lower in the patients with Guamanian ALS/PDC (8.3% and 11.8% respectively). This observation suggests a protective effect on ALS risk, which would be consistent with the role of APOE in Alzheimer disease.

In summary, APOE is one of the most frequently studied candidate genes for ALS. The only association replicated by several, although not all, studies is a more rapid disease progression for APOE-4 carriers. A potentially protective effect of the APOE-2 allele was only supported by small-scale studies of the Chamorro population. Outside this population, none of the studies performed to date have been able to demonstrate an APOE-2 associated decrease or an APOE-4 associated increase in ALS risk, leaving a definitive comparison of the role of APOE in ALS, Alzheimer, and Parkinson diseases open to further research.

Vascular Endothelial Growth Factor

Some surprising and exciting findings from ALS association studies of the vascular endothelial growth factor (VEGF) have been reported very recently. VEGF is an essential cytokine for angiogenesis and vasculogenesis. A large study of almost 600 ALS patients and more than 1000 controls proposed that it may be a susceptibility gene for ALS (67). A mouse model of VEGF regulation and functional studies of SNPs in the promoter and $5'$ untranslated region of VEGF further supported this observation. The study showed that homozygous carriers of two particular VEGF haplotypes had an almost twofold risk of ALS ($p < 0.0001$) and that these at-risk haplotypes lowered circulating VEGF levels by influencing expression of the VEGF gene. One of the three SNPs included in the associated haplotype impaired translation of a large isoform of VEGF. Treatment with *Vegf* was shown to fully protect the at-risk motor neurons of wild-type mice from damage after extended spinal cord ischemia. This study has opened new avenues for ALS research and treatment (68), and independent replication studies of the particular polymorphisms implicated by this report are an obvious next step. In addition, VEGF receptors, including VEGFR-2 and NRP1, their signaling effectors, and upstream regulators such as the hypoxia-induced factors HIF1A and HIF2A should also be examined.

Phenotypic Modifiers

It should be noted that genes might have a major influence on the course of ALS and other phenotypic characteristics, such as age or site of onset and extent of disability, even if they do not increase the disease risk per se. Recent studies in ALS as well as

Alzheimer and Parkinson disease have demonstrated genetic contributions to age at onset, but not necessarily risk (58,63,69–71). For ALS, a small study in Sardinia (72) suggested that individuals with a specific monoamine oxidase B (MAO-B) allele had a later average age at onset than carriers of other alleles. Another report suggested that MAO-B is overexpressed in ALS patients, possibly due to an increase in reactive astrocyte types (73). The *MAO-B* gene has also been found to be associated with PD risk in some, but not all studies (74,75). Interestingly, the hypothesis that MAO-B may influence the risk of neurodegenerative disorders by regulating levels of reactive astrocyte types was supported by the successful prevention of the effects of MPTP-intoxication in a mouse model of PD through immunization to Copaxone (76), which is believed to cause an increase in the astrocytic T cell influx.

Gene–Environment Interaction

The hypothesis that gene–environment (G×E) interaction may be an important component of ALS etiology is strongly supported by studies of isolated geographic regions with a 50- to 100-fold increased prevalence of ALS. As mentioned previously, two neurodegenerative conditions have been observed at elevated frequency in the Chamorro population of the Western Pacific islands, including Guam and Rota: ALS (locally known as "lytico") and a unique PDC (locally known as "bodig"). The two conditions often occur together in the same patient and co-segregate in families. A neuropathological hallmark of Guamanian ALS/PDC is intraneuronal neurofilamentous aggregation. Up until recently, a striking environmental characteristic of this particular island population was a high consumption of cycad nuts, either as a component of homemade cycad flour or indirectly through consumption of fruit bats, which were typically boiled in coconut milk and considered a delicacy for special occasions. Since the bats feed on cycad nuts and eat twice their body weight every night, their tissue can accumulate much higher levels of toxic nut components than cycad flour. This observation gave rise to the hypothesis that the combination of diet and genetic predisposition to neurofilamentous accumulation may explain the increased incidence of ALS/PDC. An increased prevalence of specific polymorphisms in the *tau* and the *CYP2D6* genes in the Chamorro population has been reported (77,78) and may partially account for the genetic susceptibility to environmental toxins. Interestingly, cycasin, a component of cycad nuts, was shown to cause persistent up-regulation of *tau* mRNA expression (79), giving further support to G×E interaction as the potential underlying cause of the increased ALS/PDC prevalence. A decrease in the consumption of traditional food due to a shift towards a more Western diet is believed to have contributed to the decreased incidence of ALS/PDC in Guam over the past 40 years (80). Similar, but less-well studied ALS clusters were also reported in two areas of the Japanese Kii peninsula and in a coastal population of former West Papua New Guinea (now Indonesia).

A possible role of G×E interaction in ALS susceptibility was also implicated by recent reports of an approximately twofold increase in ALS risk observed for deployed Gulf War (GW) veterans, relative to both non-deployed GW veterans (81) and to age-specific incidence rates in the general population (82). Both studies suggested the possibility that an unknown environmental component in the Persian Gulf region may have acted as a trigger in genetically susceptible individuals. However, a more recent study (83) reported that veterans in general, not just those deployed to the Gulf War, might have an increased ALS risk. The authors suggested that studies of a larger set of environmental exposures that may be more common in military than civilian populations may provide some insight into the reasons for these disturbing findings. The broader implication for genetic association studies is that "environmentally responsive genes" that are likely to influence the effect of environmental exposure on disease risk should be evaluated as potential ALS candidates in the context of an individual's environmental exposure history. The Environmental Genome Project currently funded by the National Institutes of Health (http://www.niehs.nih.gov/envgenom/) provides extensive information about validated polymorphisms in such environmentally responsive genes and will be a very useful resource for planning such studies.

SUMMARY

Candidate gene association studies have so far been of limited success in dissecting the etiology of sporadic ALS, notable exceptions being VEGF and possibly APOE. However, many plausible candidate genes derived from the different hypotheses of ALS pathogenesis have yet to be examined in sufficiently large samples of patients and controls in order to more definitively confirm or rule out their involvement in the more common forms of this devastating disorder. In addition to examining larger sample sizes, investigators may also have to evaluate strong biological candidate genes in the context of an individual's environmental exposure history to achieve better success with genetic association studies.

REFERENCES

1. Vance JM, Ben Othmane K. Methods of genotyping. In: Haines JL, Pericak-Vance MA, eds. Approaches to Gene Mapping in Complex Human Diseases. New York: Wiley-Liss, 1998:213–228.
2. Penrose LS. The general purpose sib-pair linkage test. Ann Eugen 1953; 18:120–124.
3. Thomas DC. Statistical Methods in Genetic Epidemiology. New York: Oxford University Press, 2004.
4. Elston RC. Algorithms and Inferences: the challenge of multifactorial disease. Am J Hum Genet 1997; 60:255–262.
5. Haines JL, Pericak-Vance MA. Approaches to Gene Mapping in Complex Human Diseases. New York, N Y: Wiley Inc., 1998.
6. Lander E, Kruglyak L. Genetic dissection of complex traits: guidelines for interpreting and reporting linkage results. Nat Genet 1995; 11(3):241–247.
7. Bonifati V, Rizzu P, van Baren MJ, Schaap O, Breedveld GJ, Krieger E, Dekker MC, Squitieri F, Ibanez P, Joosse M, van Dongen JW, Vanacore N, Van Swieten JC, Brice A, Meco G, Van Duijn CM, Oostra BA, Heutink P. Mutations in the DJ-1 gene associated with autosomal recessive early-onset parkinsonism. Science 2003; 299(5604): 256–259.
8. Kitada T, Asakawa S, Hattori N, Matsumine H, Yamamura Y, Minoshima S, Yokochi M, Mizuno Y, Shimizu N. Mutations in the parkin gene cause autosomal recessive juvenile parkinsonism. Nature 1998; 392(6676):605–608.
9. Valente EM, Abou-Sleiman PM, Caputo V, Muqit MM, Harvey K, Gispert S, Ali Z, Del Turco D, Bentivoglio AR, Healy DG, Albanese A, Nussbaum R, Gonzalez-Maldonado R, Deller T, Salvi S, Cortelli P, Gilks WP, Latchman DS, Harvey RJ, Dallapiccola B, Auburger G, Wood NW. Hereditary early-onset Parkinson's disease caused by mutations in PINK1. Science 2004; 304(5674):1158–1160.

10. Oliveira SA, Scott WK, Martin ER, Nance MA, Watts RL, Hubble JP, Koller WC, Pahwa R, Stern MB, Hiner BC, Ondo WG, Allen FH, Jr., Scott BL, Goetz CG, Small GW, Mastaglia F, Stajich JM, Zhang F, Booze MW, Winn MP, Middleton LT, Haines JL, Pericak-Vance MA, Vance JM. Parkin mutations and susceptibility alleles in late-onset Parkinson's disease. Ann Neurol 2003; 53(5):624–629.

11. Aharon-Peretz J, Rosenbaum H, Gershoni-Baruch R. Mutations in the glucocerebrosidase gene and Parkinson's disease in Ashkenazi Jews. N Engl J Med 2004; 351(19):1972–1977.

12. Ardlie KG, Kruglyak L, Seielstad M. Patterns of linkage disequilibrium in the human genome. Nat Rev Genet 2002; 3(4):299–309.

13. Risch N, Merikangas K. The future of genetic studies of complex human disorders. Science 1996; 273(5281):1516–1517.

14. Spielman RS, McGinnis RE, Ewens WJ. Transmission test for linkage disequilibrium: the insulin gene region and insulin-dependent diabetes mellitus (IDDM). Am J Hum Genet 1993; 52:506–516.

15. Martin ER, Monks SA, Warren LL, Kaplan NL. A test for linkage and association in general pedigrees: the pedigree disequilibrium test. Am J Hum Genet 2000; 67: 146–154.

16. Martin ER, Bass MP, Hauser ER, Kaplan NL. Accounting for linkage in family-based tests of association with missing parental genotypes. Am J Hum Genet 2003; 73(5): 1016–1026.

17. Rothman KJ, Greenland S. Modern Epidemiology. 2nd ed. Philadelphia: Lippincott-Raven, 1998.

18. Risch N, Teng J. The relative power of family-based and case-control designs for linkage disequilibrium studies of complex human diseases : DNA pooling. Genome Res 1998; 8:1273–1288.

19. Gauderman WJ. Sample size requirements for association studies of gene-gene interaction. Am J Epidemiol 2002; 155(5):478–484.

20. Gauderman WJ. Sample size requirements for matched case-control studies of gene-environment interaction. Stat Med 2002; 21(1):35–50.

21. Schaid DJ. Case-parents design for gene-environment interaction. Genet Epidemiol 1999; 16(3):261–273.

22. Weinberg CR, Wilcox AJ, Lie RT. A log-linear approach to case-parent-triad data: assessing effects of disease genes that act either directly or through maternal effects and that may be subject to parental imprinting. Am J Hum Genet 1998; 62:969–978.

23. Gibbs RA. The International HapMap Consortium. The International HapMap Project. Nature 2003; 426(6968):789–796.

24. Hauser MA, Li YJ, Takeuchi S, Walters R, Noureddine M, Maready M, Darden T, Hulette C, Martin E, Hauser E, Xu H, Schmechel D, Stenger JE, Dietrich F, Vance J. Genomic convergence: identifying candidate genes for Parkinson's disease by combining serial analysis of gene expression and genetic linkage. Hum Mol Genet 2003; 12(6): 671–677.

25. Scott WK, Nance MA, Watts RL, Hubble JP, Koller WC, Lyons K, Pahwa R, Stern MB, Colcher A, Hiner BC, Jankovic J, Ondo WG, Allen FH, Jr., Goetz CG, Small GW, Masterman D, Mastaglia F, Laing NG, Stajich JM, Slotterbeck B, Booze MW, Ribble RC, Rampersaud E, West SG, Gibson RA, Middleton LT, Roses AD, Haines JL, Scott BL, Vance JM, Pericak-Vance MA. Complete genomic screen in Parkinson disease: evidence for multiple genes. JAMA 2001; 286(18):2239–2244.

26. Andersen PM, Nilsson P, Keranen ML, Forsgren L, Hagglund J, Karlsborg M, Ronnevi LO, Gredal O, Marklund SL. Phenotypic heterogeneity in motor neuron disease patients with CuZn-superoxide dismutase mutations in Scandinavia. Brain 1997; 120(Pt 10):1723–1737.

27. Jackson M, Al Chalabi A, Enayat ZE, Chioza B, Leigh PN, Morrison KE. Copper/zinc superoxide dismutase 1 and sporadic amyotrophic lateral sclerosis: analysis of 155 cases and identification of a novel insertion mutation. Ann Neurol 1997; 42(5):803–807.

28. Jones CT, Swingler RJ, Simpson SA, Brock DJ. Superoxide dismutase mutations in an unselected cohort of Scottish amyotrophic lateral sclerosis patients. J Med Genet 1995; 32(4):290–292.

29. Veldink JH, Van den Berg LH, Cobben JM, Stulp RP, de Jong JM, Vogels OJ, Baas F, Wokke JH, Scheffer H. Homozygous deletion of the survival motor neuron 2 gene is a prognostic factor in sporadic ALS. Neurology 2001; 56(6):749–752.

30. Gamez J, Barcelo MJ, Munoz X, Carmona F, Cusco I, Baiget M, Cervera C, Tizzano EF. Survival and respiratory decline are not related to homozygous SMN2 deletions in ALS patients. Neurology 2002; 59(9):1456–1460.

31. Corcia P, Mayeux-Portas V, Khoris J, de Toffol B, Autret A, Muh JP, Camu W, Andres C. Abnormal SMN1 gene copy number is a susceptibility factor for amyotrophic lateral sclerosis. Ann Neurol 2002; 51(2):243–246.

32. Al Chalabi A, Scheffler MD, Smith BN, Parton MJ, Cudkowicz ME, Andersen PM, Hayden DL, Hansen VK, Turner MR, Shaw CE, Leigh PN, Brown RH, Jr. Ciliary neurotrophic factor genotype does not influence clinical phenotype in amyotrophic lateral sclerosis. Ann Neurol 2003; 54(1):130–134.

33. Rouleau GA, Clark AW, Rooke K, Pramatarova A, Krizus A, Suchowersky O, Julien JP, Figlewicz D. SOD1 mutation is associated with accumulation of neurofilaments in amyotrophic lateral sclerosis. Ann Neurol 1996; 39(1):128–131.

34. Lariviere RC, Julien JP. Functions of intermediate filaments in neuronal development and disease. J Neurobiol 2004; 58(1):131–148.

35. Al Chalabi A, Andersen PM, Nilsson P, Chioza B, Andersson JL, Russ C, Shaw CE, Powell JF, Leigh PNDeletions of the heavy neurofilament subunit tail in amyotrophic lateral sclerosis. Hum Mol Genet 1999; 8(2):157–164.

36. Tomkins J, Usher P, Slade JY, Ince PG, Curtis A, Bushby K, Shaw PJ. Novel insertion in the KSP region of the neurofilament heavy gene in amyotrophic lateral sclerosis (ALS). Neuroreport 1998; 9(17):3967–3970.

37. Figlewicz DA, Krizus A, Martinoli MG, Meininger V, Dib M, Rouleau GA, Julien JP-Variants of the heavy neurofilament subunit are associated with the development of amyotrophic lateral sclerosis. Hum Mol Genet 1994; 3(10):1757–1761.

38. Skvortsova V, Shadrina M, Slominsky P, Levitsky G, Kondratieva E, Zherebtsova A, Levitskaya N, Alekhin A, Serdyuk A, Limborska S. Analysis of heavy neurofilament subunit gene polymorphism in Russian patients with sporadic motor neuron disease (MND). Eur J Hum Genet 2004; 12(3):241–244.

39. Gros-Louis F, Lariviere R, Gowing G, Laurent S, Camu W, Bouchard JP, Meininger V, Rouleau GA, Julien JP. A frameshift deletion in peripherin gene associated with amyotrophic lateral sclerosis. J Biol Chem 2004; 279(44):45951–45956.

40. Rothstein JD, Dykes-Hoberg M, Pardo CA, Bristol LA, Jin L, Kuncl RW, Kanai Y, Hediger MA, Wang Y, Schielke JP, Welty DF. Knockout of glutamate transporters reveals a major role for astroglial transport in excitotoxicity and clearance of glutamate. Neuron 1996; 16(3):675–686.

41. Rothstein JD, Van Kammen M, Levey AI, Martin LJ, Kuncl RW. Selective loss of glial glutamate transporter GLT-1 in amyotrophic lateral sclerosis. Ann Neurol 1995; 38(1):73–84.

42. Aoki M, Lin CL, Rothstein JD, Geller BA, Hosler BA, Munsat TL, Horvitz HR, Brown RH, Jr. Mutations in the glutamate transporter EAAT2 gene do not cause abnormal EAAT2 transcripts in amyotrophic lateral sclerosis. Ann Neurol 1998; 43(5): 645–653.

43. Kawahara Y, Ito K, Sun H, Aizawa H, Kanazawa I, Kwak S. Glutamate receptors: RNA editing and death of motor neurons. Nature 2004; 427(6977):801.

44. Bruijn LI, Miller TM, Cleveland DW. Unraveling the mechanisms involved in motor neuron degeneration in ALS. Annu Rev Neurosci 2004; 27:723–749.

45. Howland DS, Liu J, She Y, Goad B, Maragakis NJ, Kim B, Erickson J, Kulik J, DeVito L, Psaltis G, DeGennaro LJ, Cleveland DW, Rothstein JD. Focal loss of the glutamate

transporter EAAT2 in a transgenic rat model of SOD1 mutant-mediated amyotrophic lateral sclerosis (ALS). Proc Natl Acad Sci USA 2002; 99(3):1604–1609.

46. Emerit J, Edeas M, Bricaire F. Neurodegenerative diseases and oxidative stress. Biomed Pharmacother 2004; 58(1):39–46.

47. Simpson EP, Henry YK, Henkel JS, Smith RG, Appel SH. Increased lipid peroxidation in sera of ALS patients: a potential biomarker of disease burden. Neurology 2004; 62(10):1758–1765.

48. Carri MT, Ferri A, Cozzolino M, Calabrese L, Rotilio G. Neurodegeneration in amyotrophic lateral sclerosis: the role of oxidative stress and altered homeostasis of metals. Brain Res Bull 2003; 61(4):365–374.

49. Urushitani M, Shimohama S. The role of nitric oxide in amyotrophic lateral sclerosis. Amyotroph Lateral Scler Other Motor Neuron Disord 2001; 2(2):71–81.

50. Mattson MP. Metal-catalyzed disruption of membrane protein and lipid signaling in the pathogenesis of neurodegenerative disorders. Ann NY Acad Sci 2004; 1012:37–50.

51. Yasui M, Ota K, Garruto RM. Concentrations of zinc and iron in the brains of Guamanian patients with amyotrophic lateral sclerosis and parkinsonism-dementia. Neurotoxicology 1993; 14(4):445–450.

52. van der Walt JM, Nicodemus KK, Martin ER, Scott WK, Nance MA, Watts RL, Hubble JP, Haines JL, Koller WC, Lyons K, Pahwa R, Stern MB, Colcher A, Hiner BC, Jankovic J, Ondo WG, Allen FH Jr, Goetz CG, Small GW, Mastaglia F, Stajich JM, McLaurin AC, Middleton LT, Scott BL, Schmechel DE, Pericak-Vance MA, Vance JM. Mitochondrial polymorphisms significantly reduce the risk of Parkinson disease. Am J Hum Genet 2003; 72(4):804–811.

53. Mancuso M, Conforti FL, Rocchi A, Tessitore A, Muglia M, Tedeschi G, Panza D, Monsurro M, Sola P, Mandrioli J, Choub A, Delcorona A, Manca ML, Mazzei R, Sprovieri T, Filosto M, Salviati A, Valentino P, Bono F, Caracciolo M, Simone IL, La B, V, Majorana G, Siciliano G, Murri L, Quattrone A. Could mitochondrial haplogroups play a role in sporadic amyotrophic lateral sclerosis?. Neurosci Lett 2004; 371(2–3):158–162.

54. Ro LS, Lai SL, Chen CM, Chen ST. Deleted 4977-bp mitochondrial DNA mutation is associated with sporadic amyotrophic lateral sclerosis: a hospital-based case-control study. Muscle Nerve 2003; 28(6):737–743.

55. Corbo RM, Scacchi R. Apolipoprotein E (APOE) allele distribution in the world. Is APOE*4 a 'thrifty' allele? Ann Hum Genet 1999; 63(pt 4):301–310.

56. Corder EH, Saunders AM, Strittmatter WJ, Schmechel DE, Gaskell PC, Small GW, Roses AD, Haines JL, Pericak-Vance MA. Gene dose of apolipoprotein E type 4 allele and the risk of Alzheimer's disease in late onset families. Science 1993; 261(5123):921–923.

57. Corder EH, Saunders AM, Risch N, Strittmatter WJ, Schmechel DE, Gaskell PC, Rimmler JB, Locke PA, Conneally PM, Schmader KE, Small GW, Roses AD, Haines JL, Pericak-Vance MA. Apolipoprotein E type 2 allele decreases the risk of late onset Alzheimer disease. Nat Genet 1994; 7:180–184.

58. Li YJ, Hauser MA, Scott WK, Martin ER, Booze MW, Qin XJ, Walter JW, Nance MA, Hubble JP, Koller WC, Pahwa R, Stern MB, Hiner CB, Jankovic J, Goetz CG, Small GW, Mastaglia F, Haines JL, Pericak-Vance MA, Vance JA. Apolipoprotein E controls the risk and age at onset of Parkinson Disease. Neurology 2004; 62(11):2005–2009.

59. Al-Chalabi A, Enayat ZE, Bakker MC, Sham PC, Ball DM, Shaw CE, Lloyd CM, et al. Association of apolipoprotein E ε4 allele with bulbar-onset motor neuron disease. Lancet 1996; 347:159–160.

60. Moulard B, Sefiani A, Laamri A, Malafosse A, Camu W. Apolipoprotein E genotyping in sporadic amyotrophic lateral sclerosis: evidence for a major influence on the clinical presentation and prognosis. J Neurol Sci 1996; 139(suppl):34–37.

61. Smith RG, Haverkamp LJ, Case S, Appel V, Appel SH. Apolipoprotein E epsilon 4 in bulbar-onset motor neuron disease. Lancet 1996; 348(9023):334–335.

62. Siddique T, Pericak-Vance MA, Caliendo J, Hong ST, Hung WY, Kaplan J, McKenna-Yasek D, Rimmler JB, Sapp P, Saunders AM, Scott WK, Siddique N, Haines JL, Brown RH. Lack of association between apolipoprotein E (APOE) genotype and sporadic amyotrophic lateral sclerosis (ALS). Neurogenetics 1998; 1:213–216.

63. Li YJ, Pericak-Vance MA, Haines JL, Siddique N, McKenna-Yasek D, Hung WY, Sapp P, Allen CI, Chen W, Hosler B, Saunders AM, Dellefave LM, Brown RH Jr, Siddique T. Apolipoprotein E is associated with age at onset of amyotrophic lateral sclerosis. Neurogenetics 2004; 5(4):209–213.

64. Haasdijk ED, Vlug A, Mulder MT, Jaarsma D. Increased apolipoprotein E expression correlates with the onset of neuronal degeneration in the spinal cord of G93A-SOD1 mice. Neurosci Lett 2002; 335(1):29–33.

65. Waring SC, O'Brien PC, Kurland LT, Thibodeau SN, Tsai MS, Petersen RC, Esteban-Santillan CEApolipoprotein E allele in Chamorros with amyotrophic lateral sclerosis/ parkinsonism-dementia complex. Lancet 1994; 343(8897):611.

66. Buee L, Perez-Tur J, Leveugle B, Buee-Scherrer V, Mufson EJ, Loerzel AJ, Chartier-Harlin MC, Perl DP, Delacourte A, Hof PRApolipoprotein E in Guamanian amyotrophic lateral sclerosis/parkinsonism-dementia complex: genotype analysis and relationships to neuropathological changes. Acta Neuropathol (Berl) 1996; 91(3):247–253.

67. Lambrechts D, Storkebaum E, Morimoto M, Del Favero J, Desmet F, Marklund SL, Wyns S, Thijs V, Andersson J, van M, I, Al Chalabi A, Bornes S, Musson R, Hansen V, Beckman L, Adolfsson R, Pall HS, Prats H, Vermeire S, Rutgeerts P, Katayama S, Awata T, Leigh N, Lang-Lazdunski L, Dewerchin M, Shaw C, Moons L, Vlietinck R, Morrison KE, Robberecht W, Van Broeckhoven C, Collen D, Andersen PM, Carmeliet P VEGF is a modifier of amyotrophic lateral sclerosis in mice and humans and protects motoneurons against ischemic death. Nat Genet 2003; 34(4):383–394.

68. Lambrechts D, Storkebaum E, Carmeliet P. VEGF: necessary to prevent motoneuron degeneration, sufficient to treat ALS? Trends Mol Med 2004; 10(6):275–282.

69. Li YJ, Scott WK, Hedges DJ, Zhang F, Gaskell PC, Nance MA, Watts RL, Hubble JP, Koller WC, Pahwa R, Stern MB, Hiner BC, Jankovic J, Allen FA, Jr., Goetz CG, Mastaglia F, Stajich JM, Gibson RA, Middleton LT, Saunders AM, Scott BL, Small GW, Nicodemus KK, Reed AD, Schmechel DE, Welsh-Bohmer KA, Conneally PM, Roses AD, Gilbert JR, Vance JM, Haines JL, Pericak-Vance MA. Age at onset in two common neurodegenerative diseases is genetically controlled. Am J Hum Genet 2002; 70(4):985–993.

70. Li YJ, Oliveira SA, Xu P, Martin ER, Stenger JE, Hulette C, Scherzer CR, Hauser MA, Scott WK, Small GW, Nance MA, Watts RL, Hubble JP, Koller WC, Pahwa R, Stern MB, Hiner BC, Jankovic J, Goetz CG, Mastaglia F, Middleton LT, Roses AD, Saunders AM, Welsh-Bohmer KA, Schmechel DE, Gullans SR, Haines JL, Gilbert JR, Vance JM, Pericak-Vance MA. Glutathione S-transferase omega-1 modifies age-at-onset of Alzheimer disease and Parkinson disease. Hum Mol Genet 2004; 13(5):573.

71. Kolsch H, Linnebank M, Lutjohann D, Jessen F, Wullner U, Harbrecht U, Thelen KM, Kreis M, Hentschel F, Schulz A, von Bergmann K, Maier W, Heun RPolymorphisms in glutathione S-transferase omega-1 and AD, vascular dementia, and stroke. Neurology 2004; 63(12):2255–2260.

72. Orru S, Mascia V, Casula M, Giuressi E, Loizedda A, Carcassi C, Giagheddu M, Contu L. Association of monoamine oxidase B alleles with age at onset in amyotrophic lateral sclerosis. Neuromuscul Disord 1999; 9(8):593–597.

73. Jossan SS, Ekblom J, Aquilonius SM, Oreland L. Monoamine oxidase-B in motor cortex and spinal cord in amyotrophic lateral sclerosis studied by quantitative autoradiography. J Neural Transm Suppl 1994; 41:243–248.

74. Costa-Mallen P, Afsharinejad Z, Kelada SN, Costa LG, Franklin GM, Swanson PD, Longstreth WT, Jr., Viernes HM, Farin FM, Smith-Weller T, Checkoway H. DNA sequence analysis of monoamine oxidase B gene coding and promoter regions in Parkinson's disease cases and unrelated controls. Mov Disord 2004; 19(1):76–83.

75. Parsian A, Racette B, Zhang ZH, Rundle M, Perlmutter JS. Association of variations in monoamine oxidases A and B with Parkinson's disease subgroups. Genomics 2004; 83(3): 454–460.

76. Benner EJ, Mosley RL, Destache CJ, Lewis TB, Jackson-Lewis V, Gorantla S, Nema-chek C, Green SR, Przedborski S, Gendelman HE. Therapeutic immunization protects dopaminergic neurons in a mouse model of Parkinson's disease. Proc Natl Acad Sci (USA) 2004; 101(25):9435–9440.

77. Poorkaj P, Tsuang D, Wijsman E, Steinbart E, Garruto RM, Craig UK, Chapman NH, Anderson L, Bird TD, Plato CC, Perl DP, Weiderholt W, Galasko D, Schellenberg GD. TAU as a susceptibility gene for amyotropic lateral sclerosis-parkinsonism dementia complex of Guam. Arch Neurol 2001; 58(11):1871–1878.

78. Chen X, Xia Y, Gresham LS, Molgaard CA, Thomas RG, Galasko D, Wiederholt WC, Saitoh T. ApoE and CYP2D6 polymorphism with and without parkinsonism-dementia complex in the people of Chamorro, guam. Neurology 1996; 47(3):779–784.

79. Esclaire F, Kisby G, Spencer P, Milne J, Lesort M, Hugon J. The Guam cycad toxin methylazoxymethanol damages neuronal DNA and modulates tau mRNA expression and excitotoxicity. Exp Neurol 1999; 155(1):11–21.

80. Plato CC, Garruto RM, Galasko D, Craig UK, Plato M, Gamst A, Torres JM, Wieder-holt W. Amyotrophic lateral sclerosis and parkinsonism-dementia complex of Guam: changing incidence rates during the past 60 years. Am J Epidemiol 2003; 157(2):149–157.

81. Horner RD, Kamins KG, Feussner JR, Grambow SC, Hoff-Lindquist J, Harati Y, Mit-sumoto H, Pascuzzi R, Spencer PS, Tim R, Howard D, Smith TC, Ryan MA, Coffman CJ, Kasarskis EJ. Occurrence of amyotrophic lateral sclerosis among Gulf War veterans. Neurology 2003; 61(6):742–749.

82. Haley RW. Excess incidence of ALS in young Gulf War veterans. Neurology 2003; 61(6):750–756.

83. Weisskopf MG, O'Reilly EJ, McCullough ML, Calle EE, Thun MJ, Cudkowicz M, Ascherio A. Prospective study of military service and mortality from ALS. Neurology 2005; 64(1):32–37.

21

ALS: A Protein Aggregate Disease?

A. Radunović, A. Dawson, J. M. Gallo, and Peter Nigel Leigh
Department of Clinical Neuroscience, Institute of Psychiatry, King's College London, London, U.K.

INTRODUCTION

Accumulation of various proteins within cells or in the extracellular space of the central or peripheral nervous system is a feature of many neurodegenerative diseases (Table 1). Indeed, accumulation of β-amyloid protein in senile plaques of Alzheimer's disease (AD), detected using classic pathological stains and only later identified specifically as containing a specific protein, provided the key to understanding the molecular basis of this disease by providing a target for genetic studies that in turn pointed back to the key role of the amyloid precursor protein. Likewise, the presence of prion protein in the extracellular plaques in transmissible spongiform encephalopathies (TSE) provided a link between a characteristic feature of the pathology in sporadic and inherited forms of TSE and prion gene mutations that were identified in familial forms of TSE (1,2). As in AD, this provided the key to understanding the relationship between altered processing of a specific protein and progressive neurodegeneration in apparently sporadic diseases. In monogenic conditions such as Huntington's disease and the hereditary ataxias, identification of gene defects led to the finding of accumulations of the gene product (3).

Although extracellular protein deposits provided important clues on pathogenesis in AD and TSE, intracellular accumulations or deposits have proven equally seminal in linking the relatively rare familial (monogenic) forms of neurodegeneration with the much more common "sporadic" forms of neurodegenerative disease (Table 1). This holds true for AD, Parkinson's disease (PD), frontotemporal dementias (FTDs), and other tauopathies including progressive supranuclear palsy (PSP) and corticobasal degeneration (CBD). It may also be true for ALS, but this remains to be proven.

Apart from providing pathways from pathology to genetics, protein accumulation may be harmful to cells. In order to understand how accumulation of normal or abnormal proteins could cause or contribute to neurodegeneration, definition of terms is required. First, accumulation does not imply any specific abnormality of protein structure or processing. Ligation of peripheral axons leads to accumulation of neurofilaments (NFs) and microtubules on either side of the block, but accumulated proteins disappear if the obstruction is reversed and the neuron is undamaged.

Table 1 Neurodegenerative Diseases and Proteins

Disease	Pathogenic mechanism	Pathological hallmarks	Proteins associated with inclusions
AD	Familial AD mutations in APP, PS1, PS2 genes	Neurofibrillary tangles (IC)	Tau Ubiquitin
	Sporadic AD ApoE E4 allele Unknown	Senile plaques (EC)	β-amyloid α-synuclein
	Down syndrome Extra copy of APP ApoE E4 allele	Prion plaques (EC)	Prion β-amyloid
TSE	Genetic TSE Prion gene mutations Sporadic TSE Infectious TSE		
PD	Familial PD α-synuclein parkin DJ-1 PINK-1	Lewy bodies (IC)	α-synuclein Ubiquitin NFs αβ-crystallin Dorfin & VCP
	Sporadic PD Unknown	Pale bodies (?LB precursors) (IC)	Ubiquitin NEDD8 NFs
MSA	Sporadic MSA Unknown	Glial cell cytoplasmic inclusions (Papp-Lantos bodies) (IC)	α-sunuclein Tau Ubiquitin Dorfin & VCP

"Tauopathies"			
FTD	Tau gene mutations	Neurofibrillary tangles (IC)/Tau accumulation in astrocytes	Tau
PSD	H1 tau haplotype		Tau
CBD	H1 tau haplotype		Tau
Huntington's disease	Huntingtin gene mutations	Huntingtin inclusions (IC & IN)	Huntingtin, Ubiquitin, Dorfin, NEDD8
Kennedy's disease (spinal bulbar muscular atrophy)	Androgen receptor gene mutations	Androgen receptor inclusions (IN)	Androgen receptor
ALS	Familial ALS, SOD1 gene mutations	UBIRIs (IC)	Ubiquitin, SOD1, Dorfin & VCP
	Alsin, sentaxin & VAPB gene mutations	?	?
	Sporadic ALS	Bunina bodies (IC), UBIRIs (IC)	Cystatin C (?), Ubiquitin, Dorfin & VCP, NFs, Peripherin
	Unknown	LBLIs (IC)	

Abbreviations: AD, Alzheimer's disease; TSE, transmissible spongiform encephalopathies; PD, Parkinson's disease; MSA, multiple system atrophy; FTD, fronto-temporal dementia; PSP, progressive supranuclear palsy; CBD, corticobasal degeneration; APP, amyloid precursor protein; PS1, presenilin 1; PS2, presenilin 2; ApoE, apolipoprotein E; IC, intracellular; EC, extracellular; IN, intranuclear; NFs, neurofilaments; NEDD8, neural precursor cell expressed developmentally down-regulated 8; SOD1, superoxide dismutase 1; VAPB, vesicle-associated protein-B; UBIRIs, ubiquitin immunoreactive inclusions; LBLIs, Lewy body like inclusions.

Accumulation of NFs, for example, is prominent in proximal motor axons of transgenic mice over-expressing human neurofilament heavy chain proteins, but is not necessarily associated with neuronal death (4–7). On the other hand, in other situations, NF accumulation is associated with neuronal damage and death (8). In the latter situation, some molecular and cellular changes apart from the simple protein accumulation must be occurring.

Accumulation of apparently normal proteins may, however, be harmful. For example, gene duplications associated with Charcot-Marie-Tooth Disease (HMSN type 1A), triplication of the APP gene in trisomy 21, and duplication or triplication of the α-synuclein gene in rare familial forms of PD suggest that over-expression of normal proteins may lead to progressive neurodegeneration (9–12). Nevertheless, because protein accumulations are dynamic structures, even "normal" proteins are likely to change in terms of their phosphorylation state, ubiquitination, and interactions with other cellular (or extracellular) proteins. An example in ALS is the occasional finding of accumulations of apparently inappropriately phosphorylated NFs in the perikarya of spinal motor neurons (13–15). Chance events that trigger changes in protein structure that are then propagated may be important in many forms of neurodegeneration.

The term aggregate, however, implies that a protein has formed abnormal structures that have biochemical characteristics that differ from the non-aggregated protein. Aggregation may be inferred from immunocytochemical studies but must be confirmed by immunoblotting—indeed, aggregation may or may not be detectable by immunocytochemistry. Aggregates of specific proteins can be detected through the appearance of high molecular weight complexes forming an immunoreactive smear on Western blots after separation by SDS-PAGE. In some cases, aggregates are SDS-insoluble and do not enter the gels. Using this approach, high molecular weight forms of SOD1 have been detected in spinal cord samples from transgenic mice expressing the G93A mutation (16). Aggregated proteins can also be detected by using an very elegant method, referred to as filter trap assay, originally devised to detect aggregates of polyglutamine-expanded proteins. In this method, a cell or tissue extract is filtered through a cellulose acetate membrane that retains insoluble proteins only. The protein of interest is then detected using specific antibodies, as for Western blots (17). The filter trap assay has been used successfully to detect insoluble SOD1 in brain and spinal cord tissue form transgenic mice expressing several human mutations (18).

There is increasing evidence that protein aggregates in neurodegenerative disease reflect the production of aberrant or misfolded proteins. At the most simplistic level, such aggregates might, for example, impair cellular viability by interfering with transport of other proteins and organelles from the Perikaryon to the axon. In truth, the processes by which protein aggregation damages neurons are likely to be much more complex, and at present little understood. Nevertheless, some components of the story are clear.

WHY DO PROTEINS AGGREGATE?

Many proteins associated with neurodegenerative disease are not folded in their normal state (19), but become misfolded as a result of a mutation, post-translational change, or by a stochastic event that triggers a "chain reaction" by which the abnormal structure is propagated indefinitely, until the molecular consequences (mediated through extracellular or intracellular mechanisms, or both) impact on cell viability. Typical examples include TSE and AD. In both, the native proteins (prion and amyloid precursor protein-APP, respectively) are modified to form β-pleated sheets with the characteristics of amyloid (20,21). In TSE and AD, as in many other neurodegenerative disorders, this transformation may result from, or be enhanced by, various factors. These include mutations of the prion or APP gene, mutations in other genes implicated in shared molecular pathways (e.g., presenilin 1 or 2 genes in AD), polymorphisms that influence the stochastic events leading to amyloid formation (e.g., the codon 129 polymorphism in the prion gene; the apolipoprotein apoE4 polymorphism in AD), altered splicing (e.g., FTD associated with mutations in the tau gene), or increased synthesis of protein (e.g., gene triplication in PD; an extra copy of the APP gene in Down syndrome). Altered production of processing of proteins may also result form haplotype variations, as in PSP and CBD that are associated (in about 80% of cases) with the H1 tau haplotype (22–24). Epigenetic factors may also influence these events. The best-documented examples are kuru and variant CJD (2,25). The role of systemic infection, trauma, physical activity, toxins of various kinds, and other environmental triggers for neurodegeneration, including ALS, remains speculative (26). Ageing is a common factor in neurodegeneration and intrinsic influences such as free radical damage may provide a common mechanism linking ageing and environmentally related damage to neuronal systems.

Amyloid formation is central to the pathogenesis of AD and TSE but it is not certain that this applies to other neurodegenerative diseases, although formation of amyloid-like aggregates by mutant huntingtin has also been demonstrated in HD models (27–30). The characteristic intracellular inclusions of the α-synucleinopathies (PD and multiple system atrophy, MSA), tauopathies (including some forms of FTD and syndromes associated with tau gene mutations, PSP, and CBD), FTD associated with "ubiquitin-only" inclusions (31,32), "neurofilament inclusion body disease," (33,34) serpinopathies (35,36), the trinucleotide repeat disorders and the hereditary ataxias (37,38), and ALS, are not associated with the typical features of amyloid by way of staining with way of Congo red birefringence under polarized light or thioflavine staining, although β-sheet formation has been identified experimentally in aggregates formed by several of the abnormal proteins that comprise these inclusions. Nevertheless, in all cases there is evidence that proteins undergo altered processing through ubiquitination, phosphorylation, and/or nitration and that they form abnormal filaments of various kinds, sometimes with β-sheet formation, but seldom with formation of classical amyloid. Understanding the molecular components of these inclusions and the processes leading to their formation is likely to provide important insights into mechanisms of disease and to reveal many variations in the pathways leading to protein aggregation and cell damage. The notion that intracellular inclusions (glial or neuronal) represent detritus of little pathogenic significance is no longer tenable. On the other hand, the assumption that inclusions are inherently harmful may be inaccurate.

PROTEIN AGGREGATION IN ALS AND OTHER MOTOR NEURON DISORDERS

Abnormalities of the cytoskeleton have been recognized for many years (Chap. 16). Swellings of proximal axons (spheroids) are a prominent but non-specific feature of ALS pathology (39–42,15). Bunina bodies (43), on the other hand, do seem to be specific for ALS, although their significance at the molecular level remains obscure, and they are only detectable in about 70% of cases. The only molecular marker of Bunina bodies is cystatin C (44) the significance of which is uncertain. Likewise, Lewy body-like inclusions (LBLIs) are relatively scarce, being present in about 20% of cases. Hyaline bodies, a term applied by some to the structures similar to LBLIs, but also including much larger masses of hyaline-appearing NFs (sometimes referred to as conglomerates) within spinal motor neurons, are distinctly rare in our experience (45,46). They may be more common in familial cases (13). Basophilic inclusions are less common than either Bunina bodies or LBLIs (47).

The hallmark of ALS pathology, however, is the characteristic ubiquitin-immunoreactive inclusion (UBIRI) (48–50). These inclusions take various forms within spinal and brain stem motor neurons. They are occasionally seen in pyramidal neurons of the primary motor cortex, and UBIRIs are also found in dentate granule cells of the hippocampus, and (usually in patients who have developed dementia) in neurons of the frontal and temporal cortex (31,32). They are occasionally seen in the substantia nigra and in the neostriatum (50). Most commonly UBIRIs take the form of filamentous bundles and masses in the cytoplasm of brain stem and spinal motor neurons (chap. 3), sometimes extending for some distance into the dendrites, and, perhaps fancifully, described as skein-like inclusions, because they often have the appearance of tangled skeins of thread or wool (48). The second type of UBIRI is the dense body, in the form of a rounded or oblong inclusion. These correspond to LBLIs. Skein-like and LBLIs are often present in the same individual, and may even coexist in the same neuron. UBIRI in one or other form (or both) are present in virtually all cases examined (45,50). Ultrastructurally, UBIRIs comprise amorphous and filamentous structures (51).

Although the typical intracellular inclusions of other neurodegenerative diseases (Table 1) are also labeled by antibodies to ubiquitin, ubiquitin has not been consistently associated with other cytoskeletal proteins in ALS (45), with the possible exception that neurofilament antibodies sometimes label LBLIs, whereas they do not identify skein-like inclusions. Similarly, peripherin may frequently colocalize with ubiquitin in LBLIs (52). This is particularly interesting in the light of mutations in the peripherin gene identified in a few individuals with ALS (53,54). Furthermore, peripherin does not seem to colocalize with skein-like inclusions, so presumably the latter arise from different molecular events, or contain cytoskeletal elements that are more altered or degraded than those present in LBLIs. One can speculate, therefore, that LBLIs represent an earlier stage in the evolution of intraneuronal inclusions and protein aggregates in ALS.

PROTEIN AGGREGATION AND THE MOLECULAR PATHOLOGY OF FAMILIAL ALS

The SOD1 gene is, as yet, the only gene linked with certainty to typical familial ALS, by which we mean ALS that clearly conforms to Charcot ALS and the El Escorial criteria of clinically definite or probable ALS, has a rapidly progressive course, and is pathologically indistinguishable from sporadic ALS. There are, of course, marked variations in the phenotype of SOD1-associated ALS both within and across families (55), but overall the pattern of familial ALS is very similar to that of sporadic ALS. These criteria cannot be met by the syndromes associated with mutations of the alsin or senataxin genes (56–58). Mutations of the vesicle-associated protein-B (VAPB) gene have been described in 24 individuals from 7 families in Brazil (59). We do not yet know whether this form of familial motor neuron disease is associated with neuronal inclusions, nor whether VAPB protein is present in UBIRIs of typical sporadic ALS, but altered function of VAPB may prove relevant to protein aggregation as it is implicated in intracellular trafficking (59). Although neurofilament heavy chain gene mutations have been implicated as a risk factor in ALS, they have not been shown to be causally linked to the disease (60), and the molecular pathology associated with these mutations is unknown.

UBIRIs in SOD1 ALS transgenic mice are immunoreactive with anti-SOD1 antibodies (61). In human SOD1 related familial ALS, UBIRIs may be labeled by anti-SOD1 antibodies, although this is variable (45,62). Neurofilaments (NFs) are often components of LBLIs and form the main substance of conglomerate inclusions, as noted above. Such conglomerates may be harmful, but conversely they may be protective, acting as a protective phosphorylation "sink" for Cdk-5 activity (63) since, in transgenic models, large accumulations of NF proteins are not necessarily lethal for motor neurons (6).

It is somewhat perplexing that not all cases of familial ALS due to SOD1 gene mutations show SOD1 aggregates. This may reflect differences in the sensitivity and specificity of the antibodies used, or the fact that in some instances very little mutant protein or microaggregate is present. For example, frame shift mutations yield truncated SOD1 proteins that are highly unstable, with low CNS tissue levels (55,64,65). In the case of the G127insTGGG mutation, which leads to a truncated protein with five novel amino acids following G127, SOD1 levels in one case were very low compared to those in controls in brain and spinal cord, but UBIRIs were present in motor neurons and some of these were labeled by an antibody specific for the mutant SOD1 protein (65). Virtually all mutant SOD1s in brain and spinal cord were present as aggregated protein.

A variety of other proteins have been associated with inclusions in familial and sporadic ALS. These include the neural precursor cell expressed developmentally down-regulated 8 (NEDD8) protein, a ubiquitin-like protein which plays a key role in the activation of SCF (Skp-cullin-1-F-box) ubiquitin ligase through the recruitment of UB E2 enzyme to the SCF complex (66,67). The presence of NEDD8 is far from specific, however, as it is present also in the characteristic inclusions of many other disorders (67). Similarly, dorfin, an E3 ligase, colocalizes with UBIRIs, but also with the inclusions of PD and MSA (68).

Furthermore, mutant SOD1 protein seems to be preferentially associated with brain and spinal cord mitochondria isolated from postmortem material and in several different SOD1 transgenic mice (69). Why this mislocalization occurs, and how it leads to cell death is uncertain, but a possible mechanism is suggested by the finding that mutant SOD1 binds the proapoptotic protein Bcl-2 both in human and mouse spinal cord, and that Bcl-2 binds to high molecular weight SOD1 aggregates that are present in spinal cord (but not liver) mitochondria (70). Copper chaperone for superoxide dismutase (CCS) colocalizes with SOD1 in hyaline inclusions in the spinal cord of five SOD1-FALS although CCS does not appear to be a consistent partner to ubiquitin in sporadic ALS (71,72). Hyaline inclusions in neurons and in astrocytes have also been associated with advanced glycation end-products (AGEs) in a familial ALS case caused by an A4V SOD1 gene mutation (73,74). The AGEs colocalized with phosphorylated NFs, SOD1, and ubiquitin.

IN VITRO EVIDENCE FOR SOD1 AGGREGATION

SOD1 protein is a 32-kDa homodimer with a highly conserved amino acid sequence, and it contains one copper and one zinc binding site, as well as a disulfide bond in each of its subunits, which are rich in β-sheet structure thus providing it with exceptional stability and specificity of fold and assembly (75). It is, therefore, expected that changes in the structure could have profound effects on structural architecture and stability of the protein. Indeed, not long after SOD1 mutations were discovered it was shown that several mutated SOD1 proteins denature under milder conditions and have shorter half lives than wild-type SOD1 protein (76). More than 100 SOD1 mutations have been identified (see www.alsod.org), predominantly single amino acid substitutions and only few deletions and truncations. They are dispersed throughout the protein sequence and are found in β-barrel, intermonomer interface, loop regions, disulfide bonds, and both copper and zinc sites.

Dimer destabilization of mutant SOD1 protein leads to increased aggregation propensity. The crystal structures of A4V and I113T SOD1 mutants as well as their X-ray solution-scattering profiles reveal a significant reorientation of the subunits at the monomer–monomer interface (77). Such instability of the A4V SOD1 promotes filamentous aggregation under acidic conditions (78). Electron microscopy indicates that A4V SOD1 can exist as a dimer, pore-like structures that resemble "amyloid-pores" formed by β-amyloid and α-synuclein or large spherical structures (79) (Fig. 1). Similar pore-like structures have been reported in SOD1 mutants G85R and G37R, which do not involve rearrangements at the dimer interface (80). Reduction of the intrasubunit bond C57-C146 abolishes dimerization (81). Aggregation of A4V SOD1 was also prevented by introduction of an engineered intrasubunit disulfide bond in the form of double mutant A4V/V148C (79). Stabilization of dimers has been proposed as a therapeutic intervention (82).

Aggregation of mutant SOD1 protein appears to be also dependent on the increase in the demetallated monomer formation. Motor neuron degeneration in SOD1-associated ALS transgenic mice is independent of copper loading via CCS, copper chaperone for SOD1 (83) and metal-free apo-state of the mutant SOD1 protein is highly unstable (84). Metal deficient SOD1 mutants crystalize in higher-order assemblies of aligned β-sheets that give rise to amyloid-like filaments and water-filled nanotubules (85). Large amorphous aggregates that are composed of smaller globular particles, reminiscent of inclusion bodies, are seen under atomic force microscope in oxidation-exposed zinc-deficient SOD1 and SOD1 mutants (86). Interestingly, the same group has claimed that oxidative damage could cause wild-type SOD1 to dissociate to aggregation-prone monomers in vitro, although at much higher concentration than seen with SOD1 mutants (87). This is an attractive suggestion that could provide a mechanistic link between sporadic and SOD1-associated ALS.

THE UBIQUITIN-PROTEASOME SYSTEM AND ALS

The ubiquitin-proteasome system (UPS) promotes non-lysosomal degradation of short-lived regulatory proteins but also damaged and misfolded proteins within the cell (88,89). This action is coordinated by many enzymes and protein complexes, including the E1 ubiquitin-activating enzyme, 20 to 40 different E2 conjugating enzymes, and hundreds of different E3 ubiquitin ligases, which are responsible for formation of polyubiquitin chain and its attachment to a given substrate protein.

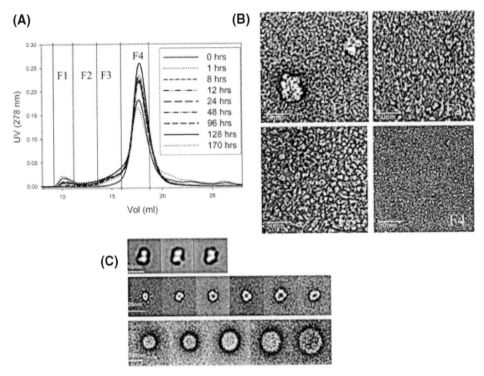

Figure 1 (**A**) Aggregation of A4V followed by size-exclusion chromatography (Superdex 200) as a function of time at 37°C. The appearance of aggregates corresponded with the loss of dimer. (**B**) Negative-staining electron microscopy of A4V aggregate fractions collected after 175 hours. The vertical bars drawn on the chromatography profile (*panel a*) indicate each fraction. (**C**) Averaged EM images show three morphological types: dimers (*top panels*), pore-like structures (*middle panels*), and large spherical aggregates (*bottom panels*). *Source*: From Ref. 79.

Polyubiquitin chain is recognized by the 19S regulatory complexes located on the 20S proteolytic core of the 26S proteasome complex. The 19S regulatory complexes unfold the polyubiquitinated substrate and facilitate its entrance into the 20S proteasome, where the substrate protein is degraded into small peptides and polyubiquitin chains cleaved and recycled into monomeric ubiquitin by different deubiquitinating enzymes (Fig. 2). For a more detailed description of the UPS pathways, see Ref. 90, and references therein.

Aberrations in the UPS have been implicated in a number of neurodegenerative diseases including ALS (90). There is now direct evidence that defects in the UPS can lead to neurodegeneration. Progressive sensory ataxia occurs in the gracile axonal dystrophy (*gad*) mouse due to a mutation in the gene coding for ubiquitin C-terminal hydrolase (91). In human disease, the evidence is becoming more compelling, although it is not conclusive. In familial PD, for example, parkin is one of the members of the ubiquitin-protein ligase (E3) system, which controls the specificity of substrate selection by ubiquitination together with a ubiquitin-activation enzyme (E1) and a ubiquitin-conjugating enzyme (E2) (92). Furthermore, the ubiquitin carboxy terminal-hydrolase gene (UCH-L1) has also been implicated in familial PD, although this association is not proven (93,94). Thus aggregation of abnormal

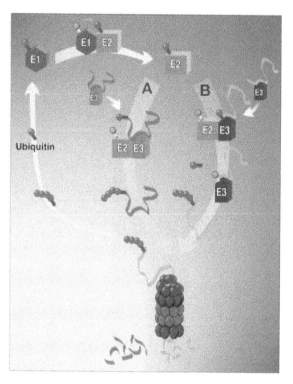

Figure 2 The Ubiquitin-Proteasome System. Ubiquitin is first activated by the ubiquitin-activating enzyme E1, to a high-energy thiol ester intermediate. It is then transferred, still as a high-energy intermediate, to a member of the ubiquitin-carrier proteins family of enzymes, E2 [known also as a ubiquitin-conjugating enzyme (UBC)]. From E2, it can be transferred directly to the substrate that is bound specifically to a member of the ubiquitin ligase family of proteins, E3 (**A**). This occurs when the E3 belongs to the RING finger family of ligases. In the case of an homologous to the E6-AP C Terminus (HECT) domain-containing ligase (**B**), the activated ubiquitin moiety is transferred first to the E3, to generate yet another high-energy thiol ester intermediate, before it is transferred to the E3-bound target substrate. Additional ubiquitin moieties are added successively to the previously conjugated one in a similar mechanism to generate a polyubiquitin chain. The polyubiquitinated substrate binds specifically to the 26S proteasome complex: the substrate is degraded to short peptides, and free and reusable ubiquitin is released via the activity of deubiquitinating enzymes. *Source*: From Ref. 90.

proteins, dysfunctional ubiquitin-mediated degradation process, or both, may be important in the pathogenesis of PD.

Aside from the examples quoted above, most of the evidences for the involvement of the UPS come from the accumulation of ubiquitin in the inclusion bodies. In the case of ALS, ubiquitinated SOD1 aggregates appeared as a component of the cytoplasmic inclusion bodies in motor neurons and in some cases within the surrounding astrocytes in SOD1-mediated FALS transgenic mice and in the spinal cords from patients with FALS (61,95). Proteinaceous aggregates of mutant SOD1 have also been found in the cytoplasm of cultured primary motor neurons expressing several different SOD1 mutants (96). SOD1 immunoreactive neuronal and astrocytic inclusions in G85R SOD1 transgenic mice were early indicators of the disease and increased markedly as disease progressed while there were no such inclusions in mice expressing wild-type human SOD1 (61). Sodium dodecyl sulphate resistant SOD1 insoluble protein complexes (IPCs) were present in the spinal cord of G93A SOD1 transgenic mice that lack microscopic SOD1 inclusion bodies and disease pathology (16). The SOD1 IPCs were also present in G85R and G93A transfected HEK293 cells and colocalized with GFP-CFTR and centrosomal marker pericentrin suggesting that mutant SOD1s accumulated in the aggresome, a distinct pericentriolar structure that is rich in intermediate filament protein vimentin (16), and is formed in response to the overproduction of aggregation-prone misfolded proteins by dynein-dependent retrograde transport of abnormal proteins along micortubules (97). These oligomers may be the most toxic form of mutant SOD1, similar to observed toxicity of oligomeric intermediates of Aβ peptide (98). Exposure to N-acetyl-leucyl-leucyl-norleucinal, a UPS inhibitor, increased the tendency for mutant SOD1 to form aggresome in transgenic cells (16). Lactacystin, another proteasome inhibitor, enhanced aggregation of mutant A4V SOD1 in PC12 cells, but interestingly had no effect on the death of PC12 cells (99). However, two other studies have shown lactacystin-enhanced cell death in cells expressing mutant SOD1 (100,101).

Dorfin, an E3 ubiquitin ligase, colocalized with ubiquitin in motor neurons of both SOD1 associated FALS and SALS, as well as in G93A SOD1 transgenic mice (102). Coexpression of dorfin with either G93A SOD1 or G85R SOD1 enhances polyubiquitylation of these mutants in both HEK293 and Neuro2a cells, and protected cell viability (103). This action of dorfin is dependent on binding with valosin-containing protein (VCP) (103). VCP is required for recognition of polyubiquitinated proteins and their translocation to the 26S proteasome for processive degradation through the VCP-Np14-Ufd1 complex (104).

These findings do not suggest that there are pathogenic links between the UPS and the formation of UBIRIs, although altered processing of misfolded and aberrant proteins may nonetheless contribute to cell damage. At present, we lack direct (biochemical) evidence that ubiquitin or other related proteins are bound to SOD1 or other cellular proteins.

INADEQUATE CELLULAR DEFENSE

In addition to the accumulation of mutant SOD1 that may be resistant to degradation by the UPS or simply overwhelms its capacity, a lack of adequate protective function by certain cellular proteins may contribute to the toxicity of mutant SOD1-containing aggregates. Normally, various physiological stresses activate a response through the UPS, lysosome-mediated autophagy, and recruitment of molecular chaperones. Molecular chaperones are highly conserved proteins that transiently stabilize and mediate the folding or assembly of unfolded protein substrates but also regulate other cellular processes, including targeting, transport, autophagy, and signal transduction (105). Temperature elevation activates a cellular program, known as the heat shock response, which is characterized by up-regulation of heat shock proteins (HSPs). There are six main families of HSPs, based on their molecular mass, HSP100, HSP90, HSP70, HSP60, HSP40, and 10 small HSPs with molecular mass less than 40 kDa that contain a conserved C-terminal α-crystallin domain. A mutation in the gene that encodes the B subunit of α-crystallin is responsible for accumulation of aggregates of intermediate filament protein desmin in desmin-related myopathy (106). Mutations in another small HSP, HSP27, that causes Charcot-Marie-Tooth and distal hereditary motor neuropathy, interfere with neurofilament assembly (107). Many more mutations have been identified in HSPs causing number of diseases including hereditary spastic paraplegia, which has been associated with a mutation in a mitochondrial form of HSP60 (108).

Activity of HSPs in SOD1 associated ALS has been studied in cell models and transgenic mice (Table 2). Primary motor neuron NIH 3T3 cells that stably expressed mutant G41S and G93A SOD1 had chronically elevated levels of HSP70, HSP27, and αB-crystallin (109). HSP70, HSP40, and αB-crystallin coimmunoprecipitated with mutant SOD1 from both G93A and G41S expressing NIH3T3 cell lines and were distributed mainly in the detergent-insoluble fraction (110). Binding of HSP70 and HSP25 leads to the formation of sedimentable aggregates in G37R and G41D transfected Neuro2a cells (111). HSP25 and αB-crystallin were found to specifically cofractionate with insoluble SOD1 in the transgenic mouse models and in human ALS tissues (112). Survival of G93A SOD1 transfected NIH 3T3 cells was prolonged when HSP70 was over-expressed. In addition, formation of SOD1 aggregation was reduced (109). If HSP70 is over-expressed in the combination with its co-chaperone, HSP40, both intracytoplasmic aggregation of mutant G93A SOD1-EGFP fusion proteins and cell death are suppressed in transiently transfected Neuro2a cells (113). HSP70 and HSP25 block transfer of demetallated mutant SOD1 into the mitochondria of mutant G37R and G41D SOD1 transfected Neuro2a cells and G93A transgenic mouse liver cells (111).

Upregulation of the HSPs is an early feature in SOD1 transgenic mice. HSP27 is localized in the nucleus of the ventral neurons and glial cells in presymptomatic and early symptomatic G93A SOD1 animals and later on in the disease process appeared together with αB-crystallin in the cytoplasm of the reactive glial cells (114). Expression of HSP70 and HSP90 to lesser extent has also been shown to be

Table 2 Effect of Chaperones on SOD1 Cell and Transgenic Mouse Models of ALS

Model	Chaperone	Endpoint	Effect	Reference
NIH3T3 cells	HSP70, HSP27, αB-crystallin	Viability Formation of aggregation	Prolonged Reduced	109
Neuro2a cells	HSP70, HSP40	Aggregation of SOD1-EGFP fusion protein and cell death	Suppressed	113
Neuro2a cells	HSP25, HSP27, HSP70	Uptake of demetallated mutant SOD1 in mitochondria	Blocked	111
G93A SOD1 mice[a]	HSP70, HSP90	Neuronal loss Motor function Survival	Slowed down Improved Extended by 22%	115

[a]G93A SOD1 mice were treated with arimoclomol, an inducer of phosphorylation of the heat shock transcription factor-1 (HSF-1) that lead to an increase in the expression of HSP70 and HSP90.

Note: NIH3T3 primary motor neurons, Neuro2a cells neuroblastoma cells, HSF-1 heat shock transcription factor-1.

increased in G93A SOD1 transgenic mice, and interestingly, the immunoreactivity was further increased by treatment of mice with arimoclomol, resulting in an improved motor function, slowing of neuronal loss, and prolongation of lifespan by 22% (115). Arimoclomol induced the phosphorylation of the heat shock transcription factor-1 (HSF-1) leading to an increase in the expression of HSP70 and HSP90. It is possible that HSF-1 could up-regulate other cochaperones such as HSP40, CHIP, and BAG1 (116). Polyglutamine disease pathology and phenotype are improved when HSP70 transgenic mice are crossed with a mouse model of SCA1 (117). Over-expression of HSP70 in a mouse model of Kennedy's disease also causes a dose-dependent improvement in motor coordination and degradation of mutant androgen receptor (118). Similar effects could be expected if HSP transgenic mice were crossed with SOD1 transgenic mice, but this type of a study has not been reported yet.

PROPOSED MECHANISM OF SOD1 AGGREGATION IN ALS

Under normal conditions the equilibrium between production and clearance of intracellular proteins exists. This dynamic balance can be interrupted by various means, including over-expression of normal or mutant proteins, UPS dysfunction, underactivity of chaperones, excitotoxic insult, oxidative and nitrosative stress, mitochondrial injury, synaptic failure, altered metal homeostasis, and failure of axonal and dendritic transport.

Structural data using X-ray crystallography and X-ray scattering have shown that a subset of SOD1 mutations leads to the destabilization of the dimeric interface, thus indicating that dimer dissociation may be the first step in the process of mutant SOD1 aggregation. Other post-translational events such as disulfide formation and metallation of the protein may also increase unfolding rates and therefore increase the propensity of mutant SOD1 to aggregate. Electron microscopy and atomic force microscopy studies have shown that an assembly process that follows dimer dissociation and/or the increase in the demetallated monomer formation results in the production of three morphological structures: mutant dimers, pore-like oligomers, and large spherical structures. Mutant SOD1 pore-like oligomers resemble amyloid pores formed by α-synuclein and β-amyloid, which have been proposed to be crucial for toxicity (119,120). Recently, an antibody has been generated that reacts with oligomeric, but not monomeric or fibrillar forms of polyglutamine, α-synuclein, β-amyloid, and prion protein implying that a common structure of soluble intermediates may lead to common mechanisms of pathology (121). The SOD1 intermediate forms are further exposed to oxidative and nitrosylation stress or excitotoxic insult, and subsequently actively transported along microtubules to the aggresome, where they are met by the components of the UPS, HSPs, ubiquitin, and mitochondria (possibly for the provision of ATP) for degradation and clearance (Fig. 3). The evidence above suggests that the UPS and HSPs are involved in the degradation of mutant SOD1 in ALS up to their maximum capacity. However, once that capacity is exceeded the mutant SOD1 oligomers form IPCs and become refractory to further intracellular proteolysis. It has been suggested that Lewy bodies in PD are failed aggresomes (122) and it is possible that inclusions seen in SOD1 associated ALS are the result of a similar process, thus representing a marker of a failed cellular defence system. The lack of adequate protection, however, may leave the cell vulnerable to damage by other dangerous proteins that would normally be strictly regulated, or may lead to

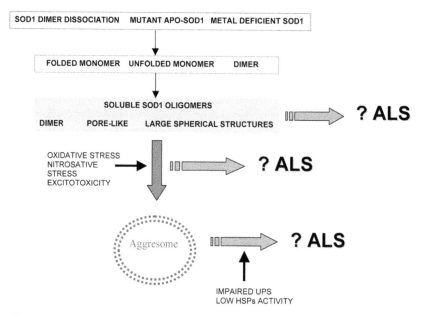

Figure 3 Proposed mechanism of mutant SOD1 aggregation and toxicity in ALS. Dimer dissociation, disulfide reduction and demetallation increase unfolding rates of mutant SOD1. Electron microscopy and atomic force microscopy studies have shown that an assembly process that follows dimer dissocation, disulfide reduction and/or the increase in the demetallated monomer formation results in the production of three morphological structures: mutant dimers, pore-like oligomers and large spherical structures. Soluble SOD1 oligomers may be toxic to cells in similar fashion to β-amyloid intermediates. The SOD1 intermediate forms are transported along microtubules to the aggresome where they are met by the components of the UPS, HSPs, ubiquitin, and mitochondria (possibly for the provision of ATP) for degradation and clearance. Before they are taken into the aggresome they can be further damaged by oxidative and nitrosative stress or excitotoxicity and could subsequently cause damage to cellular organelles. If proteolysis of mutant SOD1 fails in the aggresome, as a result of impaired UPS or low activity of HSPs and other chaperones, inclusions are formed that are likely to be toxic rather than just a by-product of degeneration.

inadequate degradation of regulatory proteins, such as cyclins, cyclin-dependent kinases, and transcriptional factors. Microtubule-dependent axonal transport could also be disrupted as mutant SOD1 would compete with other substrates that are essential for neuronal viability. Mutant SOD1 aggregates could crowd mitochondrial import channels and inhibit outer mitochondrial membrane components. Or they can act as irritants and cause a chronic inflammatory reaction. All the above mechanisms may, of course, operate at the same time.

CONCLUDING REMARKS

In patients with SOD1-associated FALS and in transgenic mouse models of the disease, the death of motor neurons is preceded by the formation of cytoplasmic inclusions containing ubiquitin and aggregated mutant SOD1 protein. Inclusion bodies containing ubiquitin-immunoreactive protein aggregates are also a feature of sporadic disease. Evidence points to a putative toxic role of protein aggregation in the pathogenesis of ALS, although the underlying mechanism remains unclear. Perhaps environmental factors in sporadic ALS converge on a pathway initiated by the SOD1 genetic mutation in FALS that leads to the loss of motor neurons via a common mechanism mediated by or resulting from protein aggregation. Understanding this mechanism should lead to the development of rational therapy, perhaps aimed at directly reducing the level of abnormal protein within the cells or enhancing cellular defence systems, ultimately ameliorating, if not halting or reversing, the progress of this devastating disease.

REFERENCES

1. Forman MS, Trojanowski JQ, Lee VM-Y. Neurodegenerative diseases: a decade of discoveries paves the way for therapeutic breakthroughs. Nat Med 2004; 10:1055–1063.
2. Collins SJ, Lawson VA, Maters CL. Transmissible spongiform encephalopathies. Lancet 2004; 363:51–61.
3. DiFiglia M, Sapp E, Chase KO, Davies SW, Bates GP, Vonsattel JP, Aronin N. Aggregation of huntingtin in neuronal intranuclear inclusions and dystrophic neurites in Brain. Science 1997; 277:1990–1993.
4. Couillard-Despres S, Meier J, Julien JP. Extra axonal neurofilaments do not exacerbate disease caused by mutant Cu, Zn superoxide dismutase. Neurobiol Dis 2000; 7:462–470.
5. Beaulieu JM, Jacomy H, Julien JP. Formation of intermediate filament protein aggregates with disparate effects in two transgenic mouse models lacking the neurofilament light subunit. J Neurosci 2000; 15:5321–5328.
6. Julien JP. Amyotrophic lateral sclerosis: unfolding the toxicity of the misfolded. Cell 2001; 104:581–591.
7. Robertson J, Kriz J, Nguyen MD, Julien JP. Pathways to motor neuron degeneration in transgenic mouse models. Biochimie 2002; 84:1151–1160.
8. Bruijn LI, Cleveland DW. Mechanisms of selective motor neuron death in ALS: insights from transgenic mouse models of motor neuron disease. Neuropathol Appl Neurobiol 1996; 22:373–387.
9. Singleton AB, Farrer M, Johnson J, Singleton A, Hague S, Kachergus J, Hulihan M, Peuralinna T, Dutra A, Nussbaum R, et al. α-Synuclein locus triplication causes Parkinson's disease. Science 2003; 302:841.
10. Chartier-Harlin MC, Kachergus J, Roumier C, Mouroux V, Douay X, Lincoln S, Levecque C, Larvor L, Andrieux J, Hulihan M, et al. α-Synuclein locus duplications a cause of familial Parkinson's disease. Lancet 2004; 364:1167–1169.
11. Ibanez P, Bonnet AM, Debarges B, Lohmann E, Tison F, Pollak P, Agid Y, Durr A, Brice A. Causal relation between α-synuclein gene duplication and familial Parkinson's disease. Lancet 2004; 364:1169–1171.
12. Antonarakis SE, Lyle R, Dermitzakis ET, Reymond A, Deutsch S. Chromosome 21 and down syndrome: from genomics to pathophysiology. Nat Rev Genet 2004; 5: 725–738.
13. Hirano A, Nakano I, Kurland LT, Mulder DW, Holley PW, Saccommo G. Fine structural study of neurofibrillary changes in a family with amyotrophic lateral sclerosis. J Neuropath Exp Neurol 1984; 43:471–480.
14. Hirano A. Cytopathology of amyotrophic lateral sclerosis. Adv Neurol 1991; 56:91–101.
15. Leigh PN, Dodson A, Swash M, Brion JP, Anderton BH. Cytoskeletal abnormalities in motor neuron disease. An immunocytochemical study. Brain 1989; 112:521–535.
16. Johnston JA, Dalton MJ, Gurney ME, Kopito RR. Formation of high molecular weight complexes of mutant Cu, Zn-superoxide dismutase in a mouse model for familial amyotrophic lateral sclerosis. Proc Natl Acad Sci USA 2000; 97:12571–12576.

17. Wanker EE, Scherzinger E, Heiser V, Sittler A, Eickhoff H, Lehrach H. Membrane filter assay for detection of amyloid-like polyglutamine-containing protein aggregates. Methods Enzymol 1999; 309:375–386.

18. Wang J, Xu G, Borchelt DR. High molecular weight complexes of mutant superoxide dismutase 1: age-dependent and tissue-specific accumulation. Neurobiol Dis 2002; 9:139–148.

19. Uversky VN. Protein folding revisited. A polypeptide chain at the folding-misfolding-nonfolding cross-roads: which way to go? Cell Mol Life Sci 2003; 60:1852–1871.

20. Selkoe DJ. Cell biology of protein misfolding: the examples of Alzheimer's and Parkinson's diseases. Nat Cell Biol 2004; 6:1054–1061.

21. Soto C. Diagnosing prion diseases: needs, challenges and hopes. Nat Rev Microbiol 2004; 2:809–819.

22. Baker M, Litvan I, Houlden H, Adamson J, Dickson D, Perez-Tur J, Hardy J, Lynch T, Bigio E, Hutton M. Association of an extended haplotype in the tau gene with progressive supranuclear palsy. Hum Mol Genet 1999; 4:711–715.

23. de Silva R, Weiler M, Morris HR, Martin ER, Wood NW, Lees AJ. Strong association of a novel Tau promoter haplotype in progressive supranuclear palsy. Neurosci Lett 2001; 311:145–148.

24. Houlden H, Baker M, Morris HR, MacDonald N, Pickering-Brown S, Adamson J, Lees AJ, Rossor MN, Quinn NP, Kertesz A, et al. Corticobasal degeneration and progressive supranuclear palsy share a common tau haplotype. Neurology 2001; 56:1702–1706.

25. Will RG. Acquired prion disease: iatrogenic CJD, variant of CJD, kuru. Br Med Bull 2003; 66:255–265.

26. Al-Chalabi A, Leigh PN. Trouble on the pitch: are professional football players at increased risk of developing amyotrophic lateral sclerosis? Brain 2005; 128:451–453.

27. Scherzinger E, Lurz R, Turmaine M, Mangiarini L, Hollenbach B, Hasenbank R, Bates GP, Davies SW, Lehrach H, Wanker EE. Huntingtin-encoded polyglutamine expansions form amyloid-like protein aggregates in vitro and in vivo. Cell 1997; 90: 549–558.

28. Scherzinger E, Sittler A, Schweiger K, Heiser V, Lurz R, Hasenbank R, Bates GP, Lehrach H, Wanker EE. Self-assembly of polyglutamine-containing huntingtin fragments into amyloid-like fibrils: implications for Huntington's disease pathology. Proc Natl Acad Sci USA 1999; 96:4604–4609.

29. Huang CC, Faber PW, Persichetti F, Mittal V, Vonsattel JP, MacDonald ME, Gusella JF. Amyloid formation by mutant huntingtin: threshold, progressivity and recruitment of normal polyglutamine proteins. Somat Cell Mol Genet 1998; 24:217–233.

30. Wightman G, Anderson VE, Martin J, Swash M, Anderton BH, Neary D, Mann D, Luthert P, Leigh PN. Hippocampal and neocortical ubiquitin-immunoreactive inclusions in amyotrophic lateral sclerosis with dementia. Neurosci Lett 1992; 139:269–274.

31. Okamoto K, Murakami N, Kusaka H, Yoshida M, Hashizume Y, Nakazato Y, Matsubara E, Hirai S. Ubiquitin-positive intraneuronal inclusions in the extramotor cortices of presenile dementia patients with motor neuron disease. J Neurol 1992; 239:426–430.

32. Cairns NJ, Grossman M, Arnold SE, Burn DJ, Jaros E, Perry RH, Duyckaerts C, Stankoff B, Pillon B, Skullerud K, et al. Clinical and neuropathologic variation in neuronal intermediate filament inclusion disease. Neurology 2004; 63:1376–1384.

33. Cairns NJ, Lee VM-Y, Trojanowski JQ. The cytoskeleton in neurodegenerative diseases. J Pathol 2004; 204:438–449.

34. Lomas DA, Carrell RW. Serpinopathies and the conformational dementias. Nat Rev Genet 2002; 3:759–768.

35. Onda M, Belorgey D, Sharp LK, Lomas DA. Latent Ser49Pro neuroserpin forms polymers in the dementia familial encephalopathy with neuroserpin inclusion bodies. J Biol Chem 2005; 280:13,735–13,741.

36. Everett CM, Wood NW. Trinucleotide repeats and neurodegenerative disease. Brain 2004; 127:2385–2405.

37. Taroni F, DiDonato S. Pathways to motor incoordination: the inherited ataxias. Nat Rev Neurosci 2004; 5:641–655.
38. Wohlfart G. Regenerative phenomena in muscles in connection with poliomyelitis and amyotrophic lateral sclerosis. Nord Med 1955; 54:1075–1078.
39. Carpenter S. Proximal axonal enlargement in motor neuron disease. Neurology 1968; 18:841–851.
40. Delisle MB, Carpenter S. Neurofibrillary axonal swellings and amyotrophic lateral sclerosis. J Neurol Sci 1984; 63:241–250.
41. Leigh PN, Swash M. Cytoskeletal pathology in motor neuron diseases. In: Rowland LP, ed. Amyotrophic Lateral Sclerosis and Other Motor Neuron Diseases. New York: Raven Press, 1991:115–124.
42. Bunina TL. On intracellular inclusions in familial amyotrophic lateral sclerosis. Zh Nevropatol Psikhiatr Im S S Korsakova. 1962; 62:1293–1299.
43. Okamoto K, Hirai S, Amari M, Watanabe M, Sakurai A. Bunina bodies in amyotrophic lateral sclerosis immunostained with rabbit anti-cystatin C serum. Neurosci Lett 1993; 162:125–128.
44. Leigh PN, Whitwell H, Garofalo O, Buller J, Swash M, Martin JE, Gallo J-M, Weller RO, Anderton BH. Ubiquitin-immunoreactive intraneuronal inclusions in amyotrophic lateral sclerosis. Brain 1991; 114:775–788.
45. Katayama S, Watanabe C, Noda K, Ohishi H, Yamamura Y, Nishisaka T, Inai K, Asayama K, Murayama S, Nakamura S. Numerous conglomerate inclusions in slowly progressive familial amyotrophic lateral sclerosis with posterior column involvement. J Neurol Sci 1999; 171:72–77.
46. Chou SM. Pathology of motor system disorder. In: Leigh PN, Swash M, eds. Motor Neuron Disease: Biology and Management. London: Springer Verlag, 1995:53–118.
47. Leigh PN, Anderton BH, Dodson A, Gallo J-M, Swash M, Power DM. Ubiquitin deposits in anterior horn cells in motor neuron disease. Neurosci Lett 1988; 93:197–203.
48. Lowe J, Lennox G, Jefferson D, Morrell K, McQuire D, Gray T, Landon M, Doherty FJ, Mayer RJ. A filamentous inclusion body within anterior horn neurones in motor neuron disease defined by immunocytochemical localisation of ubiquitin. Neurosci Lett 1988; 94:203–210.
49. Piao YS, Wakabayashi K, Kakita A, Yamada M, Hayashi S, Morita T, Ikuta F, Oyanagi K, Takahashi H. Neuropathology with clinical correlations of sporadic amyotrophic lateral sclerosis: 102 autopsy cases examined between 1962 and 2000. Brain Pathol 2003; 13:10–22.
50. Maekawa S, Cotter D, Landau S, Parnavelas J, Kibble M, Everall I, Al-Sarraj S, Leigh PN. Cortical selective vulnerability in motor neuron disease: a morphometric study. Brain 2004; 127:1237–1251.
51. Lowe J, Mayer RJ, Landon M. Ubiquitin in neurodegenerative diseases. Brain Pathol 1993; 3:55–65.
52. He CZ, Hays AP. Expression of peripherin in ubiquinated inclusions of amyotrophic lateral sclerosis. J Neurol Sci 2004; 217:47–54.
53. Leung CL, He CZ, Kaufmann P, Chin SS, Naini A, Liem RK, Mitsumoto H, Hays AP. A pathogenic peripherin gene mutation in a patient with amyotrophic lateral sclerosis. Brain Pathol 2004; 14:290–296.
54. Gros-Louis F, Lariviere R, Gowing G, Laurent S, Camu W, Bouchard JP, Meininger V, Rouleau GA, Julien JP. A frameshift deletion in peripherin gene associated with amyotrophic lateral sclerosis. J Biol Chem 2004; 279:45951–45956.
55. Andersen PM, Sims KB, Xin WW, Kiely R, O'Neill G, Ravits J, Pioro E, Harati Y, Brower RD, Levine JS, et al. Sixteen novel mutations in the Cu/Zn superoxide dismutase gene in amyotrophic lateral sclerosis: a decade of discoveries, defects and disputes. Amyotroph Lateral Scler Other Motor Neuron Disord 2003; 2:62–73.
56. Yang Y, Hentati A, Deng HX, Dabbagh O, Sasaki T, Hirano M, Hung WY, Ouhchi K, Yan J, Azim AC, et al. The gene encoding alsin, a protein with three guanine-nucleotide

exchange factor domains, is mutated in a form of recessive amyotrophic lateral sclerosis. Nat Genet 2001; 29:160–165.

57. Hadano S, Hand CK, Osuga H, Yanagisawa Y, Otomo A, Devon RS, Miyamoto N, Showguchi-Miyata J, Okada Y, Singaraja R, et al. A gene encoding a putative GTPase regulator is mutated in familial amyotrophic lateral sclerosis 2. Nat Genet 2001; 29: 166–173.

58. Chen Y-Z, Bennett CL, Huynh HM, Blair IP, Puls I, Irobi J, Dierick I, Abel A, Kennerson ML, Rabin BA, et al. DNA/RNA helicase gene mutations in a form of juvenile amyotrophic lateral sclerosis (ALS4). Am J Hum Genet 2004; 74:1128–1135.

59. Nishimura AL, Mitne-Neto M, Silva HCA, Richieri-Costa A, Middleton S, Cascio D, Kok F, Oliveira JRM, Gillingwater T, Webb J, et al. A mutation in the vesicle-trafficking protein VPB causes late-onset spinal muscular atrophy and amyotrophic lateral sclerosis. Am J Hum Genet 2004; 75:822–831.

60. Al-Chalabi A, Andersen PM, Nilsson P, Chioza B, Andersson JL, Russ C, Shaw CE, Powell JF, Leigh PN. Deletions of the heavy neurofilament subunit tail in amyotrophic lateral sclerosis. Hum Mol Genet 1999; 8:157–164.

61. Bruijn LI, Houseweart MK, Kato S, Anderson KL, Anderson SD, Ohama E, Reaume AG, Scott RW, Cleveland DW. Aggregation and motor neuron toxicity of an ALS-linked SOD1 mutant independent from wild-type SOD1. Science 1998; 281: 1851–1854.

62. Shibata N, Hirano A, Kobayashi M, Siddique T, Deng HX, Hung WY, Kato T, Asayama K. Intense superoxide dismutase-1 immunoreactivity in intracytoplasmic hyaline inclusions of familial amyotrophic lateral sclerosis with posterior column involvement. J Neuropathol Exp Neurol 1996; 55:481–490.

63. Nguyen MD, Lariviere RC, Julien JP. Deregulation of Cdk5 in a mouse model of ALS: toxicity alleviated by perikaryal neurofilament inclusions. Neuron 2001; 30:135–147.

64. Watanabe Y, Kato S, Adachi Y, Nakashima K. Frameshift, nonsense and non amino acid altering mutations in SOD1 in familial ALS: report of a Japanese pedigree and literature review. Amyotroph Lateral Scler Other Motor Neuron Disord 2000; 1:251–258.

65. Jonsson PA, Ernhil K, Andersen PM, Bergemalm D, Brannstrom T, Gredal O, Nilsson P, Marklund SL. Minute quantities of misfolded mutant superoxide dismutase-1 cause amyotrophic lateral sclerosis. Brain 2004; 127:73–88.

66. Podust VN, Brownell JE, Gladysheva TB, Luo RS, Wang C, Coggins MB, Pierce JW, Lightcap ES, Chau V. A Nedd8 conjugation pathway is essential for proteolytic targeting of p27Kip1 by ubiquitination. Proc Natl Acad Sci USA 2000; 97:4579–4584.

67. Mori F, Nishie M, Piao YS, Kito K, Kamitani T, Takahashi H, Wakabayashi K. Accumulation of NEDD8 in neuronal and glial inclusions of neurodegenerative disorders. Neuropathol Appl Neurobiol 2005; 31:53–61.

68. Hishikawa N, Niwa J, Doyu M, Ito T, Isigaki S, Hashizume Y, Sobue G. Dorfin localizes to the ubiquitylated inclusions in Parkinson's disease, dementia with Lewy bodies, multiple system atrophy, and amyotrophic lateral sclerosis. Am J Pathol 2003; 163:609–619.

69. Liu J, Lillo C, Jonsson A, Velde CV, Ward CM, Miller TM, Subramaniam JR, Rothstein JD, Marklund S, Andersen PM, et al. Toxicity of familial ALS-linked SOD1 mutants from selective recruitment to spinal mitochondria. Neuron 2004; 43: 5–17.

70. Pasinelli P, Belford ME, Lenno N, Bacskai BJ, Hyman BT, Trotti D, Brown RH Jr. Amyotrophic lateral sclerosis-associated SOD1 mutant proteins bind and aggregate with Bcl-2 in spinal cord mitochondria. Neuron 2004; 43:19–30.

71. Kato S, Sumi-Akamaru H, Fujimura H, Sakoda S, Kato M, Hirano A, Takikawa M, Ohama E. Copper chaperone for superoxide dismutase co-aggregates with superoxide dismutase 1 (SOD1) in neuronal Lewy body-like hyaline inclusions: an immunohistochemical study on familial amyotrophic lateral sclerosis with SOD1 gene mutation. Acta Neuropathol (Berl) 2001; 102:233–238.

72. Watanabe M, Dykes-Hoberg M, Culotta VC, Price DL, Wong PC, Rothstein JD. Histological evidence of protein aggregation in mutant SOD1 transgenic mice and in amyotrophic lateral sclerosis neural tissues. Neurobiol Dis 2001; 8:933–941.

73. Shibata N, Hirano A, Kato S, Nagai R, Horiuchi S, Komori T, Umahara T, Asayama K, Kobayashi M. Advanced glycation endproducts are deposited in neuronal hyaline inclusions: a study on familial amyotrophic lateral sclerosis with superoxide dismutase-1 mutation. Acta Neuropathol (Berl) 1999; 97:240–246.

74. Kato S, Horiuchi S, Nakashima K, Hirano A, Shibata N, Nakano I, Saito M, Kato M, Asayama K, Ohama E. Astrocytic hyaline inclusions contain advanced glycation endproducts in familial amyotrophic lateral sclerosis with superoxide dismutase 1 gene mutation: immunohistochemical and immunoelectron microscopical analyses. Acta Neuropathol (Berl) 1999; 97:260–266.

75. Getzoff ED, Tainer JA, Stempien MM, Bell GI, Hallewell RA. Evolution of CuZn superoxide dismutase and the Greek key barrel structural motif. Proteins: Struct Funct Genet 1989; 5:322–336.

76. Borchelt DR, Lee MK, Slunt HS, Guarnieri M, Xu Z-S, Wong P-C, Brown RH Jr, Price DL, Sisodia SS, Cleveland DW. Superoxide dismutase 1 with mutations linked to familial amyotrophic lateral sclerosis possesses significant activity. Proc Natl Acad Sci USA 1994; 91:8292–8296.

77. Hough MA, Grossmann JG, Antonyuk SV, Strange RW, Doucette PA, Rodriguez JA, Whitson LJ, Hart PJ, Hayward LJ, Valentine JS, et al. Dimer destabilization in superoxide dismutase may result in disease-causing properties: structures of motor neuron disease mutants. Proc Natl Acad Sci USA 2004; 101:5976–5981.

78. DiDonato M, Craig L, Huff ME, Thayer MM, Cardoso RMF, Kassmann J, Lo TP, Bruns CK, Powers ET, Kelly JW, et al. ALS mutants of human superoxide dismutase form fibrous aggregates via framework destabilization. J Mol Biol 2003; 332:601–615.

79. Ray SS, Nowak RJ, Strokovich K, Brown RH Jr, Walz T, Lansbury PT Jr. An inter-subunit disulfide bond prevents in vitro aggregation of a superoxide dismutase-1 mutant linked to familial amyotrophic lateral sclerosis. Biochemistry 2004; 43:4899–4905.

80. Chung J, Yang H, de Beus MD, Ryu CY, Cho K, Colon W. Cu/Zn superoxide dismutase can form pore-like structures. Biochem Biophys Res Commun 2003; 312:873–876.

81. Lindberg MJ, Normark J, Holmgren A, Oliveberg M. Folding of human superoxide dismutase: disulfide reduction prevents dimerization and produces marginally stable monomers. Proc Natl Acad Sci USA 2004; 101:15,893–15,898.

82. Ray SS, Lansbury PT Jr. A possible therapeutic target for Lou Gehrig's disease. Proc Natl Acad Sci USA 2004; 101:5701–5702.

83. Subramaniam JR, Lyons WE, Liu J, Bartnikas TB, Rothstein J, Price DL, Cleveland DW, Gitlin JD, Wong PC. Mutant SOD1 causes motor neuron disease independent of copper chaperone-mediated copper loading. Nat Neurosci 2002; 5:301–307.

84. Lindberg MJ, Tibell L, Oliveberg M. Common denominator of Cu/Zn superoxide dismutase mutants associated with amyotrophic lateral sclerosis: decreased stability of the apo state. Proc Natl Acad Sci USA 2002; 99:16,607–16,612.

85. Elam JS, Taylor AB, Strange R, Antonyuk S, Doucette PA, Rodriguez JA, Hasnain SS, Hayward LJ, Valentine JS, Yeates TO, et al. Amyloid-like filaments and water-filled nanotubules formed by SOD1 mutant proteins linked to familial ALS. Nat Struct Biol 2003; 10:461–467.

86. Rakhit R, Cunningham P, Furtos-Matei A, Dahan S, Qi X-F, Crow JP, Cashman NR, Kondejewski LH, Chakrabartty A. Oxidation-induced misfolding and aggregation of superoxide dismutase and its implications for amyotrophic lateral sclerosis. J Biol Chem 2002; 277:47,551–47,556.

87. Rakhit R, Crow JP, Lepock JR, Kondejewski LH, Cashman NR, Chakrabartty A. Monomeric Cu,Zn-superoxide dismutase is a common misfolding intermediate in the oxidation models of sporadic and familial amyotrophic lateral sclerosis. J Biol Chem 2004; 279:15,499–15,504.

88. Sherman MY, Goldberg AL. Cellular defences against unfolded proteins: a cell biologist thinks about neurodegenerative diseases. Neuron 2001; 29:15–32.
89. Glickman MH, Ciechanover A. The ubiquitin-proteasome proteolytic pathway: destruction for the sake of construction. Physiol Rev 2002; 82:373–428.
90. Ciechanover A, Brundin P. The ubiquitin proteasome system in neurodegenerative diseases: sometimes the chicken, sometimes the egg. Neuron 2003; 40:427–446.
91. Saigoh K, Wang YL, Suh JG, Yamanishi T, Sakai Y, Kiyosawa H, Harada T, Ichihara N, Wakana S, Kikuchi T, et al. Intragenic deletion in the gene encoding ubiquitin carboxy-terminal hydrolase in gad mice. Nat Genet 1999; 23:47–51.
92. Hershko A, Heller H, Elias S, Ciechanover A. Components of ubiquitin-protein ligase system. Resolution, affinity purification, and role in protein breakdown. J Biol Chem 2003; 258:8206–8214.
93. Lincoln S, Vaughan J, Wood N, Baker M, Adamson J, Gwinn-Hardy K, Lynch T, Hardy J, Farrer M. Low frequency of pathogenic mutations in the ubiquitin carboxy-terminal hydrolase gene in familial Parkinson's disease. Neuroreport 1999; 10:427–429.
94. Harhangi BS, Farrer MJ, Lincoln S, Bonifati V, Meco G, De Michele G, Brice A, Durr A, Martinez M, Gasser T, et al. The Ile93Met mutation in the ubiquitin carboxy-terminal-hydrolase-Ll gene is not observed in European cases with familial Parkinson's disease. Neurosci Lett 1999; 270:1–4.
95. Bruijn LI, Becher MW, Lee MK, Anderson KL, Jenkins NA, Copeland NG, Sisodia SS, Rothstein JD, Borchelt DR, Price DL, et al. ALS-linked SOD1 mutant G85R mediates damage to astrocytes and promotes rapidly progressive disease withSOD1-containing inclusions. Neuron 1997; 18:327–338.
96. Durham HD, Roy J, Dong L, Figlewicz DA. Aggregation of mutant Cu/Zn superoxide dismutase proteins in culture model of ALS. J Neuropathol Exp Neurol 1997; 56:523–530.
97. Johnston JA, Ward CL, Kopito RR. Aggresomes: a cellular response to misfolded proteins. J Cell Biol 1998; 143:1883–1898.
98. Walsh DM, Klyubin I, Fadeeva JV, Rowan MJ, Selkoe DJ. Amyloid-beta oligomers: their production, toxicity and therapeutic inhibition. Biochem Soc Trans 2002; 30:552–557.
99. Lee JP, Gerin C, Bindokas VP, Miller R, Ghadge G, Roos RP. No correlation between aggregates of Cu/Zn superoxide dismutase and cell death in familial amyotrophic lateral sclerosis. J Neurochem 2002; 82:1229–1238.
100. Hyun DH, Lee M, Halliwell B, Jenner P. Proteasomal inhibition causes the formation of protein aggregates containing wide range of proteins, including nitrated proteins. J Neurochem 2003; 86:363–373.
101. Aquilano K, Rotilio G, Ciriolo MR. Proteasome activation and nNOS down-regulation in neuroblastoma cells expressing a Cu,Zn superoxide dismutase mutant involved in familial ALS. J Neurochem 2003; 85:1324–1335.
102. Niwa JI, Ishigaki S, Hishikawa N, Yamamoto M, Doyu M, Murata S, Tanaka K, Taniguchi N, Sobue G. Dorfin ubiquitylates mutant SOD1 and prevents mutant SOD1-mediated neurotoxocity. J Biol Chem 2002; 277:36793–36798.
103. Ishigaki S, Hishikawa N, Niwa J, Iemura S, Natsume T, Hori S, Kakizuka A, Tanaka K, Sobue G. Physical and functional interaction between dorfin and valosin-containing protein that are colocalized in ubiquitylated inclusions in neurodegenerative disorders. J Biol Chem 2004; 49:51376–51385.
104. Dai RM, Li CC. Valosin-containing protein is a multi-ubiquitin chain-targeting factor required in ubiquitin-proteasome degradation. Nat Cell Biol 2001; 3:740–744.
105. Muchowski PJ, Wacker JL. Modulation of neurodegeneration by molecular chaperones. Nat Rev Neurosci 2005; 6:11–22.
106. Fardeau M, Vicart P, Caron A, Chateau D, Chevallay M, Collin H, Chapon F, Duboc D, Eymard B, Tome FM, et al. Familial myopathy with desmin storage seen as a

granul-filamentar, electron-dense material with mutation of the αB-crystallin gene. Rev Neurol (Paris) 2000; 156:497–504.

107. Evgrafov OV, Mersiyanova I, Irobi J, Van Den Bosch L, Dierick I, Leung CL, Schagina O, Verpoorten N, Van Impe K, Fedotov V, et al. Mutant small-heat shock protein 27 causes axonal Charcot-Marie-Tooth disease and distal hereditary motor neuropathy. Nat Genet 2004; 36:602–606.

108. Hansen JJ, Durr A, Cournu-Rebeix I, Georgopoulos C, Ang D, Nielsen MN, Davoine CS, Brice A, Fontaine B, Gregersen N, et al. Hereditary spastic paraplegia SPG13 is associated with a mutation in the gene encoding the mitochondrial chaperonin HSP60. Am J Hum Genet 2002; 70:1328–1332.

109. Bruening W, Roy J, Giasson B, Figlewicz DA, Mushynski WE, Durham HD. Up-regulation of protein chaperones preserves viability of cells expressing toxic Cu/Zn-superoxide dismutase mutants associated with amyotrophic lateral sclerosis. J Neurochem 1999; 72:693–699.

110. Shinder GA, Lacourse M-C, Minotti S, Durham HD. Mutant Cu/Zn-superoxide dismutase proteins have altered solubility and interact with heat shock/stress proteins in models of amyotrophic lateral sclerosis. J Biol Chem 2001; 276:12,791–12,796.

111. Okado-Matsumoto A, Fridovich I. Amyotrophic lateral sclerosis: a proposed mechanism. Proc Natl Acad Sci USA 2002; 99:9010–9014.

112. Wang J, Slunt H, Gonzales V, Fromholt D, Coonfield M, Copeland NG, Jenkins NA, Borchelt DR. Copper-binding-site-null SOD1 causes ALS in transgenic mice: aggregates of non-native SOD1 delineate a common feature. Hum Mol Genet 2003; 12:2753–2764.

113. Takeuchi H, Kobayashi Y, Yoshihara T, Niwa J, Doyu M, Ohtsuka K, Sobue G. Hsp70 and Hsp40 improve neurite outgrowth and suppress intracytoplasmic aggregate formation in cultured neuronal cells expressing mutant SOD1. Brain Res 2002; 949:11–22.

114. Vlemnickx V, Van Damme P, Goffin K, Delye H, Van Den Bosch L, Robberecht W. Upregulation of HSP27 in a transgenic model of ALS. J Neuropath Exp Neurol 2002; 61:968–974.

115. Kieran D, Kalman B, Kick JRT, Riddoch-Contreras J, Burnstock G, Greensmith L. Treatment with arimoclomal, a coinducer of heat shock proteins, delays disease progression in ALS mice. Nat Med 2004; 10:402–405.

116. Benn SC, Brown RH Jr. Putting the heat on ALS. Nat Med 2004; 10:345–346.

117. Cummings CJ, Sun Y, Opal P, Antalffy B, Mestril R, Orr HT, Dillmann WH, Zoghbi HY. Over-expression of inducible HSP70 chaperone suppresses neuropathology and improves motor function in SCA1 mice. Hum Mol Genet 2001; 10:1511–1518.

118. Adachi H, Katsuno M, Minamiyama M, Sang C, Pagoulatos G, Angelidis C, Kusakabe M, Yoshiki A, Kobayashi Y, et al. Heat shock protein 70 chaperone overexpression ameliorates phenotypes of the spinal and bulbar muscular atrophy transgenic mouse model by reducing nuclear-localized mutant androgen receptor protein. J Neurosci 2003; 23:2203–2211.

119. Walsh DM, Klyubin I, Fadeeva JV, Cullen WK, Anwyl R, Wolfe MS, Rowan MJ, Selkoe DJ. Naturally secreted oligomers of amyloid beta protein potently inhibit hippocampal long-term potentiation in vivo. Nature 2002; 416:535–539.

120. Volles MJ, Lee SJ, Rochet JC, Shtilerman MD, Ding TT, Kessler JC, Lansbury PT Jr. Vesicle permeabilization by protofibrilar α-synuclein: implications for the pathogenesis and treatment of Parkinson's disease. Biochemistry 2001; 40:7812–7819.

121. Kayed R, Head E, Thompson JL, McIntire TM, Milton SC, Cotman CW, Glabe CG. Common structure of soluble oligomers implies common mechanism of pathogenesis. Science 2003; 300:486–489.

122. Olanow CW, Perl DP, DeMartino GN, McNaught KStP. Lewy-body formation is an aggresome-related process: a hypothesis. Lancet Neurol 2004; 3:496–503.

22

Neuroinflammation

Albert A. Yen, Ericka P. Simpson, and Stanley H. Appel
Department of Neurology, Methodist Neurological Institute, Houston, Texas, U.S.A.

INTRODUCTION

Neuroinflammation is a key event in the pathogenesis of amyotrophic lateral sclerosis (ALS), although our understanding of its cause and significance is incomplete. ALS researchers have long recognized that inflammatory cells and mediators are present in the areas of degenerating motor neurons. However, a debate has centered on whether these inflammatory cells are only an epiphenomenon of motor neuronal loss, or if the immune cells actively contribute to the processes that determine motor neuron survival. Recent studies have provided increasing support for the importance of neuroinflammation as a participant in the mechanisms of motor neuron injury in ALS.

In the 1970s and 1980s, the central nervous system (CNS) was widely considered to be an immunoprivileged site—that is, the CNS and immune system are strictly separate structures. This viewpoint has shifted over the years, as experimental evidence has clearly shown that the CNS is under constant immune surveillance and that the CNS and immune system can interact extensively under certain conditions. It is notable, however, that inflammatory processes in the CNS can differ from those of systemic inflammation. Unlike the rapid, cellular infiltration seen in systemic inflammation, inflammatory responses to a noxious stimulus in the CNS can be less dramatic and may include the activation of the innate immune system, the resident microglial cells, as well as the release of cytokines and chemokines, the gradual entry of immune cells from the peripheral circulation, the localized proliferation of dendritic cells, and the induction of tissue repair enzymes. The initial response to an acute insult (trauma, ischemia, and infection) is directed at limiting cellular damage and enhancing repair. However, under chronic insult or a continuing stimulus, a long-lasting inflammatory response may cause additional injury to CNS tissue. In other words, the cells and signaling molecules of neuroinflammation may comprise a "double-edged sword"—sometimes protective and reparative to neurons, and sometimes injurious. Indeed, increasing evidence support a dual role of immune activation in several CNS diseases, based upon the timing and duration of immune activation, degree and type of injury, intercellular communication, and genetic modifiers (1–3). Ongoing research to decipher the nature of this dual role has been both challenging and exciting.

This excitement is shared by researchers in other fields. The interrelationships between neurology and immunology have been studied extensively in multiple sclerosis, the prototypical CNS autoimmune disease. More recently, the role of neuroinflammation has been evaluated in other neurodegenerative conditions, including Alzheimer's disease and Parkinson disease (4–7). Lessons learned from those conditions has provided valuable clues to ALS researchers.

This chapter will describe the cellular and biochemical evidence of neuroinflammation in ALS tissues and in animal models, review the evidence that immune activation may be capable of initiating disease, delineate the studies which support a prominent role for neuroinflammation in dictating motor neuron survival, and characterize what is currently believed about the "dual role" of neuroinflammation. The importance of the timing, degree, and profile of inflammatory mediators will be emphasized. Mention will be made of the limitations of previous immunosuppressive therapies, future directions of neuroimmunology research, and how new findings may impact ALS therapy.

CELLULAR AND BIOCHEMICAL EVIDENCE OF NEUROINFLAMMATION

Evidence of neuroinflammation in ALS has been provided by examination of CNS tissues from ALS patients and rodent models. Techniques utilized in these studies include immunohistochemistry, semiquantitative and real-time RT-PCR, gene chip microarrays, and ELISA. Following is a description of these findings.

In Humans

The main cellular evidence of neuroinflammation in ALS is the accumulation of activated microglia and macrophages in areas of motoneuron degeneration (8–11). These cells are seen in ALS spinal cord—in the anterior horn area and along the anterior and lateral corticospinal tracts. A lesser cellular reaction is also seen in ALS motor cortex. In contrast to resting microglia, which have long, highly branched processes, activated microglia have hypertrophied soma and thickened, retracted processes, as first described by del Rio-Hortega (12). Reactive microglia express surface markers indicative of their activated state. These include the complement receptor, CD11b; leukocyte common antigen (LCA); and major histocompatibility complex (MHC) class-II glycoproteins, such as human leukocyte antigen DR (HLA-DR). Immunohistochemical staining of microglia with antibodies to any of these antigens reveals a similar morphological staining pattern. In addition to serving a phagocytic function, activated microglia may also communicate and affect the function of cells in the local environment, by expressing a broad array of cytokines, chemokines, proteases, and other effector molecules (13,14).

Reactive astrocytes are also prevalent in ALS tissues. Staining intensely for the intermediate filament, glial fibrillary acidic protein (GFAP), these reactive astrocytes have a hypertrophied appearance and can be observed throughout the areas of degeneration. Presumably, these astrocytes continue to support nearby neurons, but the precise function of reactive astrocytes is unclear. It is likely that they interact extensively with neurons, microglia, and other cells in the local environment (15).

In addition to these resident CNS components, cells that originate in the periphery can also be found. Leukocytes can be observed marginating in postcapillary venules, and some of them can be seen entering the tissue. They express CD45, also known as LCA, a cell marker present on all hematopoeitic cells. The majority of the marginating leukocytes are T8 lymphocytes, although a few are T4 cells. The functional contribution of these few T cells to ALS pathogenesis is still a matter of debate. It has been argued by some that these T cells are an end result of chronic degeneration and immune activation. Proponents of this theory point to the scarcity of T cells in end-stage tissues and to minimal biochemical evidence of elevated T cell-related gene expression (8,10). An alternative view is that T lymphocytes need not be present in large numbers to signal instructions for neuronal repair or cytotoxicity at different stages of disease. Soluble proteins can move from the CNS parenchyma into the cerebrospinal fluid. These soluble proteins can then be transported through lymphatic channels to peripheral lymph nodes, where they provide antigenic stimulation to naïve or memory T cells (15). The memory T cells travel to the CNS, where they may encounter antigen and become further stimulated. These stimulated T cells are a sole potential source of γ-interferon, a potent activator of microglia and leukocytes. Clearly, T cells are capable of coordinating an early immune response without even being present in the CNS in large numbers.

The other bone-marrow-derived cells adjacent to the CNS endothelial cells are monocytes and macrophages, and they express many of the same surface markers as the resident microglia cells (mentioned above). If provided with proper stimulus, some of these infiltrating mononuclear cells have the potential to differentiate into full-fledged, antigen-presenting dendritic cells (17). Indeed, abundant numbers of both immature and activated/mature dendritic cells have been detected in ALS spinal cords (11).

Numerous biochemical markers of neuroinflammation have also been found in ALS tissue. A partial list is included in Table 1. The families of compounds include cytokines, chemokines, complement proteins, prostaglandins, interleukins, interferons, integrins, acute phase reactants, apolipoproteins, and proteases. Many of these biochemical markers have also been found in Alzheimer's disease tissues, suggesting that the inflammatory response in both conditions may be similar (18,19).

Some of the inflammatory mediators enhance the entry of leukocytes from the periphery into the areas of degeneration (16). For instance, the leukocytes that are observed in the postcapillary venules express leukocyte function antigen 1 (LFA-1), a surface molecule which gives activated leukocytes the ability to adhere to endothelial cells and migrate into CNS tissue. This binding involves a specific interaction between LFA-1 and intercellular adhesion molecule-1 (ICAM-1), an adhesion molecule that is upregulated on endothelial cells in areas of inflammation (20). Another molecule that is upregulated in ALS tissue is matrix metalloproteinase-9 (MMP-9) (21). MMP-9 is a proteolytic enzyme that is released by leukocytes and reactive astrocytes to degrade proteins of the extracellular matrix and enhance the entry of leukocytes into areas of inflammation.

Other inflammatory molecules in Table 1 are related to the synthesis of prostaglandins, a family of molecules with both pro- and anti-apoptotic actions in specific neuronal models (22–25). In the first step of prostaglandin production, membrane lipids are broken down by phospholipase A_2 to arachidonic acid. Interestingly, phospholipase A_2 has been identified in activated glial cells in areas of neurodegeneration (26). Next, cyclooxygenase (COX) catalyzes the rate-limiting step of prostaglandin synthesis, the conversion of arachidonic acid to prostaglandin G2 (PGG2). Two distinct COX isoenzymes, COX-1 and COX-2, can mediate this reaction, and they are 65% homologous. COX-1 is constitutively expressed in most

Table 1 Proteins Associated with the Inflammatory State Observed in ALS Tissues

LCA (leukocyte common antigen, CD45)	Membrane-bound protein tyrosine phosphatase; expressed by all hematopoeitic cells
LFA-1 (leukocyte function antigen 1, CD11a/CD18 integrin)	Appears on all leukocytes; promotes intercellular adhesion
ICAM-1 (intracellular adhesion molecule 1, CD54)	Cell surface or matrix molecule; promotes binding to LFA-1
GFAP (glial fibrillary acidic protein)	Intermediate filament protein highly expressed by activated astrocytes
Phospholipase A2	Breaks down membrane lipids to form arachidonic acid
COX-1 (cyclooxygenase-1)	Converts arachidonic acid into prostaglandin H2; rate-limiting step in prostaglandin synthesis
COX-2 (cyclooxygenase-2)	Converts arachidonic acid into prostaglandin H2; rate-limiting step in prostaglandin synthesis; inducible expression
PGE2 (prostaglandin E2)	Member of prostaglandin family; may have both pro- and anti-apoptotic actions
FcγR-1 (immunoglobulin Fc region receptor 1)	Receptor on phagocytes for IgG bound to an antigen
HLA-DR (human leukocyte antigen DR)	Antigen-presenting surface molecule on immunocompetent cells
IL-6 (interleukin 6)	Inflammatory cytokine released by activated astrocytes and microglia
MCP-1 (monocyte chemoattractant protein-1)	Chemokine that attracts monocytes and myeloid dendritic cells
M-CSF (macrophage-colony stimulating factor)	Growth factor cytokine that acts on monocytes and macrophages to cause them to differentiate
MMP-9 (matrix metalloproteinase-9)	Proteolytic enzyme that can degrade components of the extracellular matrix
C3d (complement C3 fragment d)	Degradation product of activated C3
C4d (complement C4 fragment d)	Degradation product of activated C4
CD-11b (complement receptor 3)	Phagocyte surface receptor recognizing an activated complement fragment from C3

tissues, while COX-2 is constitutively expressed in the kidney, stomach, and CNS. However, COX-2 expression is strongly inducible and can be significantly upregulated by several cellular factors, including multiple growth factors, interleukin-1β, tumor necrosis factor-α, lipopolysaccharide (LPS), phorbol ester, and elevated intracellular calcium concentration. A marked increase in COX-2 levels has been seen in ALS spinal cords, consistent with the previous reports of increased levels of prostaglandin E_2 (PGE_2), a further product of prostaglandin synthesis (27). Both mRNA and protein levels of COX-2 were elevated in ALS spinal cords and in pathologically affected areas (28,29). The implications of elevated COX-2 levels will be discussed later in this chapter.

Additionally, immunoglobulin G (IgG) is present in motor neurons in ALS spinal cords, and also in pyramidal cells of the motor cortex (30). The significance of intraneuronal IgG, if any, is unclear at this time.

In Animal Models

Mirroring the findings in human tissue, immunohistochemical studies of spinal cords from mutant SOD1 mice have revealed similar evidence of immune activation. One advantage of studying animal models is that the tissues may be examined at earlier disease stages and prior to the onset of motor weakness. Increased ICAM-1, IgG, and Fc receptor (FcR) for immunoglobulin have been observed at 40 days of age (presymptomatic) (31). Several groups have independently demonstrated the presence of activated microglia, as early as 80 days of age (early symptomatic stage) (32). In general, the development of these inflammatory changes precedes the onset of motor signs, and their increasing levels parallel disease progression.

Multiple studies have confirmed an elevation of pro-inflammatory molecules in the presymptomatic mSOD1 mouse, including mediators such as TNF-α, COX-2, inducible nitric oxide synthase (iNOS), interleukin-1α, interleukin-1β, IL-1 receptor antagonist (IL1RA), CD86, CD200R, and growth-related oncogene-α (Gro-α) (28,33–39).

Evidence of neuroinflammation has also been found in other animal models of motor neuron degeneration. For example, microglial activation was observed in the Wobbler mouse, a finding that has been confirmed by several groups (40–42). Elevated TNF-α levels were found in the brain and spinal cord of the *mnd* mouse (43). It appears that the other murine models of motor neuron degeneration share some neuroinflammatory features with the mSOD1 model.

Summary

In summary, the cellular evidence for neuroinflammation in ALS consists of activated microglia, reactive astrocytes, macrophages, and a few T cells seen marginating along postcapillary venules. The biochemical evidence consists of the presence of cytokines, chemokines, components of prostaglandin synthesis, and other pro-inflammatory molecules that have been found in Alzheimer's disease and other neurodegenerative conditions. Similar findings have been documented in both human ALS tissue and in animal models of motor neuron disease.

EVIDENCE FOR A ROLE IN INITIATING DISEASE

The pathology of ALS suggest the activation of both innate and adaptive arms of the immune system, involving antigen capture and presentation, leukocyte migration and trafficking, and microglial activation. Whether these processes are sufficient to initiate motor neuron injury in ALS is unknown, but early studies that searched for an initiating role of an immune response against "self" epitopes (autoimmunity) raised some intriguing possibilities (44,45). For example, an animal model of a primary, immune-mediated motor neuron disease was developed by inoculating guinea pigs with bovine motor neurons.

Clinical features of this experimental autoimmune motor neuron disease animal included muscle weakness, electrophysiologic and morphologic evidence of denervation, loss of motoneurons in the spinal cord, and clinical improvement with immunosuppression (46–49). Others have documented a motor neuron disease phenotype in transgenic mice that overexpress interleukin-3 (IL-3) (50). These studies documented that a primary immune process is capable of initiating motor neuron disease, but it was still unknown whether autoimmunity was playing a role in ALS.

Although the higher incidence of autoimmune diseases and paraproteinemias in ALS patients continues to suggest a link between dysimmunity or paraimmunity and motor neuron disease (51,52), the evidence that ALS is a primary, autoimmune disease remains circumstantial.

The possibility that ALS pathogenesis is initiated by a secondary immune response to a primary infectious agent has also been considered, especially in regards to viral exposure. The "viral etiology" hypothesis for ALS is based on the finding that neural cells are selectively vulnerable to infection by certain viruses, particularly poliovirus and some enteroviruses (53). In this scenario, infected neural cells would be targeted for removal by the immune system. However, early studies attempting to detect viruses in ALS tissue were uniformly negative (54,55), and even with the application of more sensitive detection techniques in later studies, the results were conflicting (56–59). Following the onset of the HIV/AIDS epidemic, renewed interest in this theory arose with reports of several cases of HIV-associated motor neuron disease (60–67).

Compared to classic ALS, HIV-associated ALS occurs in younger patients, progresses more rapidly, and improves with antiretroviral therapy—this response suggests that HIV virus is the etiologic factor in motor neuron dysfunction in these cases. Further studies indicated that the HIV retrovirus is not neurotropic. Instead, it infects and replicates within macrophage/microglia cell populations and seems to exert its neurotoxic effects indirectly via Tat, a transcriptional regulator viral protein. The Tat protein affects the functional state of infected microglial cells by stimulating them to secrete neurotoxic molecules, differentially regulating chemokine expression within the brain, and disrupting pathways regulating intracellular calcium and ion channel expression (68,69). Both in vitro models and pathological studies suggest that the HIV-infected/activated microglia and macrophages may selectively damage susceptible neurons, leading to neuropathology (70,71). This indirect, microglia-mediated mechanism of neurotoxicity may apply to other viral infections as well (72,73). Although direct neurotoxic effects on motor neurons are still contributors to HIV-associated neurodegenerative diseases (74,75), the significant neuroinflammatory state mediated by the secondary activation of microglia/macrophages appears to play the predominant role in these conditions.

Additional support for an association between retroviruses, immune activation, and ALS is provided by a murine neurotropic retrovirus, which can cause motor neuron degeneration in mice (76), and the human T-cell lymphotrophic virus type I (HTLV-1) retrovirus, which predominantly causes myelopathy/tropical spastic paraparesis but has caused an ALS-like syndrome in rare cases (77). Of note, HTLV-1 can also cause lymphoma, and lymphoproliferative disorders have an increased incidence in ALS patients (78). On the basis of this information, it has been proposed that an immune response directed against retroviral proteins induces a chronic neuroinflammatory state that leads to motor neuron degeneration. In accord with this, antibodies against HTLV-1 viral proteins have been reported in some ALS patients, as well as increased reverse transcriptase activity in ALS sera (79,80). Furthermore, this process may not even require infection and active replication by an exogenous retrovirus. A recent study showed that an immune response can be directed against retroviral proteins produced by activation of endogenous retrovirus sequences that are normally present in the human genome. In that study, the researchers reported that 56% of sporadic ALS patients had IgG antibodies reactive to a protein encoded by the endogenous retroviral sequence, HML-2/Herv-K, and that this immune response was identified in ALS patients more than five times as frequently as in Alzheimer's disease or healthy controls (81). Furthermore, 11% of the sporadic ALS patients had IgM reactivity to HML-2, suggesting that the anti-body response occurred in the same time frame as neurological symptoms in those patients. Together, these findings raise the possibility that the activation of endogenous retroviruses can perpetuate and drive ongoing inflammatory events, at least in a subset of ALS patients.

In summary, there is no conclusive evidence that a primary immune, or auto-immune, mechanism is involved in the initiation of ALS. The association of viruses, such as HIV and HTLV-1, with a motor neuron disease phenotype does suggest that a secondary immune response can cause motor neuron injury and dysfunction, without direct toxicity from the primary infection. Whether a secondary immune response is a predominant mechanism in typical ALS is not clear. The ineffectiveness of standard immunosuppressive therapies—steroids, high-dose intravenous immu-noglobulin, plasma exchange, cyclophosphamide, azathioprine, and total lymphoid irradiation (82–87)—in significantly altering the clinical disease course would suggest otherwise. Still, these treatment failures should not rule out the importance of the immune inflammatory response, because therapeutic efficacy may have been limited by several factors. These factors include the timing of treatment, access to the CNS, specificity of therapeutic target(s), and side effect profile.

In the absence of these limitations, immunomodulatory treatments have been modestly effective in animal models (88–91). Another consideration is that, like the HIV-associated ALS syndrome, immune inflammation in ALS may be a second-ary response, and effective treatment may require the suppression or elimination of the primary insult(s), in addition to immune modulation.

EVIDENCE FOR A ROLE IN AMPLIFYING DISEASE

Although the evidence that CNS inflammatory events can initiate disease is still questionable, a growing consensus among ALS researchers is that inflammatory cells and mediators play an integral role in affecting motor neuron survival. In addition to the activated microglia, dendritic cells, immunoglobulins, and inflammatory proteins mentioned earlier, we recently documented increased levels of monocyte chemo-attractant protein-1α (MCP-1α) in ALS spinal cords (11), and that the MCP-1α is expressed mainly by glial cells. MCP-1α, a chemokine that attracts myeloid dendritic cells, macrophages, and activated T cells, is also elevated in the CSF and serum of ALS patients, compared to controls (92,93). This elevation may reflect a local inflam-matory response that results in an active transmigration of cellular constituents from the periphery into the CNS. Overall, the presence of T cells, immunoglobulins, and dendritic cells suggests that the immune inflammatory response in ALS is not merely involved in scavenging cellular debris, nor is it primarily an innate response resulting in tissue damage (94). Instead, it is likely a complex, acquired response that is involved in the regulation of inflammatory processes directed at tissue injury or repair.

The first line of evidence to support that the immune response in ALS is directed towards the motor axis comes from studies investigating the effects of ALS sera and immunoglobulins on motor neurons and the neuromuscular junction. Independent groups have shown that the intraperitoneal administration of IgG from ALS patients, in contrast to disease control IgG, causes a myriad of functional and pathological alterations at the level of the neuromuscular junction and spinal cord of mice. These include alterations in calcium homeostasis and synaptic organelle ultrastructure (95–97), motor neuron degeneration (98,99), functional changes of voltage dependent calcium channels (100–103), and microglial activation and recruitment in the ventral horn of the spinal cord (104). Autoantibodies have been identified in ALS sera that are reactive against different neural components; together, they do not clearly point towards a common pathway(s) but may still be relevant to disease pathogenesis (105–111). In regards to specific effects on motor neurons, we have shown that ALS IgG is cytotoxic to primary motor neuron cultures through FcR dependent microglial activation; this effect was not observed with disease control IgG (112).

The most salient evidence concerning the role of the immune response in ALS pathogenesis comes from studies in the transgenic mutant SOD1 mouse model for ALS (113). As mentioned previously, multiple studies have documented an upregulation of immune/inflammatory genes in mutant SOD1 spinal cords at presymptomatic stages of disease (28,33–39). These data support that immune activation in mouse model is not solely due to the presence of damaged, nonviable motor neurons, but occurs prior to any demonstrable neuronal degeneration or clinical weakness; thus, it is an early response to changes occurring within relevant neural tissue. In ALS tissues, one of the upregulated, inflammatory markers is MCP-1 (11,93), a chemoattractant protein involved in the activation and recruitment of immune cells to sites of injury. This provides further support that the entry of immune cells from the periphery may contribute to disease propagation.

Further support for the concept that motor neurons do not die alone comes from recent studies in which the mutant SOD1 transgene was expressed in specific neural and glial cell populations.

Interestingly, when the mutation was solely expressed in neurons, it did not result in pathologic or clinical disease; this finding was confirmed by two separate studies (114,115). An earlier study showed that restricted expression in astrocytes, although causing astrocytic proliferation, did not result in motor neuron degeneration or clinical weakness (116). These studies demonstrate that expression of the mutant SOD1 gene, in either the motor neuron or astrocyte population alone, fails to cause disease. Expression of mSOD1 within multiple cell populations is apparently necessary for the initiation and progression of disease.

However, concern was expressed that a decreased number of mSOD1 transcripts in motor neurons could have explained the lack of motor neuron injury and disease. Nevertheless, the concept that motor neurons do not die alone in mSOD1 transgenic mice was supported by elegant experiments by Clement et al. (117). Clement et al. developed chimeric mice in which mSOD1 was expressed in varying numbers of cells across transgenic lines. They showed a delay in disease onset and an extension of disease duration, and both changes were proportional to the percentage of wild-type cells present. Furthermore, they determined that mSOD1-expressing neurons survived longer when surrounded by wild-type glial cells than when they were surrounded by mSOD1-expressing glial cells. This study suggests a potential protective role of glial and immune cells in motor neuron injury. A greater understanding of the role of neuroinflammation in ALS in terms of injury and repair may help to identify new targets for therapy.

EVIDENCE FOR A ROLE IN REPAIR AND PROTECTION

A traditional viewpoint has been that inflammatory cells and mediators are neurotoxic, and that inhibition of inflammation will delay or prevent neuronal loss.

Indeed, therapeutic trials of immunomodulatory agents in the mutant SOD1 mouse has supported this concept (88,89,91,118). However, neuroinflammation is composed of multiple processes, working in series and parallel, which cumulatively can limit cellular injury and promote regeneration, or cause tissue damage and worsen cell loss. An example of this is the dual role of prostaglandins, products of the COX-2 enzyme, in promoting either neuronal survival or apoptotic death. Determining factors may include the target cell and tissue environment, the profile of specific prostaglandin(s), and the dose-dependent cellular response to the inflammatory mediators (1). In the mSOD1 mouse model, increases in COX-2 and PGE2 parallel motor neuron loss, and selective inhibition prolongs survival (27,119), implying that COX-2 activation contributes to neuronal degeneration. However, looking at the cellular constituents rather than the biochemical effectors involved may provide greater insight into these processes.

Microglia are able to respond promptly to signals of stress or injury originating within or outside the CNS and direct their responses for purposes of tissue repair and activation of immune responses. This appears to be regulated by neuron–astrocyte–microglia interactions, which can either have stimulatory or inhibitory influences in shaping microglial and overall immune response (120). Further, microglia produce cytokines and molecules with both inflammatory (TNF-α, IL-6, etc.) and anti-inflammatory (TGF-β, IL-10, neurotrophins, etc.) activity, and the balanced interplay between the two is crucial in the propagation or resolution of the inflammatory cascade (121,122). Certain factors which may determine the outcome of this interplay include the ability of microglia to function as antigen presenting cells, their interaction with antigen-specific T cells, the cytokine milieu, and their ability to sustain T cell growth (121). Although there is insufficient evidence to confirm that neuroinflammatory responses in ALS are also directed at repair, there is evidence from other CNS inflammatory models, which may provide direction in understanding the relevance of these processes in ALS.

In models of mechanical nerve injury, T lymphocytes have been shown to protect neurons, as evidenced by a greater loss of facial motorneurons after nerve transection in severe combined immunodeficient (*scid*) mice that lack T and B cells (123). This protection is mediated by the T-cell generation of neurotrophic factors, such as brain-derived neurotrophic factor and neurotrophin-3 (124). Furthermore, this neuroprotective effect is significantly boosted by myelin-specific T cells (125). This suggests that the ability to withstand the consequences of CNS axonal injury is governed by the ability to mount an endogenous Th1 cell-mediated protective response (126). In animal models, this neuroprotective response can be achieved safely with low-affinity activation of T cells with synthetic altered myelin basic peptides, or with copolymer 1, a synthetic compound of myelin basic protein (90,127,128). Importantly, the beneficial T cell-mediated effect is dependent upon the early activation of microglia and their differentiation into efficient, antigen presenting cells (129). Furthermore, the beneficial reparative effects may be directly mediated by microglial or astroglial release of neurotrophic factors, and indirectly mediated by T cell or dendritic cell signaling to glia.

In ALS, it is unknown whether a significant neuroprotective immune response is present, or if it plays a role in determining populations at risk, disease onset, or rate of progression. The paucity of activated T lymphocytes in end stage ALS tissue may not adequately reflect what transpires at earlier stages of disease, where immune inflammatory processes may play a significant role. Moreover, the relative lack of T cells in end stage ALS tissue may reflect the high incidence of T-cell apoptosis that occurs during CNS inflammation (130,131), or it may be that a large number of T cells are not necessary to mount a significant response, as stated previously. Furthermore, dendritic cells may well dictate the protective repair or toxic functions of both innate and adaptive immune systems. Clearly, the potential roles of T-cell-, dendritic cell-, and microglia-mediated neuroprotection in neurodegenerative disease, including ALS, may become future targets of therapy and should be investigated. Indeed, in the mSOD1 mouse model, copolymer 1 has already been shown to delay disease onset, improve life span, and improve motor activity (90), and a therapeutic trial in ALS patients is strongly indicated.

CONCLUSION

Our concept of neuroinflammation in ALS has changed in recent years. Once viewed as an epiphenomenon of motor neuron degeneration, neuroinflammatory changes are now considered to play an integral role in disease pathogenesis. A better understanding of how the cellular and biochemical components of this response affect motor neuron survival will enable us to develop new, immunomodulatory therapies. These novel therapies should be directed at amplifying those pathways involved in neuroprotection, while downregulating those pathways leading to motor neuron injury.

REFERENCES

1. Consilvio C, Vincent AM, Feldman EL. Neuroinflammation, COX-2, and ALS—a dual role? Exp Neurol 2004; 187:1–10. Review.
2. Morganti-Kossmann MC, Rancan M, Stahel PF, Kossmann T. Inflammatory response in acute traumatic brain injury: a double-edged sword. Curr Opin Crit Care 2002; 8: 101–105. Review.
3. Minagar A, Shapshak P, Fujimura R, Ownby R, Heyes M, Eisdorfer C. The role of macrophage/microglia and astrocytes in the pathogenesis of three neurologic disorders: HIV-associated dementia, Alzheimer disease, and multiple sclerosis. J Neurol Sci 2002; 202:13–23. Review.
4. Mhatre M, Floyd RA, Hensley K. Oxidative stress and neuroinflammation in Alzheimer's disease and amyotrophic lateral sclerosis: common links and potential therapeutic targets. J Alzheimers Dis 2004; 6:147–157.
5. McGeer PL, McGeer EG. Local neuroinflammation and the progression of Alzheimer's disease. J Neurovirol 2002; 8:529–538. Review.
6. Moore AH, O'Banion MK. Neuroinflammation and anti-inflammatory therapy for Alzheimer's disease. Adv Drug Deliv Rev 2002; 54:1627–1656. Review.
7. Hunot S, Hirsch EC. Neuroinflammatory processes in Parkinson's disease. Ann Neurol 2003; 53(suppl 3):S49–S58; discussion S58–S60. Review.
8. Kawamata T, Akiyama H, Yamada T, McGeer PL. Immunologic reactions in amyotrophic lateral sclerosis brain and spinal cord tissue. Am J Pathol 1992; 140:691–707.
9. Lampson LA, Kushner PD, Sobel RA. Major histocompatibility complex antigen expression in the affected tissues in amyotrophic lateral sclerosis. Ann Neurol 1990; 28:365–372.
10. Troost D, Van den Oord JJ, Vianney de Jong JM. Immunohistochemical characterization of the inflammatory infiltrate in amyotrophic lateral sclerosis. Neuropathol Appl Neurobiol 1990; 16:401–410.

11. Henkel JS, Engelhardt JI, Siklos L, Simpson EP, Kim SH, Pan T, Goodman JC, Siddique T, Beers DR, Appel SH. Presence of dendritic cells, MCP-1, and activated microglia/macrophages in amyotrophic lateral sclerosis spinal cord tissue. Ann Neurol 2004; 55:221–235.

12. del Rio-Hortega P. El tercer elemento de los centros nerviosos. Poder fagocitario y movilidad de la microglia. Bol Soc Esp Biol 1920; 9:154.

13. Cross AK, Woodroofe MN. Immunoregulation of microglial functional properties. Microsc Res Tech 2001; 54:10–17. Review.

14. Gonzalez-Scarano F, Baltuch G. Microglia as mediators of inflammatory and degenerative diseases. Annu Rev Neurosci 1999; 22:219–240. Review.

15. Liberto CM, Albrecht PJ, Herx LM, Yong VW, Levison SW. Pro-regenerative properties of cytokine-activated astrocytes. J Neurochem 2004; 89:1092–1100. Review.

16. Ransohoff RM, Kivisakk P, Kidd G. Three or more routes for leukocyte migration into the central nervous system. Nat Rev Immunol 2003; 3:569–581. Review.

17. Reichmann G, Schroeter M, Jander S, Fischer HG. Dendritic cells and dendritic-like microglia in focal cortical ischemia of the mouse brain. J Neuroimmunol 2002; 129: 125–132.

18. Eikelenboom P, van Gool WA. Neuroinflammatory perspectives on the two faces of Alzheimer's disease. J Neural Transm 2004; 111:281–294. Review.

19. McGeer EG, McGeer PL. Inflammatory processes in Alzheimer's disease. Prog Neuropsychopharmacol Biol Psychiatry 2003; 27:741–749. Review.

20. McGeer PL, McGeer EG, Kawamata T, Yamada T, Akiyama H. Reactions of the immune system in chronic degenerative neurological diseases. Can J Neurol Sci 1991; 18(suppl 3):376–379. Review.

21. Lim GP, Backstrom JR, Cullen MJ, Miller CA, Atkinson RD, Tokes ZA. Matrix metalloproteinases in the neocortex and spinal cord of amyotrophic lateral sclerosis patients. J Neurochem 1996; 67:251–259.

22. Takadera T, Yumoto H, Tozuka Y, Ohyashiki T. Prostaglandin E(2) induces caspase-dependent apoptosis in rat cortical cells. Neurosci Lett 2002; 317:61–64.

23. Bezzi P, Carmignoto G, Pasti L, Vesce S, Rossi D, Rizzini BL, Pozzan T, Volterra A. Prostaglandins stimulate calcium-dependent glutamate release in astrocytes. Nature 1998; 391:281–285.

24. Kawamura T, Horie S, Maruyama T, Akira T, Imagawa T, Nakamura N. Prostaglandin E1 transported into cells blocks the apoptotic signals induced by nerve growth factor deprivation. J Neurochem 1999; 72:1907–1914.

25. Qin ZH, Wang Y, Chen RW, Wang X, Ren M, Chuang DM, Chase TN. Prostaglandin A(1) protects striatal neurons against excitotoxic injury in rat striatum. J Pharmacol Exp Ther 2001; 297:78–87.

26. Stephenson D, Rash K, Smalstig B, Roberts E, Johnstone E, Sharp J, Panetta J, Little S, Kramer R, Clemens J. Cytosolic phospholipase A2 is induced in reactive glia following different forms of neurodegeneration. Glia 1999; 27:110–128.

27. Almer G, Teismann P, Stevic Z, Halaschek-Wiener J, Deecke L, Kostic V, Przedborski S. Increased levels of the pro-inflammatory prostaglandin PGE2 in CSF from ALS patients. Neurology 2002; 58:1277–1279.

28. Almer G, Guegan C, Teismann P, Naini A, Rosoklija G, Hays AP, Chen C, Przedborski S. Increased expression of the pro-inflammatory enzyme cyclooxygenase-2 in amyotrophic lateral sclerosis. Ann Neurol 2001; 49:176–185.

29. Yasojima K, Tourtellotte WW, McGeer EG, McGeer PL. Marked increase in cyclooxygenase-2 in ALS spinal cord: implications for therapy. Neurology 2001; 57:952–956.

30. Engelhardt JI, Appel SH. IgG reactivity in the spinal cord and motor cortex in amyotrophic lateral sclerosis. Arch Neurol 1990; 47:1210–1216.

31. Alexianu ME, Kozovska M, Appel SH. Immune reactivity in a mouse model of familial ALS correlates with disease progression. Neurology 2001; 57:1282–1289.

32. Hall ED, Oostveen JA, Gurney ME. Relationship of microglial and astrocytic activation to disease onset and progression in a transgenic model of familial ALS. Glia 1998; 23:249–256.

33. Hensley K, Fedynyshyn J, Ferrell S, Floyd RA, Gordon B, Grammas P, Hamdheydari L, Mhatre M, Mou S, Pye QN, Stewart C, West M, West S, Williamson KS. Message and protein-level elevation of tumor necrosis factor alpha (TNF alpha) and TNF alpha-modulating cytokines in spinal cords of the G93A-SOD1 mouse model for amyotrophic lateral sclerosis. Neurobiol Dis 2003; 14:74–80.

34. Hensley K, Floyd RA, Gordon B, Mou S, Pye QN, Stewart C, West M, Williamson K. Temporal patterns of cytokine and apoptosis-related gene expression in spinal cords of the G93A-SOD1 mouse model of amyotrophic lateral sclerosis. J Neurochem 2002; 82:365–374.

35. Elliott JL. Cytokine upregulation in a murine model of familial amyotrophic lateral sclerosis. Brain Res Mol Brain Res 2001; 95:172–178.

36. Yoshihara T, Ishigaki S, Yamamoto M, Liang Y, Niwa J, Takeuchi H, Doyu M, Sobue G. Differential expression of inflammation- and apoptosis-related genes in spinal cords of a mutant SOD1 transgenic mouse model of familial amyotrophic lateral sclerosis. J Neurochem 2002; 80:158–167.

37. Almer G, Vukosavic S, Romero N, Przedborski S. Inducible nitric oxide synthase up-regulation in a transgenic mouse model of familial amyotrophic lateral sclerosis. J Neurochem 1999; 72:2415–2425.

38. Hensley K, Floyd RA, Gordon B, Mou S, Pye QN, Stewart C, West M, Williamson K. Temporal patterns of cytokine and apoptosis-related gene expression in spinal cords of the G93A-SOD1 mouse model of amyotrophic lateral sclerosis. J Neurochem 2002; 82:365–374.

39. Chen L, Smith AP, Ben Y, Zukic B, Ignacio S, Moore D, Lee NM. Temporal gene expression patterns in G93A/SOD1 mouse. Amyotroph Lateral Scler Other Motor Neuron Disord 2004; 11:1–8.

40. Boillee S, Viala L, Peschanski M, Dreyfus PA. Differential microglial response to progressive neurodegeneration in the murine mutant Wobbler. Glia 2001; 33:277–287.

41. Schlomann U, Rathke-Hartlieb S, Yamamoto S, Jockusch H, Bartsch JW. Tumor necrosis factor alpha induces a metalloprotease-disintegrin, ADAM8 (CD 156): implications for neuron-glia interactions during neurodegeneration. J Neurosci 2000; 20:7964–7971.

42. Rathke-Hartlieb S, Schmidt VC, Jockusch H, Schmitt-John T, Bartsch JW. Spatiotemporal progression of neurodegeneration and glia activation in the wobbler neuropathy of the mouse. Neuroreport 1999; 10:3411–3416.

43. Ghezzi P, Bernardini R, Giuffrida R, Bellomo M, Manzoni C, Comoletti D, Di Santo E, Benigni F, Mennini T. Tumor necrosis factor is increased in the spinal cord of an animal model of motor neuron degeneration. Eur Cytokine Netw 1998; 9:139–144.

44. Smith RG, Siklos L, Alexianu ME, Engelhardt JI, Mosier DR, Colom L, Habib Mohamed A, Appel SH. Autoimmunity and ALS. Neurology 1996; 47(4 suppl 2): S40–S45; discussion S45–S46. Review.

45. Appel SH, Smith RG, Engelhardt JI, Stefani E. Evidence for autoimmunity in amyotrophic lateral sclerosis. J Neurol Sci 1993; 118:169–174. Review.

46. Engelhardt JI, Appel SH, Killian JM. Experimental autoimmune motoneuron disease. Ann Neurol 1989; 26:368–376.

47. Engelhardt JI, Appel SH, Killian JM. Motor neuron destruction in guinea pigs immunized with bovine spinal cord ventral horn homogenate: experimental autoimmune gray matter disease. J Neuroimmunol 1990; 27:21–31.

48. Garcia J, Engelhardt JI, Appel SH, Stefani E. Increased MEPP frequency as an early sign of experimental immune-mediated motoneuron disease. Ann Neurol 1990; 28: 329–334.

49. Tajti J, Stefani E, Appel SH. Cyclophosphamide alters the clinical and pathological expression of experimental autoimmune gray matter disease. J Neuroimmunol 1991; 34:143–151.

50. Chavany C, Vicario-Abejon C, Miller G, Jendoubi M. Transgenic mice for interleukin 3 develop motor neuron degeneration associated with autoimmune reaction against spinal cord motor neurons. Proc Natl Acad Sci USA 1998; 95:11354–11359.

51. Haverkamp LJ, Appel V, Appel SH. Natural history of amyotrophic lateral sclerosis in a database population. Validation of a scoring system and a model for survival prediction. Brain 1995; 118:707–719.

52. Gordon PH, Rowland LP, Younger DS, Sherman WH, Hays AP, Louis ED, Lange DJ, Trojaborg W, Lovelace RE, Murphy PL, Latov N. Lymphoproliferative disorders and motor neuron disease: an update. Neurology 1997; 48:1671–1678. Review.

53. Johnson RT. Selective vulnerability of neural cells to viral infections. Brain 1980; 103: 447–472.

54. Rosener M, Hahn H, Kranz M, Heeney J, Rethwilm A. Absence of serological evidence for foamy virus infection in patients with amyotrophic lateral sclerosis. J Med Virol 1996; 48:222–226.

55. Andrews WD, Al-Chalabi A, Garson JA. Lack of evidence for HTLV tax-rex DNA in motor neurone disease. J Neurol Sci 1997; 153:86–90.

56. Walker MP, Schlaberg R, Hays AP, Bowser R, Lipkin WI. Absence of echovirus sequences in brain and spinal cord of amyotrophic lateral sclerosis patients. Ann Neurol 2001; 49:249–253.

57. Nix WA, Berger MM, Oberste MS, Brooks BR, McKenna-Yasek DM, Brown RH Jr, Roos RP, Pallansch MA. Failure to detect enterovirus in the spinal cord of ALS patients using a sensitive RT-PCR method. Neurology 2004; 62:1372–1377.

58. Berger MM, Kopp N, Vital C, Redl B, Aymard M, Lina B. Detection and cellular localization of enterovirus RNA sequences in spinal cord of patients with ALS. Neurology 2000; 54:20–25.

59. Giraud P, Beaulieux F, Ono S, Shimizu N, Chazot G, Lina B. Detection of enteroviral sequences from frozen spinal cord samples of Japanese ALS patients. Neurology 2001; 56:1777–1778.

60. Hoffman PM, Festoff BW, Giron LT Jr, Hollenbeck LC, Garruto RM, Ruscetti FW. Isolation of LAV/HTLV-III from a patient with amyotrophic lateral sclerosis. N Engl J Med 1985; 313:324–325.

61. Sher R. AIDS—overview. Nurs RSA 1988; 3:9–10, 13.

62. Verma RK, Ziegler DK, Kepes JJ. HIV-related neuromuscular syndrome simulating motor neuron disease. Neurology 1990; 40:544–546.

63. Huang PP, Chin R, Song S, Lasoff S. Lower motor neuron dysfunction associated with human immunodeficiency virus infection. Arch Neurol 1993; 50:1328–1330.

64. Simpson DM, Tagliati M. Neurologic manifestations of HIV infection. Ann Intern Med 1994; 121:769–785. Review.

65. Casado I, Gomez M, Carmona C, Garcia-Castanon I, Martin C, Sanchez JF. Motor neuron disease and HIV. Rev Neurol 1997; 25:552–554. Spanish.

66. MacGowan DJ, Scelsa SN, Waldron M. An ALS-like syndrome with new HIV infection and complete response to antiretroviral therapy. Neurology 2001; 57:1094–1097.

67. Moulignier A, Moulonguet A, Pialoux G, Rozenbaum W. Reversible ALS-like disorder in HIV infection. Neurology 2001; 57:995–1001.

68. Minghetti L, Visentin S, Patrizio M, Franchini L, Ajmone-Cat MA, Levi G. Multiple actions of the human immunodeficiency virus type-1 Tat protein on microglial cell functions. Neurochem Res 2004; 29:965–978.

69. D'Aversa T, Yu K, Berman J. Expression of chemokines by human fetal microglia after treatment with the human immunodeficiency virus type 1 protein Tat. J Neurovirol 2004; 10:86–97.

70. Yi Y, Lee C, Liu QH, Freedman BD, Collman RG. Chemokine receptor utilization and macrophage signaling by human immunodeficiency virus type 1 gp120: Implications for neuropathogenesis. J Neurovirol 2004; 10(suppl 1):91–96. Review.

71. Kolson DL, Sabnekar P, Baybis M, Crino PB. Gene expression in TUNEL-positive neurons in human immunodeficiency virus-infected brain. J Neurovirol 2004; (10 suppl 1): 102–107.

72. Baszler TV, Zachary JF. Murine retroviral neurovirulence correlates with an enhanced ability of virus to infect selectively, replicate in, and activate resident microglial cells. Am J Pathol 1991; 138:655–671.

73. Zachary JF, Baszler TV, French RA, Kelley KW. Mouse Moloney leukemia virus infects microglia but not neurons even though it induces motor neuron disease. Mol Psychiatry 1997; 2:104–106. Review.

74. Thomas FP, Chalk C, Lalonde R, Robitaille Y, Jolicoeur P. Expression of human immunodeficiency virus type 1 in the nervous system of transgenic mice leads to neurological disease. J Virol 1994; 68:7099–7107.

75. Fischer CP, Jorgen G, Gundersen H, Pakkenberg B. Preferential loss of large neocortical neurons during HIV infection: a study of the size distribution of neocortical neurons in the human brain. Brain Res 1999; 828:119–126.

76. Gardner MB, Henderson BE, Officer JE, Rongey RW, Parker JC, Oliver C, Estes JD, Huebner RJ. A spontaneous lower motor neuron disease apparently caused by indigenous type-C RNA virus in wild mice. J Natl Cancer Inst 1973; 51:1243–1254.

77. Matsuzaki T, Nakagawa M, Nagai M, Nobuhara Y, Usuku K, Higuchi I, Takahashi K, Moritoyo T, Arimura K, Izumo S, Akiba S, Osame M. HTLV-I-associated myelopathy (HAM)/tropical spastic paraparesis (TSP) with amyotrophic lateral sclerosis-like manifestations. J Neurovirol 2000; 6:544–548.

78. Gordon PH, Rowland LP, Younger DS, Sherman WH, Hays AP, Louis ED, Lange DJ, Trojaborg W, Lovelace RE, Murphy PL, Latov N. Lymphoproliferative disorders and motor neuron disease: an update. Neurology 1997; 48:1671–1678. Review.

79. Ferrante P, Westarp ME, Mancuso R, Puricelli S, Westarp MP, Mini M, Caputo D, Zuffolato MR. HTLV tax-rex DNA and antibodies in idiopathic amyotrophic lateral sclerosis. J Neurol Sci 1995; 129 (Suppl 1):140–144.

80. Andrews WD, Tuke PW, Al-Chalabi A, Gaudin P, Ijaz S, Parton MJ, Garson JA. Detection of reverse transcriptase activity in the serum of patients with motor neurone disease. J Med Virol 2000; 61:527–532.

81. Hadlock KG, Miller RG, Jin X, Yu S, Reis J, Mass J, Gelinas DF, McGrath MS. Elevated rates of antibody reactivity to HML-2/Herv-K but not other endogenous retroviruses in ALS. 56th annual meeting of the American Academy of Neurology, San Francisco, CA, Apr 24–May 1, 2004.

82. Drachman DB, Chaudhry V, Cornblath D, Kuncl RW, Pestronk A, Clawson L, Mellits ED, Quaskey S, Quinn T, Calkins A, et al. Trial of immunosuppression in amyotrophic lateral sclerosis using total lymphoid irradiation. Ann Neurol 1994; 35:142–150.

83. Meucci N, Nobile-Orazio E, Scarlato G. Intravenous immunoglobulin therapy in amyotrophic lateral sclerosis. J Neurol 1996; 243:117–120.

84. Dalakas MC, Stein DP, Otero C, Sekul E, Cupler EJ, McCrosky S. Effect of high-dose intravenous immunoglobulin on amyotrophic lateral sclerosis and multifocal motor neuropathy. Arch Neurol 1994; 51:861–864.

85. Smith SA, Miller RG, Murphy JR, Ringel SP. Treatment of ALS with high dose pulse cyclophosphamide. J Neurol Sci 1994; 124 (Suppl 1):84–87.

86. Appel SH, Stewart SS, Appel V, Harati Y, Mietlowski W, Weiss W, Belendiuk GW. A double-blind study of the effectiveness of cyclosporine in amyotrophic lateral sclerosis. Arch Neurol 1988; 45:381–386.

87. Brown RH Jr, Hauser SL, Harrington H, Weiner HL. Failure of immunosuppression with a 10- to 14-day course of high-dose intravenous cyclophosphamide to alter the progression of amyotrophic lateral sclerosis. Arch Neurol 1986; 43:383–384.

88. Kriz J, Nguyen MD, Julien JP. Minocycline slows disease progression in a mouse model of amyotrophic lateral sclerosis. Neurobiol Dis 2002; 10:268–278.

89. Keep M, Elmer E, Fong KS, Csiszar K. Intrathecal cyclosporin prolongs survival of late-stage ALS mice. Brain Res 2001; 894:327–331.

90. Angelov DN, Waibel S, Guntinas-Lichius O, Lenzen M, Neiss WF, Tomov TL, Yoles E, Kipnis J, Schori H, Reuter A, Ludolph A, Schwartz M. Therapeutic vaccine for acute and chronic motor neuron diseases: implications for amyotrophic lateral sclerosis. Proc Natl Acad Sci USA 2003; 100:4790–4795.

91. Kirkinezos IG, Hernandez D, Bradley WG, Moraes CT. An ALS mouse model with a permeable blood-brain barrier benefits from systemic cyclosporine A treatment. J Neurochem 2004; 88:821–826.

92. Simpson EP, Henry YK, Henkel JS, Smith RG, Appel SH. Increased lipid peroxidation in sera of ALS patients: a potential biomarker of disease burden. Neurology 2004; 62:1758–1765.

93. Wilms H, Sievers J, Dengler R, Bufler J, Deuschl G, Lucius R. Intrathecal synthesis of monocyte chemoattractant protein-1 (MCP-1) in amyotrophic lateral sclerosis: further evidence for microglial activation in neurodegeneration. J Neuroimmunol 2003; 144: 139–142.

94. McGeer PL, McGeer EG. Inflammatory processes in amyotrophic lateral sclerosis. Muscle Nerve 2002; 26:459–470.

95. Engelhardt JI, Siklos L, Appel SH. Altered calcium homeostasis and ultrastructure in motoneurons of mice caused by passively transferred anti-motoneuronal IgG. J Neuropathol Exp Neurol 1997; 56:21–39.

96. Obal I, Siklos L, Engelhardt JI. Altered calcium in motoneurons by IgG from human motoneuron diseases. Acta Neurol Scand 2002; 106:282–291.

97. Appel SH, Smith RG, Alexianu M, Siklos L, Engelhardt J, Colom LV, Stefani E. Increased intracellular calcium triggered by immune mechanisms in amyotrophic lateral sclerosis. Clin Neurosci 1995–1996; 3:368–374. Review.

98. Pullen AH, Demestre M, Howard RS, Orrell RW. Passive transfer of purified IgG from patients with amyotrophic lateral sclerosis to mice results in degeneration of motor neurons accompanied by Ca^{2+} enhancement. Acta Neuropathol (Berl) 2004; 107:35–46.

99. Alexianu ME, Mohamed AH, Smith RG, Colom LV, Appel SH. Apoptotic cell death of a hybrid motoneuron cell line induced by immunoglobulins from patients with amyotrophic lateral sclerosis. J Neurochem 1994; 63:2365–2368.

100. Carter JR, Mynlieff M. Amyotrophic lateral sclerosis patient IgG alters voltage dependence of Ca^{2+} channels in dissociated rat motoneurons. Neurosci Lett 2003; 353:221–225.

101. Fratantoni SA, Weisz G, Pardal AM, Reisin RC, Uchitel OD. Amyotrophic lateral sclerosis IgG-treated neuromuscular junctions develop sensitivity to L-type calcium channel blocker. Muscle Nerve 2000; 23:543–550.

102. Offen D, Halevi S, Orion D, Mosberg R, Stern-Goldberg H, Melamed E, Atlas D. Antibodies from ALS patients inhibit dopamine release mediated by L-type calcium channels. Neurology 1998; 51:1100–1103.

103. Mosier DR, Baldelli P, Delbono O, Smith RG, Alexianu ME, Appel SH, Stefani E. Amyotrophic lateral sclerosis immunoglobulins increase Ca^{2+} currents in a motoneuron cell line. Ann Neurol 1995; 37:102–109.

104. Obal I, Jakab JS, Siklos L, Engelhardt JI. Recruitment of activated microglia cells in the spinal cord of mice by ALS IgG. Neuroreport 2001; 12:2449–2452.

105. Sengun IS, Appel SH. Serum anti-Fas antibody levels in amyotrophic lateral sclerosis. J Neuroimmunol 2003; 142:137–140.

106. Ilzecka J, Stelmasiak Z. Anti-annexin V antibodies in the cerebrospinal fluid and serum of patients with amyotrophic lateral sclerosis. Neurol Sci 2003; 24:273–274.

107. Niebroj-Dobosz I, Jamrozik Z, Janik P, Hausmanowa-Petrusewicz I, Kwiecinski H. Anti-neural antibodies in serum and cerebrospinal fluid of amyotrophic lateral sclerosis (ALS) patients. Acta Neurol Scand 1999; 100:238–243.

108. Couratier P, Yi FH, Preud'homme JL, Clavelou P, White A, Sindou P, Vallat JM, Jauberteau MO. Serum autoantibodies to neurofilament proteins in sporadic amyotrophic lateral sclerosis. J Neurol Sci 1998; 154:137–145.

109. Okuyama Y, Mizuno T, Inoue H, Kimoto K. Amyotrophic lateral sclerosis with anti-acetylcholine receptor antibody. Intern Med 1997; 36:312–315.

110. Banati RB, Gehrmann J, Kellner M, Holsboer F. Antibodies against microglia/brain macrophages in the cerebrospinal fluid of a patient with acute amyotrophic lateral sclerosis and presenile dementia. Clin Neuropathol 1995; 14:197–200.

111. Engelhardt JI, Siklos L, Komuves L, Smith RG, Appel SH. Antibodies to calcium channels from ALS patients passively transferred to mice selectively increase intracellular calcium and induce ultrastructural changes in motoneurons. Synapse 1995; 20:185–199.

112. Zhao W, Xie W, Le W, Beers DR, He Y, Henkel JS, Simpson EP, Yen AA, Xiao Q, Appel SH. Activated microglia initiate motor neuron injury by a nitric oxide and glutamate-mediated mechanism. J Neuropathol Exp Neurol 2004; 63:964–977.

113. Gurney ME, Pu H, Chiu AY, Dal Canto MC, Polchow CY, Alexander DD, Caliendo J, Hentati A, Kwon YW, Deng HX, et al. Motor neuron degeneration in mice that express a human Cu,Zn superoxide dismutase mutation. Science 1994; 264:1772–1775.

114. Pramatarova A, Laganiere J, Roussel J, Brisebois K, Rouleau GA. Neuron-specific expression of mutant superoxide dismutase 1 in transgenic mice does not lead to motor impairment. J Neurosci 2001; 21:3369–3374.

115. Lino MM, Schneider C, Caroni P. Accumulation of SOD1 mutants in postnatal motoneurons does not cause motoneuron pathology or motoneuron disease. J Neurosci 2002; 22:4825–4832.

116. Gong YH, Parsadanian AS, Andreeva A, Snider WD, Elliott JL. Restricted expression of G86R Cu/Zn superoxide dismutase in astrocytes results in astrocytosis but does not cause motoneuron degeneration. J Neurosci 2000; 20:660–665.

117. Clement AM, Nguyen MD, Roberts EA, Garcia ML, Boillee S, Rule M, McMahon AP, Doucette W, Siwek D, Ferrante RJ, Brown RH Jr, Julien JP, Goldstein LS, Cleveland DW. Wild-type nonneuronal cells extend survival of SOD1 mutant motor neurons in ALS mice. Science 2003; 302:113–117.

118. Van Den Bosch L, Tilkin P, Lemmens G, Robberecht W. Minocycline delays disease onset and mortality in a transgenic model of ALS. Neuroreport 2002; 13:1067–1070.

119. Pompl PN, Ho L, Bianchi M, McManus T, Qin W, Pasinetti GM. A therapeutic role for cyclooxygenase-2 inhibitors in a transgenic mouse model of amyotrophic lateral sclerosis. FASEB J 2003; 17:725–727.

120. Aloisi F. Immune function of microglia. Glia 2001; 36:165–179.

121. Aloisi F, Ria F, Adorini L. Regulation of T-cell responses by CNS antigen-presenting cells: different roles for microglia and astrocytes. Immunol Today 2000; 21:141–147. Review.

122. Tabakman R, Lecht S, Sephanova S, Arien-Zakay H, Lazarovici P. Interactions between the cells of the immune and nervous system: neurotrophins as neuroprotection mediators in CNS injury. Prog Brain Res 2004; 146:387–401. Review.

123. Serpe CJ, Kohm AP, Huppenbauer CB, Sanders VM, Jones KJ. Exacerbation of facial motoneuron loss after facial nerve transection in severe combined immunodeficient (scid) mice. J Neurosci 1999; 19:RC7.

124. Hammarberg H, Lidman O, Lundberg C, Eltayeb SY, Gielen AW, Muhallab S, Svenningsson A, Linda H, van Der Meide PH, Cullheim S, Olsson T, Piehl F. Neuroprotection by encephalomyelitis: rescue of mechanically injured neurons and neurotrophin production by CNS-infiltrating T and natural killer cells. J Neurosci 2000; 20:5283–5291.

125. Kipnis J, Mizrahi T, Hauben E, Shaked I, Shevach E, Schwartz M. Neuroprotective autoimmunity: naturally occurring CD4+CD25+ regulatory T cells suppress the ability to withstand injury to the central nervous system. Proc Natl Acad Sci USA 2002; 99: 15620–15625.

126. Schwartz M, Kipnis J. Multiple sclerosis as a by-product of the failure to sustain protective autoimmunity: a paradigm shift. Neuroscientist 2002; 8:405–413. Review.

127. Kipnis J, Schwartz M. Dual action of glatiramer acetate (Cop-1) in the treatment of CNS autoimmune and neurodegenerative disorders. Trends Mol Med 2002; 8:319–323.

128. Monsonego A, Beserman ZP, Kipnis J, Yoles E, Weiner HL, Schwartz M. Beneficial effect of orally administered myelin basic protein in EAE-susceptible Lewis rats in a model of acute CNS degeneration. J Autoimmun 2003; 21:131–138.

129. Shaked I, Porat Z, Gersner R, Kipnis J, Schwartz M. Early activation of microglia as antigen-presenting cells correlates with T cell-mediated protection and repair of the injured central nervous system. J Neuroimmunol 2004; 146:84–93.

130. Bauer J, Bradl M, Hickley WF, Forss-Petter S, Breitschopf H, Linington C, Wekerle H, Lassmann H. T-cell apoptosis in inflammatory brain lesions: destruction of T cells does not depend on antigen recognition. Am J Pathol 1998; 153:715–724.

131. Kohji T, Tanuma N, Aikawa Y, Kawazoe Y, Suzuki Y, Kohyama K, Matsumoto Y. Interaction between apoptotic cells and reactive brain cells in the central nervous system of rats with autoimmune encephalomyelitis. J Neuroimmunol 1998; 82:168–174.

23

The Potential of Gene Therapy for Motor Neuron Diseases

Cédric Raoul and Patrick Aebischer
Integrative Biosciences Institute, Ecole Polytechnique Fédérale de Lausanne (EPFL), Lausanne, Switzerland

Motor neuron diseases (MND) are clinically distinct neurodegenerative diseases sharing a primary disorder involving the motor system. MND encompass motor syndromes of amyotrophic lateral sclerosis (ALS), spinal muscular atrophy, X-linked spinobulbar muscular atrophy (Kennedy's disease), hereditary spastic paraplegia, and postpolio muscular atrophy. MND are often lethal and incurable diseases that arise from relentless dysfunction of upper (motor cortical), lower (brainstem and spinal) or both motor neurons. Extensive research over the last decade has provided new insights into the genetic of a variety of motor neuron syndromes. A better understanding of the molecular events leading to motor neuron death has stimulated new therapeutic concepts including gene therapy. The development of transgenic animal models, which clinically recapitulate human MND, also provided more relevant targets to test novel therapeutic approaches. Due to the molecular complexity of these diseases and the challenging wide distribution of motor neurons, various therapeutic approaches have been developed in order to address these issues. The present chapter concentrates its scope to gene transfer technology. Our main emphasis will be on ALS, since animal models of this disease have been the most wildly used for gene therapy approaches.

THERAPEUTIC CONTEXT

Therapeutic interventions for MND have to come up against a broad spectrum of etiologic, neuropathologic, neuroanatomic, and physiologic hindrances. Etiologically, MND are heterogeneous since different factors including inheritance of mutated genes, exposure to endogenous or exogenous agents, and genetic-environmental interactions contribute to the development of motor neuron disorders. A multifactoriality that complicates the task for devising appropriate and effective treatments. Pathologically, the temporal sequence between the initial pathogenic events and the endpoint of massive motor neuron loss shows that MND are multisystem disorders involving complex molecular pathogenic mechanisms and interplay of neuronal and non-neuronal cells. Despite a growing repertoire of genetic and proteomic technologies, the gain for targeting specific neuropathologic events is restricted since molecular mechanisms underlying neuronal degeneration remain poorly understood. What must be also considered in therapeutic protection of motor neurons is their disseminated anatomical distribution. Upper motor neurons located in the premotor and motor cortex connect lower motor neurons in the brainstem or the spinal cord. This unique broad distribution within the central nervous system complicates the development of bio-based therapeutics. Neuroprotective treatments that make use of either small compound molecules or recombinant proteins have to take into account the presence of blood–brain barrier and the short half life of many molecules. Gene therapy has the potential to obviate some of these difficulties. Basically, gene therapy is the transfer of genetic material in a therapeutic goal. Gene therapy strategies include straight delivery of viral vector encoding neuroprotective genes or graft of genetically engineered cells that deliver therapeutic agents in the target tissue. The prerequisite for designing novel approaches for therapy is the generation of animal models that reproduce the major electrophysiological, histopathological, and clinical features of MND. Spontaneous and genetic models of motor neuron disorders provided *per se* exciting opportunities for testing gene-based therapeutic approach.

Preclinical Models for ALS Therapy

Several strains of mice showing phenotypes of motor neuron degeneration and motor impairment have been described, but for most of them, causal genes are not identified (1). Nevertheless, these animal models have proven to play a pivotal role in elucidating specific molecular pathogenic mechanisms and advancing new therapeutic treatments (1–3). An extensive review of these different models can be found in Nagai et al. (Chapter 25 in this volume). Herein, we will limit our discussion to selected mouse mutations in SOD1, the wobbler mice, and progressive motor neuronopathy (*pmn*) mice, as these three have been utilized for gene therapies.

Animal Models of Familial Amyotrophic Lateral Sclerosis

The major breakthrough in the genetic of ALS, and subsequently in MND therapy, came with the finding of missense mutations in the gene encoding for the ubiquitously expressed enzyme Cu/Zn superoxide dismutase (SOD1) in familial ALS (FALS) pedigrees (4). ALS-linked SOD1 mutations are dominantly inherited with the exception of the D90A mutation reported as homozygous in patients (5). So far, over 100 mutations have been found in SOD1 accounting for 10% to 20% of FALS. The generation of transgenic experimental models quickly followed the genetic identification of the MND. Phenotypically, mutant rodents develop severe motor impairment starting in the hindlimbs that progress rostrally over weeks or months resulting in death (6–12). Apparition of motor symptoms, duration and survival of mutant mice and rats depend not only on the nature of the mutation but also on the level of expression of the mutated form of SOD1. Compelling evidences from studies of different transgenic mice suggest that neurodamaging effects are attributable to a novel toxic gain-of-function rather than a reduced enzymatic activity. Despite considerable efforts, the molecular basis of the acquired toxic property(ies) remains elusive. Several mechanisms have been proposed for SOD1-mediated toxicity. These include aberrant free radical chemistry, glutamate excitotoxicity, neurofilament disorganization, mutant SOD1 aggregation, mitochondrial defects, or susceptibility to external death triggers (2,13,14). Potentially, each one of them may participate at variable degrees in pathogenesis in mutant SOD1 animal models. Although these multiple transgenic lines contrast with some recognized features of motor pathology in human, they represent to date the best models for therapeutic screens.

Pmn and Wobbler Mice

Historically, MND models including wobbler or *pmn* mice have greatly contributed in pioneer therapeutic works for MND. However, they do not have human counterpart. Wobbler mice are models of axonopathy presenting muscle weakness, tremor followed by muscular atrophy (15). The genetic origin of this motor neuron disorder is still unknown but inheritance is an autosomal recessive. Axonopathy is predominant in the cervical region. Muscle denervation followed by atrophy of the forelimbs is observed at seven to eight weeks. Motor defects slowly progress and mice survival is about 1.5 years. Wobbler mice present astrocytosis and degeneration of motor neurons encompassing different forms of cell death (16). Wobbler mice also present neuropathologic signs in vestibular nucleus and cerebellum. *Pmn* mice display a caudo-rostral evolution of atrophy and muscle weakness leading to death in six to seven weeks (17). This dying-back motoneuronopathy is genetically caused by a spontaneous recessive mutation in tubulin-specific chaperone e gene (18). *Pmn* mice are characterized by a loss of myelinated axons fiber as well as spinal and facial motor neurons. Prior to the identification of ALS-linked mutations in SOD1 and the generation of transgenic animal models, *pmn* and wobbler have been initially used to evaluate therapeutic benefit of small compound molecules or neuroprotective proteins.

Protein-Based Therapy of ALS

Whereas pharmacotherapy can deal with an infinite palette of *de novo* synthesized compounds, gene-based therapy has to deal with a less impressive but certainly more biologically documented choice of compounds. This disparity is well reflected in the number of ALS clinical trials involving pharmacological agents (19). Numerous chemical agents have been evaluated in clinical trials and range from antioxidants, glutamate antagonists, immunomodulatory or anti-inflammatory, antimicrobial agents, energy metabolism supplements, to calcium homeostasis regulators (19,20). Unfortunately these agents were of no or at best of moderate benefits for ALS patients (21). The discovery in the late 1980s of neurotrophic factors (NTF) generated a lot of excitement for the treatment of neurodegenerative diseases including ALS.

NTF are a broad class of polypeptides that can promote motor neuron survival in vitro, axon growth-regeneration, and have trophic influences on motor neurons by preventing neuronal atrophy and death during the period of naturally occurring cell death (22–24). Trophic support originates from various cell types including skeletal muscle fibers, glial cells, Schwann cells, or neuronal cells themselves (24). Survival-promoting effects of NTF can arise from muscle targets through retrograde transport, afferent inputs or through local paracrine or autocrine mechanisms. The classic in vivo paradigm of sciatic or facial nerve transection, ventral root avulsion, or spinal cord transection have put in epigraph NTF as therapeutic agents for MND according to their neuroprotective properties and the widespread expression of NTF receptors in the CNS. NTF including glial cell-line derived neurotrophic factor (GDNF), brain-derived neurotrophic factor (BDNF), ciliary neurotrophic factor (CNTF), or Insulin-like growth factor-1 (IGF-1) rescue axotomized neonatal motor neurons (25–28). As illustrated in Table 1, NTF have been evaluated in animal models of MND. Mainly, wobbler and ALS-linked mutated SOD1 transgenic mice have been

Table 1 Therapeutic Benefits of Systemically Delivered Recombinant NTFs

NTF	Model	Therapeutic impact	Administration	References
CNTF	Wobbler	Slowed disease progression, improved muscle strength and decreased motor neuron loss	s.c	100, 101
BDNF	Wobbler	Slowed disease progression, diminished muscle denervation and delayed motor dysfunction	s.c	102
CNTF + BDNF	Wobbler	Synergistic trophic effect that slowed considerably disease progression	s.c	103
IGF-1	Wobbler	Slowed motor dysfunction and increased muscle fiber diameters	s.c	104
IL-6 + sIL-6R	Wobbler	Diminished muscle denervation, prevented motor impairment and delayed progression of the motor neuron disease	s.c	105
CT-1	Wobbler	Slowed motor dysfunction with a modest effect on motor neuron survival	s.c	106
bFGF	Wobbler	Improved muscle function, retarded muscle atrophy and motor neuron loss	s.c	107
LIF	Wobbler	Slowed progression of muscle deterioration, retarded disease progression and delay reduction of muscle strength	s.c	108
LIF	hSOD1 G93A	Authors observed a better mobility and less paralysis. LIF also prevented motor neuron loss	i.p	109
LIF	hSOD1 G93A	No beneficial effects on motor function, motor neuron survival and disease progression independently of the route of delivery	l.m.d,s.c or i.t	110
GDNF	hSOD1 G93A	Prevented loss of large motor neurons without clinical improvement	i.m	111
BMP-7	hSOD1 G93A	No effect on mean survival and duration of the disease	i.c	112

Abbreviations: CNTF, Ciliary neurotrophic factor; BDNF, brain derived neurotrophic factor; IGF-1, Insulin-like growth factor-1; IL-6, interleukin-6; sIL-6R, soluble IL-6 receptor; CT-1, cardiotrophin-l; bFGF, basic fibroblast growth factor; LIF, leukemia inhibitory factor; GDNF, Glial cell-derived neurotrophic factor; BMP-7, bone morphogenetic protein-7; s.c, subcutaneous; i.p, intraperitoneal; l.m.d, local muscle delivery (by means of calcium alginate rods); i.t, intrathecal; i.m, intramuscular; i.c, intracisternal.

used for systemic delivery of NTF. Interestingly, most of them show positive effects on several aspects of motor neuron disorders (Table 1). On the basis of these positive preclinical results, several clinical trials have been designed. Systemic administration of NTF, including CNTF (29), BDNF (30), and IGF-1 (31,32) has been evaluated in ALS patients. Each of them responds to criteria of potential therapeutic value, i.e., promotes survival of motor neuron *in vitro*, prevent motor neuron degeneration *in vivo* following axonal injury in animal models of MND (Table 1). However, the outcome of these clinical trials was disappointing. Hence, none of these NTF have shown unequivocal efficacious effects (33). Discrepancy between experimental paradigms of MND and clinical trials might be explained by a late administration in the course of the disease or for limiting side effects which blurred clinical evaluations (34). Retrospectively, these clinical failures stimulated further questioning regarding the pharmacological use of NTF especially the route of delivery.

From a therapeutic view, transgenic mice provided opportunity to elucidate some patho-mechanistic aspects of the disease and give rise subsequently to multiple potential therapeutic targets. Counteracting some intracellular pathogenic processes offers an attractive way to prevent or slow disease onset or progression. There is a body of evidences, emerging mainly from genetic approaches, that the targeting of some intrinsic pathogenic mechanisms may represent a new therapy issue. Potential therapeutic intrinsic values is supported by the neuroprotective effect observed in double transgenic animals with enforced expression of the anti-apoptotic B-cell leukemia-2 (Bcl) protein (35), a caspase-1 dominant negative (36), the X-linked inhibitor of apoptosis XIAP and the viral broad spectrum caspase inhibitor protein p35 (37), the glial transporter EAAT2 (38). The therapeutic challenge with the delivery of these potential therapeutic molecules is related to their cell-intrinsic nature, an issue where gene transfer technology may represent a potential solution.

GENE TRANSFER TECHNOLOGY FOR MND THERAPY

One of the main challenges regarding gene therapy for MND is how to deliver a potential therapeutic gene in target cells via efficient and safe vector systems. Due to their capacity to introduce and express their genetic material into recipient cells, viruses arise as obvious potential gene therapy agents. Moreover, according to the limited efficiency to transduce both mitotic and postmitotic cells and limited transgene persistence observed with non-viral methods (injection of naked DNA, "gene gun," electrotransfer of DNA, and liposome coated genes), viral vectors rapidly became promising tools for gene transfer in the field of neuroscience in general. For clinical application, viral vectors need to be (i) non-replicative to avoid cell damage and viral spreading, (ii) non-immunogenic, in order to avoid cellular immune response against transduced cells, (iii) non-toxic via viral protein or viral gene expression, and (iv) conserve their capacity to efficiently transduce cells to deliver and express their genetic information in a long-term manner. Usually, these assignments can be achieved by deleting the coding regions of viral genome and replacing them by the desired expression cassette. The minimal *cis*-acting sequences conserved are non-coding regions that flank the viral genome at each side (the terminal repeats). Sequences required for packaging, replication or integration of viral genome into the host genome are then brought in *trans* through helper functions during production of non-replicative recombinant virus.

Recombinant Viral Vectors as Carriers of Therapeutic Instructions

The commonly used virally derived vectors for gene therapy approaches in MND (as well as in other neurodegenerative diseases) are adenovirus (AdV), adeno-associated virus (AAV) and lentivirus (LV). Their main advantage is their ability to efficiently transduce non-dividing cells that are refractory to classical retroviral vectors and to drive long-lasting expression of the gene of interest in a large variety of cell types. Moreover, the technology is scalable to produce human grade materials. Since motor neurons are defined by their terminal projection fields, the skeletal muscles fibers, mainly two compartments have been targeted. The former consist in muscle through the use of AdV and AAV. The latter consist in the spinal cord through the use of AAV and LV.

Adenoviral Vectors

AdV have a 36 kb linear double stranded DNA genome packaged within an 80 nm diameter icosahedral capsid. The viral genome is flanked by two inverted terminal repeats (ITR) and contains a set of early expressed genes before DNA replication and late genes encoding mainly structural proteins. To date, over 50 human serotypes have been identified and the *in vivo* tropism (the infection spectrum) of AdV serotypes can vary considerably. Most of these viruses present an affinity for the primary virus attachment receptor, the coxsackie-adenovirus receptor (CAR). The broad distribution of CAR and $\alpha_V\beta_{3/5}$ integrins required for virus internalization, enable AdV to efficiently transduce a wide range of mitotic and postmitotic cells including components of the motor unit, motor neurons, glial cells, Schwann cells, and muscles (39–42). Upon infection and internalization of the virus in clathrin-coated vesicles, the nucleocapsid is released from endosomes into cytoplasm and transported to the nucleus in which the replication cycle is divided in three phases of viral gene expression: early genes with five early transcripts (E1A, E1B, E2, E3, and E4), delayed early genes (transcript IX and Iva2) and L-gene (a primary transcript spliced into 18 distinct mRNA) (43). Several generations (mainly derived from the human serotypes 2 and 5) of recombinant AdV have been generated by different deletions of early genes (44,45). More recently, a generation of recombinant replication-defective AdV called "gutted" or helper-dependent adenoviral vector has been designed (45). By deletion of all viral genes, "gutted" AdV present a cloning capacity that can reach 35 kb. Gutted vectors present a reduced intrinsic toxicity, since the production of viral gene product has been eliminated, and generate a reduced host immune response compared to the E1-deleted first generation of recombinant AdV. Furthermore, gutted vectors can achieve a long-lasting expression ranging from weeks to months, although, the gene delivered by AdV is not integrating into the host genome (46,47). However, important issues in the use of adenoviral vector are the degree of transduction efficiency of mature muscle fibers and the degree of elicited immune response. The reported reduced transducibility of mature muscle involves the loss of mitotically active and fusing myoblast that acts as intermediary carrier in viral transduction as observed in neonatal myofibers and lower expression level of CAR in mature fibers. Another impediment is the restricted area near the injection site that is mainly attributable to the extracellular matrix that acts as a physical barrier for a large size viral vector (48,49).

Adeno-Associated Viral Vectors

AAV are parvovirus with a single stranded DNA linear genome containing two open reading frames (*rep* and *cap*) encapsidated into an icosahedral capsid of about 20 nm. The coding region, flanked on each side by two 145 nucleotide ITR, generates four replication proteins (Rep40/52/68/78) and three capsid proteins (VP1/2/3).

To date, eight primate AAV serotypes have been identified (50). Once in cells, AAV single strand DNA is converted into double strand DNA that is able to integrate into the host genome, most frequently on chromosome 19q (51). One concern relates to the fact that approximately 99% of AAV viral genome persists primarily as large and small episomal concatemers in muscle fibers (52). ITRs are the only *cis*-acting elements required for replication, packaging, and integration of the viral genome. Replication defective recombinant AAV carrying a gene expression cassette flanked by the two ITRs can be generated if *rep* and *cap* are present in *trans* in the presence of helper functions from an AdV (53). The main advantages of AAV are the possibility to produce high titer AAV free of replication competent AdV contaminant and its lack of innate pathogenicity. The main inconvenient of recombinant AAV vectors is a cloning capacity that reaches at best 5 kb. As depicted in Table 2, all therapeutic schemes that have been considered in different mice models of MND make use of AAV serotype 2 (AAV-2). AAV-2 tropism is defined by its binding to heparan sulfate proteoglycan (HSPG) working in conjunction with $\alpha_V\beta_5$ integrin or basic fibroblast growth factor coreceptors (54,55). Replication-defective AAV infect both dividing and non dividing cells and promote a long-term expression that ranges from months to a year (56,57). Components of the motor unit can also be efficiently transduced with AAV (58–61). The stable introduction of genes into muscle fibers via the use of AAV-2 has been proved particularly helpful for MND therapeutic applications. Hence, AAV-2 transduces very efficiently mature postmitotic muscle fibers independently of myoblast mediation as reported for AdV and lead to a long-lasting expression in an increased number of transduced mature muscles. Furthermore, when administered intramuscularly AAV was reported to be less immunogenic than AdV (62–64).

Lentiviral Vectors

LV are retroviruses encompassing primate LV; human immunodeficiency virus-1 and -2 (HIV-1 and HIV-2), simian immunodeficiency virus (SIV) and non-primate LV; feline immunodeficiency virus (FIV), bovine immunodeficiency virus (BIV), or the equine infectious anemia virus (EIAV). LV are enveloped viruses of about 100 nm of size carrying two copies of a single-strand positive RNA. The length of the provirus is about 9–10 kb. Two homologous regions of 600 to 900 nucleotides flank the viral genome, the long-terminal repeats (LTR). LTR are required for virus replication, integration, and expression. Most recombinant lentiviral vectors used for CNS applications are derived from HIV-1 and are often encapsidated by the envelope protein of the vesicular stomatitis virus G protein (VSV-G). VSV-G pseudotyping confers a higher stability, helpful for recombinant viral production and a broad-spectrum host cell infectivity as it involves interaction with phosphatidylserine (65). LV can transduce motor neurons, glial cells including Schwann cells and with less efficiency muscle cells (58,61,66–68). Following attachment of VSV-G pseudotyped LV to the target cell, fusion of the virus envelope to the cell membrane occurs upon acidification of endocytic vesicles, penetration of the nucleocapsid into the cell, reverse transcription of the viral RNA genome, integration of the viral DNA, and ultimately expression of the transgene. An important property of LV is that they integrate into the host genome leading to a stable transduction and a long-lasting expression of the transgene. LV integrate randomly into the host genome with some potential integration hotspots (69). LV are complex retroviruses that contain the prototypical *gag*, *pol*, and *env* genes. *Gag* encodes matrix, capsid, and nucleocapsid

Table 2 Delivery of Therapeutic Genes by Viral Vectors

Therapeutic factor	Transfer vector	Mice model	Route of delivery	Therapeutic impact	References
NT-3	AdV	*pmn*	i.m	50% increase in mean life span. Protective effect against the loss of myelinated phrenic nerve fibers. Improved muscular function	73, 74
CNTF	AdV	*pmn*	i.m	25–30% increase in mean life span. Protective effect against axonal degeneration of phrenic nerve	73, 74
NT-3 and CNTF	AdV	*pmn*	i.m	No additive effect on mean survival, but pronounced protective effect on axonal degeneration	73
CNTF	AdV	*pmn*	i.v	25% increase in mean life span. Increased number of phrenic nerve fibers	74
CNTF	AdV	*pmn*	i.c.v	No effect on mean survival. No effect on the number of phrenic nerve fibers	74
CT-1	AdV	hSOD1 G93A	i.m	Delayed motor deficit onset by 20% and prolonged mean survival by 8%. Improved neuromuscular function and reduced axonal degeneration	113
GDNF	AdV	hSOD1 G93A	i.m	Delayed motor deficit onset by 10% and prolonged mean survival by 12%. Protective effect on large motor neuron and improved motor function	114
GDNF	AAV-2	hSOD1 G93A	i.m	Delayed motor deficit onset and prolonged mean survival by 13%. Duration of disease unchanged. Prevented motor neuron atrophy and degeneration	72
GDNF	AAV-2	hSOD1 G93A	i.m	Delayed onset of motor neuron disease by 18% and	61

Factor	Vector	Transgene	Route	Effect	References
GDNF	LV[a]	hSOD1 G93A	i.sp, i.f	increased mean survival by 6%. No effect on disease onset and life span for spinal targeting. Increased size of motor neurons in facial nucleus	68
IGF-1	AAV-2	hSOD1 G93A	i.m	Delayed onset of motor neuron disease by 34%. Prolonged mean survival by 30% and 18% when lately administrated. Promoted motor neuron survival and improved motor performance	61
IGF-1	LV[a]	hSOD1 G93A	i.m	Delayed mean survival by 7%	61
VEGF	LV[b]	hSOD1 G93A	i.m	Delayed onset of motor neuron disease by 30%. Prolonged mean survival by 30% and 15% when lately administrated. Delayed loss of motor performances. Increased survival of facial and spinal motor neurons	82
GDNF	LV[b]	hSOD1 G93A	i.m	Delayed mean survival by 5%	82
Bcl-2	AAV-2	hSOD1 G93A	i.sp	Delayed onset of the disease by 10%. No effect on mean life span. Prevented motor neuron degeneration and improved muscular function	60
Bcl-2	AdV	hSOD1 G93A	i.m	Protected again motor neuron degeneration. Delayed cytochrome c release, decreased caspase-1 activation and inhibited vacuolar formation	76, 77
RNA interference	LV[a,b]	hSOD1 G93A	i.sp[a], i.m[b]	Delayed disease onset by 21[a]–115%[b] and life span by 77%[b]. Prevented motor neuron degeneration and improved motor performance	79,87

[a]vesicular stomatitis virus G protein (VSV-G)-pseudotyped HIV-derived lentivirus.

[b]rabies-G pseudotyped equine infectious anaemia virus (EIAV).

Abbreviations: NT-3, neurotrophin-3; VEGF, vascular endothelial growth factor; Bcl-2, B-cell leukemia/lymphoma protein; Ad, adenovirus; AAV-2, adeno-associated virus serotype 2; i.m, intramuscular; i.v, intravenous; i.c.v, intracerebroventricular; i.sp, intraspinal; i.n; intranucleus (facial nucleus); GDNF, Glial cell-derived neurotropic factor; CNTF, ciliary neurotropic factor; IGF-1, Insulin-like growth factor-1.

proteins. *Pol* gives rise to viral protease, reverse transcriptase, and integrase. *env* encodes for the envelope glycoproteins. LV also present additional accessory genes encoding regulatory elements involved in different stage of the viral life cycle. LV encodes six accessory proteins, vif, vpr, vpu, tat, rev, nef, and vpx playing a role in infection, integration of the viral genome, transcriptional events, and intracellular compartment transport of RNA. Solely rev and tat are required for virus replication. Tat acts as a transcriptional transactivator increasing transcription of the viral genome and rev by interacting with the rev responsive element (RRE) promote nuclear export. Development of vector production system for a gain of biosafety includes, deletion of pathogenic features mainly accessory elements, reduction of risk of generation of replication-competent retroviruses, e.g., by the use of self-inactivating (SIN) vectors in which a specific region of the 3'LTR has been deleted in order to create inactive LTR following integration in the host genome (70). Several conceptual generations of recombinant lentiviral vectors defective for viral replication have been reported and are based on transient transfection of three or four plasmids. Typically, the transfer vector is a SIN vector that retains packaging signals allowing vector encapsidation. For viral propagation, viral structure components including at least gag-pol and rev and VSV-G envelope are supplied by transfection of plasmids or by using packaging cell lines.

Cellular and Molecular Targets: The Delivery Issue

According to the position of motor neuron soma within the central nervous system, whereas the target muscles are distal in periphery, mainly two *modi operandi* have been proposed to deliver the therapeutic genes (Table 2). Delivery of viral vectors into muscles offers several advantages: (1) retrograde transport of a soluble therapeutic factor (e.g., NTF) directly accessible by motor neurons, (2) retrograde transport of viral particles and transduction of the projecting motor neurons, and (3) systemic delivery of the therapeutic factor allowing motor neurons located distally from the site of injection to benefit from protective properties. On the other hand, gene transfer to spinal cord offers the possibility to drive expression of intrinsic factors directly to motor neurons as well as non-neuronal cell that cannot be transduced by retrograde transport-based mechanism.

The Muscle as a Therapeutic Platform

NTF delivery through gene transfer into skeletal muscles has been evaluated in mice models of MND. Intramuscular injections of virus carrying genetic information for GDNF, CNTF, NT-3, IGF-1, or vascular endothelial growth factor (VEGF) have shown impressive neuroprotective effects (Table 2). More interestingly from a clinical point of view, following a single injection of viral vectors, transduced muscle fibers led to a significant long-lasting expression of NTF that can reach at least 10 months (71). Sustained expression of NTF is indeed a desired goal due to the chronic nature of MND. Ideally, virally transduced muscles should provide a deep-rooted tightly-regulated source of a therapeutic message avoiding repeated systemic administration of recombinant proteins.

   Physiological mechanisms of neuroprotection conferred by muscle-derived biologically active NTF can involve several non-exclusive scenari. Neuroprotective effects of NTF are mainly based on their retrograde axonal transport from targets to the cell bodies where NTF could directly elicitate survival signals in neurons. Experimental evidences suggest that GDNF acts mainly through a target-derived pathway (71,72). Interestingly, intraspinal delivery of GDNF has no effect on motor neuron degeneration in ALS mice models, which emphasize the idea that GDNF acts as a peripheral factor (68). NTF synthesized by muscle fibers can also stimulate sprouting of motor neurons and enhance reinnervation as it has been described for NT-3 in *pmn* mice (73). A bilateral neuroprotective effect in unilaterally injected mice suggest that NT-3 and CNTF can also act systemically (73,74). Viral vectors may also gain access to the spinal cord to transduce motor neurons that acts in turn as intraspinal sources of NTF (61,74). AdV and AAV can be taken up at the level of nerve endings, transported back through axonal transport to reach cell bodies (61,74–77). This route of delivery is being discussed for AAV as several groups failed to observe such retrograde transport of viral vectors and suggest a more muscle-based source of NTF at the origin of the neuroprotective effects (42,71,72). In conclusion, muscle-derived NTF can act (1) through a target-derived, autocrine or more distal and systemic pathway, (2) directly at the neuromuscular junction by stimulating sprouting, reinnervation, and/or preservation of terminal innervation pattern, (3) through transduction of motor neurons following retrograde transport of viral vectors, and (4) a combination of these different routes of delivery depending both on the NTF as well as the viral vector used.

Delivery of Therapeutic Messages to the Spinal Cord

When administrated directly into the spinal cord or facial nucleus by sophisticated stereotaxic techniques, LV promote long-lasting expression of the gene of interest in motor neurons, interneurons, and glial cells (60,68,78). This route of delivery has the advantage of targeting all cell types potentially involved in the pathogenesis. It does not restrict gene therapy approach solely to soluble factors but permits neuroprotective agents with intracellular mode of actions, such as Bcl-2, to be studied (60). More recently, intraspinal delivery of LV that promote silencing of mutated SOD1 mutant through RNA interference has also been successfully applied (79). Furthermore, the ability to deliver viral vectors in precise spinal sites allow for the targeting of motor neuron populations that control vital muscles such as those controlling breathing.

Lentiviral vectors can be pseudotyped with a broad range of heterologous envelope glycoproteins (80,81). Replacement of the natural envelope of LV confers novel properties to the vector ranging from transduction efficiency, different tropism and distribution by mean of access to retrograde transport pathways. Recently, an EIAV vector pseudotyped with rabies-G envelope glycoprotein was reported to enhanced gene transfer capacity based on the retrograde transport of viral particles that are delivered to selected populations of motor neurons (82,83). When injected intramuscularly, rabies-G pseudotyped EIAV gain entry into the spinal compartment. When injected intraspinally several connected population of neurons were transduced including sensory neurons in dorsal root ganglions, neurons in the brainstem and motor cortex and commissural interneurons that project from the contralateral part to the injected side (83,84). Mechanisms of retrograde transport of the capsid are not well understood, but could imply a microtubule motor-dependent transport from neuromuscular junctions to projecting neuronal cell bodies following internalization mediated by viral receptors (for instance p75 low affinity NGF receptor or nicotinic acetylcholine receptor for rabies-G glycoprotein) (85,86). Recently, it has been shown that delivery of Vascular endothelial growth factor (VEGF) through rabies-G pseudotyped EIAV led to an impressive therapeutical benefit in an ALS

mouse model, similar to that obtained with IGF-1 (Table 2) (61,82). A viral transfer
of Bcl-2 through retrograde transport of adenoviral vectors has also been evaluated
in restricted populations of neurons in ALS mice models with promising results
(76,77). By giving access to motor neurons, this gene transfer approach that required
simple intramuscular administration of viruses offers per se interesting therapeutic
perspectives.

Ex Vivo Gene Therapy

A promising approach to overcome some drawbacks of viral-mediated gene transfer
(elicited immune response against viral vector or transduced cells, viral toxicity,
potentially harmful viral integration in the host genome) consists in *ex vivo* gene
therapy. Basically, allogenic or even xenogenic cells are engineered to secrete a therapeutic factor *in vitro* and implanted at the appropriate site of therapeutic intervention. Although this innovative approach to gene therapy is restricted to diffusible
molecules, its clinical feasibility has already been demonstrated *in vivo* in human
patients including ALS patients (88–90).

The Cerebro-Spinal Fluid as a Therapeutic Source

Xenogenic or allogenic genetically engineered cells can be encapsulated into polymer-
based membranes that serve as immuno-isolation devices. Semi-permeable membranes allow diffusion of oxygen, nutrients, and specific bioactive substances, but
restrict inward diffusion of larger molecules and cells, thus isolating the transplanted
encapsulated cells from the host immune system. Bioartificial devices are mainly of two
kinds (1) microspheres of semi-permeable polyelectrolyte-based membranes ranging
from 300 to 1500 μm of diameter and (2) hollow fibers-based macrocapsules. Pre-
formed hollow fibers made of various thermoplastic are loaded with cells and extremities sealed with photopolymerisable glue. Hollow fibers-based macrocapsules are
preferred for clinical application due to their retrievability. Hollow fiber diameter typically varies between 500 and 900 μm with a membrane thickness comprised between 50
and 100 μm. The length of the capsule; ranging from 0.5 cm for rodents to 5 cm for
human; is directly dependent on the cell number loaded, implantation site and the type
of host. An extracellular matrix, usually polyvinyl alcohol or collagen, is introduced
within the fiber to ensure an optimal cell survival of anchorage depending cells.

   Delivery of NTF by encapsulated genetically modified cells has already been
evaluated in rodents, sheep, primates, and humans. CNTF released by genetically
modified encapsulated cells was reported to increase the life span of *pmn* mice and
to decrease motor neuron loss in facial nerve lesion paradigms (91,92). Interestingly,
biodevice-delivered CNTF show a higher efficiency than CNTF delivered by classical
subcutaneous administration (93). A phase-I study was designed to assess the therapeutic potential of this ex vivo approach. Five centimeter long hollow fibers fabricated from polyethersulfone and loaded with xenogenic fibroblasts genetically
modified to human CNTF were implanted in the lumbar intrathecal space of six
ALS patients (90). Encapsulated cells provided a continuous source of hCNTF
exclusively in the vicinity of motor neurons as demonstrated by the presence of
CNTF in patient's cerebrospinal fluid and not in blood. Unfortunately, the small
number of patients and the short observation period did not allow any conclusion
about the use of this *ex vivo* therapy in the treatment of ALS. Importantly, limiting
side effects such as body weight loss, asthenia and cough associated with systemic

delivery of the recombinant protein were not observed. This innovative therapeutic approach allows a safe route of delivery that potentially avoids side effects associated with systemic administration of recombinant NTF.

Graft of Genetically Modified Cells

Alternatively, intramuscular secretion of NTF can be obtained by grafted genetically remodeled myoblasts. The technical feasibility of this approach has already been shown in clinical trials for treatment of Duchenne muscular dystrophy, a muscle-specific disorder (94). Interestingly, a proportion of grafted myoblasts can fuse with host myofibers and become incorporated in muscle tissue that ideally transforms muscle fibers as a secretory source of therapeutic compounds. In a mouse model of ALS, primary autologous myoblast retrovirally modified to release GDNF were grafted in hindlimb muscles. GDNF-secreting myoblasts that achieved a sustained expression of the transgene provided a beneficial effect on the MND. Moreover, a portion of surviving implanted myoblasts fused with host muscle fibers and transformed muscles as a potential source of GDNF (95). Nevertheless, direct graft of autologous genetically engineered cells presents some limitations, such as immune rejection and poor survival of implanted cells (96). Neural transplantation appeared also as an alternative therapeutic approach. The intraspinal graft of neuron-like cells into the spinal cord of mouse model of ALS has led to an improvement of motor function (97). Conceptually, graft of neural stem cells that can give rise to glial and neuronal cells is rapidly emerging as a promising therapeutic tool with the aim to restore and/or prevent neuronal cell loss in MND and other neurodegenerative diseases (98,99).

CONCLUSION

The challenge of gene therapy lies not solely in the knowledge of genetic aspects of human MND, but also in the identification of cellular protagonists that will represent relevant targets for therapy. MND animal models play an undeniable role in the understanding of the molecular and cellular pathogenic mechanisms from which arose an impressive number of therapeutic trials. Nevertheless, a discrepancy between encouraging preclinical and disappointing clinical trials outcomes remains. Clinical trials can involve patients with sporadic and FALS. Although sporadic and FALS cases are claimed to be clinically indistinguishable at the cellular and molecular level, pathogenic mechanisms are certainly sufficiently different to explain that most of the therapeutic treatment failed in providing robust improvement of the disease. Hence, this concern raises several questions about the validity of present FALS/MND models as the Rosetta stone of ALS clinical trials. For the majority of ALS forms, the causes of the disease remain unknown. In order to find efficient therapies there is an important need to identify underlying causes of human MND and to replicate these human pathologies in animal models.

Moreover, gene therapists are developing safe and efficient means to deliver the appropriate therapeutic instructions in accordance with the chronic aspect of MND. Over the past two decades, an impressive enrichment of knowledge in viral vectors has comforted the rational of gene therapy for MND. Nevertheless, some drawbacks continue to veil the gene therapy field in general. It concerns the requirement of long-term expression of transgene that must be ensured for years to decades due to the human life span; although it is of less concern for neurons, the oncogenic potential of viral vehicles remains a concern for glial cells that have the potential to divide. Others issues concern the inherent toxicity and immunogenicity of viral vectors that may lead to adverse side effects such as immune sensitization limiting the effectiveness; related to viral vector productions, the generation of replication competent recombinant viruses bearing unpredictable properties and also viral proteins may activate latent endogenous virus. Major efforts are currently devoted in order to overcome these concerns.

We strongly believe that, according to the accumulating heartening results in the field of MND, gene therapy should emerge as a *bona fide* treatment of motor neuron disorders in the not too distant future.

REFERENCES

1. Nicholson SJ, Witherden AS, Hafezparast M, Martin JE, Fisher EM. Mice, the motor system, and human motor neuron pathology. Mamm Genome 2000; 11:1041–1052.
2. Cleveland DW, Rothstein JD. From Charcot to Lou Gehrig: deciphering selective motor neuron death in ALS. Nat Rev Neurosci 2001; 2:806–819.
3. Newbery HJ, Abbott CM. Of mice, men and motor neurons. Trends Genet 2001; 17:S2–S6.
4. Rosen DR, Siddique T, Patterson D, Figlewicz DA, Sapp P, Hentati A, Donaldson D, Goto J, O'Regan JP, Deng HX, Rahmani Z, Krizus A, McKenna-Yasek D, cayabyab A, Gaston SM, Berger R, Tanzi RE, Halperin JJ, Herzfeldt B, Van Den Bergh R, Hung WY, Bird T, Deng G, Mulder DW, Smyth C, Laing NG, Soriano E, Pericak-Vance M, Haines JL, Rouleau G, Gusella JS, Horvitz HR, Brown RH. Mutations in Cu/Zn superoxide dismutase gene are associated with familial amyotrophic lateral sclerosis. Nature 1993; 362(6415):59–62.
5. Andersen PM, Nilsson P, Ala-Hurula V, Keranen ML, Tarvainen I, Haltia T, Nilsson L, Binzer M, Forsgren L, Marklund SL. Amyotrophic lateral sclerosis associated with homozygosity for an Asp90Ala mutation in CuZn-superoxide dismutase. Nat Genet 1995; 10(1):61–66.
6. Gurney ME, Pu H, Chiu AY, Dal Canto MC, Polchow CY, Alexander DD, Caliendo J, Hentati A, Kwon YW, Deng HX, Chen W, Zhai P, Sufit RL, Siddique T. Motor neuron degeneration in mice that express a human Cu,Zn superoxide dismutase mutation. Science 1994; 264(5166):1772–1775.
7. Dal Canto MC, Gurney ME. Development of central nervous system pathology in a murine transgenic model of human amyotrophic lateral sclerosis. Am J Pathol 1994; 145:1271–1279.
8. Wang J, Xu G, Gonzales V, Coonfield M, Fromholt D, Copeland NG, Jenkins NA, Borchelt DR. Fibrillar inclusions and motor neuron degeneration in transgenic mice expressing superoxide dismutase 1 with a disrupted copper-binding site. Neurobiol Dis 2002; 10(2):128–138.
9. Ripps ME, Huntley GW, Hof PR, Morrison JH, Gordon JW. Transgenic mice expressing an altered murine superoxide dismutase gene provide an animal model of amyotrophic lateral sclerosis. Proc Natl Acad Sci USA 1995; 92:689–693.
10. Wang J, Slunt H, Gonzales V, Fromholt D, Coonfield M, Copeland NG, Jenkins NA, Borchelt DR. Copper-binding-site-null SOD1 causes ALS in transgenic mice: aggregates of non-native SOD1 delineate a common feature. Hum Mol Genet 2003; 12(21):2753–2764.
11. Nagai M, Aoki M, Miyoshi I, Kato M, Pasinelli P, Kasai N, Brown RH, Jr., Itoyama Y. Rats expressing human cytosolic copper-zinc superoxide dismutase transgenes with amyotrophic lateral sclerosis: associated mutations develop motor neuron disease. J Neurosci 2001; 21(23):9246–9254.

12. Howland DS, Liu J, She Y, Goad B, Maragakis NJ, Kim B, Erickson J, Kulik J, DeVito L, Psaltis G, DeGennaro LJ, Cleveland DW, Rothstein JD. Focal loss of the glutamate transporter EAAT2 in a transgenic rat model of SOD1 mutant-mediated amyotrophic lateral sclerosis (ALS). Proc Natl Acad Sci U S A 2002; 99(3):1604–1609.

13. Vila M, Przedborski S. Targeting programmed cell death in neurodegenerative diseases. Nat Rev Neurosci 2003; 4:365–375.

14. Bruijn LI, Miller TM, Cleveland DW. Unraveling the mechanisms involved in motor neuron degeneration in ALS. Annu Rev Neurosci 2004; 27:723–749.

15. Duchen LW, Strich SJ. An hereditary motor neurone disease with progressive denervation of muscle in the mouse: the mutant 'wobbler'. J Neurol Neurosurg Psychiatry 1968; 31:535–542.

16. Boillee S, Peschanski M, Junier MP. The wobbler mouse: a neurodegeneration jigsaw puzzle. Mol Neurobiol 2003; 28:65–106.

17. Schmalbruch H, Jensen HJ, Bjaerg M, Kamieniecka Z, Kurland L. A new mouse mutant with progressive motor neuronopathy. J Neuropathol Exp Neurol 1991; 50: 192–204.

18. Martin N, Jaubert J, Gounon P, et al. A missense mutation in Tbcc causes progressive motor neuronopathy in mice. Nat Genet 2002; 32:443–447.

19. Turner MR, Leigh N. Disease-modifying therapies in motor neuron disorders: the present position and potential future developments. In: Shaw PJ, Strong MJ, eds. Motor Neuron Disorders. Vol. 28. Butterworth-Heinemann, 2003:497–544.

20. Morrison KE. Therapies in amyotrophic lateral sclerosis-beyond riluzole. Curr Opin Pharmacol 2002; 2:302–309.

21. Carter GT, Krivickas LS, Weydt P, Weiss MD, Miller RG. Drug therapy for amyotrophic lateral sclerosis: Where are we now? IDrugs 2003; 6:147–153.

22. Sendtner M, Pei G, Beck M, Schweizer U, Wiese S. Developmental motoneuron cell death and neurotrophic factors. Cell Tissue Res 2000; 301:71–84.

23. Lewin GR, Barde YA. Physiology of the neurotrophins. Annu Rev Neurosci 1996; 19:289–317.

24. Oppenheim RW. Neurotrophic survival molecules for motoneurons: an embarrassment of riches. Neuron 1996; 17:195–197.

25. Henderson CE, Phillips HS, Pollock RA, Davies AM, Lemeulle C, Armanini M, Simmons L, Moffet B, Vandlen RA, Koliatos VE, Rosenthal A. GDNF: a potent survival factor for motoneurons present in peripheral nerve and muscle. Science 1994; 266(5187):1062–1064.

26. Li L, Oppenheim RW, Lei M, Houenou LJ. Neurotrophic agents prevent motoneuron death following sciatic nerve section in the neonatal mouse. J Neurobiol 1994; 25: 759–766.

27. Iwasaki Y, Ikeda K. Prevention by insulin-like growth factor-I and riluzole in motor neuron death after neonatal axotomy. J Neurol Sci 1999; 169:148–155.

28. Vejsada R, Tseng JL, Lindsay RM, Acheson A, Aebischer P, Kato AC. Synergistic but transient rescue effects of BDNF and GDNF on axotomized neonatal motoneurons. Neuroscience 1998; 84:129–139.

29. Group TACTS. A double-blind placebo-controlled clinical trial of subcutaneous recombinant human ciliary neurotrophic factor (rHCNTF) in amyotrophic lateral sclerosis. ALS CNTF Treatment Study Group. Neurology 1996; 46:1244–1249.

30. III TBSGP. A controlled trial of recombinant methionyl human BDNF in ALS. Neurology 1999; 52:1427–1433.

31. Lai EC, Felice KJ, Festoff BW, Gawel MJ, Gelinas DF, Kratz R, Murphy MF, Natter HM, Norris FH, Rudnicki SA. Effect of recombinant human insulin-like growth factor-I on progression of ALS. A placebo-controlled study. The North America ALS/IGF-I Study Group. Neurology 1997; 49(6):1621–1630.

32. Borasio GD, Robberecht W, Leigh PN, Emile J, Guiloff RJ, Jerusalem F, Silani V, Vos PE, Wokke JH, Dobbins T. A placebo-controlled trial of insulin-like growth

factor-I in amyotrophic lateral sclerosis. European ALS/IGF-I Study Group. Neurology 1998; 51(2):583–586.

33. Turner MR, Parton MJ, Leigh PN. Clinical trials in ALS: an overview. Semin Neurol 2001; 21:167–175.

34. Miller RG, Bryan WW, Dietz MA, Munsat TL, Petajan JH, Smith SA, Goodpasture JC. Toxicity and tolerability of recombinant human ciliary neurotrophic factor in patients with amyotrophic lateral sclerosis. Neurology 1996; 47(5):1329–1331.

35. Kostic V, Jackson-Lewis V, de Bilbao F, Dubois-Dauphin M, Przedborski S. Bcl-2: prolonging life in a transgenic mouse model of familial amyotrophic lateral sclerosis. Science 1997; 277:559–562.

36. Friedlander RM, Brown RH, Gagliardini V, Wang J, Yuan J. Inhibition of ICE slows ALS in mice. Nature 1997; 388:31.

37. Inoue H, Tsukita K, Iwasato T, Suzuki Y, Tomioka M, Tateno M, Nagao M, Kawata A, Saido TC, Miura M, Misawa H, Itohara S, Takahashi R. The crucial role of caspase-9 in the disease progression of a transgenic ALS mouse model. Embo J 2003; 22(24): 6665–6674.

38. Guo H, Lai L, Butchbach ME, Stockinger MP, Shan X, Bishop GA, Lin CL. Increased expression of the glial glutamate transporter EAAT2 modulates excitotoxicity and delays the onset but not the outcome of ALS in mice. Hum Mol Genet 2003; 12(19):2519–2532.

39. Romero MI, Rangappa N, Garry MG, Smith GM. Functional regeneration of chronically injured sensory afferents into adult spinal cord after neurotrophin gene therapy. J Neurosci 2001; 21:8408–8416.

40. Joung I, Kim HS, Hong JS, Kwon H, Kwon YK. Effective gene transfer into regenerating sciatic nerves by adenoviral vectors: potentials for gene therapy of peripheral nerve injury. Mol Cells 2000; 10:540–545.

41. Millecamps S, Mallet J, Barkats M. Adenoviral retrograde gene transfer in motoneurons is greatly enhanced by prior intramuscular inoculation with botulinum toxin. Hum Gene Ther 2002; 13:225–232.

42. Martinov VN, Sefland I, Walaas SI, Lomo T, Nja A, Hoover F. Targeting functional subtypes of spinal motoneurons and skeletal muscle fibers in vivo by intramuscular injection of adenoviral and adeno-associated viral vectors. Anat Embryol (Berl) 2002; 205:215–221.

43. Meier O, Greber UF. Adenovirus endocytosis. J Gene Med 2004; 6(suppl 1):S152–S163.

44. Imperiale MJ, Kochanek S. Adenovirus vectors: biology, design, and production. Curr Top Microbiol Immunol 2004; 273:335–357.

45. Kochanek S, Schiedner G, Volpers C. High-capacity 'gutless' adenoviral vectors. Curr Opin Mol Ther 2001; 3:454–463.

46. Morsy MA, Gu M, Motzel S, Zhao J, Lin J, Su Q, Allen H, Franlin L, Parks RJ, Graham FL, Kochanek S, Bett AJ, Caskey CT. An adenoviral vector deleted for all viral coding sequences results in enhanced safety and extended expression of a leptin transgene. Proc Natl Acad Sci U S A 1998; 95(14):7866–7871.

47. Schiedner G, Morral N, Parks RJ, Wu Y, Koopmans SC, Langston C, Graham FL, Beaudet AL, Kochanek S. Genomic DNA transfer with a high-capacity adenovirus vector results in improved in vivo gene expression and decreased toxicity. Nat Genet 1998; 18(2):180–183.

48. Cao B, Mytinger JR, Huard J. Adenovirus mediated gene transfer to skeletal muscle. Microsc Res Tech 2002; 58:45–51.

49. Cao B, Pruchnic R, Ikezawa M, Xiao X, Li J, Wickham TJ, Kovesdi I, Rudert WA, Huard J. The role of receptors in the maturation-dependent adenoviral transduction of myofibers. Gene Ther 2001; 8(8):627–637.

50. Grimm D, Kay MA. From virus evolution to vector revolution: use of naturally occurring serotypes of adeno-associated virus (AAV) as novel vectors for human gene therapy. Curr Gene Ther 2003; 3:281–304.

51. Kotin RM, Siniscalco M, Samulski RJ, Zhu XD, Hunter L, Laughlin CA, McLaughlin S, Muzyczka N, Rocchi M, Berns KI. Site-specific integration by adeno-associated virus. Proc Natl Acad Sci U S A 1990; 87(6):2211–2215.

52. Schnepp BC, Clark KR, Klemanski DL, Pacak CA, Johnson PR. Genetic fate of recombinant adeno-associated virus vector genomes in muscle. J Virol 2003; 77:3495–3504.

53. Blouin V, Brument N, Toublanc E, Raimbaud I, Moullier P, Salvetti A. Improving rAAV production and purification: towards the definition of a scaleable process. J Gene Med 2004; 6(suppl 1):S223–S228.

54. Qing K, Mah C, Hansen J, Zhou S, Dwarki V, Srivastava A. Human fibroblast growth factor receptor 1 is a co-receptor for infection by adeno-associated virus 2. Nat Med 1999; 5:71–77.

55. Summerford C, Bartlett JS, Samulski RJ. AlphaVbeta5 integrin: a co-receptor for adeno-associated virus type 2 infection. Nat Med 1999; 5:78–82.

56. Passini MA, Watson DJ, Wolfe JH. Gene delivery to the mouse brain with adeno-associated virus. Methods Mol Biol 2004; 246:225–236.

57. Tenenbaum L, Chtarto A, Lehtonen E, Velu T, Brotchi J, Levivier M. Recombinant AAV-mediated gene delivery to the central nervous system. J Gene Med 2004; 6(suppl 1): S212–S222.

58. Fleming J, Ginn SL, Weinberger RP, Trahair TN, Smythe JA, Alexander IE. Adeno-associated virus and lentivirus vectors mediate efficient and sustained transduction of cultured mouse and human dorsal root ganglia sensory neurons. Hum Gene Ther 2001; 12:77–86.

59. Blits B, Oudega M, Boer GJ, Bartlett Bunge M, Verhaagen J. Adeno-associated viral vector-mediated neurotrophin gene transfer in the injured adult rat spinal cord improves hind-limb function. Neuroscience 2003; 118:271–281.

60. Azzouz M, Hottinger A, Paterna JC, Zurn AD, Aebischer P, Bueler H. Increased motoneuron survival and improved neuromuscular function in transgenic ALS mice after intraspinal injection of an adeno-associated virus encoding Bcl-2. Hum Mol Genet 2000; 9:803–811.

61. Kaspar BK, Llado J, Sherkat N, Rothstein JD, Gage FH. Retrograde viral delivery of IGF-1 prolongs survival in a mouse ALS model. Science 2003; 301:839–842.

62. Xiao X, Li J, Samulski RJ. Efficient long-term gene transfer into muscle tissue of immunocompetent mice by adeno-associated virus vector. J Virol 1996; 70:8098–8108.

63. Fisher KJ, Jooss K, Alston J, Yang Y, Haecker SE, High K, Pathak R, Raper SE, Wilson JM. Recombinant adeno-associated virus for muscle directed gene therapy. Nat Med 1997; 3(3):306–312.

64. Pruchnic R, Cao B, Peterson ZQ, Xiao X, Li J, Samulski RJ, Epperly M, Huard J. The use of adeno-associated virus to circumvent the maturation-dependent viral transduction of muscle fibers. Hum Gene Ther 2000; 11(4):521–536.

65. Schlegel R, Tralka TS, Willingham MC, Pastan I. Inhibition of VSV binding and infectivity by phosphatidylserine: is phosphatidylserine a VSV-binding site? Cell 1983; 32:639–646.

66. Cisterni C, Henderson CE, Aebischer P, Pettmann B, Deglon N. Efficient gene transfer and expression of biologically active glial cell line-derived neurotrophic factor in rat motoneurons transduced wit lentiviral vectors. J Neurochem 2000; 74:1820–1828.

67. Ericson C, Wictorin K, Lundberg C. Ex vivo and in vitro studies of transgene expression in rat astrocytes transduced with lentiviral vectors. Exp Neurol 2002; 173:22–30.

68. Guillot S, Azzouz M, Deglon N, Zurn A, Aebischer P. Local GDNF expression mediated by lentiviral vector protects facial nerve motoneurons but not spinal motoneurons in SOD1 (G93A) transgenic mice. Neurobiol Dis 2004; 16:139–149.

69. Schroder AR, Shinn P, Chen H, Berry C, Ecker JR, Bushman F. HIV-1 integration in the human genome favors active genes and local hotspots. Cell 2002; 110:521–529.

70. Zufferey R, Dull T, Mandel RJ, et al. Self-inactivating lentivirus vector for safe and efficient in vivo gene delivery. J Virol 1998; 72:9873–9880.

71. Lu YY, Wang LJ, Muramatsu S, Ikeguchi K, Fujimoto K, Okada T, Mizukami H, Matsushita T, Hanazono Y, Kume A, Nagatsu T, Ozawa K, Nakano I. Intramuscular injection of AAV-GDNF results in sustained expression of transgenic GDNF, and its delivery to spinal motoneurons by retrograde transport. Neurosci Res 2003; 45(1):33–40.

72. Wang LJ, Lu YY, Muramatsu S, Ikeguchi K, Fujimoto K, Okada T, Mizukami H, Matsushita T, Hanazono Y, Kume A, Nagatsu T, Ozawa K, Nakano I. Neuroprotective effects of glial cell line-derived neurotrophic factor mediated by an adeno-associated virus vector in a transgenic animal model of amyotrophic lateral sclerosis. J Neurosci 2002; 22(16):6920–6928.

73. Haase G, Kennel P, Pettmann B, Vigne E, Akli S, Revah F, Schmalbruch H, Kahn A. Gene therapy of murine motor neuron disease using adenoviral vectors for neurotrophic factors. Nat Med 1997; 3(4):429–436.

74. Haase G, Pettmann B, Bordet T, Villa P, Vigne E, Schmalbruch H, Kahn A. Therapeutic benefit of ciliary neurotrophic factor in progressive motor neuronopathy depends on the route of delivery. Ann Neurol 1999; 45(3):296–304.

75. Baumgartner BJ, Shine HD. Neuroprotection of spinal motoneurons following targeted transduction with an adenoviral vector carrying the gene for glial cell line-derived neurotrophic factor. Exp Neurol 1998; 153:102–112.

76. Yamashita S, Mita S, Kato S, Okado H, Ohama E, Uchino M. Effect on motor neuron survival in mutant SOD1 (G93A) transgenic mice by Bcl-2 expression using retrograde axonal transport of adenoviral vectors. Neurosci Lett 2002; 328:289–293.

77. Yamashita S, Mita S, Kato S, Okado H, Ohama E, Uchino M. Bcl-2 expression using retrograde transport of adenoviral vectors inhibits cytochrome c-release and caspase-1 activation in motor neurons of mutant superoxide dismutase 1 (G93A) transgenic mice. Neurosci Lett 2003; 350:17–20.

78. Hottinger AF, Azzouz M, Deglon N, Aebischer P, Zurn AD. Complete and long-term rescue of lesioned adult motoneurons by lentiviral-mediated expression of glial cell line-derived neurotrophic factor in the facial nucleus. J Neurosci 2000; 20:5587–5593.

79. Raoul C, Abbas-Terki T, Bensadoun JC, Guillot S, Haase G, Szulc J, Henderson CE, Aebischer P. Lentiviral-mediated silencing of SOD1 through RNA interference retards disease onset and progression in a mouse model of ALS. Nat Med 2005; 11(4):423–428.

80. Mochizuki H, Schwartz JP, Tanaka K, Brady RO, Reiser J. High-titer human immunodeficiency virus type 1-based vector systems for gene delivery into nondividing cells. J Virol 1998; 72:8873–8883.

81. Stitz J, Buchholz CJ, Engelstadter M, Uckert W, Bloemer U, Schmitt I, Cichutek K. Lentiviral vectors pseudotyped with envelope glycoproteins derived from gibbon ape leukemia virus and murine leukemia virus I0AI. Virology 2000; 273(1):16–20.

82. Azzouz M, Ralph GS, Storkebaum E, Walmsley LE, Mitrophanous KA, Kingsman SM, Carmeliet P, Mazarakis ND. VEGF delivery with retrogradely transported lentivector prolongs survival in a mouse ALS model. Nature 2004; 429(6990):413–417.

83. Mazarakis ND, Azzouz M, Rohll JB, Ellard FM, Wilkes FJ, Olsen AL, Carter EE, Barber RD, Baban DF, Kingsman SM, Kingsman AJ, O'Malley K, Mitrophanous KA. Rabies virus glycoprotein pseudotyping of lentiviral vectors enables retrograde axonal transport and access to the nervous system after peripheral delivery. Hum Mol Genet 2001; 10(19):2109–2121.

84. Kingsman SM. Lentivirus: a vector for nervous system applications. Ernst Schering Res Found Workshop 2003; 43:179–207.

85. Tuffereau C, Benejean J, Blondel D, Kieffer B, Flamand A. Low-affinity nerve-growth factor receptor (P75NTR) can serve as a receptor for rabies virus. Embo J 1998; 17:7250–7259.

86. Gastka M, Horvath J, Lentz TL. Rabies virus binding to the nicotinic acetylcholine receptor alpha subunit demonstrated by virus overlay protein binding assay. J Gen Virol 1996; 77(Pt 10):2437–2440.

87. Ralph GS, Radollffe PA, Day DM, Carthy JM, Leroux MA, Lee DC, Wong LF, Bilsland LG, Greensmith L, Kingsman SM, Mitrophanous KA, Mazarakis ND, Azzouz M. Silencing mutant SOD1 using RNAi protects against neurodegeneration and extends survival in an ALS model. Nat Med 2005; 11(4):429–433.

88. Tseng JL, Aebischer P. Encapsulated neural transplants. Prog Brain Res 2000; 127: 189–202.

89. Hottinger AF, Aebischer P. Treatment of diseases of the central nervous system using encapsulated cells. Adv Tech Stand Neurosurg 1999; 25:3–20.

90. Aebischer P, Schluep M, Deglon N, Joseph JM, Hirt L, Heyd B, Goddard M, Hammang JP, Zurn AD, Kato AC, Regli F, Baetge EE. Intrathecal delivery of CNTF using encapsulated genetically modified xenogeneic cells in amyotrophic lateral sclerosis patients. Nat Med 1996; 2(6):696–699.

91. Sagot Y, Tan SA, Baetge E, Schmalbruch H, Kato AC, Aebischer P. Polymer encapsulated cell lines genetically engineered to release ciliary neurotrophic factor can slow down progressive motor neuronopathy in the mouse. Eur J Neurosci 1995; 7:1313–1322.

92. Sagot Y, Tan SA, Hammang JP, Aebischer P, Kato AC. GDNF slows loss of motoneurons but not axonal degeneration or premature death of pmn/pmn mice. J Neurosci 1996; 16:2335–2341.

93. Tan SA, Deglon N, Zurn AD, Baetge EE, Bamber B, Kato AC, Aebischer P. Rescue of motoneurons from axotomy-induced cell death by polymer encapsulated cells genetically engineered to release CNTF. Cell Transplant 1996; 5(5):577–587.

94. Gussoni E, Pavlath GK, Lanctot AM, Sharma KR, Miller RG, Steinman L, Blau HM. Normal dystrophin transcripts detected in Duchenne muscular dystrophy patients after myoblast transplantation. Nature 1992; 356(6368):435–438.

95. Mohajeri MH, Figlewicz DA, Bohn MC. Intramuscular grafts of myoblasts genetically modified to secrete glial cell line-derived neurotrophic factor prevent motoneuron loss and disease progression in a mouse model of familial amyotrophic lateral sclerosis. Hum Gene Ther 1999; 10:1853–1866.

96. Skuk D, Tremblay JP. Myoblast transplantation: the current status of a potential therapeutic tool for myopathies. J Muscle Res Cell Motil 2003; 24:285–300.

97. Garbuzova-Davis S, Willing AE, Milliken M, Saporta S, Sowerby B, Cahill DW, Sanberg PR. Intraspinal implantation of hNT neurons into SOD1 mice with apparent motor deficit. Amyotroph Lateral Scler Other Motor Neuron Disord 2001; 2(4): 175–180.

98. Jakel RJ, Schneider BL, Svendsen CN. Using human neural stem cells to model neurological disease. Nat Rev Genet 2004; 5:136–144.

99. Svendsen CN, Langston JW. Stem cells for Parkinson disease and ALS: replacement or protection? Nat Med 2004; 10:224–225.

100. Ikeda K, Wong V, Holmlund TH, Greene T, Cedarbaum JM, Lindsay RM, Mitsumoto H. Histometric effects of ciliary neurotrophic factor in wobbler mouse motor neuron disease. Ann Neurol 1995; 37(1):47–54.

101. Mitsumoto H, Ikeda K, Holmlund T, Greene T, Cedarbaum JM, Wong V, Lindsay RM. The effects of ciliary neurotrophic factor on motor dysfunction in wobbler mouse motor neuron disease. Ann Neurol 1994; 36(2):142–148.

102. Ikeda K, Klinkosz B, Greene T, Cedarbaum JM, Wong V, Lindsay RM, Mitsumoto H. Effects of brain-derived neurotrophic factor on motor dysfunction in wobbler mouse motor neuron disease. Ann Neurol 1995; 37(4):505–511.

103. Mitsumoto H, Ikeda K, Klinkosz B, Cedarbaum JM, Wong V, Lindsay RM. Arrest of motor neuron disease in wobbler mice cotreated with CNTF and BDNF. Science 1994; 265:1107–1110.

104. Hantai D, Akaaboune M, Lagord C, Murawsky M, Houenou LJ, Festoff BW, Vaught JL, Rieger F, Blondet B. Beneficial effects of insulin-like growth factor-I on wobbler mouse motoneuron disease. J Neurol Sci 1995; 129:122–126.

105. Ikeda K, Kinoshita M, Tagaya N, Shiojima T, Taga T, Yasukawa K, Suzuki H, Okano A. Coadministration of interleukin-6 (IL-6) and soluble IL-6 receptor delays progression of wobbler mouse motor neuron disease. Brain Res 1996; 726(1-2):91–97.

106. Mitsumoto H, Klinkosz B, Pioro EP, Tsuzaka K, Ishiyama T, O'Leary RM, Pennica D. Effects of cardiotrophin-1 (CT-1) in a mouse motor neuron disease. Muscle Nerve 2001; 24(6):769–777.

107. Ikeda K, Kinoshita M, Iwasaki Y. Basic fibroblast growth factor has neuroprotective effects on axotomy-induced spinal motoneuron death and wobbler mouse motoneuron disease. Muscle Nerve 1996; 19:794–795.

108. Ikeda K, Iwasaki Y, Tagaya N, Shiojima T, Kinoshita M. Neuroprotective effect of cholinergic differentiation factor/leukemia inhibitory factor on wobbler murine motor neuron disease. Muscle Nerve 1995; 18:1344–1347.

109. Azari MF, Galle A, Lopes EC, Kurek J, Cheema SS. Leukemia inhibitory factor by systemic administration rescues spinal motor neurons in the SOD1 G93A murine model of familial amyotrophic lateral sclerosis. Brain Res 2001; 922:144–147.

110. Feeney SJ, Austin L, Bennett TM, Kurek JB, Jean-Francois MJ, Muldoon C, Byrne E. The effect of leukaemia inhibitory factor on SOD1 G93A murine amyotrophic lateral sclerosis. Cytokine 2003; 23(4–5):108–118.

111. Manabe Y, Nagano I, Gazi MS, Murakami T, Shiote M, Shoji M, Kitagawa H, Abe K. Glial cell line-derived neurotrophic factor protein prevents motor neuron loss of transgenic model mice for amyotrophic lateral sclerosis. Neurol Res 2003; 25(2):195–200.

112. Dreibelbis JE, Brown RH Jr, Pastuszak KA, Smith ER, Kaplan PL, Cudkowicz ME. Disease course unaltered by a single intracisternal injection of BMP-7 in ALS mice. Muscle Nerve 2002; 25:122–123.

113. Bordet T, Lesbordes JC, Rouhani S, Castelnau-Ptakhine L, Schmalbruch H, Haase G, Kahn A. Protective effects of cardiotrophin-1 adenoviral gene transfer on neuromuscular degeneration in transgenic ALS mice. Hum Mol Genet 2001; 10(18):1925–1933.

114. Acsadi G, Anguelov RA, Yang H, Toth G, Thomas R, Jani A, Wang Y, Ianakova E, Mohammad S, Lewis RA, Shy ME. Increased survival and function of SOD1 mice after glial cell-derived neurotrophic factor gene therapy. Hum Gene Ther 2002; 13(9): 1047–1059.

24

Experimental Models of Motor Neuron Diseases

Makiko Nagai
Department of Neurology, Columbia University, New York, New York, U.S.A.

Hitoshi Kikuchi
Department of Neurology, Columbia University, New York, New York, U.S.A., and Department of Neurology, Neurological Institute, Graduate School of Medical Sciences, Fukuoka, Japan

Serge Przedborski
Departments of Neurology and Pathology and the Center for Neurobiology and Behavior, Columbia University, New York, New York, U.S.A.

INTRODUCTION

The populations of neurons responsible for carrying the impulse that leads to the execution of a voluntary movement are the upper and lower motor neurons. The cell bodies of the upper motor neurons are located in the motor cortex from where their axons project downward to connect with the lower motor neurons within the motor nuclei of the brainstem and the anterior horn of the spinal cord. While the upper motor neurons are contained entirely within the CNS, the axons of the lower motor neurons exit to make connections with the striated muscles.

In a variety of pediatric- and adult-onset neurological diseases, either upper or lower motor neurons or both are degenerating, consistently leading to muscle wasting and paralysis. It is unquestionable that over the past decade some significant strides have been made toward clarifying how and why motor neurons are dying in these pathological situations. Yet investigators are still relying heavily on experimental models of motor neuron diseases to acquire a more definitive understanding of the actual etiology and pathogenesis of these devastating neurological disorders. As one may see from the literature, these models also serve to test experimental therapies in order to preclinically identify neuroprotective strategies.

These experimental models appear in different flavors and are found in different animal species, although those found in rodents outnumber any others. In this chapter, we review the different in vivo vertebrate models of motor neuron diseases, which will be categorized based on their mode of induction, meaning genetic, toxic, or infection. Even if several of the included in vivo models are not clearly linked to a known human disease, they all represent models of motor pathway degeneration, and as such they may all provide important insights into the actual mechanisms of neurodegeneration in amyotrophic lateral sclerosis (ALS) and other human motor neuron diseases.

GENETICALLY BASED MODELS OF MOTOR NEURON DISEASES

Although useful models of motor neuron diseases can be produced by an array of means, genetically based models are by far the most popular and the most numerous. They emanate from either spontaneous mutations or transgenic/knockout interventions. A third group of genetically based models originated from mutations introduced in genes for initial reasons unrelated to neurological diseases and which, by serendipity, led to motor neuron death.

Models of Motor Neuron Diseases Due to Spontaneous Mutations

Before the techniques of making transgenic and knockout animals were established and popularized, motor neuron disease models due to spontaneous mutations were extensively used to investigate the mechanism of motor neuron death and new therapies. From the literature, it appears that the number of such models is quite large. Among these, many, however, remained at the level of more or less detailed case reports, while some others were better characterized and exploited by investigators to address pathogenic and therapeutic questions relevant to motor neuron degeneration. It seems quite clear that the most studied spontaneous mutation models include the wobbler, the progressive motor neuropathy, *mnd*, *mnd-2*, and hereditary canine spinal muscular astrophy models. Therefore, we will limit our discussion to these specific animal models.

The Wobbler Mouse Model

The wobbler mutant mouse is linked to a recessively inherited neurological disease characterized by degeneration of motor neurons, most prominent in the cervical spinal cord (1). Mutant mice can be distinguished from their wild-type littermates three to four weeks of age, by their smaller size and the presence of limb tremor and atrophy of forelimb muscles. The wobbler gene defect has been mapped to mouse chromosome 11, close to the region encoding for the enzyme glutamine synthetase (2,3). The main site of neuropathology associated with the wobbler mutation is the ventral horn of the cervical spinal cord. In presymptomatic wobbler mice, many spinal cord motor neurons appear enlarged and filled with achromatic lacunar vacuoles with an absence of overt neuronal loss (1,4). Electron micrographs of the abnormal motor neurons showed that these vacuolar changes corresponded to gross dilatation of Golgi elements and endoplasmic reticulum (5). In addition to these neuropathological features, by the time wobbler mice become symptomatic (i.e., paretic), motor neuron loss is clearly observable (1,4). Like many other models of motor neurons disease, astrocytosis is also a prominent feature in affected wobbler mice (6). In these animals, especially at an advanced stage of the disease, signs of neurodegeneration are also found in the thalamus, deep cerebellar nuclei, and brain stem (7). The actual mode of neuronal death in the wobbler mouse has not been thus far well studied. Some investigations utilizing techniques such as terminal deoxynucleotidyl transferase-mediated dUTP-biotin nick end-labeling (TUNEL) show no evidence of DNA fragmentation in motor neurons (8), whereas others have reported transient, massive DNA alterations in presymptomatic wobbler mice (9). These latter data suggest the possibility that during the course of the disease, motor neurons may be the site of activation of the apoptotic machinery.

Prior to the development of transgenic mice expressing mutant superoxide dismutase-1 (SOD1), the wobbler mice were regarded as the best animal model of motor neuron diseases. As of yet, neither the nature of the gene defect nor the mechanism by which neurodegeneration occurs in this model have been elucidated. Still, wobbler mice have been and continue to be used as a preclinical tool to test experimental treatments such as neurotrophic factors (10,11), nitric oxide synthase inhibitor (12,13) hyperbaric oxygen therapy (14), and progesterone (15).

The Progressive Motor Neuropathy Mouse Model

Due to the onset of motor abnormalities at an early age, the progressive motor neuropathy (*pmn*) mouse is proposed as a model for spinal muscular atrophy (SMA). These mutant mice develop a hereditary neurogenic muscle atrophy transmitted as an autosomal recessive trait. As early as 14 to 20 days after birth, these animals begin to develop weakness of the hindlimbs, which rapidly progresses to profound paralysis in only two to three weeks (16). Usually these mice die by the age of 50 to 55 days (16).

Neuropathological changes in these mice appear to be restricted to the lower motor neuron pathway, as the brain is intact even in end-stage *pmn* mice. Muscle histology indicates either small group atrophy with angulated fibers or large group atrophy with many small round, and a few slightly hypertrophic, fibers. Observation of the peripheral nerves suggests a dying-back neuronopathy starting at the motor endplates (16). The number of spinal cord motor neurons, as assessed by counting the number of myelinated fibers in the ventral roots of these mice was initially reported to be unaffected (16). However, subsequent studies revisited this question by using the retrograde fluorescent tracer fluorogold (17). This work found a significant loss of neuronal fluorogold-labeling in the spinal cord of symptomatic mice and led to the conclusion that the *pmn* mutation does cause the demise of motor neurons (17). Yet, immunohistochemical studies looking at glial fibrillary acidic protein (GFAP) labeling failed to identify any evidence of gliosis in *pmn* mice (16). The lack of obvious gliosis suggests that the actual neuronal loss in *pmn* mice has to be quite subtle to not induce any detectable glial response. Consequently, the marked reduction in fluorogold-labeling likely reflects an impairment in the retrograde transport machinery rather than a gross neuronal loss.

The *pmn* locus was mapped to mouse chromosome 13 (18), and the *pmn* mutation was identified as a Trp524Gly substitution of the last amino acid residue of the tubulin-specific chaperone E (*Tbce*) (19,20). The protein encoded by the *Tbce* gene (Cofactor E) is known to play the role of tubulin-specific chaperone which binds to α-tubulin and helps in its assembly with β-tubulin. It has thus been speculated that *Tbce* mutations, by ablating the normal function of the encoded protein, may impair the proper assembly of microtubules.

As discussed above, the *pmn* mouse does not show massive motor neuron degeneration. Accordingly, it is our opinion that it may represent an excellent model of axonopathy, but not of SMA as initially advertised. This fact should not however undermine the usefulness of this mouse model for the testing of new neuroprotective agents. In this view, it is worth citing the work done in *pmn* mice, which were crossed with transgenic mice expressing high levels of the antiapoptotic bcl-2 gene (21) or treated with encapsulated cells producing glial cell-derived neurotrophic factor (GDNF) (22).

Unexpectedly, both of these studies showed that these two interventions did mitigate the loss of spinal cord motor neurons in *pmn* mice but failed to protect against either axonal degeneration or worsening of symptoms. These findings suggest that the molecular basis of axonal destruction may be distinct to that of cell body destruction, a notion that has already been put forward by Raff and collaborators (23). Along this line, it is also worth mentioning that upon crossing mice carrying a triplication of the gene that protects from rapid Wallerian degeneration, Wld (24) with *pmn* mice, axonal degeneration was markedly attenuated and lifespan was significantly extended (25). This study demonstrates that slowing Wallerian degeneration overwrites the deleterious consequence of *pmn* mutation and stresses the critical link between axonal integrity and the expression of the diseases in this mouse model.

The mnd Mouse Model

The *mnd* model is an adult-onset hereditary neurological condition found in mice characterized by motor abnormality arising around six months of age and progressing to severe spastic paralysis and premature death by approximately 10 to 12 months of age (26). The *mnd* gene mutation has been mapped to mouse chromosome 8 (27) and corresponds to a 1 bp insertion (267–268insC) to the *Cln8* gene, predicting a frameshift and a truncated protein (28). The *Cln8* gene is the mouse homologue for human CLN8, which upon mutation does not give rise to a motor neuron disease, but rather to progressive epileptic syndrome with mental retardation (28,29). Yet, as the clinical phenotype of mnd is known to depend on the genetic background (30), the different phenotypes in human and mouse may also be due to the presence of modifier genes.

Pathologically, there is a dramatic degeneration of spinal cord motor neurons in the lumbar spinal cord of affected animals (31). Among the neurons, there are variable neuropathological changes including distorted plasma membranes, eccentric nuclei, chromatolysis, and swelling. These pathological cells are seen in the lower cranial nerves, which include the hypoglossal nucleus and dorsal motor nucleus of the vagus, and, to a lesser extent, the facial and motor trigeminal nuclei. Pathologic neurons were also seen in the red nucleus, reticular formation of the pons and medulla, and restricted areas of the cerebral cortex. Degenerating motor neurons demonstrate a loss of Nissl substance and increases in lipofuscin and cytoplasmic inclusions (31,32). These inclusions are associated with the accumulation of subunit c of mitochondrial ATP synthase (33). Autofluorescence provoked by the deposits of lipofuscin can be seen as early as the first month of life and progressively increases (34). These neuronal ceroid lipofuscinosis (NCL)-like inclusions are very similar to those found in human NCL (33,35). Retinal degeneration also begins in the first month (34). The *mnd* mouse is typically recognized as a murine model of Batten's disease, but sometime it is also used as a model of motor neuron disease.

The mnd-2 Mouse Model

The *mnd-2* mouse model was identified as a spontaneous, recessively inherited mutation that arose on the C57BL/6J inbred background (36). Phenotypically, the *mnd-2* mouse exhibits muscle-wasting, neurodegeneration, involution of the spleen and thymus, and dies by the age of 40 days. The earliest symptoms are altered gait and cessation of normal weight gain, followed by ataxia, repetitive movement, and paucity of spontaneous motor activity. Degeneration of striatal neurons, with astrocytosis and microglia activation, begins at around three weeks of age, and other neurons including motor neurons are affected at later stages (36,37). The neuronal degeneration combines features of necrosis with features of apoptosis including nuclear condensation, TUNEL staining, and DNA laddering (37). Early degeneration of mitochondria is also noted. The *mnd-2* gene is mapped on mouse chromosome 6 (38), and its mutation was identified as the missense mutation Ser276Cys in the protease domain of the nuclear-encoded mitochondrial serine protease Omi (HtrA2 or Prss25) (39). Protease activity of Omi is greatly reduced in tissues of the *mnd-2* mouse. Loss of Omi protease activity increases the susceptibility of mitochondria to induction of the permeability transition. Although the mnd-2 story is quite fascinating, it is unclear what is the current contribution of this model to the understanding of the pathogenesis of motor neuron diseases such as ALS or SMA. Also, it is unclear as to how useful this model would be as a preclinical tool.

The Hereditary Canine Spinal Muscular Atrophy Model

The hereditary canine spinal muscular atrophy model (HCSMA) was originally described in a male Brittany spaniel dog as an autosomal dominant trait (40). Affected animals demonstrate progressive weakness with fasciculation and muscle atrophy. The progression of muscular wasting began from proximal and caudal to more distal and rostral muscles. There are three phenotypic variants: accelerated, intermediate, and chronic. Animals affected with the accelerated type (homozygous) developed weakness by 1.5 months and are quadriparetic by three months (41). The motor neurons of selected brainstem nuclei and ventral horns of the spinal cord are characterized by chromatolysis and by neurofibrillary abnormalities in perikarya, dendrites, and most strikingly, proximal axons (42). Intermediately affected dogs show only mild weakness by six months of age and become quadriparetic several years later. The differences among phenotypes parallel the severity in neuronal abnormalities such as chromatolysis, the presence of neurofilamentous accumulations in the perikaryon and dendrites, and the frequency of axonal swelling. The age of onset in the chronic form is more than one year, and pathological studies revealed evidence of neurogenic atrophy of muscles but no abnormality in the central nervous system (41). To our knowledge this interesting model has not been the topic of investigations beyond that reviewed above. This situation closely resembles that of the equine model of motor neuron disease (43,44), which, aside from limited number of publications, never gained prominence among experimental models of motor neuron diseases. Perhaps the underlying reason for this stems from the difficulty to perform studies that require a significant number of large animals, such as dogs and horses, as opposed to smaller animals such as rodents.

Transgenic and Knockout Models of Motor Neuron Diseases

Models Linked to Copper/Zinc Superoxide Dismutase

Approximately 5% to 10% of ALS cases are familial, and of these, roughly 15% to 20% are linked to mutations in the gene encoding for SOD1. By now, more than 100 different SOD1 mutations have been associated with the development of an autosomal dominant form of adult-onset motor neuron disease (http://alsod.org). Several of these pathogenic mutations have been introduced in rodents and likewise produce an adult-onset motor neuron disease in these animals. In only a few years, transgenic animals expressing human mutant SOD1 have become the gold standard among ALS models, both for exploring pathogenic mechanisms and testing experimental therapies for this fatal disease.

Transgenic Rodents Expressing Human Mutant SOD1 Driven by the SOD1 Endogenous Promoter. Several lines of transgenic animals expressing human mutant SOD1 have been developed, and their most salient characteristics are summarized in Table 1. The first reported line of transgenic mice ubiquitously expressing high levels of human SOD1 mutant turned out to be a breakthrough for the field of modeling. Indeed, these animals successfully recapitulated most of the clinical and neuropathological hallmarks of ALS by carrying the SOD1 point mutation Gly93A1a ($SOD1^{G93A}$) (45). Worth noting, in the same report transgenic mice that expressed high levels of the SOD1 mutant AVa4Val, which is the most frequent and most aggressive in humans, did not develop motor neuron disease (45). Also not affected were transgenic mice expressing comparable high levels of human wild-type SOD1 (45), supporting the notion that the mutant protein exerts its cytotoxicity via a gain-of-function effect. Subsequently, several lines of transgenic mice expressing distinct pathogenic SOD1 mutants were also produced, and all of these mice developed a similar adult-onset paralytic disorder as seen in the transgenic $SOD1^{G93A}$ mice (46–48). Over time, the need for larger animals to perform specific biochemical analyses and therapeutic tests which were difficult or impossible to achieve in mice became obvious and prompted investigators to develop transgenic rats (49,50).

Although the age at onset and the duration of SOD1-linked ALS varied depending on the mutation (51), the natural course of the disease in transgenic mutant SOD1 animals was also modulated by the level of mutant protein expression. For instance, among the different lines of transgenic $SOD1^{G37R}$ mice, the highest expressing lines (12.3 times endogenous mouse SOD1 in spinal card) are markedly affected by 3.5 to 4 months of age, while the lowest expressing lines (5.0 times endogenous mouse SOD1) only become symptomatic by six to eight months of age (47). Likewise, the age of symptom onset for the transgenic $SOD1^{G93A}$ line G1H with 25 transgene copies is approximately four months, whereas the transgenic $SOD1^{G93A}$ line G1L with less than 18 transgene copies is about six to seven months. If the level of mutant protein expression appears critical to the expression of disease in these transgenic animals, the enzymatic activity of the mutant protein seems irrelevant to the cytotoxic process. In fact, whether human SOD1 activity is elevated as in transgenic $SOD1^{G93A}$ (45) or $SOD1^{G37R}$ mice (47) or decreased as in transgenic $SOD1^{H46R}$ rats (49), the same motor neuron disease develops. Further support to this notion are the demonstrations that inactivation of SOD1, (mutant and wild-type) by ablating the copper chaperone of SOD1 or by mutating SOD1, copper binding sites, appears to have no impact on the deleterious effects of mutant SOD1 in both mice and cultured cells (52,53).

Although the age at onset and the length of survival differ, also worth mentioning is the fact that independently of the rate of progression, the actual symptoms are quite similar among the different lines of transgenic mutant SOD1 animals. As initially reported in the G1H mice, the very first motor abnormality is a fine tremor in one or more limbs, which in these mice occurs at around 90 to 100 days of age (54,55). Many investigators have complained that this fine tremor is not a clear-cut feature, especially in the transgenic rats. For that reason, onset of symptoms is becoming more often defined as the first sign of limb paresis. Other investigators have conducted various behavioral tests in these animals to identify the means of reliably and reproducibly detecting early signs of motor deficit (56). In transgenic rats, the demonstration of difficulty in extending one hind limb upon lifting the

Table 1 The Lines of Transgenic Animals with Mutant SOD1

	Mutation	Line	Background	Copy number	Protein*	SOD Activity*	Life span	Reference
Mouse	hG93A	G1H	C57BL/6xSJL	25	4.1 ± 0.54^a	42.6 ± 2.1^a	4–5 mo	45,54
		G1L	C57BL/6xSJL	18			6–7 mo	45,55,57
		G5/G5	C57BL/6xSJL	10	1.3 ± 0.21^a	27.0 ± 2.9^a	>400 days	57
		G20	C57BL/6xSJL	2	0.7 ± 0.06^a	16.9 ± 0.4^a	>300 days	55
	hG37R	42	C57BL/6xC3H/HeJ	ND	12.3	14.5	3.5–4 mo	47
		9	C57BL/6xC3H/HeJ	ND	6.2	9	5–6 mo	47
		106	C57BL/6xC3H/HeJ	ND	5.3	7.2	5.5–7.5 mo	47
		29	C57BL/6xC3H/HeJ	ND	5	7	6–8 mo	47
	hG85R	148	ND	15	1	1	8–10 mo	48
		74	ND	ND	0.2	1	12–14 mo	48
	mG86R	M1	FVB/N	ND	ND	1.0 (Brain)	3–4 mo	46
	hH46R/H48Q	139	C3H/HeJxC57BL/6J	ND	High	1	4–6 mo	61
		67	C3H/HeJxC57BL/6J	ND	ND	ND	8–10 mo	61
		58	C3H/HeJxC57BL/6J	ND	Low	ND	10–12 mo	61
Rat	hH46R	4	Sprague-Dawley	25	6	0.21	5 mo	49
	hG93A	39	Sprague-Dawley	10	2.5	3	4–4.5 mo	49
		26H	Sprague-Dawley	64	8.6	ND	3–4 mo	50

*Protein and SOD activity is relative to controls.

[a]Calculations are: [Protein] Human SOD (ng)/total protein (µg) and [SOD Activity] SOD (Unit)/total protein (µg).

Abbreviations: h, human; m, mouse; ND, not determined.

animal by the tail has been proposed to be a satisfactory early detection test (49). In most lines, weakness and muscle atrophy gradually developed from one hindlimb to the other and then to the forelimbs. When lightly tapped on the knee or ankle, muscle reflexes are brisk, suggesting a spastic paresis and supporting the involvement of the upper motor neurons. Motor deficit is usually more evident in the hindlimbs (Fig. 1A), but in some transgenic SOD1^{G93A} rats, weakness arose first in the forelimbs (Fig. 1B). These rats hardly supported their weight and used their nose instead of forelimb to stand, but easily fell, and their disease duration is short. In the same litter, forelimb-onset and hindlimb-onset rats mingled.

Pathological analysis in end-stage transgenic animals showed four main alterations, primarily but not exclusively in the ventral horns of the lumbar, thoracic, and cervical spinal cord (55,57). These are loss of motor neurons, presence of numerous membrane-bound vacuoles and proteinaceous inclusions, and gliosis. As in humans, motor neurons with a diameter $>25\,\mu m$ were degenerating much more than those with a diameter $<25\,\mu m$ (58). Several of the spared large motor neurons were filled with phosphorylated neurofilaments (NFs) (45). Vacuoles are of various sizes and appeared more abundant in the early course of neurodegeneration than at end-stage (58). By electron microscopy, these vacuoles are bounded by a single bilayer membrane, which corresponds mainly to dilated mitochondria (57,58). Relevant to this finding is the fact that wild type and mutant SOD1 accumulated in swollen and vacuolated mitochondria (59,60). By comparing the various transgenic lines, it appears that those with high mutant SOD1 expression seem to be more prompt in developing vacuoles than those with lower levels of expression. This is likely why ALS patients carrying a SOD1 mutation, and who have much lower expression levels of the mutant protein, do not show similar vacuoles. In G93A lower expressing lines (G20 and G5/G5), G85R, and H46R mutant mice (61), there are ubiquitinated hyaline inclusions in neurons. These proteinaceous inclusions have an eosinophilic dense core and show a clear halo, but are evenly immunostained with antineurofilament, SOD1, and ubiquitin antibodies (62–64). Ultrastructural studies of these aggregates show that they contain granule-associated fibrils similar to those seen in familial ALS patients. In most lines these inclusions are primarily found in neurons, but in the G85R line they are abundantly found in glial cells (48). Fragmentation of the Golgi apparatus was also found in the early, preclinical stage in transgenic SOD1^{G93A} mice (65), and its severity did correlate with the formation of proteinaceous inclusions

(A)   **(B)**

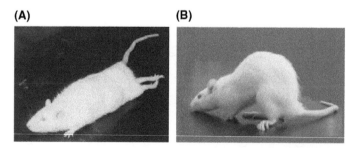

Figure 1   Transgenic rats with Mutant SOD1. **(A)** The rat shows spastic paraplegia, in which the paws of the hindlimbs are extended; the animal can still, however, grab the floor with forelimbs and can crawl. **(B)** This rat shows weakness in the forelimbs and shoulders, and uses its nose instead of forelimbs to stand. The atrophied muscles of the shoulder are also a prominent feature, making it difficult to raise its head.

and the progression of the disease (66). Gliosis in these animals is made of reactive astrocytes and activated microglial cells, and in some places images of neurophagia can be seen (67). Correlation between progression of the motor deficit and neuronal loss in transgenic SOD1^{G93A} mice reveals that the rapid decline in muscle strength coincides with maximal phase of vacuole formation, not with the loss of motor neurons (58). It is only when animals are markedly weak that further deterioration parallels the loss of large motor neurons (58). This suggests that the motor deficit is primarily the reflection of a loss of neuronal functionality or of end-plate denervation that occurs well before the motor neuron somata and axons actually degenerate.

As in other neurodegenerative situations, neuropathology is not restricted to one subpopulation of neurons, even if it is the main target of the disease. Indeed, in all transgenic mutant SOD1 lines, conspicuous histological abnormalities can be detected in brain regions other than spinal cord, including striatum, thalamus, hypothalamus, pyriform cortex, olfactory bulb, brainstem reticular formation, and choroid plexus (55,57,68). The severity of the extra-spinal pathology appears to be linked to the level of expression as low expressing lines show much milder changes.

Since the development of these transgenic animals, they have been used extensively as the most critical ingredient of a large number of studies geared toward unraveling the cytotoxic mechanism of mutant SOD1 or toward testing experimental therapies for ALS. Although this animal model is not perfect, it is fair to say that currently it is the gold standard for these two purposes (69).

Transgenic Mice Expressing SOD1 Driven by Cell-Specific Promoters. In the transgenic lines described above, mutant SOD1 is expressed in every cell. To determine whether it is sufficient to express the mutant protein in motor neurons in order to recapitulate the ALS-like phenotype, two types of transgenic mice in which mutant SOD1 expression is controlled by neuronal-specific promoters were generated. The first one carried SOD1^{G37R} driven by the NF light (NF-L) chain promoter (70). The highest level of human mutant SOD1 protein was 4.3 times endogenous mouse SOD1 in the spinal cord, and mutant SOD1 localized specifically in large neurons in the ventral horn (70). In this study, neither motor deficit nor degeneration of the ventral root could be detected (70). The second set of transgenic mouse line expressed either mutant SOD1^{G85R} or SOD1^{G93A} using a mouse Thy 1.2 expression cassette (71), which drives high constitutive expression of the transgene in postnatal mouse neurons (72). The levels of human mutant SOD1 protein in the lumbar cord were between 58 and 85% of that of the G1H mouse (G93A). Transgenic transcripts did accumulate in large ventral horn neurons and in layer-5 motor cortex projection neurons. Despite this apparent high level of transgene expression, none of these mice showed detectable signs of motor deficit or neuropathology (72). Crossing the Thy-1-SOD1^{G93A} with the G1H mice did not affect the natural course of the disease in this latter line of animals (72).

In an alternative strategy, it was also assessed whether expression of the mutant protein in astrocytes could cause neurodegeneration in this model. Here, the expression of SOD1^{G86R} was controlled by the GFAP promoter to express the mutant protein specifically in astrocytes (73). These mice did develop signs of gliosis, evidenced by hypertrophy of astrocytes and increased GFAP immunoreactivity in the nervous system, including the spinal cord (73). Yet, these mice developed normally and did not exhibit any motor deficits, neurodegeneration or activation of microglia with increasing age (73). Assuming that the levels of mutant protein expression were sufficient in all of these cell-specific lines, these studies would argue that mutant SOD1 must be expressed simultaneously in several cell types and not only in neurons or astrocytes for the disease to occur. The question of non-cell autonomy in the neurodegenerative process in ALS is discussed by Dr. Elliot and collaborators in this book.

Genetic Models Related to Cytoskeleton Abnormalities

Abnormal accumulation of the intermediate filaments in the perikaryon and axon of motor neurons is a common neuropathological feature of human ALS. Why intermediate filaments accumulate and whether this cytoskeleton perturbation causes motor neuron degeneration in ALS remain unknown. To examine these fascinating questions, several animal models have been constructed with the range including transgenic and knockout NFs, peripherin and dynein mice. Each provides quite distinct and complementary information regarding the molecular puzzle underlying the cytoskeleton-related mechanism of motor neuronal death.

Neurofilament-Based Models. The neuronal cytoskeleton is composed of three interconnected filaments including actin microfilaments, microtubules, and intermediate filaments. NFs are the major type of intermediate filament in adult motor neurons. NFs comprise three distinct subunits: NF-L (61 kDa), medium (NF-M, 90 kDa), and heavy (NF-H, 115 kDa) proteins. As already mentioned, NF accumulations are frequently detected in motor neurons of sporadic and familial ALS (74).

Ablation of any of the three NF subunit genes is associated with no developmental problem in mice (75). Yet, mutant mice lacking NF-L had a scarcity of intermediate filament structures and exhibited a severe axonal hypotrophy without motor neuron loss (76). In this model, NF-M and NF-H accumulated as proteinaceous aggregates in spinal cord motor neurons (76). The mutant mice deficient in NF-M showed reduction in NF-L content and axonal atrophy (77). Knockout mice deficient in NF-H did not show evidence of motor neuron loss, but the lack of NF-M subunit did result in the sequestering of unassembled NF-L proteins in neuronal perikarya and in a reduction of axonal caliber equivalent to the NF-L null mice (78). Collectively, these data indicate that heterodimerization of NF-L to NF-M or NF-H subunits is required to achieve a proper assembly and translocation of NFs into the axonal compartment.

Transfer of the NF-L null mutation in transgenic mutant SOD1^{G85R} mice slowed the symptom onset and prolonged survival (79). In NF-L-deficient mice, the contents of NF-M and NF-H were markedly reduced in axons, but were elevated in motor neuron cell bodies (79). This finding suggests that NF-L is the main mediator of cytotoxicity upon alterations in NF assembly and that accumulation of the other two NF subunits in the cell body may not be as harmful to motor neurons as initially thought.

Transgenic mice that express wild-type human NF-H developed symptoms consistent with motor neuron disease, characterized by onset of weakness at four to five months of age (80). The transgenic human NF-H mice exhibit severe atrophy of motor axons, axonal transport defects, and altered axonal conductances (80). Ultrastructural analysis of degenerating axons revealed a paucity of cytoskeletal elements, smooth endoplasmic reticulum, and especially mitochondria (80). However, no overt motor neuron loss was seen in this model (80,81). Paradoxically, overexpression of human NF-H subunits in transgenic SOD1^{G37R} mice prolonged survival rather then exacerbating the phenotype (82). Moreover, while massive neurodegeneration occurs in one-year-old transgenic SOD1^{G37R} mice, spinal cord motor neurons and their corresponding myelinated neurons were remarkably spared in transgenic SOD1^{G37R} overexpressing human NF-H (82). These findings are consistent with the view that excess NF-H disrupts the normal stoichiometric assembly of NF, leading to axonal morphology and functional alterations. Yet, it is not cytotoxic per se and may even hamper the accumulation of SOD1^{G37R} in the axonal compartment, whereby mitigating mutant SOD1 neurotoxicity.

Overexpression of wild-type murine NF-L induces massive accumulation of neurofilaments in the motor neurons and causes axonal degeneration and skeletal muscle atrophy (83). However, spinal cord motor neuron loss is not a feature seen in these animals. In contrast, transgenic mice not expressing wild-type but expressing mutant NF-L with a proline instead of leucine in codon 394 develop progressive forelimb and hindlimb weakness beginning at two to three weeks of age (84). Axonal spheroids were prominent in the ventral root exit zones and anterior horn regions of the spinal cord (84).

Peripherin. This protein is another intermediate filament detected in the majority of proteinaceous inclusions found in the motor neurons of ALS (85) and which, upon mutation, appears to be associated with the development of an ALS-like syndrome in humans (86,87). Peripherin is a 58-kDa type-III intermediate filament protein, which is expressed mostly in the peripheral nervous system and only at low levels in selected neuronal populations of the CNS in adult mammals (88,89). Peripherin is co-expressed with NF within axons of the ventral horns, posterior horns, posterior columns, and spinal roots. Sustained overexpression of wild-type peripherin in mice provokes massive and selective degeneration of motor axons during aging, a feature that can be exacerbated by the deficiency of NF-L (90). The formation of peripherin immunoreactive aggregates and the selective loss of motor neurons were evident in this model. By analyzing NF-L null mice that co-express both peripherin and NF-H transgenes, NF-H overexpression rescued the peripherin-mediated degeneration of motor neurons, which induced a reorganization of peripherin inclusions and prevented the massive loss of spinal motor neurons (91). In addition, Per 61, a splice variant form of peripherin, proved to be distinctly neurotoxic, being assembled incompletely and inducing degeneration of motor neurons in culture (92). Per 61 expressions was detected in both motor neurons of transgenic SOD1^{G37R} mice and in some familial ALS cases, but not in transgenic mice expressing wild-type SOD1 or peripherin (92). On the other hand, neither upregulation nor ablation of wild-type peripherin had any effect on the age at onset, survival, or loss of motor neurons in transgenic SOD1^{G37R} mice (93). These results indicate that peripherin is the crucial intermediate filament for motor neurons, but at the same time it seems that peripherin is not a key component in SOD1^{G37R}-mediated motor neuron degeneration.

Dynein. Cytoplasmic dynein is a molecular motor responsible for minus-end-directed movement along microtubules. In neurons, dynein has an essential role in fast retrograde axonal transport (94). Dynactin is a required activator of cytoplasmic dynein whose mutation has been proposed as a risk factor for ALS (95). Overexpression of dynamitin, which is a subunit of the microtubule-dependent motor complex, was found to disassemble dynactin, resulting in an inhibition of retrograde axonal transport. Mice overexpressing dynamitin demonstrate a late-onset progressive motor neuron degenerative disease characterized by decreased strength and endurance, motor neuron degeneration, and denervation of muscle (96). Hafezparast et al., however, showed that missense point mutations in the cytoplasmic dynein heavy chain (*Dnchc1*) gene result in progressive motor neuron degeneration in heterozygous mice, which in homozygotes this is accompanied by the formation of proteinaceous inclusion bodies. These mutations exclusively perturb neuron-specific functions of dynein (97).

Genetic Models Targeting the Survival Motor Neuron Protein

SMA is one of the most common neuromuscular diseases of infants and children, and it is genetically heterogeneous. Werdnig-Hoffmann disease (type-I SMA) is characterized by severe, generalized muscle weakness, and hypotonia at birth or within the first six months, and they die within the first two years. Type-II and -III SMA children are less severe, as they are able to sit, although they cannot stand or walk unaided. At the genomic level, the presence of a gene dosage effect in type I but not in type-III SMA has suggested that type-I SMA is caused by deletion of the *survival motor neuron* (*SMN*) gene, whereas type III was associated with a conversion event of *SMN* into the *SMN2* gene leading to an increased number of *SMN2* genes. The SMN protein level could thus depend on *SMN2* copy numbers in patients, identifying *SMN2* as a modifyer gene in SMA.

In the experimental models, mice carrying homozygous deletions of *SMN* plus the human *SMN2* transgene developed a phenotype depending on the number of *SMN2* transgenes (98). Mutant mice deficient in SMN, which carry a low copy number of *SMN2*, developed a severe phenotype leading to death either in utero or in the first days after birth (98). At end-stage, these mice displayed motor defect associated with a moderate loss of motor neurons in the spinal cord (98). On the other hand, mutant mice deficient in SMN, which carry a high copy number of the *SMN2* transgene had almost no phenotypic abnormality (98). These studies demonstrate that *SMN2* is able to prevent the embryonic lethality of *SMN* deficiency and that an increased copy number of *SMN2* reduced the severity of the disease phenotype.

Thus far, this mouse model has not been used very often, but recently it was reported that intra-muscular injections of an adenoviral vector expressing cardiotrophin-1 succeeded in delaying motor defect in these mutant mice (99). This result supports the suitability of this mouse model to search for effective neuroprotective agents for SMA.

In addition, exon 7 of *SMN* is the most frequent mutation found in SMA patients. Another mouse line carrying two loxP sequences flanking *SMN* exon 7 (*SMNF7*) has been established through homologous recombination. Neuronal Cre-mediated deletion of *SMN* exon 7 mice displayed severe motor defect leading to complete paralysis and death at a mean age of 4 weeks associated with severe muscle denervation (100,101). This observation supports the cell-autonomous nature of *SMN*-related toxicity.

Mutations Causing Motor Neuron Disease of Unknown Pathogenic Significance in Human Paralytic Diseases

In the last few years, the number of transgenic lines developed to examine the effects of all sorts of genes or gene mutations has increased exponentially. From time to time some of these mutant animals unexpectedly develop abnormalities of the nervous system including spinal cord motor neuron degeneration. The actual link between the gene alterations leading to the death of motor neurons in these animals and the etiopathogenesis of motor neuron diseases such as SMA and ALS is unknown. Nevertheless, it is still worth studying these serendipitous models, as they can teach us useful things about the mechanism of neuronal death.

Vascular Endothelial Growth Factor Knockout Mice

Vascular endothelial growth factor (VEGF) a hypoxia-inducible, angiogenesis-promoting protein, is implicated in tumor growth and revascularization of ischemic tissues. Presumably, VEGF inhibits the production of reactive oxidative species, reduces glutamate excitotoxicity in cultured hippocampal neurons, and modulates the apoptotic machinery. Homozygous VEGF-null mice produced by deleting the hypoxia-response element from the VEGF promoter developed a syndrome resembling ALS (102). This was manifested by limb weakness, neurogenic muscle atrophy, electrophysiological evidence of muscle denervation and reinnervation, and loss of motor neurons from the anterior horn of the spinal cord and brainstem (102). The transfer of this VEGF null mutation in transgenic $SOD1^{G93A}$ mice greatly exacerbated the ALS-like phenotype (103). Conversely, a single injection of a VEGF-expressing lentiviral vector into various muscles of transgenic $SOD1^{G93A}$ mice did delayed onset and slowed progression of symptoms in these mice (104). These findings indicate that while VEGF mutations are not known to be associated with any form of motor neuron disease in humans, VEGF appears to be a critical factor to motor neuron survival. In keeping with this view, it would be important to determine if VEGF supplementation is beneficial to transgenic mutant SOD1 mice or to patients with ALS.

Transgenic Tau Mice

Filamentous Tau aggregates are hallmarks of tauopathies including frontotemporal dementia with parkinsonism linked to mutations in chromosome 17 (FTDP-17) and ALS/parkinsonism–dementia complex (ALS/PDC). Transgenic mice expressing the smallest Tau protein isoform, specifically in neurons, showed weakness and age-dependent brain pathology similar to FTDP-17 and ALS/PDC (105). These transgenic mice developed axonal degeneration in the brain and spinal cord associated with insoluble, hyperphosphorylated Tau, and argyrophilic intraneuronal inclusions formed by Tau-immunoreactive filaments (105). Interestingly, when these transgenic mice were crossed with mutant mice deficient in NF-L, there was a dramatic decrease in the total number of Tau-positive spheroids in the spinal cord and brainstem (106). These combined mutant mice showed delayed accumulation of insoluble Tau protein, increased viability, reduced weight loss, and improved behavioral phenotype when compared with the plain transgenic Tau mice (106).

A transgenic line specifically expressing not the smallest but the longest isoform of human Tau protein in the neurons developed axonal degeneration in the brain and spinal cord. The line also developed astrocytosis and ubiquitinated protein accumulation without the formation of intraneuronal neurofibrillary tangles (107).

Mutant Mice Deficient in Ciliary Neurotrophic Factor

Ciliary neurotrophic factor (CNTF) plays an important role in the maintenance and regeneration of the adult nervous system. It prolongs neuronal survival in various culture systems and also improves survival in the *pmn* and wobbler mutant mouse models of motor neuron disease (108). Inactivation of the *CNTF* gene leads to a loss of 15% to 20% of the motor neurons in postnatal mice (109). This loss appears well tolerated, and, despite a mild reduction of muscle strength, the mice appear healthy and reach normal age in the absence of any signs of motor neuron disease. In the human *CNTF* gene, a guanine to adenine substitution in the splice acceptor site of exon 2 has been described, resulting in a truncated protein without biological activity.

This homozygous mutation is found at a similar frequency of 2% in both healthy individuals and in patients with neurological disorders (110). Giess et al. (111) have crossed transgenic SOD1^{G93A} mice with *CNTF*-deficient animals. They found that by nullifying CNTF, transgenic SOD1^{G93A} mice exhibited an earlier symptom onset, but not a shortened disease duration (111). This finding supports *CNTF* in a role of disease-modifying gene in familial ALS linked to SOD1 mutations. However, there was no difference in age of onset, clinical presentation, rate of progression, or disease duration in ALS patients carrying one or two copies of the *CNTF* null allele (112), casting doubt about the signifance of CNTF in human sporadic ALS.

MODELS OF MOTOR NEURON DISEASE DUE TO NEUROTOXINS

Toxins of various chemical structures and modes of action have been used for a long time to kill neurons and to try to recapitulate the neuropathological hallmarks of prominent neurological diseases. Motor neuron diseases do not escape the list of neurological disorders that are modeled by neurotoxins. Moreover, the enthusiasm for the use of neurotoxins to produce motor neuron degeneration stems also from the fact that according to some authorities in the field, certain forms of ALS may have a toxic etiology.

β,β'-Iminodipropionitrile (IDPN)

β,β'-IDPN causes hyperactivity in rodents characterized by the "waltzing" (continuous circling and head rolling) syndrome and progressive paralysis. Arrays of abnormally oriented NF accumulate in spheroids and, to a lesser extent, in cell bodies (113). Swollen axons are filled with SOD1-immunoreactive material (114). The spheroids are denuded of myelin and distal axons become atrophic, resembling the alterations seen in both sporadic and familial ALS. Proximal axons show swelling that also resembles that seen in ALS. β, β'-IDPN is thought to impair the slow transportation of NF proteins, perhaps because the toxin dissociates NF from microtubules (115).

Cycad Seed Products (Cycas Circinals)

For more than 150 years, Chamorro natives of the Mariana Islands in the Western Pacific Ocean have developed fatal paralysis in middle and later life. The causes of which might be exposure to seeds of the indigenous cycad and presumably the motor pathway alterations might be due to ingestion of the cycad neurotoxin, β-*N*-methylamino-L-alanine (BMAA). However, recent studies identified the most toxic types of molecules contained in washed cycad as a sterol glucoside whose actions in vitro included the excitotoxic release of glutamate and an abnormal increase in the activity of various protein kinases (116). In addition, the mice that were fed with washed cycad flour had a temporal sequence of behavioral deficits that correlated with neural death in appropriate regions of the CNS including spinal cord motor neurons (117). Readers interested in this question will find an in-depth review of the topic and most recent experimental data about the cycad-related neurotoxicity in the chapter written by Dr. Shaw and collaborators in this book.

Aluminum

Administration of aluminum salts caused accumulations of NF in perikarya and proximal processes of nerve cells, including motor neurons (118). Local intraparenchymal administration of aluminum chloride at the level of hypoglossal neurons induced the formation of neurofibrillary change in 90% to 100% of the rabbit hypoglossal neurons (119). Chronic repeated injections of aluminum results in signs of chronic myelopathy with widespread argentophilic inclusions in cell bodies and axons that are morphologically reminiscent to what is seen in ALS (120). Ubiquitin-positive, skein-like inclusions occurred in spinal cord motor neurons and are diffusely distributed in non-motor neurons in the brainstem of these aluminum-treated animals. The distribution of the affected area is mainly upper motor neurons in this model (120). Recent studies show that aluminum inhibits the normal dephosphorylation-dependent reversal of NF-H, which indicates post-translational abnormalities of NF processing and impaired slow axonal transport in the animal models (121). In another study, a chronic aluminum exposure in rats was reported as causing motor neuron degeneration, neurofibrillary tangle formation, chromatolysis, and abnormal localization of the nuclei in swollen perikarya (122). Although more studies are probably needed to better characterize the effects of aluminum on the motor pathway, the data summarized above indicate that a chronic exposure to this metal may well represent a toxic means to produce a form of motor neuron disease somewhat reminiscent of ALS.

IMMUNE-MEDIATED MODELS OF MOTOR NEURON DISEASES

Experimental allergic motor neuron disease (EAMND) is a motor neuron syndrome induced in guinea pigs by the inoculation of purified bovine motor neurons with Freund's adjuvant (123). These animals developed weight loss, sluggish movement, limb weakness, and foot drop. Electromyography showed a decreased number of firing motor units, but not fibrillation potentials. Pathologic studies showed group atrophy and fiber type grouping consistent with chronic neurogenic muscle atrophy. Anterior horn cell loss and neurophagia are seen in the spinal cord. Experimental autoimmune gray matter disease (EAGMD) is a more acute disorder involving lower and upper motor neurons induced in guinea pigs by the inoculation of spinal cord ventral horn homogenates (124). EAGMD is clinically characterized by the relatively rapid onset of weakness (two weeks after second immunization) as well as bulbar signs. Pathological studies revealed loss of large pyramidal cells in the motor cortex, as well as spinal cord motor neurons.

INFECTION-MEDIATED MODELS OF MOTOR NEURON DISEASES

Viral infection has been one of the oldest hypotheses to explain the cause of ALS. As a result of poliovirus infection in neurons in the anterior horn of the spinal cord, motor cortex, and brainstem, severe paralytic or, less frequently, fatal disease occurs that mimics ALS. Direct inoculation of the poliovirus into mouse brains causes poliomyelitis (125,126). Most poliovirus strains infect only primates, and thus monkeys have been used for an experimental animal model (127). The transgenic mouse carrying the human poliovirus receptor gene was susceptible to poliovirus and showed paralytic disease (128,129).

In contrast to the poliovirus, several retroviruses do infect mice and cause hind-limb paralysis in these animals (130,131). The neonatal mouse inoculated with a murine leukemia virus showed hindlimb paralysis within four weeks of inoculation. A marked spongy degeneration occurs in endothelial and glial cells but not in neurons. Inflammation is not seen. Neuronal degeneration appears to be indirect and not the result of neuron infection. The viral infection perhaps blocks neurotrophic receptor sites (132).

Sindbis virus is an alphavirus that causes acute encephalomyelitis in mice. A neuro-adapted strain of the Sindbis virus causes severe, often fatal encephalomyelitis in adult animals that is accompanied by prominent hindlimb paralysis (133). Pathological studies revealed neuronal changes such as hyperchromatism and chromatolysis and were most striking in the ventral horns of the thoracic and lumbar cord. Glial changes and mononuclear cell infiltration were present. Motor neurons degenerated without features typical of apoptosis (134). A recent study has used Sindbis virus-infected rats as recipients of neuronal-differentiated stem cells grafted into spinal cords (135), thus demonstrating the usefulness of this model for investigations geared toward assessing repair strategies.

CONCLUSION

It is quite clear that motor neurons, especially lower motor neurons, degenerate in a variety of paralytic human diseases in response to a host of distinct etiological factors. As we have tried to illustrate in this chapter, investigators currently have in hand a full panoply of experimental models, primarily produced in rodents, that can be utilized to search for the intimate cellular and molecular mechanisms implicated in the demise of motor neurons. Of these, some have also been used to preclinically test new drugs with potential neuroprotective actions. Although in the past, the wobbler or the *pmn* mouse models were often used for that purpose, now it is fair to say that transgenic rodents expressing human mutant SOD1 have received the lion's share of attention. It is important, however, to remember that none of the models described above is a true copy of any human disease, even if it is very close. Furthermore, it is our opinion that among the "good" models of motor neuron diseases, none must be considered consistently as the best model, as all are frowned on with some glaring imperfections from the human disease they are supposed to mimic. It is thus crucial for the investigator to be aware of the shortcomings of each of the different models and to select the one most suitable among these on the basis of the experimental question to be tested. Despite all these precautions, it remains to be established what are the actual predictive values of many if not all of these models.

Retrospectively, it seems that many of these experimental models, especially the transgenic rodents expressing human mutant SOD1, have been quite valuable in shedding light onto the pathogenic mechanism underlying the death of motor neurons. It is undeniable that, thanks to these models, we now have a much better understanding of the different factors that compose the pathogenic cascade in ALS and, to a lesser extent, in SMA, as well as in which sequence these factors are acting within the pathogenic cascade. On the other hand, it is too early to have a real feel about how good these models are in predicting whether interventions with protective activities in animals will turn out to be effective in humans with motor neuron diseases. Perhaps one central problem in the use of these experimental models is to determine whether the human conditions they model are homogeneous diseases or heterogeneous syndromes. For instance, investigators who use transgenic animals that express mutant SOD1 to study ALS assume that any pathogenic mechanism found in this model is de facto relevant to all other forms of ALS, including the large and probably mixed group of sporadic cases which is, of course, unknown. Nevertheless, while waiting to resolve these important issues, it is our position to continue to use these rodent models to screen and test putative neuroprotective agents prior to embarking on human clinical trials.

Apart from the debate on the validity of experimental models, the success of translating research efforts is also related to the need to pay attention to the pharmacology and pharmacokinetics of selected drugs before embarking on their testing in humans. Indeed, often the protocol of drug administration used in clinical trial is a direct translation from that previously used in animals. This is an aberration, as, unless proven otherwise, one cannot assume that the pharmacology of a given drug characterized in mice is the same in humans. Furthermore, almost all published mouse studies began the administration of the drug under investigation in pre-symptomatic animals, while in clinical trials we are only able to treat patients when they already have symptoms. Thus, maybe drugs that continue to be effective in animals that are more advanced in the clinical course, which probably would better mimic the situation encountered in patients with motor neuron diseases, should be our prime candidates for clinical trial testing.

In light of the above discussion, it is our opinion that future directions in motor neuron modeling would primarily establish the predictive values of popular models such as transgenic animals expressing mutant SOD1, both with respect to pathogenesis and experimental therapies. In response of the growing number of laboratories involved in pre-clinical testing of new therapies, standardization of experimental designs, and protocols may emerge as a central issue if the community wishes to be able to compare and explain some inevitable discrepancies among studies. Finally, pre-clinical studies using animal models may be rendered more efficient by using high-throughput techniques, as discussed by Henderson and collaborators in this book, to identify in a short period of time the most promising compounds for subsequent animal model testing.

ACKNOWLEDGMENTS

The authors wish to thank Mr. Matthew Lucas for his assistance in preparing the manuscript. The authors are supported by NIH/NINDS Grants RO1 NS38586 and NS42269, P50 NS38370, and P01 NS11766–27A2, the US Department of Defense Grant (DAMD 17-99-1-9474 and DAMD 17-03-1), the Parkinson Disease Foundation (New York, USA), the Lowenstein Foundation, the Lillian Goldman Charitable Trust, the MDA, and the Wings Over Wall Street. Dr. Nagai is a recipient of the David A. Gardner Neuromuscular Research Fellowship from the MDA.

REFERENCES

1. Duchen LW, Strich SJ. An hereditary motor neurone disease with progressive denervation of muscle in the mouse: the mutant "wobbler." J Neurol Neurosurg Psychiat 1968; 31:535–542.

2. Kaupmann K, Simon-Chazottes D, Guenet JL, Jockusch H. Wobbler, a mutation affecting motoneuron survival and gonadal functions in the mouse, maps to proximal chromosome 11. Genomics 1992; 13:39–43.

3. Des Portes V, Coulpier M, Melki J, Dreyfus PA. Early detection of mouse wobbler mutation: a model of pathological motoneurone death. Neuroreport 1994; 5:1861–1864.

4. Baulac M, Rieger F, Meininger V. The loss of motorneurons corresponding to specific muscles in the wobbler mutant mouse. Neurosci Lett 1983; 37:99–104.

5. Mitsumoto H, Bradley WG. Murine motor neuron disease (the wobbler mouse): degeneration and regeneration of the lower motor neuron. Brain 1982; 105(pt 4):811–834.

6. Hantaz-Ambroise D, Blondet B, Murawsky M, Rieger F. Abnormal astrocyte differentiation and defective cellular interactions in wobbler mouse spinal cord. J Neurocytol 1994; 23:179–192.

7. Rathke-Hartlieb S, Schmidt VC, Jockusch H, Schmitt-John T, Bartsch JW. Spatiotemporal progression of neurodegeneration and glia activation in the wobbler neuropathy of the mouse. Neuroreport 1999; 10:3411–3416.

8. Popper P, Farber DB, Micevych PE, Minoofar K, Bronstein JM. TRPM-2 Expression and tunel staining in neurodegenerative diseases: studies in wobbler and rd mice. Exp Neurol 1997; 143:246–254.

9. Blondet B, Ait-Ikhlef A, Murawsky M, Rieger F. Transient massive DNA fragmentation in nervous system during the early course of a murine neurodegenerative disease. Neurosci Lett 2001; 305:202–206.

10. Mitsumoto H, Ikeda K, Klinkosz B, Cedarbaum JM, Wong V, Lindsay RM. Arrest of motor neuron disease in wobbler mice cotreated with CNTF and BDNF. Science 1994; 265:1107–1110.

11. Ikeda K, Wong V, Holmlund TH, Greene T, Cedarbaum JM, Lindsay RM, Mitsumoto H. Histometric effects of ciliary neurotrophic factor in wobbler mouse motor neuron disease. Ann Neurol 1995; 37:47–54.

12. Henderson JT, Javaheri M, Kopko S, Roder JC. Reduction of lower motor neuron degeneration in wobbler mice by N-acetyl-L-cysteine. J Neurosci 1996; 16:7574–7582.

13. Ikeda K, Iwasaki Y, Kinoshita M. Neuronal nitric oxide synthase inhibitor, 7-nitroindazole, delays motor dysfunction and spinal motoneuron degeneration in the wobbler mouse. J Neurol Sci 1998; 160:9–15.

14. Dave KR, Prado R, Busto R, Raval AP, Bradley WG, Torbati D, Perez-Pinzon MA. Hyperbaric oxygen therapy protects against mitochondrial dysfunction and delays onset of motor neuron disease in Wobbler mice. Neuroscience 2003; 120:113–120.

15. Gonzalez Deniselle MC, Lopez-Costa JJ, Saavedra JP, Pietranera L, Gonzalez SL, Garay L, Guennoun R, Schumacher M, De Nicola AF. Progesterone neuroprotection in the Wobbler mouse, a genetic model of spinal cord motor neuron disease. Neurobiol Dis 2002; 11:457–468.

16. Schmalbruch H, Jensen HJ, Bjaerg M, Kamieniecka Z, Kurland L. A new mouse mutant with progressive motor neuronopathy. J Neuropathol Exp Neurol 1991; 50:192–204.

17. Sagot Y, Rosse T, Vejsada R, Perrelet D, Kato AC. Differential effects of neurotrophic factors on motoneuron retrograde labeling in a murine model of motoneuron disease. J Neurosci 1998; 18:1132–1141.

18. Brunialti AL, Poirier C, Schmalbruch H, Guenet JL. The mouse mutation progressive motor neuronopathy (PMN) maps to chromosome 13. Genomics 1995; 29:131–135.

19. Martin N, Jaubert J, Gounon P, Salido E, Haase G, Szatanik M, Guenet JL. A missense mutation in Tbce causes progressive motor neuronopathy in mice. Nat Genet 2002; 32:443–447.

20. Bommel H, Xie G, Rossoll W, Wiese S, Jablonka S, Boehm T, Sendtner M. Missense mutation in the tubulin-specific chaperone E (*Tbce*) gene in the mouse mutant progressive motor neuronopathy, a model of human motoneuron disease. J Cell Biochem 2002; 159:563–569.

21. Sagot Y, Dubois-Dauphin M, Tan SA, De Bilbao F, Aebischer P, Martinou J-C, Kato AC. Bcl-2 overexpression prevents motoneuron cell body loss but not axonal degeneration in a mouse model of a neurodegenerative disease. J Neurosci 1995; 15:7727–7733.

22. Sagot Y, Tan SA, Hammang JP, Aebischer P, Kato AC. GDNF Slows loss of motoneurons but not axonal degeneration or premature death of PMN/PMN mice. J Neurosci 1996; 16:2335–2341.

23. Raff MC, Whitmore AV, Finn JT. Axonal self-destruction and neurodegeneration. Science 2002; 296:868–871.

24. Coleman MP, Conforti L, Buckmaster EA, Tarlton A, Ewing RM, Brown MC, Lyon MF, Perry VH. An 85-kb tandem triplication in the slow Wallerian degeneration (Wlds) mouse. Proc Natl Acad Sci USA 1998; 95:9985–9990.

25. Ferri A, Sanes JR, Coleman MP, Cunningham JM, Kato AC. Inhibiting axon degeneration and synapse loss attenuates apoptosis and disease progression in a mouse model of motoneuron disease. Curr Biol 2003; 13:669–673.

26. Messer A, Flaherty L. Autosomal dominance in a late-onset motor neuron disease in the mouse. J Neurogenet 1986; 3:345–355.

27. Messer A, Plummer J, Maskin P, Coffin JM, Frankel WN. Mapping of the motor neuron degeneration (*MND*) gene, a mouse model of amyotrophic lateral sclerosis (ALS). Genomics 1992; 13:797–802.

28. Ranta S, Zhang Y, Ross B, Lonka L, Takkunen E, Messer A, Sharp J, Wheeler R, Kusumi K, Mole S, et al. The neuronal ceroid lipofuscinoses in human EPMR and mnd mutant mice are associated with mutations in CLN8. Nat Genet 1999; 23: 233–236

29. Hirvasniemi A, Lang H, Lehesjoki AE, Leisti J. Northern epilepsy syndrome: an inherited childhood onset epilepsy with associated mental deterioration. J Med Genet 1994; 31:177–182.

30. Messer A, Plummer J, MacMillen MC, Frankel WN. Genetics of primary and timing effects in the mnd mouse. Am J Med Genet 1995; 57:361–364.

31. Messer A, Strominger NL, Mazurkiewicz JE. Histopathology of the late-onset motor neuron degeneration (MND) mutant in the mouse. J Neurogenet 1987; 4:201–213.

32. Mazurkiewicz JE, Callahan LM, Swash M, Martin JE, Messer A. Cytoplasmic inclusions in spinal neurons of the motor neuron degeneration (MND) mouse. I. Light microscopic analysis. J Neurol Sci 1993; 116:59–66.

33. Pardo CA, Rabin BA, Palmer DN, Price DL. Accumulation of the adenosine triphosphate synthase subunit C in the MND mutant mouse. A model for neuronal ceroid lipofuscinosis. Am J Pathol 1994; 144:829–835.

34. Messer A, Plummer J. Accumulating autofluorescent material as a marker for early changes in the spinal cord of the MND mouse. Neuromusc Disord 1993; 3:129–134.

35. Bronson RT, Lake BD, Cook S, Taylor S, Davisson MT. Motor neuron degeneration of mice is a model of neuronal ceroid lipofuscinosis (Batten's disease). Ann Neurol 1993; 33:381–385.

36. Jones JM, Albin RL, Feldman EL, Simin K, Schuster TG, Dunnick WA, Collins JT, Chrisp CE, Taylor BA, Meisler MH. MND-2: a new mouse model of inherited motor neuron disease. Genomics 1993; 16:669–677.

37. Rathke-Hartlieb S, Schlomann U, Heimann P, Meisler MH, Jockusch H, Bartsch JW. Progressive loss of striatal neurons causes motor dysfunction in MND-2 mutant mice and is not prevented by Bcl-2. Exp Neurol 2002; 175:87–97.

38. Weber JS, Jang W, Simin K, Lu W, Yu J, Meisler MH. High-resolution genetic, physical, and transcript map of the MND-2 region of mouse chromosome 6. Genomics 1998; 54:107–115.

39. Jones JM, Datta P, Srinivasula SM, Ji W, Gupta S, Zhang Z, Davies E, Hajnoczky G, Saunders TL, Van Keuren ML, et al. Loss of Omi mitochondrial protease activity causes the neuromuscular disorder of MND-2 mutant mice. Nature 2003; 425:721–727.

40. Cork LC, Griffin JW, Munnell JF, Lorenz MD, Adams RJ. Hereditary canine spinal muscular atrophy. J Neuropathol Exp Neurol 1979; 38:209–221.

41. Sack GH Jr, Cork LC, Morris JM, Griffin JW, Price DL. Autosomal dominant inheritance of hereditary canine spinal muscular atrophy. Ann Neurol 1984; 15:369–373.

42. Cork LC, Griffin JW, Choy C, Padula CA, Price DL. Pathology of motor neurons in accelerated hereditary canine spinal muscular atrophy. Lab Invest 1982; 46:89–99.

43. Divers TJ, Mohammed HO, Cummings JF. Equine motor neuron disease. Vet Clin North Am Equine Pract 1997; 13:97–105.

44. Weber PE, King JM, Cummings JF, de Lahunta A, Divers TJ, Mohammed HO. Quantitative assessment of motor neuron loss in equine motor neuron disease (EMND). Equine Vet J 1998; 30:256–259.

45. Gurney ME, Pu H, Chiu AY, Dal Canto MC, Polchow CY, Alexander DD, Caliendo J, Hentati A, Kwon YW, Deng H-X, et al. Motor neuron degeneration in mice that express a human Cu, Zn superoxide dismutase mutation. Science 1994; 264:1772–1775.

46. Ripps ME, Huntley GW, Hof PR, Morrison JH, Gordon JW. Transgenic mice expressing an altered murine superoxide dismutase gene provide an animal model of amyotrophic lateral sclerosis. Proc Natl Acad Sci USA 1995; 92:689–693.

47. Wong PC, Pardo CA, Borchelt DR, Lee MK, Copeland NG, Jenkins NA, Sisodia SS, Cleveland DW, Price DL. An adverse property of a familial ALS-linked SOD1 mutation causes motor neuron disease characterized by vacuolar degeneration of mitochondria. Neuron 1995; 14:1105–1116.

48. Bruijn LI, Becher MW, Lee MK, Anderson KL, Jenkins NA, Copeland NG, Sisodia S, Rothstein JD, Borchelt DR, Price DL, et al. ALS-Linked SOD1 mutant G85R mediated damage to astrocytes and promotes rapidly progressive disease with SOD1-containing inclusions. Neuron 1997; 18:327–338.

49. Nagai M, Aoki M, Miyoshi I, Kato M, Pasinelli P, Kasai N, Brown RH Jr, Itoyama Y. Rats expressing human cytosolic copper-zinc superoxide dismutase transgenes with amyotrophic lateral sclerosis: associated mutations develop motor neuron disease. J Neurosci 2001; 21:9246–9254.

50. Howland DS, Liu J, She Y, Goad B, Maragakis NJ, Kim B, Erickson J, Kulik J, DeVito L, Psaltis, et al. Focal loss of the glutamate transporter EAAT2 in a transgenic rat model of SOD1 mutant-mediated amyotrophic lateral sclerosis (ALS). Proc Natl Acad Sci USA 2002; 99:1604–1609.

51. Cudkowicz ME, McKenna-Yasek D, Sapp PE, Chin W, Geller B, Hayden DL, Schoenfeld DA, Hosler BA, Horvitz HR, Brown RH. Epidemiology of mutations in superoxide dismutase in amyotrophic lateral sclerosis. Ann Neurol 1997; 41:210–221.

52. Subramaniam JR, Lyons WE, Liu J, Bartnikas TB, Rothstein J, Price DL, Cleveland DW, Gitlin JD, Wong PC. Mutant SOD1 causes motor neuron disease independent of copper chaperone-mediated copper loading. Nat Neurosci 2002; 5:301–307.

53. Wang J, Slunt H, Gonzales V, Fromholt D, Coonfield M, Copeland NG, Jenkins NA, Borchelt DR. Copper-binding-site-null SOD1 causes ALS in transgenic mice: aggregates of non-native SOD1 delineate a common feature. Hum Mol Genet 2003; 12:2753–2764.

54. Chiu AY, Zhai P, Dal Canto MC, Peters T, Kwon YH, Prattis SM, Gurney ME. Age-dependent penetrance of disease in a transgenic mouse model of familial amyotrophic lateral sclerosis. Mol Cell Neurosci 1995; 6:349–362.

55. Dal Canto MC, Gurney ME. Neuropathological changes in two lines of mice carrying a transgene for mutant human Cu, Zn SOD, and in mice overexpressing wild type human SOD: a model of familial amyotrophic lateral sclerosis (FALS). Brain Res 1995; 676:25–40.

56. Barneoud P, Lolivier J, Sanger DJ, Scatton B, Moser P. Quantitative motor assessment in FALS mice: a longitudinal study. Neuroreport 1997; 8:2861–2865.

57. Dal Canto MC, Gurney ME. A low expressor line of transgenic mice carrying a mutant human Cu, Zn superoxide dismutase (SOD1) gene develops pathological changes that

most closely resemble those in human amyotrophic lateral sclerosis. Acta Neuropathol (Berl) 1997; 93:537–550.

58. Kong J, Xu Z. Massive mitochondrial degeneration in motor neurons triggers the onset of amyotrophic lateral sclerosis in mice expressing a mutant SOD1. J Neurosci 1998; 18:3241–3250.

59. Jaarsma D, Rognoni F, van Duijn W, Verspaget HW, Haasdijk ED, Holstege JC. CuZn superoxide dismutase (SOD1) accumulates in vacuolated mitochondria in transgenic mice expressing amyotrophic lateral sclerosis-linked SOD1 mutations. Acta Neuropathol (Berl) 2001; 102:293–305.

60. Higgins CM, Jung C, Ding H, Xu Z. Mutant Cu, Zn superoxide dismutase that causes motoneuron degeneration is present in mitochondria in the CNS. J Neurosci 2002; 22:RC215.

61. Wang J, Xu G, Gonzales V, Coonfield M, Fromholt D, Copeland NG, Jenkins NA, Borchelt DR. Fibrillar inclusions and motor neuron degeneration in transgenic mice expressing superoxide dismutase 1 with a disrupted copper-binding site. Neurobiol Dis 2002; 10:128–138.

62. Johnston JA, Dalton MJ, Gurney ME, Kopito RR. Formation of high molecular weight complexes of mutant Cu, Zn-superoxide dismutase in a mouse model for familial amyotrophic lateral sclerosis. Proc Natl Acad Sci USA 2000; 97:12571–12576.

63. Shibata N, Hirano A, Kobayashi M, Dal Canto MC, Gurney ME, Komori T, Umahara T, Asayama K. Presence of Cu/Zn superoxide dismutase (SOD) immunoreactivity in neuronal hyaline inclusions in spinal cords from mice carrying a transgene for Gly93Ala mutant human Cu/Zn SOD. Acta Neuropathol (Berl) 1998; 95:136–142.

64. Tu PH, Raju P, Robinson KA, Gurney ME, Trojanowski JQ, Lee VMY. Transgenic mice carrying a human mutant superoxide dismutase transgene develop neuronal cytoskeletal pathology resembling human amyotrophic lateral sclerosis lesions. Proc Natl Acad Sci USA 1996; 93:3155–3160.

65. Mourelatos Z, Gonatas NK, Stieber A, Gurney ME, Dal Canto MC. The Golgi apparatus of spinal cord motor neurons in transgenic mice expressing mutant Cu, Zn superoxide dismutase becomes fragmented in early, preclinical stages of the disease. Proc Natl Acad Sci USA 1996; 93:5472–5477.

66. Stieber A, Gonatas JO, Gonatas NK. Aggregation of ubiquitin and a mutant ALS-linked SOD1 protein correlate with disease progression and fragmentation of the Golgi apparatus. J Neurol Sci 2000; 173:53–62.

67. Almer G, Vukosavic S, Romero N, Przedborski S. Inducible nitric oxide synthase upregulation in a transgenic mouse model of familial amyotrophic lateral sclerosis. J Neurochem 1999; 72:2415–2425.

68. Kostic V, Gurney ME, Deng H-X, Siddique T, Epstein CJ, Przedborski S. Midbrain dopaminergic neuronal degeneration in a transgenic mouse model of familial amyotrophic lateral sclerosis. Ann Neurol 1997; 41:497–504.

69. Przedborski S. Molecular targets for neuroprotection. ALS and other MNDs 2004; ; 5(suppl 1):1–5.

70. Pramatarova A, Laganiere J, Roussel J, Brisebois K, Rouleau GA. Neuron-specific expression of mutant superoxide dismutase 1 in transgenic mice does not lead to motor impairment. J Neurosci 2001; 21:3369–3374.

71. Caroni P. Overexpression of growth-associated proteins in the neurons of adult transgenic mice. J Neurosci Meth 1997; 71:3–9.

72. Lino MM, Schneider C, Caroni P. Accumulation of SOD1 mutants in postnatal motoneurons does not cause motoneuron pathology or motoneuron disease. J Neurosci 2002; 22:4825–4832.

73. Gong YH, Parsadanian AS, Andreeva A, Snider WD, Elliott JL. Restricted expression of G86R Cu/Zn superoxide dismutase in astrocytes results in astrocytosis but does not cause motoneuron degeneration. J Neurosci 2000; 20:660–665.

74. Rouleau GA, Clark AW, Rooke K, Pramatarova A, Krizus A, Suchowersky O, Julien JP, Figlewicz D. SOD1 mutation is associated with accumulation of neurofilaments in amyotrophic lateral sclerosis. Ann Neurol 1996; 39:128–131.
75. Robertson J, Kriz J, Nguyen MD, Julien JP. Pathways to motor neuron degeneration in transgenic mouse models. Biochimie 2002; 84:1151–1160.
76. Zhu Q, Couillard-Despres S, Julien JP. Delayed maturation of regenerating myelinated axons in mice lacking neurofilaments. Exp Neurol 1997; 148:299–316.
77. Elder GA, Friedrich VL Jr, Bosco P, Kang C, Gourov A, Tu PH, Lee VM, Lazzarini RA. Absence of the mid-sized neurofilament subunit decreases axonal calibers, levels of light neurofilament (NF-L), and neurofilament content. J Cell Biochem 1998; 141:727–739.
78. Jacomy H, Zhu Q, Couillard-Despres S, Beaulieu JM, Julien JP. Disruption of type IV intermediate filament network in mice lacking the neurofilament medium and heavy subunits. J Neurochem 1999; 73:972–984.
79. Williamson TL, Bruijn LI, Zhu Q, Anderson KL, Anderson SD, Julien JP, Cleveland DW. Absence of neurofilaments reduces the selective vulnerability of motor neurons and slows disease caused by a familial amyotrophic lateral sclerosis-linked superoxide dismutase 1 mutant. Proc Natl Acad Sci USA 1998; 95:9631–9636.
80. Collard JF, Cote F, Julien JP. Defective axonal transport in a transgenic mouse model of amyotrophic lateral sclerosis. Nature 1995; 375:6561–6564.
81. Beaulieu JM, Jacomy H, Julien JP. Formation of intermediate filament protein aggregates with disparate effects in two transgenic mouse models lacking the neurofilament light subunit. J Neurosci 2000; 20:5321–5328.
82. Couillard-Despres S, Zhu Q, Wong PC, Price DL, Cleveland DW, Julien JP. Protective effect of neurofilament heavy gene overexpression in motor neuron disease induced by mutant superoxide dismutase. Proc Natl Acad Sci USA 1998; 95:9626–9630.
83. Xu Z, Cork LC, Griffin JW, Cleveland DW. Increased expression of neurofilament subunit NF-L produces morphological alterations that resemble the pathology of human motor neuron disease. Cell 1993; 73:23–33.
84. Lee MK, Marszalek JR, Cleveland DW. A mutant neurofilament subunit causes massive, selective motor neuron death: implications for the pathogenesis of human motor neuron disease. Neuron 1994; 13:975–988.
85. He CZ, Hays AP. Expression of peripherin in ubiquinated inclusions of amyotrophic lateral sclerosis. J Neurol Sci 2004; 217:47–54.
86. Gros-Louis F, Lariviere R, Gowing G, Laurent S, Camu W, Bouchard JP, Meininger V, Rouleau GA, Julien JPA frameshift deletion in peripherin gene associated with amyotrophic lateral sclerosis. J Biol Chem 2004; 279(44):45951–45956.
87. Leung LC, He CZ, Kaufmann P, Chin SS, Naini A, Liem RKH, Mitsumoto H, Hays AP. A pathogenic peripherin gene mutation in a patient with amyotrophic lateral sclerosis. Brain Pathol 2004; 14:290–296.
88. Brody BA, Ley CA, Parysek LM. Selective distribution of the 57 kDa neural intermediate filament protein in the rat CNS. J Neurosci 1989; 9:2391–2401.
89. Parysek LM, Goldman RD. Distribution of a novel 57 kDa intermediate filament (IF) protein in the nervous system. J Neurosci 1988; 8:555–563.
90. Beaulieu JM, Nguyen MD, Julien JP. Late onset death of motor neurons in mice overexpressing wild-type peripherin. J Cell Biol 1999; 147:531–544.
91. Beaulieu JM, Julien JP. Peripherin-mediated death of motor neurons rescued by overexpression of neurofilament NF-H proteins. J Neurochem 2003; 85:248–256.
92. Robertson J, Doroudchi MM, Nguyen MD, Durham HD, Strong MJ, Shaw G, Julien JP, Mushynski WE. A neurotoxic peripherin splice variant in a mouse model of ALS. J Cell Biol 2003; 160:939–949.
93. Lariviere RC, Beaulieu JM, Nguyen MD, Julien JP. Peripherin is not a contributing factor to motor neuron disease in a mouse model of amyotrophic lateral sclerosis caused by mutant superoxide dismutase. Neurobiol Dis 2003; 13:158–166.

94. Hirokawa N, Sato-Yoshitake R, Yoshida T, Kawashima T. Brain dynein (MAP1C) localizes on both anterogradely and retrogradely transported membranous organelles in vivo. J Cell Biochem 1990; 111:1027–1037.

95. Munch C, Sedlmeier R, Meyer T, Homberg V, Sperfeld AD, Kurt A, Prudlo J, Peraus G, Hanemann CO, Stumm G, Ludolph AC. Point mutations of the p150 subunit of dynactin (DCTN1) gene in ALS. Neurology 2004; 63:724–726.

96. LaMonte BH, Wallace KE, Holloway BA, Shelly SS, Ascano J, Tokito M, Van Winkle T, Howland DS, Holzbaur EL. Disruption of dynein/dynactin inhibits axonal transport in motor neurons causing late-onset progressive degeneration. Neuron 2002; 34: 715–727.

97. Hafezparast M, Klocke R, Ruhrberg C, Marquardt A, Ahmad-Annuar A, Bowen S, Lalli G, Witherden AS, Hummerich H, Nicholson S, et al. Mutations in dynein link motor neuron degeneration to defects in retrograde transport. Science 2003; 300:808–812.

98. Monani UR, Sendtner M, Coovert DD, Parsons DW, Andreassi C, Le TT, Jablonka S, Schrank B, Rossol W, Prior TW, et al. The human centromeric survival motor neuron gene (SMN2) rescues embryonic lethality in SMN(−/−) mice and results in a mouse with spinal muscular atrophy. Hum Mol Genet 2000; 300:333–339.

99. Lesbordes JC, Cifuentes-Diaz C, Miroglio A, Joshi V, Bordet T, Kahn A, Melki J. Therapeutic benefits of cardiotrophin-1 gene transfer in a mouse model of spinal muscular atrophy. Hum Mol Genet 2003; 12:1233–1239.

100. Hsieh-Li HM, Chang JG, Jong YJ, Wu MH, Wang NM, Tsai CH, Li H. A mouse model for spinal muscular atrophy. Nat Genet 2000; 24:66–70.

101. Frugier T, Tiziano FD, Cifuentes-Diaz C, Miniou P, Roblot N, Dierich A, Le Meur M, Melki J. Nuclear targeting defect of SMN lacking the C-terminus in a mouse model of spinal muscular atrophy. Hum Mol Genet 2000; 9:849–858.

102. Oosthuyse B, Moons L, Storkebaum E, Beck H, Nuyens D, Brusselmans K, Van Dorpe J, Hellings P, Gorselink M, Heymans S, et al. Deletion of the hypoxia-response element in the vascular endothelial growth factor promoter causes motor neuron degeneration. Nat Genet 2001; 28:131–138.

103. Lambrechts D, Storkebaum E, Morimoto M, Del Favero J, Desmet F, Marklund SL, Wyns S, Thijs V, Andersson J, van M, et al. VEGF is a modifier of amyotrophic lateral sclerosis in mice and humans and protects motoneurons against ischemic death. Nat Genet 2003; 34:383–394.

104. Azzouz M, Ralph GS, Storkebaum E, Walmsley LE, Mitrophanous KA, Kingsman SM, Carmeliet P, Mazarakis ND. VEGF delivery with retrogradely transported lentivector prolongs survival in a mouse ALS model. Nature 2004; 429:413–417.

105. Ishihara T, Hong M, Zhang B, Nakagawa Y, Lee MK, Trojanowski JQ, Lee VM. Age-dependent emergence and progression of a tauopathy in transgenic mice overexpressing the shortest human tau isoform. Neuron 1999; 24:751–762.

106. Ishihara T, Zhang B, Higuchi M, Yoshiyama Y, Trojanowski JQ, Lee VM. Age-dependent induction of congophilic neurofibrillary tau inclusions in tau transgenic mice. Am J Pathol 2001; 158:555–562.

107. Spittaels K, Van den Haute C, Van Dorpe J, Bruynseels K, Vandezande K, Laenen I, Geerts H, Mercken M, Sciot R, Van Lommel A, et al. Prominent axonopathy in the brain and spinal cord of transgenic mice overexpressing four-repeat human tau protein. Am J Pathol 1999; 155:2153–2165.

108. Mitsumoto H, Ikeda K, Holmlund T, Greene T, Cedarbaum JM, Wong V, Lindsay RM. The effects of ciliary neurotrophic factor on motor dysfunction in wobbler mouse motor neuron disease. Ann Neurol 1994; 36:142–148.

109. Masu Y, Wolf E, Holtmann B, Sendtner M, Brem G, Thoenen H. Disruption of the CNTF gene results in motor neuron degeneration. Nature 1993; 365:27–32.

110. Takahashi R, Yokoji H, Misawa H, Hayashi M, Hu J, Deguchi T. A null mutation in the human CNTF gene is not causally related to neurological diseases. Nat Genet 1994; 7:79–84.

111. Giess R, Holtmann B, Braga M, Grimm T, Muller-Myhsok B, Toyka KV, Sendtner M. Early onset of severe familial amyotrophic lateral sclerosis with a SOD-1 mutation: potential impact of CNTF as a candidate modifier gene. Am J Hum Genet 2002; 70:1277–1286.

112. Al-Chalabi A, Scheffler MD, Smith BN, Parton MJ, Cudkowicz ME, Andersen PM, Hayden DL, Hansen VK, Turner MR, Shaw CE, et al. Ciliary neurotrophic factor genotype does not influence clinical phenotype in amyotrophic lateral sclerosis. Ann Neurol 2003; 54:130–134.

113. Clark AW, Griffin JW, Price DL. The axonal pathology in chronic IDPN intoxication. J Neuropathol Exp Neurol 1980; 39:42–55.

114. Nishiyama K, Kwak S, Murayama S, Watanabe M, Goto J, Asayama K, Kanazawa I. Increased Cu/Zn superoxide dismutase-like immunoreactivity in the swollen axons of rats intoxicated chronically with beta,beta'-iminodipropionitrile. Neurosci Lett 1995; 194:205–208.

115. Griffin JW, Hoffman PN, Clark AW, Carroll PT, Price DL. Slow axonal transport of neurofilament proteins: impairment of beta,beta'-iminodipropionitrile administration. Science 1978; 202:633–635.

116. Khabazian I, Bains JS, Williams DE, Cheung J, Wilson JM, Pasqualotto BA, Pelech SL, Andersen RJ, Wang YT, Liu L, et al. Isolation of various forms of sterol beta-D-glucoside from the seed of Cycas circinalis: neurotoxicity and implications for ALS-parkinsonism dementia complex. J Neurochem 2002; 82:516–528.

117. Wilson JM, Khabazian I, Wong MC, Seyedalikhani A, Bains JS, Pasqualotto BA, Williams DE, Andersen RJ, Simpson RJ, Smith R, et al. Behavioral and neurological correlates of ALS-parkinsonism dementia complex in adult mice fed washed cycad flour. Neuromol Med 2002; 1:207–221.

118. Troncoso JC, Price DL, Griffin JW, Parhad IM. Neurofibrillary axonal pathology in aluminum intoxication. Ann Neurol 1982; 12:278–283.

119. Bizzi A, Crane RC, Autilio-Gambetti L, Gambetti P. Aluminum effect on slow axonal transport: a novel impairment of neurofilament transport. J Neurosci 1984; 4:722–731.

120. Strong MJ, Garruto RM. Chronic aluminum-induced motor neuron degeneration: clinical, neuropathological and molecular biological aspects. Can J Neurol Sci 1991; 18:428–431.

121. Gaytan-Garcia S, Kim H, Strong MJ. Spinal motor neuron neuroaxonal spheroids in chronic aluminum neurotoxicity contain phosphatase-resistant high molecular weight neurofilament (NFH). Toxicology 1996; 108:17–24.

122. Tanridag T, Coskun T, Hurdag C, Arbak S, Aktan S, Yegen B. Motor neuron degeneration due to aluminium deposition in the spinal cord: a light microscopical study. Acta Histochem 1999; 101:193–201.

123. Engelhardt JI, Appel SH, Killian JM. Experimental autoimmune motoneuron disease. Ann Neurol 1989; 26:368–376.

124. Engelhardt JI, Appel SH, Killian JM. Motor neuron destruction in guinea pigs immunized with bovine spinal cord ventral horn homogenate: experimental autoimmune gray matter disease. J Neuroimmunol 1990; 27:21–31.

125. Miller JR. Persistent infection by poliovirus: experimental studies. Adv Neurol 1982; 36:311–316.

126. Jubelt B. Motor neuron diseases and viruses: poliovirus, retroviruses, and lymphomas. Curr Opin Neurol Neurosurg 1992; 5:655–658.

127. John TJ, Nambiar A, Samuel BU, Rajasingh J. Ulnar nerve inoculation of poliovirus in bonnet monkey: a new primate model to investigate neurovirulence. Vaccine 1992; 10:529–532.

128. Ren RB, Costantini F, Gorgacz EJ, Lee JJ, Racaniello VR. Transgenic mice expressing a human poliovirus receptor: a new model for poliomyelitis. Cell 1990; 63:353–362.

129. Koike S, Taya C, Kurata T, Abe S, Ise I, Yonekawa H, Nomoto A. Transgenic mice susceptible to poliovirus. Proc Natl Acad Sci USA 1991; 88:951–955.

130. Gardner MB, Officer JE, Rongey RW, Charman HP, Hartley JW, Estes JD, Huebner RJ. C-type RNA tumor virus in wild house mice (Mus musculus). Bibl Haematol 1973; 39:335–344.

131. Jolicoeur P, Rassart E, DesGroseillers L, Robitaille Y, Paquette Y, Kay DG. Retrovirus-induced motor neuron disease of mice: molecular basis of neurotropism and paralysis. Adv Neurol 1991; 56:481–493.

132. Westarp ME, Westphal KP, Clausen J, Rasmussen HB, Hoff-Jorgensen R, Fohring B, Kornhuber HH. Retroviral interference with neuronotrophic signaling in human motor neuron disease? Clin Physiol Biochem 1993; 10:1–7.

133. Jackson AC, Moench TR, Griffin DE, Johnson RT. The pathogenesis of spinal cord involvement in the encephalomyelitis of mice caused by neuroadapted Sindbis virus infection. Lab Invest 1987; 56:418–423.

134. Havert MB, Schofield B, Griffin DE, Irani DN. Activation of divergent neuronal cell death pathways in different target cell populations during neuroadapted sindbis virus infection of mice. J Virol 2000; 74:5352–5356.

135. Harper JM, Krishnan C, Darman JS, Deshpande DM, Peck S, Shats I, Backovic S, Rothstein JD, Kerr DA. Axonal growth of embryonic stem cell-derived motoneurons in vitro and in motoneuron-injured adult rats. Proc Natl Acad Sci USA 2004; 101:7123–7128.

25

Screening for ALS Drugs

Thierry Bordet and Rebecca Pruss
Trophos, S.A., Marseille, France

Christopher E. Henderson
Departments of Pathology and Neurology, Columbia University Medical Center, New York, New York, U.S.A.

THE DRUG SCREENING PROCESS TODAY

High-throughput Screening: Principles and Practice

High-throughput screening is the random testing of large numbers of compounds on a biological system in order to identify those that affect the system in a desired way. In principle, a compound can be a small organic molecule, a natural product extract, a polypeptide, cDNA, siRNA, or other reagent that can provide the clues necessary to advance the hypothesis or objective in mind. The drug-screening process could include all of these strategies. However, this chapter is focused on the screening of small organic molecules with the objective of discovering and developing an orally bioavailable drug that can be taken chronically by patients suffering from ALS or other neurodegenerative diseases. The challenge is to develop a relevant biological system that has the potential to identify small molecules with activities likely to intervene in the disease process. Following that, the goal is to transform these chemical entities into safe and effective drugs.

Up until the mid1980s, drug discovery was by trial and observation of the effects plant, animal, or mineral extracts might have. Alchemists, apothecaries, pharmacists, midwives, and physicians in various cultures were responsible for drug discovery and development up until the mid 1850s, when organic chemistry began to attempt the synthesis of natural product therapeutics from building blocks present in petrochemicals [for an interesting account of the origins of industrial organic chemistry giving rise to both the dye and pharmaceutical industries, see Ref. (1)].

Only in the second half of the twentieth century would it be recognized that specific molecular targets like protein receptors or enzymes were responsible for actions of these compounds (haloperidol, dopamine, and dopamine receptors; insulin and insulin receptors; aspirin and cyclooxygenases; penicillin and porins). When the natural products were small molecules, synthetic organic chemists were easily able to synthesize analogs and test them without knowledge of the specific molecular target. When the natural product was a peptide, like a hormone or neuropeptide, designing potent nonpeptide ligands was and remains a challenge. While chemistry

551

still tended to be rationally directed using the peptide sequence as a template, the shift from in vivo to in vitro testing using tissue extracts or cell lines containing the targeted biological activity meant that the testing capacity exceeded the pace of chemists to synthesize new chemical entities using a rational approach.

At this point, drug companies began to consider random screening of their historical chemical collections as a way to identify an unexpected lead for chemical optimization. At first, collections of finished compounds provided more than enough molecules for manual biological testing on the available targets. Evidence that the screening process could accelerate lead identification [e.g., identification of the first non-peptide NK1 receptor antagonist (2)] convinced companies to invest in automation and target production to exploit this strategy. Real high-throughput screening came into being with the ability to clone and express the cDNA coding for the biomolecular target. This meant that the quantities of target were not the limiting factor and soon the number of available targets and screening capacity exceeded the number of finished molecules available to screen. With the sequencing of the entire human genome, bioinformatics made it possible to identify all the potential drugable targets and their orthologs in mice, flies, worms, and yeast. The drive to identify novel compounds for all these new targets inspired pharmaceutical companies to add to their screening collections not only finished medicinal chemistry products but building blocks, synthetic intermediates, and even compounds coming from other branches of their parent chemical companies. When even these had been explored, massive combinatorial compound libraries were produced by arranged marriages between molecules in never-before-seen mixtures on the basis of their compatible reactive groups. The industrialization, automation, miniaturization, and innovations in fluorescence-based response detection methods have grown up around the needs of industry to screen the large chemical collections they have assembled, rapidly and as economically as possible. These technologies are now being adopted by academic labs, and the new disciplines of chemical biology, chemical genomics, or chemical genetics are based on recognition that high-throughput screening has provided biologists with a plethora of novel chemical entities that have provided valuable pharmacological tools to dissect and study signal transduction pathways. Although we are yet to see the impact of this technology in the form of new therapeutics, this will certainly come; drug discovery and development is a long and laborious process and potent interaction with a molecular target is not all that is necessary for a chemical compound to become a safe and effective drug.

So what is needed to apply high-throughput screening to the development of novel therapeutics to treat ALS? This chapter focuses only on the challenges to discover drugs to intervene in the fundamental processes controlling survival of motor neurons themselves. However, ALS is a complex disease and secondary health problems resulting from muscle degeneration and even symptomatic relief are important medical needs of ALS patients and their care givers. While these issues will not be covered, it is important to realize that a drug, even if highly effective in promoting motor neuron survival, may not be a magic bullet capable of arresting all the events underlying or resulting from motor neuron disease. Such a compound would nevertheless represent a huge step forward in the understanding of the disease process, even if only offering incremental benefit to patients at first.

The following is a brief overview of the basic elements needed to set up the high-throughput screening process. We will then consider how these screening approaches can be applied to ALS. These are equally applicable to chemical biology strategies to probe into the disease mechanism itself or to the discovery of potential drug candidates.

Chemical Libraries

Natural products were the original sources of chemical libraries and continue to provide innovative new drugs. Analgesics, antibiotics, and cancer chemotherapeutics derived essentially from observations and later screening of the effects of natural compounds. The major difficulties in the exploitation of natural compounds as new therapeutics are: (i) the identification of the active principle in the mixture extracted from some natural source; (ii) the ability of the natural source to reproduce this substance consistently; (iii) the abundance of the natural source to supply the quantities necessary. This explains the effort devoted to finding synthetic routes to the natural product itself, once it is identified or active parts of the structure. Even in cases where the complete synthesis of a natural product cannot be performed at the industrial scale due to the number of reactions, the number of possible stereoisomers and poor overall yield, chemical synthesis does allow exploration of the various parts of the molecule for potential activity and variations not produced by the natural source. Up to now the pharmaceutical industry has shunned natural products, including antibody and protein therapeutics, because of their manufacturing difficulties as well as the need to develop delivery systems for therapeutics that cannot be taken orally.

The major breakthroughs in human therapeutics by biotechs over the last 20 years have clearly shown that these technical difficulties are not insurmountable and can provide real benefit to patients who have serious and sometimes rare diseases (cyclosporine A, erythropoietin, and interferon). The activity of natural products, usually identified in complex phenotypic assays (see below) can eventually lead to the identification of specific targets which can then be exploited through screening synthetic chemical libraries. This is important because despite the potentially infinite number of natural products available from soil-derived fungi, marine organisms, tropical plants, etc., the difficulties associated with their collection, extraction, storage, and retrieval means that the actual number of natural products available for screening is limited.

What size of chemical library is necessary to enable the screening process? As described above, the pharmaceutical industry has continuously increased the size of its collections. Even though the number of pharmacologically active molecules that have been successfully developed into drugs may be rather small (about 2000), industrial chemical collections have now reached several million screenable compounds. The size of these collections has led to new theoretic and informatic approaches to designing, classifying, comparing, and managing them, along with the notion of "chemical space" and methods to calculate chemical diversity and similarity. Associated biological activity, protein–protein interaction maps, and 3D structural information will be needed to intelligently combine theories of biology with chemical space. Has the assembly of such large collections increased the potential for identifying new drug candidates? This question will remain open for decades until there is time to be able to retrospectively analyze the origins of the new drugs that come to market.

So how many molecules should one have available to screen? While it is easy to respond "more is better," the drive to screen more compounds leads inevitably to the design of simpler assay systems. For the development of "me-too" drugs where the target has been validated and a simple primary screening assay can be developed, it is definitely better to assure that the lead molecule is sufficiently different from ones already described. In the case of ALS or other neurodegenerative disorders,

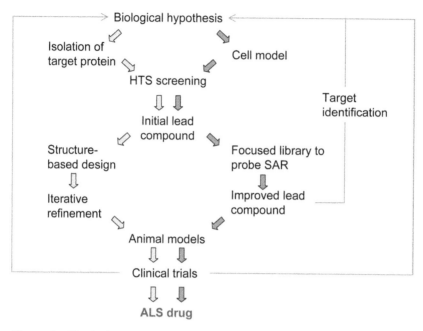

Figure 1 Classical and phenotypic screening: parallel pathways to the same goal. Although often contrasted, classical screening on an identified target and "black-box" screening based on phenotypic outcome have many points in common. In addition, initial phenotypic screening can lead to target identification and subsequent, more classical, screens.

where the mechanisms and targets remain to be validated, the size of the compound library to screen will depend on the screening assay itself. Using cancer drug discovery as an example, screening came up with innovative new drugs using whole cell-based phenotypic screens based on cell lines derived from tumors themselves (Fig. 1). If we use this as a model for ALS drug discovery, phenotypic screening using the neurons affected in the disease will have a finite capacity to screen compounds since the biological target is in limiting supply, unlike tumor cell lines. Is there a middle ground? Various alternatives for ALS drug discovery will be discussed below.

Identification of a "hit" or active compound is only the first step. In drug discovery, in contrast to chemical biology, it is rare that simply identifying the most active compound in a collection will select the best chemical family for optimization into a drug candidate. Absorption, metabolism, elimination, secondary pharmacological actions, toxicity, potential dependence, or loss of efficacy with repeated administration are all factors that enter into the final equation. While we now know that genetic variations in drug-metabolizing enzymes need to be considered, there are few general filters available to automatically classify drugs for their potential to be orally absorbed, cross the blood–brain barrier, or ensure they will be safe and nontoxic. As a shortcut or as a way to avoid risk, most companies, if presented with a selection of hits coming from a high-throughput screen, prefer to work on the development of compounds where they have information and experience on the types of problems that have been encountered and overcome in the past. One extension of this reasoning is the idea to screen previously marketed drugs on new assays or targets reasoning that these molecules already have sufficient oral absorption and safety data in man so their development for other indications will be relatively fast. However, it must be kept in mind what doses have been shown to be safe, and for how long, and in what age group. Moreover, it is important to consider whether the known pharmacological action of the drug will lead to intolerable side effects with long-term administration at the dose needed for a new indication. For CNS disorders, it is also important to consider whether the drug crosses the blood–brain barrier since drugs developed for non-CNS indications often have poor CNS penetration. Indeed, CNS-penetrating compounds are often actively avoided for peripheral indications. For ALS and other chronic CNS disorders these are important issues that have limited the development of therapeutics like trophic factors that are predicted to show clinical benefit on the basis of animal models.

All drug companies have developed checklists of drug-like properties that they use to guide the selection and optimization of molecules regardless of how they are discovered: screening, rational design, or me-too approaches. These rules, developed from experience of success (or more often failure), help to exclude or improve the characteristics of compounds prior to investing time and money in their clinical development. However, even compounds that fail in the clinic have a value. In the best case they can allow examination of the role the targeted mechanism plays in the disease process and potentially validate the approach or estimate the degree of benefit the patient may expect. This can then be used to justify continuing efforts to improve the characteristics of the compound through a backup or follow-up molecule. In the worst case, toxicity or safety in man limits the clinical trial before proof of principle can be evaluated. Unfortunately, safety and toxicity are the main causes of drugs failing to reach the market and these are often seen only when large numbers of patients have been exposed to the drug. If safety problems occur only in a few percent of the population, these problems may not be detected until the drug has been on the market for several years. This may reflect problems with a chemical class or a metabolite found only in the affected population (clozepine). Alternatively, the mechanism itself may be the culprit, bringing down other compounds in its wake (Vioxx).

Biological Readouts for Screening

In order to cope with the mass screening demanded to exploit the compound collections available, biological assays have been greatly miniaturized over the past 10 years. First, filtering stations permitted processing of multiple samples for binding or immunoassays. These were miniaturized to allow reactions to occur in 96-well microplates and this format was adapted to nonradioactive assays like ELISAs, and spectrophotometric assays to replace radioactivity. Today, fluorescence has enabled a wide range of biochemical, immunological, and functional assays to be performed in smaller and smaller volumes in denser and denser plate formats. In fact, the 96-well plate seems like a dinosaur in most screening labs where the majority of tests are run using standard automation equipment in 384-well format and some in 1526-well plates. Beyond this, specialized or dedicated liquid handling equipment is required. Miniaturization accelerates the screening process and reduces consumption of laboriously cloned and/or purified biological reagents (receptors, enzymes, etc.) and of the chemical collection. To ensure a biological signal in these reduced volumes, the targets are often cloned and re-expressed in micro-organisms or easily manipulated cell lines to amplify the quantity of target present in cell-free extracts used for enzyme or receptor binding assays. With the sequencing of the human genome and bioinformatics tools it is probably safe to say that the whole "drugable" genome has been selected, cloned, expressed, and will be screened by the pharmaceutical industry in the next few years.

The first aim is to explore and validate the function of new genes and their potential role as a drug targets. Thus, the industry will rapidly "deorphan" receptors, characterize properties of new channel subunits, create model organism knock-outs and knock-ins, develop knock-down models using siRNA both in vivo and in vitro, and use crystallography, NMR and various protein–protein interaction and proteomic methods. Subsequently, it will still be necessary to find modulators of these activities and develop them as potential drugs.

After converting the molecular target approach to drug discovery, most screening assays were tuned to the specific molecular target. In this context, the higher the affinity or the greater the potency of the hit, the better it was considered. Chemical optimization with this as a goal could produce subnanomolar compounds that then failed to show functional activity using second messenger assays or other functional assays in cell lines, isolated organ preparations, or whole animals. Over the last five years, this hurdle has triggered an important change in screening strategy, meaning that cell-based functional assays now account for the majority of screening assays in most companies. In most cases these assays are still designed to be target-specific. Such assays use recombinant cell lines engineered to express the target or a modified form of the target that amplifies or stabilizes its activity or converts the normal signal into something more easily measured (familial mutations in presenilin or APP, receptors fused to G-protein alpha subunits, complementing fragments of β-galactosidase, DNA binding domains of transcription factors, or fluorescent proteins as just some examples). Reporter gene assays are used to detect activation or inhibition of a wide range of drug targets by harnessing cAMP-, nuclear hormone-, or drug-regulated transcription factors to suitable luminescence- or fluorescence-generating proteins.

Model organisms (yeast, *C. elegans*, Drosophila, and zebrafish) in which a human gene replaces that of an endogenous ortholog necessary for survival or function have also been used for screening. These remain off the list of the approaches used by traditional pharmaceutical companies as primary screening assays but are finding a place as secondary functional assays. One difficulty in these systems is compound delivery.

Animals like rats and mice are used occasionally in screening when either the precise molecular target is unknown or the biological endpoint is not easily mimicked in vitro (antithrombotics might be an example) but, apart from ethical considerations, their use is prohibitively costly in terms of the amount of compound required.

Although target-based assays are favored today, some notable exceptions can be cited in the fields of oncology and anti-infectives. In these therapeutic areas, the primary screens are based on phenotype: cell survival, proliferation, morphological correlates of mitosis, or death (Fig. 1). This "black box" approach has identified most of the current drugs, and only secondarily the molecular targets they affect. Other types of cell-based phenotypic screening are gaining in popularity and acceptance by industrial screening groups because of development of the infrastructure necessary to use live cells in assays and to screen hundreds of thousands or even millions of compounds in the same time as other assays. Such demands led to the development of automated cell culture robots that can maintain several cell lines at a time, split them, harvest them, count them, and distribute them into microtiter plates as needed with little manual intervention. The first plate reader dedicated to cell-based assays, the Molecular Devices FLIPR, enabled measurements of intracellular calcium or membrane potential in populations of live cells using fluorescent dyes designed for these purposes. These functional responses, observed in real time measured in only a few minutes per plate initiated a revolution in screening. The response to a substance could be measured independent of knowledge about its target and new targets, e.g., putative G-protein receptors identified solely by bioinformatics methods could be expressed and screened to identify natural or surrogate ligands. Other types of fluorescence plate readers have since been developed that permit measurements in single cells (FMAT from Applied Biosystems, Molecular Devices Discovery-1, Zeiss/Cellomics ArrayScan) and the last two can even detect changes at the subcellular level in protein or organelle distribution. Multicolor fluorescence allows multiplexing and ratiometric assays. Thus, cell-based phenotypic screening is a real possibility for drug discovery.

SPECIFIC CONSIDERATIONS IN SCREENING FOR ALS

ALS occupies a special position in the field of drug development for neurodegenerative disease (3). On one hand, it presents particular difficulties linked to uncertainties about disease mechanism. On the other, because of the relative ease of organizing predictive clinical trials, it has been considered as the best entry point into the field of neurodegeneration, even for compounds aimed at larger markets such as Alzheimer's disease.

The obstacles to rational drug screening and design are multiple. First, the majority of cases are sporadic, and it is not known to what extent the disease mechanism in these patients reflects that in the familial forms, or in related diseases characterized by motor neuron degeneration. Indeed, given the variety of genetic mutations that can give rise to selective motor neuron loss, it remains possible that different sporadic cases of ALS may result from different causes. Second, the disease mechanism is known to involve at least three cell types: lower motor neurons, upper motor neurons, and astrocytes. It may be necessary to target each of these cell types independently in order to obtain a complete cure. Third, and in common with many human neurodegenerative diseases, ALS is a disease that affects the oldest cells in the body; motor neurons are never replaced during the 50 years that separate their birth from the onset of disease. Such cells may have specific properties that cannot be modeled by any experimental system. Taken together, these considerations make it impossible at present to define a perfectly validated molecular target or a predictive animal model for most cases of ALS.

In spite of these hurdles, there are reasons to believe that the field may move forward over the coming years. First, recent studies of SOD mutant mice and human patients have provided a wealth of molecular and cellular clues that are beginning to provide a rational basis for drug screening strategies. Second, much progress has been made in creating cellular and animal models that, even though they do not perfectly mimic the disease, should be useful in identifying drug candidates. Lastly, there is a growing realization that, even from a purely commercial perspective, ALS represents a market of sufficient size to interest even larger companies. In this section, we discuss some of the approaches currently available and outline some of the needs for the coming years.

Screening on Specific Targets Vs. Phenotypic Screens

What makes a validated molecular target in a disease such as ALS? The enzyme or protein should in principle be known to be involved at a specific stage in the disease mechanism, whether this be in triggering the disease during progressive degeneration,

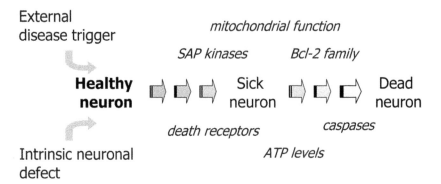

External
disease trigger

mitochondrial function

SAP kinases   *Bcl-2 family*

Healthy neuron   Sick neuron   Dead neuron

death receptors   *caspases*

Intrinsic neuronal defect   *ATP levels*

Figure 2 The degenerating neuron as a black box containing multiple relevant targets. Between the initiation of the degeneration process and the final steps of cell death, a process that may take years, lie many molecular events (arrows) that represent potential sites of intervention, i.e., therapeutic targets. Many of these remain unknown today, but a few examples of known targets are shown. Slowing or stopping the degeneration process at any of these levels is likely to be of potential therapeutic benefit.

or at later stages of neuronal cell death (Fig. 2). Ideally, pharmacologic or genetic modulation of the target should be shown to slow or stop disease progression. Mutant SOD itself is a clear target for familial cases with gain-of-function mutations in this gene.

However, given the constraints outlined above, there currently exists no validated target for sporadic ALS. Nevertheless, studies in SOD mice have provided proof-of-principle indications for the use of molecules affecting a wide range of cellular phenomena—inflammation, excitotoxicity, free radicals, kinase activation, programmed cell death, heat shock response—that may be of general use for targeting all ALS patients (4).

Therefore, the most reasonable approach at present would seem to be to target some strategies at the only validated target (mutant SOD1), others at the basic cellular phenomena involved in the disease [axonal degeneration, cell death (5), and inflammation] and, lastly, others at general cytotoxic mechanisms that have been implicated in disease progression [excitotoxicity and oxidative stress (6)] (Fig. 1). In any case, it is likely that a cure for ALS will require the use of more than one drug, even if each will first need to show its efficacy and safety in patients when used alone. This combination of target-oriented and phenotypic screens is indeed the strategy adopted by the academic Neurodegeneration Drug Screening Consortium sponsored by NINDS together with, for ALS, the ALS Association (7,8).

Molecular and Cellular Screens Focused on Mutant SOD

Although mutations in SOD1 account for only a small fraction of total ALS cases, its unique position as a validated target, the availability of excellent mouse models, and general interest in the biological mechanisms that lead mutant SOD1 to trigger selective motor neuron degeneration have resulted in focus on SOD-related screens. Unfortunately, persistent controversy and uncertainty about the ways in which point mutations in SOD trigger neurodegeneration make even this a risky venture, and mean that few strategies have targeted the SOD protein itself. Effort has been focused on SOD aggregation and SOD toxicity.

SOD1 Aggregation

Although the exact role of SOD aggregation and the formation of inclusion bodies in the disease process is not clear, there is general agreement that screening for compounds capable of preventing formation of aggregates of SOD represent a potential avenue. As previously done for Huntington's disease (9), methods are being developed to allow for more rapid screening of compounds that work in this way. As an alternative strategy, it has been proposed that compounds that enhance SOD1 dimerization might reduce aggregation (10).

SOD1 Toxicity

Although the mechanisms by which this occurs are not clear, the gain of toxic function associated with most mutant forms of SOD1 clearly justifies the use of cell models in which mutant, but not normal, SOD1 leads to increased susceptibility. There is some disagreement concerning the degree to which expression of mutant huSOD1 by mouse motor neurons leads to increased susceptibility to glutamate (11,12). However, this and other triggers (e.g., nitric oxide) may provide valid means to activate key elements of the disease pathway in cultured cells.

The human and strategic considerations that justify therapeutic strategies aimed only at this restricted group of patients are clear. The identification of an effective treatment for SOD-linked FALS would be an immense stimulus for the field and, depending on the strategy employed, might also lead directly to a treatment for sporadic disease. However, given the potential mechanistic diversity of ALS, it is important to remember that no direct link has been established between FALS and the sporadic disease. For this reason, the authors of this chapter strongly believe that the SOD mouse model should not be on the critical path for all drug discovery in the ALS field. Activity in these mice provides good proof of bioactivity in vivo. However, failure to prolong the life of SOD mice may tell us nothing about potential efficacy in sporadic ALS.

Importance of Screening Using Cell Types Related to the Disease Process

As discussed above, growing use of high-throughput procedures for drug screening created a tendency to use models based on immortalized cell lines which are easier to grow reproducibly in large quantities, and in which specific targets can be more easily over-expressed in a stable manner. We discuss below the usefulness of specific cell lines in motor neuron research. However, it is likely that such systems may not fully reflect the biology of degeneration and death of postmitotic neurons, or of mature astrocytes. This means that primary screening procedures based solely on cell lines may eliminate potentially useful compounds, even when more biologically relevant models are included as secondary screens.

We will illustrate this concept in the context of the motor neuron, but similar considerations almost certainly apply to astrocytes. First, and most generally, a motor neuron represents a cellular context (specific transcription factors, growth factor receptors, signaling pathways, and organelle properties) that is probably unique (see chapter by T.M. Jessell). A given compound may thus have quite different actions in motor neurons and in other cell types. During the long period when neurobiologists were searching for the elusive "motor neuron trophic factor" predicted by the experiments of Hamburger and Levi-Montalcini, it was only the development and use of cultures of purified primary motor neurons that finally permitted rapid progress (13–15). More recently, reports of a "motor neuron-specific" signaling pathway leading to cell death provided a striking example of the ways in which motor neurons may differ even from other neurons (12). Another illustration is provided by fact that mitochondria purified from spinal cord differ from brain mitochondria in their interactions with mutant SOD1 (16,17).

In reality, the biology of the motor neuron is still more complex in ways that are not yet integrated into screening strategies. In ALS patients, there is a well-known variation in the groups of motor neurons that are targeted in the disease. Some groups are nearly always spared, others can be initially affected in some patients but not others and, finally, certain specific groups are intimately linked to the outcome (e.g., phrenic motor neurons). This must reflect molecular and functional differences between individual motor pools, about which we are beginning to understand more. This raises the possibility that a given compound will have different effects on different motor pools. Similar considerations may apply for astrocytes, which are known to show marked regional differences (18). This cellular diversity even within neuronal classes represents a therapeutic challenge for which there is no easy solution (Section "Need for New Cell Models Directly Related to ALS").

Existing Cell Models for Motor Neuron Screening

Here, we will briefly review the cellular models available for using motor neurons as screening tools, either for primary high-throughput screening or for more specific secondary screens. Motor neurons represent only a small fraction of the total cells in the spinal cord. Therefore, if they are to be studied in culture, they either need to be purified to eliminate other cell types or to be identified so that they can be observed in presence of other cells. These approaches are complementary; each has its own advantages and drawbacks.

Purified Embryonic Motor Neurons

Pioneering studies in this field first used retrograde labeling of motor neurons by tracers injected in the limb followed by fluorescence-activated cell sorting. These techniques provided valuable initial insights but were too work-intensive to serve as the basis of a screening procedure. Since then, several laboratories, including our own, have developed reproducible techniques for dissociating, purifying, and culturing motor neurons from rat, mouse, and chicken spinal cord (19–21). The purification techniques are based on two characteristic properties of motor neurons: large size and expression of specific surface antigens allowing for purification by immunoaffinity procedures. Depending on the species and the age, the resulting preparations are highly enriched for motor neurons (>80–90%) and yield numbers of cells (10^5–10^6) that are reasonable for cell-based assays but often limiting for biochemical studies. This system has already been validated by the biotech Trophos as a primary screening tool (Section "Existing Cell Models for Motor Neuron Screening").

Purified motor neuron cultures retain several key properties of motor neurons in vivo. Indeed, they have proven to be remarkably predictive for the identification of polypeptide neurotrophic factors involved in keeping motor neurons alive during development. Approximately 15 different motor neuron trophic factors have been identified based on their survival-promoting actions for purified motor neurons in culture (13–15). All of those tested have subsequently been shown to enhance motor neuron survival in vivo in different experimental paradigms.

However, this approach also has certain drawbacks. First, it is currently only possible to purify motor neurons at embryonic stages, meaning that links with the ALS disease process still have to be established. Second, although the purity of the preparations means that any compound active must be acting on motor neurons, mechanisms involving interactions with other cell types in the spinal cord (e.g., astrocytes) are not modeled.

Organotypic Slice Cultures of Spinal Cord

At the other extreme of the spectrum, organotypic slice cultures have their own specific advantages. First, although many afferent and efferent axons are severed during preparation of slices, they maintain far more of the cellular architecture and interactions within the spinal cord than do purified motor neurons. Moreover, they can be obtained at later developmental stages than is currently possible for dissociated neurons, meaning that they may provide a closer simulation of the adult human spinal cord. To quantify effects on survival or growth, motor neurons can be identified within the explants on the basis of their position and morphology, helped by the use of selective immunological markers.

One of the most frequently used protocols, initially developed by J.R. Rothstein and collaborators (22), creates a chronic excitotoxic lesion to trigger motor neuron degeneration in explants of postnatal spinal cord. This technique has provided clear demonstration of the efficacy (or not) of several factors and compounds subsequently tested in SOD1 mutant mice. In an alternative approach, screening of FDA-approved compounds for their ability to upregulate glutamate transporters in this model led to the identification of β-lactam antibiotics as therapeutic candidates (23). Models using adult spinal cord from SOD1 mutant mice are currently under development (Pettmann and Gage, personal communication) and should model even more closely the pathologic cellular environment.

This technique too has its drawbacks. First, the great variation between motor pools at different rostro-caudal levels implies a biological and statistical variability between cultures that is currently hard to control for. Second, mixed systems such as this will detect compounds with both direct and indirect actions on motor neurons. While the latter may be clinically valuable, the degree to which the underlying indirect mechanism may be preserved in patients is not known.

Mixed Spinal Cord Cultures Containing Identified Motor Neurons

One solution to the problems of sampling posed by organotypic cultures is the use of mixed cultures of dissociated spinal cord, of which equivalent aliquots can be seeded in a large number of wells. Motor neurons can be identified in these cultures by a variety of techniques: morphology in long-term cultures, immunolabeling with specific markers, and retrograde labeling from the muscle. Mixed cultures in which motor neurons were microinjected provided some of the first evidence for altered properties of mutant SOD in primary motor neurons (24,25), but are not adapted for primary screening. More recently, the development of mouse cell lines expressing the fluorescent protein EGFP under control of a motor neuron-specific enhancer has considerable simplified such approaches (26). Once coupled to automatic detection of the fluorescent cells, this creates one of the least technically demanding systems for motor neuron-based screening. However, it shares with the techniques outlined above the drawback that active compounds may not be acting directly on motor neurons.

Motor Neuron-like Cell Lines

Motor neurons are postmitotic cells whose cellular fate can still be affected by external factors at the stage of the last division of their precursors during embryogenesis (27,28). This means that, even using standard viral genes for cell immortalization, there can be no such thing as a "motor neuron cell line" comparable to lines of fibroblasts, hepatocytes, or cancer cells, for instance. Two approaches have been taken to bring to motor neuron biology the recognized advantages of cell lines: quantity, reproducibility, and comparability between laboratories. The first, discussed here, involves fusion of postmitotic neurons with replication-competent partners. The second, discussed in the next section, aims to reconstruct the differentiation pathway of motor neurons from their biological precursors.

In the early 1990s, two groups demonstrated the feasibility of forming hybridomas with some of the properties of motor neurons in primary neurons from ventral spinal cord and mouse neuroblastoma lines (29,30). More recently, similar lines produced by fusion of purified motor neurons with neuroblastoma cells were shown to express some of the transcription factors characteristic of motor neurons (Henderson and Sanes, unpublished results). The NSC34 line produced by Cashman and collaborators (29) has proven useful in a series of studies, since it grows well in culture and is easily transfected (31).

Such models do present drawbacks for some types of screen: the presence of the non-motor neuroblastoma genome is a potential hindrance, and the fact that by definition such cell lines have an altered response to cell death signals excludes them from screens focused on this aspect of pathology. However, one may argue that their full potential in modeling steps of development and pathology that do not involve cell death, such as gene regulation, synapse stabilization, or axonal growth and dysfunction, has yet to be explored.

Motor Neurons Derived from Embryonic Stem Cells

Embryonic stem cells (ES cells) are derived by culture of cells from the inner cell mass of early embryos. Although their exact correspondence to an embryonic cell type is the subject of debate, they are in principle capable of generating all cell types in the embryo. A large number of mouse ES cell lines that have retained their full developmental capacity are now available. Moreover, technological developments mean that it is now routinely possible to derive ES cell lines from different mutant mouse strains. Undifferentiated ES cells can be expanded and grown in considerable quantities. It is therefore tempting to consider these as the source of large quantities of motor neurons (and other neuronal classes) for screening. Following an initial report that neurons with the molecular and morphological characteristics could be developed by in vitro differentiation of ES cells (32), systematic procedures for their differentiation into motor neurons and purification have been developed (26). The resulting cells have many of the functional properties of motor neurons (33) and, when grafted into chicken embryos, can innervate muscle targets in an apparently normal manner (26).

Such models represent an exciting resource whose potential is only beginning to be tapped. More needs to be done to characterize the degree to which ES cell-derived motor neurons are equivalent to primary cells, but their untransformed nature and the availability of lines from mutant genetic backgrounds will definitely provide an important thrust for future screening strategies.

Techniques for Screening Using Motor Neurons

Although classically considered technically difficult to work with, motor neurons may now be manipulated in culture by a variety of different techniques accessible to many laboratories.

Measurements of Survival, Growth, and Death

These are the three cellular readouts most directly related to the mechanism of ALS as we understand it, and so have naturally been the focus of most screening strategies. We will consider survival/death separately from growth. In fact, in models involving dissociated motor neurons, it is rarely useful to quantify dying cells per se. This is because nearly all dead or dying cells detach from the culture dish; a reduction in the number of TUNEL-positive neurons may therefore represent either a slowing or an acceleration of the cell death process. Quantification of surviving cells is relatively simple in purified motor neuron cultures. A vital dye such as AM-calcein (Molecular Probes) will label only living cells and, since essentially all cells are motor neurons, this provides a robust automatic readout for screening procedures. Survival measurement in mixed cultures requires the coupling of the marker that allows identification of the motor neuron with another, often morphologic, that provides an indication as to the health of the cell. This technique has been automated by Trophos for mixed cultures from mice with motor neuron-specific expression of EGFP.

Automated measurements of neuronal growth have become recently available in a form suited to screening procedures. It is now technically possible using a combination of an automated plate reader and image analysis software to rapidly and objectively quantify growth in a large number of culture wells. Such software quantifies the total amount of neurite growth in a well by subtracting the surface area of cell bodies from total cell area. Alternatively, other programs automatically identify individual cell bodies and their neurites, and quantify growth as a mean of such values for all the cells in the culture. Moreover, both dendritic and axonal growth and degeneration are of relevance in studying development and disease; this requires the use of specific markers such as MAP-2 to measure individually the two cell compartments. With the increasing interest in the axonal aspects of ALS and related disorders (34,35), it is to be anticipated that such techniques will play a progressively more important role over the coming years.

Gain-of-function Approaches

In the context of a screening platform, it can be extremely useful to express in motor neurons either a disease-triggering gene (e.g., mutant SOD1), a therapeutic target gene or a reporter gene construct for pathways or specific genes affected in the disease. Primary motor neurons are hard to transfect by classical methods developed for non-neuronal cell lines. However, a wide variety of approaches is now available to the investigator. First, purified motor neurons can be transduced at high efficacy using adenoviral or lentiviral vectors (36,37). Second, electroporation of suspensions of freshly purified motor neurons using cDNA vectors gives cultures in which 50% to 70% of surviving neurons are transfected (12). Although many neurons die upon electroporation, the resulting neurons are morphologically normal and respond in culture in a similar manner to untreated controls. Lastly, motor neuron-like cell lines are in general easy to transfect (31).

Loss-of-function Approaches

Although only rare cases of ALS have so far been linked to loss-of-function in known genes, the creation of "knock-down" models is a potentially interesting tool for creating dysfunctional neurons for screening purposes. Moreover, for strategies aiming at reducing levels of toxic SOD1 mutants, it is important to create in vitro models that replicate and validate the strategy to be tested in vivo. Antisense approaches have been used in cultured motor neurons with some success (36,38), and much current effort is devoted to developing techniques based on RNA interference. However, these techniques are currently far from routine and probably difficult and expensive to develop as primary screening tools.

Models for Screening in Astrocytes

The potential importance of screening in astrocytes in human ALS is suggested by a series of indicators. First, riluzole, the only approved treatment for the disease, does not have direct survival-promoting activity on motor neurons. However, when applied to cultured astrocytes, it induces them to secrete higher levels of unidentified trophic factors for motor neurons (39). Second, current evidence indicates that mutant SOD1 must be expressed in both motor neurons and astrocytes to induce the disease (40). Lastly, characteristic changes in astrocytes and microglia are associated with ALS pathology (41). To date, however, astrocytes have not figured prominently in screening strategies. This will probably change as the molecular mechanisms of their contribution to ALS become clearer, making it easier to define relevant biological readouts.

Need for New Cell Models Directly Related to ALS

Our knowledge of the molecular mechanisms underlying ALS is constantly expanding. In principle, each new mechanism may potentially be validated as a therapeutic target. In the current context, as alluded to in section "The Drug Screening Process Today," it seems likely that over the coming years much validation of both targets and lead compounds will be performed in the academic context. The risks and difficulties of drug development for a disease such as this mean that increasing pressure is being brought on biotech companies and even midsized pharmaceutical companies to identify targets or molecules that have a reasonable chance of leading to successful clinical trials. An experimental model that has already demonstrated its ability to identify compounds that are bioactive in vivo has considerably higher chances of being acquired by an industrial partner, or of serving as the basis for a new start-up. It is also more likely to justify the high revenue now expected by universities for intellectual property. Fortunately, this corresponds to the rapid expansion in academia of chemical genetics, screening platforms, and relevant animal models of disease (42). Given current interest in this field, identification of lead compounds in such a context represents a win–win situation: high-level publications and patents for the academic partner, lower risk and clearer development strategy for the industrial partner.

It is not possible in a chapter such as this to predict future developments reliably. We have therefore chosen to briefly discuss some aspects of ALS that seem ripe for screening, but for which much development remains to be done.

ES Cell-derived Human Motor Neurons

For any given target, it is not simple to determine the importance of screening on the human molecule as opposed to the rodent homolog. Fortunately, the high degree of homology often observed has allowed drugs to be developed on the basis of their activity in model systems. For motor neurons in particular, despite pioneering attempts, the culture of motor neurons from human embryos motor neurons is subject to too many variables to be of clear usefulness, and this in itself poses ethical questions. The advent of human ES cells and unpublished reports of the possibility of differentiating them into motor neurons have changed this picture. More work still undoubtedly has to be done to validate human ES cell-derived motor neurons as robust screening tools, and the relative slowness of all differentiation steps will be a hindrance for high-throughput screening. However, the availability of human cells with motor neuron-like properties cannot fail to profoundly influence screening strategies.

Screens Based on Mitochondrial Dysfunction

One of the emerging themes in ALS research is the role of the mitochondrion and its interactions with mutant SOD1 (16,17,43,44). As mentioned above, these interactions appear to be tissue-specific. Therefore, drugs that target interactions between motor neuron mitochondria and disease-triggering proteins have great potential interest. The availability of new ES cell-derived models may for the first time allow such phenomena to be addressed in a high-throughput manner.

Targeting the Cortical Motor Neuron

Despite much study, it is still not clear to what degree "saving" lower motor neurons will also cure the upper motor neuron deficit in ALS patients (45). Given the significant differences between human and rodent corticospinal circuitry, no current screen specifically targets this population. However, the advent of human cultures, linked to availability of specific markers for cortical motor neurons, may in the future allow the biology and pathology of these neurons to be probed in culture.

Targeting Specific Pools of Lower Motor Neurons

Throughout the disease course, different groups ("pools") of motor neurons are affected at different rates in different patients. Nevertheless, most patients die from respiratory failure, when phrenic and intercostal motor neurons are no longer able to maintain sufficient function. Paradoxically, in spite of some key papers, these are some of the motor neurons whose molecular and cellular development has been the least studied (46). It is quite conceivable that phrenic motor neurons respond differently than others to potential ALS drugs. Devising screening systems in which they are specifically targeted could therefore be of major benefit.

Differences Between Embryonic and Adult Motor Neurons

One of the major characteristics of ALS and other neurodegenerative diseases is that they occur in late adulthood. Moreover, it is clear that the molecular and survival characteristics of motor neurons change with age, even though some embryonic markers are still expressed by certain motor neurons in the adult. Nevertheless, virtually no experimental model of ALS concerns motor neurons older than six months, and many are considerably younger.

It is not conceivable that long-term cultures will per se significantly narrow this gap. It will therefore be important to study and model the differences between adult and juvenile motor neurons, and to incorporate the most significant changes into available models for drug screening.

DRUG DISCOVERY FOCUSED ON THE MOTOR NEURON: TROPHOS AS AN EXAMPLE

All three authors have commercial links with a start-up company called Trophos, based in Marseille, France. It is not our aim here to defend either the screening strategy or the compounds that have emerged from it. However, since Trophos represents one of the few examples of technology transfer focused on motor neurons, we believe that a short first-hand account of the screening strategy will be of interest to the reader.

Trophos is a biopharmaceutical company employing 35 people, committed to the discovery and development of novel therapeutic compounds for the treatment of neurodegenerative disorders. Its clinical targets are the motor neuron diseases ALS and SMA, and Huntington's disease. The screening strategy adopted since 1999 arises directly from many of the biological and technological arguments reviewed above. There are no validated molecular targets for ALS, and successful drugs will need to cross several biological barriers. This makes it an obvious target for the "black box" cell-based screening approach outlined in section "The Drug Screening Process Today" (Fig. 1). A compound active in such a model has already demonstrated activity in a relatively physiological context, and shown its capacity to cross the cell membrane and resist metabolic degradation.

A Screening Platform Based on Primary Neurons

Although polypeptide neurotrophic factors are not themselves ideal drugs, they have many of the properties that one would hope for in a chemical drug candidate for neurodegenerative disease. A survey of the literature concerning their initial discovery shows that, in nearly every case, it was the use of primary neuronal cultures that allowed detection of their biological activity.

Indeed, in many cases, the cultures used were purified preparations of specific neuronal classes. This pointed to such cultures as starting points for drug discovery, but raised technical problems of reproducibility and quantity.

The initial decision was to target the motor neuron, the prime target in ALS and SMA. Although the purification procedure for embryonic motor neurons is relatively long and complex, it is possible for a team of two to four persons to generate sufficient cells from E14 rat embryos to conduct a screening campaign (Fig. 3). Quality control procedures are vital at this and all other steps of the screen in order to maximize reproducibility and eliminate preparations or measurements that are substandard.

Motor neurons are seeded into 96-well plates and induced to die by different means (see below). Chemical compounds are assayed for their ability to prevent cell death. One initial challenge was to assay neuronal survival at a speed compatible

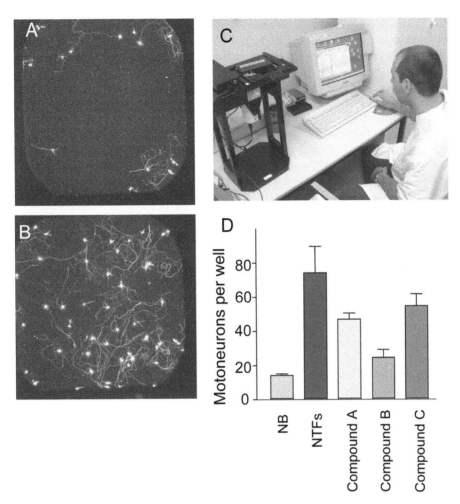

Figure 3 Automated screening for compounds that enhance motor neuron survival. Purified motor neurons can be grown in microplate culture wells and submitted to treatments that mimic pathology. (**A**) When living cells are visualized in such wells using fluorescent dyes a few days later, only few remain. (**B**) In wells treated with neurotrophic factors or candidate chemical compounds, many more motor neurons survive. (**C**) The number of surviving motor neurons can be quantified automatically in about 20 samples per minute. (**D**) The resulting data provide quantitative means for comparing the efficacy of different chemical compounds (compound A, B, C) between themselves and with controls. In the example shown, the negative control (NB) is a culture of motor neurons grown in Neurobasal medium alone, and the positive control (NTFs) is a culture of motor neurons grown in the same medium, but with the addition of a cocktail of polypeptide neurotrophic factors. (*See color insert.*)

with screening. It is not feasible to use biochemical or ELISA methods to accurately measure the small number (*ca.* 100) of motor neurons in each well and, traditionally, all investigators in this field have used direct counting of surviving neurons as the most reliable endpoint. Trophos therefore devised a fluorescence-based high-throughput image analyzer called the Flash Cytometer that rapidly takes pictures of whole culture wells, at a resolution sufficient to distinguish neurites but not growth cones or filopodia. Living neurons are stained with AM-calcein

(Section "Specific Consideration in Screening for ALS") and identified by their size; in this manner, both particulate debris and large cellular aggregates are eliminated from the counts. Automated counting gives results indistinguishable from those obtained manually, but in a fraction of the time. When coupled to appropriate software, the Flash Cytometer can also be used to quantify neurite outgrowth, calcium transients, or immunofluorescence (Fig. 3).

It is important that every cell preparation and each individual 96-well plate be validated before the data are considered acceptable to be incorporated into the database. Robotic cell handling and the use of multiple replicates, together with the fact that every cell in the dish is counted, considerably reduce the scatter of results inherent in primary cultures. In spite of this, only *ca.* 70% of plates provide data that pass the different quality control procedures.

Mimicking the Disease Process in the Culture Dish

A pathologic process of neuronal degeneration and cell death may occur over a period of years. It is thought to involve an initial phase in which there is loss of function followed by a second phase during which the sick neuron gradually undergoes cell death (Fig. 2). Apart from the disease triggers in some cases, we know extremely little about the molecular steps involved at any level. It is likely that even the programmed cell death mechanisms bear little resemblance to the rapid apoptosis much studied in non-neuronal cell lines. One major target of research on neurodegenerative diseases is to characterize the degeneration process in molecular and cellular terms. In the meantime, it is perhaps best to consider the process itself as an array of potentially important clinical targets that can be screened in parallel. The challenge then becomes to recreate this array in the culture dish.

Different neuronal types die by different mechanisms, and even a given neuronal system may activate different death pathways depending on the nature of the external death trigger. Therefore, we argue that the best approach to modeling disease in the dish is provided by cultures of neurons of the same class as those affected in the disease (motor neurons for ALS) exposed to conditions that mimic the disease triggers as closely as possible. For genetic diseases such as Huntington's disease, this may involve overexpression of a mutant protein. For ALS, one possibility is overexpression of mutant SOD. In reality, Trophos exposes motor neurons to two stresses with some potential link to the disease mechanism: removal of neurotrophic factors, or exposure to excitotoxic agents.

The endpoint in all assays is motor neuron survival or death. The advantage of phenotypic assays such as this is that they may potentially select compounds acting upstream close to the initiation of the degeneration phase as well as others more involved in the cell death process.

From Hit Compound to Drug Candidate

Once hit compounds with reproducible and significant biological activity have been identified by primary screening, the "black box" approach is not adapted to the classical procedures of structure-based optimization, since no 3D structure for the target exists. Two parallel solutions to this problem can be adopted: activity-based optimization, and target identification. In the first, focused chemical libraries synthesized initially at random around the initial building block can progressively provide information about the types of modification that can lead to improved lead activity.

Subsequently, testing in animal models and preclinical regulatory safety data are performed in a standardized manner by external contractors.

Target identification can be a long process; only in rare cases will the chemical structure of the lead compound give direct clues as to its mode of action. While not strictly required for testing a new drug with functional rationale in ALS, indications as to the mechanism are nevertheless valuable both to regulatory authorities and practicing clinicians. The most general approaches are to screen the lead compound for binding activity against a wide range of recombinant protein targets, or to synthesize analogs with biotinyl or reactive moieties that can label the binding site on the target.

RECENT APPROACHES IN DRUG DISCOVERY AND CLINICAL TRIALS

Drug discovery for ALS has led to testing of over 50 compounds in clinical trials and to the launch of the only drug currently available for the treatment of ALS, riluzole. Unfortunately, the therapeutic benefits for patients with ALS still remain modest: riluzole prolongs survival by approximately two to three months without a clear effect on muscle strength. Thus, ALS definitely represents an unmet medical need for effective drugs. Fortunately, progress in our understanding of the disease and development of new techniques mean that drug discovery in ALS is now moving from testing previously identified neuroprotective agents to the design of specific high-throughput strategies focused on ALS.

Review of Recent Clinical Trials

Since ALS does not represent a large or growing market, only relatively few companies are engaged specifically in the field. However, some big pharmaceutical companies have been attracted to ALS as a first step toward larger markets. Riluzole (Aventis) provides an example of this, since it is now being evaluated in Phase-III trials for Parkinson's disease, and Phase-II trials for Alzheimer's and Huntington's diseases. Understandably, such compounds target general pathogenic processes such as oxidative stress, glutamate excitotoxicity, and neurotrophic support. Other "known" compounds, already approved for other indications, have also been evaluated or are still under evaluation in clinical trial as potential ALS therapeutics, on the basis of evidence of activity in in vitro or in animal models. Most of them are natural products or nutritional supplements (Vitamin E) or FDA-approved products (celebrex, tamoxifen). These approaches have given rise to a large number of double-blind, placebo-controlled trials in ALS, involving several thousand patients. Results (in some cases preliminary) from the most recent trials are summarized in Table 1.

Antioxidants

Oxidative stress is classically proposed as a key determinant in the cascade of neuronal damage in ALS. Several antioxidant compounds have been evaluated. Among them, the antioxidant Vitamin E (α-tocopherol) was shown to improve the motor function of transgenic SOD1 G93A mouse model of familial ALS (47). However, two large clinical trials conducted in Europe, in add-on therapy with riluzole, have failed to show significant benefit in ALS patients (48,49). Coenzyme Q10, another endogenous antioxidant, prolongs survival in the mouse model of ALS and has shown promise in a clinical trial of Parkinson's disease (50,51). A clinical trial of high dose of CoQ10 was recently launched after completion of a safety pilot study.

Table 1 Recent Large Clinical Trials for Amyotrophic Lateral Sclerosis

Drug	Rationale	Phase	Number of patients	Duration	Outcome
Vitamin E (α-tocopherol)	Antioxidant	III	289	12	No survival benefit. Significantly more patients remained in a milder disease state after 12 months add-on therapy with riluzole (48)
Coenzyme Q10	Prolongs SOD1 mouse survival (47) Mitochondrial cofactor Endogenous antioxidant Prolongs SOD1 mouse survival (51)	III III	160 —	18 9	No benefit of high-dose Vitamin E (49) High-dose study. Enrollment planned October 2004
Celebrex	FDA-approved treatment for arthritis COX-2 inhibitor Prolongs SOD1 mouse survival by 25% (55)	II	300	12	No benefit on the rate of progression in ALS (800 mg/day, no side effects) (52)
Topiramate	FDA-approved treatment for epilepsy Protects motor neurons from glutamate toxicity in organotypic spinal cord cultures (59)	II	296	12	Faster rate of decline in muscle strength and adverse events at a dose of 800 mg/day (60)
IGF-1 (Myotrophin) Xaliproden (SR557746A)	Neurotrophic factor Neurotrophic factor enhancer	III III	300 867	24 18	Enrollment open summer 2003 Benefit on vital capacity at the dose of 2 mg/day
	Promotes motor neuron survival in vitro & in PMN mice (68,69)	III	1210	18	Trend for improved survival at the 1 mg dose in add-on therapy with riluzole (71)
Creatine	Mitochondrial protection Prolongs SOD1 mouse survival by 18% (72)	II	104	6	No significant benefit (73)

Drug	Description	Phase			
Minocycline	FDA-approved treatment for arthritis Antiapoptotic agent, inhibits microglial activation (97,98) and prolongs SOD1 mouse survival (78)	III	400	13	Enrollment open in November 2003
Pentoxifylline (EHT001, Ikomio®)	FDA-approved treatment for arterial vasodilatation Phosphodiesterase & TNF-α inhibitor	III	400	18	No effect on motor function (Meininger V, 15th International Symposium on ALS/MND 2004)
Tamoxifen	FDA-approved treatment for breast cancer Mild form of ALS in patient receiving Tamoxifen for breast cancer Retards onset of symptoms in a model of motor neuron degeneration (79)	II	100	12	Dose-ranging study still in progress (Brooks B, 15th International Symposium on ALS/MND 2004)

Abbreviations: ALS, amylotrophic lateral sclerosis; MND, motor neuron diseases; SOD1, superoxide dismutase; IGF-1, insulin-like growth factor-1.

Recently, Cudkowicz et al. (52) reported the negative results of a large 12-month study with Celebrex, a cyclooxygenase-2 (COX-2) inhibitor, FDA-approved for the treatment of arthritis. This is in spite of much preclinical evidence for a beneficial effect of COX-2 inhibitors: (i) strong upregulation of COX-2 mRNA has been observed in ALS spinal cord (53), (ii) COX-2 inhibition provided significant protection against loss of spinal motor neurons in organotypic spinal cord cultures (54), and (iii) Celebrex prolongs SOD1 survival by 25% when administered before symptom onset (55).

Antiglutamate Compounds

In addition to riluzole, many antiglutamate agents, including gabapentin, have been evaluated without success in ALS patients (56,57). Topiramate, an FDA-approved agent for epilepsy, was the most recent antiglutamate compound to be tested. This AMPA receptor antagonist diminishes glutamate release from neurons (58) and protects motor neurons from chronic glutamate toxicity in organotypic spinal cord cultures (59). However, at the maximum tolerated dose of 800 mg/day, topiramate did not have a beneficial effect for patients with ALS (60). Furthermore, high-dose topiramate treatment was associated with a faster rate of decline in muscle strength and several adverse effects, precluding any other study at that dose in ALS patients.

Neurotrophic Agents

Several neurotrophic factors (BDNF, CNTF, and GDNF) that enhance motor neuron survival in vitro and in vivo have undergone clinical trials as potential ALS treatments. Unfortunately, none of them demonstrated efficacy (61–63). The most recent to be tested was IGF-1 (Myotrophin®), a neurotrophic factor essential for normal development of the nervous system that promotes motor neuron survival and nerve regeneration (64,65). Clinical trials of IGF-1 in ALS patients in the US and in Europe led to conflicting conclusions with promising results in US and negative results in Europe, most likely due to differences in study design (66,67). A third study was launched in summer 2003, including 300 patients and designed to detect a 30% difference in manual muscle testing score (MMT) over a two-year-treatment period.

To counteract some of the problems with the use of exogenous neurotrophic factors, interest has been shown in orally active compounds that can stimulate their synthesis. Xaliproden (SR57746A), a 5-HT$_{1A}$ agonist developed by Sanofi-Synthelabo, was the first neurotrophic factor enhancer investigated in clinical studies. Here too, preclinical and clinical data were initially optimistic. Xaliproden promotes mouse motor neuron survival in vitro (68) and in the *pmn* mouse (69). In a first Phase-II study, patients with 2 mg/day xaliproden had a slower rate of deterioration in vital capacity than placebo-treated patients (70). On the basis of these findings, two other large Phase-III trials with xaliproden as monotherapy or as add-on with riluzole were undertaken for an 18-month period. The drug was well tolerated and demonstrated a trend for improved survival (71). These effects were judged not to be sufficient to justify its use in the clinic.

Other Targets

The role of mitochondrial dysfunction in ALS has been reinforced by many recent studies, suggesting that treatments aimed at protection and stabilization of mitochondria may have a role in ALS. Creatine treatment, for example, resulted in a dose-related increase in survival of up to 26 days in the SOD mice (72). However, a six-month study on 104 patients with ALS did not show any beneficial effect of creatine at 5 g/day (73). Minocycline, an antibiotic currently approved for the treatment of rheumatoid arthritis, has demonstrated impressive efficacy in slowing down ALS progression in SOD1 mouse models, alone or in combination with other compounds (74–78). Although its mechanism of action remains uncertain (blockade of inflammatory mechanisms, mitochondrial protection, and inhibition of caspase activation, inhibition of p38 kinase), its efficacy is currently being tested in a large Phase-III 13-month trial involving 400 participants.

Based on its inhibitory effect on PDE4 (phosphodiesterase-4) and on TNF-α, Exonhit Therapeutics selected pentoxifylline (EHT001, Ikomio®), an FDA-approved compound for the treatment of arterial vasodilatation, as a drug candidate for treatment of ALS. Its efficacy was recently evaluated in addition to riluzole in an 18-month study enrolling about 400 ALS patients. However, preliminary analysis of the study failed to demonstrate any effect (V Meininger, 15th ALS/MND Symposium, Philadelphia 2004).

More encouraging results come from an ongoing randomized multiple dose-ranging clinical trial of tamoxifen in add-on therapy with riluzole (B Brooks, 15th ALS/MND Symposium, Philadelphia 2004). Interest in tamoxifen began when clinicians at the University of Wisconsin-Madison noted that an ALS patient receiving tamoxifen for breast cancer had an unusually mild form of ALS. This clinical observation was followed by the demonstration that tamoxifen delayed to some extent the onset of symptoms in a mouse model of motor neuron degeneration induced by viral infection (79). Recent preliminary results from the ongoing clinical trial demonstrated a four- to six-month increase in survival by the end of the two years in the groups taking the higher doses of tamoxifen. No significant side effects were observed. Additional clinical trials with larger groups of patients will be needed to confirm this potentially promising observation.

Reasons of Failure

Except for the riluzole trials and potentially that of tamoxifen, all clinical trials have led to disappointing results. Reasons for failure probably differ from one trial to another and are difficult to identify. Historically, the design of clinical trials may have been a problem. Indeed, the ALS community recognizes that many of the earlier clinical trials in ALS included few subjects for a short treatment period that there was very little chance of finding a beneficial effect. However, recent trials in ALS were larger powered placebo-controlled studies on about 400 patients, for periods greater than 12 months.

New Drugs for ALS

High-throughput screening may increase the likelihood of success. In parallel with a better understanding of the physiopathology of ALS, in vitro miniaturized models can be developed for screening of thousands of small molecules in a rapid, reliable, and less expensive way. This drug discovery process normally used by pharmaceutical companies is now available for the research of new therapeutic compounds in ALS and the first optimized molecules produced by combinatorial chemistry or high-throughput screenings are now moving forward (Table 2).

Table 2 Compounds in Development for ALS

Drug	Company	How discovered	Rationale	Status
TCH-346 (CGP 3466)	Novartis	Analog of R-(-)-deprenyl	Antiapoptotic agent Prolongs PMN mouse survival (83)	Ph.2b
ONO-2506	ONO Pharmaceuticals	Analog of valproic acid	An astrocyte modulator (85)	Ph.2
AEOL 10150	Aeolus Pharmaceuticals Inc	Analog of metalloporphyrins	Antioxidant with potent superoxide dismutase activity Prolongs survival in SOD1 mouse (90)	Ph.1
PYM50018 (Myogane®)	Phytopharm plc	Synthetic analog of a natural compound purified from plant extracts	Antioxidant Antiexcitotoxic Antiapoptotic Prolonged survival in SOD1 mouse	Orphan drug status Ph.1b
BN82,451	Ipsen Beaufour	Analog of phenolic thiazoles	MAO, lipid peroxidation and NOS inhibitor Mitochondrial protection Prolongs survival in SOD1 mouse (93)	Ph.1
TRO19622	Trophos SA	HTS on rat embryonic motor neurons	Promotes motor neuron survival in vitro and in facial nerve axotomy Stimulates regeneration of peripheral nerve Modulates opening of the MPTP Prolongs survival in SOD1 mouse (T. Bordet, 15th ALS/MND Symposium 2004)	Ph. 1
Ceftriaxone	NINDS, ALSA consortium	Screen of 1040 FDA-approved drugs on organotypic spinal cord cultures	Enhances GLT1 expression Inhibits motor neuron degeneration induced by glutamate toxicity	Preclinical
Scriptaid & DPD	Harvard Medical School	HTS on mutant SOD-GFP aggregation in COS1 cells	Prolongs survival in SOD1 mouse (23) Inhibits assembly of large SOD1 aggresomes (95)	Preclinical

Abbreviations: MPTP, mitochondrial permeability transition pore; MAO, monoamine oxidase; NOS, nitric oxide synthase.

Combinatorial Chemistry

Combinatorial chemistry has been extensively used to modify compounds already known to have effects in the CNS. This is the case of most of the new chemical entities currently under preclinical or Phase-I studies for ALS (Table 2). For example, TCH346 (Novartis) which is being evaluated in ALS in a multicenter Phase-III clinical trial enrolling about 500 patients, is a structural analog of deprenyl. Deprenyl was first developed for Parkinson's disease, but has already been tested with no apparent effect in 10 patients suffering from ALS (80). Clinical effects of deprenyl were disappointing due to problems of metabolism, lack of neuroprotection, and adverse cardiovascular effects of the deprenyl metabolites amphetamine and methamphetamine. THC346 (previously labeled CGP3466B) was developed to overcome these metabolic complications. It exhibits neuroprotective properties in cellular and animal models of PD that are about 100-fold more potent than those of deprenyl (81). TCH346 was shown to directly interact with GAPDH to possibly mediate its antiapoptotic action (82). In vivo, TCH346 enhances survival in the PMN mouse (83) but has no effects on survival in G93A SOD mutant mice (84).

Similarly, ONO Pharmaceuticals developed ONO-2506, a new analog of the antiepileptic agent valproic acid (85). Originally, valproic acid was shown to restore GABA-A receptor function in reactive astrocytes suggesting that it might have wider neuroprotective effects (86). After investigating 161 structural analogs of valproic acid in an in vitro model of cultured reactive astrocytes, ONO-2506 was selected on the basis of its ability to reduce infarct volume (87). Furthermore, in contrast to valproic acid, ONO-2506 does not seem to possess teratogenic activity. ONO-2506 is under development for the potential treatment of stroke, as well as Alzheimer's and Parkinson's diseases. Since March 2002, Phase-II trials for ALS are underway in Europe although no evidence of activity on motor neurons has been reported. Results are expected by the end of year 2005.

Aeolus Pharmaceuticals, Inc. (previously called Incara Pharmaceuticals Corp.) has developed catalytic antioxidants by chemical modification of previously described metalloporphyrin compounds (88). Of these analogs, AEOL 10150 has potent superoxide dismutase and catalase activity in vitro and is protective in the MCAO model (89). When orally administered to SOD mice, AEOL improved survival by 38% as compared to controls (90). On the basis of these encouraging results, Phase-I clinical trials have exceptionally been initiated directly in ALS patients without any safety, tolerability, and pharmacokinetics data in healthy volunteers. PYM50018 (Myogane™) is a result of the neurodegeneration program of Phytopharm. This program arose from the discovery of a single chemical purified from an Asian plant which demonstrated a significant improvement in cognitive function in patients with mild to moderate senile dementia. This has led to the development of a large library of synthetic compounds that share the same mode of action. Phytopharm reported protective effects of PYM50018 in in vitro models of neuronal damage and after orally administration into a transgenic mouse model of ALS (unpublished data). The Phase-1 study is underway to evaluate the safety, tolerability, and pharmacokinetic profile of PYM50018 associated with repeated daily dosing in healthy volunteers. The drug has recently received Orphan Drug designation and Fast Track approval from the FDA. Lastly, Ipsen Beaufour is developing novel analogs of phenolic thiazol which have been shown to inhibit monoamine oxidase, lipid peroxidation, and modulate Na^+ channels. One of these, BN82,451, displays antioxidant activity in vitro and is neuroprotective in in vivo models of mitochondrial respiratory chain

intoxication (91). Moreover, it has been shown to provide increased survival in a transgenic mouse model of Huntington's disease (92) and in ALS model mice (93).
BN82,451 recently completed its Phase-1 development.

Although all these compounds are new chemical entities and have enhanced
activity as compared to their parent compounds, none of them was specifically
designed for ALS.

High-throughput Screening

Currently few high-throughput screens specifically dedicated to ALS have been
reported. In a joint effort by the ALS Association, the National Institute of Neurologic Disorders and Stroke, the Hereditary Disease Foundation, and the Huntington's
Disease Society of America, a consortium of 26 academic laboratories screened
1040 FDA-approved drugs using different in vitro models of neurodegenerative diseases including eight ALS assays (7,94). Ceftriaxone, a β-lactam antibiotic, is the first
drug to come from this program (23).

Identified by screening on organotypic spinal cord slice cultures, ceftriaxone
increases the expression of the glutamate transporter GLT1 (also known as EAAT2),
thus reducing glutamate neurotoxicity in ischemic injury and motor neuron degeneration in in vitro models. When administered to G93A mice at disease onset stage,
ceftriaxone delayed loss of muscle strength and increased overall survival of the mice
by 10 days. As ceftriaxone was developed first as an antibiotic, long-term safety data
in animals will be needed before moving to clinical trials in ALS.

A larger screen was conducted by Liu et al. at the Harvard Medical School for
small molecules that inhibit mutant SOD1 aggresome-like formation (95). By screening 20,000 compounds on COS cells expressing G85RSOD-GFP, cardiac glycosides
and two structurally different compounds sharing a mechanism of action were identified: scriptaid, a known histone deacetylase inhibitor (96) and DPD (5-(3-Dimethyl
amino-propylamino)-3,10-dimethyl-10*H*-pyrimidol[4,5-*b*]quinoline-2,4-dione), a flavin
analog. By affecting the interaction of misfolded mutant SOD-GFP proteins with the
dynein/dynactin machinery, these compounds inhibit assembly of SOD into large
aggresomes, although formation of microaggregates was not abolished. Experiments
are currently underway to test these compounds in ALS transgenic mice.

Finally, Trophos, with the support of the French patient foundation AFM
(Association Française contre les Myopathies), recently presented the results of its
high-throughput screening on the survival of primary motor neurons (EU ALS
Symposium Nice 2004; 15th ALS/MND Symposium Philadelphia 2004). Through
screening of 40,000 small molecules on embryonic motor neurons deprived of trophic
factors, TRO19622 was identified as the best lead compound. This new chemical
entity is as effective as a cocktail of three neurotrophic factors in keeping motor
neurons alive in culture. TRO19622 also enhances survival of striatal neurons in a
cell-based model of Huntington's disease and displays antiapoptotic properties for
other types of primary neurons. In vivo, TRO19622 increases survival of motor
neurons following facial nerve axotomy in neonatal rats, accelerates regeneration
following a nerve crush injury in adult mice, prolongs life in a transgenic mouse
model of SMA, and increases mean survival of SOD1 G93A by 13 days. By a process
of reverse engineering, Trophos scientists found that TRO19622 interacts with the
mitochondrial permeability transition pore (MPTP) preventing the release of apoptotic factors and increasing the calcium buffering capacities of mitochondria. The
molecule has satisfactorily completed regulatory safety studies. An oral formulation

has been developed for clinical trials and Phase-1 studies in healthy volunteers started in December 2004. A Phase-II clinical study in patient with ALS is expected to commence at the end of 2005.

PERSPECTIVES

Interest in developing therapeutics for ALS has never been higher. Strategies currently envisioned include not only small-molecule drugs but also gene therapy and cell therapy that have shown promise in animal models. Each of these will need to be evaluated individually. However, it is likely that, in order to have a strong effect on the disease course, it will be necessary to administer combinations of drugs, or to combine classical drugs with gene therapy. The number of candidate compounds and strategies is a source for reasoned optimism but creates practical and ethical problems of its own. It will become increasingly urgent to establish and validate predictive animal models and to standardize protocols for preclinical studies both in terms of functional outcome and pharmacokinetics. This should in theory allow the most promising compounds and their range of active concentrations in the spinal cord to be better selected.

REFERENCES

1. ALS CNTF Treatment Study Group. A double-blind placebo-controlled clinical trial of subcutaneous recombinant human ciliary neurotrophic factor (rHCNTF) in amyotrophic lateral sclerosis. ALS CNTF Treatment Study Group. Neurology 1996; 46:1244–1249.
2. Andreassen OA, Dedeoglu A, Friedlich A, Ferrante KL, Hughes D, Szabo C, Beal MF. Effects of an inhibitor of poly(ADP-ribose) polymerase, desmethylselegiline, trientine, and lipoic acid in transgenic ALS mice. Exp Neurol 2001; 168:419–424.
3. Arce V, Garces A, de Bovis B, Filippi P, Henderson C, Pettmann B, deLapeyriere O. Cardiotrophin-1 requires LIFRbeta to promote survival of mouse motoneurons purified by a novel technique. J Neurosci Res 1999; 55:119–126.
4. Bachoo RM, Kim RS, Ligon KL, Maher EA, Brennan C, Billings N, Chan S, Li C, Rowitch DH, Wong WH, DePinho RA. Molecular diversity of astrocytes with implications for neurological disorders. Proc Natl Acad Sci U S A 2004; 101:8384–8389.
5. Barbeito LH, Pehar M, Cassina P, Vargas MR, Peluffo H, Viera L, Estevez AG, Beckman JS. A role for astrocytes in motor neuron loss in amyotrophic lateral sclerosis. Brain Res Brain Res Rev 2004; 47:263–274.
6. Barnham KJ, Masters CL, Bush AI. Neurodegenerative diseases and oxidative stress. Nat Rev Drug Discov 2004; 3:205–214.
7. Beal MF. Coenzyme Q10 as a possible treatment for neurodegenerative diseases. Free Radic Res 2002; 36:455–460.
8. Bloch-Gallego E, Huchet M, el M'Hamdi H, Xie FK, Tanaka H, Henderson CE. Survival in vitro of motoneurons identified or purified by novel antibody-based methods is selectively enhanced by muscle-derived factors. Development 1991; 111:221–232.
9. Borasio GD, Robberecht W, Leigh PN, Emile J, Guiloff RJ, Jerusalem F, Silani V, Vos PE, Wokke JH, Dobbins T. A placebo-controlled trial of insulin-like growth factor-I in amyotrophic lateral sclerosis. European ALS/IGF-I Study Group.. Neurology 1998; 51:583–586.
10. Bowler RP, Sheng H, Enghild JJ, Pearlstein RD, Warner DS, Crapo JD. A catalytic antioxidant (AEOL 10150) attenuates expression of inflammatory genes in stroke. Free Radic Biol Med 2002; 33:1141–1152.

11. Briscoe J, Ericson J. Specification of neuronal fates in the ventral neural tube. Curr Opin Neurobiol 2001; 11:43–49.
12. Brooks BR, Szurek PF, Vann JM. Tamoxifen delays disease onset and progression in a mouse model of amyotrophic lateral sclerosis. Abstr Soc Neurosci Poster 2001; 628(8).
13. Bruijn LI, Miller TM, Cleveland DW. Unraveling the mechanisms involved in motor neuron degeneration in ALS. Annu Rev Neurosci 2004; 27:723–749.
14. Camu W, Henderson CE. Purification of embryonic rat motoneurons by panning on a monoclonal antibody to the low-affinity NGF receptor. J Neurosci Methods 1992; 44:59–70.
15. Cashman NR, Durham HD, Blusztajn JK, Oda K, Tabira T, Shaw IT, Dahrouge S, Antel JP. Neuroblastoma x spinal cord (NSC) hybrid cell lines resemble developing motor neurons. Dev Dyn 1992; 194:209–221.
16. Chabrier PE. In vivo pharmacological properties of BN82451: a multitargeting neuro-protective agent. Amyotroph Lateral Scler Other Motor Neuron Disord 2004; 5.
17. Chabrier PE, Roubert V, Harnett J, Cornet S, Delafotte S, Charnet-Rousillot C, Spinnewyn B, Auget M. New neuroprotective agents are potent inhibitors of mitochon-drial toxins: in vivo and in vitro studies. Soc. Neurosci. Abstr. 2001; 27:530.
18. Cisterni C, Henderson CE, Aebischer P, Pettmann B, Deglon N. Efficient gene transfer and expression of biologically active glial cell line-derived neurotrophic factor in rat motoneurons transduced wit lentiviral vectors. J Neurochem 2000; 74:1820–1828.
19. Clement AM, Nguyen MD, Roberts EA, Garcia ML, Boillee S, Rule M, McMahon AP, Doucette W, Siwek D, Ferrante RJ, Brown RH, Jr., Julien JP, Goldstein LS, Cleveland DW. Wild-type nonneuronal cells extend survival of SOD1 mutant motor neurons in ALS mice. Science 2003; 302:113–117..
20. Corcoran LJ, Mitchison TJ, Liu Q. A novel action of histone deacetylase inhibitors in a protein aggresome disease model. Curr Biol 2004; 14:488–492.
21. Cudkowicz ME, Shefner JM, Schoenfeld D, Rothstein J, Drachman DB, Northeast ALS. Consortium NEALS. Clinical trial of celecoxib in subjects with amyotrophic lateral sclerosis. Amyotroph Lateral Scler Other Motor Neuron Disord 2004; 25(5 Suppl 1).
22. Cudkowicz ME, Shefner JM, Schoenfeld DA, Brown RH, Jr., Johnson H, Qureshi M, Jacobs M, Rothstein JD, Appel SH, Pascuzzi RM, Heiman-Patterson TD, Donofrio PD, David WS, Russell JA, Tandan R, Pioro EP, Felice KJ, Rosenfeld J, Mandler RN, Sachs GM, Bradley WG, Raynor EM, Baquis GD, Belsh JM, Novella S, Goldstein J, Hulihan J. A randomized, placebo-controlled trial of topiramate in amyotrophic lateral sclerosis. Neurol-ogy 2003; 61:456–464.
23. de Paulis T. ONO-2506. Ono. Curr Opin Investig Drugs 2003; 4:863–867.
24. Desnuelle C, Dib M, Garrel C, Favier A. A double-blind, placebo-controlled randomized clinical trial of alpha-tocopherol (vitamin E) in the treatment of amyotrophic lateral sclerosis. ALS riluzole-tocopherol Study Group. Amyotroph Lateral Scler Other Motor Neuron Disord 2001; 2:9–18.
25. Drachman DB, Frank K, Dykes-Hoberg M, Teismann P, Almer G, Przedborski S, Rothstein JD. Cyclooxygenase 2 inhibition protects motor neurons and prolongs survival in a transgenic mouse model of ALS. Ann Neurol 2002; 52:771–778.
26. Drachman DB, Rothstein JD. Inhibition of cyclooxygenase-2 protects motor neurons in an organotypic model of amyotrophic lateral sclerosis. Ann Neurol 2000; 48:792–795.
27. Duong F, Fournier J, Keane PE, Guenet JL, Soubrie P, Warter JM, Borg J, Poindron P. The effect of the nonpeptide neurotrophic compound SR 57746A on the progression of the disease state of the pmn mouse. Br J Pharmacol 1998; 124:811–817.
28. Duong FH, Warter JM, Poindron P, Passilly P. Effect of the nonpeptide neurotrophic compound SR 57746A on the phenotypic survival of purified mouse motoneurons. Br J Pharmacol 1999; 128:1385–92.
29. Dupuis L, di Scala F, Rene F, de Tapia M, Oudart H, Pradat PF, Meininger V, Loeffler JP. Up-regulation of mitochondrial uncoupling protein 3 reveals an early muscular metabolic defect in amyotrophic lateral sclerosis. Faseb J 2003; 17:2091–3.

30. Durham HD, Roy J, Dong L, Figlewicz DA. Aggregation of mutant Cu/Zn superoxide dismutase proteins in a culture model of ALS. J Neuropathol Exp Neurol 1997; 56:523–530.
31. Ericson J, Briscoe J, Rashbass P, van Heyningen V, Jessell TM. Graded sonic hedgehog signaling and the specification of cell fate in the ventral neural tube. Cold Spring Harb Symp Quant Biol 1997; 62:451–466.
32. Garfield S. "Mauve: how one man invented a color that changed the world.". : Faber & Faber, 2000.
33. Graf M, Ecker D, Horowski R, Kramer B, Riederer P, Gerlach M, Hager C, Ludolph AC, Becker G, Osterhage J, Jost WH, Schrank B, Stein C, Kostopulos P, Lubik S, Wekwerth K, Dengler R, Troeger M, Wuerz A, Hoge A, Schrader C, Schimke N, Krampfl K, Petri S, Zierz S, Eger K, Neudecker S, Traufeller K, Sievert M, Neundorfer B, Hecht M. High dose vitamin E therapy in amyotrophic lateral sclerosis as add-on therapy to riluzole: results of a placebo-controlled double-blind study. J Neural Transm. 2004.
34. Greer JJ, Allan DW, Martin-Caraballo M, Lemke RP. An overview of phrenic nerve and diaphragm muscle development in the perinatal rat. J Appl Physiol 1999; 86:779–786.
35. Group TBS. A controlled trial of recombinant methionyl human BDNF in ALS: The BDNF Study Group (Phase III). Neurology 1999; 52:1427–1433.
36. Gurney ME. The use of transgenic mouse models of amyotrophic lateral sclerosis in preclinical drug studies. J Neurol Sci 1997; 152(Suppl 1):S67–73.
37. Gurney ME, Cutting FB, Zhai P, Doble A, Taylor CP, Andrus PK, Hall ED. Benefit of vitamin E, riluzole, and gabapentin in a transgenic model of familial amyotrophic lateral sclerosis. Ann Neurol 1996; 39:147–157.
38. Heemskerk J. High throughput drug screening. Amyotroph Lateral Scler Other Motor Neuron Disord 2004; 1(5 Suppl):19–21.
39. Heemskerk J, Tobin AJ, Bain LJ. Teaching old drugs new tricks. Meeting of the Neurodegeneration Drug Screening Consortium, 7–8 April 2002, Washington, DC USA. Trends Neurosci 2002; 25:494–496.
40. Heemskerk J, Tobin AJ, Ravina B. From chemical to drug: neurodegeneration drug screening and the ethics of clinical trials. Nat Neurosci2002(5 Suppl):1027–1029.
41. Heiser V, Engemann S, Brocker W, Dunkel I, Boeddrich A, Waelter S, Nordhoff E, Lurz R, Schugardt N, Rautenberg S, Herhaus C, Barnickel G, Bottcher H, Lehrach H, Wanker EE. Identification of benzothiazoles as potential polyglutamine aggregation inhibitors of Huntington's disease by using an automated filter retardation assay. Proc Natl Acad Sci U S A 2002; 4(99 Suppl):16400–6.
42. Henderson CE. Role of neurotrophic factors in neuronal development. Curr Opin Neurobiol 1996; 6:64–70.
43. Jablonka S, Wiese S, Sendtner M. Axonal defects in mouse models of motoneuron disease. J Neurobiol 2004; 58:272–286.
44. Jossan SS, Ekblom J, Gudjonsson O, Hagbarth KE, Aquilonius SM. Double blind cross over trial with deprenyl in amyotrophic lateral sclerosis. J Neural Transm Suppl 1994; 41:237–241.
45. Kaufmann P, Pullman SL, Shungu DC, Chan S, Hays AP, Del Bene ML, Dover MA, Vukic M, Rowland LP, Mitsumoto H. Objective tests for upper motor neuron involvement in amyotrophic lateral sclerosis (ALS). Neurology 2004; 62:1753–1757.
46. Kiaei M, Kipiani K, Petri S, Chen J, Calingasan NY, Crow JP, Beal MF. A novel catalytic antioxidant, manganese (AEOL 10150) slows disease progression and extends lifespan in transgenic mouse model. Amyotroph Lateral Scler Other Motor Neuron Disord 2004; 90(5 Supp 2).
47. Kirkinezos IG, Bacman SR, Hernandez D, Oca-Cossio J, Arias LJ, Perez-Pinzon MA, Bradley WG, Moraes CT. Cytochrome c association with the inner mitochondrial membrane is impaired in the CNS of G93A-SOD1 mice. J Neurosci 2005; 25:164–172.
48. Klivenyi P, Ferrante RJ, Gardian G, Browne S, Chabrier PE, Beal MF. Increased survival and neuroprotective effects of BN82451 in a transgenic mouse model of Huntington's disease. J Neurochem 2003; 86:267–272.

49. Klivenyi P, Ferrante RJ, Matthews RT, Bogdanov MB, Klein AM, Andreassen OA, Mueller G, Wermer M, Kaddurah-Daouk R, Beal MF. Neuroprotective effects of creatine in a transgenic animal model of amyotrophic lateral sclerosis. Nat Med 1999; 5:347–350.

50. Kragten E, Lalande I, Zimmermann K, Roggo S, Schindler P, Muller D, van Oostrum J, Waldmeier P, Furst P. Glyceraldehyde-3-phosphate dehydrogenase, the putative target of the antiapoptotic compounds CGP 3466 and R-(-)-deprenyl. J Biol Chem 1998; 273:5821–5828.

51. Kriz J, Gowing G, Julien JP. Efficient three-drug cocktail for disease induced by mutant superoxide dismutase. Ann Neurol 2003; 53:429–436.

52. Kriz J, Nguyen MD, Julien JP. Minocycline slows disease progression in a mouse model of amyotrophic lateral sclerosis. Neurobiol Dis 2002; 10:268–278.

53. Lacomblez L, Bensimon G, Douillet P, Doppler V, Salachas F, Meininger V. Xaliproden in amyotrophic lateral sclerosis: early clinical trials. Amyotroph Lateral Scler Other Motor Neuron Disord 2004; 5:99–106.

54. Lai EC, Felice KJ, Festoff BW, Gawel MJ, Gelinas DF, Kratz R, Murphy MF, Natter HM, Norris FH, Rudnicki SA. Effect of recombinant human insulin-like growth factor-I on progression of ALS. A placebo-controlled study. The North America ALS/IGF-I Study Group. Neurology 1997; 49:1621–1630.

55. Lariviere RC, Julien JP. Functions of intermediate filaments in neuronal development and disease. J Neurobiol 2004; 58:131–148.

56. Lewis ME, Neff NT, Contreras PC, Stong DB, Oppenheim RW, Grebow PE, Vaught JL. Insulin-like growth factor-I: potential for treatment of motor neuronal disorders. Exp Neurol 1993; 124:73–88.

57. Liu J, Lillo C, Jonsson PA, Vande Velde C, Ward CM, Miller TM, Subramaniam JR, Rothstein JD, Marklund S, Andersen PM, Brannstrom T, Gredal O, Wong PC, Williams DS, Cleveland DW. Toxicity of familial ALS-linked SOD1 mutants from selective recruitment to spinal mitochondria. Neuron 2004; 43:5–17.

58. Maragakis NJ, Jackson M, Ganel R, Rothstein JD. Topiramate protects against motor neuron degeneration in organotypic spinal cord cultures but not in G93A SOD1 transgenic mice. Neurosci Lett 2003; 338:107–10.

59. Meininger V, Bensimon G, Bradley WR, Brooks B, Douillet P, Eisen AA, Lacomblez L, Leigh PN, Robberecht W. Efficacy and safety of xaliproden in amyotrophic lateral sclerosis: results of two phase III trials. Amyotroph Lateral Scler Other Motor Neuron Disord 2004; 5:107–117.

60. Menzies FM, Cookson MR, Taylor RW, Turnbull DM, Chrzanowska-Lightowlers ZM, Dong L, Figlewicz DA, Shaw PJ. Mitochondrial dysfunction in a cell culture model of familial amyotrophic lateral sclerosis. Brain 2002; 125:1522–1533.

61. Miles GB, Yohn DC, Wichterle H, Jessell TM, Rafuse VF, Brownstone RM. Functional properties of motoneurons derived from mouse embryonic stem cells. J Neurosci 2004; 24:7848–7858.

62. Miller RG, Moore DH, 2nd, Gelinas DF, Dronsky V, Mendoza M, Barohn RJ, Bryan W, Ravits J, Yuen E, Neville H, Ringel S, Bromberg M, Petajan J, Amato AA, Jackson C, Johnson W, Mandler R, Bosch P, Smith B, Graves M, Ross M, Sorenson EJ, Kelkar P, Parry G, Olney R. Phase III randomized trial of gabapentin in patients with amyotrophic lateral sclerosis. Neurology 2001; 56:843–848.

63. Miller RG, Petajan JH, Bryan WW, Armon C, Barohn RJ, Goodpasture JC, Hoagland RJ, Parry GJ, Ross MA, Stromatt SC. A placebo-controlled trial of recombinant human ciliary neurotrophic (rhCNTF) factor in amyotrophic lateral sclerosis. rhCNTF ALS Study Group. Ann Neurol 1996; 39:256–260.

64. Miller RG, Shepherd R, Dao H, Khramstov A, Mendoza M, Graves J, Smith S. Controlled trial of nimodipine in amyotrophic lateral sclerosis. Neuromuscul Disord 1996; 6:101–104.

65. Neff NT, Prevette D, Houenou LJ, Lewis ME, Glicksman MA, Yin QW, Oppenheim RW. Insulin-like growth factors: putative muscle-derived trophic agents that promote motoneuron survival. J Neurobiol 1993; 24:1578–1588.

66. Nilsson M, Hansson E, Ronnback L. Interactions between valproate, glutamate, aspartate, and GABA with respect to uptake in astroglial primary cultures. Neurochem Res 1992; 17:327–332.

67. Nishimune H, Vasseur S, Wiese S, Birling MC, Holtmann B, Sendtner M, Iovanna JL, Henderson CE. Reg-2 is a motoneuron neurotrophic factor and a signalling intermediate in the CNTF survival pathway. Nat Cell Biol 2000; 2:906–914.

68. Oppenheim RW. Neurotrophic survival molecules for motoneurons: an embarrassment of riches. Neuron 1996; 17:195–197.

69. Pasinelli P, Belford ME, Lennon N, Bacskai BJ, Hyman BT, Trotti D, Brown RH, Jr. Amyotrophic lateral sclerosis-associated SOD1 mutant proteins bind and aggregate with Bcl-2 in spinal cord mitochondria. Neuron 2004; 43:19–30.

70. Peluffo H, Estevez A, Barbeito L, Stutzmann JM. Riluzole promotes survival of rat motoneurons in vitro by stimulating trophic activity produced by spinal astrocyte monolayers. Neurosci Lett 1997; 228:207–211.

71. Raoul C, Estevez AG, Nishimune H, Cleveland DW, deLapeyriere O, Henderson CE, Haase G, Pettmann B. Motoneuron death triggered by a specific pathway downstream of Fas potentiation by ALS-linked SOD1 mutations. Neuron 2002; 35:1067–1083.

72. Ray SS, Nowak RJ, Strokovich K, Brown RH, Jr., Walz T, Lansbury PT, Jr. An intersubunit disulfide bond prevents in vitro aggregation of a superoxide dismutase-1 mutant linked to familial amytrophic lateral sclerosis. Biochemistry 2004; 43:4899–4905.

73. Renoncourt Y, Carroll P, Filippi P, Arce V, Alonso S. Neurons derived in vitro from ES cells express homeoproteins characteristic of motoneurons and interneurons. Mech Dev 1998; 79:185–197.

74. Rothstein JD, Bristol LA, Hosler B, Brown RH, Jr., Kuncl RW. Chronic inhibition of superoxide dismutase produces apoptotic death of spinal neurons. Proc Natl Acad Sci U.S.A. 1994; 91:4155–4159.

75. Rothstein JD, Kuncl RW. Neuroprotective strategies in a model of chronic glutamate-mediated motor neuron toxicity. J Neurochem 1995; 65:643–651.

76. Rothstein JD, Sarjubhai P, Regan MR, Haenggeli C, Huang YH, Bergles DE, Jin L, Dykes Hoberg M, Vidensky S, Chung DS, Vang Toan S, Bruijn LI, Su Z-Z, Gupta P, Fisher PB. Beta-Lactam antibiotics offer neuroprotection by increasing glutamate transporter expression. Nature 2005; 433:73–77.

77. Roy J, Minotti S, Dong L, Figlewicz DA, Durham HD. Glutamate potentiates the toxicity of mutant Cu/Zn-superoxide dismutase in motor neurons by postsynaptic calcium-dependent mechanisms. J Neurosci 1998; 18:9673–84.

78. Sagot Y, Toni N, Perrelet D, Lurot S, King B, Rixner H, Mattenberger L, Waldmeier PC, Kato AC. An orally active anti-apoptotic molecule (CGP 3466B) preserves mitochondria and enhances survival in an animal model of motoneuron disease. Br J Pharmacol 2000; 131:721–728.

79. Salazar-Grueso EF, Kim S, Kim H. Embryonic mouse spinal cord motor neuron hybrid cells. Neuroreport 1991; 2:505–508.

80. Sendtner M, Pei G, Beck M, Schweizer U, Wiese S. Developmental motoneuron cell death and neurotrophic factors. Cell Tissue Res 2000; 301:71–84.

81. Shefner JM, Cudkowicz ME, Schoenfeld D, Conrad T, Taft J, Chilton M, Urbinelli L, Qureshi M, Zhang H, Pestronk A, Caress J, Donofrio P, Sorenson E, Bradley W, Lomen-Hoerth C, Pioro E, Rezania K, Ross M, Pascuzzi R, Heiman-Patterson T, Tandan R, Mitsumoto H, Rothstein J, Smith-Palmer T, MacDonald D, Burke D. A clinical trial of creatine in ALS. Neurology 2004; 63:1656–1661.

82. Sheng H, Enghild JJ, Bowler R, Patel M, Batinic-Haberle I, Calvi CL, Day BJ, Pearlstein RD, Crapo JD, Warner DS. Effects of metalloporphyrin catalytic antioxidants in experimental brain ischemia. Free Radic Biol Med 2002; 33:947–961.

83. Shinder GA, Lacourse MC, Minotti S, Durham HD. Mutant Cu/Zn-superoxide dismutase proteins have altered solubility and interact with heat shock/stress proteins in models of amyotrophic lateral sclerosis. J Biol Chem 2001; 276:12791–12796.

84. Shults CW, Oakes D, Kieburtz K, Beal MF, Haas R, Plumb S, Juncos JL, Nutt J, Shoulson I, Carter J, Kompoliti K, Perlmutter JS, Reich S, Stern M, Watts RL, Kurlan R, Molho E, Harrison M, Lew M. Effects of coenzyme Q10 in early Parkinson disease: evidence of slowing of the functional decline. Arch Neurol 2002; 59:1541–1550.

85. Skradski S, White HS. Topiramate blocks kainate-evoked cobalt influx into cultured neurons. Epilepsia 2000; 41(Suppl 1):S45–7.

86. Snider RM, Constantine JW, Lowe JA, 3rd, Longo KP, Lebel WS, Woody HA, Drozda SE, Desai MC, Vinick FJ, Spencer RW, et al. A potent nonpeptide antagonist of the substance P (NK1) receptor. Science 1991; 251:435–437.

87. Stockwell BR. Exploring biology with small organic molecules. Nature 2004; 432: 846–854.

88. Su GH, Sohn TA, Ryu B, Kern SE. A novel histone deacetylase inhibitor identified by high-throughput transcriptional screening of a compound library. Cancer Res 2000; 60:3137–3142.

89. Tateishi N, Mori T, Kagamiishi Y, Satoh S, Katsube N, Morikawa E, Morimoto T, Matsui T, Asano T. Astrocytic activation and delayed infarct expansion after permanent focal ischemia in rats. Part II: suppression of astrocytic activation by a novel agent (R)-(-)-2-propyloctanoic acid (ONO-2506) leads to mitigation of delayed infarct expansion and early improvement of neurologic deficits. J Cereb Blood Flow Metab 2002; 22:723–734.

90. Tikka T, Fiebich BL, Goldsteins G, Keinänen R, Koistinaho J. Minocycline, a tetracycline derivative, is neuroprotective against excitotoxicity by inhibiting activation and proliferation of microglia. J Neurosci 2001; 21:2580–2588.

91. Tikka T, Vartiainen NE, Goldsteins G, Oja SS, Andersen PM, Marklund SL, Koistinaho J. Minocycline prevents neurotoxicity induced by cerebrospinal fluid from patients with motor neurone disease. Brain 2002; 125:722–731.

92. Van Den Bosch L, Tilkin P, Lemmens G, Robberecht W. Minocycline delays disease onset and mortality in a transgenic model of ALS. Neuroreport 2002; 13:1067–1070.

93. Vila M, Przedborski S. Targeting programmed cell death in neurodegenerative diseases. Nat Rev Neurosci 2003; 4:365–375.

94. Waldmeier PC, Boulton AA, Cools AR, Kato AC, Tatton WG. Neurorescuing effects of the GAPDH ligand CGP 3466B. J Neural Transm Suppl 2000:197–214.

95. Wichterle H, Lieberam I, Porter JA, Jessell TM. Directed differentiation of embryonic stem cells into motor neurons. Cell 2002; 110:385–397.

96. Yasojima K, Tourtellotte WW, McGeer EG, McGeer PL. Marked increase in cyclooxygenase-2 in ALS spinal cord: implications for therapy. Neurology 2001; 57:952–956.

97. Zhang W, Narayanan M, Friedlander RM. Additive neuroprotective effects of minocycline with creatine in a mouse model of ALS. Ann Neurol 2003; 53:267–270.

98. Zhu S, Stavrovskaya IG, Drozda M, Kim BY, Ona V, Li M, Sarang S, Liu AS, Hartley DM, Wu du C, Gullans S, Ferrante RJ, Przedborski S, Kristal BS, Friedlander RM. Minocycline inhibits cytochrome c release and delays progression of amyotrophic lateral sclerosis in mice. Nature 2002; 417:74–78.

26
Clinical Trial Methodology

Paul H. Gordon
Neurological Institute, Columbia University, New York, New York, U.S.A.

INTRODUCTION

In progressive disorders such as amyotropic lateral sclerosis (ALS), new therapies can be studied adequately only in the context of randomized controlled trials, which not only determine if a treatment is effective but also increase our overall understanding of the disorder. Rapid innovation at the bench and in trial design have led to a number of recent sophisticated multicenter clinical trials. Yet, despite great strides in both the basic and clinical sciences, progress in ALS research has not so far translated into practical clinical applications. Riluzole remains the only medication approved for use in ALS, nearly a decade after its introduction.

Past trials have provided valuable experience, but the outcome of many has been hampered by various difficulties inherent in the study of a rapidly progressive heterogeneous disease like ALS. Some of the problems facing clinical trialists in ALS include lack of consensus in using the transgenic mouse model, and whether the murine model fully represents an effective drug screen for human sporadic ALS; incomplete definition of dosage and route in early phase human trials; inadequate sample size and statistical planning in later phase trials; variability in data collection and outcome at different trial sites; and higher than expected subject dropout.

Many questions remain in the search for effective treatments, including which preclinical screens to use, which clinical assessments are the best outcome measures, and how trials should be designed to minimize variability of data and reduce subject dropout. In 1995, the World Federation of Neurology (WFN) Subcommittee on Motor Neuron Disease has established ALS Clinical Trial Guidelines (1), and while clinical trials are planned and executed with great care, the evolution in trial design continues. This chapter is devoted to the process of introducing new drugs into the clinical arena, and includes discussions of trial design and methodology.

DRUG DEVELOPMENT AND TRANSLATIONAL RESEARCH

Clinical trials are the final stage of the complex process of drug development, which begins with basic science research and ends in large-scale human trials. A strong scientific rationale must be present before embarking on an expensive clinical trial, but consensus guidelines that define which model is the best estimator of human response have not been defined. Preclinical research includes pathological, pharmacokinetic, toxicity, and efficacy studies, which test the effects of a new drug in in vitro and in vivo models. In vitro models such as motor neuron and spinal cord tissue culture, provide rapid results, and have been used for high throughput screening, but may not reflect complex in vivo pathophysiology. The transgenic mouse model is probably the most widely accepted means of establishing the scientific merit of an investigational agent. Questions remain, however, such as the timing of administration (late presymptomatic phase vs. early symptomatic phase), how best to define dose and pharmacokinetics that translate well into human trials, and what degree of improvement in the murine model is meaningful. Survival differs depending on the strain used, and brain drug levels are difficult to measure. Past trials have begun with or without supporting murine data. As more potential agents become available, expert consensus is needed to establish criteria for preclinical testing.

Human clinical trials begin once the basic science investigations are complete and a drug is considered to have suitable scientific rationale for use in ALS. The United States Food and Drug Administration (FDA) has formulated guidelines for developing new drugs for human consumption (http://www.fda.gov/cber/ind/indpubs.htm). The FDA oversees all clinical trials under an Investigational New Drug (IND) Application. The investigation is headed by an academician with independent funding, or by a pharmaceutical company. The FDA has designated ALS as an "orphan" disease because it affects only a small proportion of the population, having a prevalence of less than 200,000 individuals in the United States. The FDA promotes the rapid development of orphan drugs and has procedures for the use of investigational drugs in the treatment of immediately life-threatening diseases and serious illnesses, such as ALS. A "treatment IND" allows original drugs that are still in the final stages of clinical trials to be given to patients when there are no satisfactory alternative treatments (2). Riluzole and insulin-like growth factor (IGF-I) were both prescribed using a treatment IND while drug approval was under evaluation at FDA.

The clinical trials process includes several phases. Phase-I studies test pharmacokinetic characteristics and clinical safety and toxicity of the drug for the first time, usually in less than 100 human subjects, often healthy volunteers. In certain terminal diseases, such as cancer and AIDS, affected patients may participate in the phase-I investigation, which then provides an early test of efficacy. Past studies of neurotrophic factors used this approach in ALS (3,4).

Phase-II studies explore dose regimen, safety and toxicity, feasibility, and early evidence of efficacy, and generally include up to several 100 patients. The phase-II study seeking early evidence of efficacy, however, risks being an underpowered phase-III trial. Innovative pilot designs are needed that act as efficient screens for proceeding to efficacy trials, possibly testing multiple medications at once. One potential design is the futility study, in which a medication is tested against a minimum accepted effect level, while at the same time establishing optimal dose and regimen. Those drugs, for which "non-futility" is shown, could then be tested for efficacy.

The phase-III trial is the final test of efficacy and safety and is usually undertaken in several 100 to several 1000 patients. The outcome measure best establishing efficacy has yet to be determined. There are no biomarkers that enable the investigator to directly measure a drug's effect on the motor neuron. Traditionally, survival has been considered the gold standard, but as different interventions emerge, surrogates have been sought, including functional scales and strength measures (see below). Phase-IV studies are occasionally conducted once a drug has received marketing approval, with the goal of detecting low frequency, serious side effects that may have escaped detection in earlier phase studies.

CHOOSING TRIAL CANDIDATES: PATIENT INCLUSION AND EXCLUSION CRITERIA

Inclusion and exclusion criteria (Table 1) for clinical trials are chosen to balance the needs, to test the medication in those with the greatest likelihood of response (i.e., those with early ALS in whom a neuroprotective agent may have most benefit), to minimize subject dropout in order to maintain quality of data, and to obtain results generalizable to the greater population of ALS patients. The most fundamental criterion is the accuracy of the diagnosis. As there are no diagnostic biomarkers for ALS, the diagnosis depends on accepted clinical guidelines, such as the El Escorial diagnostic criteria (5), though some consider these to be too limiting. Other subsets of motor neuron disease, such as progressive muscular atrophy, are usually excluded from ALS trials because they may have different causes, respond differently to a

Table 1 Example Inclusion and Exclusion Criteria for Clinical Trials in ALS

Inclusion criteria
A clinical diagnosis of ALS, according to modified El Escorial criteria
Age 21–85 years
Disease duration generally <3–5 years
Functional level: best FVC <60–75%, or ALSFRS >16–20
Patients on stable dose riluzole
Women of childbearing age must be nonlactating and surgically sterile or using an effective
    method of birth control and have a negative pregnancy test (adequate birth control
    includes use of intra-uterine device or oral contraceptives plus a barrier method,
    e.g., condom and diaphragm)
Willing and able to give signed informed consent that has been approved by your IRB
Exclusion criteria
Requirement for tracheotomy ventilation (or non-invasive ventilation >23 hr/day)
Diagnosis of other neurodegenerative diseases (Parkinson's disease, Alzheimer's disease, etc.)
FVC <60–75% of predicted
A clinically significant history of unstable medical illness (unstable angina, advanced cancer,
    etc.) over the last three years
Subjects with ALS in a first-degree relative (parent, sibling, and child) (FALS)
Treatment with any medications with side effect profile similar to drug under investigation
Pregnancy or lactation
Women with the potential to become pregnant who are not practicing effective birth control
Allergy to class of medications of drug under investigation
Limited mental capacity rendering the subject unable to provide written informed consent or
    comply with evaluation procedures
History of recent alcohol or drug abuse or noncompliance with treatment or other
    experimental protocols
Use of any investigational drug within the past 30 days

Abbreviations: ALS, amyotropic lateral sclerosis; FVC, forced vital capacity; ALSFRS, amyotropic lateral sclerosis functional rating scale; IRB, Institutional Review Board; FALS, familial amyotropic lateral sclerosis.

drug, and have different rates of progression. Similarly, those patients with familial ALS, patients with active neurological diseases other than ALS, and patients with ALS of long duration (>5 years) may be different from typical ALS (6), and are also generally excluded. A certain amount of arbitrariness may be unavoidable in determining the clinical category for a given patient.

ALS functional scales or muscle strength testing are used to screen patients for inclusion and exclusion. Recent trials have included patients with early ALS and with no or only minor respiratory failure (7). These subjects are most likely to be able to complete the trial, to be able to tolerate minor adverse events induced by the drug, and thus to provide the most complete data. Those with more advanced ALS may be excluded because of the low likelihood of response, and the high risk of dropout. Patients having active, unstable concomitant diseases, recent major surgery, or a history of significant medical diseases are also excluded. These patients are not assumed to respond to experimental treatment in ways similar to sporadic ALS, and their illnesses may confound interpretation of adverse events occurring during the study.

Patients may be allowed to take other medications or not, depending on their potential impact on the disease, and on the medication under investigation. Although this has not always been the case in past trials, other investigational agents are usually excluded from the study to ensure clarity of results. The investigator then runs the risk of having some patients who secretly take other drugs hoping for benefit, but possibly disrupting the validity of the trial. Riluzole, FDA-approved for treatment of ALS, is ordinarily allowed in trials, despite its modest effect, and subjects are randomized according to its use. Some "off-label drugs" (FDA-approved drugs for diseases other than ALS) cause relatively minor side effects and may not interfere with the main purpose of the investigation. The decision to include or exclude patients receiving such drugs may depend on the nature of the medication to be tested. When a test drug is expected to have side effects similar to those of a concomitant medication, or if one drug may mask the side effects of the other, the concomitant medication is discontinued. Some medications, however, are often crucial because they provide symptomatic relief for patients. It may not be appropriate, for instance, to discontinue antidepressants, muscle relaxants, and antisialorrhea agents unless there are clear safety reasons for doing so.

The effects of investigational drugs on a fetus or on breast-fed infants are usually unknown, so women of childbearing age undergo pregnancy testing and are instructed to use birth control during the trial. A recent trial of IGF-I excluded all women of childbearing age, causing ethical concerns (8). Some trials have also asked men to use birth control because of potential effects on sperm. The last criterion is the ability of study subjects to understand and sign the consent form.

ASSESSMENTS AND OUTCOME MEASURES

An outcome measure is any measurement that is used for assessing the effect of an intervention. The primary outcome measure is defined during the design phase and used to calculate the sample size required for ensuring that the study has sufficient power. As there are no biomarkers of disease progression in ALS, investigators must use potential surrogate markers, which measure disease progression, if not the drug's direct impact on motor neurons. A variety of outcome measures have been used in clinical trials (9,10). Louwerse et al. (11) listed 12 requirements for measurement techniques used in clinical trials for ALS, including relevance, validity, reliability, simplicity, and sensitivity to change, among others. Other considerations in choosing the outcome measures include expense, degree of variability, and ease of administration. The most common currently used outcome measures are described below.

Primary and Secondary Outcomes

Outcomes in ALS trials are chosen to detect impact in several ways: (i) symptomatic improvement, (ii) reduced rate of deterioration, and (iii) prolonged survival time (12). In ALS, measurement of muscle strength, motor function, respiratory function, or survival are usually chosen as primary outcomes. Secondary outcomes are related to the primary outcomes but are considered of less clinical or medical importance (13).

The primary outcome measure should be clinically relevant to the patient, and ideally, effects of the treatment on the primary outcome should impact medical practice. Riluzole, e.g., has been shown to extend survival by several months, an outcome that many patients and their doctors do not find clinically meaningful, so that approximately 40% of patients in the United States do not take it, and the Canadian health system will not cover the cost.

The outcomes should be defined before the start of a trial, incorporated into the statistical planning and clinical hypotheses, and reported accordingly at the end of the study, whether or not they are statistically or clinically significant. Selective reporting, in which only the desirable findings of the study are presented, detracts from scientific knowledge, and may hinder future trial design. Results of post-hoc analysis may be difficult to interpret; often the only defense against selective reporting is to determine whether the relationships make clinical sense. Thus, all results should be reported accurately, completely, and in context. To ensure accurate data reporting, investigators need to have full access to data from industry sponsored trials (14). What degree of improvement or deterioration is clinically meaningful to patients has yet to be determined. Studies are underway that assess the clinical meaningfulness of changes in outcome measures.

Survival

Survival has been a standard outcome measure in past clinical trials (15), and may be the definitive outcome in a disorder in which death is an early manifestation. There are disadvantages, however, to using survival as a primary outcome measure. Varying patterns of practice at different centers influence survival (16,17), and adequate power for study requires large long studies. Longevity in ALS depends, in part, on other external health factors (18), which include not only the level of general medical care and the presence or absence of other systemic diseases, but also qualities of the caregiver and the administration of palliative care (19). The use of non-invasive mechanical ventilation, gastrostomy, antibiotics for bronchitis or presumed aspiration pneumonia, and opioid treatments vary from center to center and may all impact survival. Tracheostomy for permanent ventilator care clearly postpones death, as can prolonged daily non-invasive ventilation, and thus both are considered as equivalent to death in defining an outcome in survival analysis (20).

The strongest argument against using death as the primary outcome may be the greater length of the study required. Adequate numbers of events must occur in order to detect differences in placebo and intervention groups. The median duration of survival in ALS ranges from 23 to 52 months, with 50% survival somewhere near three years after the onset of disease. Sufficient power may require study of at least

1000 subjects over three years, greatly increasing cost and the time to obtain results. A recent trial of creatine, however, used continuous data monitoring, stopping the trial once the statistical ability to detect efficacy was impossible, thus reducing its length and cost (21).

ALS Global Scales and Other Scales

ALS Functional Rating Scale/R. The ALS Functional Rating Scale (ALSFRS), which measures activities of daily living (ADL), was first designed to augment the standard outcome measures of mortality, muscle strength, and pulmonary function in clinical trials of ALS (22). It was modeled after the ALS Severity Scale (23), which was patterned after the Unified Parkinson Disease Rating Scale (24). All 12 activities of the revised scale (ALSFRS-R), consisting of three bulbar functions, three respiratory functions, two upper extremity functions (cutting food and dressing), two lower-extremity functions (walking and climbing), and two other functions (dressing-hygiene and turning in bed), are relevant in ALS. Each activity is recorded to the closest approximation from a list of five choices, scored 0 to 4, with the total score ranging from 48 (normal function) to 0 (unable to attempt any task).

Prior to use in clinical trials, the ALSFRS was validated in two preliminary studies (25). The ALSFRS was shown to have high internal consistency, reliability, validity in comparison to other measures, and responsiveness to change. It was then assessed in a large clinical trial of CNTF (3,26). The test–retest reliability and internal consistency (correlation coefficient = 0.95) were confirmed in the 245 patients in the placebo group. The baseline ALSFRS score correlated strongly with muscle strength, Schwab and England ADL scores, and with survival. Patients whose ALSFRS scores were 30 or above had a greater than 90% survival during the nine months study, and those below 30 had a 76% survival (26). Change in ALSFRS over time closely paralleled change in other measures, including muscle testing, forced vital capacity (FVC), Schwab and England scale, and global clinical impression reports.

One weakness of the original scale was that it disproportionately weighted limb and bulbar function over respiratory function. During the course of a clinical trial of brain-derived neurotrophic factor (BDNF) (27), three additional questions were developed and tested, which evaluate the progression of respiratory dysfunction in ALS. The addition of the respiratory symptom ratings resulted in a scale that was better able to predict survival and more sensitive to change than the original ALSFRS (28). In that study, baseline ALSFRS-R scores ranked only behind age and prestudy FVC% as the strongest predictor of survival.

A recent retrospective study of a clinic population of 267 patients validated the ALSFRS-R as a surrogate for survival beyond the constraints of clinical trials. The association of the ASLFRS-R score at baseline with mortality was examined using Cox proportional hazards models, which showed the baseline score was a strong predictor of death or tracheostomy independently of FVC. Patients with a total ALSFRS-R score below the median had a 4.4-fold increased risk of death or tracheostomy compared to those who scored above the median (29).

One advantage of using a functional rating scale over other primary outcome measures is the ease of administration, theoretically reducing subject dropout from trials. Disease progression may make it impossible to perform strength or respiratory function testing properly, when subjects and their caregivers are still fully able to complete a questionnaire. To magnify this benefit, a recent study compared the ALSFRS-R administered in person and over the telephone. Use of standardized procedures for the interview minimized errors between clinic and telephone administration (30).

The ALSFRS-R is easy to administer, inexpensive, sensitive, clinically meaningful, and reliable. The scale reports patients' functional abilities, and correlates with physiological measures of progress and survival. The first major trials using the ASLFRS-R as the primary outcome are starting to enroll patients now.

Appel ALS Scale. The Appel ALS scale integrates pulmonary function and manual muscle testing (MMT) (31,32). The scale consists of 16 tests and three subjective evaluations. One possible shortcoming of this scale is the use of MMT, a technique that may be insensitive to changes over time unless administered to large numbers of muscles by trained therapists (see below). Sensitivity may also be reduced in patients whose scores reach more than 100 (range 30–160) (9). However, in one study the standard deviation of the Appel scores at 12 months was smaller than that of the Norris scale, suggesting that the Appel scale might allow smaller sample sizes in standard placebo-controlled studies to detect the effectiveness of a drug over 12 months. Several clinical trials of IGF-1 have used this scale as the primary outcome measure (8).

Norris Scale. The Norris scale, proposed in 1979 (33) and modified in 1990, uses 28 clinical tests and six subjective evaluations (e.g., chewing, bowel/bladder pressure, and feeding) to measure neurologic function. The Norris scale is simple and feasible, and has been used in clinical trials (15,34,35), but it has disadvantages (9,36). The arm subscore is weighted more heavily than other subscores, including the respiratory score, and variables such as bladder pressure and reflexes, which have little clinical bearing, are considered equivalent to major variables, weakening the scale's ability to predict progression.

Schwab and England Global Rating Scale. Schwab and England (37) developed a global measure of ADL in evaluating surgical outcomes in Parkinson's disease. This scale consists of 11 points and assesses ADL function from 100 (normal) to 0 (vegetative functions only). The ALS CNTF Treatment Study Group (22) analyzed the validity of the scale and found it to be highly correlated with ALSFRS and sensitive to changes over time. A 1-point change in the Schwab and England scale is roughly equivalent to a 3-point change in the ALSFRS.

Ashworth Scale. The Ashworth scale (38) is a semi-quantitative measurement of spasticity, but the scale has no quantitative measurements to test upper motor neuron signs. This scale has been used as a secondary outcome measure in past trials in ALS.

Pseudobulbar Lability Scale. Several scales are available that measure emotional lability. A recently published clinical trial used the pseudobulbar lability scale to monitor changes in lability over time. The scale can be self-administered (39). A separate emotional lability questionnaire has been modified for ALS patients, but has not yet been tested in clinical trials (40).

Muscle Strength Testing

Manual Muscle Testing. MMT has been used in most neuromuscular treatment trials, often in conjunction with maximum voluntary isometric contraction (MVIC), and is a global assessment of strength. MMT of 34 muscle groups was recently shown to be more sensitive than MVIC in detecting changes in strength with proper evaluator training in a population of ALS patients (41). In that study test reliability was compared between MMT and MVIC scores among 14 institutions and test validity was examined by comparing change in scores over time. Sixty-three subjects were examined at 3-month intervals for 12 months. MMT was more sensitive in detecting change over time in patients with ALS, had a more favorable coefficient of variation, was less expensive, and consumed less examiner time.

MMT has several disadvantages (42). MMT produces ordinal scores, which require non-parametric, statistically less powerful analyses. The ordinal scores on the medical research council (MRC) score are also not uniformly distributed. The MRC score is characterized by a loss of sensitivity, particularly at the higher end of the scale (42). The scores of grade 4 (overcomes passive resistance) and grade 5 (normal) reflect at least 40% and sometimes as much as 97% of the patient's muscle strength (9,43). The high degree of precision necessary to perform MMT requires trained physical therapist evaluators. MMT will be used as a primary outcome for the first time in a trial of IGF-1, now enrolling.

Maximum Voluntary Isometric Contraction. MVIC is a quantitative measure of isometric muscle strength. The technique was developed as part of the tufts quantitative neuromuscular evaluation (TQNE) (44). MVIC requires a strain gauge (a force displacement transducer), a strap to hold the limb being tested, a special examining table to position the patient's joints and to fix the strain gauge at a proper angle, and a computer to process the data. This technique has been used in many trials during the past 10 years (26,27,45). MVIC satisfies most of the important requirements for measurement techniques, and its range and sensitivity have been validated by several natural history studies (9,18,46,47). However, reliability may be low unless the examiner is well trained, and the need for complex and expensive equipment reduces its simplicity. There has been variability of data between sites and high dropout because of the difficulty the patients with advanced ALS have in performing the test (45,48).

While MMT allows ordinal scores of different muscles to be compared, raw scores from MVIC must first undergo z-score transformation to standardize raw scores relative to a reference population by comparison to those from a normative population (18,46,47). Once the raw scores are standardized, individual z-scores can be averaged by region (right or left arm, arms, right or left leg, or legs) to form a "megascore." MVIC has been the primary outcome measure in recent clinical trials of CNTF, gabapentin, and topiramate, but MVIC may not be considered the ideal primary outcome measure it once was, because of the needed equipment and space, the expense entailed, and the high degree of associated dropout.

Hand-Held Dynamometer. Hand-held dynamometry is inexpensive, portable, provides quantitative, reproducible data, and has been used as a secondary outcome measure in clinical trials (49). Variability in data collection may occur, however, because the technique partly depends on the examiner's muscle strength. Simple outcomes such as dynamometry may regain favor as large trials seek greater numbers of patients at diverse centers.

Pulmonary Function

Respiratory function tests such as negative inspiratory pressure (NIP), sometimes called maximum inspiratory pressure (MIP), and FVC assess diaphragm strength. The FVC (percent predicted) produces linear and reliable data in longitudinal studies of ALS patients (48). Although FVC was used as the primary endpoint in the BDNF trial (27) and one of the coprimary endpoints in a trial of xaliproden (unpublished), and has always been used as a secondary outcome measure, it is difficult to administer accurately, requiring special training, and provides a limited assessment of only one function.

Quantitative Neuromuscular Testing

Tufts Quantitative Neuromuscular Evaluation. The TQNE (18,44,49) includes the MVIC; pulmonary function tests; timed bulbar function tests, such as syllable repetition; and timed upper extremity function tests, such as the time to dial a 7-digit phone number; and the time to transfer a set of pegs to a Purdue pegboard. In the TQNE, these quantitative tests are grouped into five major categories (megascores), which have been analyzed extensively in ALS patients producing normative data to compute the z-scores. Despite a long record of accomplishment, the complexity of equipment, expense, and training required have made the TQNE a less attractive outcome currently.

Other Quantitative Measurements. Timed function tests of the leg include the time required to walk 5 m. Quantitative bulbar function tests have been used, but their utility is limited. The time to drink 5 oz. of water, e.g., is difficult to perform because of the potential risk of aspiration. Bulbar muscle strength has been assessed by testing bite pressure, lip closure, and tongue muscle strength (9,50). The changes of these tests have been correlated with MVIC in limb muscles (9,42), but standardization is difficult and data is often variable.

Electrophysiologic Testing

Motor Unit Number Estimation. Electrodiagnostic studies can provide information on disease progression not readily available from measurement of muscle strength or clinical scales. Over the past decade, the field of motor unit number estimation (MUNE) has become increasingly sophisticated. MUNE provides a quantitative assessment of lower motor neuron survival and loss, by estimating the number of functioning motor units (51). It has been applied to untreated populations of ALS patients in a number of studies, resulting in natural history data on motor unit deterioration (52,53). Of the several methods available, the most sensitive and reliable has yet to be determined.

MUNE is increasingly being used as a secondary outcome measure in clinical trials of ALS. MUNE was performed in 80 patients during the clinical trials with CNTF, and in more recent trials of creatine and topiramate, the number of the motor units declined predictably in both treated patients and controls (26,54).

Neurophysiological Index. The neurophysiological index (NI) is calculated as the compound muscle action potential amplitude divided by the distal motor latency multiplied by the F frequency percent, and has been correlated with strength (55). In one study of a small number of patients, the NI had a smaller coefficient of variation, and decreased more markedly during the course of one year than other physiological measures (55). It has been shown to have small variance and high reliability. The NI is simple, takes very little time, is quite inexpensive, and is available using standard electrophysiological equipment. Nevertheless, the NI still needs to be studied in larger numbers of patients before it can be considered a standard outcome measure.

Quality-of-Life Assessments

Quality of life (QOL) is important in patients who suffer from chronic, debilitating diseases (56,57), and its assessment is helpful in making clinical decisions. Whether or not a new drug improves QOL is an important factor in ascertaining its value. In trials, investigators may seek medications that slow the progression of ALS or reduce mortality. A prolongation in life, however, without an impact on QOL, may not be considered meaningful. For this reason, the WFN Subcommittee on

Motor Neuron Disease now recommends that all clinical trials include a QOL assessment. The sickness impact profile and SF-36 have both been used in recent trials, but there are multiple facets of QOL, and these scales may correlate more with strength in ALS than with true QOL (57). QOL measures that are heavily focused on disease functionality do not sufficiently assess existential and spiritual QOL, which may be maintained despite functional deterioration (57). At present there is no single, uniformly accepted or widely used instrument, and no validated ALS-specific QOL scale. Simple and objective QOL assessment techniques, which fulfill requirements for clinical measurement, still need to be developed.

Biomarkers

Biomarkers, laboratory measures of the disease process, are undergoing study in ALS. Potential markers of upper motor neuron function, including transcranial magnetic stimulation, magnetic resonance imaging, and spectroscopy are discussed elsewhere. Biochemical markers are also being increasingly studied as secondary outcomes in trials of ALS. Potential biomarkers include indices of DNA oxidative injury (58), protein oxidation (59), lipid peroxides (60), and serum levels of matrix metalloproteinase-9 (61) and transforming growth factor-1 (62). However, Most are not specific to ALS and have low sensitivity. Proteomics and metabolomics, studies of proteins and small molecules, are just now being investigated in ALS.

STUDY DESIGN

One of the most important aspects of studying new interventions is the trial design itself. Successful trials are those that provide valid, easily interpretable data. A trial should be appealing to patients, so that enrollment does not lag, and dropout is minimal, but validity cannot be sacrificed for the sake of patient interests. Several different designs have been used in past trials of ALS, with varying degrees of success.

The Open-Label Study

An open-label study is one in which all subjects receive the active medication. Open-label studies are very desirable to patients who often wish to try any potentially beneficial medication in the face of a devastating disease. However, unless the drug produces an overwhelming impact, a study without a control group is often uninterpretable, and the data is usually not acceptable as evidence of efficacy (63). Even in patients with ALS, an otherwise ineffective drug may produce placebo effects lasting as long as three or four months (63,64). Furthermore, if side effects of an experimental drug mimic symptoms produced during the natural course of ALS (weakness, fatigue, weight loss, or respiratory failure) (39), they may not be identified correctly as adverse effects of the medication. Thus, open-label trials are currently considered for only early phase studies.

Several methods have been proposed to improve the interpretability of data from open-label trials. The comparison of changes in endpoints reported during the open trials with those obtained from natural historical controls is one method (65), but questions regarding the reliability of natural history data have not been fully answered. The treated patients in a randomized trial often differ from patients in previous natural history studies (63). Control patients in randomized studies are a specifically selected population (by inclusion and exclusion criteria) and may not represent the general ALS population. In fact, the megaslopes summarizing the decline in muscle strength of control patients who participated in the CNTF studies were different from those constituted with natural history data derived from the Wisconsin–Colorado database (63). Finally, as palliative care evolves in ALS, natural history databases may lose relevance to current patients.

A separate method is to use patients as their own controls. Patients may be followed for a period of 3 to 6 months to identify the rate of disease progression (a lead-in period) and then receive an open-label drug in the study period. The changes in measured variables between the lead-in period and the treatment period are compared statistically. Questions remain, however, regarding the impact of placebo effect, and whether the lead-in period and the treatment period are medically and biologically comparable. This type of study is also limited by the absence of a control group.

The Randomized, Double-Blind, Placebo-Controlled, Cross-Over Study

A cross-over study provides active medication to all subjects, although not in the same sequence. Patients are randomly assigned to either schedule I (placebo to active drug) or schedule II (active drug to placebo), so all participants receive the active drug in either the first or the second phase. Although this design may appeal more to patients, it has disadvantages (66). The carry-over effect in schedule II (that is, an effect from the active drug that lasts into the placebo stage) adds an element of uncertainty, making the evaluation of the placebo in the second stage potentially less valid as in schedule I, in which patients are naive to the study drug. Furthermore, it is not yet clear whether the disease can be considered biologically identical during the early and later stages. The biology may change as the disease progresses, causing the response to the medication to be different in schedules I and II.

The Randomized, Double-Blind, Placebo-Controlled, Parallel Study

This design remains the gold standard, offers data simplest to interpret, and would be required before FDA approval of any new medication (66). Typically, in this study design, patients are randomly assigned to one of two groups. One group of patients receives the drug to be tested, while the other group receives placebo (or the standard treatment). Both the patients and investigators are blinded to the assignments, which can be made from random number tables by computer generation.

The effects of different dose levels may be investigated concurrently, and multiple parallel groups can be included in a double-blind, placebo-controlled design. The strengths of this design include the ability to randomize patients at the same stage of the disease for direct prospective comparison, and negation of the placebo effect because both blinded groups presumably experience the placebo effect to the same degree.

Potential Problems with the Double-Blind Study

The prospective, randomized, double-blind, controlled design is not fool-proof. Potential pitfalls include, e.g., finding no difference in a study with low power and concluding that the two groups are equivalent, when in fact they are not. Such studies are not negative but inconclusive; not enough data were collected to detect a clinically important difference even if one existed. Statistical planning prior to study roll out is necessary to reduce problems of under-powering.

When an active drug produces obvious side effects or adverse reactions, it may be difficult to carry out a blinded study. Such a phenomenon has been observed in several controlled clinical studies and creates an inherit limitation to double-blind, controlled studies (64,67,68). In one controlled study an "active" placebo (norepinephrine) was given to mimic the side effects produced by the drug (64).

If the groups of patients are not comparable at study outset, then changes occurring in the clinical trial may not be due to the medication, but result instead from imbalance in patient characteristics between treatment groups. A well-designed randomization scheme ensures balance between the treatment groups at the entry.

Need for Innovation

The Single Arm Futility Design

In this era of increasingly productive bench research, it has become necessary to efficiently select which drugs will be moved into expensive and time-consuming phase-III trials. One potential means of drug screening is the phase-II-futility design. In the futility design, the null hypothesis is reversed and states that a drug effect is greater than a minimally acceptable outcome (69). If the null hypothesis is rejected, futility of the therapy is established. If futility is not shown within a cohort, then the study proceeds to a phase-III efficacy study. The rationale for this design is to ascertain futility with a minimum number of subjects in a one-sample design, thereby avoiding exposure of large numbers of patients to a potentially futile treatment.

Patient Adherence and Maintenance of Accrual

Adherence is an important factor in the success of any therapeutic regimen. The higher the overall quality of data at the end of the study, the more valid the conclusions. For this reason, investigators who conduct treatment trials must consider and deal with a variety of adherence issues (70). Patients with ALS are generally motivated, but the situation may change when expected benefits do not occur and side effects develop. Patients may become depressed and lose interest in the trial as their disease advances. They may dropout of a trial to participate in a new and recently publicized study, or they may secretly use other available investigational agents. During clinical trials, it is important to monitor adherence and to implement effective adherence-improving strategies (70). Treatment of depression and other palliative measures should be pursued aggressively. Study nurses and physicians should spend time personally with patients, discussing various issues and difficulties patients face while participating in the study. A discussion of the importance of scientific research and the need for complete data in testing medications prior to enrollment may help patients understand their vital role in the process. The principal investigator of a trial may contact sites frequently and use advertising as means to maintain interest in the trial. Outcomes may be chosen that enhance complete participation by patients.

BIOSTATISTICAL SUPPORT

In any formal clinical trial, biostatisticians should be involved from the early planning stages. Obtaining biostatistical help for the first time at the completion of the study may reveal serious flaws that invalidate the study and its results (66). Biostatistical consultation involves several key areas: control of bias through study design, sample size estimation, database management, data analysis, and interpretation of results.

Before estimating sample size, it is necessary to determine how many groups are involved in the trial, whether the trial aims to look at differences in absolute measures between the beginning and the end of the study, whether it will look at the rate of change in measures during the study, and how much of a difference in these measures is expected to occur between groups. If expected differences are large, testing differences in absolute measures may require a relatively short study, whereas examining the rate of change requires a longer study because the longer the analysis, the more reliable the regression curve over time. Summarizing data collected over time as a slope of the line through the data has some advantages because the calculation of slope uses all available follow-up data and can be less variable than simply evaluating two data points at the beginning and end of the study. The slope as an overall rate of change also provides a way of using the data from all patients, not simply those who finish the study, because slope can incorporate data from patients lost to follow up and even patients who do not complete the study. Slope has disadvantages, however, because it assumes that changes are linear during the study period. Moreover, the question of how to analyze data from patients who die during the study or drop out of the study, especially in the early stages, may be problematic.

Sample Size Estimation

Sample size requirements differ based on the study design, the degree of improvement sought, within- and between-patient variability of the outcome measures, the length of follow up, the spacing of measurements over time, the length of the trial, the α-level, the required statistical power, and the estimated dropout rate (71). Two general types of measurement of the primary outcome are considered: (i) a continuous variable (i.e., measured on an interval scale, such as ALSFRS, MVIC, and FVC, or (ii) a categorical variable, such as number of deaths or major disability.

Past trials have often been powered to detect an effect of between 35% and 50% (46,49), an outcome that may be unrealistic in a disorder as complex as ALS. Current studies, modeled after trials in other fields, are powered to detect sizes between 15% and 30%. Different outcome measures require different sample sizes to detect a significant change. When a categorical outcome, such as death, is used, the sample size may be lower. In contrast, when the time to an event such as survival time or time to respiratory failure is used, the sample size increases.

Statistical Analyses

Two types of statistical errors, types I and II, can occur in testing the hypothesis of a clinical trial (72). A type I error is committed when one concludes that a treatment is effective when, in fact, it is not. Typical acceptable rates of type-I errors are 0.05 or 0.01, usually referred to as the α-level of the study. This error rate can increase rapidly when multiple statistical tests are performed through data dredging or unplanned exploring, because the more variables analyzed, the more likely one is to find a difference by chance alone. Multiple comparison procedures such as the Bonferroni technique are helpful for protecting against this error rate increase, but careful planning with predefined endpoint and analysis plans are sounder.

A type-II error occurs when one concludes incorrectly that a treatment is not effective. In planning a study, the acceptable probability of this type of error is referred to as the β-level (typically, 0.2, 0.1, or 0.05). Statistical power, the probability of finding a treatment effective when in fact it is effective, is equal to $1-β$ (72). The error rates, $α$ and $β$, are set as low as possible. When the result of a clinical trial is negative, it is crucial that there be sufficient power to conclude that the study is in fact negative and not merely inconclusive (73).

Dropouts and the Intent-To-Treat-Analysis

Patients withdraw from trials for many reasons, and the probable dropout rate is an important component of sample size estimation (72). Past dropout rates have ranged from 30% to nearly 80% for the study period, rates that may invalidate trial results.

Patients who drop out during a study may do so because of adverse events or ineffectiveness of the intervention. Analysis that excludes those that dropout may result in a skewed sample and cause false results. Excluding data from analysis introduces bias and threatens validity. In contrast, the intent-to-treat analysis includes all patients once they are randomly assigned to a treatment arm, is the most robust means of assuring valid conclusions, and is now considered the gold standard in trial primary analysis. This technique increases type-II error (probability of not finding an effect that really exists), but provides realistic results, like those that would be seen if the medication were prescribed to a clinic population with ALS.

The best solution is prevention of dropout. A recent Dutch study had no loss of data due to dropouts other than death (21). Investigators traveled to patients' houses when necessary to collect data. Future U.S. trials will emphasize methods of reducing dropout, including easy-to-administer outcomes, infrequent patient visits, and home visits if necessary.

REGULATORY OVERSIGHT

The safety and ethical conduct of clinical trials is overseen by a number of governmental and center regulatory bodies, including the FDA, a data and safety monitoring board (DSMB) if the study is funded by the National Institutes of Health, and the individual center's Institutional Review Board (IRB). The investigator is responsible for maintaining close interaction with all oversight organizations, and notifying them of any changes in the trial and any serious adverse events that occur (66).

The Institutional Review Board, Informed Consent and Protection of Human Subjects

All clinical research must be approved by the IRB at the institution where the research is to take place. The IRB consists of various professionals such as physicians, lawyers, biomedical ethicists, and members of the lay community. Its primary objectives are to protect patients from unethical clinical research, as defined by The World Medical Association Declaration of Helsinki in 1979 (74) and to ensure the scientific quality of the study. Its secondary objective is to protect the investigators and institution. Institutions are mandated to train their research personnel in appropriate ethical conduct during clinical research, including impartiality in choosing subjects with regard to sex and ethnicity, informed consent at the time of enrollment, concern for the welfare of subjects with safety monitoring and administration of the best treatment available. Patients must understand the potential risks and alternatives to participation, and their data must be handled confidentially.

All subjects must sign the IRB-approved consent form, written in plain language. The investigator must also verbally explain the content of the consent form. Patients must understand its content fully before signing. Those who are unable to sign (e.g., because of hand weakness) may sign by proxy.

Data and Safety Monitoring Board

NIH and FDA-funded studies require an independent DSMB and a safety monitor to review data periodically for safety and toxicity (75). Adverse events are reported to all sites for their individual IRBs and to the FDA. A coordinating center oversees the day-to-day conduct of the trial, and a data management center collects data and prepares it for analysis. Sites are monitored to ensure that good clinical practice parameters are met during the trial.

Food and Drug Administration

The FDA maintains direct oversight of all trials, whether investigator initiated or pharmaceutical company sponsored. No trial begins without an IND application. Annual reports are sent to the FDA summarizing the trial status, and all severe adverse events are submitted to the FDA within seven days of their occurrence. The FDA selects certain trials for audit to ensure that good clinical practice guidelines are being met, and that patients are being properly informed at the time of consent to participate.

ORGANIZATIONAL STRUCTURE

As ALS is a rare disease, enrolling adequate numbers of patients in relatively short periods of time requires multicenter consortia. The larger the sample size, the greater the number of clinical centers required to ensure that the needed number of subjects are entered into the study during an acceptable time period. Multicenter studies are relatively new in ALS. The national TRH study in 1989 involved 14 centers and was the first large-scale multicenter study in ALS (73). All recent well-powered studies have involved multiple sites, whether industry sponsored or investigator initiated. In investigator-initiated studies, typically one center will coordinate the trial with the assistance of a Steering Committee. Data management may occur at the Coordinating Center or a separate center. Ideally, one blinded statistician will oversee data acquisition, management, and analysis, while a second independent unblinded statistician may assist data monitoring agencies in interim data analyses.

ETHICAL ISSUES

The Ethics of Clinical Research

The objective of the clinical trial is not to deliver therapy; rather it is to answer scientific questions about the safety and efficacy of a drug, and in the process, learn more about the disease (76). In ALS, one drug, riluzole, has been proved efficacious, but there is no cure, and there is a strong need to investigate better treatments. Unless trials are pursued aggressively, an effective medication may not be identified (77). However, regardless of study design, the study is ethical only when there is genuine uncertainty in the expert medical community about the efficacy of the treatment. Withholding a drug known to benefit patients with ALS to accomplish a placebo-controlled design clearly violates the ethics of clinical trials. Thus, the ethics of controlled studies require *equipoise*—a state of genuine uncertainly on the part of the clinical investigator regarding the comparative therapeutic merits of each arm in a trial (76). Another issue is the use of resources. Large multicenter trials are very expensive and need large numbers of eligible patients. The trial undertaken must be well designed and have appropriate scientific rationale (19,66).

There is little doubt that the randomized, double-blind clinical trial is a powerful technique because of the efficiency and credibility associated with treatment comparisons involving randomly assigned concurrent controls. When studies are properly carried out with informed consent, clinical equipoise, and a design adequate to answer the questions posed, randomized clinical trials protect physicians and their patients from therapies that are ineffective or toxic.

The Ethics of Clinical Investigators

Randomized clinical trials require doctors to act simultaneously as physicians and as scientists (78). Physicians engaged in clinical trials do so for the good of patients in the future. Many physicians prescribe a cocktail of unproved therapies, with the intention of either providing some benefit or providing hope to the patient. The argument is that physicians have a personal obligation to use their best judgment and recommend the best therapy, no matter how tentative or inconclusive the data on which that judgment is based (79). The use of unproven therapies, however, detracts from enrollment in clinical trials, and probably offers the patients less hope than the honest analysis that only through clinical trials will the eventual inroads be made.

Clinical investigators have other ethical responsibilities. Conflict of interest must be avoided in any study. Investigators who have financial interests in a drug company that supports a drug trial should not participate. Investigators must also adhere to the protocol; that is, no deviation is allowed from the original research plan, unless the study protocol is formally changed after the approval of the IRB and the FDA. There is a legal responsibility to maintain "good clinical practice" and to record all events related to patient care in the medical record and report forms. Investigators are responsible for reporting all major adverse events, including death, to their own IRB and to their sponsoring agency.

Patient Obligations

Patients who participate in clinical studies have no ethical responsibilities but they do incur some obligations. In the past several years, patients have adopted an activist mode (80). They use the Internet to share information (and sometimes misinformation) on investigational drugs and often advocate multiple medication usage. Patients continue to seek new, ostensibly more effective clinical trials. Under these circumstances, establishing and maintaining a study population becomes increasingly difficult.

Most consent forms do not emphasize the patients' obligations in the clinical trials. No patient can be forced to continue in a trial, but the importance of continuing participation adherent to the protocol and follow up should be stressed at the time of recruitment and throughout the trial (81). Ideally, investigators are very honest with their patients about the lack of effect of current therapies, and the need for good trials. Through open and honest conversations, we may see a future where all ALS patients will be enrolled in clinical trials.

SUMMARY

Therapeutic trials are important not only in developing an effective treatment for ALS, but also in increasing our understanding. Sophisticated design with appropriate statistical planning ensures that the time and expense are well spent.

Consensus in which preclinical models provide the best scientific rationale to proceed to human trials, and innovative trial designs to test multiple medications more reliably and efficiently are needed. While patient inclusion and exclusion criteria determine the study population, a balance must be struck between ensuring that the diagnosis is correct and that the majority of patients complete the trial, and having a range of patients included. Until a definite biomarker is identified, the ALSFRS and survival are currently considered to be the most important outcome measures.

Our ultimate goal as clinical investigators is to find therapeutic agents that relieve the suffering of patients, that improve the quality of their lives and that slow the progress of the illness. To do so, clinical trials must be carried out in an ethical, scientific, and statistically sound fashion.

REFERENCES

1. The World Federation of Neurology Research Group on Neuromuscular Diseases Subcommittee on Motor Neuron Disease: Airlie House Guidelines. Therapeutic trials in amyotrophic lateral sclerosis. J Neurol Sci 1995; 129(suppl 1):1–10.
2. Young FE, Norris JA, Levitt JA, Nightingale SL. The FDA's new procedures for the use of investigational drugs in treatment. JAMA 1988; 25:2267–2270.
3. A phase I study of recombinant human ciliary neurotrophic factor (rHCNTF) in patients with amyotrophic lateral sclerosis. The ALS CNTF treatment study (ACTS) phase I–II study group. Clin Neuropharmacol 1995; 18:515–532.
4. Ochs G, Penn RD, York M, Giess R, Beck M, Tonn J, Haigh J, Malta E, Traub M, Sendtner M, Toyka KV. A phase I/II trial of recombinant methionyl human brain derived neurotrophic factor administered by intrathecal infusion to patients with amyotrophic lateral sclerosis. Amyotroph Lateral Scler Other Motor Neuron Disord 2000; 1:201–206.
5. Brooks BR, Miller RG, Swash M, Munsat TL, for the world federation of neurology research group on motor neuron diseases. El Escorial revisited: revised criteria for the diagnosis of amyotrophic lateral sclerosis. Amyotroph Lateral Scler Other Motor Neuron Disord 2000; 1:293–299.
6. Kondo K, Hemmi I. Clinical statistics in 515 fatal cases of motor neuron disease. Neuroepidemiology 1984; 3:129–148.
7. Gordon PH, Moore DH, Gelinas DF, Qualls C, Meister ME, Werner J, Mendoza M, Mass J, Kushner G, Miller RG. Placebo Controlled Phase I/II studies of minocycline in amyotrophic lateral sclerosis. Neurology 2004; 62:1845–1847.

8. Lange D. Experience with myotrophin. In: Armon C, Rowland LP, eds. Clinical Issues in ALS Trials: Update, Consensus and Controversies. Minneapolis: American Academy of Neurology, 1995:27–28.

9. Brooks BR, Sufit RL, DePaul R, Tan YD, Sanjkak M, Robbins J. Design of clinical therapeutic trails in amyotrophic lateral sclerosis. Adv Neurol 1991; 56:521–546.

10. Bromberg MB. Diagnostic criteria and outcome measurement of amyotrophic lateral sclerosis. Adv Neurol 2002; 88:53–62.

11. Louwerse ES, de Jong VJMB, Kuether G. Critique of assessment methodology in amyotrophic lateral sclerosis. In: Rose FC, ed. Amyotrophic Lateral Sclerosis. New York: Demos, 1990:151–179.

12. Guiloff RJ, Goonetilleke A. Longitudinal clinical assessments in motor neurone disease. Relevance to clinical trials. In: Rose FC, ed. ALS—From Charcot to the Present and into the Future. London: Smith-Gordon, 1994:73–82.

13. Meinert CL. Clinical Trials. New York: Oxford University Press, 1986.

14. Rosenberg RN, Aminoff M, Boller F, Soerensen PS, Griggs RC, Hachinski V, Hallett M, Johnson RT, Kennard C, Lang AE, et al. Reporting clinical trials: full access to all the data. Brain 2002; 125:i–ii.

15. Lacomblez L, Bensimon G, Leigh PN, Guillet P, Meininger V. Dose-ranging study of riluzole in amyotrophic lateral sclerosis. Amyotrophic lateral sclerosis/riluzole study group II. Lancet 1996; 347:1425–1431.

16. Mitsumoto H, Davidson M, Moore D, Gad N, Brandis M, Ringel S, Rosenfeld J, Shefner JM, Strong MJ, Sufit R, et al. ALS CARE Study Group. Percutaneous endoscopic gastrostomy (PEG) in patients with ALS and bulbar dysfunction. Amyotroph Lateral Scler Other Motor Neuron Disord 2003; 4:177–85.

17. Cedarbaum JM, Stambler N. Disease status and use of ventilatory support by ALS patients. BDNF Study Group. Amyotroph Lateral Scler Other Motor Neuron Disord 2001; 2:19–22.

18. Munsat TL, Andres PL, Finison L, Conlon T, Thibodeaur L. The natural history of motoneuron loss in amyotrophic lateral sclerosis. Neurology 1988; 38:409–413.

19. Steiner TJ. Clinical trials. In: Williams AC, ed. Motor Neuron Disease. London: Chapman & Hall Medical, 1994:701–724.

20. Drachman DB, Chaudhry V, Cornblath D, Kuncl RW, Pestronk A, Clawson L, Mellits ED, Quaskey S, Quinn T, Calkins A. Trial of immunosuppression in amyotrophic lateral sclerosis using total lymphoid irradiation. Ann Neurol 1994; 35:142–150.

21. Groeneveld GJ, Veldink JH, van der Tweel I, Kalmijn S, Beijer C, de Visser M, Wokke JH, Franssen H, van den Berg LH. A randomized sequential trial of creatine in amyotrophic lateral sclerosis. Ann Neurol 2003; 53:437–445.

22. The ALS CNTF Treatment Study (ACTS) Phase I-II Study Group. The amyotrophic lateral sclerosis functional rating scale. Assessment of activities of daily living in patients with amyotrophic lateral sclerosis. Arch Neurol 1996; 53:141–147.

23. Hillel Ad, Miller RM, Yorkston K, McDonald E, Norris FH, Konikow N. Amyotrophic lateral sclerosis severity scale. Neuroepidemiology 1989; 8:142–150.

24. Fahn S, Elton RL, Members of the UPDRS Development Committee. Unified Parkinson's disease rating scale. In: Fahn S, Marsden CD, Calne D, Goldstein M, eds. Recent Developments in Parkinson's Disease. Vol. 2. Florham Park, NJ: Macmillan Healthcare Information, 1987:153–164.

25. Cedarbaum JM, Stambler N. Performance of the amyotrophic lateral sclerosis functional rating scale (ALSFRS) in multicenter clinical trials. J Neurol Sci 1997; 152(suppl 1): S1–S9.

26. ALS CNTF Treatment Study (ACTS) Study Group. A double-blind placebo-controlled clinical trial of subcutaneous recombinant human ciliary neurotrophic factor (rHCNTF) in amyotrophic lateral sclerosis. Neurology 1996; 46:1244–1249.

27. A controlled trial of recombinant methionyl human BDNF in ALS: the BDNF study group (phase III). Neurology 1999; 52:1427–1433.

28. Cedarbaum JM, Stambler N, Malta E, Fuller C, Hilt D, Thurmond B, Nakanishi A. The ALSFRS-R: a revised ALS functional rating scale that incorporates assessments of respiratory function. BDNF ALS Study Group (Phase II/III). J Neurol Sci 1999; 169: 13–21.

29. Kaufmann P, Levy G, Thompson JLP, DelBene ML, Battista V, Gordon PH, Rowland LP, Levin B, Mitsumoto M. The ALSFRSr predicts mortality in an ALS clinic population. Neurology 2005; 64:38–43.

30. Florence JM, Moore DH, Mendoza M, Mass J, Renna R, Malinowski L, Parnell J, Roelke K, Gelinas DF, Brooks BR, et al. Validation of telephonic administration of the ALSFRS-R. Neurology 2004; 62(suppl 5):A134.

31. Appel V, Stewart SS, Smith G, Appel SH. A rating scale for amyotrophic lateral sclerosis: description and preliminary experience. Ann Neurol 1987; 22:328–333.

32. Haverkamp LJ, Appel V, Appel SH. Natural history of amyotrophic lateral sclerosis in a database population. Validation of a scoring system and a model for survival prediction. Brain 1995; 118:707–719.

33. Norris FH Jr, U KS, Sachais B, Carey M. Trial of baclofen in amyotrophic lateral sclerosis. Arch Neurol 1979; 36:715–716.

34. The Italian ALS Study Group. Branched-chain amino acids and amyotrophic lateral sclerosis: a treatment failure? Neurology 1993; 43:2466–2470.

35. Olarte MR, Shaffer, SQ. Levamisole is ineffective in the treatment of amyotrophic lateral sclerosis. Neurology 1985; 35:1063–1066.

36. Brooks BR. The Norris ALS score: Insight into the natural history of amyotrophic lateral sclerosis provided by Forbes Norris. In: Rose FC, ed. ALS—From Charcot to the Present and into the Future. London: Smith-Gordon, 1994:21–29.

37. Schwab R, England A. Projection technique for evaluating surgery in Parkinson's disease. In: Gillingham J, Donaldson L, eds. Third Symposium on Parkinson's Disease. Edinburgh: Livingstone, 1969:152–157.

38. Ashworth B. Trial of carisoprodol in multiple sclerosis. Practitioner 1964; 192:540–542.

39. Smith RA, Berg JE, Pope LE, Thisted RA. Measuring pseudobulbar affect in amyotrophic lateral sclerosis. Amyotroph Lateral Scler Other Motor Neuron Disord 2004; 5(Suppl 1):99–102.

40. Newsom-Davis IC, Abrahams S, Goldstein LH, Leigh PN. The emotional lability questionnaire: a new measure of emotional lability in amyotrophic lateral sclerosis. J Neurol Sci 1999; 169:22–25.

41. Sorenson E. A Comparison of muscle strength testing techniques in amyotrophic lateral sclerosis. Presented at the 12th International Symposium on ALS/MND, Oakland, CA, Oct 2001.

42. Andres PL, Skerry LM, Thornell B, Portney LG, Finison LJ, Munsat TL. A comparison of three measures of disease progression in ALS. J Neurol Sci 1996; 139(Suppl 1):64–70.

43. Van der Ploeg RJO, Oosterhuis HJGH, Reuvekamp J. Measuring muscle strength. J Neurol 1984; 231:200–203.

44. Andres PL, Finison LJ, Conlon T, Thibodeau LM, Munsat TL. Use of composite scores (megascores) to measure deficit in amyotrophic lateral sclerosis. Neurology 1988; 38: 405–408.

45. Cudkowicz ME, Shefner JM, Schoenfeld DA, Brown RH Jr, Johnson H, Qureshi M, Jacobs M, Rothstein JD, Appel SH, Pascuzzi RM, et al. Northeast ALS Consortium. A randomized, placebo-controlled trial of topiramate in amyotrophic lateral sclerosis. Neurology 2003; 61:456–464.

46. Brooks BR, Lewis D, Rawling J, Sanjak M, Belden D, Hakim H, de Tan Y, Sufit R, Gaffney J, Depaul R. The natural history of amyotrophic lateral sclerosis. In: Williams AC, ed. Motor Neuron Disease. London: Chapman & Hall Medical, 1994:131–169.

47. Ringel SP, Murphy JR, Alderson MK, Bryan W, England JD, Miller RG, Petajan JH, Smith SA, Roelofs RI, Ziter F. The natural history of amyotrophic lateral sclerosis. Neurology 1993; 43:1316–1322.

48. Miller RG, Moore DH 2nd, Gelinas DF, Dronsky V, Mendoza M, Barohn RJ, Bryan W, Ravits J, Yuen E, Neville H, et al. Western ALS Study Group. Phase III randomized trial of gabapentin in patients with amyotrophic lateral sclerosis. Neurology 2001; 56: 843–848.

49. Guiloff FJ, Goonetilleke A. Longitudinal conical assessments in motor neurone disease. Relevance to clinical trials. In: Rose FC, ed. ALS—from Charcot to the Present and into the Future. London: Smith-Gordon, 1994:73–82.

50. Barlow SM, Abbs JH. Force transducers for the evaluation of labial, lingual, and mandibular motor impairments. J Speech Hearing Res 1983; 26:616–621.

51. McComas AJ, Fawcett PRW, Campbell MJ, Sica REP. Electrophysiological estimation of the number of motor units within a human muscle. J Neurol Neurosurg Psychiatr 1971; 34:121–131.

52. Kadrie HA, Yates SK, Milner-Brown HS, Brown WF. Multiple point electrical stimulation of ulnar and median nerves. J Neurol Neurosurg Psychiatr 1976; 39:973–985.

53. Gooch CL, Harati Y. Motor unit number estimation, ALS and clinical trials. Amyotroph Lateral Scler Other Motor Neuron Disord 2000; 1:71–82.

54. Wang FC, Bouquiaux O, De Pasqua V, Delwaide PJ. Changes in motor unit numbers in patients with ALS: a longitudinal study using the adapted multiple point stimulation method. Amyotroph Lateral Scler Other Motor Neuron Disord 2002; 3:31–38.

55. de Carvalho M, Scotto M, Lopes A, Swash M. Clinical and neurophysiological evaluation of progression in amyotrophic lateral sclerosis. Muscle Nerve 2003; 28:630–633.

56. Guyatt GH, Feeny DH, Patrick DL. Measuring health-related quality of life. Ann Intern Med 1993; 118:622–629.

57. Robbins RA, Simmons A, Bremer BA, Walsh SM, Fischer S. Quality of life in ALS is maintained as physical function declines. Neurology 2001; 56:442–444.

58. Bogdanov M, Brown RH, Matson W, Smart R, Hayden D, O'Donnell H, Flint Beal M, Cudkowicz M. Increased oxidative damage to DNA in ALS patients. Free Radic Biol Med 2000; 29:652–658.

59. Beal MF, Ferrante RJ, Browne SE, Matthews RT, Kowall NW, Brown RH Jr. Increased 3-nitrotyrosine in both sporadic and familial amyotrophic lateral sclerosis. Ann Neurol 1997; 42:644–654.

60. Simpson E, Henkel J, Henry Y, Smith R, Appel S. Elevated levels of 4-HNE in the sera of patients with ALS. Neurology 2003; 60:A242.

61. Beuche W, Yushchenko M, Mader M, Maliszewska M, Felgenhauer K, Weber F. Matrix metalloproteinase-9 is elevated in serum of patients with amyotrophic lateral sclerosis. Neuroreport 2000; 11:3419–3422.

62. Houi K, Kobayashi T, Kato S, Mochio S, Inoue K. Increased plasma TGF-beta1 in patients with ALS. Acta Neurol Scand 2002; 106:299–301.

63. Bradley WG. The need for double-blind controlled trials in amyotrophic lateral sclerosis. In: Rose FC, ed. ALS—From Charcot to the Present and into the Future. London: Smith-Gordon, 1994:263–265.

64. Mitsumoto H, Salgado ED, Negroski D, Hanson MR, Salanga VD, Wilber JF, Wilbourn AJ, Breuer AC, Leatherman J. Amyotrophic lateral sclerosis: effects of acute intravenous and chronic subcutaneous administration of thyrotropin-releasing hormone in controlled trials. Neurology 1986; 36:152–159.

65. Pradas J, Finison L, Andres PL, Thornell B, Hollander D, Munsat TL. The natural history of amyotrophic lateral sclerosis and the use of natural history controls in therapeutic trials. Neurology 43; 1993:751–755.

66. Mitsumoto H, Chad DA, Pioro EP. Treatment trials. Amyotrophic Lateral Sclerosis. Philadelphia: FA Davis Co, 1998:329–354.

67. Haynes RB, Dantes R. Patient compliance and the conduct and interpretation of therapeutic trials. Control Clin Trial 1987; 8:12–19.

68. Altman DG. Practical Statistics for Medical Research. London: Chapman & Hall, 1991.

69. Palesch YY, Tilley BC. Value of a single-arm futility design for Phase II clinical trial of acute stroke therapy. American Academy of Neurology Meeting. Honolulu, HI, April 2003.
70. Kurtzke JF. Neuroepidemiology. Part II: assessment of therapeutic trials. Ann Neurol 1986; 19:311–319.
71. Lachin JM. Introduction to sample size determination and power analysis for clinical trials. Control Clin Trial 1981; 2:93–113.
72. Fleiss JL, Levin B, Paik MC. Statistical Methods for Rates and Proportions. 3rd ed. New Jersey: Wiley, 2003.
73. The National TRH Study Group. Multicenter controlled trial: no effect of alternate-day 5 mg/kg subcutaneous thyrotropin-releasing hormone (TRH) on isometric-strength decrease in amyotrophic lateral sclerosis [abstr]. Neurology 1989; 39(Suppl 1):322.
74. The World Medical Association Declaration of Helsinki. In: Beauchamp TL, Childress JF, eds. Principles of Biomedical Ethics. New York: Oxford University Press, 1979: 289–293.
75. Slutsky AS, Lavery JV. Data safety and monitoring boards. N Engl J Med 2004; 350: 1143–1147.
76. Lilford RJ. Ethics of clinical trials from a Bayesian and decision analytic perspective: whose equipoise is it anyway? BMJ 2003; 326:980–981.
77. Marshall FJ, Kieburtz K, McDermott M, Kurlan R, Shoulson I. Clinical research in neurology. From observation to experimentation. Neurol Clin 1996; 14:451–466.
78. Hellman S, Hellman D. Sounding board of mice but not men. Problems of the randomized clinical trial. N Engl J Med 1991; 342:1585–1589.
79. Passamani E. Clinical trials—are they ethical? N Engl J Med 1991; 324:1589–1592.
80. Miller RG, Munsat TL, Swash M, Brooks BR. Consensus guidelines for the design and implementation of clinical trials in ALS. World Federation of neurology committee on research. J Neurol Sci 1999; 169:2–12.
81. McKhann GM. Clinical trials in a changing era. Ann Neurol 1994; 36:683–687.

27

The Multidisciplinary Care Clinic: The Principles and an International Perspective

Hiroshi Mitsumoto
*Eleanor and Lou Gehrig MDA/ALS Research Center, Department of Neurology,
Columbia University Medical Center, The Neurological Institute,
New York, New York, U.S.A.*

Gian Domenico Borasio
*Interdisciplinary Center for Palliative Medicine and Department of Neurology,
Motor Neuron Disease Research Group, Munich University Hospital,
Grosshadern, Munich, Germany*

Angela L. Genge
Montreal Neurological Hospital, Montreal, Quebec, Canada

Orla Hardiman
Richmond Institute of Neurology, Beaumont Hospital, Dublin, Ireland

Peter Nigel Leigh
*Department of Clinical Neuroscience, Institute of Psychiatry, King's College London,
London, U.K.*

Vincent Meininger
Fédération de Neurolgie Mazarin, Hôpital Salpétrière, Paris, France

Wim Robberecht
*Department of Neurology, School of Medicine, University Hospital Gasthuisberg,
University of Leuven, Leuven, Belgium*

Toyokazu Saito
*Departments of Neurology and Rehabilitation, Kitasato University Higashi Hospital and
Kitasato University School of Allied Health Science, Sagamihara, Kanagawa, Japan*

Markus Weber
Department of Neurology, Kantonsspital St. Gallen, St. Gallen, Switzerland

INTRODUCTION

The care of patients with amyotrophic lateral sclerosis (ALS) is especially challenging
and differs from the care of patients with other neurodegenerative disorders because

- the disease progresses rapidly and is terminal,

605

- its course is predictably short in most cases,
- majority of patients maintain normal mental function, and
- to date, no effective curative treatment.

In caring for ALS patients, we take a holistic approach. As Thompson (1) states, "ALS requires a commitment on the part of the patient, family, and health-care providers to collaborate in a way that can bring meaning and hope to circumstances that make no sense, and a sense of wholeness in the face of relentless physical disintegration." Therefore, to provide effective care for patients with ALS, special skills and experience are essential (2–5).

Table 1 lists the general principles of caring for patients with ALS (3). Probably the most important factor for successful care is that the patient's decisions concerning his or her care are central to the overall care plan. Care and treatment decisions should not be driven by the desires of the health care providers or family. To achieve this, health care professionals keep in mind that patients have significant difficulties in making such decisions because they are emotionally stressed and in most cases, lack medical knowledge of any sort, particularly when they initially receive the diagnosis. One of our key tasks is to respect, to provide support, and to educate our patients and their families so that they can make informed decisions. Successful care also requires the treating physician to have a clinical interest in ALS and a commitment to treating patients with ALS. In addition, with the advent of information technology and free access to the World Wide Web, the neurologist needs to understand, contextualize, and explain the significance of clinical and scientific advances in disease pathogenesis and treatment.

Once they have received the diagnosis, patients are closely followed so that impending problems in mobility, communication, nutrition, or respiration are quickly detected. The neurologist is responsible for all the issues summarized in Table 2 (3). Whenever patients need to make a treatment decision, the neurologist and allied health team members provide the necessary information and invite questions from the patient and family to help ensure they have a good understanding of the issues involved in the decision. At some point, it is crucial to discuss advance directives related to nutritional and respiratory care (2).

The needs of patients with ALS and their family caregivers are not only medical, neurological, or physical and rehabilitative in nature. The disease has an impact on all aspects of life. Patients and families also confront psychosocial, financial, and ethical issues. The ALS clinic has the capability both to provide initial multidisciplinary support from clinical professionals and to direct patients and their

Table 1 General Principles of Care for the Patient with ALS

Care is driven by the patient's decisions
Patient and caregiver receive education about the disease and its treatment
The neurologist and allied health professionals should have a thorough understanding of ALS
The neurologist must be strongly committed to caring for patients with ALS
Care is provided via a holistic and team approach at an MDC ALS clinic
Aggressive symptomatic treatment is provided
Patients have the opportunity to participate in clinical trials
Home care and hospice care are used effectively
Close communication exists between patients, caregivers, and health-care providers
Advance directives and end-of-life decision-making are discussed with the patient and family
Palliative care is provided during the final stages

Abbreviations: ALS, amyotrophic lateral sclerosis; MDC, Multidisciplinary care.

Table 2 Responsibilities of the Neurologist

Performs medical and neurological evaluation
Explains the diagnosis and disease
Explains treatment modalities
Provides maximum symptomatic treatment
Makes recommendations based on recommendations from the MDC team
Discusses progress in research
Evaluates and explains treatment trials
Discusses advance directives
Directs the MDC ALS clinic
Educates the public about ALS

Abbreviations: MDC, Multidisciplinary care; ALS, amyotrophic lateral sclerosis.

families to services and support structures that extend beyond the traditional confines of medical practice. Ideally, the medical, psychosocial, and social services collaborate to develop individualized care plans for patients and their families (3).

THE MULTIDISCIPLINARY CARE CLINIC

The multidisciplinary care (MDC) clinic is not a new concept—it is an approach that is well established at many muscular dystrophy clinics. Such services also have been developed for patients with ALS at many centers throughout the world (6). For example, the Muscular Dystrophy Association (MDA) and the ALS Association in the United States and many similar ALS or motor neuron disease (MND) associations in other countries have certified ALS clinics or centers, which provide expertise in diagnosis, management, and research of ALS (7–10). The MDC clinic has several advantages over the regular neurology office setting. Allied health-care professionals working at such a center can develop expertise in ALS much faster and in greater depth than therapists elsewhere because of concentrated experience with many ALS patients. Because all the members are available at the same clinic site, the patient's and family's questions and concerns can be effectively and quickly answered, particularly when the patient's problems cross-over a number of different disciplines. Patients need not travel from one office to another to see different therapists, conserving energy and time, and so preventing unnecessary physical fatigue. Also, the approach to ALS treatment can be holistic, and the ALS clinic setting is conducive to such an approach. A recent study in Ireland has indicated that patients who are cared for in an MDC setting survive significantly longer (11), suggesting this may be the best approach currently available for providing treatment in ALS.

Some shortcomings exist as well. Seeing many therapists in succession over many hours may be exhausting for patients (this is also true for therapists seeing many ALS patients). Also, the time allocated for appointments with each therapist may be insufficient when patients present with complex or multiple problems, so sometimes patients will have to return for further evaluation and treatment. One of the most serious issues is the high cost to the clinic (see below).

Table 3 lists the team members of a typical multidisciplinary ALS clinic (3). All the services provided by the members are important and ideally are available at the clinic site. The format of the clinic, however, may vary, depending on the availability of certain services, characteristics of the individual institutions, the director's philosophy, and the

Table 3 Members of the ALS Multidisciplinary Clinic

On-site members	On-call members
Neurologist	Research nurse coordinator
ALS nurse coordinator	Pulmonologist
Physical therapist	Physiatrist
Occupational therapist	Gastroenterologist
Dietitian	Psychiatrist or psychologist
Speech pathologist	Orthotist
Social worker	Prosthodontist
Patient service coordinator from voluntary disease organizations	

unique nature of each clinic's development. Most clinics are directed by neurologists who have special expertise in ALS, but occasionally they are run by physiatrists or a physician who is not a neurologist. Some clinics see only follow-up patients, that is, patients who already have an established diagnosis, whereas other clinics see a mixture of new patients and established patients. Regardless of these differences, access to necessary acute medical and neurological care, all required diagnostic laboratories, such as electromyography, neuroradiology, and neuropathology, and participation in clinical research (including clinical trials) are key to a successful MDC.

The MDC Clinic Members

The Neurologist

The neurologist is responsible for patient's care (Table 2) although in some centers, a physiatrist may be responsible (3). He or she directs the ALS MDC clinic and therefore is responsible for care provided by the individual health care professionals. Neurologists make orders based on recommendations given by the team members and prescribe appropriate equipment and braces. Ideally, MDC care commences at diagnosis. As is discussed in Chapter 9, although ALS is fatal, it is possible to deliver the diagnosis in a manner that does not exclude hope. The diagnosis is given in a relaxed setting with enough time for questions and initial patient education. The neurologist explains the disease, the purposes and side effects of all treatments and medications, and progress in ALS research. At regular follow-up visits, the possibilities of pro-active treatment, such as enteral feeding and noninvasive positive-pressure ventilation (NIPPV) can be discussed, as can the future need for advance directives.

The topics that the neurologist discusses with patients and their families may overlap those of the nurse coordinator and other therapists, but such repetition by different team members usually helps patients and families to understand more fully, not only because they hear the information again but because each team member will have his or her own individual educational style. Neurologists, along with the ALS nurse or social workers, also discuss preparation of a living will and durable power of attorney for health-care.

The ALS Nurse

We define an ALS nurse as an experienced nurse who has special expertise and interest in ALS and provides care for patients with ALS. The ALS nurse most often is an

Table 4 Responsibilities of the ALS Nurse

Coordinates the clinic team
Explains the disease
Provides informative literature
Provides emotional and psychological support and discusses advance directives
Teaches patients how to maximize functional ability and quality of life
Assesses general medical status, including respiratory and weight status
Evaluates current medications
Suggests participation in a support group
Reviews care path and suggests changes as the disease progresses
Acts as a liaison to other therapists and the clinical research team
Coordinates home care and placing of patients at alternative care sites
Educates the home care staff about ALS symptoms
Educates the public about ALS
Engages in nursing research regarding quality of life and patient satisfaction
Acts as a patient advocate

Abbreviation: ALS, amyotrophic lateral sclerosis.

advanced nurse practitioner or a registered nurse specializing in ALS. The ALS nurse usually has a key role in the MDC clinic, having many responsibilities, including coordinating the activities of the health professionals, directing nursing care, and co-ordinating home care or hospice care, as well as being an educator and advocate for the patients. At the end of the clinic, the nurse coordinator moderates the team conference (Table 4) (3).

An important function of the ALS nurse is to help patients understand the concept and structure of the MDC clinic. Because the neurologist may be perceived as an authority figure, making personal decisions difficult for some patients, the nurse is in a unique position in explaining the purpose of the MDC and the care path to the patient and family. Once the patient and family understand the concept of the MDC clinic, they know how, when, and why treatment is given—such an understanding will help to ensure patient compliance and satisfaction. At the first clinic visit, the patient receives an information packet that includes ALS literature published by voluntary disease organizations, such as the MDA, ALS Association, or the National Institutes of Health (in the U.S.A.). Many ALS MDC clinics prepare a packet that includes the clinic's own ALS literature. The ALS nurse explains the information provided and schedules the next appointment. Overall the nurse is responsible for ensuring good communication between patients and families and team members.

The Physical and Occupational Therapists

At the MDC clinic, physical therapists most frequently evaluate lower-extremity muscle strength, trunk muscle function (ability to maintain a stable head and neck posture), and motor skills. They develop individualized exercise programs for each patient, and to maintain the patient's existing motor function, they evaluate the need for leg braces (such as the ankle-foot orthosis), neck braces, and wheelchairs. Physi-cal therapists also work closely with occupational therapists to recommend home equipment for patient safety and mobility. Chapter 31 describes the physical therapy that ALS patients require.

Occupational therapists address the skilled motor functions that enable patients to engage in activities of daily living. In the MDC clinic, they often work closely with physical therapists to evaluate hand and arm function. On the basis of the assessment, they give recommendations for splinting and adaptive devices. They also discuss activity modification, energy conservation, and work simplification with the patient.

The Dietitian or Nutritionist

Careful assessment of nutritional status and appropriate recommendations through-out the disease course are important for patients with bulbar dysfunction. At the MDC, a dietitian or nutritionist follows the patient's nutritional status by regularly evaluating the patient's appetite and weight and determining whether the patient is at risk for poor nutrition. In the United States, the American Academy of Neurology ALS Practice Parameter Guidelines (1999) serves as the foundation for care of patients with ALS (12). The dietitian often works with a speech pathologist to deter-mine the degree of dysphagia and will recommend strategies to modify swallowing and alternative methods to prepare food. Early oral supplementation is important when appetite or weight begins to decline. The dietitian also helps to determine whether enteral feeding is required. For those patients who undergo percutaneous endoscopic gastrostomy (PEG) or radiologically inserted gastrostomy (RIG), the dietitian selects an enteral feeding formula based on the patient's daily caloric, pro-tein, and fluid requirements before the procedure, immediately afterward, and for the remainder of the disease course. Chapter 32 reviews dietary therapy in detail.

The Speech Pathologist

Speech pathologists are responsible for evaluating bulbar function in patients with ALS. When office evaluation at the MDC is not sufficient to determine the degree of swallowing impairment, speech pathologists request a modified barium-swallowing test or videofluoroscopy, which helps to identify less obvious dysfunction as well as silent aspiration. Because these procedures more precisely identify swallowing impairments, they also present an excellent opportunity to educate patients about dysphagia and how to swallow food of various textures. Speech pathologists work closely with dietitians to recommend effective treatment strategies and to teach patients how to compensate for progressive dysphagia. They also counsel patients in regard to augmentative and other communication devices (see Chapter 31).

The Social Worker

The social worker assesses health insurance coverage and assists the patient in apply-ing for disability payments. Social workers provide referrals for financial resources, community resources, ALS Association chapters, and support groups. When the dis-ease progresses to a stage at which patients require home or hospice care, the social worker makes the necessary arrangements and applications for patients. In addition, the social worker discusses advance directives, durable power of attorney for health-care, and preparation of a living will. Although they evaluate and discuss nonmedical issues with patients and their families, they also often provide emotional and psychological support.

Voluntary Disease Organization Service Coordinator

Voluntary disease organizations often send a patient service coordinator representa-tive to their certified ALS clinic to provide educational literature and information about the many services they offer, including equipment loans and patient transportation services. They often organize patient and caregiver support groups. The support that these groups provide can be quite important to patients and their families, particularly because they meet and talk with others who are going through the same experience.

Consultants

Pulmonologist

A pulmonologist usually sees patients who have an impending respiratory problem or if the neurologist suspects they need a thorough pulmonary evaluation. The pulmonologist may not be a regular on-site member of the MDC team. However, because respiratory muscle weakness occurs in ALS, impending respiratory impairment may develop, and pulmonary consultation will be necessary, sometimes urgently. Thus, a pulmonologist should be readily available for consultation, and the neurologist should develop a close consulting relationship with this pulmonologist. If impending respiratory distress develops, NIPPV devices are used when appropriate. Occasionally, respiratory support will be required when a patient undergoes gastrostomy, and in such cases the pulmonologist works closely with the gastroenterologist or radiologist performing the gastrostomy. For those patients who have decided to undergo permanent ventilatory support, a pulmonary consultation is obtained long before respiratory distress develops.

The Gastroenterologist and Interventional Radiologist

The gastroenterologist is consulted when enteral feeding is necessary and the patient agrees to PEG. Gastroenterologists evaluate the patient's gastrointestinal status and obtain informed consent for the PEG. The procedure is performed in an outpatient endoscopy suite, and patients whose respiratory status is unstable before the procedure may stay overnight for observation. According to the American Academy of Neurology Practice Parameter guidelines, patients with ALS who undergo PEG should have an FVC better than 50% of predicted (12). However, in reality, it is not uncommon that patients whose FVC falls far below 50% wish to have enteral tube feeding. In such cases, an interventional radiologist may be consulted to perform a radiologically guided gastrostomy, which requires only a local anesthetic and is somewhat less invasive. When a patient's FVC is below 50%, a pulmonologist also is usually consulted. Both the gastroenterologist and dietitian follow the patient during the immediate postprocedure period (details are discussed in chap. 32).

The Psychiatrist and Psychologist

Depression secondary to the disease is prevalent in patients with ALS, but if the depression is properly managed, psychiatric consultation usually is unnecessary. However, an overwhelming catastrophic reaction to the disease, stress-induced adjustment problems, or marital problems stemming from stress may become serious issues. A psychiatry or clinical psychology referral is essential for these patients. Endogenous major depression or frank psychosis is rare in patients with ALS but can occur and also requires such consultation. In general, all members of the ALS clinic attempt to provide psychosocial support to patients and their families.

The Orthotist

An orthotist is available either in or outside of the hospital setting. Patients with ALS most frequently need an ankle-foot orthosis. For those who develop a relatively restricted paraspinal muscle weakness as manifested by the head-droop posture with well-preserved extremity strength, a neck brace may be needed. Orthotists and biomechanical engineers may need to work together to design and fabricate a customized neck brace because the commercially available neck braces are disappointingly ineffective (see Chap. 31).

The Prosthodontist

When patients have predominantly paretic bulbar palsy and velopharyngeal incompetence, a palatal prosthesis (the palatal lift) may improve paretic dysarthria that is caused by air leakage. After evaluation by the speech pathologist, the patient is referred to a prosthodontist, who will fabricate the prosthesis (13).

The Chaplain

The importance of pastoral or spiritual care for patients, families, and even for health care professionals who staff the ALS clinic is increasingly being recognized (see Chap. 34). In the United States, the availability of chaplaincy and spiritual care is still limited at ALS clinics in general but is expanding.

The ALS Team Meeting

At the end of each MDC clinic, the team members discuss the patients seen that day. Usually the ALS nurse or neurologist facilitates the discussion, and the team reviews the issues and recommendations. The problems and concerns of each patient and family are addressed, and necessary solutions and suggestions are presented. The team will also discuss specific treatment plans, including symptomatic medical treatment, clinical trial participation, necessary consultations, home care, and hospice referral. The nurse records the key points, and the team decides on a treatment plan for each patient, which the nurse then prepares. The nurse or the appropriate individual team members arrange to discuss the recommendations with the patient. Neurologists are asked to write necessary letters to various outside agencies.

This meeting gives the team members the opportunity to discuss patient issues that are of concern to all. Furthermore, unrecognized or innovative ideas and suggestions are frequently raised because of the meeting's collaborative nature. Psychologically, the meeting is also important for team members because it can foster camaraderie, provide hope, and boost morale after working with patients afflicted by a devastating disease.

The ALS Care System

Ideally, each MDC clinic develops a care path individualized for each patient and his or her caregiver. The ALS nurse or social worker at the MDC clinic usually coordinates the complex care needed for the patients and so is responsible for the overall coordination of the care path. This coordination includes

- providing information for outpatient therapy, home care, and hospice services and

- identifying suitable services specifically for the patients based on their insurance coverage, geographic location and need completing medical necessity forms connecting patients with other resources.

At the MDC clinic, the health care providers should determine whether the care path is working for the patients and informal caregivers, how well the patient is following the care path, and whether the care path requires modification. MDC team members and patients have used e-mail to effectively communicate between clinic visits; however, in the United States, newly enacted health care privacy regulations (Health Insurance Portability & Accountability Act–HIPAA) appear to make this nearly impossible unless secured encryption technology is used and a legally acceptable confidentiality statement is included.

Difficulties Facing MDC Clinics

The costs to operate an MDC clinic are high because multiple health care professionals need to be on site. In the United States, Medicare (the principle government insurance for the elderly or disabled) does not pay for therapy given by allied health-care professionals at the doctor's office on the same day. The reimbursement is allowed when such therapy is done at a formally designated therapy facility. Because commercial medical insurance generally follows the government Medicare guidelines, the physician can charge for only a regular follow-up fee even after the patients have been seen and examined by multiple health care professionals at the MDC clinic. Essentially, none of allied health care services will be reimbursed by the insurance payer. This lack of reimbursement imposes an enormous financial burden on most MDC clinics. Financially, the existence of the ALS MDC clinic appears to be endangered in the United States.

The MDA provides financial support to their designated MDA/ALS clinics, now 34 clinics throughout the United States. However, this financial support is contingent on including treatment for more than 40 other neuromuscular diseases. The MDC arrangement is a prerequisite for ALS Association certification of an ALS clinic. Unfortunately, the ALS Association currently can only provide modest financial support to their certified clinics. Locally, more support may exist for some ALS clinics because a number of prominent MDC clinics are closely associated with local ALS foundations, receive direct support from strong local ALS chapters, or have a strong focus on fund-raising. Although the MDC concept and structure seem to be widely accepted and promoted, operating the clinics is costly, and additional financial support is necessary beyond what the voluntary disease organizations and foundations can provide.

Not all ALS MDC clinics are run identically. The structure and service may vary between clinics, depending not only on the level of financial support that the clinic receives, but also on each clinic's philosophy and development of innovative ideas. Specifying one uniform structure or team composition for all MDC clinics is not useful because it does not allow for unique services or care systems that function efficiently within the larger health care structure in which the clinic operates. The key to effective treatment is to structure and operate an MDC clinic in the way that allows us to care for patients with ALS and their family caregivers in the ways that they need most. The difficulties we face in the United States are perhaps unusual compared to other countries. Generating new ideas not only to sustain MDC clinics in the United States, but also to allow them to thrive is absolutely essential. In this respect, the experiences of our international colleagues may serve to stimulate innovative thinking in our search for a solution.

INTERNATIONAL PERSPECTIVES

In the remainder of the chapter, international experts describe the health systems and insurance coverage that are unique to their countries and may directly or indirectly affect ALS patient care and the ALS MDC clinic structure. Gaining insights as to how our international colleagues are maintaining and growing the MDC concept and specifically what they have found works well and not so well will improve all ALS MDC clinics and thus, overall ALS care.

Germany and the ALS/MND Clinic in Munich

The ALS/MND outpatient clinic at the Department of Neurology, Munich University Hospital—Grosshadern, founded in 1991, is one of the largest ALS clinics in Germany, with about 70 to 80 new patients annually (8). The clinic is part of the Munich Neuromuscular Center, which is part of the German Society for Neuromuscular Disorders (DGM). The clinic aims to provide:

- Early, accurate, and appropriate diagnosis of ALS and other MNDs
- Coordinated interdisciplinary care provided by professionals in each discipline for patients with ALS and related diseases, and for their families as well
- An information resource for patients and their families, as well as for health-care and related professionals
- An active research program spanning the molecular, clinical, and palliative care aspects of ALS
- A link between the neurological and palliative care communities

The clinic has been funded largely by sponsored research trials, research grants, and to a small extent, by private donations. The DGM provides for the part-time services of a social worker and a physiotherapist for ALS outpatients. The University Hospital and the Department of Neurology support the clinic through infrastructure (clinic space, nursing and medical support, neurological beds, etc.), and through the involvement of other specialized units (pulmonology and gastroenterology). No funding so far has been provided by either the government or other medical insurance programs. The ALS clinic liaises with the Departments of Gastroenterology and Pulmonology in the University Hospital, as well as with the Division for Home Mechanical Ventilation of the Pulmonological Hospital in Gauting (near Munich), where our patients are referred for evaluation and initiation of noninvasive ventilation.

The clinic is active in clinical trials, laboratory research, and clinical research. A main research focus concerns the palliative care of patients with ALS and care for their families; issues include giving bad news, mechanical ventilation (including ethical issues such as withdrawal of ventilation), advance directives, psychosocial care during the terminal phase, and quality-of-life issues, including sexuality, spirituality, and caregiver needs (15–17). Research at our clinic has shown that the natural course of the terminal phase in ALS is generally peaceful (18), and we were major contributors to the first books published on palliative are in ALS (19) and in neurology (20). In Germany, the Munich ALS clinic has pioneered the use of noninvasive mechanical ventilation and disease-specific advance directives for ALS. In addition, it has established close links with the local, national, and international palliative care communities, and this has led to increased recognition that palliative care for neurological disorders (with ALS as a paradigm disease) will be a major focus for research and care programs in the future.

In 2004, the University of Munich inaugurated a new Interdisciplinary Center for Palliative Medicine, which is run jointly by the Departments of Anesthesiology, Neurology, and Oncology. The center has a dedicated 10-bed inpatient unit, which is open to all patients requiring palliative care. Admission is possible for symptom control, initiation of noninvasive ventilation, and respite care of patients with ALS. The aim is to discharge the patient home in a stable condition with a care plan that the family caregivers manage and sustain. To this end, we cooperate closely with local home hospice services and give them in-depth training in caring for patients in the advanced stages of ALS. The spiritual needs of the patients are attended to through direct involvement of members of the hospital chaplaincy. This service is also available for outpatients with ALS. The cooperation between the Palliative Care Center and Neurology Department is a hallmark of our clinic and has brought great benefits to patients, families, and staff.

Canada and the ALS Clinic at Montreal Neurological Hospital, McGill University

The ALS clinic at the Montreal Neurological Hospital is a multidisciplinary clinic that has existed in its current form since 1998. During 2003, 179 patients were followed. The clinic is held on each Monday; 12 to 20 patients are seen, and all staff members are available. Every patient referred to us is seen within three weeks of our receiving the referral. The current staff consists of a neurologist, ALS clinical nurse specialist, respiratory therapist, physiotherapist, occupational therapist, social worker, dietitian, speech therapist, pastoral care counselor, orthotics technician, secretary/coordinator, and pet therapy volunteer. A pulmonologist and gastroenterologist are available for consultation during clinic hours. Patients and caregivers are seen by all staff initially. At each follow-up visit, at least the neurologist, nurse, respiratory therapist, and physiotherapist or occupational therapist will see them, although frequently they are seen by all the staff. We meet on Monday mornings before the clinic and again on the following morning after the clinic to review issues that have arisen and further develop or alter care plans as necessary for each patient seen at the clinic that week.

After the diagnosis has been made, patients are seen, whenever possible, monthly for three months to deal with all the issues, both physical and emotional, that arise as a result of the diagnosis, and to clinically establish the rate of progression via strength testing, ALS functional rating scale (ALSFRS), weight and respiratory parameters, including the percent predicted FVC. Thereafter, patients are seen once every three months unless urgent issues arise, particularly with respect to nutritional and respiratory status. Careful attention is paid to the caregivers as the patient's ability to remain in the home depends on adequate support for people providing the care. Although ALS support group meetings are offered, our experience suggests that individual attention provided to the caregivers during clinic visits is the most effective way to troubleshoot problems, alleviate anxieties, and help with the universal emotional issues that arise. Meetings may also be set up during clinic visits that include the community service personnel who work with the individual patients.

In-hospital care is provided at the Montreal Neurological Hospital when appropriate or at a community hospital with the direct involvement of the ALS clinic staff. All planning for percutaneous gastrostomies, noninvasive ventilation trials, sleep studies, and planned tracheotomies are done before admission to minimize the length of hospital stays. Whenever possible, noninvasive ventilation trials are done during weekend overnight stays.

At-home and end-of-life care is coordinated by the clinic staff, particularly the neurologist, nurse, and social worker. Community-based resources are provided in part by a provincial network of community clinics [Centre Locale de Sante Communitaire (CLSC)] in combination with private care paid for by the patient or insurance plans. A major goal of the ALS team is to coordinate this care and educate the care providers in the ever-evolving management of the patients. Therefore, team members are available to give advice to both patients and CLSC providers at all times. Other key services include a monthly wheelchair clinic which is run in conjunction with a rehabilitation center and a provincially supported home ventilation program that assists patients at home who are using either noninvasive or permanent mechanical ventilation.

Fortunately the Montreal Neurological Hospital views the care of the ALS patient population as part of its responsibility. Therefore, all financial support required for staffing of the clinic is provided by the hospital, save for the pastoral services personnel, the orthotics technician, and the neurologist. Canada has a universal health care system that is under provincial jurisdiction, and therefore each province determines how it will provide coverage within certain guidelines and, more specifically, exactly what equipment and services are covered. In Quebec, major shortfalls occur in financial coverage for equipment (particularly ventilation equipment) and caregivers. Home renovation for ramps and elevators is included in the provincial plans; however, government delay in disbursing the funds is frequently sufficient to force patients to do these renovations outside of the health-care system.

All clinical research occurs in conjunction with the Clinical Research Unit of the Montreal Neurological Institute, and a research coordinator who is part of the ALS team staff covers all ALS-related clinical trials and functions. All nursing and other support required to run a clinical trial is coordinated through the Clinical Research Unit, an approach that has permitted research nurse responsibilities and ALS team nurse responsibilities to be completely separate, allowing the team nurse more time for patient education and care.

Like other ALS clinics in other countries, psychosocial support is an essential component of our care. We have found pastoral care to be invaluable, not only for the patients and their families but also for the staff. Recognizing the importance of this aspect of patient care has helped the staff as much as the patients in coping with the constant loss encountered in an ALS clinic. The support provided by pastoral services must be culturally sensitive and supportive of all faiths. Our clinic, being located in a city as culturally diverse as Montreal, has emphasized strategies to support patients from every background. We have also added a pet therapy program to help patients and there families cope with the length of time and the anxiety connected with clinic visits. Currently a golden retriever and his owner visit the clinic every week. Being able to interact with the dog makes the visit more informal and seems to break down emotional walls between patients and their caregivers. Hugging the dog is easier for some patients than hugging us, and I think this enables some of the serious discussion to occur between patients and family and patients and the staff. Thus far, this has been welcome addition.

Voluntary organizations also provide additional support to the Clinic. The clinic interacts with the ALS Quebec division of ALS Canada primarily through referrals and equipment needs. There is also an annual information day organized through the ALS Society of Canada in conjunction with the Canadian Congress of Neurological Sciences where the local chapter invites speakers and sets up workshops that are open to the public as well as the allied health care professionals.

Our biggest problem appears to be community-based support. The CLSCs are underfunded and cannot provide the level of assistance that the home caregivers require. The CLSC home ventilation program has a waiting list of several years and so is not always available to our patients, leaving the ALS team to manage ventilator issues. The availability of home palliative care can also be a problem. However, we have had minimal turnover in staff with an extraordinary degree of commitment on everyone's part. We would also like to increase clinical research activities but need a clinical scientist to participate in more research activities. Further growth within our institution will come, as the longstanding tradition of basic and clinical research in ALS at the Montreal Neurological Institute becomes further integrated and expanded with overall research activities in other fields. We hope that, as more effective therapies are developed, we will be able to meet the changing needs of the population.

Ireland and the MDC Clinic in Dublin

The model of ALS care in Ireland is based on a single centralized specialist MDC clinic in Dublin that has strong links to the Irish Motor Neurone Disease Association (IMNDA) and health care professionals in the community (9). The Dublin clinic is associated with the Beaumont Hospital and works closely with health professional staff at the hospital. The primary aim of the MDC is to provide ongoing and regular access to hospital-based neurology, physiotherapy, occupational therapy, speech and language therapy, psychology, social services, and nutritional therapy. In addition, close liaison between hospital-based and community-based services is essential for optimal delivery of care, given the structure of health-care in Ireland. The clinic is staffed by a consultant neurologist, a clinical nurse specialist, the Director of the IMNDA, an occupational therapist, a speech and language therapist, a nutritionist, a physiotherapist, and a respiratory technologist or physiologist. All the clinical professionals have extensive experience in ALS.

Approximately 40% of all patients with ALS in the Republic of Ireland attend the MDC. Patients who do not regularly attend the specialist MDC clinic can consult with the clinical nurse specialist, who also acts as a liaison for patients under the care of neurologists at other hospitals. Data from the Irish Register of Motor Neurone Disease indicate that those who regularly attend the MND clinic with full access to MDC have an enhanced life expectancy of up to nine months in comparison to those who attend nonspecialist clinics run by primary physicians (11).

Despite the need for an interdisciplinary approach to ALS and other chronic neurological diseases, the commitment by the Irish health administrators to this model of good practice has been limited. This reluctance is in part due to the limited development and funding of services in neurology in general: the ratio of neurologists to the general population is currently 1:280,000 in Ireland. The Irish ALS clinic has therefore been developed primarily through research funding, with core funding provided by the hospital for the consultant neurologist and specialist nurse. All the clinical professionals involved in the clinic also engage in clinical research in ALS, and accordingly, a portion of their salaries are paid from research funds.

The Irish health care system is based on the premise that all patients have a community-based general practitioner who operates as a gatekeeper for secondary and tertiary hospital-based services. Public hospital outpatient and inpatient care is provided free of charge, but waiting lists are long. However, urgent neurological review of patients with potentially serious illnesses such as ALS can be "fast-tracked" through appropriate representations by a general practitioner or other doctor to the MDC neurologist or specialist nurse. Despite this provision, the inexperience of general practitioners in diagnosing and managing neurological disease as well as the nihilistic attitude of some nonneurological specialists toward neurological disease often results in long delays before diagnosis, and poorly coordinated care and support of those who are not referred for neurological review.

Although community-based services are essential, unfortunately they are very limited in Ireland in terms of patient care for ALS. General practitioners work independently in solo or group practices, and provide a mixture of public (the free General Medical Service) and private (fee for service) care. A state-funded network of public health nurses and regional occupational therapists operate independently of both the hospital-based system and general practitioners. However, community-based physiotherapists are not available in some parts of the country, and community-based speech and language therapists, psychologists, and social workers primarily work in pediatric services. A limited number of clinical professionals are in private practice; however, waiting lists are long and consultations are expensive.

Automatic entitlement to the General Medical Service and community services, such as they exist, is means-tested, but with an income ceiling of approximately €100 per week, more than 60% of the general population is effectively excluded from accessing community-based services, given the costs. Discretionary provision of free General Medical Service care is occasionally made on grounds of serious illness, such as cancer. However, the guidelines are poorly defined, and decisions are generally made on a case-by-case basis. Private insurance is of limited usefulness, as the majority of third-party providers neither cover the costs of outpatient-based private medicine, nor do they consistently cover the fees of private nonphysician clinical professionals such as physiotherapists and occupational therapists.

Patients attending our ALS MDC clinic are seen every six weeks. For those who are unable to regularly attend the specialist MDC clinic, the specialist nurse is available to consult over the phone, and he or she also acts as a liaison for patients who are under the care of neurologists at other hospitals. The specialist nurse coordinates the MDC clinic, provides home visits, if possible, and ensures that the community services are made available to patients on the basis of need. This is achieved by advocating for individual ALS patients for free community-based care through the General Medical Service, and on occasion, by directly liaising with general practitioners and community-based clinical professionals.

Each patient's equipment needs are assessed by the hospital-based occupational therapist, who may also liaise with his or her counterpart in the community. Once recommended by the occupational therapist, all equipment is provided free of charge by the IMNDA. The availability of the IMNDA equipment bank minimizes the delay that patients would otherwise encounter in the Irish health-care system. The service ensures that the equipment requested is appropriate to the needs of the patient when it is delivered, and that patients of limited financial means can obtain equipment without the anxiety of incurring debt. NIPPV systems and feeding pumps for patients with gastrostomy are provided by the national government free of charge.

In Ireland, patients with ALS usually prefer home-based care during the later stages of disease when they are too ill to continue attending the MDC. The nurse specialist remains in telephone contact and conducts home visits at regular intervals. In 2003 in Ireland, 64% of patients with ALS died at home. Home care in the terminal stages is achieved by detailed planning with the family and constructing a comprehensive care plan to include "duty rotes." These incorporate a limited community-based (state-funded) home help service and private care attendants. The IMNDA underwrites the cost of care attendants, and facilitates the introduction of hospice home care teams when needed.

As the patient enters the final phase, hospice home care or day care services are included to alleviate distressing symptoms and maintain quality of life. In Ireland, this service is provided free of charge. Of the 64% of Irish patients with ALS who died at home in 2003, about one quarter used the hospice home care service. A proportion of patients (18%) elect acute hospital care during the terminal stage. Patients are more likely to choose this option if they have rapidly progressive disease, have not had access to the multidisciplinary service, or have a limited number of caregivers or have caregivers who are unable to provide adequate care at this stage. A smaller but growing proportion of patients (12%) elect hospice-based terminal care.

Discussions concerning end-of-life decisions usually take place before the patient enters the terminal stage. These discussions are frequently initiated by the nurse specialist, who has a close relationship with the patient and caregiver and can help the patient and family plan for the final stages. Such planning, although painful, permits the open discussion of options such as whether the patient desires to be resuscitated in the event of respiratory or cardiac arrest, or desires permanent mechanical ventilation if respiratory failure occurs. Clear decisions regarding these eventualities obviate the need for emergency room admission at the time of crisis and the imperative for full mechanical ventilation under such circumstances. Furthermore, frank discussion of the terminal stages can alleviate anxieties about how the patient will die, particularly with respect to the fear of choking and asphyxiation, as the availability and role of the hospice and home-based palliative care services can be explored.

In Ireland, our practice is to discuss end-of-life decisions in advance and to obtain a clear directive from the patient and caregiver as to their wishes. Of the approximately 350 patients attending our MDC clinic over the past nine years, only one has undergone full mechanical ventilation—this was an emergency measure after an unexpected respiratory arrest. Moreover, only 2 of about 900 patients on the Register of Motor Neurone Disease have committed suicide, and no patient has discussed or requested euthanasia.

The United Kingdom and the King's MND Care Center

Until the mid-1990s, care for patients with ALS or other MNDs in the UK was somewhat haphazard. This situation developed in part because, during the 1970s and 1980s, many neurologists served populations of between 200,000 and 500,000 and thus had no time to create a multidisciplinary approach to the care of patients with progressive neurological disorders. With the exception of a few major research centers, the role of the neurologist was seen primarily as that of a diagnostician. Once diagnosed, patients were often left to work with their general practitioner to organize physiotherapy, occupational therapy, speech and language therapy, dietetics, and so on. All too often the vagaries of local services were such that "needs-led" care was simply not available. Similarly, although St. Christopher's Hospice in London had begun a palliative care program in ALS in the 1970s, it was only in the late 1980s that a substantial proportion of local hospices and palliative care teams began to take an interest in ALS.

The MND Association of England, Wales, and Northern Ireland (MNDA), a patient support group, was formed in 1979 through the action of people affected by ALS, and increasing pressure from this organization, together with growing awareness among neurologists with an interest in neuromuscular diseases and ALS, provided the impetus to establish MND clinics that provide MDC. This pressure, coinciding with a renewed interest in multidisciplinary neurological rehabilitation and palliative care, led the MNDA to develop a policy to create MND care centers throughout England, Wales, and Northern Ireland. The need for such centers was also perceived in Scotland, although the patient support group in Scotland is a separate organization (the Scottish MND Association). The MNDA therefore advanced a strategy for encouraging neurologists and other key health and social care professionals to develop a coordinated and multidisciplinary approach to providing care for people with MND. To provide a framework for approved centers, the MNDA developed standards of care against which the services could be assessed and evaluated (the standards can be seen at www.mndassociation.org). These standards of care were created to achieve a better quality of life for people affected by ALS or other MNDs and covered the diagnostic process and all aspects of subsequent care.

In 1993, the MNDA invited bids for MNDA Care Centers. Applicants were asked to show that they provided MDC at a single location, with appropriate audit systems and plans for further developing the quality of care in collaboration with local and national representatives of the MNDA. Following peer review, the first center recognized was the King's MND Care and Research Center, which began to evaluate patients in 1995 (7,10). Subsequently, the MNDA has recognized 13 MND Care Centers with plans to establish an additional four or five to ensure equitable geographical distribution and access throughout England, Wales, and Northern Ireland. In addition, the MNDA works closely with the MND Care Center in Dublin (directed by Dr Orla Hardiman) and with colleagues in Scotland. The potential for the Care Center program to influence the standards of MND care nationally has long been recognized and is being built upon through a partnership between the centers and the MNDA. We are also working with the MNDA to develop educational activities, management guidelines, care pathways, and models of good practice.

The reminder of this section describes the structure, organization, and patient care activities of the King's MND Care and Research Center. The care model differs slightly in each center depending on local resources and history, but the care approach is similar and all endeavor to provide services that fulfill the MNDA standards of care. At least once annually, the Center Directors and Coordinators and the MNDA's Regional Care Advisers meet for a day to discuss strategy and new developments, and the development of the Centers remains a high priority for the Association. The aim is to create an effective regional network of centers through which advances in care can be rapidly introduced.

The King's MND Care and Research Center was developed through research funding, including funding for clinical trials. The philosophy of the King's team is to ensure that care and research are fully integrated so that patients who attend primarily to participate in research (e.g., clinical trials) receive excellent care, and patients who attend primarily for diagnosis and care receive information about, and the benefits of, an active research program. With the creation of the South East Regional

Table 5 Main Contributors to the King's MND Care Center Team

Care coordinator	Palliative care team
Nurse specialist	Consultant respiratory physician
Speech and language therapist	Interventional radiologist (for RIG)
Occupational therapist	Gastroenterologist (for PEG)
Physiotherapist	Psychology support team
Dietitian	Family and child counseling service
Social worker	Neuropsychologist
Clinical electrophysiologist	Neuropsychiatrist
Consultant neurologist	Voluntary association staff (e.g., Motor Neurone Disease Association)
Clinical research fellows and residents	Other volunteers[a]
Consultant in rehabilitation	

[a]Volunteers from British MND Association come to the Center and provide invaluable assistance in areas such as accompanying patients and caregivers and assisting them for some emotional support.
Abbreviations: RIG, radiologically inserted gastrostomy; PEG, percutaneous endoscopic gastrostomy.

Neurosciences Center at the King's Center, it was possible to establish a weekly MDC clinic involving physical therapists, occupational therapists, speech and language therapists, dietitians, a psychology support team, pulmonologists, and others (Table 5). Two elements were key to the success of this initiative. First, King's College Hospital signed a service-level agreement committing health-care providers to work with MND patients and to be present at the MDC clinic once a week. Second, the MNDA funded a team coordinator for the Center who is a single point of contact for patients and their families and integrates the activities of the team members. The team coordinator is responsible for arranging weekly meetings of the multidisciplinary team, meetings with community health workers, and quarterly meetings for the whole team, including laboratory and clinical researchers. The coordinator is also responsible for representing the team at the South East MND Forum, a network of community health care teams throughout southeast England who meet regularly to share information, develop skills and expertise, and develop health policy in relation to MND. These community care teams address care needs for all MND patients. The Regional MNDA Care Adviser is involved in these activities, and often the national MNDA office is also represented. Finally, the hospital funds a nurse specialist who, working closely with the coordinator, is responsible for interdisciplinary liaison on the ward (particularly with respect to gastrostomy and noninvasive ventilation) and in the clinic.

The King's MND Care and Research Center has a management committee composed of a director, deputy director, consultant neurologists (currently four), the team coordinator, the nurse specialist, a clinical manager for neurosciences, and the clinical director at St. Christopher's Hospice. We maintain strong links with St. Christopher's Hospice, and we have recently established the King's Center for Palliative Care in Neurology in collaboration with the Department of Palliative Care and Policy at Guy's, King's, and St. Thomas' School of Medicine.

Ideally, we would hold two weekly MDC clinics, but at present the resources are not available. Our MDC clinic is therefore restricted to one morning each week during which we see 8 to 12 patients. The clinic is covered by two neurologists (one consultant and one experienced trainee). The team also receives support from clinical research fellows who receive training in all aspects of MND care and are pursuing their own clinical or laboratory projects. Recently, a consultant from the palliative care team at Guy's, King's, and St. Thomas' School has joined us in the clinic, as has our consultant pulmonologist so that end-of-life issues and respiratory symptoms can be more easily addressed within the clinic period. A consultant gastroenterologist from King's College does not attend the MDC clinic but is available for consultation. Visits are preplanned so that patients have access to all the services appropriate to their needs. Mental health counselors are available at the Center, but most appointments for counseling are outside clinic hours. To facilitate mental health counseling, the needs of both patients and caregivers are assessed by the coordinator at each visit. A consultant neurologist from the MND team is always on call outside of the formal MDC clinic hours to address medical queries and liaise with other health workers.

At present there are 400 follow-up interviews each year for approximately 100 patients. There is multidisciplinary feedback at the end of each clinic, and further discussion among the team members during the following week, with preparation for the next week's clinic. Therapists are responsible for liaising with their community counterparts to maintain needed therapies outside the Center, and the coordinator ensures that appropriate records are kept and queries are efficiently dealt with.

The MND Care and Research Center receives about 200 new referrals through the clinic every year. In addition, 30 to 50 patients are referred directly by consultant colleagues who cover the southeast of England (a population of approximately 3.5 million). Thus the Center deals with about 250 new patients each year. Some of these patients will not have an MND, and one of the main functions of our outpatient service is to perform a thorough diagnostic assessment on patients who have been referred to us. Patients with MND or suspected MND are "fast-tracked" for diagnostic evaluation according to an agreed upon care pathway.

The beds of the King's Regional Clinical Neurosciences Center are available for patients who require admission for gastrostomy (mainly radiologically inserted gastrostomy) and for assessment for assisted ventilation. All admitted patients are evaluated by the palliative care and MND teams. For patients with suspected cognitive dysfunction, neuropsychological, and neuropsychiatric evaluation is available. The psychology support team and the chaplaincy are available for inpatients.

Apart from direct clinical care, the team is responsible for developing care pathways, treatment protocols and guidelines, and for auditing the service. The team has also developed patient satisfaction questionnaires and is about to launch a survey of patient and caregiver experiences at the time of diagnosis. Our guidelines for gastrostomy and noninvasive ventilation have been widely disseminated and seem to be useful in day-to-day practice. We also have prepared guidelines concerning delivery of the diagnosis for ALS. In the United Kingdom, a wide variety of patient education materials are available, some of which we have produced and many developed and provided by the MNDA and other support organizations. Team members are frequently involved in meetings with patient support groups throughout the southeast of England, and with national and international meetings of the MNDA. Rightly, patients and caregiver education is seen by the Association as a key activity for their Care Centers.

To conduct research in familial cases of ALS, the King's Center established the King's Database in 1990, and we have (with IRB approval) maintained this and built up a large DNA and tissue bank through the Medical Research Council-funded Institute of Psychiatry Brain Bank. Currently the Brain Bank holds frozen and fixed tissue more than 100 brain and spinal cord samples, with appropriate controls. The Brain Bank also has extensive tissue samples from patients with Alzheimer's disease and other neurodegenerative conditions.

Despite all these developments, care is still unsatisfactory for many people affected by MND in the United Kingdom. Community care varies widely, and local coordination is equally variable. The South-East MND Forum is helping to drive improvements in care provision, with the appointment of local coordinators and local nurse specialists. At present radiologically inserted gastrostomy for MND is provided only at King's Center, and noninvasive ventilation is, likewise, unavailable in many districts. However, some districts are appointing nurse specialists with an interest in assisted ventilation, and it is the aim of our Center, in collaboration with colleagues throughout the southeast of England, to develop an effective service for noninvasive ventilation so that all patients who might benefit have the opportunity to try it.

It will be important to develop care pathways and protocols that will be common to all the centers, as the MNDA is developing evidence-based guidelines that will inform local protocols. An exciting development is the increasing involvement of palliative care teams and hospices with early referral for palliative care for patients with ALS or other MNDs. The development of the Center for Palliative Care in Neurology at King's should spur research into the needs of patients with MND (and other long-term neurological conditions) as well as being an impetus to develop prospective studies and randomized, controlled trials of established and evolving therapies.

Finally, there is a strong international perspective to these developments through links with other Centers throughout Europe and North America. The European ALS Consortium is now closely linked with the European Federation of Neurological Societies, and actively collaborates in many aspects of clinical care and basic science research. The Consortium is developing brief but rigorous evidence-based guidelines in collaboration with the MNDA and has held a number of workshops on key issues (e.g., noninvasive ventilation, clinical trial design, epidemiology, and databases) sponsored by the European Neuromuscular Center (ENMC; www.enmc.org). In addition, the Center has also developed the database (www.alsod.org). This database registers patients with the SOD1 gene mutation and summarizes clinical and pathological information relating to the mutation. The database has been expanded to allow new ALS genes to be tracked in the same way. Finally, in collaboration with Professor Irene Higginson and her colleagues at Palliative Care Medicine at King's College, we have developed a user website (www.build.org) for people affected by ALS or other MNDs, but it is also used by health professionals and others with an interest in ALS. We value our links with North American centers and hope to strengthen those over the next few years.

France and the ALS Center at Salpétrière and Regional ALS Centers

In France, a multidisciplinary approach has been developed through constant cooperation between the academic neurology clinics that treat patients with ALS and the French ALS association, the Association pour la Recherche sur la Sclérose Latérale Amyotrophique (ARS). The first clinic was formally created in 1989 in Paris by an agreement between the ARS and the Assistance Publique-Hôpitaux de Paris, which oversees the administration of the Paris hospitals. The ALS center, initially located at Hôtel Dieu de Paris, moved in 1994 to the Salpétrière. This center developed rapidly and contributed significantly to what has become the basis of the multidisciplinary approach in France for patients with ALS. The center is also a leader in clinical trials, contributing to the design of large international trials such as the riluzole and the xaliproden trials, in collaboration with the Salpétrière Department of Pharmacology.

The center cares for patients in Paris and the surrounding region (which has a population of nearly 12 million) and has also a key role as the "last advice" center for all patients in France with ALS. The center sees approximately 920 patients annually, with nearly 35 new patients each month. Follow-up visits are scheduled for every three months, but may be more frequent, especially when a patient is experiencing increasing respiratory problems. Most patients are seen during a one-day clinic that is held weekly. We have also seven beds available for patients who require hospitalization for PEG, adaptation to the nasal interface mask for noninvasive ventilatory support, or end-of-life care. The team is composed of four neurologists, one pulmonologist, one gastroenterologist, two referent nurses, one physiotherapist, two speech therapists, one psychomotricist (a person with training in both psychology and physiotherapy who deals with mind-body issues), one dietitian, one psychologist, and one ergotherapist.

Under pressure from the ARS, the French Ministry of Health has created regional centers and provided permanent funding (5.2 million Euros annually) for personnel to staff 16 regional centers as well as the national center located at Salpétrière. These centers cover approximately the entire national territory, ensuring that each patient with ALS has the same opportunity to receive care that meets specific guidelines in regard to both the provision and quality of the care. The national center coordinates the activity of the regional centers, particularly in respect to developing processes to ensure that a uniform multidisciplinary approach to care takes place throughout the entire disease course, from diagnosis to the end of life. Funding was also provided for this coordination process. Various strategies to coordinate activity between the regional centers currently are being developed through consensus during annual meetings of all the multidisciplinary team members from all the centers, including the representatives of the ARS.

Although each regional center adapts to provide care according to the needs of its patients, the basis of care remains the same throughout all the centers. Each has a multidisciplinary team with a neurologist in charge of managing the team and who leads the entire care process. An ARS representative is also present at each center. We are formalizing standard-of-care operational procedures for each member of the team and for each point at which the team has to give the patient bad news (e.g., diagnosis, PEG, assisted ventilation, and end of life). Video recordings have been made by the national center to allow intradisciplinary discussion during our meetings concerning patient issues and management plans. A dossier that will be used at all the centers currently is being tested at the national center. This dossier is given to the patient and provides all the basic information that is necessary for him or her and for all the members of the team in charge of the patient at home. All 16 centers are working together to achieve this objective. We are also developing tools to evaluate physical, psychosocial, and financial issues involved in care at the regional centers. A future goal is to design clinical and basic science research components within the framework of the regional ALS centers.

Belgium and the NMRC of the University Hospital Gasthuisberg in Leuven

In Belgium, MDC for patients with ALS was initiated by the Belgian Minister of Health several years ago. Experts in neuromuscular disease and nongovernmental neuromuscular disease organizations had significant roles in the planning of care centers. Today, six neuromuscular centers (NMRCs) are located throughout the country, and they provide MDC care for patients of all ages with any type of neuromuscular disease. In a country with a population of little more than 10 million, this means that patients with neuromuscular diseases have little difficulty accessing MDC care. In general, the centers are attached to the country's main university hospitals, and several, such as the Leuven NMRC, have ALS research teams, so patients can participate in clinical trials. Several years ago, national reimbursement to the centers was implemented so that they are now financed through the national health care system, resulting in no or very low costs for the patients. Thus, care is readily accessible to patients with neuromuscular disease because the number of centers is adequate for the population and costs to patients are minimal. Overall, our program has been working well, both in terms of providing care and maintaining the clinics financially.

The NMRC of the University Hospital Gasthuisberg in Leuven is coordinated by a neurologist with specific expertise in neuromuscular diseases, in collaboration with a rehabilitation physician. The center provides mostly outpatient care. A nurse specialist with expertise in ALS care coordinates the care for individual patients. An administrative manager organizes the clinic visits and makes sure that the patient is seen by team members as requested by the patient or caregivers, the nurse specialist, the neurologist, or rehabilitation physician. Our neuromuscular disease clinic is held once a week for all neuromuscular patients, and we see about eight patients (both new and follow-up cases) with ALS each week.

A physical therapist, occupational therapist, speech therapist, dietitian, and social worker as well as psychologist are permanent members of the team. The social worker plays a key role in connecting the patients and their families with various social services available within the health care system, while the psychologist is available for both patients and caregivers to help them cope with stress and other mental health issues that may arise. The occupational therapist visits patients at home when necessary. The occupational therapist and social worker also take charge of preparing the paperwork necessary for the patient to apply for assistive equipment, additional financial support, etc.

The MDC team also closely collaborates with a variety of specialists who have a special interest in the medical complications of neuromuscular diseases. Of these specialists, the pulmonologist is consulted most frequently and is involved to the greatest extent. He or she assesses respiratory function, discusses options when ventilatory issues arise for patients and caregivers, and provides guidance and education when they are considering noninvasive or invasive ventilatory support. An ophthalmologist and cardiologist are also associated with the NMRC, but their services are used on an as-needed basis. A genetics team works closely with the NMRC to identify cases of familial ALS. A gastroenterologist performs PEG, but the decision for PEG is made by the patient and her or his caregiver, the nurse, the dietitian, speech therapist, and neurologist. We admit patients for this procedure, not only for safety, but also to ascertain that the patient and caregiver feel comfortable with the feeding system once PEG has been performed.

The MDC team consults with care providers in the community for certain services. Day-to-day physical, occupational and speech therapy is provided by local community therapists, with whom the team interacts both in writing and by telephone. Most patients visit the MDC clinic four to six times a year. The multidisciplinary team has weekly team meetings after the clinic, and the team prepares a written report on each patient. The MDC system undoubtedly has significantly improved care for ALS patients because such MDC was not available before. The multidisciplinary approach and the coordinated nature of the activities are also of substantial help to the professional caregivers themselves because it promotes clear and coordinated communication about each patient between all the health care providers.

Although we have found that our approach and clinic structure have worked well, there are areas in that need improvement. A visit to the team requires the patient to travel to the NMRC, and even in a small country such as Belgium, this requires quite an effort from patients. Visits to multidisciplinary teams are tiring for both patients and caregivers. Physicians play a pivotal role in referring their patients to an NMRC. However, the Internet allows many patients to locate specialized care independently of their general physician. The fact that the Leuven NMRC is attached to an ALS research group has the advantage that patients remain updated about progress in ALS research and can easily participate in clinical research. In addition, at the Leuven clinic, the lack of space has become a problem, since we cannot hire additional health care professionals who can further contribute to MDC.

Japan and the Kitasato University Higashi Hospital

For the past 20 years in Japan, most patients with ALS received permanent mechanical ventilation at the onset of respiratory failure. This approach differs from that in the rest of the world and has had a significant impact on how ALS treatment has developed in Japan. Thus, we would like to begin by explaining how this practice became common. In the 1970s, the Japanese Ministry of Health and Welfare adopted a law to protect those who had terminal diseases, including intractable neurological diseases, such as ALS, Parkinson's disease, Huntington's disease, spinocerebellar atrophy, multisystem atrophy, multiple sclerosis, and myasthenia gravis. Medical research and patient care were fully funded by this act, so patients who were diagnosed with these diseases received free medical care at any hospital in Japan. Traditionally in Japan, physicians would not tell their patients that they had a terminal disease, but they would tell the family. However, the family also would not share such information with their loved one. Thus, physicians did not have to discuss the prognosis or decisions regarding end-of-life care. Rather, with the advent of permanent mechanical ventilation, they simply chose permanent ventilatory support for their patients with ALS, and the costs were covered by the intractable disease act. Therefore, most patients with ALS received a tracheostomy with permanent ventilation and stayed in the hospital for an extended period. Although this practice might have helped patients and families because it relieved the families of caring for the patient at home, the hospitals (particularly in teaching hospitals where ALS expertise is available) gradually suffered from a lack of beds for other patients because a number of ventilated patients with ALS remained hospitalized until they died. Moreover, at the same time a nursing shortage developed that was exacerbated by the long-term hospitalization of ventilated patients with ALS because care for these patients requires enormous time.

In the past decade, however, major changes in the Japanese health care system have taken place because of changes in Japanese economy. Following the American health care system, shorter hospital stays are now the norm, and long-term hospitalization is not possible for ventilated patients. Another impetus for changes in ALS care derives from the consideration of the quality of life for those with long-term permanent ventilation who are hospitalized for months or even years. At the same time, attitudes toward the importance of the patient's right to self-determination have shifted, and physicians now directly discuss the diagnosis and end-of-life issues with their patients. Therefore, more patients with ALS now openly discuss the diagnosis as well as their options and choices for medical treatment, including tracheostomy and permanent ventilation. Finally, because long-term hospitalization is no longer possible, a greater number of patients with ALS must be cared for at home, implying that family members are becoming the primary caregivers for their family member. These changes have resulted in a rapid transition from tracheostomy with permanent ventilation as the main treatment in the advanced stages of ALS to an emphasis on palliative care. The introduction of NIPPV has accelerated this shift. Another factor that prevents patients from choosing permanent ventilation is that removal or stopping permanent ventilatory support is a criminal offense because it is considered to be physician-assisted suicide. Therefore, even if patients wish to discontinue ventilation with or without advance directives, stopping ventilatory support is impossible. A study in 2004 indicated that among 5711 active patients with ALS registered in the Japanese ALS Database, only 1530 (26.8%) received permanent ventilation whereas in the past almost all patients who required ventilatory support would have received permanent ventilation. At our hospital, approximately 15% of patients with ALS are ventilated via tracheostomy.

As a result of these changes in health care, the Japanese community has adopted a unique program that provides home care for those with intractable neurological diseases. Many local communities have established close working relationships with nearby major teaching or community hospitals that have expertise in ALS and other intractable neurological diseases and have developed systems for both emergency care and routine home care visits from the network hospitals. For example, our hospital, Kitasato University Higashi Hospital, located in a prefecture neighboring Tokyo, has been one of the pioneers in developing a community-based home-care system. Those patients who are receiving permanent ventilatory support have a monthly home care visit by a team consisting of the family doctor or neurologist, social worker, biomedical technicians, pharmacists, and nutritionists, and others depending on the patient's needs. In the interim, every two weeks, a team without the physicians also makes a home visit to evaluate the ventilator and other equipment. The Japanese government pays only the physicians for the home visits; the other health care professionals are not paid. We have estimated the costs of the monthly and twice-monthly visits and found that they are high because of the manpower and time involved. However, changing this system to reduce costs will be difficult because patients and community government alike take it for granted. Home care for invasive or noninvasive ventilation is covered by all health insurance, and patients have the option of receiving permanent ventilatory care at home. Although everyone in Japan must have health insurance, either governmental or private, patients with intractable diseases receive additional support from the national government. Although the overall rate of ventilator use appears to have diminished in recent years, we cannot predict whether this decrease will continue.

Our hospital also provides respite service for the families of our ventilated patients for as long as two weeks (the current average hospital stay for all diseases is 17 to 19 days). While the patients are admitted to this respite service, respiratory, nutritional, and other medical issues are fully evaluated necessary. We have asked the community government to increase the annual budget to support ventilated patients with ALS and area hospitals to allocate more beds for respite care; however, these changes have yet to occur, and the rapid changes in the overall health care system in Japan makes it hard to predict what will happen.

The concept of the multidisciplinary clinic for ALS is relatively new in Japan, but a clear trend toward such clinics exists, particularly at teaching and large national hospitals. At our hospital, the ALS clinic is held once a week for the whole day. Usually 8 to 10 patients are seen and follow-up generally occurs monthly. The team members consist of neurologists, nutritionists, speech pathologists, occupational therapists, and various volunteers. Gastroenterologists are available for same-day evaluation of patients for PEG as are pulmonologists for assessment of patients for noninvasive and invasive ventilation. Our clinical research focuses on prospective analysis of quality of life in the outpatient population. We have found it helpful to have hospital volunteers accompany the patients while they are evaluated at the clinic. In our region, the general community also helps patients with basic tasks. For example, community volunteers may transport patients to their clinic appointments and some private taxi companies have modified their taxis so they can transport disabled patients, including those with ALS. Our community government issues taxi vouchers for those who need transportation.

The size of our ALS Clinic is more or less similar to other ALS clinics in Japan, although multidisciplinary ALS clinics still constitute a small minority of neurology outpatient services. Furthermore, large centralized ALS clinics are still rare because it is still a new concept for patients to travel long distances to seek advice from specialists. The Japanese government (Health and Welfare Ministry) has extensively supported ALS research and patient care for the past three decades. The Japanese Neurological Society recently published the ALS Practice Guidelines (in Japanese), a counterpart of the American Academy of Neurology ALS Practice Parameter Guidelines. A number of Japanese ALS specialists have developed an educational and information website in Japanese for patients with ALS and their families.

At present, many issues exist in Japan concerning patient care and management in ALS. Although the ALS care guidelines were published, health care professionals have strongly differing opinions as to how physicians should provide care for patients with ALS, particularly in regard to breaking the news of the diagnosis, the use of permanent ventilation, and aggressive symptomatic treatment. The Japanese health-care system is also evolving, and the rapid changes in how we think about health-care and terminal disease sometimes can make it difficult for both patients and health professionals to predict the future direction. Despite these problems, we believe that the MDC clinic concept will expand to result in more effective care for patients with ALS.

Switzerland and the MND Clinic in St. Gallen

Not until 2001 were patients with ALS followed regularly at one of the major hospitals in Switzerland. The Kantonsspital in St. Gallen was the first Swiss hospital to implement such follow-ups. Initially, only a resident and a supervising physician who was an ALS specialist saw the patients. Referrals to other onsite health care professionals and physicians were made as needed. This structure had many shortcomings, but fortunately this changed fundamentally when the Kantonsspital St. Gallen provided space and the infrastructure for a specialized MND clinic. The Swiss ALS foundation donated furniture for the clinic. In spring 2003, the ALS clinic in St. Gallen was officially founded. Since then the core staff has consisted of an ALS nurse, a resident in neurology and a consultant neurologist who is an ALS specialist. Other on-site members of the team are a physiotherapist, occupational therapist, speech therapist, and a social worker. We have rapidly developed excellent collaborations with the departments of pulmonology, gastroenterology, and the palliative care unit so that patients are quickly evaluated for specific difficulties—for instance, all patients can obtain polysomnography within two weeks. A four-bed unit for the initiation of noninvasive ventilation will be established in the near future.

In addition to support from the hospital, funding is provided by the Swiss Society of Muscular Disorders (SGMK), the pharmaceutical industry, the Swiss ALS foundation, and private donors. Neither the government nor medical insurance provides financial support. The external funding covers only the costs associated with the part-time ALS nurse, whereas the hospital fully covers the physician's and other team members' salaries and time devoted to ALS patient care. In the Swiss health care system, medical insurance can be billed for physical, speech, and occupational therapy when the patient is seen in an outpatient setting. In addition, the hospital pays for all prescribed medications. As long as the patients are employed, disability insurance (Invalidenversicherung) covers any type of assistive aid, such as braces, wheelchairs, and necessary alterations to the home. This is not the case, however, if the patient receives a pension, usually after the age of 65. In these cases it is quite often a struggle to obtain financial support from the pension plan or medical insurance for assistive devices.

Currently, the MND clinic in St. Gallen cares for 80 to 90 patients who are followed at three-month intervals. Less than half of them live in the province of St. Gallen, and the others come from various parts of Switzerland. Many patients are seen initially at the St. Gallen clinic for a second opinion, but are then also followed at the St. Gallen clinic because to date it is the only MND clinic in Switzerland. When patients can no longer attend the ALS clinic, the ALS nurse organizes home visits (usually herself and one of the ALS physicians). Contact with a social worker and community services is established early in the disease.

Finding health-care professionals with experience in ALS is a major problem for patients who do not live in the vicinity of St. Gallen. Although most health-care professionals in Switzerland may have seen one or a few ALS patients a year, they lack education and experience with the disease, most likely because the country's population is small (approximately seven million) and therefore there are relatively few patients with ALS. In 2004, the first Swiss ALS Day was held for neurologists and allied health-care professionals. One of its goals was to start to address this problem by devoting half the day's program to the education of health care professionals about ALS. Although this is a good first step, an organized network and access to health care professionals with a profound knowledge of ALS is urgently needed. To enhance public awareness and education, an annual Swiss ALS Symposium has been established and was first held in 2002. World-renowned speakers and ALS researchers have contributed to the symposium, making it a state-of-the-art event. The MND clinic in St. Gallen also organizes meetings for relatives of patients with ALS so we can better understand and address their needs. Additionally, this year we are implementing training in caregiving that is aimed at primary caregivers and consists of several modules.

The MND clinic is involved in a clinical trial of TCH346 (Novartis), which has become a major source of funding. In parallel, a multicenter substudy to explore the value of neurophysiological measurements to follow disease progression has been initiated by the St. Gallen clinic. The clinic has also received a grant from the American ALS Association for a pilot study of treatment for cramps. The clinic also collaborates nationally and internationally in research in clinical neurophysiology, genetics, and gene profiling in human motoneurons.

In our experience, the success of a MND clinic depends on the motivation and engagement of the MND team members. Within a short time, the ALS clinic in St. Gallen has become the major referral center for ALS patients in Switzerland, offering multidisciplinary patient care as well as engaging in ALS research. Patients and their relatives soon become aware that the ALS team members give their hearts and souls to their patients. Such dedication ensures not only a growing number of referrals but also support from the patients, families, and patient organizations.

CHALLENGES AND CONCLUSIONS

In the first part of this chapter, we described the concept of the multidisciplinary ALS clinic, the function of each team member, and potential issues involved with such an approach, largely based on Eleanor and Lou Gehrig MDA/ALS Research Center at Columbia University (14). Different clinics in the United States offer a more or less comprehensive approach based on needs and financial support. In the latter half of the chapter, clinic directors from throughout the world described their ALS clinics to illustrate the diversity in MDC clinic structure and approach to care. It is helpful to know how other clinics have developed, how they are run, and whether similar problems exist and how these difficulties have been solved. The multidisciplinary concept and clinic is relatively new in Japan, but they have developed an effective home-care system. In Switzerland, a new clinic has succeeded rapidly and influenced other neurologists in Switzerland. The ALS Care Center first established in the U.K. appears to have become a leader worldwide in comprehensive care. In France and Belgium, the national governments have formed unique and highly successful regional multidisciplinary clinics. In contrast, a single comprehensive centralized MDC clinic has been established in Ireland in order to work skillfully within the structure of the Irish health care system. In Montreal, pet therapy has been found to enhance patient and caregiver comfort during the clinic, adding a unique aspect to their comprehensive MDC clinic. Each clinic demonstrates original ideas and structures that are skillfully adapted to each country's health care system, societal customs, and the patient's and family's needs. In developing ideas for the multidisciplinary ALS clinic, voluntary disease organizations have provided strong support in each country. We hope this chapter helps not only to further improve each existing ALS clinic, but also provides ideas for those who wish to establish multidisciplinary ALS clinics in their regions.

ACKNOWLEDGMENTS

Tricia Holmes, MND Association, provided invaluable information on the status of ALS patient care in the U.K.

REFERENCES

1. Thompson B. Amyotrophic lateral sclerosis: integrating care for patients and their families. Am J Hosp Pall Care 1990; 7:27–32.
2. Mitsumoto H, Bromberg M, Johnston W, Tandan R, Byock I, Lyon M, Miller RG, Appel SH, Benditt J, Bernat JL, Borario GD, Carver AC, Clawson L, Del Bene ML, Kasarskis EJ, LeGrand SB, Mandler P, McCarthy J, Munsat T, Newman D, Sufit RL,

Versenyi A. Promoting excellence in end-of-life care in ALS. Amyotroph Lateral Scler Other Motor Neuron Dis (in press).

3. Mitsumoto H, Chad DA, Pioro EP. Comprehensive care. In: Mitsumoto H, Chad DA, Pioro EP, eds. Amyotrophic Lateral Sclerosis. Contemporary Neurology Series No. 49. New York: Oxford University Press, 1998:303–320.

4. Mitsumoto H, Del Bene M. Improving the quality of life for people with ALS: the challenge ahead. Amyotroph Lateral Scler Other Motor Neuron Disord 2000; 1:329–336.

5. Mitsumoto H, Munsat TL, eds. Amyotrophic Lateral Sclerosis. Patient and Family Guide to Management and Care. New York: Demos, 2001.

6. Norris FH, Smith RA, Denys EH. Motor neurone disease: towards better care. Br Med J 1985; 291:259–262.

7. Leigh PN. ALS Center Report: The King's MND Care and Research Centre, London, UK. Amyotroph Lateral Scler Other Motor Neuron Disord 1999; 1:53–54.

8. Wasner M, Borasio GD. ALS center reports. Amyotroph Lateral Scler Other Motor Neuron Disord. 2001; 2:109–211.

9. Hardiman O, Traynor BJ, Corr B, Frost E. Models of care for motor neuron disease: setting standards. Amyotroph Lateral Scler Other Motor Neuron Disord 2002; 3: 182–185.

10. Leigh PN, Abrahams S, Al-Chalabi A, Ampong MA, Goldstein LH, Johnson J, Lyall R, Moxham J, Mustfa N, Rio A, Shaw C, Willey E. King's MND Care and Research Team. The management of motor neurone disease. J Neurol Neurosurg Psychiatry 2003; 74(suppl 4):32–47.

11. Traynor BJ, Alexander M, Corr B, Frost E, Hardiman O. Effect of a multidisciplinary amyotrophic lateral sclerosis (ALS) clinic on ALS survival: a population based study, 1996–2000. J Neurol Neurosurg Psychiatry 2003; 74:1258–1261.

12. Miller RG, Rosenberg JA, Gelinas DF, Mitsumoto H, Newman D, Sufit R, Borasio GD, Bradley WG, Bromberg MB, Brooks BR, Kasarskis EJ, Munsat TL, Oppenheimer EA. and the ALS practice Parameters Task Force. Practice parameters: an evidence-based review. Neurology 1999; 52:1311–1323.

13. Esposito SJ, Mitsumoto H, Shanks M. Use of palatal lift and palatal augmentation prostheses to improve dysarthria in patients with amyotrophic lateral sclerosis: a cases series. J Prosthet Dent 2000; 83:90–98.

14. Mitsumoto H. ALS Center Report: the Eleanor and Lou Gehrig MDA/ALS Center, New York, USA. Amyotroph Lateral Scler Other Motor Neuron Disord 1999; 1:51–52.

15. Borasio GD, Voltz R, Miller RG. Palliative care in amyotrophic lateral sclerosis. In: Palliative Care, Carver A, Foley K, eds. Neurol Clin 2001; 19:829–847.

16. Wasner M, Bold U, Vollmer TC, Borasio GD. Sexuality in patients with amyotrophic lateral sclerosis and their partners. J Neurol 2004; 251:445–448.

17. Kaub-Wittemer D, von Steinbüchel N, Wasner M, Laier-Groeneveld G, Borasio GD. Quality of life and psychosocial issues in ventilated patients with amyotrophic lateral sclerosis and their caregivers. J Pain Symptom Manage 2003; 26:890–896.

18. Neudert C, Oliver D, Wasner M, Borasio GD. The course of the terminal phase in patients with amyotrophic lateral sclerosis. J Neurol 2001; 248:612–616.

19. Oliver D, Borasio GD, Walsh D, eds. Palliative Care in Amyotrophic Lateral Sclerosis (Motor Neurone Disease). Oxford: Oxford University Press, 2000.

20. Voltz R, Bernat J, Borasio GD, Maddocks I, Oliver D, Portenoy R, eds. Palliative Care in Neurology. Oxford: Oxford University Press, 2004.

28

The ALS Patient CARE Program—North American Patient CARE Database

Robert G. Miller
Department of Neurosciences, California Pacific Medical Center, San Francisco, California, U.S.A.

Fred Anderson, Neelam Gowda, and Wei Huang
Department of Surgery, Center for Outcomes Research, University of Massachusetts Medical School, Worcester, Massachusetts, U.S.A.

Walter G. Bradley
Department of Neurology, University of Miami School of Medicine, Miami, Florida, U.S.A.

Benjamin R. Brooks
Department of Neurology, University of Wisconsin Medical School, Madison, Wisconsin, U.S.A.

Hiroshi Mitsumoto
Eleanor and Lou Gehrig MDA/ALS Research Center, Department of Neurology, Columbia University Medical Center, The Neurological Institute, New York, New York, U.S.A.

Dan H. Moore
Research Institute, California Pacific Medical Center, San Francisco, California, U.S.A.

Steve Ringel
Department of Neurology, University of Colorado Health Sciences Center, Denver, Colorado, U.S.A.

Linda Boynton De Sepulveda
ALS Haven, Montecito, California, U.S.A.

Laura Coker
Department of Public Health Sciences, Wake Forest University School of Medicine, Winston-Salem, North Carolina, U.S.A.

Noah Lechtzin
Department of Medicine & Neurology, Johns Hopkins University School of Medicine, Baltimore, Maryland, U.S.A.

Mark Ross
Department of Neurology, Mayo Clinic, Scottsdale, Arizona, U.S.A.

INTRODUCTION

Evidence-based medicine has begun to make a major impact in the field of neurology and neuromuscular diseases. The American Academy of Neurology has published an extensive series of practice parameters to integrate evidence-based recommendations into patient management. The Cochran Collaboration, a global network of volunteers developing evidence-based systematic reviews, has completed a growing body of meta-analyses for therapies in neurology and neuromuscular disease. In the field of ALS, the first systematic review on riluzole was published five years ago and now there are 20 reviews either published or in preparation. One major shortcoming in the field of evidence-based medicine is the ability to track adherence to practice parameters and to examine the health outcomes resulting from those recommendations. In ALS, there have been efforts to track adherence to the practice parameters and evaluate outcomes, and to our knowledge these represent the first such efforts in neuromuscular diseases (1–4). As new therapies become available for patients with ALS, evidence-based recommendations are needed to provide optimal utilization of these new therapies.

Without uniform evidence-based standards, the utilization of these therapies will continue to depend upon clinician opinion, advice from mentors, and anecdotal experience. One example of the high degree of variance in utilization of beneficial treatments was published in a recent clinical trial of brain-derived neurotrophic factor in ALS (5). There was a large variance in the utilization of non-invasive mechanical ventilation for patients in this trial from zero at one center to as high as 48% at another of the 39 centers participating in the trial.

The ALS CARE database was developed with the hope of standardizing the use of effective therapies for patients with ALS and tracking outcomes to raise the overall standard of care (6,7). Observational databases enable both the patients and physicians to become more fully informed about management and to assess health outcomes in an effort to provide optimal patient management. In many neurological diseases, other databases have been developed to help evaluate outcomes and to direct future efforts at standardizing therapies for diseases including epilepsy, Alzheimer's disease, Parkinson's disease, fascioscapulohumeral (FSH) muscular dystrophy, myotonic dystrophy, ataxia, and hereditary neuropathy.

One other goal for the ALS Patient CARE database was the possibility of gathering sufficient data for hypothesis generation and to provide preliminary data for future research. In this chapter, we will summarize some of the successes and failures of these efforts and also document temporal trends in the management of patients with ALS.

METHODS

Background

The ALS Patient Care Database was developed by an advisory board of experts in ALS including neurologists, nurses, statisticians, and a representative from the ALS Association, a national patient advocacy group. To ensure the credibility and integrity of the database, the advisory board established laws covering issues such as publication of data, confidentiality, and the role of a corporate sponsor. The advisory board controls these data and has sole discretion regarding their dissemination. The board has established a university-based Study Coordinating Center, which mails quarterly reports to physicians, protects the confidentiality of patients, neurologists and ALS clinics, and supports the publication of data.

Data Collection

All neurologists practicing in North America are eligible to join the database, regardless of their practice setting (i.e., ALS clinic, community hospital, academic medical center, or private practice). Participating clinical sites are encouraged to enroll all of their ALS patients, including both incident and prevalent cases. Data are collected in the following domains: diagnosis, prognostic factors, natural history, and therapeutic interventions. In addition to data reported by neurologists, self-reports are collected from patients and their caregivers (Table 1).

Health Professional Form

Neurologists enroll patients with confirmed or suspected ALS by completing a Health Professional Form, which records the clinical findings at each clinic visit. The physician or designee completes this two-page form, which takes only 5 to 10 minutes. Data are collected on a number of clinical variables, including disease severity and current management. Patients are assigned to a diagnostic classification based on the El Escorial criteria, which were revised in 2001 by the World Federation of Neurology Subcommittee on Motor Neuron Diseases (8). Disease severity is assessed by both forced vital capacity and the ALS Functional Rating Scale (ALSFRS)—a reproducible and objective means to describe the degree of functional impairment due to ALS (9).

Table 1 Variables Collected in the ALS Patient Care Database

Patient reported	Physician reported
Demographic information	Date of diagnosis
Type of insurance	Diagnostic criteria
Employment status	Diagnostic tests performed
Annual income	Atypical features
Number of ALS-related visits to physician/year	Region affected by ALS
Satisfaction with medical care	ALS functional rating scale score
Duration of symptoms	Forced vital capacity
Initial diagnosis	ALS-related conditions
Capacity to perform ADL	Disease-specific medications
Self-reported health status	Feeding modalities
Symptoms and satisfaction with symptomatic treatments	Respiratory interventions
Non-pharmacological interventions	End-of-life measures
General health status	Caregiver-reported
	Relationship to patient
	Source of payments (if any) for care giving
	General health status
	Impact of care giving on psychosocial status
Concomitant medications	Employment status

Patient Form

Patients complete a six-page form, which takes approximately 15 minutes; the patient caregiver or clinic staff may provide assistance if necessary. The Patient Form incorporates information on demographics, therapeutic interventions, and two quality-of-life (QOL) measures: the Short Form (SF-12^{TM}) Health Survey—a generic instrument that allows patients to report their health-related quality-of-life, and the ALSA-Q5, a more disease-specific instrument. The SF-12^{TM} Health Survey consists of 12 questions designed to rate a number of aspects of the patient's mental and physical functioning (10). The SF-12^{TM} was designed so that a physical or mental component score of 50 represents the functional status of an average individual in the general U.S. population (10). The ALS/SIP-19 is an ALS-specific complement to the SF-12^{TM}, consisting of 19 questions from the Sickness Impact Profile (SIP^{TM}), which is a general functional status instrument comprising 136 items. Experts in ALS selected 19 items from the SIP that represent issues of particular importance to patients with ALS. The ALS/SIP-19 was recently validated in ALS and was strongly correlated with changes in both quantitative muscle strength and pulmonary function (11). The ALSA-Q5 is an ALS-specific complement to the SF-12^{TM}, consisting of five questions from the ALSA-Q40, which are incorporated in five scales (physical mobility, activities of daily living/independence, eating and drinking, communication, and emotional functioning). Each question is followed by five responses, $0 =$ Never to $4 =$ Always or cannot do at all. The ALSAQ-5 summary scores are reported in a range from $0 =$ best and $100 =$ worst.

Patient Caregiver Form

The primary caregiver is asked to complete a two-page form, which takes approximately five minutes. The general health of the caregiver is surveyed along with the financial and psychological impact of caring for a patient with ALS. The Caregiver Form incorporates the Caregiver Burden Scale, comprising 17 questions that have been validated in a number of chronic conditions (12).

Completion Form

This single-page form is completed by the neurologist or designee and includes documentation of either the date that ALS was excluded or the circumstances surrounding the patient's death.

All forms except the Completion Form are completed at the time of patient enrollment. Follow-up data are collected at intervals of between three and six months. The Study Coordinating Center sends a monthly reminder to participating neurologists that lists patients who are due for an interval follow-up.

All forms were revised to more completely track adherence to the ALS practice parameter in 2001.

Study Coordinating Center

Data management and support of publications is based at the Center for Outcomes Research at the University of Massachusetts Medical School, located in Worcester, Massachusetts. The Study Coordinating Center manages the data, performs analyses, and protects the confidentiality of participants, including patients, neurologists, and clinical sites. Systems to maintain confidentiality are strictly enforced. The Study

Coordinating Center assigns enrolling neurologists an identification (ID) number that is used to encode their data. Physician names are kept in a locked file, and quarterly reports are created by the Study Coordinating Center and mailed to participating neurologists in sealed envelopes that are marked *confidential*. Patient names are not used in the database; the individual clinic or neurologist assigns a patient ID number to each patient. Initials identify patient caregivers. The provisions for protecting the rights of physicians and patients participating in this project have been reviewed and approved by the Institutional Review Board (IRB) of the University of Massachusetts Medical School. Quarterly reports sent to neurologists include aggregate North American data as well as physician-specific data on over 100 variables relating to physician practices, caregiver burden, patient-reported QOL, and issues arising in the terminal phase of the disease.

Positive Feedback for Clinicians

By participating in the ALS CARE Database, clinicians, patients, and caregivers can all make a contribution to improving our understanding of ALS and to increasing available data regarding the management of this disease. Collecting data on their patients and submitting to the database, a clinician can receive feedback about the nature of the decision-making process and about the outcomes of their patients. Participating clinicians receive reports about their own patients and compare them with the aggregate data of all patients in the North American database. This feedback permits the clinician to make detailed comparisons of their practice patterns and outcomes, and how they differ from those of colleagues throughout North America. These results are completely confidential but they do provide clinicians with feedback that may guide improvement in practice to optimize their standard of care. The data for each patient is confidential and anonymous but each clinician may receive feedback about the level of satisfaction of their patients with their overall neurological care for ALS and compare this with the North American aggregate. They get feedback about the degree of education and information that their patients are receiving, the cost of their illness, and therapies as compared to the national norm. Moreover, important data about the socio-economic and psychosocial impact of the disease on both patients and caregivers is provided.

RESULTS

Overview

Enrollment

Since inception in September 1996, there have been more than 5603 patients diagnosed with ALS who have enrolled in the database across North America. About 387 neurologists representing 107 clinical sites have enrolled patients. Approximately 2/3 of enrolled sites are affiliated with academic medical centers, however over 90% of patients have been enrolled in academic centers. Thus, the majority of patients in this database represent care provided in large tertiary ALS clinics. A major challenge for the database has been obtaining continuing follow-up data at 6, 12, 18, and 24 months. The number of patients fitting into these follow-up categories are 1838, 1334, 736, and 682, respectively (Health Professional Forms).

Table 2 Diagnostic Studies Performed at the Time of Enrollment

Study	Patients % ($n = 3,333$)
EMG/nerve conduction studies	87.4
MRI (spine)	56.8
Thyroid function	50.8
SIEP/SPEP	47.2
MRI (brain)	50.4
GM$_1$ antibody	38.1
Heavy metal screen	31.2
Lumbar puncture	19.7

Abbreviations: EMG, electromyography; MRI, magnetic resonance imaging; GM$_1$, ganglioside antibody; SIEP, serum immunoelectropheresis; SPEP, serum electropheresis.

Demographic Features

Ninety-three percent of patients in the database were Caucasian and 61% were male with a mean age of 58 ± 13.2 years (range 20–100 years). Ninety-four percent of patients had sporadic ALS and only 6% had familial ALS. At the time of enrollment, 77% of patients were employed full-time. Enrollment of veterans in the database has been substantial. The annual percentage of patients enrolled in the database who were veterans has varied between 21% and 35%.

Diagnostic Testing

A variety of diagnostic tests were utilized to establish a diagnosis of ALS (Table 2). Electrodiagnostic studies (electromyography and nerve conduction studies) were the most frequent, performed in 87% of patients. Neuroimaging studies were widely used (57%) substantially more than lumbar puncture (20%) and muscle biopsy (10%).

Atypical features, considered insufficient to rule out ALS, included distal sensory loss (5.1%), cognitive changes (3.4%), ataxia (1.5%), sphincter impairment (1.8%), and extrapyramidal features (1.4%). A second opinion was obtained in 86% of cases. Based on El Escorial diagnostic criteria, 47% of patients were diagnosed as having definite ALS, 33% had probable ALS, 12% possible ALS, and 5% suspected ALS.

Disease Severity: At the time of enrollment, symptoms of weakness attributable to ALS had been present for a mean of 2.4 ± 2.7 years (range: 0 to 44 years). Mean delay between the first symptom of ALS and diagnosis of ALS was 9.2 months in 1997 with a slow increase to a mean of 11 months in 2003. Approximately 50% of patients enrolled in the database were diagnosed with ALS within six months of symptom onset. Mean forced vital capacity was 75% of predicted (SD $\pm 26\%$, range 0% to 200%). The mean score on the ALSFRS was 28 (SD 7.9%, range 0 [worst] to 40 [best]). These data indicate that the average patients was somewhere in the middle of their disease course.

Self-reports indicated that 16% of patients could perform less than 10% of activities of daily living (ADL), while 40% could independently perform more than 90% of ADL. Common ALS-related condition reported by patients: included falls, depression, choking, and disturbed sleep were reported frequently.

Health-related quality-of-life: Patients ratings of disease severity indicated a broad range of illness. There was a weak positive correlation between physician-recorded ALSFRS scores and patient-recorded SF-12^{TM} physical component summary scores ($r^2 = 0.43$). The mean SF-12^{TM} Physical and Mental Component Scores at enrollment were 38 and 49 respectively (0 = worst, 100 = best). The ALSA-Q5 documented at enrollment is: physical mobility 43.4., independence 50.9, eating and drinking 25.7, communication 39.8 and emotional functional 37.1.independence 50.9, eating and drinking 25.7, communication 39.8, and emotional functional 37.1

Patient Satisfaction

Patient's level of satisfaction with their general level of ALS care was generally high with 89% of patients being either satisfied or extremely satisfied, 8% were slightly satisfied, and 3% were dissatisfied with the medical care they received for ALS. Over the past six years the proportion of patients dissatisfied with their care ranged between 0.6% and 3%. Patients have obtained information from a variety of sources. Forty-six percent found the ALS Clinic to be their most valuable source of information, 39% the ALS Association, and 15% the Muscular Dystrophy Association (MDA). In the last four years, the ALS Clinic has become the most valuable source of information for an increasing percentage of patients; most recently up to 70% compared with 23% for the ALS Association and 8% for MDA.

Therapy

ALS-specific treatments included riluzole (52%), gabapentin (14%), creatine 39%, high-dose vitamins or antioxidants (48%), non-traditional medications (15%), or other unspecified medication (42%). Over the past seven years, utilization of riluzole has increased from a low of 45% in 1998 to a high of 61% in 2002 ($p < 0.001$). At the time of enrollment, 26% of patients were enrolled in a formal ALS clinical trial.

On the basis of patient self-reports, symptomatic therapies for constipation, cramps, depression, disturbed sleep, spasticity, and sialorrhea were generally effective. Since only a minority of patients was treated for ALS symptoms, these data suggest that additional patients might benefit from symptomatic pharmacotherapy. A broad array of non-pharmacological therapies was utilized (Table 3). At the time of enrollment approximately 80% of patients were taking two or less symptomatic medications. The level of patient satisfaction with specific non-pharmacological and pharmacological interventions was generally high; 89% of patients reported that they were satisfied with their medical care. There has been a steady increase in the

Table 3 Use of Non-pharmacological Interventions at the Time of Enrollment

Intervention	Patients (%) ($n = 5,097$)
Physical therapy	47.0
Occupational therapy	39.0
Speech therapy	35.0
Home nurse	30.6
Dietary(nutrition)	30.0
Socialwork	30.6
Psychology/psychiatry	29.0

number of patients taking medication for sialorrhea from a low of 12% in 1999 to a high of 25% in 2002 ($p < 0.0001$).

Adherence to ALS Practice Parameters

Evidence-based practice parameters for the management of ALS, sponsored by the American Academy of Neurology and developed by an appointed task force, were published in 1999 (13). On the basis of data obtained from the ALS CARE Program, we published an analysis of the management of patients with ALS in the three years prior to the publication of the practice parameter (1). The results indicated that a number of areas of the management of patients with ALS fell below the evidence-based standards. This was particularly evident in the under-utilization of percutaneous endoscopic gastrostomy, non-invasive positive pressure ventilation, and symptomatic therapies. Shortly, thereafter, the data collection forms were redesigned to obtain more in depth information about the adherence to the evidence-based practice parameter and to develop preliminary insights into reasons for gaps in adherence. The goal of the most recent study was to examine the impact of the publication of the practice parameter upon practice patterns across North America as recorded in the ALS CARE database. A secondary goal was to try to understand what progress has been made and the reasons for persistent problem areas.

The data for this comparative study were extracted from the forms of 646 patients with ALS collected from May 2001 to November 2002 and from 465 forms completed by caregivers for patients who died during that period. These data were compared with previous forms obtained from the database between 1996 and May 1999.

One of the five major areas addressed in the practice parameters was the delivering of the news about the diagnosis and prognosis of ALS. The diagnosis was shared with 46% of patients by a neurologist at a specialized ALS center and by 41% of patients with a community neurologist. In 96% of cases the diagnosis was given in person but in 3% it was given over the telephone. In 78% of interviews, the people who were considered most important to the patient were present when the diagnosis was given. Although 65% of patients reported satisfaction with the presentation of the diagnosis, 11% described the presentation as insensitive and 17% felt that too little information was provided. No sense of hope was provided to 16% of patients and 4% reported insufficient understanding of what was being said. Seventy percent of patients received information about ALS advocacy organizations that provide resources for patients. The fraction of patients who reported receiving enough information about the disease increased from 78% to 87% within the first six months after diagnosis, a figure, which has improved since the publication of the practice parameter.

Symptomatic Treatment

One of the major disturbing symptom for patients is excessive saliva (sialorrhea) with drooling. Treatment of this symptom was addressed in the evidence-based practice parameter and recommendations were made for management. Seventy-five percent of patients with moderate-to-marked sialorrhea were offered medications in the period after publication of the practice parameter compared to 54% prior to publication ($p = 0.0085$).

Another very disturbing symptom is pseudobulbar affect, or excessive emotionality, a common symptom in patients with bulbar involvement with ALS. Most patients with this excessive emotionality respond to antidepressant medication, which is recommended by the practice parameter. The proportion of patients treated for pseudobulbar affect rose from 29% prior to the practice parameter to 44% in the period after publication ($p < 0.0001$). Thus, the symptomatic treatment for both sialorrhea and pseudobulbar affect increased substantially in the period following publication of the practice parameter according to data from the ALS CARE database.

Percutaneous Endoscopic Gastrostomy

The practice parameter recommendation is that patients who develop symptomatic dysphagia should receive percutaneous endoscopic gastrostomy (PEG) soon after symptom onset and before the vital capacity falls below 50% of predicted in order to reduce the risk of PEG placement. The proportion of patients receiving PEG when the vital capacity was less than 50% of predicted rose from 12% to 22% following the practice parameter ($p < 0.0001$). Approximately 43% of patients for whom a gastrostomy was recommended went ahead and had it inserted. Thus, a substantial number of patients did not accept the recommendations of the practice parameter. The reasons included: 31% of patients thought their swallowing was still adequate, 16% reported of not liking the concept of PEG, 4% received insufficient information to make a decision, and 20% recorded a series of other reasons. There was no correlation between household income and type of health insurance with the decision to have PEG.

To try and better understand the under-utilization of PEG, another study examined the characteristics of patients in the ALS CARE database, with and without PEG, in terms of their ALS functional rating scale bulbar sub scores and also their health outcomes (14).

There was a strong correlation between PEG use and declining ALSFRS bulbar scores. Demographic characteristics of the two groups were not significantly different but ALSFRS composite scores as well as the bulbar and arm subscale scores were all lower in patients with PEG compared to those without ($p < 0.0001$). Patients with PEG used significantly more assistive devices, multidisciplinary care, home care nurses and aids, and had more frequent physician and emergency department visits as well as hospital admissions ($p < 0.0001$). Patients with PEG also had lower overall health status based on the mini-SIP survey ($p = 0.0047$). There was a marked variation in PEG utilization between ALS clinics. The range of PEG utilization was 0% to 52% in nine different centers. PEG use was only 20% among patients with mild bulbar score abnormalities and the percentage increased to a peak of 88% in those with the most severe impairment of bulbar function (14).

With follow-up study, in patients who had or did not have PEG, a positive impact of PEG was documented in 79% of patients with PEG. However, in only 37% of patients who received PEG later in their disease course, was there a similar beneficial impact. Overall, there was no demonstrable survival advantage associated with PEG in the database. These data suggest that PEG may have been performed too late to impact survival in this database. More studies are needed to determine the beneficial impact of earlier intervention with PEG.

Non-Invasive Positive Pressure Ventilation

The practice parameter recommended non-invasive positive pressure ventilation (NIPPV) for patients who are symptomatic with respiratory insufficiency and whose forced vital capacity is less than 50% of predicted (15,16). The proportion of patients with FVC less than 40% of predicted, who received NIPPV, rose from 9% in the pre-publication era to 21% following practice parameter publication ($p < 0.0001$) (1). For those with FVC above 40% of predicted, there was an increase from 4% to11% ($p < 0.0001$). The reasons for the under-utilization of NIPPV is not clear but nearly 50% of patients not using NIPPV tried it and could not successfully adapt to its use. A very small fraction of patients opted for tracheostomy and permanent artificial ventilation with the number stable at 3% of patients both before and after publication of the practice parameter. This option was only offered to a further 3% of patients who declined, presumably on the basis of care and financial burdens involved in tracheostomy and permanent artificial ventilation.

To better understand the impact of NIPPV, on outcomes for patients with ALS, a further study was conducted. About 1458 patients provided sufficient data for an analysis of the use of NIPPV in the ALS CARE database (17). Of these patients 16% used NIPPV and 2% used tracheostomy/invasive mechanical ventilation. Patient characteristics of those who used NIPPV indicated a significantly elevated incidence of male patients and also a higher income for those who used NIPPV compared to those who did not. Patients using NIPPV were more likely to have a PEG tube, lower vital capacity, more severe disease, bulbar involvement, and poor general health status as measured by the Sickness Impact Profile (SIP-19) and the SF-12. A multivariant analysis revealed that lower FVC use of a PEG tube and higher income were each independently associated with NIPPV use. The association with higher income raises the concern that some under-utilization of NIPPV may relate to fiscal concerns (17).

Patients with a vital capacity less than 50% of predicted at enrollment who never used NIPPV were compared with those who used NIPPV. Patients were followed until their last entry in the database or until death. About 490 patients were eligible for the analysis out of a total of 4725 patients. About 159 of these patients (32%) were NIPPV users while 331 (68%) never used NIPPV. Demographic descriptors were similar between the two groups, except that NIPPV users were more often male (68%) compared with non-users (52%) ($p < 0.002$). Users had a higher income than non-users ($p < 0.003$). More NIPPV users had PEG tubes compared with non-users and more users took riluzole ($p < 0.02$ for both comparisons). NIPPV users were less likely to report very good or excellent health (13.8% vs. 25.7%, $p < 0.02$). Five years survival was 53% in NIPPV users and 38% in non-users ($p < 0.03$ by log rank). When these data were adjusted for potential confounding variables, such as gender, riluzole use, and PEG tube use, the survival advantage was still significant (hazard ratio $= 0.66$, $p < 0.04$).

These data, which represent the first large study of NIPPV use in many sites across North America, albeit retrospective, demonstrate a positive impact of NIPPV on survival in patients with ALS. Important prognostic variables were similar between the users and non-users and five years survival was significantly longer in patients who used NIPPV. The study adds to already existing evidence, which suggests that NIPPV improves survival for patients with vital capacity below 50% of predicted.

Palliative Care

Sixty-four percent of patients died at home compared with 61% prior to the publication of the practice parameter. Sixty-three percent of these patients had used home hospice services, a moderate increase compared to the 58% who used it prior to the publication ($p = 0.02$). Data were collected from the caregiver about the quality of life in the final phase of ALS. Caregivers were asked whether the patient died peacefully and what symptoms were experienced at the end of life. Eighty-nine percent of patients were recorded as having died peacefully, although 38% were said to have had some breathing difficulties at the end of life. Pain medications were administered in 80% of patients and oxygen was given to 25% of patients in the terminal phase, values that were not significantly changed from the period prior to the practice parameter publication.

A very high proportion of patients (94%) had advance directives in place and 96% of these patients' advance directives were followed. These data reflect an extraordinarily high utilization of advanced directives compared with cancer, AIDS, and the general population.

Overall, these data provide some basis for optimism that the diagnosis of ALS was for the most part delivered in accord with the evidence-based recommendations and treatment of important symptoms such as sialorrhea and pseudobulbar affect was generally widely used. These data do however illustrate the need for increased utilization of effective therapies such as: percutaneous endoscopic gastrostomy, non-invasive mechanical ventilation, opioids, and oxygen in the final phases of the disease.

Depression

Depression was a common symptom in the ALS CARE database with 41% of patients reporting symptomatic depression. When the symptom was looked at longitudinally, patients who had symptoms for more than a year and follow-up over 18 months, the percentage of patients who were depressed was still 33%, only slightly less than the figure at enrollment. There has been very little change over the seven years since we began to gather this data with the percentage of patients who are depressed varying between 39% and 45%, with no significant increasing or decreasing trends. Patients who were depressed generally had lower scores on the SF-12 mental component portion of the quality of life scale compared to those who were not depressed ($p < 0.0001$). When patients were followed over 18 months there was very little change in the SF-12 mental component score over time. This tendency toward a relatively stable quality of life measure has been described by others (18) in spite of the declining physical score associated with the functional worsening secondary to progressive ALS. The rate of decline in the physical component score was virtually identical between patients who were depressed and those who were not, over an 18 months period. With respect to the ALS functional rating scale, there was a slightly increased rate of decline in patients who were depressed compared to those who were not during an 18 months interval ($p = 0.05$).

There has been a steady increase in the percentage of patients in the database who have received treatment for depression, with a low of 27% in 1997 to a high of 41% in 2003. When patients with only depression are considered, the percentage of patients treated with antidepressants increased from 63% to 84% over the past six years.

Caregivers

Relatively little attention has been paid to examining the stress of care giving for patients with ALS. The ALS CARE database contains a validated self-assessment questionnaire for caregivers, known as the Caregiver Burden Scale. This questionnaire includes 17 questions related to the experiences caring for an ALS patient. Recently, the data on spousal caregivers was examined with respect to living arrangements, employment status, health status, interference with social activities, assistance with care giving, perceived importance of care giving, perceived rewards of care giving (19), and also gender issues in care giving (20).

Most caregivers rated their own health as being good or very good. Only 11% of patient caregivers rated their overall health as fair or poor. The data provided by caregivers documented the stress and emotional burden of the disease upon the caregiver. This important member of the health care team appears to experience increasing distress as the disease progresses. Nevertheless, at enrollment, 93% of caregivers reported that the opportunity to participate in the care of a loved one provided a measure of satisfaction; and 92% of caregivers felt they were doing something important by caring for the patient.

The spouse was the main caregiver for 74% of patients and 65% of care giving spouses were wives. Few caregivers were paid for their services (3%). Self-reported health status was similar between care giving husbands and wives, but wives reported that their personal health problems interfered with social activities more often than husbands (63% vs. 53%, $p < 0.0001$). Wives acting as care givers were more likely to live with the patient ($p = 0.04$) and to shoulder more of the care responsibilities compared with husbands ($p < 0.0018$). Husbands were more likely to be employed ($p < 0.0001$), to receive assistance with care giving from both friends and family (52% vs. 40%, $p < 0.0001$), and to provide care to sicker patients than did wives ($p < 0.0001$). In general, caregivers who were rewarded for care giving experienced fewer burdens than caregivers who did not ($p < 0.0001$). Increasing caregiver burden was associated with female gender, increasing patient disability, assistance from family or friends, and interference with social activities.

The percentage of caregivers who provided unassisted care, declined as the illness progressed (duration less than one year —54%, duration more than four years—45%, $p < 0.034$). The majority of caregivers (80%) described their own health as good-to-excellent through the course of ALS, and most caregivers (83%) found the experience of care giving to be rewarding. The caregiver burden worsened with disease duration and also with declining caregiver self-rated health: there was a correlation between the ALS functional rating score and the caregiver burden ($r = 0.42$), and correlations were found between the time ($r = 0.49$), anxiety ($r = 0.24$), and demand burden ($r = 0.31$) subscales. The time burden subscale was most strongly correlated with the ALSFRS score ($r = 0.41$, $p < 0.001$). These data suggest that as ALS advances in severity, caregivers will require additional assistance to care for the patient with ALS (19).

Since ALS is more common in males, wives are more likely to serve as caregivers. Wives found care giving to be a greater burden, suggesting that additional resources may be needed to assist these caregivers. Further study is needed to examine the caregiver burden and to evaluate temporal trends during disease progression related to specific disease milestones (20).

Epidemiologic Studies

Veterans Vs. Non-Veterans with ALS

An increased incidence and prevalence of ALS was reported in young members of the U.S. military who were deployed in the Persian Gulf (21,22). The ALS CARE database provides an opportunity to examine outcomes for patients who are veterans developing ALS. Male veterans were significantly more prevalent than female veterans in the ALS CARE database ($p < 0.0001$). Male veterans with ALS were significantly different in age distribution from male non-veterans ($p < 0.0001$). Male veterans over the age of 60 were significantly more numerous in the database (66%) compared with male non-veterans (34%). There were no significant differences between veterans and non-veterans in the distribution of anatomic regions involved with the disease (23). There was decreased survival in veterans compared with non-veterans, but this was largely explained by the increased age differences between the two groups. Male veterans with ALS were more likely to have deafness ($p < 0.0001$), and diseases affecting the bones and joints ($p = 0.002$) when compared with male non-veterans. In contrast, lung disease, diabetes mellitus, and depression were equally represented in the two groups. Thus, the ALS CARE database offers a direct comparison of large cohorts of veterans and non-veterans with ALS. The increased prevalence of deafness and bone and joint diseases deserves further evaluation.

Pre-Existing Bone and Joint Disease

Physical trauma and large bone fractures have both been cited as potential risk factors for the development of ALS. The ALS CARE database provided an opportunity to compare patients with documented and treated bone and joint disease along with their ALS compared to patients with no joint disease. Bone and joint disease was reported by 21% of the patients in the database (24). The mean age of onset of ALS in the bone and joint disease group was 59.9 years, significantly older than the age of patients without bone and joint disease ($p < 0.001$). There were more females (57%) in the bone and joint disease group (36%, $p < 0.001$). Demographic characteristics were similar between those with and without pre-existing bone and joint disease. Surprisingly, the probability of survival for longer than four years from symptom onset was greater in patients with bone and joint disease compared with those who had no bone and joint disease and ALS. However, the Cox proportional hazards model indicated that much of the survival advantage was due to the increased age of patients with ALS who have bone and joint disease and a later age of disease onset. In fact, the age of onset of ALS symptoms was significantly later in both male and female patients with pre-existing bone and joint disease. In view of recent evidence suggesting inflammation of the nervous system in patients with ALS, increased expression of cyclo-oxygenase-2 in spinal cord of patients with ALS and preclinical data suggesting that inhibitors of cyclo-oxygenase-2 confer a survival advantage, further studies of patients with bone and joint disease appear warranted (23,24).

Limitations of the Database

There are a number of important limitations to the interpretation of large observational registries. Some of these limitations are inherent in uncontrolled trials. Others can be minimized or avoided by careful data collection and analysis. (i) Controlled, randomized clinical trials are required to demonstrate the efficacy of therapeutic interventions. The ALS Patient Care Database is not a controlled trial. It is a large observational study, designed to document practices in the management of ALS in routine clinical settings. Since patients enrolled in this database are not randomly assigned to a particular treatment, they are likely to be dissimilar across treatment groups with regard to important characteristics including age, sex, and co morbid conditions. Therefore, comparison of outcomes across treatment groups is likely to lead to inappropriate conclusions. (ii) It is also important to note that there is no independent monitoring to ensure that each data collection form accurately reflects the information in the patient's medical record or that prescribed data collection methods were followed. In addition, some clinics may not enroll all of their patients with ALS into the database. This may lead to intentional or unintentional bias. Registry data may not reflect the clinic's overall ALS patient population. (iii) There is uncertainty as to whether these patients are representative of the ALS patient population at large, and whether the conclusions are generalizable. The demographic data in this database appear to be similar to other large natural history studies (25–28), and to the populations in large clinical trials (29) with respect to gender, age, duration of symptoms, and incidence of familial disease. However, these data represent the experience of self-selected participating clinics, whose patients may not be representative of North American patients with ALS. (iv) There is no pathologic confirmation of diagnoses except in a small percentage of cases. This issue deserves further attention. (v) A majority of data is cross-sectional; major initiatives to obtain more longitudinal data are underway and will be critical to our plan to use the database to monitor practice patterns and outcomes. (vi) Observations on management practices for dysphagia, percutaneous endoscopic gastrostomies, dyspnea, mechanical ventilation, and palliative care must await additional data to provide an adequate sample size for a meaningful analysis.

Future Directions

The increased emphasis on obtaining more complete follow-up data rather than enrolling more patients should improve our ability to analyze outcomes. In particular, more complete survival information will allow for more comprehensive studies of risk factors and the effectiveness of various therapeutic interventions. As more therapies become available for ALS, the ALS CARE database is ideally positioned to track the outcomes and impact of these therapies in the real world.

A web-based version of ALS CARE is also planned which will be for the most part patient-driven as opposed to the current arrangement that depends more on neurologists in large specialized clinics to provide the impetus for enrollment and data collection. The web-based database should provide more information about the standard of care in the community than is the case currently.

REFERENCES

1. Bradley WG, Anderson F, Bromberg M, Gutmann L, Harati Y, Ross M, Miller RG. ALS CARE Study Group. Current management of ALS: comparison of the ALS CARE database and the AAN practice parameter. The American Academy of Neurology. Neurology 2001; 57:500–504.
2. Bradley WG, Anderson F, Gowda N, Miller RG, ALS CARE Study Group. Improvement in the management of ALS since 1999 publication of the practice parameter: Evidence from the ALS patient CARE database [abstr]. ALS & Other Motor Neuron Disorders 2003; 4(suppl 1):20–21.
3. Miller RG, Mitchell JD, Lyon M, Moore DH. Riluzole for amyotrophic lateral sclerosis (ALS)/motor neuron disease (MND). Cochrane Neuromuscular Disease Group Cochrane Database of Systematic Reviews 2004:2.

4. Jewitt K, Hughes RAC. Systematic reviews to help guide clinical practice in neuromuscular disease. J Neurol Neurosurg Psychiatry 2003; 74(suppl 2):43–44.
5. Cedarbaum JM, Stambler N. Disease status and use of ventilatory support by ALS patients. BDNF Study Group. ALS & Other Motor Neuron Disorders 2001; 2:19–22.
6. Miller RG, Anderson FA, Bradley WG, Brooks BR, Mitsumoto H, Munsat TL, Ringel SP, ALS CARE Study Group. The ALS patient CARE database: Goals, design, and early results. Neurology 2001; 54:53–57.
7. Miller RG, Anderson FA, ALS CARE study group. The ALS patient CARE database. In: Mitsumoto H, Munsat T, eds. Amyotrophic Lateral Sclerosis: A Guide for Patients & Families. 2d ed. New York: Demos Medical Publishing, 2001.
8. Brooks BR, Miller RG, Swash M, Munsat TL. El Escorial revisited: Revised criteria for the diagnosis of amyotrophic lateral sclerosis. ALS & Other Motor Neuron Disorders 2000; 1:293–299.
9. The ALS CNTF Treatment Study (ACTS) Phase I-II Study Group. The Amyotrophic Lateral Sclerosis Functional Rating Scale. Assessment of activities of daily living in patients with amyotrophic lateral sclerosis. Arch Neurol 1996; 53:141–147.
10. Ware JE, Kosinski M, Keller SD. SF-12: How to Score the SF-12 Physical and Mental Status Health Summary scales. 2d. Boston: The Health Institute: New England Medical Center, 1995.
11. McGuire D, Garrison L, Armon C, Barohn R, Bryan W, Miller R, Parry G, Petajan J, Ross M. Relationship of the Tufts Quantitative Neuromuscular Exam (TQNE) and the Sickness Impact Profile (SIP) in measuring progression of ALS. SSNJV/CNTF ALS Study Group. Neurology 1996; 46:1442–1444.
12. Montgomery RJV, Gonyea JG, Hooyman NR. Caregiving and the experience of subjective and objective burden. Family Relations 1985; 34:19–26.
13. Miller RG, Rosenberg JA, Gelinas DF, Mitsumoto H, Newman D, Sufit R, Borasio GD, Bradley WG, Bromberg MB, Brooks BR, et al. Practice parameter: the care of the patient with amyotrophic lateral sclerosis (an evidence-based review): report of the Quality Standards Subcommittee of the American Academy of Neurology: ALS Practice Parameters Task Force. Neurology 1999; 52:1311–1323.
14. Mitsumoto H, Davidson M, Moore D, Gad N, Brandis M, Ringel S, Rosenfeld J, Shefner JM, Strong MJ, Sufit R, et al., ALS CARE Study Group. Percutaneous Endoscopic Gastrostomy (PEG) in patients with ALS and bulbar dysfunction. ALS & Other Motor Neuron Disorders 2003; 4:177–185.
15. Aboussouan LS, Khan SU, Meeker DP, Stelmach K, Mitsumoto H. Effect of noninvasive positive-pressure ventilation on survival in amyotrophic lateral sclerosis. Ann Int Med 1997; 127:450–453.
16. Kleopa KA, Sherman M, Neal B, Romano GJ, Heiman-Patterson T. Bipap improves survival and rate of pulmonary function decline in patients with AL. J Neurol Sci 1999; 164:82–8.
17. Lechtzin N, Wiener CM, Clawson L, Davidson MC, Anderson F, Gowda N, Diette GB. Use of noninvasive ventilation in patients with amyotrophic lateral sclerosis. ALS & Other Motor Neuron Disorders 2004; 5:9–15.
18. Robbins RA, Simmons Z, Bremer BA, Walsh SM, Fischer S. Quality of life in ALS is maintained as physical function declines. Neurology 2001; 56:442–444.
19. Ross MA, Bradley WG, Heiman-Patterson T, Lyon M, Gowda N, Anderson FA, Dabbous OH, Moore DH, ALS CARE Study Group. The ALS Caregiver – new insights from the ALS patient CARE database [abstr]. ALS & Other Motor Neuron Disord 2003; 4(suppl 1):21–22.
20. Coker L, Donofrio P, Ross M, Caress J, Hege A, Ashburn C, Walker T, Gowda N. ALS CARE Study Group: Gender-related differences in spousal caregiving for patients with ALS. ALS Motor Neuron Disord 2002; 3(suppl 2):6–7.
21. Haley RW. Excess incidence of ALS in young Gulf war veterans. Neurology 2003; 61:750–756.

22. Horner RD, Kamins KG, Feussner JR, Grambow SC, Hoff-Lindquist J, Harati Y, Mitsumoto H, Pascuzzi R, Spencer PS, Tim R, et al. Occurrence of amyotrophic lateral sclerosis among Gulf war veterans. Neurology 2003; 61:742–749.

23. Brooks BR, Madison WI, Anderson FA, Gowda N, ALS CARE Study Group. Amyo-trophic Lateral Sclerosis (ALS) outcomes in US military veterans compared with non-veterans: Neuroepidemiological insights from the ALS CARE database. ALS & Other Motor Neuron Disord 2003; 4(suppl 1):114.

24. Waclawik AJ, Brooks BR, Madison WI, Anderson FA, Gowda N, ALS CARE Study Group. Onset of Amyotrophic Lateral Sclerosis (ALS) is delayed, but course is not altered in ALS patients with pre-existing bone and joint disease: Neuroepiodemiological insights from the ALS CARE database. ALS & Other Motor Neuron Disord 2003; 4(suppl 1):115–116.

25. Ringel SP, Murphy JR, Alderson MK, Bryan W, England JD, Miller RG, Petajan JH, Smith SA, Roelofs RI, Ziter F. The natural history of amyotrophic lateral sclerosis. Neurology 1993; 43:1316–1322.

26. Mitsumoto H, Chad DA, Pioro EP. Amyotrophic lateral sclerosis. Philadelphia, PA: FA Davis Company Publishers, 1998.

27. Haverkamp LJ, Appel V, Appel SH. Natural history of amyotrophic lateral sclerosis in a database population. Validation of a scoring system and model for survival prediction. Brain 1995; 118(pt 3):707–719.

28. Rosen AD. Amyotrophic lateral sclerosis. Clinical features and prognosis. Arch Neurol 1978; 35:638–642.

29. Lacomblez L, Bensimon G, Leigh PN, Guillet P, Meininger V. Dose-ranging study of riluzole in amyotrophic lateral sclerosis. Amyotrophic Lateral Sclerosis/Riluzole Study Group II. Lancet 1996; 347:1425–1431.

29

Symptomatic Pharmacotherapy: Bulbar and Constitutional Symptoms

Carlayne E. Jackson
Department of Medicine/Neurology, University of Texas Health Science Center, San Antonio, Texas, U.S.A.

Jeffrey Rosenfeld
Division of Neurology, Carolinas Neuromuscular/ALS-MDA Center, Carolinas Medical Center, Charlotte, North Carolina, U.S.A.

INTRODUCTION

ALS, once thought to be an untreatable disease, has emerged as a model highlighting the significant impact that supportive and adjunctive therapies have on the disease course. ALS results in a large constellation of disabling bulbar and constitutional symptoms for which there is effective therapy. Unfortunately, there are few randomized, controlled trials of medications or interventions addressing symptom management. As a result, physicians caring for ALS patients base their selection of specific therapies upon personal experience and anecdotal reports from colleagues and patients. While this "on the job" training is helpful, the lack of scientific data to guide therapy has led to a wide variety of management practices (1).

SYMPTOMS RELATED TO BULBAR WEAKNESS

Sialorrhea

A distressing symptom related to loss of ability to swallow is sialorrhea. In ALS, sialorrhea is caused by swallowing dysfunction resulting from pharyngeal muscle weakness rather than by increased salivary gland production. Patients frequently have to repeatedly wipe their mouth with a tissue or, in extreme cases, may need to insert a washcloth into their mouths to absorb the saliva. In addition to being socially embarrassing, sialorrhea can lead to aspiration pneumonia, the most common cause of death in ALS other than respiratory failure.

The prevalence of sialorrhea among ALS patients is estimated at 50% (2). The American Academy of Neurology practice parameter for the care of ALS patients recommends both pharmacologic interventions and non-pharmacologic approaches

Table 1 Commonly Used Medications for Sialorrhea

Medication	Dose/schedule
Amitriptyline	25–50 mg qhs
Imipramine	25–100 mg qhs
Nortriptyline	20–100 mg qhs
Atropine	0.40 mg q 4–6 hrs
	1–2 ophthalmic drops SL q 4–6 hrs
Glycopyrrolate	1–2 mg tid
Hyoscyamine sulfate	0.125–0.250 mg q 4–6 h (available as oral tabs, elixir or sublingual tabs)
Diphenydramine	25–50 mg tid
Scopolamine transdermal patch	0.5 mg applied behind ear q 3 days

Abbreviation: SL, sublingually.

such as suctioning (3). Treatment with anticholinergic medication (Table 1) is considered "first line" pharmacologic therapy; however, the benefits of this class of medication can be self-limited, requiring additional medications after an initial improvement. In addition, common side effects associated with anticholinergic therapy include: constipation, fatigue, and impotence most commonly, with urinary retention, blurred vision, tachycardia, orthostatic hypotension, confusion, and dizziness occurring in especially sensitive patients. In addition, they are relatively contraindicated in patients with a history of glaucoma, benign prostatic hypertrophy, and cardiac conduction disorders (especially bifascicular block, left bundle-branch block, and a prolonged QT interval). The frequency of anticholinergic side effects is less common with sublingual hyoscyamine sulfate and greater with the oral anticholinergic medications.

Selection of a particular medication often depends upon the severity and frequency of the drooling. Sialorrhea associated with mealtimes or a particular time of day may be treated with PRN administration of hyoscyamine with its transient benefit. Transdermal scopolamine, oral glycopyrollate, or the antidepressant medications provide a more continuous effect.

Data from the national ALS Patient CARE Database indicate that over 70% of ALS patients treated with atropine, glycopyrrolate, or amitriptyline reported that these modalities were helpful (2,4). By inference, approximately 30% of patients were not helped by these therapies (See Case Report No. 1; below). It is reasonable to try up to three different agents or several different combinations however, if the patient continues to remain symptomatic, newer, more aggressive approaches, as discussed below, should be considered. There remains, to date, no randomized trial comparing the efficacy of these different agents in the ALS population. Patients who have difficulty in swallowing medications may prefer an agent that can be given sublingually, transdermally, or is available in a liquid form that can be administered directly through a percutaneous endoscopic gastrostomy (PEG) tube. In general, all of these medications may cause or aggravate existing problems with constipation, and therefore it is recommended that a stool softener be initiated at the same time the anticholinergic agent is prescribed.

Case Report No. 1

A 70-year-old woman with a three-year history of bulbar-onset ALS presents with complaints of severe drooling that she finds so embarrassing that she has been essentially home bound for the past three months. The patient has received trials of amitriptyline, glycopyrrolate, and scopolamine patches but has been unable to tolerate these agents due to complaints of sedation, constipation, and urinary retention. The patient chokes constantly on her saliva and has to wear a bib to keep her shirt dry. Her caregiver has to use a suction machine at least once an hour throughout the night and is exhausted. What can you recommend?

Botulinum Toxin. Botulinum toxin is the newest mode of sialorrhea therapy and has, thus far, shown to have great promise in patients resistant to conventional medical therapy (5). Giess et al. (6) reported the results of injections of botulinum toxin A (Botox^{TM}) into the salivary glands of five ALS patients with disabling sialorrhea. Botox induces blockade of acetylcholine release at the cholinergic neurosecretory junction of the salivary glands. Six to twenty mouse units (MU) were injected into each parotid gland. If the clinical response was insufficient, as judged by the patient, the same dose was reinjected into each parotid gland two weeks later. The submandibular glands were only injected (5 MU each) if parotid gland injections alone were not effective. The mean total dosage injected into the parotid glands was 46 MU (range 30–72). A reduction of sialorrhea was first noticed three to five days after injection. A pronounced reduction measured by the number of paper handkerchiefs used each day was found four weeks after the last injection [before injection 11 (range 3–20); four weeks after the last injection 2.6 (range 2–3)]. Three patients showed a marked improvement of quality of life based upon a modified Dermatology Life Quality Index, one patient showed moderate improvement, and one patient did not benefit from treatment. Scintigraphy of the parotid glands two weeks after injection showed a marked reduction of radiotracer uptake. In the follow-up interval up to three months, no worsening of sialorrhea or bulbar function was seen.

Rowe et al. (7) reported the results of an open-label pilot study of intraparotid botulinum toxin A injections for the treatment of sialorrhea in ALS patients. Five patients received an injection into two sites in each parotid gland. Ten units were injected into the portion of the parotid isolated between the ascending ramus of the mandible and the mastoid process and five units into the portion of the gland over the masseter. Four of the five patients demonstrated reduction in the mean amount of saliva production with a mean reduction of 52%. There were no adverse effects reported. The duration of benefit ranged between 56 and 72 days.

These studies suggest that botulinum toxin may be a relatively safe and effective treatment for sialorrhea in ALS patients. Previous reports of botulinum toxin treatment for drooling in ALS patients, however, have cited the following adverse events: mild worsening of dysphagia (8,9) and mild chewing difficulties (8). Recurrent temporomandibular joint dislocation occurred in one patient two months after the second bilateral parotid gland injection (10). One patient experienced severe swelling of the sublingual salivary gland and base of the tongue following administration of botulinum toxin via catheters into the ducts of sublingual and parotid glands (8).

Currently a multicenter national trial using botulinium toxin for sialorrhea is underway. Optimal dosing regimens and additional safety data should be available soon.

Radiotherapy. Stalpers and Moser (11) reported the results of radiotherapy for drooling in 19 ALS patients. The prescribed radiation dose in all patients was 12 Gy in two fractions per week. The parotids on both sides were irradiated using 250 kV photons in 14 patients, or 8 to 14 MeV electrons in five patients. Doses were specified at a 1-cm surface depth. A satisfactory response was defined as a complete or partial improvement of drooling within two to three weeks as reported by the patient. Fourteen patients (74%) had a satisfactory response after initial radiation, either complete (11 patients) or partial (three patients). Four patients had a relapse and were reirradiated 1 to 15 months after the first treatment. Six patients reported pain in the parotid area, and four had complaints of dryness of the mouth. Both pain and dryness were self-limiting within several days. Harriman et al. (12) reported their experience with nine ALS patients, who underwent radiotherapy of the submandibular, sublingual glands, and the tail of the parotid gland. The authors felt that these were the most likely glands to target since 80% of salivary flow is produced by them. Patients were divided into two groups—group 1 (five patients) underwent treatment with a single fraction of 8 Gy, and group 2 (four patients) underwent two fractions of 6.25 Gy, for a total of 12.5 Gy. They were followed over the next six months and were evaluated for effectiveness and side effects. Both groups achieved effective control of their drooling and increasing the dose did not appear to influence initial control. Long-term control could not be adequately evaluated due to the patients' short life expectancy. Side effects included erythema and burning of skin from a few hours to two weeks in four patients, sore throat for a few hours to four days in two patients, and nausea for one patient for a few days. One patient felt that the saliva had become thicker post-treatment. All patients were given a prescription for prednisone to take if there was significant swelling of the skin and throat, although none of them had to take it. The use of low-dose radiotherapy, therefore, appears to provide great benefit with minimal side effects. Further studies have been suggested to determine optimal timing of this intervention and to determine optimal dosing regimens.

Thick Phlegm

Thick mucous secretions may occur independently or may coexist along with sialorrhea. Occasionally, treatment of sialorrhea can result in the production of thick phlegm as the salivary viscosity is changed as a result of the medical management. This latter problem can be exacerbated by inadequate water intake, a common sequelae in patients with dysphagia. ALS patients frequently report a sensation of something "stuck" in the back of their throat associated with the inability to clear their airway due to an ineffective cough. The symptoms are frequently misinterpreted as being related to "allergies" but generally do not respond to antihistamines or decongestants.

Pharmacologic treatments that have shown some benefit include: high-dose guaifenesin (1800–24000 mg/day), nebulized 10% acetylcysteine, nebulized saline, or beta-blockers (propranolol). An uncontrolled survey of other alternative measures include dark grape juice, papaya tablets, sugar-free citrus lozenges, and grape seed oil (13). Dietary modifications that may be beneficial including reduction of alcohol and caffeine, increased fluid intake, and the elimination of dairy products. Use of a cool mist humidifier can also be helpful.

Recently, there has been a renewed interest in evaluating the use of mechanical insufflation–exsufflation (Cough-Assist®, Emerson) for improved clearance of upper airway secretions (14). Anecdotal experience from multiple tertiary ALS treatment facilities indicates that this may ultimately be the most effective method available.

In addition, there is a randomized trial of high-flow chest wall oscillation therapy in progress (The Vest™) which has also been anecdotally reported to dramatically improve the clearance of thick phlegm in patients with cystic fibrosis (15,16).

Laryngospasm

Laryngospasm is described by patients as a sudden sensation of being unable to breathe or a feeling that their throat is constricting. The phenomenon is due to adduction of the vocal cords usually from a hyperactive gag reflex in response to aspirated liquids or saliva or acid reflux. Laryngospasm usually aborts spontaneously within several seconds and repeated swallowing while breathing through the nose may accelerate resolution of the attack. If the episodes occur frequently, pharmacologic intervention is warranted since the attacks can be extremely anxiety provoking for the patient. Liquid lorazepam in a concentrated formulation applied as few drops sublingually will generally rapidly abort the spasm. Antacids and proton pump inhibitors should also be considered, particularly if there are other symptoms suggestive of gastroesophageal reflux disease (GERD) such as heartburn, acid taste, throat irritation, or hoarseness. Since GERD may be worsened by diaphragmatic weakness and overeating, patients with decreased vital capacity and/or who use a PEG tube for feedings should especially be considered for therapy with peristaltic agents metochlorpropamide 10 mg 30 min qac and qhs) as well as either antacids or proton pump inhibitors.

SYMPTOMS RELATED TO UPPER MOTOR NEURON DEGENERATION

Emotional Lability

Signs of emotional lability are common in many neurodegenerative disorders. The characteristics of pseudobulbar affect include uncontrolled laughter or crying, often with minimal or no provocation. The syndrome was described by Charles Darwin over 130 years ago although to date an underlying etiology has not yet been confirmed. Episodes are often sudden, involuntary outbursts of emotion inappropriate to the context of the situation. Patients experiencing uncontrolled crying are more common than those with uncontrolled laughter; however, the symptoms can result in a significant disability, limiting social interactions and limiting quality of life.

Two primary theories have been proposed on the etiology of pseudobulbar affect. Wilson (17) suggested that interruption of pyramidal pathways from brain to brainstem yields a "faciorespiratory response" and loss of inhibition that results in an affective display that is dissociated from an appropriate emotion.

Privizi et al. (18) reported that reciprocal pathways between motor cortex, brainstem, and cerebellum comprise a circuit that controls emotional responses appropriate for specific cognitive and social contexts. Lesions that disrupt the circuit disconnect centers that regulate perceived emotion from those that are involved with displayed emotion.

Both theories implicate a disconnection between neuronal connectivity that imparts a balance between perceived emotion and displayed emotion. The resulting disinhibition can cause a significant social disability, negatively affecting quality of life. Fortunately, available medications can greatly impact or reverse this disabling symptom.

At present, Food and Drug Administration (FDA)-approved therapy for pseudobulbar affect is not available; however, existing selective serotonin reuptake inhibitors, tricyclic antidepressants, and some dompaminergic agents have been beneficial in selected patients (Table 2). Until recently, most available clinical trials have been small ($n < 30$) with variable results in poststroke and multiple sclerosis (MS) patient populations. Individual case reports have been more encouraging with selective dramatic effects justifying ongoing research and empiric attempts at treatment.

Table 2 Medications Used for Emotional Liability

Drug	Dose	Common side effects
SSRI antidepressants		
Paroxetine	10–50 mg qd	Sexual dysfunction, anesthesia, sleep disturbance, and anxiety
Fluoxetine	10–30 mg qd	
Fluvoxamine	50 mg qd-bid	
Sertraline	50–100 qd-bid	
Citalopram	20–60 mg qd	
Tricyclic antidepressants		
Amitryptiline	25–75 mg qhs	Dry mouth, fatigue, dizziness, urinary retention, and constipation
Nortriptyline	10–75 mg qhs	
Desipramine	25–75 mg qd	
Mirtazapine	15 mg qhs	Abnormal dreams, mild cognitive change, and constipation
Ventafaxine	37.5–75 mg bid-tid	Anorexia, constipation, weight loss, impotence, anxiety, and dizziness
Quinidine/dextromethorphan	30/30 mg 1 tab bid	Nausea, dizziness, somnolence, and loose stools

Recently a novel combination of dextromethorphan hydrobromide (30 mg) and quinidine sulfate (30 mg) (Neurodex™) has been shown to be effective in a large, phase-three, multicenter, randomized trial (19). One hundred and forty patients were randomized to receive Neurodex or placebo twice per day for four weeks. Neurodex patients reported significantly less emotional lability, improved quality of life, and improved quality of relationship scores. Similarly favorable results were reported for a more recent study in patients with multiple sclerosis. Neurodex is currently under consideration for FDA approval based upon these favorable results and a subsequent phase-four trial.

Spasticity

The etiology of spasticity in motor neuron disease likely involves loss of upper motor neuron connectivity onto cortical, brainstem, and spinal cord targets. Disinhibition of motor neurons in the ventral horn results in rigid and spastic movements, further confounding the consequences of lower motor neuron loss in patients with ALS.

Facilitation of motor neuron inhibition can be accomplished with baclofen (Lioresal™), a gamma-amino-butyric acid (GABA) analog. This is often a first-line agent and results can be dose specific. Progressive dose titration should begin at 10 mg qd-tid and increased by 10 mg every three to five days depending upon tolerance. Maximum tolerated effective doses can range from 30 to 180 mg/day and responsiveness is rather idiosyncratic. Dose-limiting side effects include weakness, fatigue, and sedation. Subjective complaints of weakness can, however, result from the absence of chronic rigidity and spasticity. Patients may report "feeling more loose" and misreport that as weakness in the setting of a normal motor examination. Slow but progressive dose titration allowing accommodation can minimize such complaints.

When the maximum tolerated dose of oral baclofen is not effective, intrathecal administration is a viable alternative (20,21). Direct administration of sterile baclofen into the cerebral spinal fluid (CSF) can dramatically minimize the dose-limiting side effects seen frequently in oral administration. The magnitude of the intrathecal dose required is approximately 1/1000th of the oral dose. One significant advantage of intrathecal administration is the availability of variable dose delivery tailored to an individual patient's daily variation in symptoms. Additional bolus doses in early morning or later in the evening can be programmed routinely. Prior to consideration of intrathecal dosing, a test bolus dose of 50 μg should be infused via lumbar puncture to access bioactivity and the possibility of drug hypersensitivity.

Dantrolene sodium (Dantrium^{TM}) is often well tolerated with significant benefits at reducing both rigidity and spasticity. Dantrolene acts by blocking calcium release at the level of the sarcoplasmic reticulum and has a theoretical benefit at reducing excess neuronal excitation. Dantrolene can be easily used in conjunction with baclofen and, although untested, in select patients there appears to be a synergistic effect of the two drugs. Dosing can be initiated at 25 mg tid and the drug has been well tolerated and effective at higher doses without apparent weakness. Maximum suggested dose is 100 mg four times per day. Liver function studies should be checked regularly, especially at higher doses.

Tizanidine (Zanaflex^{TM}), an alpha-2 agonist with inhibitory action on excitatory interneurons in the spinal cord, acts to reduce rigidity and spasticity. Tizanidine can also be easily used in conjunction with other antispasticity medication. Side effects are similar to baclofen and optimal tolerance depends upon slow dose titration. Initial dosing of 2 to 4 mg/day can be increased by 2 to 4 mg every 3 days to as much as 360 mg/day in divided doses.

Benzodiazepines have a limited role in the primary treatment of spasticity but may be effective in treating painful spasms or cramps, which can accompany spasticity. The use of benzodiazepine drugs must be weighed against the potential for sedation and respiratory suppression. Stretching exercises have also been reported to lessen or eliminate spasms and cramping often associated with spasticity (22). Tone reduction ankle-foot orthoses (AFO) bracing (posterior leaf spring) can also be beneficial in stabilizing gait and reducing the consequences of both rigidity and spasticity.

Botulinum toxin injections have been successful in reported cases of painful spasticity although not yet studied in the ALS patient population. The primary effect of botulinum toxin is to induce muscle paralysis, thereby reducing increased muscle tone rigidity, associated spasticity. This method is usually reserved for indications when all other conventional medications have not proven to be effective due to the obvious confound of inducing paralysis in a disease marked by progressive paralysis.

Bladder Urgency

Case Report No. 2

A 62-year-old female with a history of bulbar-onset ALS presents with complaints of increased urinary frequency and frequent "accidents." The patient states that over the past three months, unless the patient gets up and goes to the restroom immediately after perceiving the need to urinate, the patient wets herself before she can and is awakening three to four times a night in order to go to the bathroom. The patient has to wear pads in her underwear and has avoided social invitations due to her fear of having an "accident" in public. The patient has been treated on two separate occasions by her family practitioner with antibiotics for suspected bladder infections; however, she continues to remain symptomatic. A post-void residual performed in the clinic was 4 cm^3 and urine analysis was normal. What can you recommend?

Although classic teaching suggests that ALS patients have complete sparing of bowel and bladder function, many patients, especially those with significant lower extremity spasticity, may report symptoms of bladder urgency. Patients may report the need to void as often as every one to two hours; however, each time they are only able to void small volumes. Urinary frequency and urgency are confounded by impaired mobility with anxiety resulting from fear of not being able to reach the commode in time. The presumed etiology of these bladder symptoms involves spasm of the urinary sphincter and/or detrussor muscle.

It is imperative to rule out a urinary tract infection or prostatism if patients report symptoms of bladder urgency and/or frequency. If no other cause can be identified, an empiric trial of a spasmolytic agent should be considered. Oxybutynin (Ditropan^{TM}) 5 mg bid-tid is the least expensive and can be crushed and put through a PEG tube. Oxybutynin is also available in doses of 5, 10, and 15 mg as an extended release tablet that can be administered once a day, although it cannot be crushed. Tolterodine tartrate (Detrol^{TM}) is longer acting and can be prescribed as 1 to 2 mg bid. Recently, oxytrol patches have been released, which may be used in addition to the oral tablets in patients with refractory symptoms. Patients with mild symptoms can sometimes be managed simply by the recommendation to comply with a "voiding schedule" in which patients attempt to urinate every two to three - hours regardless of whether they have an urge in order to avoid accidents.

Jaw Quivering/Clenching

Some ALS patients may develop jaw quivering or clenching due to upper motor neuron dysfunction. These symptoms may be precipitated by noxious stimuli such as pain, anxiety, or cold. Jaw clenching, in particular, can make suctioning and/or oral hygiene difficult, if not impossible, to perform. Traditional therapies have included clonazepam 0.5 mg tid, diazepam 2.5 to 5 mg bid-qid, or lorazepam 0.5 to 1.0 mg q 8 h PRN. Botulinum toxin injected at two sites within the masseter muscles bilaterally has also been anectodally reported to be effective.

SYMPTOMS RELATED TO IMMOBILITY

Edema

Dependent edema is a common consequence of immobility. In addition, loss of skeletal muscle tone and mass results in less vascular tone, further contributing to edema in the extremities. The consequences of chronic edema and static blood flow include pain, venous thrombosis, sensory nerve damage, and impaired range of motion. Available conservative management can be highly effective in addressing signs and consequences of edema; however, diligent compliance is essential for optimal benefit.

Elevation of the legs is perhaps the simplest and most effective early intervention. Patients should be instructed that placement of pillows under the calves can facilitate drainage of distal edema and optimal position should be adopted often when patients are in reclining or recumbent positions. In patients with wheelchair dependence, proper planning is essential prior to the detection of distal edema to ensure that placement of elevating leg rests are an available option. Motorized scooters, for example, do not offer such adaptability.

When periodic elevation alone is not effective in reducing edema, specialized elastic stockings can be more effective. Many brands and variations of specialized support hose are available; however, custom fit prescription elastized support stockings are most beneficial. Stockings are prescribed based on the length required and the degree of compression. For moderate edema compression of 20 to 30 mm Hg is usually adequate. For more advanced or persistent edema, 30 to 40 mm Hg is usually recommended. Proper fitting requires accurate measurement of the calf and foot. Personnel specially trained for such fitting should be sought. Custom-made support stockings are available for patients with atypical size and proportions of the lower extremities.

Multiple other debilitating consequences of immobility are also common. Diminished range of motion can result in painful contractures, which are easily avoided by early recognition and proactive treatment. Range-of-motion exercises and massage therapy are also effective. A portable standing frame can provide adequate muscle stretch, healthy weight bearing on the bones, and a large psychological benefit to be able to stand upright in an otherwise wheelchair dependent individual. These devices can be used at home and easily integrated into the daily routine. Proper transfer devices, including a hydraulic Hoyer-type lift, can reduce the physical difficulty for caregivers in overcoming immobility. A patient's capacity to leave their home, increase their repertoire of daily activities, and maintain passive mobility is both psychologically and physically essential to optimizing quality of life and available hopeful alternatives.

Sleep Disruption

Disordered sleep patterns in patients with motor neuron disease are likely multifactorial in etiology. Respiratory weakness, difficulty repositioning in bed, anxiety, depression, and pain can interfere together with normal sleep patterns. Respiratory insufficiency, increased arousals, and decreased total sleep time have been recognized in patients with ALS (23–26). The symptomatic consequences of impaired sleep include daytime fatigue, exacerbation of respiratory compromise, weakness, and depression. Overall, impaired sleep can markedly affect quality of life and likely implicate prognosis and longevity.

Available solutions to address impaired sleep are as varied as the diverse problems causing it. Simple physical adaptations such as a power, hospital-type bed can be ideal to enhance mobility and positioning. An inexpensive alternating pressure air pad or gel overlay mattress can lessen the discomfort from limited repositioning and impaired nocturnal mobility. Noninvasive positive pressure ventilation can affect respiratory hygiene and improve sleep quality. Antidepressant medications are also effective at reducing anxiety, depression, and promoting sleep. In that regard, mirtazapine (15 mg qhs) can be especially helpful. At higher doses (>30 mg) mirtazapine may have a confounding effect due to enhancement of its noradrenergic effect. The anticholinergic action of the tricyclic antidepressant group can also be especially helpful.

Anxiolytic medications such as benzodiazepines, used specifically to induce sleep, can be helpful when used selectively. Zolpidem tartrate (10 mg qhs) is often effective and preferred due to low risk of respiratory depression. Pharmacological tolerance and withdrawal symptoms can become evident with chronic use. Addressing the underlying cause of such anxiety (depression, fear, pain, etc.) is a preferred method of treatment.

Alternative pharmacologic agents such as melatonin, passionflower, lavender, and hops have been effective for individual patients; however, their benefits are quite variable and untested.

Fatigue

Fatigue and exercise intolerance are among the most common complaints in patients with motor neuron disease. Although fatigue is not a primary consequence of motor neuron degeneration, it is often synonymous with and mistakenly interpreted as advancing weakness. Limitations in daily activity secondary to fatigue have a direct impact on quality of life. The initial challenge in treating fatigue is the identification of the primary etiology (Table 3). There are few objective criteria for use in "observing" fatigue and tremendous variability in subjective descriptions of the symptom.

Energy conservation is perhaps the first line and simplest method of treatment for complaints of fatigue. Patients with weakness may try to establish for themselves that their weakness is mild by attempting activities more appropriate for their premorbid state. Reassurance to the patient that exercise, daily activity, and travel are acceptable within the guidelines of an energy conservation protocol can be very therapeutic. Patients who are able to enjoy aerobic exercise can be told to "stop before you would otherwise need to stop exercising." This can be useful advice to reassure a patient that normal activities are possible and encouraged.

Fear for a patient that their fatigue is synonymous with weakness and this is interpreted as disease progression can be dispelled with sound advice and encourage-

Table 3 Etiologies of Fatigue in Motor Neuron Disease

Etiology	Treatment
Physical fatigue	Rest, energy conservation, adaptive equipment, possibly creatine monohydrate, and medications (Table 5)
Mental "tiredness"	Evaluate ADLs, r/o depression, encourage community/family resources, address hopeful alternatives, unexpressed fears, and increase activity as tolerated
Lack of interest and/or difficulty concentrating, and/or anxiety	Consider empiric antidepressant
Failure to feel rested after sleep	Sleep study, consider BiPAP regardless of FVC
Pain or physical discomfort	See pain section below, evaluate for etiology, if non-localizing, consider antidepressant, and increase activity as tolerated
Medication	Fatigue is a side effect of many commonly used medications. Alternatives should be sought (Table 4)

Abbreviations: ADLs, activities of daily living; BiPAP, bilevel positive airway pressure; FVC, forced vital capacity.
Source: Modified from Ref. 27.

Table 4 Commonly Used Medication Classes with Associated Fatigue

Drug class	Indication	Examples
Analgesics	Pain	Butalbital, oxycodone
Anti-spasticity	Spasms, rigidity, and spasticity	Baclofen, dantrolene sodium, tizanidine, and clonazepam
Anticonvulsants	Pain, fasciculations, anxiety, and depression	Gabapentin, carbamazepine, and divaloprex
Antidepressants	Depression	Tricyclics (amitryptilline), SSRI (sertraline, paroxetine, and others in this class)
Antihistamines	Congestion, secretion management	Diphenhydramine, loratadine, and fexofenadine
Anticholinergics	Sialorrhea	Hyocyanime, glycopyrrolate, and scopolamine

Abbreviation: SSRI, selective serotonin reuptake inhibitor.

ment. Deconditioning from the lack of exercise can be more disabling and fatigue inducing than controlled activity and exercise.

Mild to moderate nocturnal respiratory insufficiency may be significantly under recognized as a source of daytime fatigue. Standard measures of pulmonary health (forced vital capacity, negative inspiratory force, and nocturnal desaturation) are helpful but not required for a patient to benefit from bilevel positive airway pressure (BiPAP) intervention. Occasionally, when daytime fatigue results in an artificially low pulmonary function test (justifying the onset of BiPAP therapy), we have seen an improvement in both the fatigue and the pulmonary function as a result of starting BiPAP therapy.

Pharmacologic treatments of fatigue symptoms are often effective (Table 5). Response to medications can, however, be as idiosyncratic as the etiology of the fatigue. In addition, common medications taken for other reasons can contribute to fatigue symptoms and should be considered prior to addition of new drugs to manage side effects resulting from existing drugs (Table 4).

Off label use of pyridostigmine (Mestinon®, 60 mg q 3–12 PRN) can reduce complaints of weakness by facilitating the efficiency of the neuromuscular junction. In patients sensitive to this therapy, increased "energy" can result in feeling stronger and less fatigued.

Methylphenidate (10–50 mg qd) can also provide another treatment option in selected patients. Caution must be taken to monitor side effects of anorexia, restlessness, anxiety, or palpitations.

Constipation

Constipation is a frequent symptom of ALS patients, particularly when they become less mobile and/or wheelchair dependent. Constipation can be further aggravated by the prescription of anticholinergic medications for sialorrhea or the use of narcotic medications for pain or air hunger. Inadequate fluid intake due to dysphagia, arm weakness, or a desire to minimize trips to the bathroom may also contribute to the problem. In later stages of the disease, abdominal wall muscles may weaken to the point that patients are unable to "push" the stool out, even if it is soft.

Table 5 Medications Commonly Used to Treat Fatigue

Drug	Starting dose	Usual maintenance dose	Usual maximal dose	Side effects
Amantadine (Symmetrel™)	100 mg/day in the morning	100 mg twice per day	300 mg/day	Insomnia, vivid dreams
Modafinil (Provigil™)	100 mg/day in the morning	200 mg/day in the morning or 100 mg in the morning and 100 mg at lunchtime	200 mg/day (some people might respond well to higher doses)	Headache, insomnia
Pemoline (Cylert™)	18.75 mg/day in the morning	18.75–56.25 mg/day	93.75 mg/day	Irritability, restlessness, insomnia, potential liver problems
Bupropion, sustained release (Wellbutrin-XL™)	150 mg/day in the morning	150 mg/day	450 mg/day	Agitation, anxiety, and insomnia
Fluoxetine (Prozac™)	20 mg/day in the morning	20–80 mg/day	80 mg/day	Weakness, nausea, and insomnia
Venlafaxine (Effexor-XR™)	75 mg/day in the morning	75–225 mg/day	225 mg/day	Weakness, nausea, and dizziness

Source: Modified from Ref. 27.

Initial management of constipation should include the use of stool softeners such as Surfek® (240 mg bid), Pericolase® (50–300 mg per day), or Senekot® (2–4 tabs qd-bid). If these are ineffective, Milk of Magnesia® or Dulcolax® tablets can be added to the regimen. In patients with a PEG tube, lactulose (10 g/15 cc, 15–30 cc qd-bid) can be administered as long as the patient is not impacted. There are a variety of different enemas as well as magnesium citrate that can be used in urgent situations. Occasionally, simply increasing fluid intake and substituting medications with fewer anticholinergic effects can resolve the problem. A creative recipe for constipation that has been recommended is "power pudding," which consists of equal parts of prunes, prune juice, apple sauce, and bran (28). Two tablespoons with each meal and at bedtime, along with adequate fluid intake and fruits and vegetables in the diet, can be as effective as medications for constipation in many cases.

Pain

Pain affecting patients with motor neuron disease is often multifactorial and under recognized (Table 6). Complications of physical immobility and emotional distress can individually and together result in disabling pain. Although the primary pathophysiology of ALS, is recognized to spare pain pathways, signs and symptoms of pain can comprise the primary disability. Early proactive recognition of the common precipitants leading to pain is the first line of treatment.

Table 6 Causes and Treatment of Pain in Patients with ALS

Etiology	Non-pharmacologic interventions	Medications	Other treatment
Painful spasm	Stretching, passive/active range of motion	Baclofen, dantrium, gabapentin, clonazepam	Botulinum toxin
Cramping	Massage, stretching	Quinine, vitamin E, clonazepam	
Immobility	Stationary peddler, standing frame, aquatic therapy, active range of motion, part-time use hard cervical (Philadelphia type) or a Freeman or Headmaster type collar (padded wire frame collar), alternative mattress	Nonsteroidal anti-inflammatory, intracapsular injection	Surgery for release of painful contracture
Edema	Massage, elastic support hose, and elevation	Diuretic (selected cases)	Cardiac evaluation
Headache	Evaluate nocturnal ventilation, consider NIPPV, neck muscle stretch, r/o cervical radiculopathy, eval head support on chair	Nonsteroidal anti-inflammatory	

Immobility can result in a multitude of potential pain complaints. Weakness and diminished range of motion result in muscle contracture, which, if associated with spasm or increased tone, can be painful. Adhesive capsilitis is a very common source of pain often secondary to shoulder weakness. Poor vascular tone can induce painful dependent edema and, in more extreme cases, dysesthesia from sensory nerve compromise. Many noninvasive resources exist to address multiple sources of pain and these should be commonly adopted in every proactive, aggressive treatment plan.

Nonsteroidal anti-inflammatory medications (NSAIDS) are often empirically used for non-specific pain complaints. Cox-2 inhibitors (cytochrome oxidase inhibitor, type 2) are often tried alone or in conjunction with NSAIDs. Last, the use of benzodiazepines and opioids are generally safe but should be used with caution due to possible respiratory depression, increasing tolerance, and dependence/withdrawal.

SYMPTOMS RELATED TO ANXIETY AND DEPRESSION

Depression and anxiety are perhaps the most pervasive and significant clinical sequelae limiting optimal quality of life for patients with motor neuron disease (29,30). Fortunately, the number of available options for treatment is vast and often effective. The challenge in the treatment of anxiety and depression is in the recognition of subtle early clinical signs. Onset is often insidious and patients can deny significant symptoms for fear of being labeled with "another illness."

Table 7 Medications Commonly Used in Treating Anxiety and Depression

Medication class/name	Advantages	Disadvantages
Mirtazepine (Remeron™)	Ideal for depressed affect with anxiety	Sedation
	Quick onset of action	Confusion
	Effective for insomnia	
	Comes in dissolvable tab	
Selective serotonin reuptake inhibitors	Good for emotional lability, anxiety, anhedonia	Sexual dysfunction
		Gastrointestinal side effects
Tricyclic antidepressants	Inexpensive	Orthostasis
	Effective for insomnia	Sedation
	Effective for sialorrhea	Bladder retention
Venlafaxine (Effexor™)	May be activating	May raise blood pressure
	Well-tolerated	Nausea
	Available in sustained-release tab	
Bupropion (Wellbutrin™)	May be activating (causing insomnia)	Moderate anticholinergic effects
	Minimal sexual side effects	May cause seizures

Patients may adopt a "reactive depression" in response to limitations imposed by the impact of motor neuron disease on their lifestyle. By comparison with accepted clinical criteria for depression (31), patients may have fewer overt signs. Manifestations of reactive depression may include a patient rejecting available treatment alternatives while maintaining an outward appearance of resignation with an appropriate affect.

Anxiety and depression are often comorbid symptoms, each compounding the other. Clinical recognition leading to appropriate treatment of anxiety can be challenging due to similar feelings of anxiety arising from dyspnea and dependence on caregivers for regular mobility. Routine feelings of nervousness, insomnia, irritability, and restlessness are, however, readily treatable often using medications that also will address the concurrent depression.

Optimal treatment of depression and/or anxiety is dependent upon which associated clinical signs are most prominent. Response to medication is usually idiosyncratic and often selection of a specific drug is empiric based upon a secondary benefit that a specific side effect may have, such as sedation for insomnia or increased appetite for anorexia (Table 7). Most importantly, it is essential to recognize that a treatment failure should not be synonymous with a failure to treat. Medication trials, in the absence of disabling side effects, should last at least four weeks and multiple modes of medication and counseling may be required.

SUMMARY

The spectrum of available treatments, both symptomatic and adjunctive, have markedly advanced the care of patients with motor neuron disease. Once thought to be untreatable, patients with motor neuron disease today should be exposed to opportunities for multidisciplinary care. The impact of such care on the disease course, including rate of progression and mortality, can surpass the treatment effects commonly sought in current clinical drug trials. The benefit of simultaneous multiple modes of supportive care can be synergistic, supporting not only a multidisciplinary diagnostic evaluation but ongoing treatment as well.

REFERENCES

1. Forshew DA, Bromberg MB. A survey of clinicians' practice in the symptomatic treatment of ALS. Amyotroph Lateral Scler Other Motor Neuron Disord 2003; 4:258–263.
2. Sufit R, Miller R, Mitsumoto H, et al. Prevalence and treatment outcomes of sialorrhea in Amyotrophic Lateral Sclerosis patients as assessed by the ALS Patient Care Database. Ann Neurol 1999: 46:506.
3. Miller RG, Anderson FA Jr, Bradley WG, Brooks BR, Mitsumoto H, Munsat TL, Ringel SP. The ALS patient care database: goals, design, and early results. ALS CARE Study Group. Neurology 2000; 54:53–57.
4. Bradley WG, Anderson F, Bromberg M, Gutman L, Hardli Y, Ross M, Miller RG. ALS Care Group. Current management of ALS: comparison of the ALS CARE Database and the AAN Practice Parameter. The American Academy of Neurology. Neurology 2001; 57:500–504.
5. Portis M, Gamba M, Bertaccji G, Vaj P. Treatment of sialorrhea with ultrasound guided botulinium toxin type A injection in patienss with neurological disorders. J Neurol Neurosurg Psychiatry 2001:538–540.
6. Giess R, Naumann M, Werner E, Riemann R, Beck M, Puls I, Reiners L, Toyka K.V. Injections of botulinum toxin A into the salivary glands improve sialorrhoea in amyotrophic lateral sclerosis [see comment]. J Neurol Neurosurg Psychiatry 2000; 69:121–123.
7. Rowe D, Erjavec S. An open-label pilot study of intra-parotid botulinum toxin A injections in the treatment of sialorrhea in motor neuron disease. Amyotroph Lateral Scler Other Motor Neuron Disord 2003; 4:53–54.
8. Winterholler MG, Erbguth FJ, Wolf S, Kat S. Botulinum toxin for the treatment of sialorrhoea in ALS: serious side effects of a transductal approach [comment]. J Neurol Neurosurg Psychiatry 2001; 70:417–418.
9. Bhatia KP, Munchau A, Brown P. Botulinum toxin is a useful treatment in excessive drooling in saliva. J Neurol Neurosurg Psychiatry 1999; 67:697.
10. Tan EK, Lo YL, Seah A, Auchus AP. Recurrent jaw dislocation after botulinum toxin treatment for sialorrhoea in amyotrophic lateral sclerosis. J Neurol Sci 2001; 190:95–97.
11. Stalpers L, Moser E. Results of radiotherapy for drooling in amyotrophic lateral sclerosis. Neurology 2002; 58(8):1308.
12. Harriman M, Morrison M, Hay J, Revonta M, Eisen A, Lentle B. Use of radiotherapy for control of sialorrhea in patients with amyotrophic lateral sclerosis. J Otolaryngol 2001; 30:242–249.
13. Foulsum I. Secretion management in motor neuron disease., 10 International Symposium on ALS/MND, 1999. ALS and Other Motor Neuron Disorders.
14. Bach JR. Amyotrophic lateral sclerosis: prolongation of life by noninvasive respiratory AIDS [see comment]. Chest 2002; 122:92–98.
15. Arens R, Gozal D, Omlin K, Vegd J, Boyo KP, Keens TG, Wob MS. Comparison of high frequency chest compression and conventional chest physiotherapy I hospitalized patients with cystic fibrosis. Am J Respir Crit Care Med 1994; 150:1154–1157.
16. Warwick W, Hansen L. The long term effect of high frequency chest compression therapy on pulmonary complications of cystic fibrosis. Pediatr Pumonol 1991; 11: 265–271.
17. Wilson S. Some problems in neurology II. Pathological laughter and crying. J Neurol Psychopathol 1924; 4:299–333.

18. Parvizi J, Anderson S, Martin C, Damasio H, Damasio AR. Pathological laughter and crying/A link to the cerebellum. Brain 2001; 124:1708–1719.

19. Books BR, Thisted RA, Appel SH, Bradley WG, Okey RK, Berg JE, Pope LE, Smith RA. AVP-ALS study group. Treatment of pseudobulbar affect in ALS with dextromethorphan/quinidine: a randomized trial. Neurology 2004; 63:1364–1370.

20. Marquardt G, Seifert V. Use of intrathecal baclofen for treatment of spasticity in amyotrophic lateral sclerosis. J Neurol Neurosurg Psychiatry 2002; 72:275–276.

21. Stempien L, Tsai T. Intrathecal baclofen pump use for spasticity: a clinical survey. Am J Phys Med Rehabil 2000; 79:536–541.

22. Ashworth NL, Satkunam LE, Deforge D. Treatment for spasticity in amyotrophic lateral sclerosis/motor neuron disease. Cochrane Database Syst Rev 2004; 1.

23. Arnulf I, Similowski T, Salachas F, Gdrmd L, Mehiri S, Attdli V, Behin-Bellheer V, Meninger V, Dereme JP. Sleep disorders and diaphragmatic function in patients with amyotrophic lateral sclerosis. Am J Respir Crit Care Med 2000; 161:849–856.

24. Ferguson KA, Strong MJ, Ahmad D, George CF. Sleep-disordered breathing in amyotrophic lateral sclerosis. Chest 1996; 110:664–669.

25. Gay PC, Westbrook PR, Daube JR, Litchy WJ, Windebank AJ, Iverson R. Effects of alterations in pulmonary function and sleep variables on survival in patients with amyotrophic lateral sclerosis. Mayo Clin Proc 1991; 66:686–694.

26. Kimura K, Tachibana N, Kimura J, Shibasaki H. Sleep-disordered breathing at an early stage of amyotrophic lateral sclerosis [see comments]. J Neurol Sci 1999; 164:37–43.

27. Krupp L. Fatigue in Multiple Sclerosis: A Guide to Diagnosis and Management. New York: Demos, 2004.

28. Gelinas D. Treating the Symptoms of ALS. In: Mitsumoto H, Munsat TL, eds. Amyotroph Lateral Scler: A Guide Patients and Families, 2001:47–62.

29. Lou J, Reeves A, Benice T, Sexton G. Fatigue and depression are associated with poor quality of life in ALS. Neurology 2003; 60:122–123.

30. Ganzini L, Johnston WS, Hoffman WF. Correlates of suffering in amyotroph lateral sclerosis. Neurology 1999; 52:1434–1440.

31. American Psychiatric Association Task Force on Nomenclature and Statistics: Diagnostic and Statistical Manual of Mental Disorders (DSM-IV). Washington DC: American Psychiatric Association, 1994.

30

ALS Pharmacotherapy: Riluzole and Clinical Trials

Petra Kaufmann

*Department of Neurology, The Neurological Institute, Columbia University
College of Physicians and Surgeons, New York, New York, U.S.A.*

INTRODUCTION

Finding a cure for ALS is the goal of all ALS research. Recent decades have seen remarkable progress in all stages of drug development: basic laboratory research has elucidated steps in the cascade leading to motor neuron death and thus identified molecular targets for experimental treatment. Transgenic animal research has resulted in several models of ALS, facilitating preclinical testing of candidate drugs. Finally, clinical research has refined outcome measures and trial design. This allows for valid clinical experiments to assess the efficacy of new ALS treatments. Despite the remarkable progress in all areas of preclinical and clinical drug development, the glutamate antagonist riluzole remains the only drug approved by the Food and Drug Administration (FDA) for the treatment of ALS. This chapter provides an overview of riluzole's path to approval and of its impact on ALS care. This is followed by a discussion of recent randomized, controlled clinical trials in ALS. The series of negative trials that has followed riluzole's success has raised a fundamental question: Do the drugs tested truly lack benefit in ALS or have the clinical trials designed to evaluate them just failed to demonstrate their benefit? This chapter discusses the limitations and accomplishments of recent ALS trials. It is always easy to raise issues with hindsight. The intent of this chapter is not to be critical of specific ALS trials, but rather to constructively discuss what lessons could be learned from the accumulating experience.

The rationale for most trials is based on hypotheses that have been developed to explain the pathogenesis of ALS. These research hypotheses are discussed in detail in chapters 11 through 25 and include oxidative stress, mitochondrial dysfunction, glutamate excitotoxicity, neuronal rescue by neurotrophic factors, enhanced apoptosis, viral or hormonal factors, inflammation, and microglial proliferation.

RILUZOLE

Background

Increased excitatory neurotransmission may initiate or accelerate cell death in ALS and thus play an important role in ALS pathogenesis (1). Glutamate, the main excitatory transmitter in the brain, is associated with neurotoxicity in ALS (see Chapter 12). Riluzole is a benzothiazole derivative that mitigates glutamatergic neurotoxicity (2). On the basis of its neuroprotective properties, riluzole has been evaluated as possible treatment for ALS. Human trials for riluzole were initiated prior to testing in the transgenic ALS mouse model (3), but its efficacy was confirmed later in animal studies: In the transgenic mouse model of ALS, riluzole prolongs survival, but does not delay disease onset (4). In the "wobbler" mouse, high-dose riluzole slows the progression of neuromuscular impairment (5).

Randomized, Controlled Clinical Trials of Riluzole

The first randomized, double blind, placebo-controlled trial included 155 patients, stratified by the site of disease onset (limb vs. bulbar). At the end of the 12-month treatment period, 74% of those treated with 100 mg riluzole daily were still alive, compared with 58% in the placebo group. This represented a statistically significant survival benefit. The survival difference between treatment groups was larger for bulbar onset patients than for limb onset patients. At the end of the placebo-controlled observation period (median follow up 573 days), the survival benefit was smaller but continued to be significant for the entire study population and for the bulbar onset patients, but not for the limb onset patients. The rate of muscle strength deterioration was significantly slower in the riluzole group. Other functional outcomes, including quality-of-life measures, were not different between treatment groups. Adverse reactions to riluzole included asthenia, spasticity, and mild elevations in aminotransferase levels (3).

A confirmatory phase-III trial in 959 ALS patients followed. This trial tested three dose arms: 50, 100, and 200 mg daily, with tracheotomy-free survival as primary outcome. After a mean follow-up time of 18 months, 50% on placebo versus 57% receiving 100 mg riluzole daily were alive. The 100 mg dose had the most favorable efficacy and safety profile. There was no difference in the rate of decline for the secondary outcome measures including muscle strength. Common adverse events included asthenia, dizziness, gastrointestinal disorders, and increased liver enzymes (6).

A third randomized, controlled riluzole clinical trial included 168 patients who did not meet the inclusion criteria for the large, confirmatory riluzole trial (6). Patients who were elderly or had advanced stage disease were randomized to 100 mg riluzole daily or placebo and treated for 18 months. The safety profile in this sample was similar to that observed in the previous trials (3). The study could not include enough patients to reach sufficient power, and no survival difference between treatment groups was observed (7).

A fourth randomized, controlled riluzole trial in Japan involving 195 patients was negative. The primary outcome was a composite measure of disease progression. The evidence-based and systematic Cochrane review reports a meta-analysis of randomized riluzole trials with tracheotomy-free survival as primary endpoint (876 riluzole-treated and 406 placebo-treated patients) (8). For the homogeneous group included in the two initial randomized trials (3,6), 100 mg riluzole daily provided a significant survival benefit. This benefit fell short of significance when the more advanced or elderly patients from the third trial (7) were included in the analysis. On the basis of their meta-analysis, the authors concluded that riluzole at 100 mg daily is reasonably safe and prolongs survival by about two months (8).

Riluzole in Uncontrolled Studies

The long-term safety of riluzole was confirmed in an open-label, multicenter extension of the two controlled riluzole trials. Five hundred and sixteen patients who had participated in those trials were treated with riluzole at 100 mg daily for a mean follow-up time of 28.7 months and a maximum follow-up time of 81 months.

On the basis of the positive results from the controlled riluzole trials, a large uncontrolled, multicenter, multinational trial followed to assess the safety of riluzole in a broad patient population. Almost 8000 patients, over 10% of the estimated ALS population worldwide, received 100 mg riluzole daily for a mean treatment duration of about 200 days. The safety results were consistent with those observed in the controlled riluzole trials (9).

Several studies of open-label riluzole treatment have reported a survival benefit that may exceed the two months suggested by controlled trials. The retrospective study design limits the validity of these reports (10).

Riluzole serum levels may be associated with adverse events and treatment benefit. In a study of 169 patients with ALS, those with high-serum riluzole levels had fewer instances of fasciculations and muscle stiffness, but more instances of diarrhea. Current evidence from randomized clinical trials justifies treatment with a fixed 100 mg daily dose. Further research is needed to determine the benefits of increasing the riluzole dose in patients with low serum levels (11).

Efficacy

On the basis of the Cochrane review meta-analysis of controlled clinical trials, riluzole at 100 mg daily increases the probability of surviving one year by 9% (8). There was no positive effect on muscle strength, but a small beneficial effect on patient function in the Norris limb and bulbar scales. The effect on quality of life was not reported, but a post-hoc analysis of blinded data from the study by Lacomblez suggested that patients treated with riluzole remained longer in a more moderately affected health state compared with placebo treated patients (12).

The authors of the Cochrane review concluded that 100 mg riluzole daily probably prolonged life by about two months in ALS patients under the experimental conditions of the two riluzole trials [i.e., probable or definite amyotrophic lateral sclerosis, symptom duration less than five years, forced vital capacity (FVC) greater than 60% of predicted, and age less than 75 years] (8).

Safety

Riluzole is overall well tolerated. The most common adverse events observed in the controlled trials were nausea (15%) and asthenia (18%). Less common adverse events included dizziness and gastrointestinal events. Open-label studies have found the same adverse events at lower frequencies and have not uncovered any additional, unexpected adverse events.

Caution is warranted in patients with liver disease. In 10% to 15% of riluzole-treated patients, serum transaminases increased to more than three times the upper limit of normal, and additional patients developed a smaller increase in transaminases (13). Riluzole may be contraindicated in ALS patients with active liver disease and in those with elevated transaminases at the beginning of treatment. It is recommended that serum transaminases be monitored during treatment (every month during the first three months of treatment, every three months during the remainder of the first year, and periodically thereafter) (14). However, in practice many ALS experts see few clinically significant abnormalities of serum transaminases.

Impact on ALS Care

The survival benefit demonstrated in clinical trials has resulted in regulatory approval of riluzole by the FDA. Several guidelines have been issued in Europe and the United States recommending the use of riluzole in the treatment of ALS. These include a practice parameter issued by the American Academy of Neurology, which recommends riluzole treatment for patients with definite and probable ALS, symptom duration of less than five years, and FVC >60% of predicted and without tracheostomy based on class I evidence. On the basis of expert opinion, the practice parameters recommend treatment with riluzole for ALS patients with suspected or possible ALS, symptom duration of more than five years, FVC < 60% predicted, and ventilator-independent patients with tracheostomy for prevention of aspiration only. Riluzole is considered of uncertain benefit in those with tracheostomy required for ventilation, those with other incurable disease, and in patients with anterior horn cell disease other than ALS (15).

In the United Kingdom, the National Institute for Clinical Excellence (NICE), an organization that makes recommendations on treatments and care on behalf of the National Health Service using the best available evidence, issued guidelines recommending riluzole as an important and worthwhile treatment for ALS patients (16).

However, in a survey of 559 patients from 10 U.S. medical centers in 1996 (after FDA approval) only 43% of ALS patients had taken riluzole even though 90% knew about it (17). Patient-identified factors influencing their decision to start riluzole included: benefit of the drug (45%), expense (31%), opinion of ALS physician (23%), risk of side effects (14%), and opinions of family/friend (10%). Sixty-three percent of patients who took riluzole paid less than US $25 per month, compared with 12% who paid more than US $600 per month. Thirty-four percent discontinued the drug due to lack of benefit, expense, or adverse events. The probability of taking riluzole varied significantly between centers, with the percentage of patients having taken riluzole ranging from 18% to 75% at different centers. Independent risk factors that significantly influenced the probability of taking riluzole included whether the ALS physician encouraged or discouraged the patient from taking riluzole, as well as prescription drug benefit. This study suggests that physician preference and drug cost to the patient are important factors in the decision whether to begin riluzole treatment. In Ireland, for example, where the health care system provides access to prescription medication, 99% of patients cared for by ALS specialists and 61% of patients cared for by general neurologists are treated with riluzole (10,18). In contrast, the proportion of ALS patients in North America who are taking riluzole remains low. On the basis of the data from the ALS CARE Database it was 35% in 1997 and 59% in 2002 (19). It is unfortunate that ALS patients in the United States are facing this most difficult decision whether to pay for a medication that has shown efficacy in treating their disease. It seems likely that the second factor in the decision, physician preference, is largely constrained by the patient's access to riluzole. Strongly recommending riluzole to a patient who cannot afford to buy it would obviously cause distress to ALS patients and their families. Therefore, physician preference against riluzole likely reflects compassion rather than therapeutic nihilism towards a medication that is only modestly effective.

Most patients with access to riluzole choose treatment, indicating that both physicians and patients have embraced the first drug for ALS. Having an effective treatment has changed the attitude and practice of neurology when discussing the diagnosis of ALS. The first positive clinical trial has stimulated the effort to discover a second effective drug.

RECENT ALS CLINICAL TRIALS

The following list reviews key features of large randomized, controlled trials (RCTs) in ALS completed since the early 1990s. The list is incomplete, omitting many smaller trials and past trials. More extensive listings of ALS clinical trials are available elsewhere (20–22).

Targeting Oxidative Stress

Several research findings suggest that oxidative stress contributes to motor neuron degeneration in ALS (see Chapter 13). Drugs with antioxidant properties that have been studied in the treatment of ALS include vitamin E (α-tocopherol), coenzyme Q10, N-acetylcysteine, and selegiline (Tables 1 and 2). Many ALS patients are taking antioxidants with the hope of slowing disease progression. The rationale for their use is compelling, but there is no significant evidence to date to support the benefit of these antioxidants (23).

A randomized, placebo-controlled, double-blind study in 110 ALS patients of acetylcysteine 50 mg/kg subcutaneous infusion daily found no difference in tracheostomy-free survival at 12 months (24). Selegeline at 5 mg twice daily for six months was found ineffective in an RCT including 133 ALS patients. Primary endpoint was rate of change of Appel ALS total score (25).

Two clinical randomized, controlled clinical trials of vitamin E in ALS have been negative. The first trial was a randomized, placebo-controlled, double-blind study in 268 patients of vitamin E at 500 mg taken twice daily in addition to riluzole. The primary endpoint was change in functional status of each patient using the modified Norris limb scale over the 12-month follow-up time (26). The second trial was an RCT in 160 patients of 5000 mg vitamin E daily in addition to riluzole for 18 months with tracheostomy-free survival at endpoint. Both trials showed that vitamin E was well tolerated, but did not demonstrate a significant effect on the course of ALS (27).

Selegiline and acetylcysteine were evaluated as monotherapy, and vitamin E was studied in combination with riluzole as standard of care. Even though riluzole is only modestly effective, an increasing number of trials evaluate new treatments against riluzole. This, however, does not allow testing for possible interactions between the two treatments. Some of these trials may not have had sufficient power to detect a small effect size.

Additional antioxidant strategies that are currently in early clinical evaluation include edaravone (28) and manganese porphyrin (AEOL 10150). AEOL 10150 is

Table 1 Selected ALS Clinical Trials (Randomized, Controlled Phase-II/-III Trials Completed Since the Early 1990s)

Drug name	Design	Endpoint	Hypothesis	Comment
IGF-I (U.S.A.)	$n = 266$ 9 mo 0.05 or 0.1 mg/kg/day sc	Appel scores	Neurotrophic	Functional decline significantly less in high-dose group
IGF-I (Europe)	$n = 183$ 9 mo IGF-1: Placebo randomization = 2:1 0.1 mg/kg/day sc	Appel scores	Neurotrophic	Negative result. U.S. results not confirmed. Review combining both trials suggests modest effect. Third trial ongoing
CNTF (U.S.A.)	$n = 730$ Phase II/III 15 or 30 μg/kg sc TIW	QMT change	Neurotrophic	Excluded ALSFRS <16 and ALS >5 yr No benefit Side effects included anorexia, weight loss, and cough
CNTF (U.S.A.)	$n = 570$ Phase III 0.5, 2, or 5 μg/kg/day sc 3 mo lead-in + 6 mo study period	QMT and FVC change combined	Neurotrophic	Excluded ALS >3 yr, FVC <50% No benefit AE exceeded anticipated and included nausea, anorexia, and weight loss
Riluzole (Rilutek®, multinational)	$n = 959$ Follow up 18 mo	Death, tracheostomy	Antiglutamate	Positive: at 18 mo 50% of placebo-treated versus 57% in 100 mg dose arm alive
Riluzole (Rilutek®, France)	$n = 155$ Follow up 12 mo	Death	Antiglutamate	Positive: at 12 mo, 58% of placebo-treated versus 74% of riluzole-treated patients alive.
Acetylcysteine (The Netherlands)	$n = 110$ 50mg/kg/day sc Follow up 12 mo	Death, tracheostomy	Antioxidant	Negative
Nimodipine (U.S.A.)	$n = 87$	QMT and pulmonary function	Antioxidant Mitigating excitotoxicity	Negative

Verapamil (U.S.A.)	n = 72 3 mo lead-in, 6 mo treatment, 3 mo post-treatment	QMT and pulmonary function	Antioxidant Calcium channel blocker	Negative
Gabapentin (Neurontin®, U.S.A.)	n = 152 2400 mg daily 6 mo follow up	QMT in eight arm muscles	Antiglutamate	Trend toward slower decline of arm strength in gabapentin group (not significant)
Gabapentin (Neurontin®, U.S.A.)	n = 204 3600 mg daily 9 mo follow up	QMT in eight arm muscles	Antiglutamate	Negative
Selegiline (Eldepryl®, U.S.A.)		Appel total score	Antioxidant MAO-B inhibitor	Negative
Lamotrigine (Lamictal®, Sweden)	n = 30 Cross over design 6 wk dose escalation to 100 mg LTG TID for 16 wk	Norris scale	Antiglutamate	Negative
Lamotrigine (Lamictal®, Canada)	n = 67 100 mg QD 18 mo follow up	Clinical scale	Antiglutamate	Negative
BDNF (U.S.A.)	n = 1135 6 mo study period 25 or 100 µg/kg sc	6 mo FVC change and survival	Neurotrophic	Primary analysis negative, but benefit in secondary analyses Low event rate Exclusion ALSFRS <18, FVC <60%
SR 57746A (Xaliproden®, multinational)	n = 867 18 mo follow up 1 or 2 mg QD, monotherapy	Death/tracheostomy and VC	Neurotrophic	Negative, but non-significant beneficial effect on VC for 2 mg arm Excluded FVC <60%, ALS >5 yr
SR 57746A (Xaliproden®, multinational)	n = 1210 18 mo follow up 1 or 2 mg QD, plus riluzole 50 mg BID	Death/tracheostomy and VC	Neurotrophic	Overall negative, but trend towards beneficial effect of 1 mg on VC Excluded FVC <60%, ALS >5 yr

(Continued)

Table 1 Selected ALS Clinical Trials (Randomized, Controlled Phase-II/-III Trials Completed Since the Early 1990s) (*Continued*)

Drug name	Design	Endpoint	Hypothesis	Comment
Creatine (The Netherlands)	n = 175 16 mo follow up, sequential design	Death, tracheostomy	Energy metabolism	Negative
Creatine (U.S.A.)	n = 104 5 gm PO QD 6 mo follow up	MQMT in 8 arm muscles	Energy metabolism	Negative, well tolerated
Vitamin E (France)	n = 268 500 mg BID plus riluzole Follow up 12 mo	Norris limb scale	Antioxidant	No significant difference
Vitamin E (Europe)	n = 160 5000 mg QD plus riluzole Follow up 18 mo	Death or tracheostomy	Antioxidant	No significant difference between groups Well tolerated
Dextromethorphane (DM)+ Quinidine (Q) (Neurodex®, U.S.A.) Brooks BR, Thisted RA, Appel SH, Bradley WG, Olney RK, Berg JE, Pope LE, Smith RA, AVP-923 ALS Study Group. Treatment of pseudobulbar affect in ALS with dextromethorphan/quinidine: a randomized trial. Neurology 2004; 63(8):1364–1370.	n = 140 3 arms: DM, Q, and DM & Q	Center for neurologic study lability score	DM is antagonist of glutamate receptor (NMDA) Quinidine inhibits DM metabolism, increasing availability	D/Q combination effective in symptomatic treatment of pseudobulbar affect

Drug/Trial	Enrollment/Duration	Outcome measure	Mechanism	Result
Indinavir (U.S.A.) Scelsa sn, MaCGowan DJL, Mitsumoto H, imperato T, Le valley AJ, Liu MH, DelBene M, Kim MY. A pilot, double-blind, randomized, placebo-controlled trial of indinavir in patients with ALS. Neurology 2005, 64: 1298–1300	$n = 46$ Phase II 9 mo follow up	ALSFRS	Antiapoptotic, anti-viral	Negative: AE included nephrolithiasis and gastrointestinal problems
Topiramate (Topamax®, U.S.A.)	$n = 296$ 12 mo follow up	QMT in 8 arm muscles	Antiglutamate	Negative 2:1 randomization, unanticipated adverse events
Celecoxib (Celebrex®, U.S.A.) *Publication pending*	$n = 300$ 12 mo follow up	QMT in 8 arm muscles	Antiglutamate	2:1 randomization Negative
Pentoxifylline (Europe)	$N = 400$ 18 mo follow up	Death	Antiapoptotic	Negative
TCH 346 (Novartis, international)	$n = 500$ 4 mo lead in, 12 mo follow up 4 dose levels + placebo group	ALSFRS	Antiapoptotic	Negative

Abbreviations: IGF-I, Insuline-like growth factor-I; BDNF, brain-derived neurotrophic factor; CNTF, ciliary neurotrophic factor; QMT, quantitative muscle testing; FVC, forced vital capacity; (% predicted); VC, vital capacity; mo, month.

Source: From Refs. 3, 9, 24–27, 34–38, 41–43, 52, 56–59, 61, 71, 75, 83, 96, 101, 102.

Table 2 Selected Ongoing Randomized Phase-II/-III Clinical Trials

Drug	Design	Endpoint	Hypothesis	Comment
IGF-1 (U.S.A.)	n = 330 Phase III Study period 2 yr	MMT	Neurotrophic agent	Includes FVC >60% predicted, progressive motor weakness onset <24 mo
Minocycline (U.S.A.)	n = 400 Phase III 4 mo lead in 9 mo study period	ALSFRSr	Antiapoptotic (NOS)	Includes FVC >75% predicted Disease duration <3 yr
Creatine (U.S.A.)	n = 156 Phase III 10 g for 5 days, 5 g thereafter Study period 9 mo	MVIC, change in arm strength	Energy metabolism	Includes disease duration <5 yr
Coenzyme Q10 (U.S.A.)	n = 185 Phase II 9 mo study period	ALSFRSr	Mitochondrial cofactor, antioxidant	Includes FVC >60% and symptom onset <5 yr
Ceftriaxone	n = 60 in phase I n = 600 in Phase III Phases I–III in sequential, non-stop drug development design		Result of non-hypothesis driven drug screening process, antiglutamate	
Tamoxifen (U.S.A.)	n = 100 Phase II 12-wk follow up	MVIC	Hormonal hypothesis	
AEOL 10150 (U.S.A.)	n = 30 Subcutaneous	Dose finding	Antioxidant	
Ritonavir and hydroxyurea	6 mo follow up 25% patients on placebo		Antiviral	

More extensive lists are maintained and updated by patient voluntary and government organizations and available on the World Wide Web (for example From Ref. 28a)
Source: From Refs. 103, 104, 105.

promising because it prolonged survival in the transgenic mouse model of ALS, even when treatment was initiated at symptom onset, rather than in the presymptomatic phase (29).

Coenzyme Q10, an antioxidant and mitochondrial cofactor, was well tolerated in pilot studies (30) and is currently under phase-II evaluation. High-dose coenzyme Q10 is being studied in a randomized, controlled clinical trial including 185 ALS patients using an innovative two-stage design where a dose selection procedure is followed by an early efficacy test to determine whether it is justified to proceed to a phase-III clinical trial (Table 2).

Antiglutamate Strategies

An accumulating body of evidence suggests that glutamate, an excitatory neuro-transmitter, may contribute to motor neuron death in ALS (see Chapter 12). Three branched-chain amino acids can activate glutamate dehydrogenase. They have therefore been evaluated for the treatment of ALS based on the rationale that they would reduce glutamate levels. Several randomized clinical trials in Europe and the United States could not demonstrate any significant benefit for branched-chain amino acids (31–33).

A randomized, controlled, phase-II study of 2400 mg gabapentin daily in 152 ALS patients found a trend toward slower decline of arm strength in patients taking gabapentin compared with the placebo group (34). A subsequent phase-III trial of 3600 mg gabapentin daily in 204 ALS patients was unable to document a significant difference between the gabapentin and placebo groups (Table 1) (35). The primary outcome measure was the slope of the arm megascore, the average maximum volun-tary isometric strength from eight arm muscles standardized against a reference ALS population. This measure had demonstrated a non-significant treatment bene-fit in the phase-II study. However, it was associated with a high rate of missing visits and patient dropout of greater than 20%, suggesting that the testing may be too burdensome for many ALS patients. It cannot be excluded that the different dose used in the phase-II and -III trials may have contributed to the discrepancy in trial results.

The well-designed and implemented gabapentin trials have strengthened clini-cal trial infrastructure and study groups. The data have been provided to other inves-tigators to plan current ALS trials (e.g., minocycline, coenzyme Q10).

Two randomized clinical trials of lamotrigine in 30 and 67 ALS patients, respectively, did not find evidence of a functional benefit in ALS (36,37). A third medication used in the treatment of epilepsy, topiramate, was not beneficial in an ALS clinic trial (38). Patients were randomized to receive topiramate or placebo (2:1) for 12 months. There was no benefit on the primary outcome measure, the decline in arm muscle strength. However, the placebo data validated quantitative strength testing as predictor of survival, because the baseline score and the decline of strength over the initial three months were both predictive of survival (39). Patients on topiramate developed greater muscle and pulmonary impairment, and the open-label phase was discontinued because ALS patients receiving topira-mate had more deep vein thrombosis, pulmonary emboli, and renal calculi. These experiences underscored the importance of an independent data safety monitoring board. Many ALS investigators and data safety monitoring board members are now reluctant to support the practice of an open-label treatment extension in a clinical trial prior to data analysis. Overall, anti-glutamate strategies remain an important focus of ALS research, especially following the positive riluzole trials (see Section "Randomized, Controlled Clinical Trials of Riluzole").

Targeting Mitochondrial Function and Energy Metabolism

Mitochondrial impairment is thought to play an important role in the pathogenesis of ALS (see Chpater 17). Creatine, a natural compound central to energy metabolism, showed promise in the mouse model of ALS (40). However, two randomized, controlled clinical trials were negative: A well-designed study of 10 mg creatine in 175 ALS patients showed no survival benefit in a 16-month study (41). The group-sequential design was successful in allowing for the early detection of futility.

The investigators continued to monitor patients via telephone in case they were unable to travel to the trial site and achieved record follow up so that the actual survival status of all 175 participants was included in the final analysis. A second study evaluated the effect of 5 mg creatine daily on the decline in arm muscle strength and found no difference between creatine and placebo groups over a six-month follow-up period (42). This discrepancy between the positive animal studies and the negative clinical trial results raises doubts about the predictive value of animal studies in ALS. A third study in 156 ALS patients treated with 10 mg creatine for five days followed by 5 mg daily or placebo for a total follow-up period of nine months is underway in the United States (Table 2).

Neuronal Rescue by Growth Factors

Based on their survival-promoting effects on motor neurons in cell culture and animal models, neurotrophic factors that have emerged as possible treatments for ALS include insulin-like growth factor-1 (IGF-I) (43–45), brain-derived neurotrophic factor (BDNF) (46), ciliary neurotrophic factor (CNTF) (47), glial cell-line derived neurotrophic factor (GDNF) (48), and vascular endothelial growth factor (VEGF) (49,50). The preclinical studies were rapidly followed by a number of randomized, controlled clinical trials. A promising phase-I/-II trial of BDNF (51) was followed by a large randomized, controlled phase-III trial of 1135 ALS patients followed over six months that evaluated FVC change and survival in BDNF-treated patients compared to the placebo group (52). The primary analysis was negative, but secondary analyses suggested benefit. The unexpectedly low event rate may have reduced power in this study. Intrathecal BDNF was well tolerated in a phase-I/-II study in 25 ALS patients, but the study was not designed to evaluate efficacy (53). Although the BDNF trials failed to demonstrate a treatment benefit for BDNF, they resulted in the validation of a disease-specific functional rating scale, the ALS functional rating scale (ALSFRS). The validity of the ALSFRS has since been confirmed (54,55), and the ALSFRS is being used as primary outcome measure in several trials because it is easy to administer, well tolerated, and cost-effective (Table 2).

IGF-1 was studied in a randomized trial of 266 patients over nine months with a functional primary outcome (Appel scores). The study demonstrated less functional decline in the high-dose group (56). A second study in 183 ALS patients and with similar design did not confirm this result (57), but a meta-analysis of both trials suggests a modest effect (43). A third IGF-1 study is currently under way in the United States (Table 2).

CNTF was studied in two large randomized, placebo-controlled clinical trials including 730 (58) and 570 (59) patients, respectively. Adverse events were more frequent than anticipated in both trials. No treatment benefit was demonstrated in either trial, and a meta-analysis of the two trials combined found no effect of CNTF on disease progression (44).

Insufficient drug delivery to the target cells may have contributed to the failure to demonstrate a significant treatment effect of neurotrophic factors in ALS trials (44). Many of the neurotrophic factors underwent preclinical testing in the wobbler mouse model rather than in transgenic SOD1 mice. This raises doubts as to the predictive value of a successful treatment trial in the wobbler mouse model. However, this model is validated by the riluzole experience. On the basis of mouse studies, neurotrophic factors may be more effective when combined (60).

Sanofi SR57746A (Xaliproden®) is a small peptide with both neurotrophic and neuroprotective properties as well as good central nervous system (CNS) penetration. Two randomized, controlled clinical trials have been completed, one evaluating xaliproden alone, the second evaluating xaliproden in combination with riluzole. The trials were designed to have two co-primary endpoints defined as: (i) time to death, tracheostomy, or permanent-assisted ventilation (DTP) and (ii) time to VC of less than 50%.

The initial trial compared 1 or 2 mg SR57746A versus placebo in 867 ALS patients and found no significant effect on the primary outcome, but a non-significant beneficial effect on VC for the 2 mg dose arm. The subsequent trial studied SR57736A at 1 and 2 mg daily in combination with riluzole in 1210 ALS patients. The trial was overall negative but suggested a trend towards a beneficial effect of the 1 mg dose on VC (61).

Mitigating Motor Neuron Apoptosis

Evidence suggests that apoptotic pathways including the caspase group are activated in ALS contributing to motor neuron degeneration (see Chapters 11 and 15). Minocycline, a caspase inhibitor and microglial inhibitor, has shown benefit in preclinical studies (62,63). A pilot study demonstrated that minocycline was well tolerated in patients with ALS, although gastrointestinal side effects did occur (64). A phase-III clinical trial is currently under way (Table 2).

TCH346 (Novartis) binds glycareldehyde-3-phosphate dehydrogenase and prevents p53-related neuronal apoptosis. TCH346 slowed disease onset and progression in a mouse model of motor neuron disease (65), but not in the transgenic ALS mouse model (G93A) (66). A randomized, controlled, phase-II clinical trial has recently been completed following ALSFRSr scores over nine months in 500 ALS patients randomized to TCH346 or placebo after a four month lead-in period. No significant benefit for the TCH346 treated group was identified.

Antiviral Strategies

Infectious causes including viral etiologies have been implicated in the pathogenesis of ALS (see Chapter 21). In motor neuron disease associated with HIV infection, antiretroviral treatment can be associated with remarkable improvement (67–70). Scelsa and colleagues (28)b tested the benefits of indinavir in a pilot study in patients with sporadic ALS but no HIV infection. No clear benefits were found, although the number of patients was too small to make definitive conclusions. Patients who were on indinavir had more side effects such as nephrolithiasis and significant gastrointestinal symptoms.

A study of the HIV protease inhibitor ritonavir in combination with hydro-xyurea (a medication used in hematology/oncology as well as HIV multidrug treatment) is currently under way (Table 2).

Targeting Inflammation and Microglial Activation

Mounting evidence suggests that inflammatory pathways and microglia are activated in the pathogenesis of ALS (see Chapter 14). A randomized clinical trial in 300 ALS patients evaluated the efficacy of celcoxib, a cyclo-oxygenase-2 (COX-2) anagonist that had prolonged survival in transgenic ALS mice. Participants were randomized 2:1 to receive 800 mg celecoxib daily or placebo for 12 months. No difference between treatment groups was found for the primary outcome measure, i.e., the decline in muscle arm strength (71). The high frequency of missed visits and subject drop-out supported the notion that frequent quantitative muscle strength testing (MVIC) may be too burdensome for patients, and has led many investigators in the field to consider alternative outcome measures.

ONO-2506 is a glial cell-modulating factor and appears to have neuroprotecitve effects via its action on glial cells. Its neuroprotective effects have been demonstrated in animal models of brain ischemia (72) and Parkinson's disease (73). A clinical trial to evaluate ONO-2506 in the treatment of ALS is under way in Europe.

Neurovaccination strategies targeting the inflammatory processes that may contribute to motor neuron degeneration have been suggested in the treatment of ALS. Glatiramer acetate, a polypeptide mixture that has been approved by the FDA for the treatment of multiple sclerosis, has demonstrated moderate benefit in the transgenic mouse model of ALS and has recently been studied in a pilot trial at Columbia University (74).

Other Neuroprotective Strategies

The xanthine derivative pentoxyfilline (EHT 0201) is thought to have neuroprotective properties based on preclinical studies and has recently been evaluated in a phase-II trial as a potential treatment for ALS. Four hundred subjects were enrolled within four months and treated with EHT 0201 as an add-on therapy to riluzole. The study period was 18 months with patient survival regardless of tracheostomy/ventilation status as the primary efficacy endpoint. No difference was found between treatment groups (75).

Tamoxifen, an anti–breast cancer agent, is a protein kinase C inhibitor. Anecdotally, a patient with breast cancer experienced marked slowing of ALS progression when treated with tamoxifen. Abnormally activated protein kinase and abnormally phosphorylated proteins have been found in degenerating motor neurons. On the basis of promising preclinical data, tamoxifen is currently undergoing early clinical testing. The drug was overall well tolerated but was associated with frequent hot flashes. In the same study population, data from an extended follow-up period suggested that patients receiving 20 to 40 mg of tamoxifen daily had longer survival compared with patients receiving only 10 mg daily. Further evaluation is under consideration (76).

Ceftriaxone is a cephalosporine identified as candidate treatment for ALS in a non-hypothesis driven research effort. In this NINDS led initiative, 1040 FDA approved drugs were tested in over 28 in-vitro assays relevant to neurodegeneration (77). Follow up in-vitro testing suggested an effect of ceftriaxone on the astrocytic glutamate transporter, EAAT2. In addition, it is thought to have antioxidant and calcium-binding properties. Ceftriaxone penetrates the blood–brain barrier. In rodent brains, it increases EAAT2 promotor activation (78). An NIH-funded, double-blind, placebo-controlled clinical trial of Ceftriaxone in 600 ALS patients is scheduled to begin in 2005. An initial phase-I stage compares two dose levels to placebo in 60 ALS patients. If the drug is found safe, subjects will continue into an efficacy stage with survival as primary endopint after a miminum follow-up period of 12 months.

Stem cell therapy has not been evaluated in controllled clinical trials. Preliminary, small, open label trials in ALS patients have been reported at motor neuron disease conferences using allogenic hematopoietic stem cells (79) or autologous cultured bone marrow mesenchymal stem cells that were directly injected into the lumbar spinal cord (80–82). These efforts are in very early stages and require extensive basic research, animal studies, and feasibility studies before their efficacy can be evaluated.

Clinical Trials for Symptomatic Treatment of ALS

Few studies have systematically evaluated palliative pharmacotherapy in ALS. Dextromethorphan, an NMDA receptor antagonist, was initially explored as a potential curative treatment for ALS. The investigators noted that it did not significantly alter the course of ALS, but that it improved pseudobulbar symptoms (uncontrolled laughter or crying). As a result, dextromethorphan with or without concurrent quinidine (a P450 inhibitor slowing dextromethorphan metabolism) was studied in a randomized, controlled clinical trial in 140 ALS patients. The combination of dextromethorphan and quinidine significantly improved pseudobulbar symptoms as measured by a clinical scale (83).

Two randomized studies have evaluated the benefits of noninvasive positive-pressure ventilation (NIPPV). Twenty-two ALS patients receiving NIPPV survived significantly longer and had higher quality of life (QoL) scores than 19 ALS patients receiving standard care (84). A second prospective, randomized trial studied the timing of NIPPV by comparing two physiologic markers to be used as a trigger for starting NIPPV. Twenty ALS patients were randomized to receive NIPPV based upon nocturnal oxymetry with O_2 saturations <90% for one cumulative minute (early intervention), or to receive NIPPV based on FVC <50% predicted (standard of care). The results suggest that nocturnal oxymetry may be a more sensitive indicator of early respiratory insufficiency and that the early intervention may result in improved QoL (85).

A prospective study of the effects of NIPPV and nutritional care is currently under way (PI: Edward Kasarskis, University of Kentucky).

ISSUES THAT MAY HAVE NEGATIVELY AFFECTED RECENT ALS CLINICAL TRIALS

Validity of Animal Models for Drug Testing in ALS

Numerous candidate treatments for ALS have been tested in rodent models, and many have resulted in statistically significant improvement of the disease course (86). Among the drugs with positive results in animal testing, none held its promise in the clinical arena. Riluzole is the exception: it had not been tested in the transgenic mouse model prior to the positive human clinical trial, but was later found to produce a survival benefit in transgenic ALS mice and wobbler mice (4,5).

Following the discovery of mutations in SOD1 in familial ALS several transgenic rodent models have been created (87–90). Before transgenic mice were available, drugs had been tested in other motor neuron disease animal models including the wobbler, pmn, and mnd mice (see Chapter 23). The poor correlation between animal and human trials for most drugs may be due to several factors including the following:

1. *Timing*: Treatment in mouse models is often initiated in the presymptomatic phase in animal studies. In human ALS trials, patients are typically included when they have reached a specified level of diagnostic certainty. This time point usually occurs more than a year after symptom onset and probably at an even longer interval to the onset of subclinical motor neuron loss (91). Treating transgenic ALS mice after symptom onset is more challenging because of the relatively rapid disease course in some models, but has shown positive results (92).

2. *Model adequacy*: The animal model based on a genetically engineered defect in SOD1 may not be representative of the human ALS patient population, given that only 10% have familial disease, and among these, only 20% have an SOD1 mutation, and fewer harbor the specific mutation used in preclinical animal testing. With regards to tolerability, rodents and humans may differ in metabolism and toxicity for a given drug.

3. *Interpretation of benefit in a mouse model*: There are several types of transgenic mouse models, based on different mutations or variations in transgenic techniques. Some transgenic mice have several copies of the mutant gene and more rapidly progressive disease, other models progress more slowly (87,90,93). When comparing results between experiments, it is thus preferable to compare survival benefit relative to survival in a given mouse model rather than absolute differences in survival (94).

4. *Drug dose and delivery*: Daily doses used in animal studies may be higher than the equivalent doses by weight that are tolerated by humans. In animal experiments, study drug may be administered chronically in food or water rather than in two or three daily doses.

Pharmacological Properties of Candidate Drugs

Some drugs are promising in vitro or animal models, but do not cross the blood–brain barrier sufficiently in ALS patients. In parallel to preclinical research aimed at evaluating safety and toxicity, we need research on drug transport across the blood–brain barrier. This includes not only studies measuring the CNS penetrance of a specific experimental drug, but also more basic research into the properties of the blood–brain barrier and as well as research into ways to enhance transport. For those drugs without sufficient CNS penetrance, modifications can be explored to enhance transport into the CNS (including lipid-, carrier-, and receptor-mediated transport) (95).

Outcome Measures

ALS clinical trials have used a number of different outcome measures in the search for a valid primary endpoint. A suitable endpoint is one that can be reliably ascertained. Its variance in the study population has to be such that a meaningful effect can be demonstrated with a feasible sample size. When a clinical trial fails to demonstrate a difference between treatment groups, different factors may have contributed. In addition to a truly ineffective study drug, the outcome measure may not have been sensitive enough to detect change under the experimental conditions of the trial.

Validation

A clinical trial outcome measure is considered suitable when its use can demonstrate a meaningful difference between treatment groups. The riluzole trials used tracheostomy-free survival as primary outcome (3,6). The positive results leading to FDA approval validated this method and survival became the primary outcome in subsequent trials. When a series of consecutive trials was negative, researchers reconsidered their trial designs. Using a functional outcome measure, the Appel ALS scale, the US IGF-1 study was able to demonstrate a significant delay in functional deterioration in patients treated with IGF-1 (56). IGF-1 was not approved by the FDA because a European companion trial was negative (57). Pulmonary function measures were able to distinguish between the treatment and placebo groups in both SR 57746A (Xaliproden®) trials: for the 2 mg group in the initial study, a significant relative risk reduction was found for time to VC <50%. Similarly, there was a trend suggesting risk reduction in favor of the add-on 1 mg dose xaliproden for time to VC <50% (61). Quantitative MVIC demonstrated differences between treatment groups in several studies: The gabapentin-II study showed a trend towards slower arm muscle strength decline in favor of the gabapentin group (34). In the ACTS group CNTF and the topiramate trials, the primary MVIC endpoint allowed detecting a more rapid decline in the active treatment groups compared with the placebo group (38,58).

Death as Primary Endpoint

The riluzole clinical trials used death as primary endpoint (3,96). As they led to FDA approval, death has been the gold standard endpoint in subsequent clinical trials. However, death in the reality of ALS trials may not be as robust an endpoint as it is in other diseases. Death in ALS typically occurs as a result of respiratory failure and researchers have therefore used qualifiers to adjust for the use of life-extending respiratory treatment.

Time to death or tracheostomy were used as endpoint in several trials including those evaluating riluzole (3,96), creatine (41), and vitamin E (27). Tracheostomy placement typically occurs when a patient needs permanent ventilator support. In some patients, however, tracheostomy placement occurs for secretion management and may then not be associated with permanent ventilation.

Dual mortality and respiratory endpoints were the primary outcome in clinical trials evaluating BDNF (52) and SR 57746A (Xaliproden®) (61). However, dual endpoints may result in loss of power because a Bonferroni correction is needed to each of the two primary endpoints to maintain an overall type-I error rate of 0.05.

The widespread use of NIPPV has raised the question whether NIPPV dependence (defined for example as > 18 hours daily NIPPV use) should be considered as endpoint equivalent to tracheostomy. Considering time to respiratory failure and time to death as equivalent may be clinically intuitive, but takes away the main advantage of death as endpoint. Death is considered a robust endpoint because there ought not to be any measurement errors. More importantly, even when contact with a study subject has been disrupted, the investigators can usually at least ascertain survival status and when applicable to the date of death. Respiratory failure endpoints can introduce additional confounders: The practice and timing of respiratory intervention likely varies across sites. This is of particular concern in multinational trials because differences in health care access and cultural attitudes likely influence the use and timing of respiratory support. Similarly, respiratory treatment for ALS is evolving over time. The increase in NIPPV use over the last decade complicates comparisons of present and past ALS cohorts. The European pentoxifylline trial used death as endpoint in the primary analysis, without qualifiers for respiratory status (75).

Functional Outcome Measures

Ascertaining a functional outcome measure introduces issues related to measurement precision as well as intra- and inter-rater reliability. The investigators have to ensure adequate evaluator training and certification throughout the trial, which typically requires significant planning and resources. Several ALS clinical trials have used quantitative MVIC as primary outcome measure (35,38,42,71,97). This outcome measure restricts trial participation to clinical sites that have access to the expensive equipment needed and have staff trained to perform the testing. Muscle strength testing can be burdensome to disabled ALS patients who may not be able to complete the testing as required. This results in excess missing data and may have increase drop out.

Clinical Trial Design and Implementation

Center effects may confound study results. Medical care for ALS patient varies between centers and probably even more between different countries. In the phase-III riluzole study, survival curves were different comparing between North American and European sites (96). The use and timing of NIPPV, gastrostomy placement, and riluzole may vary among sites (17,98,99). When randomization is not balanced among study sites, the results may be jeopardized.

Time effects need to be considered. Some investigators have advocated the use of historical controls, in particular in phase-II trials. However, with changes in the medical management of ALS, the "natural history" in the placebo groups of clinical trials differs from one study to another (25,34,35).

The size of the expected effect may have been set too large in some trials. Given that only one medication has been FDA approved for the treatment of ALS to date, even a modest effect may be clinically meaningful.

This needs to be weighed against the feasibility of a clinical trial powered to detect a small effect size given the finite number of potential trial participants and the limited resources available for ALS research.

Missing data and loss to follow up can call clinical trial results into question. ALS trials with survival as primary endpoint have experienced relatively small amounts of missing data (3,41,52). However, clinical trials using functional primary endpoints have reported missing data from 20% or more visits (35,38). If there are differences in the amount of missing data by treatment group, the results may be invalid. The intent-to-treat principle requires that data from all patients randomized enter into the analysis, resulting in the imputation of missing data with the inherent limitations (100). It is therefore important for investigators to design ALS trials with the goal of avoiding missing data. Strategies may include patient-friendly visit schedules, allocating resources for home visits in case patients are unable to travel, and outcome measures that can be ascertained remotely (e.g., survival status, functional rating scale by telephone).

CONCLUSION

The impressive series of large, randomized, multicenter trials for ALS has resulted in the approval of rizulole, the first medication effective in the treatment of ALS. The successful riluzole trials have changed the practice of ALS care and have demonstrated that clinical trials can identify new treatments for this disease. It is unknown whether subsequent trials were negative because the drugs tested were truly ineffective, or whether the clinical trials lacked sensitivity to demonstrate their benefit. Because of this uncertainty, ALS investigators have used different trial designs and outcome measures over time. The modifications in ALS trial design have undoubtedly improved clinical trials, but have also made it more difficult to compare data across trials.

We will not be able to ultimately judge a new ALS trial design unless it is validated by a positive clinical trial. Therefore, it may be helpful to focus on what can be learned from the recent ALS trials experience: (i) Clinical trials in ALS are feasible and can lead to drug approval. Often, controlled trials did not confirm preclinical or anecdotal experience. Therefore, controlled trials are needed to evaluate the effectiveness of a new treatment in patients. (ii) In some cases, new treatments not only lacked benefit but also worsened the course of ALS due to adverse events. This underscores the difficulties of treating a patient clinically with drugs of uncertain efficacy. Instead, clinicians should educate patients on the benefits of clinical trial participation. (iii) Trial designs that include frequent and physically demanding visits may lead to excess missing data, threatening the validity of the results. (iv) The only trial that led to drug approval used a conventional time-to-event design with robust endpoint (tracheostomy-free survival). Therefore, this design should be considered in phase-III drug evaluation. (v) Recruitment has been challenging in recent trials. Therefore, ALS trials that include sites outside of large ALS centers may allow the timely recruitment of a larger proportion of ALS patients into trials.

ALS research has seen remarkable progress over the last decade. Laboratory researchers have improved our understanding of ALS pathogenesis and identified molecular targets for treatment. Advances in robotic technology have facilitated the rapid in-vitro screening of a large number of potential treatments for ALS. Animal models allow for preclinical efficacy testing. Clinical investigators have improved clinical trials methodology, strengthened collaborations, and established the infrastructure for regional and national clinical trial consortia. These advances in all areas of ALS drug development are setting the stage for the long-awaited second positive trial in ALS.

REFERENCES

1. Shaw PJ, Ince PG. Glutamate, excitotoxicity and amyotrophic lateral sclerosis. J Neurol 1997; 244(suppl 2):S3–S14.
2. Bryson HM, Fulton B, Benfield P. Riluzole. A review of its pharmacodynamic and pharmacokinetic properties and therapeutic potential in amyotrophic lateral sclerosis. Drugs 1996; 52(4):549–563.
3. Bensimon G, Lacomblez L, Meininger V. A controlled trial of riluzole in amyotrophic lateral sclerosis. ALS/Riluzole study group. N Engl J Med 1994; 330(9):585–591.
4. Gurney ME, Cutting FB, Zhai P, Doble A, Taylor CP, Andrus PK, Hall ED. Benefit of vitamin E, riluzole, and gabapentin in a transgenic model of familial amyotrophic lateral sclerosis. Ann Neurol 1996; 39(2):147–157.

5. Ishiyama T, Okada R, Nishibe H, Mitsumoto H, Nakayama C. Riluzole slows the progression of neuromuscular dysfunction in the wobbler mouse motor neuron disease. Brain Res 2004; 1019(1,2):226–236.

6. Lacomblez L, Bensimon G, Leigh PN, Guillet P, Meininger V. Dose-ranging study of riluzole in amyotrophic lateral sclerosis. Amyotrophic lateral sclerosis/riluzole study group II. Lancet 1996; 347(9013):1425–1431.

7. Bensimon G, Lacomblez L, Delumeau JC, Bejuit R, Truffinet P, Meininger V. A study of riluzole in the treatment of advanced stage or elderly patients with amyotrophic lateral sclerosis. J Neurol 2002; 249(5):609–615.

8. Miller RG, Mitchell JD, Lyon M, Moore DH. Riluzole for amyotrophic lateral sclerosis (ALS)/motor neuron disease (MND). Cochrane Database Syst Rev 2002; (2): CD001447.

9. Debove C, Zeisser P, Salzman PM, Powe LK, Truffinet P. The Rilutek (riluzole) global early access programme: an open-label safety evaluation in the treatment of amyotrophic lateral sclerosis. Amyotroph Lateral Scler Other Motor Neuron Disord 2001; 2(3):153–158.

10. Traynor BJ, Alexander M, Corr B, Frost E, Hardiman O. An outcome study of riluzole in amyotrophic lateral sclerosis—a population-based study in Ireland, 1996–2000. J Neurol 2003; 250(4):473–479.

11. Groeneveld GJ, Van Kan HJ, Kalmijn S, Veldink JH, Guchelaar HJ, Wokke JH, Van den Berg LH. Riluzole serum concentrations in patients with ALS: associations with side effects and symptoms. Neurology 2003; 61(8):1141–1143.

12. Riviere M, Meininger V, Zeisser P, Munsat T. An analysis of extended survival in patients with amyotrophic lateral sclerosis treated with riluzole. Arch Neurol 1998; 55(4):526–528.

13. Bensimon G, Doble A. The tolerability of riluzole in the treatment of patients with amyotrophic lateral sclerosis. Expert Opin Drug Saf 2004; 3(6):525–534.

14. Anonymous. Entry for rilutek tablets. Physician's Desk Reference, 2003.

15. Practice advisory on the treatment of amyotrophic lateral sclerosis with riluzole: Report of the Quality Standards Subcommittee of the American Academy of Neurology. Neurology 1997; 49(3):657–659.

16. National Institute for Clinical Excellence–Guidance on the use of riluzole (Rilutek) for the treatment of motor neurone disease. Technol Appraisal Guidance 2001:20.

17. Bryan WW, McIntire D, Camperlengo L, et al. Factors influencing the use of riluzole by ALS patients [abstract]. 8th International Sympsium on ALS/MND. J Neurol Sci 1997.

18. Traynor BJ, Alexander M, Corr B, Frost E, Hardiman O. Effect of a multidisciplinary amyotrophic lateral sclerosis (ALS) clinic on ALS survival: a population based study, 1996–2000. J Neurol Neurosurg Psychiatry 2003; 74(9):1258–1261.

19. Miller RG, Mitsumoto H, Brooks B, Gowda N, Anderson FA, Group ftAC. Temporal trends in the treatment of ALS in North America: findings from the ALS CARE patient databse 1997–2004 [abstr]. Amyotroph Lateral Scler Other Motor Neuron Disord 2004; 5(suppl 2):42.

20. Murray B, Mitsumoto H. Drug therapy in amyotrophic lateral sclerosis. Adv Neurol 2002; 88:63–82.

21. www.als.net/research/studies.

22. Gordon PH. Advances in clinical trials for amyotrophic lateral sclerosis. Curr Neurol Neurosci Rep 2005; 5(1):48–54.

23. Orrell R, Lane J, Ross M. Antioxidant treatment for amyotrophic lateral sclerosis/ motor neuron disease. Cochrane Database Syst Rev 2004; (4):CD002829.

24. Louwerse ES, Weverling GJ, Bossuyt PM, Meyjes FE, de Jong JM. Randomized, double-blind, controlled trial of acetylcysteine in amyotrophic lateral sclerosis. Arch Neurol 1995; 52(6):559–564.

25. Lange DJ, Murphy PL, Diamond B, Appel V, Lai EC, Younger DS, Appel SH. Selegiline is ineffective in a collaborative double-blind, placebo-controlled trial for treatment of amyotrophic lateral sclerosis. Arch Neurol 1998; 55(1):93–96.

26. Desnuelle C, Dib M, Garrel C, Favier A. A double-blind, placebo-controlled randomized clinical trial of alpha-tocopherol (vitamin E) in the treatment of amyotrophic lateral sclerosis. ALS riluzole-tocopherol study group. Amyotroph Lateral Scler Other Motor Neuron Disord 2001; 2(1):9–18.

27. Graf M, Ecker D, Horowski R, Kramer B, Riederer P, Gerlach M, Hager C, Ludolph AC, Becker G, Osterhage J, et al. High dose vitamin E therapy in amyotrophic lateral sclerosis as add-on therapy to riluzole: results of a placebo-controlled double-blind study. J Neural Transm 2004.

28. Yoshino H. Randomized, placebo-controlled double blind study of free radical scavenger, edavarone in amyotrophic lateral sclerosis [abstr]. ALS Other Motor Neuron Disorders 2004; 5(suppl 2):24.

28a. at mdausa.org, alsa.org, and clinicaltrials.gov.

29. Kiaei M, Kipiani K, Petri S, Chen J, Calingasan NY, Crow JP, Beal MF. A novel catalytic antioxidant, manganese porphyrin (AEOL 10150) slows disease progression and extends lifespan in transgenic mouse model [abstr]. Amyotroph Lateral Scler Other Motor Neuron Disord 2004; 5(suppl 2):90.

30. Ferrante KL, Shefner JM, Betensky RA, O'Brien ML, Taft JM, Yu H, Fantasia MI, Zhang H, Ahsburn C, Florence J, et al. Clinical trial of coenzyme Q10 in patients with amyotrophic alteral sclerosis [abstr]. ALS Other Motor Neuron Disorders 2004; 5(suppl 2):25.

31. Tandan R, Bromberg MB, Forshew D, Fries TJ, Badger GJ, Carpenter J, Krusinski PB, Betts EF, Arciero K, Nau K. A controlled trial of amino acid therapy in amyotrophic lateral sclerosis: I. Clinical, functional, and maximum isometric torque data. Neurology 1996; 47(5):1220–1226.

32. Branched-chain amino acids and amyotrophic lateral sclerosis: a treatment failure? The Italian ALS Study Group. Neurology 1993; 43(12):2466–2470.

33. Parton M, Mitsumoto H, Leigh PN. Amino acids for amyotrophic lateral sclerosis/motor neuron disease. Cochrane Database Syst Rev 2003; (4):CD003457.

34. Miller RG, Moore D, Young LA, Armon C, Barohn RJ, Bromberg MB, Bryan WW, Gelinas DF, Mendoza MC, Neville HE, et al. Placebo-controlled trial of gabapentin in patients with amyotrophic lateral sclerosis. WALS Study Group. Western Amyotrophic Lateral Sclerosis Study Group. Neurology 1996; 47(6):1383–1388.

35. Miller RG, Moore DH II, Gelinas DF, Dronsky V, Mendoza M, Barohn RJ, Bryan W, Ravits J, Yuen E, Neville H, et al. Phase III randomized trial of gabapentin in patients with amyotrophic lateral sclerosis. Neurology 2001; 56(7):843–848.

36. Ryberg H, Askmark H, Persson LI. A double-blind randomized clinical trial in amyotrophic lateral sclerosis using lamotrigine: effects on CSF glutamate, aspartate, branched-chain amino acid levels and clinical parameters. Acta Neurol Scand 2003; 108(1):1–8.

37. Eisen A, Stewart H, Schulzer M, Cameron D. Anti-glutamate therapy in amyotrophic lateral sclerosis: a trial using lamotrigine. Can J Neurol Sci 1993; 20(4):297–301.

38. Cudkowicz ME, Shefner JM, Schoenfeld DA, Brown RH Jr, Johnson H, Qureshi M, Jacobs M, Rothstein JD, Appel SH, Pascuzzi RM, et al. A randomized, placebo-controlled trial of topiramate in amyotrophic lateral sclerosis. Neurology 2003; 61(4):456–464.

39. Cudkowicz M, Zhang H, Qureshi M, Schoenfeld D. Maximum voluntary isometric contraction (MVIC). Amyotroph Lateral Scler Other Motor Neuron Disord 2004; 5(suppl 1):84–85.

40. Klivenyi P, Ferrante RJ, Matthews RT, Bogdanov MB, Klein AM, Andreassen OA, Mueller G, Wermer M, Kaddurah-Daouk R, Beal MF. Neuroprotective effects of creatine in a transgenic animal model of amyotrophic lateral sclerosis. Nat Med 1999; 5(3):347–350.

41. Groeneveld GJ, Veldink JH, van der Tweel I, Kalmijn S, Beijer C, de Visser M, Wokke JH, Franssen H, van den Berg LH. A randomized sequential trial of creatine in amyotrophic lateral sclerosis. Ann Neurol 2003; 53(4):437–445.

42. Shefner JM, Cudkowicz ME, Schoenfeld D, Conrad T, Taft J, Chilton M, Urbinelli L, Qureshi M, Zhang H, Pestronk A, et al. A clinical trial of creatine in ALS. Neurology 2004; 63(9):1656–1661.

43. Mitchell JD, Wokke JH, Borasio GD. Recombinant human insulin-like growth factor I (rhIGF-I) for amyotrophic lateral sclerosis/motor neuron disease. Cochrane Database Syst Rev 2002; (3):CD002064.

44. Bongioanni P, Reali C, Sogos V. Ciliary neurotrophic factor (CNTF) for amyotrophic lateral sclerosis/motor neuron disease. Cochrane Database Syst Rev 2004; (3): CD004302.

45. Neff NT, Prevette D, Houenou LJ, Lewis ME, Glicksman MA, Yin QW, Oppenheim RW. Insulin-like growth factors: putative muscle-derived trophic agents that promote motoneuron survival. J Neurobiol 1993; 24(12):1578–1588.

46. Henderson CE, Camu W, Mettling C, Gouin A, Poulsen K, Karihaloo M, Rullamas J, Evans T, McMahon SB, Armanini MP, Berkemeier L, Phillips HS, Rosenthal A. Neurotrophins promote motor neuron survival and are present in embryonic limb bud. Nature 1993; 363(6426):266–270.

47. Arakawa Y, Sendtner M, Thoenen H. Survival effect of ciliary neurotrophic factor (CNTF) on chick embryonic motoneurons in culture: comparison with other neurotrophic factors and cytokines. J Neurosci 1990; 10(11):3507–3515.

48. Henderson CE, Phillips HS, Pollock RA, Davies AM, Lemeulle C, Armanini M, Simmons L, Moffot B, Vandlen RA, Simpson LC, Moffet B, Vandlen RA, Koliatsas VE, Rosenthal A. GDNF: a potent survival factor for motoneurons present in peripheral nerve and muscle. Science 1994; 266(5187):1062–1064.

49. Lambrechts D, Storkebaum E, Morimoto M, Del-Favero J, Desmet F, Marklund SL, Wyns S, Thijs V, Andersson J, van Marion I, et al. VEGF is a modifier of amyotrophic lateral sclerosis in mice and humans and protects motoneurons against ischemic death. Nat Genet 2003; 34(4):383–394.

50. Zheng C, Nennesmo I, Fadeel B, Henter JI. Vascular endothelial growth factor prolongs survival in a transgenic mouse model of ALS. Ann Neurol 2004; 56(4): 564–567.

51. Bradley WG. A phase I/II study of recombinant brain-derived neurotrophic in patients with ALS [abstr]. Ann Neurol 1995; 38:971.

52. A controlled trial of recombinant methionyl human BDNF in ALS: the BDNF Study Group (Phase III). Neurology 1999; 52(7):1427–1433.

53. Ochs G, Penn RD, York M, Giess R, Beck M, Tonn J, Haigh J, Malta E, Traub M, Sendtner M, et al. A phase I/II trial of recombinant methionyl human brain derived neurotrophic factor administered by intrathecal infusion to patients with amyotrophic lateral sclerosis. Amyotroph Lateral Scler Other Motor Neuron Disord 2000; 1(3):201–206.

54. Traynor BJ, Zhang H, Shefner JM, Schoenfeld D, Cudkowicz ME. Functional outcome measures as clinical trial endpoints in ALS. Neurology 2004; 63(10):1933–1935.

55. Kaufmann P, Levy G, Thompson JL, Delbene ML, Battista V, Gordon PH, Rowland LP, Levin B, Mitsumoto H. The ALSFRSr predicts survival time in an ALS clinic population. Neurology 2005; 64(1):38–43.

56. Lai EC, Felice KJ, Festoff BW, Gawel MJ, Gelinas DF, Kratz R, Murphy MF, Natter HM, Norris FH, Rudnicki SA. Effect of recombinant human insulin-like growth factor-I on progression of ALS. A placebo-controlled study. The North America ALS/IGF-I Study Group. Neurology 1997; 49(6):1621–1630.

57. Borasio GD, Robberecht W, Leigh PN, Emile J, Guiloff RJ, Jerusalem F, Silani V, Vos PE, Wokke JH, Dobbins T. A placebo-controlled trial of insulin-like growth

factor-I in amyotrophic lateral sclerosis. European ALS/IGF-I Study Group. Neurology 1998; 51(2):583–586.

58. A double-blind placebo-controlled clinical trial of subcutaneous recombinant human ciliary neurotrophic factor (rHCNTF) in amyotrophic lateral sclerosis. ALS CNTF Treatment Study Group. Neurology 1996; 46(5):1244–1249.
59. Miller RG, Petajan JH, Bryan WW, Armon C, Barohn RJ, Goodpasture JC, Hoagland RJ, Parry GJ, Ross MA, Stromatt SC. A placebo-controlled trial of recombinant human ciliary neurotrophic (rhCNTF) factor in amyotrophic lateral sclerosis. rhCNTF ALS Study Group. Ann Neurol 1996; 39(2):256–260.
60. Mitsumoto H, Ikeda K, Klinkosz B, Cedarbaum JM, Wong V, Lindsay RM. Arrest of motor neuron disease in wobbler mice cotreated with CNTF and BDNF. Science 1994; 265(5175):1107–1110.
61. Meininger V, Bensimon G, Bradley WR, Brooks B, Douillet P, Eisen AA, Lacomblez L, Leigh PN, Robberecht W. Efficacy and safety of xaliproden in amyotrophic lateral sclerosis: results of two phase III trials. Amyotroph Lateral Scler Other Motor Neuron Disord 2004; 5(2):107–117.
62. Zhu S, Stavrovskaya IG, Drozda M, Kim BY, Ona V, Li M, Sarang S, Liu AS, Hartley DM, Wu du C, et al. Minocycline inhibits cytochrome c release and delays progression of amyotrophic lateral sclerosis in mice. Nature 2002; 417(6884):74–78.
63. Kriz J, Nguyen MD, Julien JP. Minocycline slows disease progression in a mouse model of amyotrophic lateral sclerosis. Neurobiol Dis 2002; 10(3):268–278.
64. Gordon PH, Moore DH, Gelinas DF, Qualls C, Meister ME, Werner J, Mendoza M, Mass J, Kushner G, Miller RG. Placebo-controlled phase I/II studies of minocycline in amyotrophic lateral sclerosis. Neurology 2004; 62(10):1845–1847.
65. Sagot Y, Toni N, Perrelet D, Lurot S, King B, Rixner H, Mattenberger L, Waldmeier PC, Kato AC. An orally active anti-apoptotic molecule (CGP 3466B) preserves mitochondria and enhances survival in an animal model of motoneuron disease. Br J Pharmacol 2000; 131(4):721–728.
66. Groeneveld GJ, Van Muiswinkel FL, de Leeuw van Weenen J, Blauw H, Veldink JH, Wokke JH, Van Den Berg L, Baer P. CGP 3466B has no effect on disease course of (G93A) mSOD1 transgenic mice. Amyotroph Lateral Scler Other Motor Neuron Disord 2004; 5(4):220–225.
67. Verma RK, Ziegler DK, Kepes JJ. HIV-related neuromuscular syndrome simulating motor neuron disease. Neurology 1990; 40(3 Pt 1):544–546.
68. Huang PP, Chin R, Song S, Lasoff S. Lower motor neuron dysfunction associated with human immunodeficiency virus infection. Arch Neurol 1993; 50(12):1328–1330.
69. Galassi G, Gentilini M, Ferrari S, Ficarra G, Zonari P, Mongiardo N, Tommelleri G, Di Rienzo B. Motor neuron disease and HIV-1 infection in a 30-year-old HIV-positive heroin abuser: a causal relationship? Clin Neuropathol 1998; 17(3):131–135.
70. MacGowan DJ, Scelsa SN, Waldron M. An ALS-like syndrome with new HIV infection and complete response to antiretroviral therapy. Neurology 2001; 57(6):1094–1097.
71. Cudkowicz M, Shefner JM, Schoenfeld D, Rothstein J, Drachman DB, Neals NAC. Clinical trial of celecoxib in subjects with amyotrophic lateral sclerosis [abstr]. ALS Other Motor Neuron Disorders 2004; 5(suppl 2):C35,25.
72. Mori T, Tateishi N, Kagamiishi Y, Shimoda T, Satoh S, Ono S, Katsube N, Asano T. Attenuation of a delayed increase in the extracellular glutamate level in the peri-infarct area following focal cerebral ischemia by a novel agent ONO-2506. Neurochem Int 2004; 45(2,3):381–387.
73. Kato H, Araki T, Imai Y, Takahashi A, Itoyama Y. Protection of dopaminergic neurons with a novel astrocyte modulating agent (R)-(-)-2-propyloctanoic acid (ONO-2506) in an MPTP-mouse model of Parkinson's disease. J Neurol Sci 2003; 208(1–2):9–15.
74. Angelov DN, Waibel S, Guntinas-Lichius O, Lenzen M, Neiss WF, Tomov TL, Yoles E, Kipnis J, Schori H, Reuter A, et al. Therapeutic vaccine for acute and chronic motor

neuron diseases: implications for amyotrophic lateral sclerosis. Proc Natl Acad Sci USA 2003; 100(8):4790–4795.

75. Meininger V. Presentation at 15th ALS/MND symposium, Philadelphia, 2004.

76. Brooks B. Presentation at the 15th International Symposium on ALS/MND in Philadelphia, 2004.

77. Miller TM, Cleveland DW. Medicine. Treating neurodegenerative diseases with antibiotics. Science 2005; 307(5708):361–362.

78. Rothstein JD, Patel S, Regan MR, Haenggeli C, Huang YH, Bergles DE, Jin L, Dykes Hoberg M, Vidensky S, Chung DS, et al. Beta-lactam antibiotics offer neuroprotection by increasing glutamate transporter expression. Nature 2005; 433(7021):73–77.

79. Appel SH, Engelhardt J, Henkel JS, Simpson EP, Luo Y, Brenner MK, Popat UR. Allogeneic hematopoietic stem cell transplantation in ALS. Amyotroph Lateral Scler Other Motor Neuron Disord 2004; 5(4).

80. Mazzini L, Fagioli F, Boccaletti R. Stem-cell therapy in amyotrophic lateral sclerosis. Lancet 2004; 364(9449):1936–1937.

81. Mazzini L, Fagioli F, Boccaletti R, Mareschi K, Oliveri G, Olivieri C, Pastore I, Marasso R, Madon E. Stem cell therapy in amyotrophic lateral sclerosis: a methodological approach in humans. Amyotroph Lateral Scler Other Motor Neuron Disord 2003; 4(3):158–161.

82. Silani V, Cova L, Corbo M, Ciammola A, Polli E. Stem-cell therapy for amyotrophic lateral sclerosis. Lancet 2004; 364(9429):200–202.

83. Brooks BR, Thisted RA, Appel SH, Bradley WG, Olney RK, Berg JE, Pope LE, Smith RA. Treatment of pseudobulbar affect in ALS with dextromethorphan/quinidine: a randomized trial. Neurology 2004; 63(8):1364–1370.

84. Bourke SC, Tomlinson M, Willams TL, Shaw PJ, Bullack RE, Gilson GJ. Randomized controlled trial of non-invasive ventilation in amyotrophic lateral sclerosis [abstr]. Amyotroph Lateral Scler Other Motor Neuron Disord 2004; 5(suppl 2):59.

85. Jackson CE, Rosenfeld J, Moore DH, Bryan WW, Barohn RJ, Wrench M, Myers D, Heberlin L, King R, Smith J, et al. A preliminary evaluation of a prospective study of pulmonary function studies and symptoms of hypoventilation in ALS/MND patients. J Neurol Sci 2001; 191(1,2):75–78.

86. Cleveland DW, Rothstein JD. From Charcot to Lou Gehrig: deciphering selective motor neuron death in ALS. Nat Rev Neurosci 2001; 2(11):806–819.

87. Gurney ME, Pu H, Chiu AY, Dal Canto MC, Polchow CY, Alexander DD, Caliendo J, Hentati A, Kwon YW, Deng HX, Chen W, Zhai P, Sujit RL, Siddique T. Motor neuron degeneration in mice that express a human Cu, Zn superoxide dismutase mutation. Science 1994; 264(5166):1772–1775.

88. Howland DS, Liu J, She Y, Goad B, Maragakis NJ, Kim B, Erickson J, Kulik J, DeVito L, Psaltis G, et al. Focal loss of the glutamate transporter EAAT2 in a transgenic rat model of SOD1 mutant-mediated amyotrophic lateral sclerosis (ALS). Proc Natl Acad Sci USA 2002; 99(3):1604–1609.

89. Bruijn LI, Beal MF, Becher MW, Schulz JB, Wong PC, Price DL, Cleveland DW. Elevated free nitrotyrosine levels, but not protein-bound nitrotyrosine or hydroxyl radicals, throughout amyotrophic lateral sclerosis (ALS)-like disease implicate tyrosine nitration as an aberrant in vivo property of one familial ALS-linked superoxide dismutase 1 mutant. Proc Natl Acad Sci USA 1997; 94(14):7606–7611.

90. Wong PC, Pardo CA, Borchelt DR, Lee MK, Copeland NG, Jenkins NA, Sisodia SS, Cleveland DW, Price DL. An adverse property of a familial ALS-linked SOD1 mutation causes motor neuron disease characterized by vacuolar degeneration of mitochondria. Neuron 1995; 14(6):1105–1116.

91. Aggarwal A, Nicholson G. Detection of preclinical motor neurone loss in SOD1 mutation carriers using motor unit number estimation. J Neurol Neurosurg Psychiatry 2002; 73(2):199–201.

92. Kaspar BK, Llado J, Sherkat N, Rothstein JD, Gage FH. Retrograde viral delivery of IGF-1 prolongs survival in a mouse ALS model. Science 2003; 301(5634):839–842.

93. Bruijn LI, Becher MW, Lee MK, Anderson KL, Jenkins NA, Copeland NG, Sisodia SS, Rothstein JD, Borchelt DR, Price DL, et al. ALS-linked SOD1 mutant G85R mediates damage to astrocytes and promotes rapidly progressive disease with SOD1-containing inclusions. Neuron 1997; 18(2):327–338.

94. Rothstein JD. Of mice and men: reconciling preclinical ALS mouse studies and human clinical trials. Ann Neurol 2003; 53(4):423–426.

95. Pardridge WM. Blood-brain barrier drug targeting: the future of brain drug development. Mol Interv 2003; 3(2):90–105, 151.

96. Lacomblez L, Bensimon G, Leigh PN, Guillet P, Powe L, Durrleman S, Delumeau JC, Meininger V. A confirmatory dose-ranging study of riluzole in ALS. ALS/Riluzole Study Group-II. Neurology 1996; 47(6 suppl 4):S242–S250.

97. Miller RG, Moore DH, Dronsky V, Bradley W, Barohn R, Bryan W, Prior TW, Gelinas DF, Iannaccone S, Kissel J, et al. A placebo-controlled trial of gabapentin in spinal muscular atrophy. J Neurol Sci 2001; 191(1,2):127–131.

98. Mitsumoto H, Davidson M, Moore D, Gad N, Brandis M, Ringel S, Rosenfeld J, Shefner JM, Strong MJ, Sufit R, et al. Percutaneous endoscopic gastrostomy (PEG) in patients with ALS and bulbar dysfunction. Amyotroph Lateral Scler Other Motor Neuron Disord 2003; 4(3):177–185.

99. Cedarbaum JM, Stambler N. Disease status and use of ventilatory support by ALS patients. BDNF Study Group. Amyotroph Lateral Scler Other Motor Neuron Disord 2001; 2(1):19–22.

100. Thompson JL, Levy G. ALS issues in clinical trials. Missing data. Amyotroph Lateral Scler Other Motor Neuron Disord 2004; 5(suppl 1):48–51.

101. Miller RG, Shepherd R, Dao H, Khramstov A, Mendoza M, Graves J, Smith S. Controlled trial of nimodipine in amyotrophic lateral sclerosis. Neuromuscul Disord 1996; 6(2):101–104.

102. Miller RG, Smith SA, Murphy JR, Brinkmann JR, Graves J, Mendoza M, Sands ML, Ringel SP. A clinical trial of verapamil in amyotrophic lateral sclerosis. Muscle Nerve 1996; 19(4):511–515.

103. www.clinicaltrials.gov.

104. www.mdausa.org/research.

105. www.alsa.org/patient.

31
Rehabilitation

Lisa S. Krivickas
Department of Physical Medicine and Rehabilitation, Spaulding Rehabilitation Hospital and Harvard Medical School, Boston, Massachusetts, U.S.A.

Vanina Dal Bello-Haas
School of Physical Therapy, University of Saskatchewan, Saskatoon, Saskatchewan, Canada

Suzanne E. Danforth
Department of Speech Therapy, Massachusetts General Hospital, Boston, Massachusetts, U.S.A.

Gregory T. Carter
Department of Physical Medicine and Rehabilitation, University of Washington, Centralia, Washington, U.S.A.

INTRODUCTION

Despite the explosion of research interest in amyotrophic lateral sclerosis (ALS) and the numerous clinical trials that have been conducted over the last decade, clinicians treating ALS still have only one United States Food and Drug Administration (FDA) approved drug, riluzole, that marginally slows disease progression. At the present time, aggressive rehabilitation and symptom management, which includes management of respiratory failure and dysphagia, can prolong the life of the patient with ALS longer than any currently available pharmacologic interventions (1–6). As researchers develop additional drugs that slow disease progression in ALS, life expectancy will increase and rehabilitation will become even more important.

"*Rehabilitation is the process of helping a person to reach the fullest physical, psychological, social, vocational, avocational, and educational potential consistent with his or her physiological or anatomic impairment, environmental limitations, and desires and life plans. Realistic goals are determined by the person and those concerned with his care. Thus, one is working to obtain optimal function despite residual disability, even if the impairment is caused by a pathological process that cannot be reversed*" (7). In ALS, the pathological process cannot be reversed and is progressive. Comprehensive ALS medical care should include rehabilitation that restores the patient to a level of optimal functioning in his or her normal societal environment and achieves the optimal quality of life possible throughout the course of the disease. For patients with

ALS, rehabilitation is a fluid process because of their rapidly changing physical status. Consequently, rehabilitation is more challenging than it is for patients with static functional deficits produced by events such as stroke or spinal cord injury. One of the most difficult tasks for the rehabilitation team is to predict how quickly the patient's disease will progress so that the team may stay ahead of the disease process.

Rehabilitation and symptom management in ALS may be approached in a problem-oriented manner. Rehabilitation problems addressed in this chapter are the role of exercise in patients with ALS and management of muscle weakness resulting in mobility and activity of daily living (ADL) difficulties, dysarthria, and dysphagia. Musculoskeletal pain syndromes and spasticity also are discussed because of their direct impact on the ability to exercise, maintain mobility, and perform ADLs. These problems are best addressed by a multidisciplinary team, which may consist of some or all of the following: physiatrist, neurologist, physical therapist, occupational therapist, speech therapist, nutritionist, orthotist, social worker, and nurse. The concept of the multidisciplinary team is explored in greater detail in chapter 28. Other rehabilitation and symptom management issues such as respiratory failure, sialorrhea, mood disorders, autonomic dysfunction, bowel and bladder function, cognitive impairment, caregiver burden and family distress, quality of life, and palliative care are addressed elsewhere in this book.

Rehabilitation is necessary during all stages of ALS. As the disease progresses, however, rehabilitation strategies and needs change. Most therapies will be discontinuous. For example, a patient with early ALS may be referred to a physical therapist for help with designing an appropriate aerobic exercise and strengthening program. As increasing spasticity develops, the patient may return to physical therapy for a few sessions on stretching and range of motion (ROM) exercises. If a footdrop develops and the patient is prescribed an ankle foot orthosis (AFO), the patient may again return for a few sessions of gait training with the new brace. As weakness increases, additional sessions of physical therapy may be necessary to teach the caregiver to effectively transfer the patient.

Insurance carriers will often deny coverage of continuous physical, occupational, or speech therapy to patients with ALS because they consider it maintenance therapy with no "improvements" expected. This is faulty reasoning about which health-care providers need to educate insurers. ALS is not a static disease, and as function declines, patients develop the need for new treatment interventions and additional therapy is required. In addition, therapy is sometimes required in order for the patient to maintain function or to slow decline in function.

EXERCISE

Rehabilitation should begin early in the course of ALS so that it may be used to prevent or delay the onset of disability. This concept is known as "prehabilitation" because it is a preventive form of rehabilitation. One important method of prehabilitation is exercise. There are three types of exercise that are important for all individuals, whether or not they have ALS: flexibility or stretching exercises, strengthening exercises, and aerobic exercises.

Flexibility training involves stretching and ROM exercises. While there is a paucity of scientific literature on the role of flexibility training in patients with ALS, it is widely accepted that this form of exercise helps prevent the development of painful contractures and non-pharmacologically decreases spasticity and aborts painful muscle spasms. Loss of ROM can result in a painful adhesive capsulitis and even complex regional pain syndrome (8).

Unfortunately, there are only case reports on the effect of strengthening exercises in patients with ALS (9,10). Therefore, the use of strengthening exercises in ALS is somewhat controversial. Traditionally, physicians have been reluctant to recommend strengthening exercises because they feared that overuse weakness would occur accelerating disability. This philosophy promotes the development of disuse weakness and muscle deconditioning that may compound the weakness produced by ALS itself.

Studies of patients with more slowly progressive motor neuron disease, including spinal muscular atrophy and other neuromuscular diseases such as muscular dystrophy, hereditary motor and sensory neuropathies, and postpolio syndrome, suggest that muscles that are only mildly affected by the disease process can be strengthened by a moderate resistance strengthening program (11–14). Moderate resistance exercise was defined by Aitkens et al. (11) as performing three sets of four to eight repetitions of a given exercise using a load ranging from 20% to 40% of the maximal voluntary contraction (MVC). A study of high-resistance exercise, performed with a training load equal to the 12 repetition maximum (12 RM) in a heterogeneous group of neuromuscular patients suggested that overuse weakness may develop in muscles exercised eccentrically (lengthening contraction) with high resistance (15). Furthermore, the strength gains achieved by these patients were less than those achieved in a comparable group of subjects in a moderate resistance strengthening study conducted by the same investigators (11).

We may conclude from strengthening studies in these diverse populations of neuromuscular patients that with moderate resistance training, overuse weakness and muscle damage do not occur in muscles with $\geq 3/5$ strength on the MRC scale, and strength gains can be achieved, although they are not as great as they would be in subjects without a neuromuscular disorder. In general, the strength gain is proportional to the initial muscle strength, suggesting that a strengthening program should be initiated as early as possible in the course of the disease. High-resistance eccentric exercise should be avoided as it may produce muscle damage. The ability to extrapolate these findings to patients with ALS needs to be demonstrated in well-controlled randomized trials. Furthermore, no studies of strength training in neuromuscular patients have demonstrated translation of the modest strength gains achieved into improved function in ADLs or alteration of the overall course of the disease.

For patients with ALS, we recommend beginning a strengthening program as soon as possible after diagnosis. The objective of such a program is to maximize the strength of unaffected or mildly affected muscles in an attempt to delay the time at which function becomes impaired. For example, if an elderly patient must use 90% of the strength of his leg muscles to rise from a chair before he develops ALS, he will be unable to arise from a chair after losing only 10% of his motor units. If another individual requires only 50% of her maximal leg strength to arise from a chair before developing ALS, even if the disease progresses at the same pace as in the previous individual, she will remain independent much longer. Weight training or strengthening exercise should be performed with a weight that the individual can lift 20 times; this is a simple way for the patient to select a weight that is in the 20% to 40% of maximum voluntary contraction (MVC) range. The patient should then perform two or three sets of 10 repetitions. This guideline will prevent overworking the muscles with excessively heavy weights. Another general guideline is that if an exercise regimen consistently produces muscle soreness or fatigue lasting longer than one-half hour after exercise, it is too strenuous.

The final form of exercise to be considered is aerobic exercise, which helps maintain cardiorespiratory fitness. Only one study has compared the response to aerobic exercise using a bicycle ergometer in patients with ALS and healthy controls (16). The oxygen cost of exercise, at similar intensity levels, was increased in patients with ALS. One explanation for this finding is that spasticity increases energy consumption. Plasma glucose, pyruvate, and lactate levels changed similarly in patients and controls, but free fatty acids, β-hydroxybutyrate, and carnitine did not rise as much as in control subjects suggesting either a possible defect in lipid metabolism during exercise or physical deconditioning. Overall, heart rate and ventilatory response to exercise were similar to those seen in controls.

Given the lack of any apparent contraindication, aerobic exercise training is recommended for patients with ALS as long as it can be performed safely without a risk of falling or injury. In addition to the physical benefits, this form of exercise often has a beneficial effect on mood, psychological well-being, appetite, and sleep. Pool therapy is often an ideal place for patients with ALS to do aerobic exercise, which can be as simple as walking in the water, with the water at midchest height. This is best done in a therapy pool with a flat, uniform depth floor that is heated to 92°F to 95°F. The warmth of the water will help reduce spasticity and facilitate movement.

Drory et al. (17) reported the beneficial effects of a simple, moderate home exercise program in 14 patients with ALS. They randomized 25 ALS patients to receive a moderate daily exercise program consisting of gentle aerobic activity such as walking, stationary bicycling, or swimming for 30 minutes or less ($n = 14$) or not to perform any physical activity beyond their usual daily requirements ($n = 11$). At three months, patients who performed regular exercise showed less deterioration on the ALS-FRS and Ashworth scales. At six months, there was no significant difference between groups, although a trend toward less deterioration in the treated group was observed. This study showed that a regular moderate physical exercise program has a short-lived positive effect on disability in ALS patients.

Two recent studies in the transgenic mouse model of ALS have suggested that aerobic exercise slows disease progression. Kirkinezos et al. (18) showed that 30 min/day of treadmill running 5 days/wk for 10 weeks increased life span by 8% in female mice and 4% in male mice. In a study by Veldink et al. (19) mice were exercised 45 min/day; disease onset was delayed and survival prolonged in female but not male mice. In contrast to these findings, a study of high-intensity endurance exercise in the transgenic mouse showed decreased survival in exercised male mice only (20); the mice in this study ran almost twice as fast as those in the study of Kirkinezos et al. (18). Thus, in mice, it appears that light to moderate aerobic exercise has a neuroprotective effect but heavy resistance exercise may have a deleterious effect. In addition, there appears to be a gender and exercise interaction whereby exercise is more beneficial to female mice.

MUSCLE WEAKNESS

Due to the progressive nature of ALS, at some point all patients will require compensatory interventions to manage muscle weakness. Compensatory interventions provide the patient with alternative means of carrying out functional activities with adaptive equipment and alternate methods for performing tasks and activities. In the early and early-middle stages of ALS, the task or activity may be adapted in order to achieve function. As the disease progresses, increasing environmental adaptations will be necessary. Regardless of the stage of the disease, the overall goal is to maximize function and promote independence to the highest level possible, with the least restrictive device or piece of equipment, without compromising safety. Not only should the patient's current problems be addressed, but also future problems and equipment needs should be anticipated and planned for.

Most aids, devices, and equipment, particularly those classified as durable medical equipment (DME), require a written itemized prescription and a letter of medical necessity signed by the physician, once the evaluation and recommendations by the rehabilitation team members have been completed. Reimbursement coverage varies greatly. Medicare and some managed care plans may pay for some mobility equipment, bedside commodes and hospital beds, if the need has been justified. Some third party payers will request additional justifications or deny coverage for specific items. The therapists and social worker involved in the patient's care should determine what reimbursement is available early in the planning process.

Assistive Devices—Mobility Aids

Muscle weakness, spasticity, and resultant balance problems will eventually necessitate that the patient use an aid to enhance mobility and safety. The type of assistive device recommended is determined by the degree of lower extremity (LE) and trunk weakness and spasticity, ROM and strength of the upper extremities (UE), extent and rate of progression of the disease, acceptance of the aid by the individual, and economic constraints. In addition to taking into account which device will ensure optimal function and safety, the weight of the mobility aid is an important factor to consider in decision making because individuals with ALS experience muscle fatigue.

Canes

Canes (Fig. 1A) provide the least amount of support and are usually recommended in the early stages of ALS for mild LE weakness or balance problems. A cane is carried in the hand opposite to the most affected leg, requires good UE strength, and can be used on stairs. The standard wooden cane is the least expensive, has a curved handle and can be made shorter but not longer. An adjustable aluminum cane easily adapts for various heights and is lightweight. An aluminum cane may have a curved handle or an offset handle. An offset handle allows the weight to be directed over the cane tip when in contact with the floor, rather than anteriorly, as is the case with a curved handle. Quad canes are aluminum canes with four points of floor contact. Quad canes provide greater stability than straight canes, but all tips must be in contact with the ground for stability. The size of base can vary and these canes are heavier to lift. Aluminum and quad canes come in a variety of styles and sizes of handgrips. Patients with hand muscle weakness may be better able to grip an enlarged or molded handle.

Crutches

In general, crutches (Fig. 1B) are rarely recommended for individuals with ALS because the patient must have very good UE and trunk strength, and adequate balance to use them. If crutches are recommended, Loftstrand or Canadian crutches are preferred. These crutches consist of a single upright, a forearm cuff, and a handgrip; the hands can be freed for standing tasks without having to release the crutch.

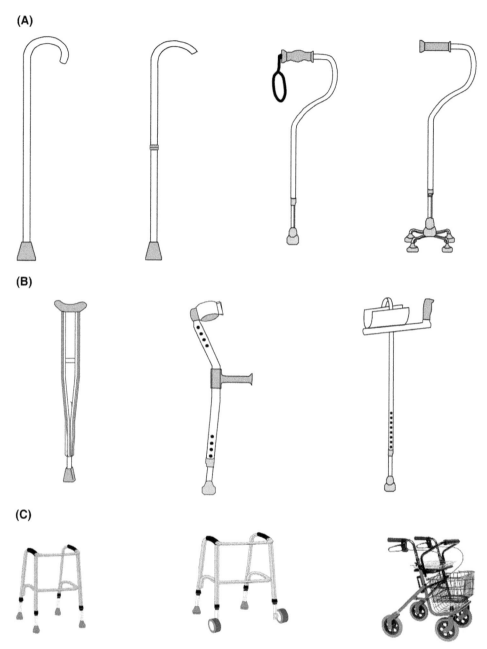

Figure 1 (**A**) Canes (*from left to right*: standard wooden, adjustable aluminum, adjustable aluminum with offset handle, four-point quad cane). (**B**) Crutches (*from left to right*: axillary, Loftstrand or Canadian crutch, platform crutch). (**C**) Walkers (*from left to right*: standard walker, wheeled walker, specialized walker).

Walkers

Walkers (Fig. 1C) provide greater support than canes and crutches, but are more bulky and may be cumbersome in confined spaces. Various types of walkers are available (e.g., folding, with or without wheels, with brakes, with seating surfaces, etc.) and some walkers can be modified to suit the individual's walking environment and needs; for example, they may be fitted with a basket, food tray or forearm trough. Standard aluminum walkers are the least expensive, very stable, and can be adjusted for various heights. However, they must be picked up and lowered during ambulation, and patients may find them heavy to lift. Walkers with wheels do not need to be lifted and they roll forward easily so they are usually recommended for patients with ALS. However, the stability of wheeled walkers is less, and they may move forward too quickly. Some walkers come equipped with brakes. Push down brakes secure a walker when the patient loads his or her weight on the walker and are preferred over squeeze type brakes for patients with hand weakness. Specialized wheeled walkers are the most expensive. They have large wheels that can move over a variety of terrains.

Orthoses

Orthoses are devices worn on a person's body designed to: (i) improve function by offering support to weakened muscles and the joints they surround; (ii) decrease the stress on compensatory muscles; (iii) minimize local or generalized muscle fatigue; (iv) prevent deformity; and/or (v) conserve energy.

Cervical Weakness

In the early stages of ALS, individuals with neck extensor muscle weakness may complain of neck stiffness, heaviness, and fatigue in holding the head up; they also notice difficulties in keeping the head upright with unexpected movements. In the later stages and in cases of severe muscle weakness, the head drops forward, the cervical spine is completely flexed, and the patient experiences severe neck pain and anterior neck muscle tightness.

Several different types of collars that can support the head, protect the weakened muscles and prevent further deformity are available. For mild to moderate weakness a soft, foam collar is usually recommended. Soft collars are usually comfortable and well tolerated, and neck movements are limited to a certain degree.

For moderate to severe weakness, a semirigid collar, such as the traditional Philadelphia® collar is required. Patients find these collars very warm, may experience discomfort at points of contact and pressure over the trachea, or may feel confined. If the individual has a tracheostomy, a Miami-J®, Aspen® or Malibu® collar that allows for anterior neck access is prescribed. Warmth, discomfort, and a sense of confinement are also common with these collars. The Headmaster®, Executive®, and Canadian® collars have an open-air design, but do not control as well for lateral instability as the Miami-J, Aspen, or Malibu collars. In our practices, we have found that the Headmaster collar is well accepted by many patients and is a compromise between providing maximal stability and comfort (Fig. 2).

Patients with combined cervical and upper thoracic weakness may benefit from a cervical-thoracic orthosis, or a sterno-occipital mandibular immobilizer (SOMI). These devices provide maximum support, but are more expensive, heavy and may be difficult to don and doff. For severe or intractable cervical or trunk weakness, referral to an orthotist or biomedical engineer for a custom-made device may be necessary.

Upper Extremity Weakness

An arm sling is an orthosis designed to support the proximal UE when muscles are weak or if the glenohumeral joint is subluxed. Slings similar to those used with

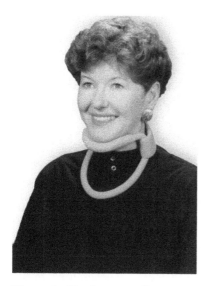

Figure 2 Headmaster collar.

patients post-stroke may decrease pain, prevent soft tissue stretching, and relieve tension on the neurovascular bundle. A pouch sling or single strap hemisling supports the elbow and wrist; however, these types of slings position the arm close to the body in adduction, internal rotation, and elbow flexion; with prolonged use, contractures may develop. The axilla roll sling ("Bobath" sling) consists of a soft roll fashioned to fit under the axilla and is secured with a figure of eight harness. This type of sling holds the humerus slightly abducted, while supporting the shoulder joint. A humeral cuff sling consists of an arm cuff on the distal humerus supported by a figure-eight harness. Studies in patients with stroke have found some supports more effective than others in reducing subluxation (21–23).

Splints are hand orthoses that are available commercially or can be custom-made. They may be static (no moving parts) or dynamic (moving parts). Splinting of the wrist or hand is indicated when improving the patient's hand function or preventing contractures are goals. Splints (Fig. 3) that may be beneficial for patients with ALS include:

Resting Hand Splint: patients with hand weakness may be at risk for developing finger flexion contractures. Resting splints are used to maintain muscle length.

Anticlaw Hand Splint: keeps the metacarpalphalangeal (MCP) joints in flexion; useful for patients with intrinsic muscle weakness to prevent "claw hand" deformity and to improve ability to grasp.

Dynamic Finger-Extension Splint: extends the MCP joints so that extended fingers can flex and grasp objects; useful for patients with finger extensor weakness, who still have adequate flexor strength.

Volar Cock-Up Splint: supports the wrist in 20° to 30° of extension and is useful for patients who have wrist extensor and finger extensor weakness, which prevents them from grasping.

Opponens Splint: designed to support the thumb in an abducted and opposed position and is useful for patients with prehension difficulties due to abductor pollucis brevis and thumb extensor muscle weakness.

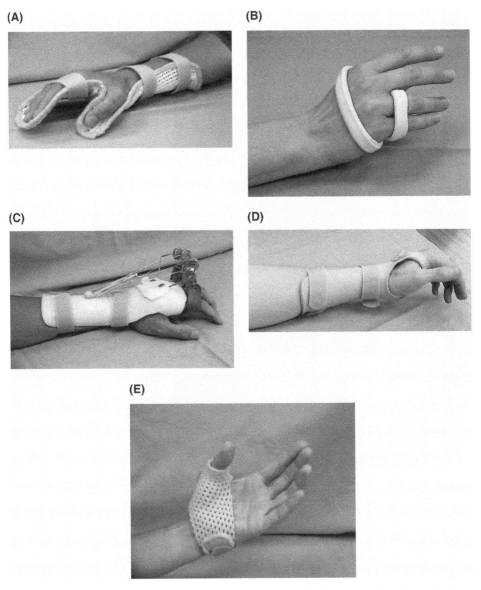

Figure 3 Hand splints. (**A**) Resting hand splint, (**B**) Anti-claw splint, (**C**) Dynamic finger extension splint, (**D**) Cock-up splint, (**E**) Opponens splint. *Source*: Photos courtesy of the Occupational Therapy Department, Royal University Hospital (Saskatoon Health Region).

Lower Extremity Weakness

Ankle–foot orthoses (AFOs) are probably the most common type of orthotic devices used by individuals with ALS (Fig. 4). Prefabricated AFOs may be purchased "off-the-shelf," or AFOs may be custom-made. Deciding between a premanu-factured versus custom orthosis is certainly dependent on the economics of the individual; however, the rate of disease progression should also be considered. For an individual with rapidly progressive ALS and who is likely to use the orthosis for limited time, a premanufactered orthosis may suffice.

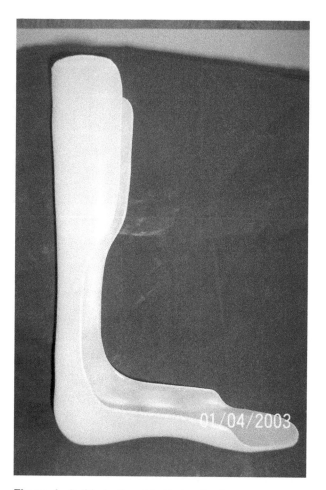

01/04/2003

Figure 4 Solid plastic ankle–foot orthosis.

A solid AFO is usually fabricated from thermoplastic material and is designed to provide maximum immobilization of the ankle–foot complex in all three planes of movement. Knee stability can be enhanced by setting the ankle angle into a few degrees of plantar flexion. Solid AFOs are a good choice for patients who have medial and lateral instability of the ankle with quadriceps weakness; however, the fixed ankle position, combined with quadriceps weakness may make sit to stand transfers and climbing stairs and inclines difficult.

A hinged AFO incorporates a mechanical ankle joint between the foot and calf portions of the orthosis. Hinged AFOs may be appropriate for the patient with adequate knee extensor strength with mild ankle dorsiflexion strength loss. A 90° plantar flexion stop mechanism can be incorporated into a hinged AFO if the prevention of excessive plantar flexion is desired. Transferring from sit to stand is easier with a hinged AFO than it is with a solid AFO.

AFOs with medial and lateral trim lines placed posterior to the midline of the malleolus are posterior leaf spring (PLS) AFOs. PLS braces are more flexible than solid AFOs and allow some plantar flexion to occur during heel strike. Push-off returns the foot to neutral during swing phase, providing dorsiflexion assistance. These AFOs may be appropriate for patients with mild spasticity and a slight footdrop.

Another alternative for patients with a mild foot drop is a carbon fiber kevlar AFO that wraps around the anterior aspect of the leg. This style of brace is less restrictive than a PLS and provides the advantage of some floor reaction, so it may be easier for the patient to become accustomed to when he or she is initially introduced to bracing. However, the cost is three to four times that of a plastic AFO, and ALS patients quickly outgrow the usefulness of this device.

For patients with severe spasticity, antispasticity features can be built into the AFO. These features include a full-foot plate, building up the area under the metatarsal heads and the medial longitudinal arch, and a peroneal ridge.

Again, it is important to consider the weight of the orthosis; it may be more fatiguing for the patient to ambulate with a heavy orthosis than to ambulate without the impairment being corrected. For this reason, metal uprights or knee–ankle–foot orthoses are not recommended.

Wheelchairs

At some time point as the disease progresses, the extent of muscle weakness or the energy requirements for ambulation will necessitate that a patient use a wheelchair for mobility. In the early or early-middle stage of ALS, a manual wheelchair, preferably lightweight or ultra-lightweight may be used for traveling long distances to conserve energy. This wheelchair should be rented on a short-term basis or borrowed from a local Amyotrophic Lateral Sclerosis Association (ALSA) or Muscular Dystrophy Association (MDA) chapter or other source because most insurance companies will only reimburse for one wheelchair purchase.

As the disease progresses, a power wheelchair system tailored to the patient's current and potential future needs should be purchased. Manual wheelchairs can have an external "add-on" power pack attached directly to the rear wheels of the wheelchair. The advantage of this system is that a specialized transportation system is not required—the power pack can be disassembled and the wheelchair folded to fit inside the trunk of a car or the back of a van. Conventional power wheelchairs resemble a manual wheelchair with large powered rear wheels and front casters. Power-base wheelchairs are designed so that the powered section is independent of the seating components and are categorized according to the placement of the drive (rear wheel drive, mid-wheel drive, and front-wheel drive).

Although power scooters may be suitable for a patient with adequate upper extremity and trunk strength in the earlier stages of ALS, the vehicle becomes limiting as the disease progresses. Most insurance companies will not pay for a power wheelchair if the patient has already been reimbursed for a scooter because the scooter is considered a power mobility device. Thus, the purchase of a scooter is usually not recommended.

The optimum wheelchair to be purchased should be one that: (i) has a high back and adequate head and neck support to support weakened trunk muscles; (ii) has a reclining or tilt-in-space seat that enables postural changes for resting and pain and pressure relief; and (iii) can be modified to add a ventilator tray or communication device.

Numerous features and options are available in a wheelchair system. Some of these features are preferred, as they better assist the individual to maintain a maximum level of independence and comfort (Table 1). Trail et al. (24) surveyed 42 patients with ALS and moderate disability, as documented on the Appel ALS Rating Scale, about the wheelchair features they found most beneficial. Sixty-one percent of patients reported that their wheelchairs allowed them to maintain their previous activity levels, and the most and least desirable features are summarized in Table 2.

Table 1 Wheelchair Components

Component	Options	Description/comment
Drives	Rear-wheel drive (RWD)	Stable; can handle gradient changes; requires more space for turning
	Mid-wheel drive (MWD)	Offer smallest, full turning radius; less stable
	Front-wheel drive (FWD)	Optimal stability; good maneuverability; good for environmental obstacles
Drive controls	Proportional control	Usually a joystick; direction and speed linked to angle and magnitude of displacement
	Microswitch control	Joystick or multiple-switch array; less responsive than proportional; each activation engages a single preset direction and speed
	Sip and puff system	Action is controlled by user sipping and puffing into a tube held in the mouth
	Scanning system	Choices presented to user one at a time, until desired choice is offered for the user to select by switch activation
Armrests	Fixed	
	Detachable	Preferred; allow greatest ease for transfers
	Swing away	Allow greater ease for transfers
	Slanted	Useful for dependent edema
	Adjustable height	Prevents subluxation of a weakened shoulder
	Full length	Run the full length of the seat
	Desk length	Shorter; allows table top access with armrests in place; may make independent transfers more difficult, as patient needs to reach back
Leg rests	Fixed	
	Swing away	Allow greater ease for transfers
	Detachable	Preferred; allow greatest ease for transfers
	Elevating	Useful for dependent edema; patients with limited knee flexion
	Adjustable length	Allows optimal hip and knee angles
	Tapered	
Footplates	Heel loops	
	Ankle straps	
	Other foot harnessing	
Tires	Pneumatic (air filled)	Require regular maintenance; provide shock absorption which improves comfort and longevity of the chair; good for outdoors
	Semipneumatic (airless inserts)	Less maintenance; good cushioning; tire wear may be a problem
	Polyurethane or rubber	Minimal maintenance; little shock absorption; heavier than air-filled
Casters	Small (e.g., 3, 5, 6 in.)	Increase turning maneuverability
	Large (8 in.)	Better for environmental obstacles, outdoors
	Pneumatic, semipneumatic	Provide some shock absorption; best for outdoors or rough surfaces
	Solid core	Best for indoor use and on smooth surfaces

(*Continued*)

Table 1 Wheelchair Components (*Continued*)

Component	Options	Description/comment
Seating	Solid–gel or foam	Preferred; promotes better posture
	Sling	Lightweight; foldable; promotes poor posture
	Adaptive	Custom molded; optimal; very expensive
Antitipping extensions		Fixed or adjustable extensions; prevent chair from tipping; needed for RWD and MWD
Wheel locks		Prevent rolling of the wheelchair at rest
Lapbelts, safety vests, and harnesses		May be necessary for patients with severely impaired postural control or who slide forward due to weakness
Wheelchair tie downs		Secure the wheelchair to the base of the vehicle; keep chairs stabilized when traveling in vans
Other	Removable lap tray	Provides a working or eating surface; may prevent shoulder subluxation
	Seat elevators	Available on some power base wheelchairs; raises height of the seating surface; assist with transfers, provide access to countertops, cupboards
	Head supports, back supports	

Because of the complex needs of patients with ALS, potential restrictive factors (e.g., accessibility into and within the home, availability of accessible transportation, the patient's financial resources), the expense of a power wheelchair system (up to $30,000), and reimbursement restrictions, the type of wheelchair system to be recommended should be carefully evaluated by the entire rehabilitation team, preferably in a specialized seating clinic.

Table 2 Desirable and Undesirable Features Cited by Manual and Motorized Wheelchair Users

	Most desirable features (in order of priority)	Least desirable features (in order of priority)
Manual wheelchair users	A lightweight frame Small turning radius High reclining back Supports for the head, trunk, and extremities	Low, sling, non-reclining back Non-motorized chair Static, non-adjustable leg rests Too heavy; too large Non-removable armrests
Motorized wheelchair users	Increased independence with mobility Maneuverability Overall comfort Tilt/recline features	Low, non-reclining back Too heavy; too large Uncomfortable seat Non-adjustable leg rests General discomfort

Source: Adapted from Ref. 24.

Home Modifications

Home modifications can range from simple, such as moving the patient's bed to the main floor, to extensive. It is beyond the scope of this chapter to explore all possible environmental situations and to describe all possible home adaptations and modifications. Physical and occupational therapists should evaluate the home for accessibility and safety. The overall goal when considering recommendations for home adaptations is to create the most safe and supportive environment for the patient, family, and caregiver. Home modifications and renovations are not reimbursable by Medicare or most private insurance companies.

For patients confined to a wheelchair, ramps are necessary to access the home's entrance. Ramps need to be sturdily built, with a grade of no more than 1 foot of height for every 12 feet of length (American National Standards Institute, Inc.). Portable ramps and vertical platform lifts are commercially available and may be an option.

Wheelchair and walker users need a door width of approximately 32 in. to allow clearance for most devices, and about three feet of space to approach a chair or commode or to turn in a semicircle. Furniture rearrangement may be a simple solution to increase in-home accessibility, and door openings can be modified by removing doors, reversing doors (to open outward), or replacing them with folding doors. Offset hinges, which provide an additional 2 in. of clearance and swing the door open clear of the door frame, can also be installed.

The bathroom is typically not adequately accessible to individuals in wheelchairs. If the doorframe prohibits clearance of a wheelchair, the patient may transfer to a commode with casters at the door. Various devices and pieces of equipment are available that enhance independent or assisted bathing and toileting (Table 3). Selection is dependent on the layout of the bathroom and the willingness to make modifications. A standard shower stall with a 3 to 4 in. rim may be made more accessible with a portable ramp if room allows. A custom-made shower area that allows the patient to enter the stall on a special shower commode, but has a raised slope that prevents water from running out also may be an option, depending on financial resources.

Inexpensive remote control units, readily available from hardware stores, can be used in any room of the house to control small appliances or lights via a portable hand-held keypad or button. Environmental control systems are more expensive and consist of a system or device that is attached to electronic or electrical equipment, such as household lighting, heating systems, appliances, the television, telephone, or stereo. The patient operates the equipment through a switch, remote-control device, or the computer.

Chair glides and stairway lifts can be recommended for those individuals with multi-level homes. These lifts are measured and custom-made for individual staircases and are very expensive. Insurance companies usually do not reimburse for stairway lifts, but some medical supply companies offer "rent-to-own" options. In addition, local ALSA and MDA chapters may have recycled lifts. Some local chapters of these organizations will also send a PT or OT to the home to evaluate safety at no charge to the patient. Whether or not this service is available depends on the finances of the local chapter.

Adaptive Devices and Equipment

A large variety of adaptive devices and equipment is available to help individuals with muscle weakness perform ADLs, but no one type of device is suitable for every patient or for every stage of the disease. Medicare does not reimburse for the cost of

Table 3 Commonly Used Adaptive Devices and Equipment

ADL area	Device/equipment	Description/comments
Food preparation, feeding, and eating	Foam tubing, enlarged handles	Increases the size of handles, making the utensils easier to grip
	Cups with modified handles or holders, extended straw, straw holder	
	Long-levered jar opener	
	Plate guard, plate with raised lip	Allows food to be scooped, prevents food from spilling
	Serrated or rocker knife	Less force is required, less likely to slip, increases ease of cutting
	"Spork"	A utensil that combines the tines of a fork and the bowl of the spoon
	Adapted cuff/universal cuff	Cuff goes around palm of the hand; has a pocket to hold the utensil when grasp is absent
	Mobile arm support	Frictionless arm support mounted to a table or attached to a table via a clamp; uses gravity in an inclined plane to assist U/E movements, when shoulder and elbow muscles are weak
	Dycem®	Stabilizes objects, prevents dishes from slipping
Self-care and bathing	Bathing bench	Padded board placed across tub; provides level transfer surface
	Bath tub seat	Relatively long seat positioned with two legs in the tub, two legs outside the tub; provides safer means for transfer
	Shower/commode chair	Can function as a shower chair, stand-alone commode or be used over the toilet
	Grab bars	Need to be securely fastened to a reinforced wall
	Raised toilet seat	
	Handheld shower head, long handled sponge, bath mitt, and sponge	
	Electric toothbrush or shaver	
	Strap-fitted hairbrush, long-handled comb	
Dressing	Zipper pull or hook, button hook	
	Long-handled shoe horn	
	Velcro® clothing closures	Eliminates need for buttons, snaps
	Elastic shoe laces	Eliminates need to tie and untie laces
	Reacher	

(Continued)

Table 3 Commonly Used Adaptive Devices and Equipment (*Continued*)

ADL area	Device/equipment	Description/comments
Writing and reading	Foam tubing, triangular pencil grip	
	Pen holder, e.g., "writing bird"	Device holds a pen and allows writing as the patient moves the device
	Book holder	
	Automatic page turner	Portable; turns pages with a slight touch on a switch
	Adjustable angle table	Has clips for holding newspapers or magazines; can be used in a chair or bed
	Mouthstick, headstick	Allow access to keyboard; patient needs good head control
Other	Key holder	Attaches to keys to provide larger gripping area
	Doorknob adapter	Converts existing doorknobs into lever-type mechanisms or increases circumference of doorknob
	Lamp extension switch	
	Personal alarm system	
	Remote control speaker phone with automatic dialing	
	Telephone holder	
	Telecommunication devices for the deaf (TDD)	Consists of a small display screen, a modem, phone connection and an input device (e.g., keyboard); sends typewritten words over telephone lines

many of the devices, but a physician's prescription may allow partial reimbursement from third party payers.

Upper Extremity Weakness

Weakness of the UE greatly impacts the patient's ability to carry out ADLs. Adaptive devices that prolong independent function are outlined in Table 3.

Lower Extremity Weakness

Those individuals with LE weakness may find it difficult to get out of a chair. Initially, difficulty rising from a seated position to standing may be addressed by placing a firm cushion, 2 to 3 in. thick, under the buttocks in the chair or by placing prefabricated blocks under the chair, so that the hips are higher than the knees.

Self-powered lifting cushions, such as the UPlift Seat Assist™, are relatively inexpensive, portable devices that provide assistance for rising to standing, using hydro-pneumatics; however, the patient must have adequate trunk control and standing balance to use the device safely. Powered seat lift recliner chairs, although much more expensive, are also available for rental or purchase. These chairs enable a person to rise to a standing position or recline by activating an electric control.

Transfer boards may be used for transfers once the individual is unable to stand. The patient can use the board alone if he has adequate arm strength and good sitting balance, or with the assistance of a caregiver. Other useful devices that assist with mobility are transfer belts and swivel cushions or seats. Transfer belts ease the burden of the transfer for the caregiver and prevent potential painful traction on the patient's UE. Swivel cushions are lightweight, cushioned seats that swivel in both directions and make getting in and out of a car easier.

Individuals who have difficulty transferring, even with the assistance of a caregiver, will require a mechanical lift, such as the Easy Pivot^{TM}, the Hoyer Lift, or the Trans-Aid Patient Lifter^{TM} (Fig. 5). Use of an electric hospital bed will also facilitate bed mobility and transfers, both for the patient and the caregiver. A variety of mattresses and mattress overlays, such as alternating air pressure pads, are available and necessary, especially in the late stages of ALS, to relieve pressure and to improve the patient's comfort when in bed.

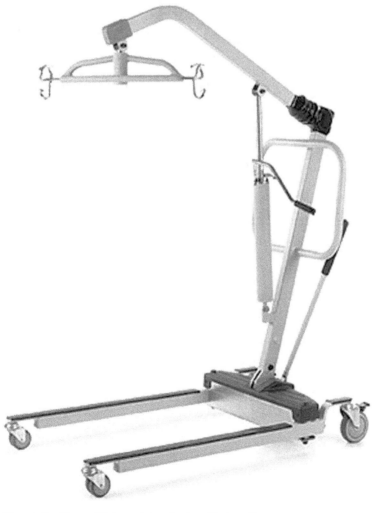

Figure 5 Hoyer lift to assist patients with transfers.

Difficulty with transferring may complicate bladder management. Although ALS primarily causes denervation of striated skeletal muscle, it may occasionally involve the urinary sphincters. Despite this, incontinence is usually not a significant clinical problem in ALS. When incontinence is a problem it is usually due to immobility and difficulty getting to the toilet in time rather than to lack of sphincter control. Patients should avoid drinking large amounts of fluids after dinner to avoid nighttime incontinence. Males may wear a condom catheter at night. Absorbent undergarments may also be used but skin should be monitored closely for maceration and protected with topically applied moisture repelling agents. Sympathomimetic agents like pseudoephedrine at 30 to 60 mg up to four times a day may help increase urinary outlet sphincter tone. However, this may also increase blood pressure and could induce urinary retention, particularly if used in conjunction with anticholinergic agents in a male with prostatic enlargement. An indwelling Foley or suprapubic catheter is a reasonable choice later in the course of the disease when alternative options have been exhausted.

MANAGEMENT OF MUSCULOSKELETAL PAIN

Although the disease process in ALS does not primarily involve pain pathways, there are a number of secondary painful musculoskeletal syndromes that can arise. The best management is pro-actively preventing the development of these, and this approach is most effective when started in the early stages of the disease.

The muscle weakness, spasticity, and the progressive loss of mobility encountered in ALS places increased stress on the musculoskeletal system, contributing to pain generation (25–27). This is enhanced by a reduction in overall functional conditioning, including reduced aerobic capacity and pulmonary function (28). As ALS advances, patients are at high risk of becoming deconditioned. Deconditioned states are usually associated with a decreased pain tolerance, which may be a factor that negatively impacts quality of life for all persons with neuromuscular disorders, including ALS (29–33). Pain may exacerbate fatigue and depression, which are also associated with poor quality of life in ALS (34–36).

Prevention of Deconditioning

The role of exercise in managing ALS has been previously discussed in this chapter. However, it is worth noting that generalized loss of cardiopulmonary fitness or "deconditioning" can lower pain tolerance and contribute to depression. Aerobic exercise helps maintain cardiorespiratory fitness and has a beneficial effect on mood, psychological well-being, appetite, and sleep (37). Although fatigue in ALS is multifactorial and due in part to impaired muscular activation, deconditioning and loss of mobility also play a significant role (38).

Adhesive Capsulitis

Patients with ALS are at high risk for developing progressive loss of ROM, particularly in the shoulders (39). If left untreated, the patient will develop a frozen shoulder (adhesive capsulitis), which can be very painful. Just as exercise may help pro-actively with maintaining mobility and preventing the development of secondary deconditioning, a good stretching program may help prevent painful musculoskeletal syndromes such as joint contracture or adhesive capsulitis. It is especially important to maintain shoulder ROM when the patient can no longer actively raise his arms overhead. Loss of ROM can result not only in a painful frozen shoulder but has also been reported to cause complex regional pain syndrome in ALS (8,40).

If a frozen shoulder develops, then more aggressive treatment may be indicated. This would include radiographs to make sure the joint cartilage space is intact and to exclude gross anatomic deformities such as a fracture; if there is severe calcification or heterotopic ossification, one should focus on pain management and not expect significant gains in ROM. An intra-articular corticosteroid injection may help reduce inflammation. This may also be accomplished with dexamethasone given via electrical current (iontophoresis), although this may be less effective in a deeper joint such as the shoulder. Topical heat and ice, given alone or sequentially (contrast therapy) may help reduce pain. If local treatment does not control the pain completely then oral pain medications should be used. Aggressive manipulation, including manipulation under anesthesia, is not indicated in ALS, given the overall prognosis of the disease.

Back and Neck Pain

Although common in the hereditary motor neuron disease spinal muscular atrophy, spinal deformities such a scoliosis or kyphosis do not occur in ALS (41). Because of immobility and neck and trunk muscle weakness leading to poor spinal support, the vast majority of ALS patients will experience some degree of back and neck pain. Spinal bracing may be used to improve sitting posture and balance. Severe neck flexor and extensor weakness can lead to a "floppy head" associated with severe neck pain and tightness. This condition may be helped by a cervical orthosis as described earlier in this chapter.

Pain from Immobility

Impaired mobility is expected with disease progression and often causes pain. Wheelchairs should have adequate lumbar support and good cushioning (gel-foam) (24). Wheelchairs and beds should be properly fitted with good pressure relief over all bony prominences to avoid pain and pressure ulcers. If the patient cannot independently perform pressure relief maneuvers, a power tilt-in-space attachment to the wheelchair is critical to protect their skin. This device, which allows the patient to tilt back the entire seat on the wheelchair, also relieves pressure on the low back. Foam wedges should be used to facilitate proper positioning. Daily passive and active-assisted ROM is also helpful in treating pain from immobility.

Pharmacological Management of Pain

We have discussed a number of physical and rehabilitative interventions designed to limit and help treat pain. However, there may well be residual pain even after all of this is done. Thus a brief discussion of pharmacological management of pain in ALS is warranted (see Chap. 29).

Initially, the use of non-steroidal anti-inflammatory (NSAID) medication, particularly if there is evidence of an active inflammatory process like tenosynovitis or arthritis, is helpful. Regular dosing of acetaminophen (1000 mg every six hours) may be used along with an NSAID or alone if NSAIDs are not tolerated. Tri-cyclic antidepressants and antiepilitic drugs (AEDs) can sometimes be helpful for pain, particularly if there is a neuropathic component, which can occur in ALS (42). One of the newer AEDs, gabapentin, also has the added benefit of some antispasticity properties (43).

Narcotic medicine should be reserved for refractory pain (44). Concern for narcotic addiction is pointless in a terminal disease. The medications should be given on a regular dosing schedule and titrated to the point of comfort. Concomitant use of the antiemetic, antihistamine hydroxyzine (Vistaril®) given along with the narcotic will enhance the effectiveness (i.e., 30 mg codeine plus 50 mg hydroxyzine every six waking hours). Unlike narcotic medications, hydroxyzine is not a cortical depressant but does have direct skeletal muscle relaxant and analgesic properties and is known to potentiate the analgesic effect of narcotic medication, although the exact mechanism is unknown. Dextromethorphan, through an NMDA-receptor mediated mechanism, may also enhance the effects of narcotics and may possess some analgesic effect of its own. Combination elixirs can be prepared by the pharmacy for ease of administration.

Oral or sublingual morphine (Roxanol®), 10 to 30 mg every four hours, is effective for comfort care and may help relieve "air hunger" in the terminal stages of the disease. Another option is taking the total dose of immediate release morphine required to alleviate pain and giving half of that every 12 hours in a controlled-release preparation such as MS Contin®. Intramuscular delivery route should be avoided due to muscle wasting. Fentanyl or morphine patches may deliver inconsistent dosing, particularly if there is excessive perspiration. A patient-controlled analgesic (PCA) pump mechanism may not work in advanced stages of ALS due to inability of the patient to control the delivery. The main problems with narcotic medication in ALS are respiratory depression and constipation (see Chap. 35).

Marijuana is a substance with many properties that may be applicable to the management of ALS (45,46). These include analgesia, muscle relaxation, bronchodilation, saliva reduction, appetite stimulation, and sleep induction. In addition, various cannabinoids have now been shown to have strong antioxidative and neuroprotective effects, which prolong neuronal cell survival in vitro in mouse models (47,48). Further investigation into the usefulness of marijuana in ALS is warranted.

SPASTICITY

Spasticity in ALS probably is induced both at the motor cortex and at the spinal cord level (49). The vast majority of patients with ALS will have spasticity, which can adversely affect mobility and contribute to pain. Despite this, treatment of spasticity in ALS has been poorly studied. The Cochrane Neuromuscular Disease Group recently reviewed this topic and was able to identify only one randomized controlled trial showing that individualized, moderate intensity walking, swimming, or cycling may help to reduce spasticity (50). Remarkably, no other medical, surgical or alternative treatment therapy has been evaluated in a randomized fashion in this patient population.

Despite this lack of data, there are a number of drugs that effectively treat spasticity in ALS. The gamma-amino-butyric acid (GABA) analog baclofen facilitates motor neuron inhibition at spinal levels and is the agent of choice. The recommended initial dose is 5 to 10 mg two to three times a day, titrating up to doses of 20 mg four times a day. Occasionally higher doses (up to 160 mg/day) are more effective but caution is advised. Side effects include weakness, fatigue, and sedation. An intrathecal baclofen pump may be beneficial to some patients with predominantly upper motor neuron symptoms (51). Tizanidine, an α_2 agonist similar to clonidine, inhibits excitatory interneurons and may also be helpful. Dosing range is 4 to 8 mg three to four times a day, with a similar side effect profile to baclofen. Baclofen and tizanidine can be effectively used together, as long as side effects, particularly increasing weakness and hypotension, are monitored. Benzodiazepines may also be helpful but can cause respiratory depression and somnolence. Dantrolene blocks Ca^{2+} release in the sarcoplasmic reticulum; it effectively reduces muscle tone but will also cause generalized muscle weakness and is not recommended for patients with ALS. Slow (30 seconds sustained), static muscle stretching may be helpful, particularly in the more symptomatic muscle groups like the gastrocnemius, and may be done in bed. Positional splinting is also a helpful adjunctive modality but skin must be monitored frequently for pressure areas.

Another option for focal spasticity that is causing positioning problems is botulinum toxin injections. These have not been studied in ALS but are effective in producing local, partial paralysis of a muscle for up to six months. Nerve blocks, using agents such as marcaine, may temporarily relieve spasticity and may be indicated as a short-term solution for a limb-positioning problem or to help facilitate a physical therapy regimen of stretching. Ice, or immersion in ice water bath, will also temporarily relieve spasticity, with the effects lasting a few hours. The mechanism involves slowing of nerve conduction and direct impairment of muscle contractility via lowered temperature. Conversely, heat provides a similar, although generally less pronounced, effect mediated by vasodilation and reflex relaxation of the muscle. Cooling and heating the limb are both short-term antispasticity measures that should be performed with physical therapy supervision to avoid thermal damage to the extremity.

DYSARTHRIA AND COMMUNICATION

Management of speech and communication changes in ALS requires anticipation of disease progression, early and accurate provision of information to the patient, and interventions designed to preserve and enhance existing function. While treating current difficulties, the speech pathologist must prepare for further decline.

Diagnosis of Dysarthria and Communication Impairments

Approximately 24% of patients with ALS present with bulbar signs and symptoms (52), and up to 80% of patients will ultimately develop bulbar signs regardless of site of onset (26). Patients develop changes in speech due to upper and/or lower motor neuron dysfunction characterized by progressive weakness and dysfunction in the lips, jaw, tongue, palate, pharynx, and larynx. Altered voice quality, slowed speaking rate and changes in diadochokinetic rates are early and easily identifiable signs of bulbar changes (53,54). In addition, patients are exquisitely sensitive to even subtle changes in speech function and will often report symptoms if they are asked about their ability to communicate in various areas of their lives. Patients may report a change in communication effectiveness (i.e., vocal fatigue after giving a presentation) even when their speech is quite normal in the clinical environment, especially during the early part of the day.

Reassessment of dysarthria should be performed at each clinic visit since changes are ongoing. Assessment is accomplished by a detailed oral motor and sensory examination of the entire speech system, including the range and rate of motion and strength of all articulators.

Intelligibility measures are often administered and can involve single-word and sentence length material that is tape-recorded and given to a blind rater for transcription. Because these measures are administered by a speech-language pathologist in a highly optimal communication environment (i.e., face to face, known context, good lighting, and quiet environment), use of a communication effectiveness assessment tool also is helpful. Social participation measures show that patients can score up to 90% intelligibility in a testing environment but report significant communication difficulties in social, vocational, and familial settings (55).

Tracking the rate of change in dysarthria and communication effectiveness is accomplished several ways. Matching the patient with the same clinician over time is a reliable perceptual way to gauge change, as is the use of rating scales, which allow the clinician to assign a numeric value to communication and speech abilities (56).

Management of Dysarthria and Communication Impairments

Patients experiencing early speech changes in ALS typically use compensatory speech strategies to enhance intelligibility. Use of adequate breath support for phrasing and over articulation often allows the patient to continue to participate in all social and communicative obligations. However, very early in the disease process, patients complain of and suffer from fatigue. Many people complain that their speech production is clear in the morning but begins to deteriorate as the day progresses. Therefore, compensatory strategies must themselves be used judiciously and in conjunction with environmental strategies. For an evening engagement, resting or napping in the afternoon or minimizing speaking during the same time can allow more efficient use of compensatory strategies later in the day.

Education of family members is a critical step in optimizing communication. If a person close to the patient has hearing loss, referral to an audiologist can assist in maximizing the communication environment, as can ensuring that partners are speaking face to face in a well-lit environment without competing noise.

For patients with diminished voice volume due to lack of breath support, use of a simple amplification device enhances communication.

Patients with lower motor neuron dysarthria may benefit from a prosthetic palatal lift. A palatal lift is an oral-device that will elevate the soft palate to occlude the nasopharyngeal port and allow build up of intraoral pressure, which can significantly improve speech quality if nasality is one of the primary features of the dysarthria. Most studies of palatal lifts do not include ALS patients. Those that do suggest that patients with nasality, but comparatively better articulation and slow disease progression, are the best candidates (57,58). The ability of patients to inhibit the gag response and tolerate the prosthesis is another key aspect to consider in fitting ALS patients with a lift.

Oral motor exercise is not well understood within the discipline of speech-language pathology, and just a handful of studies provide guidance in managing the patient with a degenerative neuromuscular disease (59). However, there are existing frameworks for identifying sound practice parameters and making practical inferences (59,60). Most patients want to preserve their ability to speak, even as they are losing it. Many either inquire about oral motor exercise for this purpose or come to the specialized clinic from a more general practice already on an oral motor exercise regime. For patients with ALS, we do not recommend oral motor strengthening programs beyond light ROM exercise. Even ROM is questionably beneficial, especially since most patients continue to "range" their speech and swallowing musculature simply by daily use. On the other hand, ROM exercise may add to the psychological well being of patients who desire to be proactive in maintaining current function and preventing further deterioration.

Even in the early stages of bulbar dysfunction in ALS, education and planning for augmentative communication is indicated. Alternative Augmentative Communication (AAC) describes any mode of communication other than speech. It includes gesture, facial expression, writing, symbol or picture boards, and devices or computers that create synthesized speech.

Most AAC use by patients with ALS occurs in the middle and late stages of the disease, when intelligibility is significantly impaired, but while patients can still access specialized devices. For patients in the middle stage of the disease, there are two primary AAC options; low technology, which does not require computer technology for operation, or high technology, which utilizes electronic or computerized devices.

Early stage patients typically rely on unaided or low technology approaches (such as writing, or indicating the first letter of a word), with increased reliance on high technology during the middle stage (i.e., speech generating device) and a return to low-technology communication methods during the late stage of the disease (61).

Even in the latest stage, when some patients have chosen permanent mechanical ventilation, most patients continue to retain some ability to communicate. Some patients utilize eye gaze or blinking and infrared technology to operate AAC devices. However, the longer a patient is ventilated, the more likely he is to become locked-in, or unable to access any reliable muscle movement for communication purposes (62). Techniques are currently being developed that will allow these patients to utilize EEG signal to operate an AAC device.

Use of high-technology AAC requires subspecialized speech-language pathology intervention. There is a surfeit of devices on the market and a specialized vocabulary; choosing a system that is appropriate for a particular individual can be challenging. Prior exposure to and comfort with use of computers tends to influences patients' choices.

One popular AAC device is the LightWRITER™ (Fig. 6). This is a simple device that many people with basic typing skills are comfortable using. For those with impaired hand function, the device can be set to scan the alphabet, and the patient can select via use of a switch. Switches are usually buttons or wands that are touch or pressure sensitive. They can be positioned so that any preserved muscular action can activate them.

Higher-level AAC technologies include use of laptop and palm or desktop computers. These utilize programs which can either be picture or text-based, and which are accessible in the same ways as described above. These devices can be mounted at the bedside or on wheelchairs. Planning for acquisition of a device should begin aggressively in the early stages of bulbar dysfunction because of the high cost of these types of AAC devices, usually between $4000 and $6000, and because they can take several months to acquire due to the slowness of the insurance approval process.

Funding the devices should first be attempted by insurance coverage. Private insurers have different policies, but tend to follow Medicare guidelines. AAC devices were in the past considered a convenience item not primarily medical in nature. Fortunately, their designation was changed to DME in January 2001. DME is equipment that can be expected to make a meaningful contribution to the treatment of

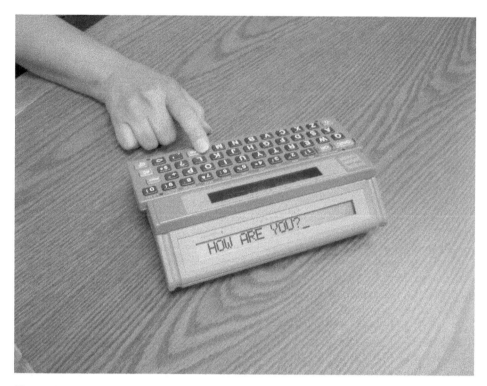

Figure 6 LightWRITER alternative augmentative communication device.

the patient's illness or injury and which is at least partially covered by Medicare. Shortfalls in funding can be made up via a one time $2000 grant from the MDA, or via local fundraising efforts. Many local chapters of the MDA and ALSA also have device loan programs.

Late stage patients and their caregivers typically revert to low technology means of communication, such as eye blinking to indicate yes or no. The most frequent use of AAC in this stage is for communication of basic needs and clarifying needs with caregivers.

In all stages of the disease, speech-language pathologists should be aware that some patients with ALS have cognitive deficits affecting word fluency, working memory, and problem solving (63); these deficits can impact the type and complexity of AAC chosen for use by the patient.

SWALLOWING AND DYSPHAGIA

As with other rehabilitation problems encountered in ALS, management of swallowing changes requires enhancement of existing function with simultaneous preparation for further decline.

Diagnosis of Dysphagia

Changes in the underlying physiological and anatomical structures involved in speaking are inextricably linked to similar changes in swallowing. Clinically, as a patient is experiencing decline in speech and communication function, swallowing changes follow a similar course. Just as assessment of dysarthria and communication must be performed anew at every clinic visit, so must dysphagia assessment. Information from the detailed oral motor and sensory examination informs the clinician as to the level of safety (aspiration or airway protection) and efficiency (nutrition and the ability to eat without undue fatigue) of the swallow, as well as the laterality of progression, which can be used to identify appropriate compensatory strategies.

A detailed clinical history should include how long it takes for the patient to eat, how many times a day he eats, how often he is coughing, and on what food consistencies. Dysphagia in ALS typically occurs with liquids prior to solids. This occurs because the deteriorating swallow is slowing, and the rapidity of the liquid bolus outpaces the rate at which laryngeal protection can occur. An examination of swallowing in the clinic is easily accomplished with use of a liquid (water), a solid (cookie), and a soft food (pudding or applesauce).

In the oral phase, the following are assessed; efficiency and pattern of chewing, ability of the patient to form boluses easily and cohesively in the mouth, presence of nasal regurgitation, and the ability to easily move the bolus around the mouth with the tongue and to move it posteriorly to trigger the swallow. Finally, checking for residue in the oral cavity is a necessary part of the bedside examination of swallowing.

In the pharyngeal-laryngeal stage of swallowing, assessment includes the briskness and fullness of laryngeal elevation (accomplished by palpation of the thyroid cartilage during swallowing) as well as the presence of indicators of overt signs of dysphagia. Overt signs of pharyngeal dysphagia include reflexive coughing or throat clearing following a swallow, the need for multiple swallows for one bite/sip and a change in voice quality, which can indicate residue in the pharynx. A unique and unstudied phenomenon in ALS patients is the presence of a noisy swallow. It tends to be present with all consistencies and can best be described as a "clunk." Atrophy in the base of the tongue and along the posterior pharyngeal wall may be responsible for the noise, since these structures, which are supposed to oppose fully to initiate the drive of the swallow, often do not meet fully during fluoroscopic examination of swallowing.

Instrumentation can be helpful in diagnosing the nature of dysphagia in this population, especially since it has been shown in stroke patients that between 42% and 50% of aspiration are missed in the clinical examination (64,65). Two primary modes are available to characterize swallowing physiology, the modified barium swallow study or video fluoroscopic swallow study (VFSS) and fiberoptic endoscopic evaluation of swallowing (FEES).

VFSS is a radiographic procedure in which the oral-pharyngeal swallow is visualized fluoroscopically. FEES are a naso-endoscopic assessment of the pharyngeal stage of swallowing. Indications for one versus the other study vary, but both essentially assess for the presence of aspiration and characterize the physiology of the swallow. Identification of tailored compensatory strategies to lessen or prevent aspiration and to increase the efficiency of eating is the goal of these studies for patients with ALS. Studies of dysphagia should be used less to determine the presence or absence of aspiration than to understand the patient's swallowing physiology to direct compensatory treatment.

The speech pathologist must also monitor the patient's weight and make early referral to a dietician. ALS patients with even a mild dysphagia have shown a tendency toward reduced caloric intake, resulting in weight loss greater than that expected from the disease process alone (66).

Management of Dysphagia

Dysphagia is best managed in a hierarchical fashion, moving from least to more restrictive strategies. Similarly, the goals of management change as the patient's disease progresses. For example, maximizing nutrition and preventing infection are early goals of dysphagia management. As the disease progresses, maximizing nutrition remains a goal only if the patient decides not to have a percutaneous endoscopic gastrostomy (PEG) tube placed. Following PEG placement, maintaining intake of food or liquid for pleasure becomes the goal. Preventing infection may not be entirely possible, even in a patient who no longer eats anything by mouth, because of aspiration of secretions (67). Also, as swallowing impairment becomes more severe, it is important to educate the patient on ways to prevent airway obstruction during eating, and to encourage caregivers to learn the Heimlich maneuver.

Typically, patients in the early stages report they are beginning to cough on thin liquids and are taking longer to eat meals. However, they usually do not self-restrict any foods because of difficulty chewing or swallowing. Early interventions include educating the patient on the need to focus on eating and drinking when engaged in the activity, turning off the television or other distracters, and educating family and friends about dysphagia. The patient should be encouraged not to speak with food in the mouth because it can overtax the muscles of deglutition in a patient with an underlying neuromuscular process. Alternating solids and liquid sips is another simple but effective strategy that aids in clearance of food from both the oral and pharyngeal cavities.

As dysphagia progresses, changes in food consistencies and presentation and the use of postural maneuvers are the predominant management strategies. Food consistency changes include use of soft moist foods (casseroles, well-cooked vegetables) that require less mastication than regular foods. Early consistency difficulties occur with meat, salads, hard breads, nuts, and mixed consistencies, such as cereal and milk. When gathering food into a cohesive bolus becomes difficult, soft moist foods that hold their own shape help in binding the food together in the oral cavity. In addition, maximizing calories without increasing volume is important in this stage. Patients often begin to eat less and less in the middle stages of the disease because of the length of time it takes to finish a meal and concomitant fatigue. Using jams, jellies, powdered milk, wheat germ, oil, and other additives can boost calories but not burden the patient with the need to eat more food. Changing from a traditional three-meal-a-day model to eating smaller amounts throughout the day is also helpful and makes eating become less of an overwhelming prospect.

Liquid consistencies may also need to be modified in this stage. Thickened liquids are available commercially either in powder form or in prethickened form. Thickening a liquid can help to slow a bolus down enough for the patterned pharyngeal response to occur in a timely fashion, helping to prevent aspiration.

The increasing weaknesses in the bulbar musculature often necessitates the addition of postural maneuvers to aid in swallowing. As muscles atrophy, the intrapharyngeal pressure necessary to drive the swallow is insufficient, leaving residue in the mouth after the swallow. Postural maneuvers are designed to increase airway protection by reducing the diameter of the laryngeal vestibule and aid in the clearance of residue from the pharynx. This is accomplished by increasing the drive of the swallow via torque or by capitalizing on lateral strengths (68).

Patients begin to have significant difficulty taking pills in the middle stage of the disease. Strategies to aid in pill-taking include taking one at a time, changing to liquid forms of medication, cutting pills with consent of the pharmacist, or placing pills in a puree consistency, like applesauce or pudding. Even so, some pills are very difficult for patients to swallow, and use of PEG tube, if one is in place, is recommended for medications.

In the latest stage of the disease, swallowing becomes profoundly impaired. If patients have a PEG tube and continue to eat for pleasure, they are usually only able to manage pureed foods and thickened liquids. Suction may be necessary at this point to clear residue in the oral cavity and pharynx, and education should be provided to the patient and caregivers regarding the risks versus the benefits of continuing to eat.

PEG tube placement will be discussed in great detail in the next chapter. However, it is worth noting the American Academy of Neurology's ALS practice parameter recommends PEG tube placement for patients with symptomatic dysphagia soon after symptom onset and that this be done while the forced vital capacity is still 50% of predicted or better to diminish the morbidity and mortality associated with the procedure (69). Since publication of the practice parameter, many ALS centers have used BiPAP assistance to successfully place PEG tubes in those with a much lower vital capacity.

Finally, aggressive mouth care is a critical aspect of management of swallowing throughout all stages of the disease. Lack of dental caries and frequency of mouth care has been shown to decrease the risk of infection when aspiration cannot be avoided (67).

Providing patients with options for continued intake of food and liquid, sharing information regarding available evidence and empiric observation, and respecting patient autonomy with regard to eating and swallowing best characterize management of dysphagia in the ALS patient.

SUMMARY

Rehabilitation is a critical component of care for the ALS patient. It helps patients maintain mobility, communication, nutrition, and independence as long as possible despite disease progression and also helps to prevent the development of pain associated with immobility. Thus, rehabilitation has the ability to significantly improve quality of life for the ALS patient. In the early stages of ALS, an exercise program may be a useful prehabilitation strategy to delay the onset of disability. Once significant muscle weakness is present, assistive mobility devices, wheelchairs, orthoses, adaptive equipment to assist with ADLs, and home modifications serve to minimize disability and help patients maintain their independence. Musculoskeletal pain, which is secondary to muscle weakness, and spasticity may further limit function in ALS patients. Both pain and spasticity respond to a combination of physical rehabilitation techniques and pharmacologic management. Appropriate speech therapy interventions allow the patient to maintain communication and maximize nutritional status. The overall goal of rehabilitation is to optimize function and quality of life.

REFERENCES

1. Aboussouan LS, Khan SU, Meeker DP, Stelmach K, Mitsumoto H. Effect of non-invasive positive pressure ventilation on survival in amyotrophic lateral sclerosis. Ann Inter Med 1997; 127:450–453.
2. Kleopa KA, Sherman M, Neal B, Romano GJ, Heiman-Patterson T. Bipap improves survival and rate of pulmonary function decline in patients with ALS. J Neurol Sci 1999; 164:82–88.

3. Aboussouan L, Khan S, Banerjee M, Arroliga A, Mitsumoto H. Objective measures of the efficacy of noninvasive positive-pressure ventilation in amyotrophic lateral sclerosis. Muscle Nerve 2001; 24:403–409.

4. Desport J, Preux P, Truong T, Vallat J, Sautereau D, Couratier P. Nutritional status is a prognostic factor for survival in ALS patients. Neurology 1999; 53:1059–1063.

5. Mazzini L, Corra T, Zaccala M, Mora G, Piano MD, Galante M. Percutaneous endoscopic gastrostomy enteral nutrition in amyotrophic lateral sclerosis. J Neurol 1995; 242:695–698.

6. Mathus-Vliegen L, Louwerse L, Merkus M, Tytgat G, Jong JVD. Percutaneous endoscopic gastrostomy in patients with amyotrophic lateral sclerosis and impaired pulmonary function. Gastrointest Endosc 1994; 40:463–469.

7. Haas J. Ethical considerations of goal setting for patient care in rehabilitation medicine. Am J Phys Med Rehabil 1993; 72:228–232.

8. deCarvalho M, Nogueira A, Pinto A, Miguens J, Luis MS. Reflex sympathetic dystrophy associated with amyotrophic lateral sclerosis. J Neurol Sci 1999; 169:80–83.

9. Bohannon R. Results of resistance exercise on a patient with ALS: a case study. Phys Ther 1983; 63:965–968.

10. DalBello-Haas V, Kloos AD, Mitsumoto H. Physical therapy for a patient through six stages of amyotrophic lateral sclerosis. Phys Ther 1998; 78:1312–1324.

11. Aitkens SG, McCrory MA, Kilmer DD, Bernauer EM. Moderate resistance exercise program: its effect in slowly progressive neuromuscular disease. Arch Phys Med Rehabil 1993; 74:711–715.

12. Einarrson G. Muscle conditioning in late poliomyelitis. Arch Phys Med Rehabil 1991; 72:11–14.

13. Lindeman E, Leffers P, Spaans F, Drukker J, Reuten J, Kerckhoff M, Koke A. Strength training in patients with myotonicndystrophy and hereditary motor and sensory neuropathy: a randomized clinical trial. Arch Phys Med Rehabil 1995; 76:612–620.

14. McCartney N, Moroz D, Garner SH, McComas AJ. The effects of strength training in patients with selected neuromuscular disorders. Med Sci Sports Exerc 1988; 20: 362–368.

15. Kilmer DD, McCrory MA, Wright NC, Aitkens SG, Bernauer EM. The effect of a high resistance exercise program in slowly progressive neuromuscular disease. Arch Phys Med Rehabil 1994; 75:560–563.

16. Sanjak M, Paulson D, Sufit R, Reddan W, Beavlieu D, Erickson L, Shug A, Brooks B. Physiologic and metabolic response to progressive and prolonged exercise in amyotrophic lateral sclerosis. Neurology 1987; 37:1217–1220.

17. Drory V, Goltsman E, Reznik J, Mosek A, Korczyn A. The value of muscle exercise in patients with amyotrophic lateral sclerosis. J Neurol Sci 2002; 191:133–137.

18. Kirkenezos I, Hernandez D, Bradley W, Moraes C. Regular exercise is beneficial to a mouse model of amyotrophic lateral sclerosis. Ann Neurol 2003; 53:804–807.

19. Veldink J, Bar P, Joosten E, Otten M, Wokke J, Berg LVD. Sexual differences in onset of disease and response to exercise in a transgenic model of ALS. Neuromuscul Disord 2003; 13:737–743.

20. Mahoney D, Rodriquez C, Devries M, Yasuda N, Tarnopolsky M. Effects of high intensity endurance exercise training in the G93A mouse model of amyotrophic lateral sclerosis. Muscle Nerve 2004; 29:656–662.

21. Brooke M, Lateur BD, Diana-Rigby G, Questad K. Shoulder subluxation in hemiplegia: effects of three different supports. Arch Phys Med Rehabil 1991; 72:582–586.

22. Moodie N, Brisbin J, Margan A. Subluxation of the glenohumeral joint in hemiplegia: evaluation of supportiv devices. Phys Can 1986; 31:151–157.

23. Zorowitz R, Idank D, Ikai T, Hughes M, Johnston M. Shoulder subluxation after stroke: a comparison of four supports. Arch Phys Med Rehabil 1995; 76:763–771.

24. Trail M, Nelson N, Van J, Appel S, Lai E. Wheelchair use by patients with amyotrophic lateral sclerosis: a survey of user characteristics and selection preferences. Arch Phys Med Rehabil 2001; 82:98–102.

25. Fowler W, Carter G, Kraft G. Role of physiatry in the management of neuromuscular disease. Phys Med Rehabil Clin 1998; 9:1–8.
26. Francis K, Bach J, DeLisa J. Evaluation and rehabilitation of patients with adult motor neuron disease. Arch Phys Med Rehabil 1999; 80:951–963.
27. Carter G, Miller R. Comprehensive management of ALS. Phys Med Rehabil Clin 1998; 9:271–284.
28. Sharma KR, Kent-Braun JA, Majumdar S, Huang Y, Mynhier M, Weiner MW, Miller RG. Physiology of fatigue in amyotrophic lateral sclerosis. Neurology 1995; 45:733–740.
29. Abresch R, Seyden N, Wineinger M. Quality of life: issues for persons with neuromuscular diseases. Phys Med Rehabil Clin 1998; 9:233–248.
30. Simmons Z, Bremer B, Robbins R, Walsh S, Fischer S. Quality of life in ALS depends on factors other than strength and physical function. Neurology 2000; 55:388–392.
31. Kiebert GM, Green C, Murphy C, Mitchell JD, O'Brien M, Burreil A, Leigh PN. Patients' health-related quality of life and utilities associated with different stages of amyotrophic lateral sclerosis. J Neurol Sci 2001; 191:87–93.
32. Mitsumoto H, Del Bene M. Improving the quality of life for people with ALS: the challenge ahead. Amyotroph Lateral Scler Other Motor Neuron Disord 2000; 1:329–336.
33. Abresch R, Carter G, Jensen M, Kilmer D. Assessment of pain and health-related quality of life in slowly progressive neuromuscular disease. Am J Hosp Palliat Care 2002; 19: 39–48.
34. Lou J, Reeves A, Benice T, Sexton G. Fatigue and depression are associated with poor quality of life in ALS. Neurology 2003; 60:122–123.
35. Trail M, Nelson ND, Van J, Appel S, Lai E. A study comparing patients with amyotrophic lateral sclerosis and their caregivers on measures of quality of life, depression, and their attitudes toward treatment options. J Neurol Sci 2003; 209:79–85.
36. Hecht M, Hillemacher T, Grasel E, Tigges S, Winterholler M, Heuss D, Hilz MF, Neundorfer B. Subjective experience and coping in ALS. Amyotroph Lateral Scler Other Motor Neuron Disord 2002; 3:225–231.
37. Kilmer DD. The role of exercise in neuromuscular disease. Phys Med Rehabil Clin N Am 1998; 9:115–125, vi.
38. Sharma KR, Miller RG. Electrical and mechanical properties of skeletal muscle underlying increased fatigue in patients with amyotrophic lateral sclerosis. Muscle Nerve 1996; 19:1391–1400.
39. Johnson E, Fowler WM. Lieberman Contractures in neuromuscular disease. Arch Phys Med Rehabil 1992; 73:807–810.
40. Shibata M, Abe K, Jimbo A, Shimuzu T, Mihara M, Sadahiro S, Yoshikawa H, Mashimo T. Complex regional pain syndrome type I associated with amyotrophic lateral sclerosis. Clin J Pain 2003; 19:69–70.
41. Carter G, Abresch R, WM Fowler J, Johnson E, Kilmer D, McDonald C. Profiles of neuromuscular diseases. Spinal muscular atrophy. Am J Phys Med Rehabil 1995; 74: S150–S159.
42. Carter G, Galer B. Advances in the management of neuropathic pain. Phys Med Rehabil Clin North Am 2001; 12:447–459.
43. deCarvalho M. Gabapentin for the treatment of spasticity in patients with amyotrophic lateral sclerosis. Amyotroph Lateral Scler Other Motor Neuron Disord 2001; 2:47–48.
44. Fields H. Relief of unnecessary suffering. In: Fields H, Liebeskind J, eds. Pharmacologic Approaches to the Treatment of Chronic Pain: New Concepts and Critical Issues. Seattle: International Association for the Study of Pain Press, 1994:1–11.
45. Carter G, Weydt P. Cannabis: old medicine with new promise for neurological disorders. Curr Opin Investig Drugs 2002; 3:437–440.
46. Carter G, Rosen B. Marijuana in the management of amyotrophic lateral sclerosis. Am J Hosp Palliat Care 2001; 18:264–270.
47. Sinor A, Irvin S, Greenberg D. Endocannabinoids protect cerebral cortical neurons from in vitro ischemia in rats. Neurosci Lett 2000; 278:157–160.

48. Panikashvili D, Simeonidou C, Ben-Shabat S, Hanus L, Breuer A, Mechoulam R, Shohami E. An endogenous cannabinoid (2-AG) is neuroprotective after brain injury. Nature 2001; 413:527–531.

49. Hunter M, Robinson I, Neilson S. The functional and psychological status of patients with amyotrophic lateral sclerosis: some implications for rehabilitation. Disabil Rehabil 1993; 15:119–126.

50. Ashworth N, Satkunam L, Deforge D. Treatment for spasticity in amyotrophic lateral sclerosis/motor neuron disease. Cochrane Database Syst Rev 2004; 1:CD004156.

51. Marquardt G, Seifert V. Use of intrathecal baclofen for treatment of spasticity in amyotrophic lateral sclerosis. J Neurol Neurosurg Psychiatry 2002; 72:275–276.

52. Norris F, Shepherd R, Denys E, U K, Mukai E, Elias L, Holden D, Norris I. Onset, natural history, and outcome in idiopathic adult motor neuron disease. J Neurol Sci 1993; 118:48–55.

53. Yorkston K, Strand E, Miller R, Hillel A, Smith K. Speech deterioration in amyotrophic lateral sclerosis: implications for the timing of intervention. J Med Speech-Lang Pathol 1993; 1:35–46.

54. Ball L, Willis A, Beukelman D, Pattee G. A protocol for identification of early bulbar signs in amyotrophic lateral sclerosis. J Neurol Sci 2001; 191:43–53.

55. Ball L, Beukelman D, Pattee G. Communication effectiveness of individuals with amyotrophic lateral sclerosis. J Commun Disord 2004; May–June; 37(3):197–215.

56. Hillel A, Miller R, Yorkston K, McDonald E, Norris F, Konikow N. Amyotrophic lateral sclerosis severity scale. Neuroepidemiology 1989; 8:142–150.

57. Esposito S, Mitsumoto H, Shanks M. Use of palatal lift and palatal augmentation prostheses to improve dysarthria in patients with amyotrophic lateral sclerosis: a case series. J Prosthet Dent 2000; 83:90–98.

58. Yorkston K, Spencer K, Duffy J, Beukelman D, Golper L, Miller R. Evidence-based practice guidelines for dysarthria: management of velopharyngeal function. J Med Speech-Lang Pathol 2001; 9:257–274.

59. Clark H. Neuromuscular treatments for speech and swallowing: a tutorial. Am J Speech-Lang Pathol 2003; 12:400–415.

60. Duchan J, Calculator S, Sonnenmeier R, Diehl S, Cumley G. A framework for managing controversial practices. Lang Speech Hear Serv Schools 2001; 32:133–141.

61. Doyle M, Phillips B. Trends in augmentative and alternative communication use by individuals with amyotrophic lateral sclerosis. AAC Augmentation Altern Commun 2001; 17:167–178.

62. Hayashi H, Oppenheimer E. ALS patients on TPPV: totally locked-in state, neurological findings and ethical implications. Neurology 2003; 61:135–137.

63. Strong M, Rowe A, Rankin R. Percutaneous gastrojejunostomy in amyotrophic lateral sclerosis. J Neurol Sci 1999; 169:128–132.

64. Splaingard M, Hutchins B, Sulton L, Chaudhuri G. Aspiration in rehabilitation patients: videofluoroscopy vs bedside clinical assessment. Arch Phys Med Rehabil 1988; 69: 637–640.

65. Smithard D, O'Neill P. The role of videofluoroscopy in the assessment of swallowing disorders. Age Ageing 1992; 21:37.

66. Slowie L, Paige M, Antel J. Nutritional considerations in the management of patients with amyotrophic lateral sclerosis (ALS). J Am Diet Assoc 1983; 83:44–47.

67. Langmore SE, Terpenning M, Schork A, Chen Y, Murray JT, Lopatin D, Loesche WJ. Predictors of aspiration pneumonia: how important is dysphagia?. Dysphagia 1998; 13:69–81.

68. Logemann J. Therapy for oropharyngeal swallowing disorders. In: Schulze-Delrieu APaK, ed. Deglutition and its Disorders: Anatomy, Physiology, Clinical Diagnosis and Management. San Diego: Singular, 1997.

69. Miller RG, Rosenberg JA, Gelinas DF, Mitsumoto H, Newman D, Sufit R, Borasio GD, Bradley WG, Bromberg MB, Brooks BR, Kasankis EJ, Munvat TL, Oppenheimer EA. Practice parameter: the care of the patient with amyotrophic lateral sclerosis (an evidence based review). Neurology 1999; 52:1311–1323.

32

Nutritional Treatment: Theoretical and Practical Issues

Lan Chi T. Luu
Department of Nutritional Sciences and Neurology, University of Kentucky, Lexington, Kentucky, U.S.A.

Edward J. Kasarskis
Department of Neurology, University of Kentucky, Lexington, Kentucky, U.S.A.

Rup Tandan
Department of Neurology, University of Vermont, Burlington, Vermont, U.S.A.

INTRODUCTION

Nutritional research in amyotrophic lateral sclerosis (ALS) has grown past its infancy into preadolescence. To understand our approach to nutrition and our recommendations for ALS patients, we first wish to examine some theoretical issues. We will review the nutritional challenges faced by ALS patients, evaluate the current knowledge of nutrition in ALS, and examine an energy balance model for the nutritional treatment in ALS. Finally, we will discuss the practical aspects of nutritional treatment for ALS including monitoring of nutritional status, managing dysphagia, optimal timing for nutritional intervention with percutaneous endoscopic gastrostomy (PEG), and use of vitamins and supplements.

The goal of nutritional management is to maintain good nutrition by matching dietary intake to meet the nutritional requirements of an individual ALS patient. What is "good nutrition"? Recommendations for good nutrition can be found in dietary guidelines set by the scientific community to advise consumers about eating habits designed to maintain health. Since the 1970s, dietary goals have been set by the U.S. Department of Agriculture and the Department of Health and Human Services. These guidelines advise healthy Americans, two years and older, about general good nutritional practices to prevent diseases. These recommendations are revised every five years, with the last edition in 2000. The guidelines are quite general and include recommendations for physical activity, a variety of food choices using the food pyramid, and moderating dietary fat, sugar, and salt. Although sensible, these recommendations are ill suited for a progressive neurodegenerative disease, where the nutritional needs are constantly changing.

Table 1 Recommended Dietary Allowances, 1989 Edition

Age (years)	Energy (kcal/day)	Protein (g/day)
Males		
11–14	2500	45
15–18	3000	59
19–24	2900	58
25–50	2900	63
51+	2300	63
Females		
11–14	2200	46
15–18	2200	44
19–24	2200	46
25–50	2200	50
51+	1900	50

In addition to these general dietary principles, specific Recommended Dietary Allowances (RDA) assist consumers to achieve certain recommended dietary goals. Table 1 illustrates some of the RDA suggestions for males and females in regard to total energy (i.e., calories, given as kcal/day) and protein intake (g/day). The goal of the RDA approach is to provide adequate nutrients for growth (in children and adolescents) and maintenance of body composition and function (in adults) to prevent deficiency diseases as a result of malnutrition. There are several pitfalls in the RDA approach. One shortcoming is that it does not provide specific recommendations for carbohydrate, total fat, saturated fat, or cholesterol. Another is that it does not give detailed recommendations for the large segment of the population older than age 51 years, or advice for other food components such as caffeine and alcohol. Also no consideration is given to energy needs associated with physical activity, which can constitute a significant proportion of daily energy expenditure. Although the RDA provides general guidance, it is not specific enough for a complex, progressive disorder like ALS.

THEORETICAL ISSUES

Nutritional Complexities in ALS and the Risk for Nutritional Insufficiency

It is understandable why the ALS patient is at risk for failure to meet even these general goals for good nutrition when considering the pathophysiology of the disease. Evolving dysphagia and progressive hand and arm weakness are both risk factors for restricted dietary intake. Less apparent are factors that lead to changing energy expenditure. These include: changing body composition, declining levels of physical activity, increasing energy expenditure to perform functional movements, and the presence of energy-wasting non-functional muscle contractions (fasciculations, cramps, spasticity, and pseudobulbar motor activities). Additional factors include the use of various therapies, most notably non-invasive positive pressure ventilation (NIPPV), which can reduce energy expenditure while simultaneously alleviating troublesome symptoms from weakness of respiratory muscles. Weighing the contributions of these individual factors to determine nutritional adequacy cannot be given at this time and is the subject of active investigation. Nevertheless, it is clear that decreasing energy intake and increasing energy expenditure can, and does, result in negative energy balance and malnutrition.

Is Weight Loss a Sensitive Indicator of Malnutrition in ALS?

One definition of malnutrition is a body weight less than 10% of the ideal body weight or a body mass index [BMI = weight (kg)/height (m^2)] below 18.5 to 20 kg/m^2 (1–4). Descriptive terms such as "cachexia," "aging anorexia," and "sarcopenia" are used to describe the phenomenon of weight loss due to malnutrition or as part of normal aging. Simple loss of body weight is not informative since it does not identify the source of tissue loss. For example, a person on a weight reduction diet will lose body weight from the fat compartment. In this situation, one can conclude that this person is losing body weight because of a negative energy balance, which is the desired effect in this circumstance. However, in ALS, weight loss can occur because of muscle wasting, making weight loss an unreliable indicator of energy (calorie) balance.

The pathophysiology of weight loss in ALS is complex and involves neurogenic muscle atrophy, depletion of fat mass if the patient is in chronic negative energy balance, and potentially catabolism of innervated muscle fibers for energy if the extent of negative energy balance is severe. This has been termed "ALS cachexia" by Denys and Norris (5). Recent studies in ALS document increased mortality and morbidity associated with malnutrition using weight loss as the criterion. The mechanism(s), whereby malnutrition increases mortality in ALS, may include impaired diaphragmatic structure and function, and muscle catabolism leading to further immobility, hypoventilation, aspiration, and pulmonary infection (6). Malnutrition appears to amplify the relative risk of death by 7.7-fold in such ALS patients (2).

The Concept of Energy Intake and Energy Expenditure

In normal persons with a stable body weight, energy intake (EI) equals the total daily energy expenditure (TDEE). This should be the goal for ALS patients as well. Quantification of EI is based on the measurement of the contents of food and beverages consumed each day. The methods of assessment vary, but include: food frequency questionnaires, 24-hour dietary recall, and three days of dietary recording and weighing of meal components. Calculation of nutrient and energy intake typically relies on the expertise of a dietician or nutritionist using one of several compendia of food compositions and their nutrient value. However, the assessment of EI is intrusive and is totally dependent on the cooperation and memory of the subject, which makes these methods inherently limited.

On the expenditure side, TDEE is comprised of three factors as shown in Eq. (1)

$$TDEE = RMR + EE_{act} + TEF \tag{1}$$

in which RMR represents the resting metabolic rate, EE_{act} is the energy expenditure as the result of physical activities, and TEF is the thermic effect of food, which is the energy cost of ingesting and absorbing food.

The RMR for healthy persons is about 5% to 15% higher than the basal metabolic rate (BMR) because of the energy cost of arousal and maintenance of muscle tone. Theoretically, BMR is the minimal energy requirement of the organism but is very difficult to measure consistently. However, RMR can be measured in the research setting using indirect calorimetry (IC) and reflects the energy requirements

Table 2 Studies of Energy Metabolism of ALS Patients

Author (Ref.)	Journal (year)	Conclusion
Slowie et al. (7)	J Am Diet Assoc (1983)	ALS patients experience weight loss and muscle atrophy. Early nutritional management may help to alleviate energy loss
Nau et al. (8)	J Neurol Sci (1995)	ALS patients do lose muscle mass but gain in fat mass due to declining physical activity
Kasarskis et al. (9)	Am J Clin Nutr (1996)	ALS patients are chronically energy deficient but appear to consume adequate protein
Kasarskis and Naville (10)	Neurology (1996)	Recommendations for nutritional management
Desport et al. (2)	Neurology (1999)	Using BMI, the study found 16.4% of 55 subjects were malnourished putting them at a 7.7-fold increase risk of death
Desport et al. (3)	ALS&MND (2000)	Between 16% and 50% of all ALS patients are malnourished. Enteral nutrition can improve respiratory status. For greatest advantage to survival, enteral support should be done before vital capacity drops below 70% and BMI below $18.5\,\mathrm{kg/m^2}$
Pessolano FA et al. (11)	Am J Phys Med Rehabil (2003)	BMI should be used with caution to evaluate nutritional status in ALS patients because it does not account for compartmental distribution of muscle and fats

for sustaining basic metabolic functions without movement upon awakening from sleep after an overnight fasting.

Energy expended during physical activity (EE_{act}) is the energy cost of muscle contraction and is the most variable component of TDEE, even in healthy persons. Quantifying EE_{act} in a free-living individual is challenging due to the variation, range, and intensity of different activities. A variety of methods estimate EE_{act} including accelerometers, actigraphy, and physical activity questionnaires.

Thermic effect of food (TEF) reflects the increase in oxygen consumption due to food ingestion, digestion, absorption, and processing of nutrients. This typically accounts for 8% to 10% of the energy content of food consumed.

Since weight change per se is not a reliable indicator of nutritional status in ALS patients, maintaining energy balance appears to be a more logical goal of nutritional management. Simply stated, a well-nourished ALS patient is one in whom daily EI meets TDEE. Theoretically both overfeeding and underfeeding can be associated with negative consequences. Underfeeding can result in loss of fat reserves and accelerated loss of innervated, functional muscle to meet TDEE if underfeeding continues for a long time. Overfeeding results in a net increase in body fat, which may increase body weight and impose an added burden for functional movement by weakened muscles. Currently, our ability to provide an accurate assessment of TDEE and EI is limited and is the subject of intense research by our group. In the absence of definitive research, what is known about the nutritional status of ALS patients? Table 2 summarizes knowledge in this area.

These studies rely on weight loss, BMI, anthropometry, bio-impedance analysis (BIA), indirect calorimetry, nitrogen balance, and dietary records to relate alterations in body composition to energy metabolism in ALS. None of these criteria or methods has been validated against the doubly labeled water (DLW) technique, the gold standard method of measuring energy balance, in ALS. Hence, the current literature on nutrition in ALS is limited and does not provide practical, accurate equations to predict TDEE.

Accurate Assessment of Energy Intake and Energy Expenditure

The most common method to quantify EI is measurement of food intake utilizing either food recall or food diaries. Under ideal circumstances, both methods are valid and reliable tools for the assessment of EI. The accuracy depends on a variety of factors, including: the dietician's training and standardization of interview questions for 24-hour food recall. In theory, three-day dietary recording of food intake should be more accurate but it is intrusive and, ipso facto, may alter eating behaviors. Accuracy depends on the instructions to the patients and families, and the attention of the person recording the components of the meal or snack. In contrast to other research methods, recording food intake occurs in the home away from supervision of the investigator. With either method, accuracy also depends on the type of dietary software used to analyze the data. Available databases include: the National Database System (NDS), the Food Intake Analysis System (FIAS), NutriBase Clinical, Food Processor SQL, and Nutritionist.

Indirect calorimetry can assess RMR, which in conjunction with the calculated TEF based on recorded dietary intake, can specify two of the components of TDEE. Indirect calorimetry estimates the amount of energy produced by biologic oxidations (energy expenditure), the type of substrates utilized (i.e., carbohydrate and lipids), and the amount oxidized by measuring respiratory gas exchange (i.e., oxygen consumption, oxygen volume, carbon dioxide production, and carbon dioxide volume). RMR represents between 60% and 75% of TDEE and has strong correlation with FFM (12,13). RMR can be measured with high precision (using IC) or calculated from fat-free mass (FFM) as determined by dual energy X-ray absorptiometry (DXA), bioelectrical impedance spectroscopy (BIS), or bioelectrical impedance analysis (BIA). Hence, TDEE can be calculated from Eq. (1) if one knows RMR (from IC), TEF (from records of food consumption), and EE_{act} (from questionnaires or quantitative methods).

However, TDEE can be determined directly using the DLW method, which is considered to be the "gold standard." It has the distinct advantage over other methods in that it determines TDEE over time (typically 10 to 14 days) in free-living ALS patients in their home environment, and without confinement to a metabolic chamber. The method has been well validated in many animal species and has been successfully used in ALS (14,15). The major disadvantage to the DLW method is extreme expense of the DLW cocktail and the requirement of a specialized mass spectroscopy facility for sample analysis. These factors limit its clinical use, but in a research setting it is a powerful tool to understand energy expenditure in ALS patients.

Identifying ALS Patients with Impending Nutritional Insufficiency

Implication of Dysphagia

Several studies measured reduced EI in ALS patients, even in the absence of bulbar weakness (16,17). This implies that the presence or absence of dysphagia is not an accurate indicator of impending nutritional insufficiency even though dysphagia serves as one criterion for intervention with PEG in the American Academy of

Neurology Practice Parameters. It appears that patients may deny swallowing difficulties because they employ adaptive swallowing techniques and food modification that enables them to complete their meals. From that perspective, they may minimize or deny the presence of dysphagia (10,16,18). It is a common anecdotal observation that family members of ALS patients appreciate prolonged meal times, while at the same time patients deny any problems with feeding. Studies in the general aging population show that prolonged meal times is associated with lower EI compared to individuals eating at a normal pace (19,20). Nutritional insufficiency in the setting of dysphagia is not universal among ALS patients based on preliminary data from our group, indicating that some ALS patients with dysphagia do, in fact, meet their TDEE. However, the presence of dysphagia does imply that bulbar weakness exists and should alert the clinician to the possibility of impending nutritional compromise.

Alterations in Body Composition

In theory, a declining fat mass as ALS progresses should imply that EI is not sufficient to meet TDEE. Hence, determining body composition could serve as a "bottom line" criterion for energy insufficiency. Several research methods are available to measure fat mass including: underwater weighing, anthropometry, DXA, BIA and BIS; and CT and MRI methods (2,3,8,10,18). Each has its own technical limitations, a discussion of which is beyond the scope of this review. All of these methods can provide an assessment of body fat, which in turn could serve as a long-term index of nutritional status. However, a single determination of body fat will not be able to provide insight into acute changes in EI or TDEE.

Predictive Equations

Many published equations predict BMR and TDEE based on height, weight, sex, age, race, fat-free mass (FFM), or a combination of these and other factors. The most popular of the predictive equations in clinical practice is the Harris-Benedict equation (HBE), which is designed to estimate BMR. Interestingly, the HBE was developed, between 1909 and 1919, based on normal fit young subjects. Equations (2) and (3) represent the two HBE and their predictive ability (r^2)

$$\text{BMR in males} = 278 + (57.5 \times \text{Wt}) + (20.9 \times \text{Ht}) - (28.3 \times \text{age}) \ (r^2 = 0.75) \quad (2)$$

$$\text{BMR in females} = 274 + (40.0 \times \text{Wt}) + (7.7 \times \text{Ht}) - (19.6 \times \text{age}) \ (r^2 = 0.53) \quad (3)$$

where Wt is weight in kg and Ht is height in cm and age is in years.

Many studies have shown that the HBE has poor predictive ability for other populations not sharing similarities with the original cohort from which the equations were developed. As may be anticipated in the case of an age-associated neurodegenerative disease such as ALS, the HBE was found to be inaccurate in estimating BMR by 20% to 40% (21,22) because it fails to take into account the heterogeneity of the population, particularly in relation to the degree of physical activity (Table 3). Developing ALS-specific predictive equations represents an important focus of our research group.

Synergism Between Nutritional and Respiratory Support

A recent evidence-based review indicates that most ALS patients develop symptomatic hypoventilation by the time forced vital capacity (FVC) falls below 50% (23).

Table 3 Validity of Estimated Energy Expenditure Against DLW Using Predictive Equations in 10 ALS Patients

Unadjusted TDEE by DLW	2785 ± 349 kcal/day
Estimated energy expenditure	
Using resting metabolic rate equations	2234 ± 301 kcal/day
Using Harris–Benedict equations	2227 ± 247 kcal/day
Difference between TDEE and equations	
Resting metabolic rate equation	567 ± 270 kcal/day; $\downarrow 20\%$
Harris–Benedict equations	550 ± 403; $\downarrow 19\%$

Early symptoms of respiratory insufficiency include frequent nocturnal arousals, nightmares, morning headaches, and excessive daytime sleepiness (24). The energy cost to maintain adequate respiration in the setting of diaphragmatic weakness, and of frequent nocturnal arousals, has not been measured. NIPPV is frequently recommended for patients with a FVC < 50% of predicted for symptomatic treatment of respiratory insufficiency. In theory, NIPPV should reduce TDEE in addition to its intended use of supporting nocturnal respiration in low-functioning ALS patients. Therefore, NIPPV may have bifunctional benefits by both supporting respiration and reducing the number of calories required. This hypothesis, as illustrated in Figure 1, has not been tested to date, but is the subject of investigation by our study group.

PRACTICAL ISSUES

Monitoring of the Nutritional State and Swallowing

Ideally, one should have knowledge of EI and TDEE to determine if a given patient is in energy balance on an ongoing basis. If the patient falls into negative energy

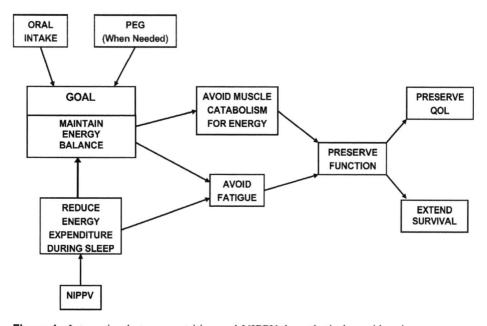

Figure 1 Interaction between nutrition and NIPPV: hypothetical considerations.

balance, a firm recommendation for PEG as an alternative route for nutrition can be given. Similarly, one could tailor nutritional recommendations to avoid overfeeding as this can have adverse consequences, especially if undertaken over a relatively short time span. This ideal situation has yet to be realized in clinical practice. However, several practical steps can be taken in the interim.

Vigilant monitoring of patients' nutritional and swallowing states, using currently available tools, followed by intervention with PEG may improve the prognosis for survival in ALS. A downward trend in body weight and/or BMI can provide some indication of the nutritional status. The ALS Functional Rating Scale (ALSFRS) is a well validated and important tool for monitoring functional status. The ALSFRS includes questions regarding bulbar weakness, swallowing difficulties, and upper limb weakness which provide an important, but indirect indications of potential deteriorating nutritional status. Other scales, such as the ALS EATS (25) scale, query appetite and the social dimensions of eating, in addition to dysphagia and upper extremity weakness and can provide additional information. The 24-hour food recall methodology can be beneficial in understanding energy, protein, and micronutrient intake but it is not generally available in a neurology or ALS clinic.

A very empiric approach is to aim for a stable body weight, recognizing that this is, at best, an indirect indicator of nutritional status in ALS. A falling body weight could result from: rapidly progressive neurogenic muscle atrophy, shrinking fat stores (due to energy insufficiency), extreme dehydration, or a combination of these factors. For whatever reason, it should prompt the clinician to activate a plan for nutritional intervention, including PEG insertion, if appropriate.

Early Nutritional Intervention

Early nutritional intervention includes changes in the kinds of food consumed, the consistencies of food, frequency and duration of meals, and incorporation of adaptive techniques to assist swallowing, using adaptive eating utensils from occupational therapists (OT), and/or PEG. The timing of these interventions depends on how quickly eating problems are detected. Vigilant monitoring of patients' eating habits, measuring body weight and body composition, and determining TDEE and EI are important for early detection. However, these goals are infrequently met in practice today.

Choking spells, excessive saliva, lengthy meal times, avoidance of eating in public, fatigue while eating, changes in dietary consistency or food choices, depression, or anorexia are practical clinical cues to institute aggressive nutritional intervention. Patients may deny that they are experiencing swallowing difficulties because they are careful when they eat or drink, resulting in longer meal times. However, redirecting the questions to inquire about length of meals, food choices and consistency, and inquiry of family members directly about the patient's ability to eat are all important strategies in recognizing the insidious appearance of nutritional inadequacy.

Other techniques can assess the mechanics of swallowing, such as a modified barium swallow, video-fluoroscopy, ultrasound evaluation, or fiberoptic endoscopic study. These tests are designed to visualize the physiological process of swallowing with the goal of rehabilitation. These functional tests may provide guidance for food choice to facilitate successful swallowing. However, in of themselves, they do not probe the totality of the eating experience (mechanical, social, affective, and appetite), all of which may be compromised in ALS. Undue dependence on a single test to guide nutritional management is to be discouraged because of the progressive and multifaceted nature of the disease.

Swallowing and Appropriate Dietary Modifications

With the onset of dysphagia, it is important to consider modifying the patient's diet and/or its consistency to maintain adequate nutrition by the oral route as long as possible. Diet changes may include

1. cooking meats, fruits, and vegetables until very tender and moist,
2. limiting raw vegetables and fruits,
3. cutting food finely,
4. using pureed and or strained foods,
5. cooking with ground meats,
6. eating foods high in water content, like gelatin, puddings, gravy, and sauces,
7. including more beverages that are thick and dense in texture, such as tomato juice, and
8. mixing commercial thickening agents to food and beverages (such as Thick-It®).

Keys to minimizing the risk of aspiration are: (i) preparing foods that are soft and moist, (ii) eating small size bites, and (iii) drinking thickened beverages. In addition to alterations in food properties, the meal size, timing, and frequency may require modification as well. Rather than the usual three meals a day, multiple smaller meals throughout the day may be better tolerated. A potential complication of these dietary changes may be constipation due to lack of dietary fiber and reduced fluid intake. Supplementation of fiber and increased consumption of fluid should be actively encouraged.

Timing is crucial to effectively manage dysphagia, and the management must emphasize early monitoring of symptoms. Education regarding specific head positioning (i.e., the chin tuck position which instructs patients to sit up straight, position the head slightly forward with the chin down to help prevent food from going down the airway, and not to breathe until food is completely swallowed) and placement of food inside the mouth to better facilitate control of the food bolus during chewing and swallowing are important first steps in managing dysphagia. Recommendations about optimal food textures, meal size and timing, and minimizing fatigue are also important in the management of ALS-associated dysphagia. However, such compensatory strategies are only temporarily effective and with disease progression, alternate routes of nutritional support will be needed (e.g., PEG).

PEG as an Alternative Route for Nutrition

Despite modifying swallowing techniques, altering food consistency, and using adaptive equipment, many ALS patients will not be able to maintain their oral intake to meet their TDEE requirements. Tube feeding or some other type of gastrostomy procedure will become the only option to deliver optimal nutrition. Three types of enteral nutrition are available: (i) nasogastric feeding, (ii) PEG, and (iii) percutaneous endoscopic jejunostomy (PEJ). At some institutions, Radiologically Inserted Gastrostomy (RIG) is an evolving technique. Although feeding through a nasogastric tube is the least invasive, it is impractical for long-term nutritional support (26,27). PEG placement is simple and relatively safe, although the risks of complications increases as the FVC declines below 50% of predicted (26,27). The feeding schedule is similar to regular oral feeding, that is, four to five times a day. Although nutritional supplementation is usually administered via PEG as bolus feeding, patients may report bloating following meals, especially in those with nutritional deprivation prior to

PEG. Patients should be instructed to bolus feed slowly or to use continuous feeding without or with a pump to minimize this complication. Many patients require titration, starting with diluted supplements until the feedings are better tolerated and the nutritional goals are met. There may be a mistaken notion that a PEG signals the end of the ability of patients to eat by mouth. It should be a point of emphasis that patients can continue to eat pleasurable foods by mouth in a social setting, while receiving the majority of their nutrition, hydration, and medications via PEG.

Studies to date document that nutritional support administered via PEG is effective in stabilizing body weight. Early placement of PEG as an alternative route for nutritional supplementation will prevent further weight loss in most cases and may be associated with improved survival (3,4,14). Some of these benefits of PEG, and the published studies to-date, are summarized in Table 4. Currently, PEG placement is recommended when the FVC is above 50% of predicted in patients with rapid weight loss and/or dysphagia. Although PEG can be successfully placed in patients with a FVC < 50%, caution is advised because studies indicate a higher morbidity and mortality in these instances.

Nutritional Formulations

There are a variety of commercial products for nutritional supplementation. Formulations range from high calorie to high protein to disease-specific compositions. If weight loss persists or progresses, it is recommended that patients augment their regular meals with additional caloric supplementation. Patients should be encouraged to focus on high calorie supplements rather than high protein, unless there are other chronic medical conditions such as diabetes mellitus or cardiovascular disease.

Supplements are easy to use in patients, and in the absence of severe dysphagia, will maintain or increase body weight. These commercially available products range in price and most health insurance plans provide coverage, particularly, for patients experiencing cachexia. Clinicians and patients are encouraged to work closely with a registered dietician or nutritionist to identify appropriate formulations for their specific need.

Over-the-Counter Dietary Supplements

A bewildering variety of natural products are sold in health food and nutrition stores in almost every shopping mall in the United States. Needless to say, none of these has been studied in ALS for safety and efficacy. Although some patients may prefer their own brand of a favorite natural food products, there is no scientific basis to recommend the use of these products. Moreover, many products purporting to be "cures" for ALS are advertised on Internet web pages. These lack scientific credibility and patients should be wary of these products.

Vitamins and Supplements

Antioxidants

One of the theories of causation of ALS is oxidative damage to motor neurons, thus making antioxidants popular with patients. Although antioxidants may, at best, have a marginal benefit in slowing progression of the disease, they are probably the most widespread form of pharmacological intervention. Historically, Lou Gehrig himself took Vitamin E back in 1939 attesting to the long-standing popularity of this

Table 4 Studies of Nutritional Evaluation in ALS Patients at Time of PEG

	Mathus-Vliegen et al., 1994 (28)	Mazzini et al., 1995 (29)	Strong et al., 1999 (30)	Chio et al. 1999 (31)	Kasarskis et al., 1999 (32)
N	68	31	73	50	36 (CNTF) 172 (BDNF)
M:F	31:24	18:13	46:27	21:29	17:19, 74:62
Age at onset (yrs)	56.4	—	63.2 (Bulbar)	59.6	—, 57.5 (Limb)
Age at PEG (yrs)	58.8	60.9	—	61.7	56.3, 59.2
Time between diagnosed of ALS and PEG (mos)	28.4	26.0	17.7 (Bulbar)	25.2	29.9 (Limb)
Weight (kg)	74.4	—	—	—	—
Weigh loss/mo	0.60%	0.65%	—	0.66%	
BMI	21.1	19.7	—	21.3	21.3, 22.2
FVC (% predicted)	45.8	30.6	—	68.9	41.6, 53.0
ALS-FRS	—	—	—	—	18.1, 22.2
Norris scale	—	51.4	—	56.1	—
Serial weights	+	+	+	+	+, +
Serial lung function	+	+	—	+	+, +
Albumin	—	+		+	+, +
Chloride	—	—		+	+, +
Stability of weight loss	+	+	?	+	+, +
Mortality after 24 hrs	1.8%	0%	0%	0%	0%, 0.7%
Mortality after 30 days	11.5%	9.7%	9.6%	0%	6.3%, 9.6%
Mean survival (day)	—	393 vs. 108	—	—	151, 260
Median survival (day)	122 vs. 92.5	300 vs. 450	660 vs. 900 (Bulbar)	720 vs. 1065 (Limb)	915 vs. 760
ALS-FRS	—	—	—	—	18.1, 22.2

Table 5 Summary of Key Concepts of Nutritional Treatment in ALS

The goal of nutritional intervention in ALS is to match nutritional intake to meet
  nutritional requirements
    Ensuring the energy (i.e., calorie) intake matches TDEE so that patients
      maintain energy balance throughout the course of their disease
    Maintaining energy balance may prolong survival, but this has not been
      shown conclusively in a prospective study
Nutritional problems are complex and arise because of:
  Changing energy intake
    Evolving dysphagia
    Progressive hand and arm weakness
  Changing energy expenditure
    Changing body composition
    Changing level of physical activity
    Presence of energy-wasting muscle contractions (fasciculations, cramps,
      spasticity, and pseudobulbar motor activity)
    Increased energy expenditure to perform functional movements
    Energy-wasting effect of respiratory dysfunction and energy-sparing effect of
      respiratory support
Nutritional needs may be met using a combination of:
  Modifying food consistency and eating patterns
  Using adaptive equipment
  PEG or other alternate routes of nutritional intake
An integrated approach of respiratory and nutritional support is desirable

approach. High dose Vitamin E (5000 IU/day) in combination with riluzole did not
show any added benefit in a recent multicenter European study in ALS patients. In
fact, a recent meta-analysis of several studies with high or low dose Vitamin E undertaken in healthy individuals and in several disease states showed greater general
mortality in patients taking higher doses and the recommendation by the authors
was that doses greater than 400 IU/day should be discouraged (33).

The following represent reasonable guidelines for antioxidants, recognizing
that these guidelines are not based on formal scientific study. Most, if not all, can
be purchased over the counter:

1. *Vitamin E*: Based on studies in Alzheimer's disease and Parkinson's
   disease, a safe dose appears to have been 400 international units (IU) three
   times per day. Some advocate 800 IU three times per day. Nevertheless,
   Vitamin E, a fat-soluble vitamin, can accumulate and become toxic if taken
   chronically in high doses (33).
2. *Vitamin C*: A reasonable dose might be 500 to 1000 mg four times per day.
   However, Vitamin C has never received scientific study in ALS.
3. *Zinc*: Zinc is not a vitamin but a mineral, which in some experimental
   situations exhibits antioxidant properties by stabilizing membranes. A reasonable preparation is zinc sulfate in a dose of 220 mg twice per day.
4. *Antioxidant–vitamin combinations*: There are many commercially available
   vitamin pills which contain Vitamin E, Vitamin C, zinc, and selenium, in
   addition to β carotene and Vitamin A.
5. *Creatine*: Creatine is another natural product that protects mitochondria and
   extends survival in transgenic SOD-1 ALS mouse models. However, creatine

administered to ALS patients at 5 to 10 g/day in two controlled studies did not retard the progression of weakness. A safe dose has not been established for ALS patients. Currently, we do not recommend creatine to patients.

Coenzyme Q10

Co-Q10 is a naturally occurring substance that improves mitochondrial function. Co-Q10 extends the lifespan of the G93A SOD-1 ALS mouse model in laboratory experiments. In a phase-II study, coadministration of Vitamin E (1200 mg/day) and Co-Q10 (2400 mg/day) appear to reduce the functional decline in the participants (34). Many ALS patients take Co-Q10. Although Co-Q10 appears to have no serious side effects, the safety and efficacy of Co-Q10 has not been formally studied in ALS.

CONCLUSION

In summary, the points listed in Table 5 are critical concepts when considering nutritional treatment of patients with ALS.

GLOSSARY

ALS	Amyotrophic Lateral Sclerosis
PEG	Percutaneous Endoscopic Gastrostomy
RDA	Recommended Dietary Allowances
NIPPV	Non-Invasive Positive Pressure Ventilation
BMI	Body Mass Index
EI	Energy Intake
TDEE	Total Daily Energy Expenditure
RMR	Resting Metabolic Rate
EE_{act}	Energy Expenditure from Physical Activities
TEF	Thermic Effect of Food
BMR	Basal Metabolic Rate
IC	Indirect Calorimetry
BIA	Bio-Impedance Analysis
NDS	National Database System
FIAS	Food Intake Analysis System
FFM	Fat-Free Mass
DXA	Dual Energy X-ray Absorptiometry
BIS	Bio-electrical Impedance Spectroscopy
DLW	Doubly Labeled Water
CT	Computed Tomography
MRI	Magnetic Resonance Imaging
HBE	Harris–Benedict Equations
Wt	Weight
Ht	Height
FVC	Forced Vital Capacity
ALSFRS	ALS Functional Rating Scale
ALS EATS	ALS Extremities Appetite Tongue and Swallowing
OT	Occupational Therapist
PEJ	Percutaneous Endoscopic Jejunostomy
IU	International Units
Co-Q10	Co-Enzyme Q10
RIG	Radiologically Inserted Gastrostomy

REFERENCES

1. Witte KA, Andrew LC. Nutritional abnormalities contributing to cachexia in chronic illness. Int J Cardiol 2002; 85:23–31.
2. Desport JC, Preux PM, Truong TC, Vallat JM, Sautereau D, Couratier P. Nutritional status is a prognostic factor for survival in ALS patients. Neurology 1999; 53(5):1059–1063.
3. Desport JC, Preux PM, Truong CT, Courat L, Vallat JM, Couratier P. Nutritional assessment and survival in ALS patients. ALS OMND 2000; 1(2):91–96.
4. Stratton RJ, Hackston A, Longmore D, Dixon R, Price S, Stroud M, King C, Elia M. Malnutrition in hospital outpatients and inpatients: prevalence, concurrent validity and ease of use of the 'malnutrition universal screening tool' (MUST) for adults. Br J Nutr 2004; 92(5):799–808.
5. Denys EH, Norris FH, Jr. Amyotrophic lateral sclerosis. Impairment of neuromuscular transmission. Arch Neurol 1979; 36(4):202–205.
6. Arora NS, Rochester DF. Respiratory muscle strength and maximal voluntary ventilation in undernourished patients. Am Rev Respir Dis 1982; 126:5–8.
7. Slowie LA, Paige MS, Antel JP. Nutritional considerations in the management of patients with amyotrophic lateral sclerosis (ALS). J Am Dietetic Assn 1983; 83:44–47.
8. Nau KL, Bromberg MB, Forshew DA, Katch VL. Individuals with amyotrophic lateral sclerosis are in caloric balance despite losses in mass. J Neurol Sci 1995; 129:47–49.
9. Kasarskis EJ, Berryman S, Vanderleest JG, Schneider AR, McClain CJ. The nutritional status of patients with amyotrophic lateral sclerosis: Relation to the proximity of death. Am J Clin Nutr 1996; 63:130–137.
10. Kasarskis EJ, Neville HE. Management of ALS: Nutritional care. Neurology 1996; 47(Suppl 2):S118–S120.
11. Pessolano F, Suarez AA, Monteiro SG, Mesa L, Dubrovsky A, Roncorni AJ, Devito EL. Nutritional assessement of patients with neuromuscular diseases. Am J Phys Med Rehabil 2003; 82(3):182–185.
12. Heymsfield S. Measurements of energy balance. Acta Diabetol 2003; 40(suppl 1):S117–S121.
13. Wang Z, Heshka S, Gallagher D, Boozer CN, Kotler DP, Heymsfield SB. Resting energy expenditure-fat-free mass relationship: new insights provided by body composition modeling. Am J Physiol Endocrinol Metab 2000; 279(3):E539–E545.
14. Westerterp KR. Body composition, water turnover and energy turnover assessment with labeled water. Proc Nutr Soc 1999; 58(4):945–951.
15. Schoeller DA. Measurement of energy expenditure in free-living humans by using doubly labeled water. J Nutr 1988; 118:1278–1289.
16. Silani V, Kasarskis EJ, Yanagisawa N. Nutritional management in amyotrophic lateral sclerosis: a worldwide perspective. J Neurol 1998; 245 Suppl 2:S13–19; discussion S29.
17. Hardiman O. Symptomatic treatment of respiratory and nutritional failure in amyotrophic lateral sclerosis. J Neurol 2000; 247:245–251.
18. Kasarskis EJ. Disease-modifying interventions. ALS OMND 2004(suppl 1):1–3.
19. Wilson M, Morley J. Aging and energy balance. J Appl Physiol 2003(95):1728–1736.
20. Morley JE, Thomas DR. Anorexia and aging: pathophysiology. Nutrition 1999; 15:499–503.
21. Kien CL, Ugrasbul F. Prediction of daily energy expenditure during a feeding trial using measurements of resting energy expenditure, fat-free mass or Harris-Benedict equations. Am J Clin Nutr 2004; 80(4):876–880.
22. Reeves MM, Capra S. Variation in the application of methods used for predicting energy requirements in acutely ill adult patients: a survey of practice. Eur J Clin Nutr 2003; 57(12):1530–1535.
23. Miller RG, Rosenberg JA, Gelinas DF, Mitsumoto H, Newman D, Sufit R, Borasio GD, Bradley WG, Bromberg MB, Brooks BR, Kasarskis EJ, Munsat TL, Oppenheimer EA.

Practice parameter: the care of the patient with amyotrophic lateral sclerosis (an evidence-based review): report of the Quality Standards Subcommittee of the American Academy of Neurology: ALS Practice Parameters Task Force. Neurology 1999; 52(7):1311–1323.

24. Krivickas L. In: Mitsumoto H, ed. Amyotrophic Lateral Sclerosis. New York: Davis; 1998:388–389.

25. Luu LC, Kasarskis EJ. ALSEATS, a comprehensive instrument for assessing the multi-dimensional nature of eating in amyotrophic lateral sclerosis patients. In: Neurology Outcomes Research, American Neurological Association, 129th Annual Meeting. Toronto; 2004.

26. Chio A, Galletti R, Finocchiaro C. Percutaneous radiological gastrostomy: a safe and effective method of nutritional tube placement in advanced ALS. J Neurol Neruosurg Psychiat 2004; 75(4):645–647.

27. Mitsumoto H, Davidson M, Moore D. ALS CARE Study Group. Percutaneous endo-scopic gastrostomy (PEG) in patients with ALS and bulbar dysfunction. ALSOMND 2003; 4(3):177–185.

28. Mathus-Vliegen LM, Louwerse LS, Merkus MP, Tytgat GN, Vianney de Jong JM. Percutaneous endoscopic gastrostomy in patients with amyotrophic lateral sclerosis and impaired pulmonary function. Gastrointest Endosc 1994; 40(4):463–469.

29. Mazzini L, Corra T, Zaccala M, Mora G, Del Piano M, Galante M. Percutaneous endo-scopic gastrostomy and enteral nutrition in amyotrophic lateral sclerosis. J Neurol 1995; 242:695–698.

30. Strong MJ, Rowe A, Rankin RN. Percutaneous gastrojejunostomy in amyotrophic lateral sclerosis. J Neurol Sci 1999; 169(1-2):128–132.

31. Chio A, Finocchiaro E, Meineri P, Bottacchi E, Schiffer D. Safety and factors related to survival after percutaneous endoscopic gastrostomy in ALS. Neurology 1999; 53(5):1123–1125.

32. Kasarskis EJ, Scarlata D, Hill R, Fuller C, Stambler N, Cedarbaum JM. A retrospective study of percutaneous endoscopic gastrostomy in ALS patients during the BDNF and CNTF trials. J Neurol Sci 1999; 169(1-2):118–125.

33. Miller ER, III, Pastor-Barriuso R, Dalal D, Riemersma RA, Appel LJ, Guallar E. Meta-analysis: high-dosage Vitamin E supplementation may increase all-cause mortality. Ann Intern Med 2005; 142:37–46.

34. Shults CW, Beal M, Song D, Fontaine D. Pilot trial of high dosages of coenzyme Q10 in patients with Parkinson's disease. Exp Neurol 2004; 188(2):491–494.

33
Respiratory Care in Amyotrophic Lateral Sclerosis

Terry Heiman-Patterson
*Neurology Control, Drexel University College of Medicine, Philadelphia,
Pennsylvania, U.S.A.*

Loutfi S. Aboussouan
*Departments of Pulmonary Critical Care and Allergy, Cleveland Clinic
Foundation Beachwood, Beachwood, Ohio, U.S.A.*

INTRODUCTION

Amyotrophic lateral sclerosis (ALS) is a progressive and uniformly fatal neuromuscular disease, with a median survival from diagnosis of about two years (1). Death is usually secondary to respiratory failure or respiratory complications (2). Riluzole, the only specific treatment for ALS, prolongs survival by about three months (3) but recent advances in the management of respiratory complications can have a major impact both on survival and quality of life underscoring the need to recognize respiratory muscle weakness and the signs of respiratory failure so that treatment can be initiated in a timely fashion. This chapter reviews normal respiratory function and the resultant changes with weakness of the respiratory muscles as ALS progresses. This is followed by a review of the general strategy for the respiratory management of patients with ALS including non-invasive management and tracheostomy with invasive ventilation.

PULMONARY PHYSIOLOGY AND PATHOPHYSIOLOGY

Physiology of Respiration

The function of respiration is the exchange of carbon dioxide for oxygen. Optimum exchange requires that the muscles of the nasopharynx function to protect the airways, the airways be patent and clear of significant secretions, the alveoli are open and respiratory muscle function is adequate. Normal respiratory muscle function includes both an inspiratory and expiratory phase. The inspiratory phase is active and requires the diaphragm and internal intercostals muscle. The expiratory phase is passive and most affected by weakness of abdominal muscles and the external intercostals. In addition, a normal cough is critical for airway clearance of secretions.

Normally the cough consists of a quick inspiration followed by expiration against a closed glottis. The glottis then opens at the end of the cough. Further protection to the airway is afforded by the presence of a gag reflex.

Respiratory Muscle Weakness

In ALS, when respiratory muscle weakness occurs, a cascade of events leading to respiratory failure can be observed. Respiratory failure initially appears as a consequence of diaphragm fatigue but involvement of both inspiratory and expiratory muscles play an important role as described below. Rarely, patients can present with acute respiratory failure and in some but not all of these patients, the involved anterior horn cells are predominantly cervical and correspond to the phrenic nuclei (4–6). Electrophysiological studies of patients with motor neuron disease presenting with respiratory failure reveal widespread denervation in limb muscles with reduced compound muscle action potentials in the phrenic nerves, and to a lesser extent, the limbs (7).

Inspiratory Muscle Weakness

Although patients often first manifest with inspiratory muscle weakness, overall, inspiratory muscle pressures tend to be better preserved than expiratory muscle strength in patients with ALS. In one study of 32 patients with ALS, maximal static inspiratory pressures (PI_{max}) were found to be higher than maximal static expiratory pressures (PE_{max}) (62% vs. 37% predicted, respectively) (8). Similarly, at the onset of respiratory insufficiency ($PaCO_2 \geq 45$ mmHg or presence of orthopnea), maximal inspiratory pressures (MIP) averaged 36% of predicted whereas maximal expiratory pressure (MEP) averaged 27% of predicted (9). Moreover, Griggs et al. (10) found that PE_{max} but not PI_{max} was markedly reduced in adult patients with neuromuscular disease.

Whether this difference between measurements of inspiratory and expiratory pressures translates into clinically significant outcomes remains to be determined. For instance, as the disease progresses, inspiratory muscle weakness remains the primary determinant of respiratory symptoms and ventilatory failure (11). The diaphragm is the primary inspiratory muscle and the earliest complaints relate to diaphragmatic fatigue. Diaphragm fatigue is due to many factors, the most important of which is reduced strength of the diaphragm. Diaphragm weakness results in inability to increase minute ventilation when required and manifests as acute shortness of breath when work of breathing increases, such as during bathing and dressing. The threshold for fatigue may be also reduced during sleep [specifically rapid eye movement (REM) sleep] and by metabolic factors such as poor nutritional states with decreased muscle energy stores, and by fever or infection, which increase metabolic and work demands on the diaphragm. In fact, upper respiratory infections (defined by the onset of symptoms of cough, fever, rhinorrhea, and sore throat) can result in symptomatic reductions in respiratory muscle strength in patients with neuromuscular diseases (12). Additionally, atelectasis may occur and contribute to a decreased in oxygen saturation. Alveolar hypoventilation and hypercapnic respiratory failure may occur as the disease progresses and minute ventilation fails to match ventilatory demands, further reducing diaphragm contractility and increasing fatigue.

Recumbency places an additional burden on the weakened diaphragm and increases the work of breathing because of the additional need for the diaphragm to displace abdominal contents in order to generate a negative pressure in the intrathoracic cavity. As the diaphragm fatigues, accessory muscles of inspiration become active. With further fatigue, the weak diaphragm begins to passively follow the outward movement of the chest wall. This produces a paradoxical pattern of movement, with the rib cage moving outward while the diaphragm moves inward. Routine pulmonary function measurements, usually conducted with the patient in a sitting position, may not be markedly abnormal, but values may fall by half in the supine position (see "Sitting and Supine Spirometry").

Expiratory Muscle Weakness

While expiration is predominantly a passive process, active expiration can occur during exercise, talking, singing, coughing, or sneezing. Expiratory muscle weakness results in inability to generate sufficient increase in air flow during coughing thereby impairing dynamic airway compression which is necessary for effective cough and clearance of secretions (11). Bulbar symptoms further compound the expiratory muscle weakness by impairing the ability to swallow and manage secretions. Therefore expiratory muscle weakness in conjunction with bulbar dysfunction contributes to the risk of aspiration, atelectasis, and pneumonia, and can precipitate respiratory failure. Decreased oral intake of fluids and food leading to dehydration and malnutrition further weakens the respiratory muscles (13).

Pattern of Restrictive Lung Impairment in ALS

Total Lung Capacity

The total lung capacity (TLC) is usually preserved until relatively late in the course of ALS (8,14). One explanation is the patchy nature of ALS that may result in a relatively preserved diaphragmatic function. For instance, as mentioned above, inspiratory muscle strength, which is a major determinant of TLC, may be preserved until later on in the course of the disease. Additionally, the shape of the relaxation pressure–volume curve of the respiratory system is such that a decrease in inspiratory muscle strength is accompanied by a comparatively much smaller decrement in TLC (8). As a result, decreases in MIP do not correlate (15), or correlate weakly (16), with changes in TLC and VC (Fig. 1).

Vital Capacity and Residual Volume

Expiratory muscle strength, which is frequently impaired in ALS, is a major determinant of residual volume and there is a good negative correlation between maximum static expiratory pressure and residual volume in ALS (8). The residual volume is therefore often increased in neuromuscular disease affecting the expiratory muscles (8,14,17). As a result, the vital capacity (VC) (the difference between TLC and residual volume) is decreased predominantly from an increase in RV, and to a lesser degree, a decrease in TLC. It also follows that VC can be reduced in ALS before a decrease in TLC is seen. This latter point is important to keep in mind as a possible exception to the American Thoracic Society interpretative strategies, which specify a decrease in TLC rather than the VC for the diagnosis of restrictive lung disease (Fig. 1) (18).

Functional Residual Capacity

The functional residual capacity (FRC) is determined by a balance of the inward elastic recoil of the lung and outward elastic recoil of the chest, and usually

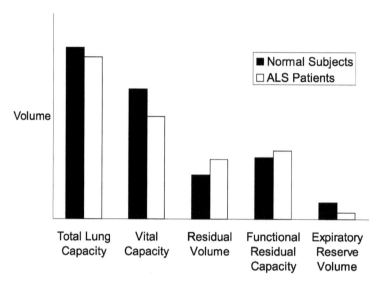

Figure 1 Changes in selected lung volumes and capacities in mild to moderately advanced ALS. Note the relatively preserved TLC, reduced VC predominantly due to an increase in residual volume, and high normal FRC. *Source*: From Ref. 14.

unaffected by neuromuscular disorders (17) and even tends to be slightly increased or at the upper limits of normal in patients with ALS (8,14), possibly because of decreased abdominal tone and passive descent of the diaphragm (8). A preserved or high-normal FRC can be a useful clue to neuromuscular disease in patients presenting with a restrictive pulmonary impairment (Fig. 1).

Pathophysiology of Sleep Disturbances in ALS

During sleep, a number of physiologic changes occur that may affect ALS patients. These include changes in body position of which the patient is unaware, but which result in diaphragm fatigue and reduced activation of accessory muscles during REM sleep, which is a state of generalized muscle atonia. Therefore, sleep, and more specifically REM sleep, may uncover respiratory disturbance events and assist in the early detection of the onset of respiratory impairment in ALS. In one case report, hypopneas with nocturnal desaturations, particularly during REM sleep, were proposed to be the initial symptoms of ALS (19). Several mechanisms underlie this observation including the normal shift of the burden of respiration to the diaphragm during REM sleep (20) and the predisposition of patients with bulbar ALS to hypopneas during REM sleep (21–23). Patients with neuromuscular disease and early diaphragmatic or bulbar involvement would therefore be particularly vulnerable to respiratory events during REM sleep, even in the absence of daytime symptoms. Nocturnal desaturation of <88% for at least five consecutive minutes has been proposed as a simple and early marker of diaphragmatic dysfunction (24) and can be seen even in individuals with VC > 50% (25).

Sleep studies indicate that in most ALS patients the overall quality of sleep is similar to that measured in normal subjects of similar age. Arousals and mild disorders of breathing occur, but are infrequently associated with clinically significant hypoxemia (PaO_2 < 80 mmHg). Kimura et al. (22) found hypopneas and central or obstructive apneas in 27% (3 of 11) of patients with bulbar ALS who had no respiratory or sleep related complaints, with predominance of events during REM sleep in one patient. Similarly, Ferguson et al. (21) reported the presence of hypopneas predominantly during REM sleep in 44% (8 of 18) of ALS patients with bulbar involvement. Several studies report essentially no significant obstructive events in patients with ALS (21,23,26), though the prevalence of obstructive sleep apnea may be higher than expected especially in the presence of bulbar symptoms (23).

One study showed a possible adaptation mechanism in the form of reduction in REM sleep in ALS patients with diaphragmatic dysfunction compared to an otherwise similar group of ALS patients without diaphragmatic dysfunction (26). That study also showed a longer REM sleep duration in some ALS patients with diaphragmatic dysfunction who were able to adapt and supplement their inspiratory muscles by preservation of a phasic inspiratory sternomastoid activation during REM (26).

In summary, nocturnal desaturation in ALS can occur because of the shift in the burden of respiration to a weakened diaphragm during sleep and the predisposition to hypopneas during REM sleep particularly in patients with bulbar symptoms. Obstructive events may depend on a complex interaction of bulbar symptoms (which may facilitate obstructive events) and diaphragmatic dysfunction (which may decrease the prevalence of sleep obstructive events by causing an inability to generate an inspiratory pressure above the closing pressure of the upper airway). This may explain the decrease in sleep events with increasing duration of the disease (23), anecdotal evidence of disappearance of snoring with disease progression, and the absence of obstructive events in patients with diaphragmatic weakness (21). Individuals without bulbar signs appear to have a higher prevalence of central apneas (23). Lastly, adaptive mechanisms to the impaired diaphragmatic dysfunction may include inspiratory support during REM sleep by persistence of sternomastoid activity during REM in some patients, and reduction in REM sleep to protect against nocturnal hypoventilation (26).

CLINICAL EVALUATION

Symptoms of Respiratory Muscle Fatigue

The slow progression of muscle weakness in ALS means that early symptoms and signs of respiratory failure frequently appear transiently as fatigue. Early symptoms of fatigue may occur only during exertion. Initially, this may be a subjective sensation of inadequate respiration felt by the patient and not associated with tachypnea, but later there is a clear increase in breathing effort. With progression of respiratory muscle weakness, even the exertion of bathing and dressing brings on respiratory fatigue. Since patients may unconsciously adjust their activity to reduce fatigue, early symptoms must be actively sought by specific questions, particularly those relating to disrupted sleep and daytime fatigue as follows.

In contrast to the greater contribution of intercostals muscles to breathing in non-REM sleep, intercostals activity in REM sleep is markedly decreased, highlighting the importance of both the intercostals muscles and the diaphragm in maintaining adequate ventilation during sleep (20). For instance, early fatigue and failure of the diaphragm and intercostals muscles may become noticeable at bedtime and during sleep resulting in the inability to lie prone or supine. Later, sleeping with additional pillows, the head of the bed steeply elevated, or even sitting up may be the most comfortable position. Due to the physiologic changes described above that occur during sleep, an occasional patient will have profound nocturnal hypoventilation and hypoxia. Some other common early symptoms of disordered sleep that should be sought in the history include: insomnia, waking up frequently at night, fatigue, morning headaches, vivid dreams, and daytime sleepiness and decreased concentration.

As respiratory muscle weakness progresses, hypoventilation results in hypoxemia and hypercapnia. The initial symptom of respiratory failure in ALS patients is more often related to hypercapnia than to hypoxemia leading to morning headaches, nightmares, daytime sleepiness, and yawning. Other factors that contribute to hypercapnia include superimposed infection with fever and underlying lung diseases such as emphysema. Ventilation is further compromised by the increased secretions and poor airway clearance as a result of bulbar involvement and decreased cough. This leads to aspiration and pneumonia as well as poor oral intake with resulting dehydration and malnutrition. Symptoms of aspiration include coughing while eating, alterations in breathing, gagging, frequent throat clearing, swallowing more than once for each bite or sip, and even a gurgly sound to the voice.

Finally, as respiratory weakness progresses, shortness of breath, and use of accessory muscles occurs even at rest and CO_2 narcosis becomes prominent. It should be kept in mind that lack of dyspnea on exertion can be deceiving since many patients will be too weak to move around. In some people with ALS, respiratory function plateaus and stabilizes.

While these respiratory symptoms typically occur later in the course of the of ALS, our experience suggests that about 7% of patients ultimately diagnosed to have ALS report subtle pulmonary symptoms as a presenting feature of their disease. Respiratory failure, usually triggered by a concurrent pulmonary infection, may also be the presenting symptom of ALS and usually portends a poor prognosis and rapid progression of the illness (4–7,27). Early pulmonary manifestations of ALS pose a particular diagnostic challenge as these patients may first present to pulmonary and critical care physicians before a diagnosis is established. Motor neuron disease is often not considered as a reason for respiratory failure, particularly when precipitating factors such as pneumonia, exacerbation of chronic obstructive pulmonary disease (COPD), heart failure, or sleep apnea are concomitantly present and considered to be the primary etiology (4). A diagnosis of motor neuron disease should therefore be entertained in the appropriate setting and proposed clinical features that may raise the suspicion for a neuromuscular disorder as a cause for respiratory insufficiency include: (i) absence of a chronic cardiopulmonary disorder, (ii) relatively normal physical exam, electrocardiogam, and chest radiograph, and (iii) rapid improvement with ventilatory support with subsequent difficulty in weaning (6,27,28). In a case report, common features in three ALS patients with an early presentation of respiratory failure and minimal motor signs included older age (over 62) and fasciculations (29).

Physical Examination

Patients may demonstrate tachypnea, paradoxical breathing, accessory muscle use (i.e., the sternocleidomastoids, scalenes, and external intercostals), low volume speech, ineffective cough, and speech difficulties. In addition there may be abdominal paradox during inspiration or sniff testing. Dyssynchronous movements of rib cage and abdomen, with breath to breath variation in the inspiratory movements of rib cage and abdomen, "respiratory alternans," are a sign of respiratory muscle fatigue, and may indicate impending respiratory failure. As bulbar muscles weaken, speech changes become obvious with dysarthria, along with atrophy and fasciculations of a decreasingly mobile tongue. If there is primarily lower motor neuron involvement the gag reflex will be reduced and a gurgly speech with pooling secretions is evident. As swallowing becomes further compromised overt drooling occurs, often noticed first at night.

The patient should be examined both upright and lying flat while observing the respiratory rate, as well as chest and abdominal movement while breathing. In patients unable to lie flat, percussion of the base of the lung in inspiration and expiration with the patient in a seated position can determine whether the excursion of either hemidiaphragm is impaired. This test is particularly useful in sequential follow-up as excursion diminishes with time. Abnormalities may be most evident when lying flat because a weak diaphragm, the major muscle of respiration, is at a disadvantage in this position. As respiratory muscle function becomes weaker, the effectiveness of both ventilation and cough is reduced.

On auscultation there may be coarse breath sounds or inspiratory crackles, particularly at the lung bases due to poor bronchial clearance, patchy atelectasis, aspiration, or infection. These findings may be masked by shallow breathing and inability to take a deep breath. Upper extremity weakness may be associated with expiratory muscle weakness and poor cough. The clinician should also note quality of speech, nutritional status, pedal edema, and signs of other problems, such as cor pulmonale.

Pulmonary Function Testing

Once diagnosed, the ALS patient requires a baseline respiratory evaluation followed by regular follow ups at least every three to four months for most patients, and every one to three months when weakness appears to be progressing rapidly (e.g., a drop in forced vital capacity, FVC >15% over three months). Other respiratory problems amenable to treatment may be identified, such as asthma or COPD. Initial pulmonary function testing should at least include spirometry with VC, airflow measurement, flow volume loop, maximal voluntary ventilation (MVV), and maximal static inspiratory and expiratory pressure measurements.

Measurement of respiratory function in ALS is especially important since the early signs of respiratory impairment are subtle and may be easily missed. For instance, in a study by Fallat et al. (30), 64% of patients with reductions in VC to less than 50% of predicted were given normal breathing scores by neurologists. Early symptoms of respiratory insufficiency include frequent nocturnal arousals, nightmares, morning headaches, and excessive daytime sleepiness (31). These symptoms may not be immediately interpreted as indicators of respiratory muscle weakness. Given the lack of mobility, exertional dyspnea may not be present. Thus, while history is important, measures of respiratory muscle strength remain a critical part of the clinical evaluation in ALS patients.

In order to discuss changes of respiratory measurements in ALS we need to review the measurements available to the clinician, their ease of use and then discuss our recommendations for the best screens in a busy clinic. Unfortunately, despite the importance of respiratory muscle function, there is no consensus regarding the single best method to serially measure pulmonary function in ALS. Proposed parameters to include in the pulmonary evaluation are listed in Table 1.

Table 1 Parameters to Include in a Pulmonary Evaluation

Parameter	Comment
Forced vital capacity (FVC)	The most important component of spirometry in ALS. Small portable spirometers are quite reliable provided they are regularly calibrated. Their regular use in neurologic clinics with readings every three to four months is recommended. Sitting spirometry with an FVC < 50% qualifies an individual with ALS for non-invasive ventilation. A greater than 10% drop in FVC between sitting and supine spirometry or a supine FVC < 75% suggest diaphragmatic weakness
Maximum voluntary ventilation (MVV)	Measures respiratory strength and endurance and is characteristically reduced in ALS. It is often difficult to perform in patients with more advanced disease
Maximal inspiratory and expiratory pressures (PI_{max}, PE_{max})	More sensitive than reduction in FVC, MVV, or ABG. Tends to have marked variability. A $PI_{max} < 60$ cm H_2O qualifies an individual with ALS for non-invasive ventilation
Assisted peak cough flows	Can be a good marker of expiratory function and ability to clear secretions. Values <2.7 L/s with failure to clear secretions identifies patients who may require tracheostomy
Arterial blood gases (ABG)	An awake $PaCO_2 \geq 45$ mmHg at the patient's usual fraction of inspired oxygen qualifies an individual with ALS for non-invasive positive pressure ventilation. Relatively insensitive as respiratory muscle weakness can be quite advanced before abnormalities in ABGs are seen
Nocturnal oximetry	A proposed sensitive marker of early diaphragmatic dysfunction. Desaturation $\leq 88\%$ for ≥ 5 consecutive minutes during nocturnal oximetry qualifies an individual with ALS for NIPPV
Sleep study	Can be used if concomitant sleep apnea is suspected as this may impact on NIPPV settings (Table 3). May also be used in titration of NIPPV for control of hypoventilation. In that regard, the titration algorithm is different than the one used for sleep apnea and usually requires monitoring of $PaCO_2$ transcutaneously or with capnography (end-tidal CO_2)

Vital Capacity

Although, as discussed above, the VC is more sensitive to progress of disease and respiratory involvement than the TLC, there is considerable difficulty in obtaining measurements that fulfill the validity criteria of the American Thoracic Society (32). Problems with the FVC include inability to obtain tests that satisfy the end-of-test criteria of the American Thoracic Society and lack of reproducibility in patients at advanced stages of their disease. For instance, in one report, 60% of patients were unable to achieve an expiratory time of six seconds or greater on the spirometric maneuver, indicating that end-of-test criteria were not met in a majority of cases, therefore resulting in possible underestimation of the FVC (9). In that same report, FVC measurements were reproducible in only 62% of the spirometry maneuvers performed in ALS patients (9).

Nevertheless, the VC remains one of the most important tools for the longitudinal follow up of pulmonary function in ALS clinics. Techniques that can be used to improve the measurement of VC include minimizing air leaks by use of a face mask to measure spirometry, and prevention of premature glottic closure by upward chin extension or allowing a gentle as opposed to a forced exhalation. The natural history of decline of VC in ALS is quite variable with some patients exhibiting a precipitous decline in lung function (30). While several studies have shown that overall, the rate of decline of lung function is linear ranging from 2.3% to 4.6% predicted points loss in FVC per month (9,30,33–35), the FVC plateaus in the months immediately prior to death (36). This is quite consistent with the pattern of a decelerating decline of FVC reported in another study (9) and may be due to longer survival of motor neurons that are most resistant to progress of the disease.

Current guidelines of the American Academy of Neurology and a consensus statement from the American College of Chest Physicians recommend counseling on the use of non-invasive ventilation with the onset of respiratory symptoms or when the FVC drops to about 50% of predicted value (24,37).

Sitting and Supine Spirometry

Sitting and supine spirometry can detect unsuspected diaphragmatic dysfunction in asymptomatic patients and should be obtained whenever technically feasible. A 5% to 10% reduction in FVC from sitting to supine positions can be expected in normals, with larger decrements in the range of 10% to 20% in obesity or unilateral diaphragmatic paralysis. Decreases larger than 20% are seen in diaphragmatic weakness as may be seen in ALS, and patients with bilateral diaphragmatic paralysis have a 40% to 50% decrement in VC between the sitting and supine positions (38).

Additionally, a supine FVC correlates highly with transdiaphragmatic pressure (Pdi) in patients with ALS ($R^2 = 0.76$) and a supine FVC cutoff of <75% was reported to be 100% specific and sensitive in predicting a Pdi <70 cm H_2O (39). This raises the possibility of using supine FVC as a more sensitive marker of early respiratory compromise than sitting FVC.

Respiratory Muscle Pressures

The maximal static inspiratory and expiratory pressures (PI_{max} and PE_{max}, respectively), sometimes called MIP and MEP, respectively, are also often reduced in ALS patients and appear to correlate with the degree of respiratory muscle impairment (8,31,34). They measure muscle force but not endurance, and are more sensitive than reductions in VC, MVV, or arterial blood gas (ABG) abnormalities. For instance, many patients with considerable respiratory muscle weakness have a normal VC but a decreased PE_{max} and PI_{max}, and ABG abnormalities may not occur until maximal static pressures have decreased to less than 30% of predicted. A reduction of MIP to less than 60 cmH$_2$O has an 86% sensitivity for the presence of a nocturnal oxygen saturation nadir of <80%, a 100% sensitivity in predicting 18 months mortality (40), and was proposed as a surrogate marker of nocturnal desaturation (24). A low PI_{max} also correlated in one study with the presence of sleep disruption (41). Additionally, a model incorporating PI_{max} and supine FVC was found to be an excellent predictor of diaphragmatic muscle weakness (39). A PI_{max} of less than 60 cmH$_2$O is one of the criteria for initiation of non-invasive ventilation in patients with a documented restrictive lung disease (24). Whereas PI_{max} measures inspiratory muscle strength and its correlates, PE_{max} measures expiratory force, necessary for effective cough. Caveats to the use of the PI_{max} and PE_{max} are the greater reduction in PE_{max} reported in several studies (8–10), and the wide inter-test variations of PE_{max} ranging from 5 mmHg to 15 mmHg, so that the test may not be useful for sequential follow-up for severely weak patients (10).

Placement of a transesophageal catheter allows measurement of esophageal (Pes, a reflection of pleural pressure) and transdiaphragmatic pressure (Pdi, the difference between gastric and esophageal pressures) for more accurate estimation of diaphragmatic muscle strength. In one study, a Pes < 30 cmH$_2$O was independently associated with increased mortality in patients with ALS (42).

Sniff nasal pressure (SNP) is a newer non-invasive measure of inspiratory pressure that can accurately reflect intrathoracic pressures and may provide a more sensitive early marker of respiratory failure in ALS patients. It decreases over time in ALS patients and changes were associated with respiratory failure (43,44). The SNP was more sensitive than either FVC or MIP in detecting respiratory failure in one study of over 81 patients (44). Additional studies will be required to determine the most sensitive non-invasive marker of respiratory failure in ALS.

Modified Vital Capacity, FEV$_6$ and FEV$_1$

In a modified (or slow) VC, the initial maximal inspiratory effort is followed by a relaxed expiration for as long as possible (as opposed to the "forced" VC) (45). The modified maneuver results in increased values for the VC compared to the forced maneuver predominantly because of an increase in expiratory time. Unfortunately, anecdotal experience suggests that it is not particularly easier to perform in patients with ALS and that the expiration time is not usually extended by the use of the modified spirometric maneuver in patients with ALS (Kevin McCarthy, personal communication).

Other methods include the use of the forced expiratory volume at six seconds (FEV$_6$). For instance, the FEV$_6$ has been proposed as a less physically demanding test for the diagnosis of airway obstruction and restriction (46). Moreover, there are now published references: values for the FEV$_6$ (47,48). Whether its use can be extended to patients with ALS remains to be determined.

There are no data concerning the use of the FEV$_1$ as a surrogate marker of restrictive lung disease in ALS, however it has been found to be reproducible in 68% of patients with ALS (compared to 62% for FVC), and the mean FEV$_1$ predicted at onset of respiratory failure is 44% compared to 41% for the FVC (9). The challenge becomes to be able to exclude the presence of associated obstructive lung disease, which can similarly decrease the FEV$_1$.

Arterial Blood Gases, Nocturnal Oximetry, Sleep Studies, and Serum Chloride

ABG measurements have been shown to remain near normal until the preterminal stage of disease (8,30). An awake PaCO$_2$ $\geq$ 45 mmHg at the patient's usual fraction of inspired oxygen is one of the criteria for initiation of non-invasive positive pressure ventilation (NIPPV) in patients with restrictive lung disease such as ALS (24). As a comparative measure, when patients with ALS are serially followed with ABGs and spirometric measures, the FVC can be seen to range from 16% to 70% (mean 44% predicted) at around the time of onset of hypercapnia (defined as a PaCO$_2$ $\geq$ 45 mmHg) or orthopnea (49). As a general guideline, ABGs need not be routinely measured but should be obtained if hypoventilation is suspected (e.g., presence of morning headaches, daytime sleepiness, and lethargy), to guide adjustments to

NIPPV support in patients already receiving it, and to justify NIPPV in patients who are unable to perform spirometry or in whom inspiratory respiratory pressures cannot be obtained.

On the basis of the pathophysiologic mechanisms of sleep disturbance discussed above, nocturnal desaturation ≤88% for ≥5 consecutive minutes has been proposed as a marker of early diaphragmatic dysfunction and as an indication for initiation of NIPPV in patients with a restrictive lung disease (24). In one study of ALS patients with symptoms suggestive of sleep-disordered breathing (frequent arousals, daytime sleepiness, or fatigue), there was no significant difference in the percentage of time with oxygen saturation <88% between individuals with FVC above versus below 50% suggesting that many symptomatic patients with nocturnal desaturation have an FVC >50% (25). More formal sleep studies can be obtained though their exact role remains to be determined. A sleep study may correlate the presence of nocturnal desaturation to REM sleep, may be helpful to adjust NIPPV settings in patient with concomitant sleep apnea, and be useful to formally titrate pressures for control of hypoventilation (Table 1).

Recently, serum chloride, a metabolic indicator of the degree of respiratory acidosis, has been identified as a prognostic factor in ALS patients. A level below the lower limit of normal indicates impending respiratory decompensation (36), but chloride levels are clearly not a helpful predictor of *early* respiratory insufficiency.

RESPIRATORY MANAGEMENT

Respiratory management of the ALS patient should be directed at optimization and prevention of complications and not simply ventilation. Respiratory intervention begins at diagnosis with a program that is aimed at the reduction of infections, improvement of function, and prediction of failure necessitating the initiation of non-invasive or invasive ventilation (Table 2). Initially baseline pulmonary function should be measured and followed at regular intervals to allow early detection of respiratory muscle weakness and failure. Symptoms of respiratory involvement may occur before the FVC declines to 50% and are indications for follow-up testing including overnight oximetry, ABGs, and an overnight full sleep study. Breathing at low tidal volumes, with a poor ability to sigh can further compromise lung function, with resulting microatelectasis and decreased compliance. As the respiratory abnormalities progress, there is a high risk of sudden life-threatening respiratory failure due to a small aspiration, some mucous plugs, a relatively minor respiratory illness, or even without any clear additional event. Finally, as bulbar involvement worsens there is dehydration and further thickening of secretions further decreasing the ability of weakened muscles to clear the airways. This is made even worse by malnutrition with further weakening of the respiratory muscles. Since many of these complicating factors can be managed medically, respiratory failure may be delayed and averted with appropriate and early intervention thereby underscoring the need to initiate an aggressive and encompassing approach to the respiratory management and assessment in patients with ALS. Table 2 outlines this approach to the management of respiratory complications in ALS.

General Care

Clinical evaluation of the ALS patient should begin with the assessment of the baseline pulmonary status (see above) and the identification of any other medical

Table 2 Considerations in the Management of Respiratory Complications of ALS

General care
  Pneumovaccine and flu vaccine
  Gastrostomy placement to maintain adequate nutrition
  Control secretions
    Decreased production: anticholinergic medications
    Thinning: fluids, nebulizers, and medications
    Mobilization: incentive spirometry, pulmonary toileting, assisted cough maneuvers, mechanical in-exsufflator, and suction devices
  Monitor for aspiration
  Treatment of acute respiratory infections
  Pulmonary consultation for FVC < 60% or early symptoms of respiratory compromise (see text)
  Improve sleep hygiene
Measurement of pulmonary function
  Baseline and every three months to evaluate for weakening and failure
  Additional studies when indicated
    Arterial blood gases
    Overnight oximetry
    Sleep studies
Identify and treat respiratory failure: non-invasive and invasive ventilation
Palliative care

condition that might contribute to respiratory problems. For example, asthma, COPD, and congestive heart failure are common and are amenable to specific therapy. Risk factors, such as cigarette smoking, secondhand smoke, dusts and fumes, and exposure to people with acute viral respiratory illness, should be identified and avoided. Pneumovax immunization and yearly influenza immunizations are advised. Bronchitis with purulent sputum or any evidence of lower respiratory tract infection should be evaluated, including chest X-ray, and treated to improve bronchial clearance of secretions, plus prompt antibiotic therapy. Patients with chronic cough should have medications and instructions available at home so that antibiotic treatment can be started without delay. In a few cases, there may be value in teaching postural drainage and percussion (beware, this can cause hypoxemia) to help clear secretions. Using an incentive spirometer at home may help prevent patchy atelectasis. The use of theophylline to improve diaphragmatic function has had mixed results (50) but can strengthen loaded respiratory muscles in ALS patients (51). As bulbar dysfunction progresses, prevention of aspiration is of primary importance and patients should be educated about eating in an upright position with the chin tucked towards the chest, taking small bites, and allowing more time for meals.

Secretion management is an important part of pulmonary care in ALS since secretions can lead to plugging, atelectasis, and infections secondary to aspiration. Treatments are directed both at decreasing and thinning the secretions as well as increasing clearance. Pharmacologic agents that decrease secretions include: Anticholinergic medications [glycopyrrolate (Robinul®), amitriptyline, and transderm scopolamine]. Botulinum toxin injection has been used by to temporarily disable salivary glands function by clinicians who have experience in applying this method, but the technique is still under investigation. If these modalities fail, irradiation of the parotid gland can be helpful. If the secretions are thickened, especially with use of anticholinergic agents, hydration, guaifenesin, propranolol, and acetylcysteine nebulizing treatments can be considered.

Peak cough flows of greater then 160 L/min are necessary to maintain clear airways (52). Once the peak cough flow declines to 270 L/min, a program to optimize secretion mobilization should be initiated (52). Interventions that facilitate the clearance of secretions consist of air stacking (52,53), assisted cough either manually or mechanically through an insufflator–exsufflator (54,55), training to improve maximum insufflation capacity (56), and use of a suction machine to remove oropharyngeal secretions that have been mobilized. Air stacking enhances cough efficacy by initiating cough at higher lung volumes, and can be achieved by glossopharyngeal breathing, which consists of stacking several gulps of air behind a closed glottis (57), or by delivery of air via a manual resuscitator or a volume limited ventilator (56). Cough efficacy can be further enhanced by an abdominal thrust timed with the cough effort (58) or by application of negative pressure though a mask. The mechanical insufflator–exsufflator (MI–E) combines elements of air stacking and cough enhancement by manual or mechanical cycling from a positive pressure to enhance lung volumes (insufflation), to a negative pressure to facilitate clearing of airway secretions (exsufflation) (54,55). High-frequency oscillation techniques have also been used to help clearance of secretions though their use and efficacy are currently under investigation.

Oxygen may be used at home to treat hypoxemia. The indication for home oxygen is a persisting $PaO_2 < 55$ mmHg, or an $SaO_2 < 88\%$ by either ABG or oximetry. However since oxygen can aggravate hypercapnia (59), and may increase the rates of pneumonia and hospitalizations (60) it should be used only with extreme care. If used, oxygen should be titrated to the lowest desirable level using a pulse oximetry target of 92% to 94% as a tentative goal, but should ideally be reserved for use concomitantly with NIPPV (to avoid hypoventilation), or in a palliative care setting.

Careful attention to swallowing and feeding is also important so as to initiate aggressive management when needed to avoid aspiration and weight loss. If dysphagia is present, the speech and swallow therapist should initiate an educational program directed at the appropriate food consistency and proper swallow technique using a chin tuck. In addition the patient should sleep with his head elevated and never lay flat following meals. As dysphagia progresses or the vital capacity drops below 50%, a percutaneous gastrostomy (PEG) tube should be recommended to maintain nutrition but the clinician must keep in mind that this does not prevent aspiration. Early intervention with PEG tube has been proposed in retrospective studies to prolong survival from two to four months, though the data is conflicting in that regard (61,62) (see also chap. 34).

Finally, since acute respiratory infections can precipitate ventilatory failure in the already compromised ALS patient, these infections must be treated aggressively. The additional secretions combined with an ineffective cough and reduced inspiratory and expiratory pressures leads to increased airway obstruction and microatelectasis with worsening hypercapnea. Thus, ALS patients with an upper respiratory infection may require hospitalization at a lower threshold for intravenous hydration, antibiotics, and aggressive secretion management and pulmonary toileting.

Treatment of Respiratory Failure

Short-Term Mechanical Ventilation

Acute respiratory failure may occur associated with pneumonia or other causes before a person is permanently unable to sustain breathing. Medical care should try to reverse the acute underlying causes and provide rehabilitation to restore the highest level of independent function. Temporary ventilator support can be given using non-invasive ventilation or by endotracheal intubation. The method chosen should reflect the experience of the medical center to achieve the safest and most effective care. If the patient is conscious and able to co-operate and cough effectively, then the non-invasive approach may be best. Some ALS patients can recover from acute respiratory failure and regain fully independent breathing for a considerable period of time; this may happen repeatedly before it is necessary to consider long-term mechanical ventilation. Alternatively, there may be a period of time when mechanical ventilation is needed for only part of the 24 hours, such as during sleep, allowing considerable "free time" off the ventilator during the day.

Non-Invasive Ventilation

As the deterioration of muscle strength and respiratory function caused by ALS progresses, the need for ventilatory assistance should be considered. In recent years, nocturnal NIPPV has become the treatment of choice for patients with chronic respiratory insufficiency secondary to ALS (63). A variety of non-invasive nasal ventilators have been developed and utilized in an attempt to avoid the complications and difficulties associated with invasive mechanical ventilation in later stages of respiratory insufficiency (64). Non-invasive ventilation can preserve oral feeding and speech, reduce risk of respiratory infections as well as reduce burden for care-givers and costs (63). The bi-level intermittent positive air pressure non-invasive ventilator is the closest to physiologic function. It is triggered by the patient's own respiratory efforts and reduces the work of breathing, improves gas exchange, sleep quality, and compliance (65,66). Thus, bi-level positive airway pressure ventilation could provide a non-invasive means of ventilatory support and prolong survival as well as improve the quality of life in ALS patients.

A number of both retrospective and prospective studies have been published demonstrating the value of NIPPV. Aboussouan et al. (49) at the Cleveland Clinic demonstrated a 3.1-fold increase in the risk for death in patients with ALS who could not tolerate NIPPV when compared to those who could tolerate it. NIPPV was offered to patients at the "onset of respiratory insufficiency" which the authors defined based upon symptoms of dyspnea on exertion, hypercarbia, orthopnea, or a FVC < 60% of predicted. The difference in survival persisted even after stratification for the presence or absence of moderate or severe bulbar symptoms, however bulbar patients were less tolerant of NIPPV (30% tolerance vs. 46% tolerance among patients with mild or no bulbar symptoms). A prospective study by Pinto et al. (67) compared survival between ten ALS patients treated with palliative management compared to 10 patients receiving NIPPV. The authors showed a significant improvement in total survival time ($p < 0.004$) and in survival from onset of diurnal disorders of gas exchange ($p < 0.006$) in the patients treated with NIPPV. They found no significant differences between the two groups with a mean FVC% of 43.9%. The authors concluded that despite the small number of patients, further studies should be performed to identify the best time for introducing NIPPV (67). The authors did not address the fact that the "palliative measures" used in the control group, including the use of morphine and oxygen, may have further suppressed the respiratory drive, accounting for the differences in survival.

A retrospective study by Kleopa et al. analyzed the results of NIPPV use in 122 patients followed at Hahnemann University (33). All patients were offered NIPPV when their FVC dropped below 50% of predicted. Group 1 ($n = 38$) used NIPPV > 4 hr/day, Group 2 ($n = 32$) used NIPPV <4 hr/day due to poor compliance, and Group 3 ($n = 52$) refused NIPPV. There was a statistically significant improvement in survival from initiation of NIPPV in Group 1 (14.2 months) compared to Group 2 (7.0 months, $p = 0.002$) or Group 3 (4.6 months, $p < 0.001$). Furthermore, Group 1 had a slower mean decline in vital capacity (-3.5% change/mo) compared to Group 2 (-5.9% change/mo, $p = 0.02$) and Group 3 (-8.3% change/mo, $p < 0.001$) (33). A recently published cohort study of 47 patients compared survival and FVC% decline in tolerant ($n = 23$) and intolerant ($n = 24$) patients (9). The median survival in intolerant patients was five months compared to 20 months in tolerant patients ($p = 0.002$), again confirming the apparent survival benefit of NIPPV. That study, in contrast to the Kleopa paper, showed that NIPPV did not change the rate of decline of FVC or FEV_1 (9). In addition, the mean change in FEV_1 due to initiation of NIPPV was –5.94% predicted points ($p = 0.07$) suggesting that NIPPV may actually have a deleterious effect on spirometric measurements (9). The authors speculate that unloading of respiratory muscles by NIPPV may result in deconditioning.

Other beneficial effects of NIPPV in patients with ALS include improvements in quality of life (9,68–71) and cognitive function (72). In one study, quality of life was examined by administering the Chronic Respiratory Index Questionnaire to eight patients pre- and post-NIPPV. There were improvements in the fatigue ($p = 0.03$) and mastery ($p = 0.07$) scores (9). Similarly, Lyall et al. (71) prospectively measured QOL using the SF36 questionnaire, ALSFRS, and Epworth sleepiness scale in 16 ALS patients with symptomatic hypoventilation. NIPPV improved scores in the "Vitality" domain by as much as 25% compared to control ALS patients without diaphragmatic weakness. Following initiation of NIPPV, the mean score fell to 4 ($p < 0.0001$) from 9.25. The only independent predictor of improved QOL with NIPPV use was compliance with the intervention (68).

Although the benefits of NIPPV are apparent even in these small observational studies, there is still no consensus as to which physiologic marker and/or clinical symptom(s) should be used to trigger the initiation of NIPPV. In addition, at the present time, there is no single test that has been shown to reliably detect early respiratory insufficiency. A recent evidence-based review of the subject pointed out that most patients with ALS are symptomatic of hypoventilation by the time VC (FVC) falls below 50% of predicted (37). The authors provided a management algorithm that suggests that NIPPV should probably be instituted when patients are symptomatic and when FVC reaches 50%. However it is important to be aware of recently established criteria by the Health Care Financing Administration (HCFA) for initial coverage of respiratory assist devices. In order for NIPPV to be covered by Medicare, the patient must have documentation of symptoms characteristic of sleep-associated hypoventilation, demonstrate an ABG $PaCO_2$ which is ≥ 45 mmHg, have nocturnal oximetry demonstrating oxygen desaturation $\leq 88\%$ for at least five continuous minutes, have a FVC <50% of predicted, or a maximum inspiratory pressure <60 cm H_2O (24). There are ongoing randomized trials of timing of NIPPV (73,74), with initial results suggesting that patients randomized to receive earlier NIPPV at the onset of nocturnal desaturation (defined as a saturation of <90% for at least one cumulative minute) had improved quality of life as measured on the vitality subscale of the SF-36 compared to those receiving NIPPV for FVC <50% (73). Similarly, in another study, ALS patients receiving early NIPPV at the onset of nocturnal desaturation had a greater survival attributed to improved

Table 3 Suggested Settings for Initiation of Bi-Level Positive Airway Pressure Ventilation

	Initial set-up	Comments
Inspiratory pressure (IPAP, cmH$_2$O)	10	Start low to facilitate adaptation. Increase as necessary for comfort first, then to ABG's, nocturnal desaturation, daytime symptoms of fatigue, or until the baseline respiratory rate falls below 20/min. In concomitant sleep apnea, baseline IPAP should be of sufficient magnitude to control hypopneas. Augmentation of tidal volume and support of hypoventilation depends on the gradient between IPAP and EPAP
Expiratory pressure (EPAP, cmH$_2$O)	5	Higher expiratory pressures can be used if auto-PEEP is suspected (as with COPD) or for control of obstructive event in patients with concomitant sleep apnea
Back up rate (mn)	10	Set below the daytime breathing rate to allow predominant triggering by the patient's effort
Mode	Spontaneous (assist)/timed (control)	Allows pressure-support ventilation responsive to the patient's effort, and a pressure-control type of ventilation in case the breathing rate drops below the back up rate
Interface	For comfort	Nasal masks, pillows or seals are most commonly used as they permit speech and eating. Oronasal masks can be used in case of mouth leaks but may interfere with coughing. Mouth pieces are excellent alternatives for patients able to maintain a seal
Accessories	Heated humidifier	Helpful to avoid nasal dryness. Over the counter nasal buffered saline can also be used for persistent symptoms
Usage	Nightly	Ability to sleep with the device on for at least four consecutive hours suggests adequate tolerance and adaptation to the device. This adaptation may take up to six weeks and may be facilitated by daytime use for short periods (1–2 hr) while awake. Daytime use can also be necessary for comfort and support of hypoventilation
Other adjustments	Depends on device	Inspiratory triggering sensitivity, rise time (0.3–0.5 sec), pressure ramping feature (0–45 min). The latter allows a slow increase in pressure to allow the patient to fall asleep before the full pressure is delivered

compliance compared to historical controls (75). Table 3 shows some proposed settings for initiation of bi-level positive airway pressure ventilation. In addition to the actual IPAP and EPAP settings, the clinician must consider the interface (mask), the use of a chin strap, the ability of the patient to communicate with the caregiver while on the ventilator, and treatment of symptoms that limit comfort on the ventilator such as nasal congestion, mucosal dryness, and claustrophobia. Once the NIPPV is initiated, the ventilator must be adjusted regularly based on the patients symptoms, evidence of increased CO_2, and prevention of nocturnal hypoxemia. Long-term use of NIPPV with avoidance of tracheostomy has been reported and depends on preserved glottic function (76). As a corollary, inability to maintain assisted peak cough flows above 160 L/min and decrease in baseline saturation that cannot be corrected by NIPPV and MI-E, may indicate a high likelihood of death within two months unless a tracheotomy is performed (52,76).

Of the different modalities of NIPPV, pressure-limited ventilation may be better tolerated than volume-limited ventilation (49), though volume-limited ventilation may be used to facilitate air stacking when needed to enhance cough efficacy (77), and to ensure delivery of higher volumes when needed to control hypoventilation. Other non-invasive ventilators include the cuirass and tank ventilators, which are based on generation of a negative pressure. Use of these ventilators is limited in ALS because of bulbar muscle involvement since the negative pressures can exacerbate airway collapse in patients with weakened bulbar musculature (78).

Ventilator Decision Making

As ALS progresses, the patient will become increasingly dependent on ventilation and ultimately, will require invasive ventilation with a tracheostomy for the control of the upper airway and secretions. The decision to proceed with tracheostomy and invasive ventilation is often difficult and is highly individual. It requires an educational process that includes the patient, family, and health-care professionals with frequent decision modifications. Long-term ventilator assistance is elected in advance by only a small minority of people with ALS. People with ALS who are most likely to electively choose home mechanical ventilation in advance are those with gradually progressive disease that has allowed incremental accommodation, who still are able to communicate and have some independent function, who have a thorough understanding of the options and a supportive family, who have financial resources and who are still actively engaged in life (Table 4) (79).

Only about 2% to 5% of ALS patients choose invasive ventilation with a tracheostomy (80,81). These choices are influenced by physician attitudes, cost, caregiver burden, and the continued progression of illness (82). The choice of a home ventilation program requires supportive families and 24-hour-a-day supervision with family members and nursing. The cost of invasive ventilation has been estimated at $153,252–$336,852 per year (80,83). The major determinant of cost is that of home nursing. While few patients chose invasive ventilation and a home program, 90% of those patients who are cared for at home were glad they chose to be ventilated and would choose to be ventilated again (81), while 72% of those patients who were in institutions would make the same choice (84).

Table 4 Characteristics that Favor Home Mechanical Ventilation

Patient is highly motivated and engaged in living
ALS is progressing slowly
Patient is able to communicate and do some ADLs
Patient and family understand the options
Family is able and wants to participate in home ventilation
Resources for equipment and caregivers are available
Experienced multidisciplinary team supports home ventilation

Termination of Ventilatory Support

If a patient expresses desire to terminate ventilatory support, a careful and thought-ful approach is necessary. First there needs to be a complete discussion of the deci-sion to terminate care and the ramifications. Counseling to assure that the patient understands the decision and attention to any depression is important. Once the decision is finalized, palliative care should be initiated as the ventilator is titrated off. The patient and family should be in a quiet setting with adequate support from the physician, nursing, and hospice personnel. For treatment of mild or intermittent dyspnea, lorazepam, inhaled opioids, or low doses of midazolam can be adminis-tered. As the dyspnea worsens, increased use of opiates, either intravenously, subcuta-neously, transdermally, or even orally, should be initiated along with benzodiazepines and chlorpromazine as needed for restlessness. If the patient is hypoxic, oxygen can be added for comfort (see also chaps. 37 and 38).

SUMMARY

Although, death from ALS predominantly occurs from respiratory failure, recent advances in pharmacologic therapies, along with inspiratory and expiratory support of respiration, may have a favorable impact on survival, quality of life, cognitive function, and hospitalization rates to the extent that a nihilistic approach is no longer acceptable. In fact, the respiratory management of ALS patients is integral to their care. Respiratory symptoms, examination, and measurement of respiratory function should be monitored and provide a guide to the clinician in order to imple-ment respiratory interventions early enough to maximize benefit.

In the initial phases of the disease, monitoring of pulmonary function can in many instances be implemented in a neuromuscular clinic with spirometry testing every three months. Patients with a FVC $\leq 50\%$ of predicted value, or those who become symptomatic with orthopnea, unexplained nocturnal arousals, morning headaches, or excessive daytime sleepiness, may need pulmonary referral for further testing. This may include measurements of maximal static inspiratory or expiratory mouth pressures (PI_{max} and PE_{max}, respectively), ABGs, and overnight oximetry (85). Other techniques to measure diaphragmatic strength are not uniformly avail-able, have the disadvantage of being invasive, and may not be well tolerated.

As prolongation of survival with NIPPV appears to exceed that of pharmaceu-tical agents such as riluzole, this should be taken into account in the design of future drug trials.

The optimal timing of NIPPV remains to be determined. Current guidelines recommend initiation of NIPPV for a VC <50%, an awake $PaCO_2$ ≥ 45 mmHg at the patient's usual fraction of inspired oxygen, sleep oximetry study demonstrating an oxygen saturation $\leq 88\%$ for at least five continuous minutes at the patient's usual fraction of inspired oxygen, or an PI_{max} <60 cm H_2O. Patients with bulbar symp-toms may still benefit from non-invasive ventilation if they are able to tolerate the intervention, although assisted peak cough flows <2.7 L/s with failure to clear secre-tions and desaturation from baseline more accurately identify patients who may require tracheostomy (52,76).

Equal attention should be paid to the use of expiratory aids to clearing secre-tions as a complement to the support of breathing, with evidence that these measures can significantly decrease the hospitalization rates and improve survival (52). Expira-tory aids consist of assisted cough, either manually or mechanically through an insufflator–exsufflator, use of high-frequency oscillation techniques, training to improve maximum insufflation capacity, and air stacking.

Lastly, the decision toward more permanent invasive mechanical ventilation via tracheostomy depends on a complex interplay of patient, caregiver, and societal factors. Choices should be discussed in advance and in an unbiased fashion. The physician must adhere to the ethical and legal principals within the community. While decisions regarding care and ventilation are ultimately those of the patient, the physician and health-care team must provide education and support throughout the process for the patient and family. Furthermore, if the patient elects not to be ventilated, compassionate palliative care should be initiated.

REFERENCES

1. Sorenson EJ, Stalker AP, Kurland LT, Windebank AJ. Amyotrophic lateral sclerosis in Olmsted County, Minnesota, 1925 to 1998. Neurology 2002; 59(2):280–282.
2. Caroscio JT, Mulvihill MN, Sterling R, Abrams B. Amyotrophic lateral sclerosis. Its natural history. Neurol Clin 1987; 5(1):18.
3. Miller RG, Mitchell JD, Lyon M, Moore DH. Riluzole for amyotrophic lateral sclerosis (ALS)/motor neuron disease (MND). Cochrane Database Syst Rev 2002; (2):CD001447.
4. Chen R, Grand'Maison F, Strong MJ, Ramsay DA, Bolton CF. Motor neuron disease presenting as acute respiratory failure: a clinical and pathological study. J Neurol Neurosurg Psychiatr 1996; 60(4):455–458.
5. de Carvalho M, Matias T, Coelho F, Evangelista T, Pinto A, Luis ML. Motor neuron disease presenting with respiratory failure. J Neurol Sci 1996; 139(suppl):117–122.
6. Fromm GB, Wisdom PJ, Block AJ. Amyotrophic lateral sclerosis presenting with respiratory failure. Diaphragmatic paralysis and dependence on mechanical ventilation in two patients. Chest 1977; 71(5):612–614.
7. Chen R, Grand'Maison F, Brown JD, Bolton CF. Motor neuron disease presenting as acute respiratory failure: electrophysiological studies. Muscle Nerve 1997; 20(4):517–519.
8. Kreitzer SM, Saunders NA, Tyler HR, Ingram RH Jr. Respiratory muscle function in amyotrophic lateral sclerosis. Am Rev Respir Dis 1978; 117(3):437–447.
9. Aboussouan LS, Khan SU, Banerjee M, Arroliga AC, Mitsumoto H. Objective measures of the efficacy of noninvasive positive-pressure ventilation in amyotrophic lateral sclerosis. Muscle Nerve 2001; 24(3):403–409.
10. Griggs RC, Donohoe KM, Utell MJ, Goldblatt D, Moxley RT III. Evaluation of pulmonary function in neuromuscular disease. Arch Neurol 1981; 38(1):9–12.
11. Polkey MI, Lyall RA, Green M, Nigel LP, Moxham J. Expiratory muscle function in amyotrophic lateral sclerosis. Am J Respir Crit Care Med 1998; 158(3):734–741.
12. Poponick JM, Jacobs I, Supinski G, DiMarco AF. Effect of upper respiratory tract infection in patients with neuromuscular disease. Am J Respir Crit Care Med 1997; 156(2 pt 1): 659–664.
13. Murciano D, Rigaud D, Pingleton S, Armengaud MH, Melchior JC, Aubier M. Diaphragmatic function in severely malnourished patients with anorexia nervosa. Effects of renutrition. Am J Respir Crit Care Med 1994; 150(6 pt 1):1569–1574.
14. Braun SR. Respiratory system in amyotrophic lateral sclerosis. Neurol Clin 1987; 5(1):9–31.
15. Rochester DF, Arora NS. Respiratory muscle failure. Med Clin North Am 1983; 67(3):573–597.
16. Mier-Jedrzejowicz AK, Brophy C, Green M. Respiratory muscle function in myasthenia gravis. Am Rev Respir Dis 1988; 138(4):867–873.
17. Ries AL. Measurement of lung volumes. Clin Chest Med 1989; 10(2):177–186.
18. Lung function testing: selection of values and interpretative strategies. American Thoracic Society. Am Rev Respir Dis 1991; 144(5):1202–1218.

19. Carre PC, Didier AP, Tiberge YM, Arbus LJ, Leophonte PJ. Amyotrophic lateral sclerosis presenting with sleep hypopnea syndrome. Chest 1988; 93(6):1309–1312.

20. Tusiewicz K, Moldofsky H, Bryan AC, Bryan MH. Mechanics of the rib cage and diaphragm during sleep. J Appl Physiol 1977; 43(4):600–602.

21. Ferguson KA, Strong MJ, Ahmad D, George CF. Sleep-disordered breathing in amyotrophic lateral sclerosis. Chest 1996; 110(3):664–669.

22. Kimura K, Tachibana N, Kimura J, Shibasaki H. Sleep-disordered breathing at an early stage of amyotrophic lateral sclerosis. J Neurol Sci 1999; 164(1):37–43.

23. Santos C, Braghiroli A, Mazzini L, Pratesi R, Oliveira LV, Mora G. Sleep-related breathing disorders in amyotrophic lateral sclerosis. Monaldi Arch Chest Dis 2003; 59(2): 160–165.

24. Clinical indications for noninvasive positive pressure ventilation in chronic respiratory failure due to restrictive lung disease, COPD, and nocturnal hypoventilation—a consensus conference report. Chest 1999; 116(2):521–534.

25. Elman LB, Siderowf AD, McCluskey LF. Nocturnal oximetry: utility in the respiratory management of amyotrophic lateral sclerosis. Am J Phys Med Rehabil 2003; 82(11): 866–870.

26. Arnulf I, Similowski T, Salachas F, Garma L, Mehiri S, Attali V, Behin-Bellhesen V, Meininger V, Derenne JP. Sleep disorders and diaphragmatic function in patients with amyotrophic lateral sclerosis. Am J Respir Crit Care Med 2003; 161(3 pt 1): 849–856.

27. Meyrignac C, Poirier J, Degos JD. Amyotrophic lateral sclerosis presenting with respiratory insufficiency as the primary complaint. Clinicopathological study of a case. Eur Neurol 1985; 24(2):115–120.

28. Czaplinski A, Strobel W, Gobbi C, Steck AJ, Fuhr P, Leppert D. Respiratory failure due to bilateral diaphragm palsy as an early manifestation of ALS. Med Sci Monit 2003; 9(5):CS34–CS36.

29. Scelsa SN, Yakubov B, Salzman SH. Dyspnea-fasciculation syndrome: early respiratory failure in ALS with minimal motor signs. Amyotroph Lateral Scler Other Motor Neuron Disord 2002; 3(4):239–243.

30. Fallat RJ, Jewitt B, Bass M, Kamm B, Norris FH Jr. Spirometry in amyotrophic lateral sclerosis. Arch Neurol 1979; 36(2):74–80.

31. Krivickas LS. Pulmonary function and respiratory failure. In: Mitsumoto H, Chad DA, Pioro EP, eds. Amyotrophic Lateral Sclerosis. Philadelphia: F.A. Davis, 1998:388–389.

32. Standardization of Spirometry, 1994 Update. American Thoracic Society. Am J Respir Crit Care Med 1995; 152(3):1107–1136.

33. Kleopa KA, Sherman M, Neal B, Romano GJ, Heiman-Patterson T. Bipap improves survival and rate of pulmonary function decline in patients with ALS. J Neurol Sci 1999; 164(1):82–88.

34. Ringel SP, Murphy JR, Alderson MK, Bryan W, England JD, Miller RG, Petajan JH, Smith SA, Roelofs RI, Ziter F, Lee MY, Brinkmann JR, Almada A, Gappmaier E, Graves J, Herbelin L, Mendoza M, Mylar D, Smith P, Yu P. The natural history of amyotrophic lateral sclerosis. Neurology 1993; 43(7):1316–1322.

35. Schiffman PL, Belsh JM. Pulmonary function at diagnosis of amyotrophic lateral sclerosis. Rate of deterioration. Chest 1993; 103(2):508–513.

36. Stambler N, Charatan M, Cedarbaum JM. Prognostic indicators of survival in ALS. ALS CNTF Treatment Study Group. Neurology 1998; 50(1):66–72.

37. Miller RG, Rosenberg JA, Gelinas DF, Mitsumoto H, Newman D, Sufit R, Borasio GD, Bradley WG, Bromberg MB, Brooks BR, Kasarskis EJ, Munsat TL, Oppenheimer EA. Practice parameter: the care of the patient with amyotrophic lateral sclerosis (an evidence-based review): report of the quality standards subcommittee of the American academy of neurology: ALS practice parameters task force. Neurology 1999; 52(7): 1311–1323.

38. Loh L, Goldman M, Davis JN. The assessment of diaphragm function. Medicine (Baltimore) 1977; 56(2):165–169.
39. Lechtzin N, Wiener CM, Shade DM, Clawson L, Diette GB. Spirometry in the supine position improves the detection of diaphragmatic weakness in patients with amyotrophic lateral sclerosis. Chest 2002; 121(2):436–442.
40. Gay PC, Westbrook PR, Daube JR, Litchy WJ, Windebank AJ, Iverson R. Effects of alterations in pulmonary function and sleep variables on survival in patients with amyotrophic lateral sclerosis. Mayo Clin Proc 1991; 66(7):686–694.
41. David WS, Bundlie SR, Mahdavi Z. Polysomnographic studies in amyotrophic lateral sclerosis. J Neurol Sci 1997; 152(suppl 1):S29–S35.
42. Vitacca M, Clini E, Facchetti D, Pagani M, Poloni M, Porta R, Ambrosino N. Breathing pattern and respiratory mechanics in patients with amyotrophic lateral sclerosis. Eur Respir J 1997; 10(7):1614–1621.
43. Chaudri MB, Liu C, Watson L, Jefferson D, Kinnear WJ. Sniff nasal inspiratory pressure as a marker of respiratory function in motor neuron disease. Eur Respir J 2000; 15(3):539–542.
44. Lyall RA, Donaldson N, Polkey MI, Leigh PN, Moxham J. Respiratory muscle strength and ventilatory failure in amyotrophic lateral sclerosis. Brain 2001; 124(pt 10):2000–2013.
45. Stoller JK, Basheda S, Laskowski D, Goormastic M, McCarthy K. Trial of standard versus modified expiration to achieve end-of-test spirometry criteria. Am Rev Respir Dis 1993; 148(2):275–280.
46. Swanney MP, Jensen RL, Crichton DA, Beckert LE, Cardno LA, Crapo RO. FEV(6) is an acceptable surrogate for FVC in the spirometric diagnosis of airway obstruction and restriction. Am J Respir Crit Care Med 2000; 162(3 pt 1):917–919.
47. Hankinson JL, Odencrantz JR, Fedan KB. Spirometric values from a sample of the general U.S. population. Am J Respir Crit Care Med 1999; 159(1):179–187.
48. Hankinson JL, Crapo RO, Jensen RL. Spirometric values for the 6-s FVC maneuver. Chest 2003; 124(5):1805–1811.
49. Aboussouan LS, Khan SU, Meeker DP, Stelmach K, Mitsumoto H. Effect of noninvasive positive-pressure ventilation on survival in amyotrophic lateral sclerosis. Ann Intern Med 1997; 127(6):450–453.
50. Moxham J. Aminophylline and the respiratory muscles: an alternative view. Clin Chest Med 1988; 9(2):325–336.
51. Schiffman PL, Belsh JM. Effect of inspiratory resistance and theophylline on respiratory muscle strength in patients with amyotrophic lateral sclerosis. Am Rev Respir Dis 1989; 139(6):1418–1423.
52. Bach JR. Amyotrophic lateral sclerosis: prolongation of life by noninvasive respiratory AIDS. Chest 2002; 122(1):92–98.
53. Lahrmann H, Wild M, Zdrahal F, Grisold W. Expiratory muscle weakness and assisted cough in ALS. Amyotroph Lateral Scler Other Motor Neuron Disord 2003; 4(1):49–51.
54. Bach JR. Mechanical insufflation–exsufflation. Comparison of peak expiratory flows with manually assisted and unassisted coughing techniques. Chest 1993; 104(5): 1553–1562.
55. Winck JC, Goncalves MR, Lourenco C, Viana P, Almeida J, Bach JR. Effects of mechanical insufflation–exsufflation on respiratory parameters for patients with chronic airway secretion encumbrance. Chest 2004; 126(3):774–780.
56. Kang SW, Bach JR. Maximum insufflation capacity. Chest 2000; 118(1):61–65.
57. Bach JR, Alba AS, Bodofsky E, Curran FJ, Schultheiss M. Glossopharyngeal breathing and noninvasive aids in the management of post-polio respiratory insufficiency. Birth Defects Orig Artic Ser 1987; 23(4):99–113.
58. Bach JR. Update and perspective on noninvasive respiratory muscle aids. Part 2: The Expiratory Aids. Chest 1994; 105(5):1538–1544.

59. Gay PC, Edmonds LC. Severe hypercapnia after low-flow oxygen therapy in patients with neuromuscular disease and diaphragmatic dysfunction. Mayo Clin Proc 1995; 70(4):327–330.

60. Bach JR, Rajaraman R, Ballanger F, Tzeng AC, Ishikawa Y, Kulessa R, Bansal T. Neuromuscular ventilatory insufficiency: effect of home mechanical ventilator use v oxygen therapy on pneumonia and hospitalization rates. Am J Phys Med Rehabil 1998; 77(1):8–19.

61. Mathus-Vliegen LM, Louwerse LS, Merkus MP, Tytgat GN, Vianney de Jong JM. Percutaneous endoscopic gastrostomy in patients with amyotrophic lateral sclerosis and impaired pulmonary function. Gastrointest Endosc 1994; 40(4):463–469.

62. Mazzini L, Corra T, Zaccala M, Mora G, Del Piano M, Galante M. Percutaneous endoscopic gastrostomy and enteral nutrition in amyotrophic lateral sclerosis. J Neurol 1995; 242(10):695–698.

63. Hillberg RE, Johnson DC. Noninvasive ventilation. N Engl J Med 1997; 337(24): 1746–1752.

64. Bach JR. Respiratory muscle aids for the prevention of pulmonary morbidity and mortality. Semin Neurol 1995; 15(1):72–83.

65. Carrey Z, Gottfried SB, Levy RD. Ventilatory muscle support in respiratory failure with nasal positive pressure ventilation. Chest 1990; 97(1):150–158.

66. Heckmatt JZ, Loh L, Dubowitz V. Night-time nasal ventilation in neuromuscular disease. Lancet 1990; 335(8689):579–582.

67. Pinto AC, Evangelista T, Carvalho M, Alves MA, Sales Luis ML. Respiratory assistance with a non-invasive ventilator (Bipap) in MND/ALS patients: survival rates in a controlled trial. J Neurol Sci 1995; 129(suppl):19–26.

68. Bourke SC, Bullock RE, Williams TL, Shaw PJ, Gibson GJ. Noninvasive ventilation in ALS: indications and effect on quality of life. Neurology 2003; 61(2):171–177.

69. Bourke SC, Gibson GJ. Non-invasive ventilation in ALS: current practice and future role. Amyotroph Lateral Scler Other Motor Neuron Disord 2004; 5(2):67–71.

70. Butz M, Wollinsky KH, Wiedemuth-Catrinescu U, Sperfeld A, Winter S, Mehrkens HH, et al. Longitudinal effects of noninvasive positive-pressure ventilation in patients with amyotrophic lateral sclerosis. Am J Phys Med Rehabil 2003; 82(8):597–604.

71. Lyall RA, Donaldson N, Fleming T, Wood C, Newsom-Davis I, Polkey MI, Leigh PN, Moxham J. A prospective study of quality of life in ALS patients treated with noninvasive ventilation. Neurology 2001; 57(1):153–156.

72. Newsom-Davis IC, Lyall RA, Leigh PN, Moxham J, Goldstein LH. The effect of non-invasive positive pressure ventilation (NIPPV) on cognitive function in amyotrophic lateral sclerosis (ALS): a prospective study. J Neurol Neurosurg Psychiatry 2001; 71(4): 482–487.

73. Jackson CE, Rosenfeld J, Moore DH, Bryan WW, Barohn RJ, Wrench M, Myers D, Heberlin L, King R, Smith J, Gelinas D, Miller RG. A preliminary evaluation of a prospective study of pulmonary function studies and symptoms of hypoventilation in ALS/ MND patients. J Neurol Sci 2001; 191(1–2):75–78.

74. Perez T, Salachas F. [Early nasal ventilation in amyotrophic lateral sclerosis: impact on survival and quality of life (the VNP-SLA study)]. Rev Mal Respir 2003; 20(4):589–598.

75. Pinto A, de Carvalho M, Evangelista T, Lopes A, Sales-Luis L. Nocturnal pulse oximetry: a new approach to establish the appropriate time for non-invasive ventilation in ALS patients. Amyotroph Lateral Scler Other Motor Neuron Disord 2003; 4(1):31–35.

76. Bach JR, Bianchi C, Aufiero E. Oximetry and indications for tracheotomy for amyotrophic lateral sclerosis. Chest 2004; 126(5):1502–1507.

77. Bach JR. Update and perspectives on noninvasive respiratory muscle aids. Part 1: the inspiratory aids. Chest 1994; 105(4):1230–1240.

78. Ellis ER, Bye PT, Bruderer JW, Sullivan CE. Treatment of respiratory failure during sleep in patients with neuromuscular disease. Positive-pressure ventilation through a nose mask. Am Rev Respir Dis 1987; 135(1):148–152.

79. Oppenheimer EA. Decision-making in the respiratory care of amyotrophic lateral sclerosis: should home mechanical ventilation be used? Palliat Med 1993; 7(suppl 4): 49–64.
80. Lechtzin N, Wiener CM, Clawson L, Davidson MC, Anderson F, Gowda N, Diette GB. ALS CARE Study Group. Use of noninvasive ventilation in patients with amyotrophic lateral sclerosis. Amyotroph Lateral Scler Other Motor Neuron Disord 2004; 5(1):9–15.
81. Moss AH, Casey P, Stocking CB, Roos RP, Brooks BR, Siegler M. Home ventilation for amyotrophic lateral sclerosis patients: outcomes, costs, and patient, family, and physician attitudes. Neurology 1993; 43(2):438–443.
82. Moss AH, Oppenheimer EA, Casey P, Cazzolli PA, Roos RP, Stocking CB, Siegler M. Patients with amyotrophic lateral sclerosis receiving long-term mechanical ventilation. Advance care planning and outcomes. Chest 1996; 110(1):249–255.
83. Albert SM, Murphy PL, Del Bene ML, Rowland LP. A prospective study of preferences and actual treatment choices in ALS. Neurology 1999; 53(2):278–283.
84. Cazzolli PA, Oppenheimer EA. Home mechanical ventilation for amyotrophic lateral sclerosis: nasal compared to tracheostomy-intermittent positive pressure ventilation. J Neurol Sci 1996; 139(suppl):123–128.
85. Lechtzin N, Rothstein J, Clawson L, Diette GB, Wiener CM. Amyotrophic lateral sclerosis: evaluation and treatment of respiratory impairment. Amyotroph Lateral Sclerosis Other Motor Neuron Disord 2002; 3(1):5–13.

34

Psychosocial Care for Patients with ALS and Their Caregivers

Gian Domenico Borasio
Interdisciplinary Center for Palliative Medicine and Department of Neurology, Motor Neuron Disease Research Group, Munich University Hospital, Grosshadern, Munich, Germany

Mark Bromberg
Department of Neurology, University of Utah, Salt Lake City, Utah, U.S.A.

Maura L. Del Bene
Department of Neurology, New York University School of Medicine, New York, New York, U.S.A.

Hiroshi Mitsumoto
Eleanor and Lou Gehrig MDA/ALS Research Center, Department of Neurology, Columbia University Medical Center, The Neurological Institute, New York, New York, U.S.A.

INTRODUCTION

The term "psychosocial" refers to the aspects of one's being and functioning that encompass the emotional, social, and intellectual realms. Studies have shown that psychosocial well-being promotes survival in ALS; patients with a low quality of life (psychological distress) are seven times more likely to die sooner than those with a high quality of life (psychological well-being), a finding that corresponds to those reported for patients with terminal cancer (1). The importance of psychosocial care is emphasized in the recent Robert Wood Johnson Initiative to Improve End-of-Life Care in ALS as well as other specific diseases (2). Psychosocial care in terminal diseases like ALS, which progress steadily without remission, is complex and requires recognition and exploration of psychosocial issues in the context of the concurrent disease.

This chapter reviews the impact of ALS on psychosocial issues for patients and their families and makes specific recommendations for intervention by health care and social service providers. Many of our references are to studies in chronic diseases other than ALS because little formal research has been conducted on psychosocial care in ALS. Regardless, data on psychosocial care from these studies are likely to be valid for ALS, although future investigations specific to ALS will provide valuable insights.

PATIENT AND CAREGIVER EDUCATION

Educating patients and their families about ALS is the first step in providing psycho-social care. Education begins with the initial evaluation of the patient and continues throughout the disease course. Disclosing the diagnosis and subsequent bad news as the disease progresses so that patients and families feel engaged, supported, and even hopeful in the face of devastating loss is an art and requires adequate patient and family education. Health care providers must respect the patient's autonomy because it is the patient who makes decisions about care at the end of life; respecting our patients' autonomy and providing education will help them make the best decisions regarding their care.

Although the care team at an ALS clinic largely focuses on physical care, the team members are also educators for their patients and families. The surveys of care-givers and patients indicate that the lack of readily available resources and medical information about the disease itself, much less research or coping with the disease, is a significant stressor (HM, personal communication based on a focus group study on caregiver issues, 2004). Although information is available on the Internet, it may be inaccurate and confusing, and accurate information is essential if our patients are to make decisions regarding their care and feel supported by the medical community. Having ALS-specific literature designed for patients and families, as well as the telephone numbers and Web sites of local voluntary organizations, is the starting point. Educational and support group sessions for patients and caregivers that are organized by the ALS Association, the Muscular Dystrophy Association, and other local or regional ALS organizations are available (3). However, their availability and frequency may vary depending on location and organizational factors.

CARE FOR INFORMAL CAREGIVERS

Traditionally, physicians' primary responsibilities are considered to be unequivocally to their patients, which is based on Western medicine's exclusive focus on the individual patient in its codes of ethics, training, and practice (4). However, family members now act as advocates for the patient, provide or manage care, serve as trusted companions during the patient's journey through illness and death, and make decisions on behalf of the incompetent patient (4). In the current health care system in the United States, patients with debilitating chronic diseases are increasingly cared for at home, except when acute medical complications occur. The financial and physical burdens of care are shifted from the hospital to the families, in part to reduce the costs of care to society. Data from the North American ALS CARE Database indicate that 56% of patients with ALS die at home and, thus, a family member (most often the spouse) usually becomes the principal caregiver (an "informal" caregiver because the caregiver is not a professional home care nurse) (5). Consequently, the home may become a place of sickness, even hospital-like, and what once was a place of relaxation and enjoyment is transformed into a place of stress for all family members.

Caregiver Burden and Distress

Primary caregivers spend a median of 11 hours daily caring for patients in various stages of ALS *despite* having home care assistance. Accordingly, primary caregivers report feeling either physically (42%) or psychologically (48%) unwell (6). A small study of ventilator-dependent patients and their informal caregivers determined that caregivers were heavily burdened and their outside activities were severely limited (7). This was confirmed in a recent study that found patients with tracheostomy had a quality of life as good as that of patients with noninvasive ventilation but that the caregivers of the tracheostomy patients had a much greater care burden (8). Goldstein et al. (9) also point out that caregivers are anxious and depressed, with the latter positively correlating with the degree of the patient's functional impairment. Analysis of the ALS CARE Database indicates that a large number of family caregivers experience significant burden during all stages of the disease (Table 1). The reasons that this stress exists are complex, but in part it occurs because, at least in the United States, formal home health care for patients with ALS often is inadequate and occurs too late to relieve the burden placed on caregivers.

Although it might appear obvious that ALS caregivers suffer, an interview-based study of 56 patients in the terminal stages of ALS and their 31 caregivers found that neither patients nor caregivers had significant psychopathology with respect to either depressive disorders or scores on depression symptom scales (10).

Table 1 Analysis of Caregiver Distress as Reported in the ALS CARE Database[a]

Question: Has assisting the patient...	Percentage of responding moderately, a lot, or a great deal (%)
Added tension to your life?	48
Restricted the vacation activities and trips you take?	44
Decreased the time you have to yourself?	43
Increased your anxiety about things?	39
Decreased the time you have to spend in recreational activities?	38
Reduced the time you have to do your own work and daily chores?	35
Increased the nervousness and depression you have concerning your relationship with him/her?	33
Decreased the time you have for friends and other relatives?	30
Increased the stress in your relationship with him/her?	26
Decreased the money available to meet the rest of your expenses?	25
Restricted personal privacy?	20
Caused you to neglect other important relationships (e.g., children and parents)?	15
Increased the number of unreasonable requests made by you?	15
Increased attempts by him/her to manipulate you?	13
Affected your ability to attend to your personal medical needs?	12
Increased demands made by him/her that are over and above what he/she needs?	10
Added to your feelings that you are being taken advantage of?	8

[a]These data are derived from an analysis of North American ALS CARE Database Question 21, which examines the caregiver's burden. Each question has five possible levels of response: (i) not at all, (ii) a little, (iii) moderately, (iv) a lot, or (v) a great deal. The numbers following each question indicate the total percentage of these caregivers who answered moderately, a lot, or a great deal. These data are based on responses from 2688 caregivers of patients who were enrolled at 97 clinical sites participating in the North American ALS Patient Care Database, from 1996 through May 2001.

Although caregivers were distressed, their perception of the amount of burden was significantly associated with finding positive meaning in caregiving. This finding suggests that clinical depression or significant depressive symptomatology in caregivers is not an inevitable outcome of caring for someone with a terminal illness. Concordance between patient and caregiver distress was high, suggesting that attending to the mental health needs of caregivers may alleviate the patient's distress as well (10).

Psychological Mechanisms of Distress from Caregiving

Understanding the mechanisms that underlie the development of distress and caregiver coping may help health care providers support the caregivers (11). In ALS, the caregiver's perception of burden has been shown to correlate with a loss of intimacy with the patient, which in turn is predicted by the degree of change in the patient's cognitive, behavioral, and communication functions (9). Changes in the patient's ability to interact socially also correlate with the extent to which caregivers feel that the illness affects other areas of their lives, the extent to which the patient dominates their thoughts, and the extent to which they can control their reactions when thinking about the patient (9). Interviews of caregivers for the elderly suggest that the stress can be explained by the concept of the "theory of the gift" as modified by negotiation (12). Gift giving involves giving, receiving, and giving back. When the balance is perceived as negative (giving, but receiving back with no negotiation to modify the process), the cycle of gift-giving breaks down. Like gift-giving, care is given, received, and returned. Accordingly, when the balance is negative, the caregiver feels trapped in a cycle of giving only and stress develops that undermines the caregiving role.

Caregiver distress is also influenced by how well the caregiver has mastered care giving. In interviews with a large number of disabled elderly informal caregivers, Yates et al. (13) explored the relationships between caregiving stressors and caregiver well-being. Tasks that were required for care of the patient (caregiving stressors) indirectly led to caregiver depression through their effect on the hours of care needed and the caregiver's resulting perception of work overload. However, caregivers who had high levels of mastery of caregiving and emotional support were at lower risk for depression, regardless of the number of primary caregiving stressors, indicating the importance of emotional support and skills training for the caregivers.

Caregiver Health and Its Effect on Distress

Among caregivers for cancer patients, those who also have physical problems of their own are at risk for psychological morbidity that may become apparent at a later time (14). Research concerning this issue in ALS should include comprehensive assessment of caregivers' physical problems as well as other major life stressors that caregivers may face. Moreover, caregivers in general who have lower subjective burden scores practice more health-promoting behaviors than those with higher subjective burden scores, which may be an important factor for caregivers who have physical difficulties themselves (15).

Schulz and Beach (16) suggest that elderly spousal caregivers may require special consideration, particularly those who experience mental or emotional strain because they are at higher risk for mortality than those who do not. Older married couples should be evaluated as a unit, both in terms of their health status as well as the caregiving demands that exist in the home. Although research is necessary, because we have no data, this association also holds true in caregivers for patients with ALS; ALS clinicians must pay close attention to the caregiver-spouse's physical well-being.

Caregiver Awareness of Dying

One of the major processes that the family caregivers go through is a development of an awareness that their loved one is dying. This awareness develops gradually and is characterized by uncertainty and anguish, followed by hope that dying will be far in the future, pretending that nothing has changed, and then preparing for the death (17). ALS health professionals should try to identify stages in the process for each family and give appropriate support. Support may include helping family caregivers to maintain hope, sustain social relationships, and prepare for the patient's death. Further research as to how family caregivers use these strategies for managing their developing awareness of dying is required in ALS (17).

Special Issues Regarding Spousal and Adult Child Caregivers

Wives and husbands differ in their selection of informal caregivers (18), with gender role norms being a main factor. Wives are only one-third as likely as husbands to select their spouses as caregivers. However, spouses, regardless of gender, who describe their mates as confidants (meaning that there is mutual trust) are three times more likely to also name them as caregivers than those who do not, suggesting that although gender role norms are important, an emotionally close marriage is an important criterion in whether the patient selects the spouse to be the caregiver. The closeness of a couple's long-term relationship also affects caregiver distress. Among middle-aged and elderly married couples, if their relationship has been communal (characterized by mutual concern for and responsiveness to one another's needs), the caregiver's restriction of activity outside the home is predicted by the degree of loss of intimacy and affection rather than by the severity of patient symptoms—the greater the loss, the greater the restriction. In turn, the loss of intimacy and affection predicts depression for the caregiver. Conversely, among caregivers in less communal relationships, activity restriction is predicted by the severity of patient symptoms rather than by loss of intimacy and affection—perhaps because the relationship has been less close, with less affection and intimacy being lost, activity restriction is influenced more by symptom severity (19).

Male spousal caregivers make up nearly 30% to 36% of all caregivers in the United States. Caregiver husbands experience significant changes in their household responsibilities, social integration, marital relationship, and well-being, but little data are available on whether there are issues that are unique compared to caregiver wives. Attention to the experience of the caregiver husband is especially important because husbands play a major role in caring for chronically ill older women, and the number of caregiver husbands is predicted to increase (20).

Dautzenberg et al. (21) and Centers (22) studied distress in middle-aged daughters providing assistance to elderly parents with diseases other than ALS. Most distressed were women who were not performing any major social role, suggesting that the lack of social roles, rather than having to perform many roles (e.g., caregiver, mother, and working outside the home), is associated with distress. For some women, acting in the caregiver role might even reduce distress if they have very few other social roles.

Use of Formal Home Health Care Services

It is plausible to postulate that the use of formal home health care services should alleviate the burden of family caregivers. However, Goldstein et al. (9) found that it alleviated neither caregiver burden nor depression. Furthermore, formal services did not reduce the amount of informal care provided but only supplemented it. Thus, although formal services may be necessary as the patient becomes more disabled, they appear to have little or no effect on family caregiver well-being (13). Several factors, including the home care service itself, may account for the lack of impact: (i) home care received by patients with ALS often is inadequate and obtained too late to relieve the burden placed on family caregivers; (ii) patients and caregivers often have no choice in selecting a designated home care nurse; (iii) home care services change personnel without telling the patients and family caregivers; and (iv) the nurses may not have much knowledge of ALS or end-of-life care (6). Furthermore, the high cost of professional home health care, which is poorly covered by insurance in the United States, can add stress. Extensive education on ALS is required for home care and hospice care agencies.

Houde (23) determined that formal home care services were used less frequently as the hours of informal care increased. Patient characteristics that were important predictors of the use of formal home care services included residence in elder housing, recent hospitalization, female sex, marked limitations in managing the activities of daily living, receiving Medicaid, older age, quantity of informal care provided, and low number of household members. Formal services were also used more often if caregivers were physically limited in their mobility outside the home, had to rearrange their work hours, or if male caregivers performed bowel and bladder care. These findings support considering both patient and caregiver characteristics when anticipating whether a family will use formal home care services. Improving caregiver support is especially important, given that expected demographic and social trends may result in a greater number of elderly caregivers and fewer other available family caregivers.

Respite Service for Family Caregivers

In the United States, respite services have not been used extensively despite the fact that Medicare pays for such care during the end of life (Susan DeGrande, personal communication, 2002). High levels of intimacy and love between the patient and caregiver are associated with less use, suggesting a key reason why respite is often requested but not used. Conversely, an absence of intimacy and love is associated with greater use (24). Hanson et al. (25) recommend broadening the concept of respite care so that respite services can be structured to also help address the family caregiver's needs for information, skills training and education, and emotional support. Although respite effectively provides immediate relief from the demands of caring, it often fails to facilitate the maintenance of socially supportive relationships that could reduce strain after the respite period has ended (26). To address this problem, a more care-centered approach could be adopted in both providing and evaluating respite service. In Japan, where hospital admission is available to patients with ALS, admission primarily for the purpose of caregiver respite occurs more often than in any other neurodegenerative disorder (T. Saito, M.D, Kitasato University). Accordingly, both social custom and the structure of the societal health care system appear to dictate the use of respite.

Financial Concerns

In interviews of almost 1000 terminally ill patients (any disease) and their caregivers, Emanuel et al. (27) found that 35% of patients needed substantial care and that their care imposed an economic burden—10% of household income was spent on health care. Patients with substantial care needs were more likely to consider euthanasia or physician-assisted suicide. Also, caregivers of the patients who needed substantial care were more likely to be depressed and to report that caring for the patients interfered with their lives. Despite the economic burden, in the United States, no financial support is available to family caregivers, unlike in other countries (27,28). The economic value of the caregiver's work has been studied only in home care situations in which the patient is on a ventilator: one estimate showed that home care was more expensive than care at a long-term care facility for as many as 37% of patients (29). Home care costs for ventilator-dependent patients are often higher than for hospitalized patients when the total economic value of the caregiver effort is considered, which includes reduced work outside the home, lost employment or educational opportunities, lost wages of both the caregiver and patient, and the extent to which the caregiver has depended on the patient financially.

Improving Caregiver Coping

Strategies are available to help caregivers and the family cope. Caregivers need to feel that they have both social and medical support. One study of ALS caregivers who were asked to predict their ability to cope found that the predicted ability positively correlated with the number of social groups to which the caregivers belonged and with their satisfaction with formal home health care (9). Further, when physicians are perceived to listen to patients' and caregivers' needs, caregivers have fewer burdens and thus may be better able to cope (27). Caregivers who depended on religious or spiritual beliefs to cope had better relationships with their patients, which in turn was associated with lower levels of depression and feelings of submersion in the caregiver role (30).

Psychotherapeutic Counseling

ALS patients and family members benefit from formal family counseling. Ideally, the family should participate in family-based therapy to assist them as a unit to understand their pre-illness coping mechanisms and how to apply them with the goal of decreasing stress. Family therapy can also help mobilize the family to maintain a sense of normalcy and develop mutual support. Referral to mental health professionals with experience in ALS is ideal, but referral to therapists who specialize in chronic or terminal illness is more realistic because few therapists will have specific ALS experience. When a patient declines psychotherapy or when access to counseling is limited by insurance reimbursement or referral availability, referral to an ALS support group is more practical. As support groups are based on peer support, they can provide significant guidance for patients and families. The value of interacting with others in the same situation should not be underestimated.

SEXUALITY AND INTIMACY

Sexuality in patients with ALS is seldom discussed. The information in this section has been previously published but is repeated here because it remains highly valid

(31). Patients with ALS experience a decrease in sexual activity as well as problems such as decreased libido and passivity that they report due to physical weakness and the loss of a positive body image (32). We cannot emphasize the need for health professionals to be ready to discuss sexuality openly and comfortably—the more open and relaxed the providers are, the more comfortable the patients and their spouses will be.

As ALS does not affect the autonomic nervous system, sexual function is thought to be well preserved. In patients with ALS, however, various medications used for symptomatic treatment may cause sexual dysfunction. For instance, baclofen (Lioresal®) can reduce libido, and the anticholinergic effects of tricyclic antidepressants may cause erectile dysfunction, decreased vaginal lubrication, and decreased clitoral enlargement. Patients with ALS who do not have side effects from medications may still experience problems with sexual function. Muscle weakness, fatigue, spasticity, communication difficulty, respiratory distress, fear, anxiety, and depression may interfere with sexual performance. The loss of a positive body image and self-esteem, fear of losing the affection of one's partner, fear of impotence, loss of interest in sex, and fear that the partner will "look elsewhere" may all be potentially serious issues (33). Also, patients often express the feeling that when everyday survival is an issue, talking about sexuality is not only a rather embarrassing but also an inappropriate subject. Pernick (34) twice surveyed patients with ALS and health professionals about sexuality. In 1981, she found that almost no health professionals had discussed ALS and sexuality; in 1988, however, more health professionals were talking about sexuality, although their attitude was essentially the same as that in 1981; many felt that it was not a pressing issue. All the patients and their partners wanted their diagnosing doctor to discuss the issue, and 75% of them also wanted nurses to discuss it. Health professionals express discomfort with the subject matter, because of inadequate knowledge, insufficient time for meaningful discussion during the clinic visit, and the dismissal of the importance of pleasurable sexual activity.

If one takes a holistic approach to health care, the issue of sexuality must not be ignored. Health professionals may begin the discussion of sexuality directly. One may refer to other patients, saying that "some patients with ALS express concern about continuing to express their sexuality. Do you have any concerns or questions?" Alternatively, the issue can be raised indirectly by providing literature containing information on the issue of sexuality in ALS. The more open the atmosphere, the more comfortable both patients and the health care professional will be.

Health care professionals must understand that patients with ALS have limited physical ability but normal sexual desire and should be able to enjoy sexual intimacy. Health care professionals can suggest role changes within the partnership, more comfortable positions during intercourse, and other ways to express affection and intimacy, such as mutual masturbation (33). One of our patients, who had moderate respiratory difficulty, developed wheezing during sexual intercourse, which frightened both the patient and spouse and resulted in abstinence. At the next ALS clinic visit, his wife hesitantly expressed her concerns, which led to a frank discussion about techniques the couple might use to continue a satisfying sexual relationship.

ADDRESSING THE NEEDS OF CHILDREN

The psychosocial effects of ALS on the family members may vary significantly. Although children are not directly involved in the care and decision-making processes, they are deeply affected emotionally by the changes occurring in the family, most obviously if the patient is a parent or grandparent whom they know well. As children often have difficulty articulating their emotions, changes in their behavior may give clues to how they are feeling and give both the family and health care providers insight as to how to give psychosocial support to the child in the present and future. Such support begins long before the death of the family member.

Children need:

- Respect and acknowledgment of their fears and emotions
- Information about what is happening. It needs to be clear, simple, truthful, and repeated often as children struggle to come to terms with what is happening and what might happen next.
- Reassurance. Children can become very frightened as they watch a parent or relative becoming dependent and perhaps emotionally labile or irrationally angry. They need explanations and to know that they did not cause the illness and cannot catch it. Children will also want reassurance about practical issues such as what is going to happen to the family and their own care after the person has died.
- Appropriate involvement in helping the patient
- A chance to talk about feelings
- Access to other adults with whom they can safely share their feelings
- Various means for self-expression, for example, drawing, writing, playing games, and, in older children, age-appropriate reading material concerning loss. Most children's literature focuses on the grief process by discussing the death of a loved one. However, books that relate to loss, aging, and the natural cycle of life will be more helpful in the time before the actual death of the family member.
- Opportunities to know that life during and after ALS goes on and that it is all right to have fun
- To know, most importantly, that they are not alone in their experience

SPIRITUALITY

Preservation of human dignity at the end of life cannot be separated from attention to the spiritual needs of the dying. For this reason, the World Health Organization (WHO) places management of spiritual issues at the same level of importance as psychosocial and physical care in its definition of palliative care (35). Unfortunately, because of a lack of knowledge and familiarity, health care professionals still largely neglect their patients' spiritual needs when providing end-of-life care. However, because patients' spiritual health affects the medical decisions they make, health care providers must discuss spiritual well-being with their patients. A recent study of 46 individuals with ALS indicated that those with greater spirituality were more likely to have completed advance directives, less likely to undergo gastrostomy, less fearful of death and dying, less likely to participate in support groups, and more likely to choose a natural death rather than mechanical ventilation (36). In this study, the Beck Hopelessness Scale score was significantly related to levels of religiousness and spirituality. The authors conclude that "although religion and spirituality may not offer a cure, they may ease adaptation to a grave diagnosis and the transitions of life that occur in the process of dying." Cases also have been reported of patients with ALS whose spiritual practices greatly enhanced their ability to cope with the disease (37).

Spirituality and Religiousness

Defining spirituality is difficult, and there is often confusion between the words "spiritual" and "religious" (38). Moreover, religious, spiritual, and psychological issues overlap. Sykes (39) defines "spiritual" as "the need to find within present existence a sense of meaning," which may or may not involve a religious framework. All people engage in this search, particularly as they approach death. Problems arise when spirituality and religiousness are confused. Spirituality, being centered on the meaning of life, cannot be assessed solely by determining adherence to defined formal practices, such as church going or praying. Conversely, data on the frequency of attendance at religious services do not necessarily correlate with spiritual well-being. This distinction must be kept in mind, and it may need to be discussed with patients because people tend to confuse the two ideas.

Roles of the Health Care Professionals and Spiritual Counselors

Health care professionals often find attending to the spiritual aspect of care to be difficult, in part due to inadequate training and insufficient time (38). However, data from recent surveys indicate that 70% of cancer patients want to discuss spiritual issues with their physicians (40). It is important to remember that spiritual care for patients and families usually is given most effectively by those individuals, regardless of their profession, who have been taking good spiritual care of themselves.

Collaboration with chaplains and other spiritual counselors is important. Cross-cultural differences in the spiritual attitudes and needs of patients from diverse ethnic and religious backgrounds must be acknowledged and responded to in sensitive ways. Sensitivity requires a basic understanding of the different ways death and dying are viewed within the major religious traditions. Hospital and hospice chaplains often have received specific training in these issues and also usually have contacts with ministers of various faiths who can be called upon when needed.

Spiritual Care for the Family

Spiritual care should not be limited to patients, but rather should involve the whole family as a means of easing bereavement. Initial data indicate that bereavement in relatives after the death of the patient with ALS may be particularly severe and prolonged (41), most likely because of the huge burden of care in the months preceding death. However, appropriate counseling is available that can ease the impact of the loss (42). It is important to acknowledge that bereavement in ALS actually starts immediately after the diagnosis is given, in the form of "anticipatory grief" (see below) and that callous delivery of the diagnosis may affect psychological adjustment to bereavement (43).

Assessing the Patient's Spiritual Needs

Table 2 describes Faith, Importance, Community, Address (FICA), which is a structured interview that can be used to assess patients' spiritual needs (44). Although the clinical efficacy of this instrument has not been formally validated in ALS, it is a

Table 2 The FICA Spiritual Assessment Instrument

Some specific questions one can use to discuss spiritual issues are:

F: What is your faith or belief?
   Do you consider yourself spiritual or religious?
   What things do you believe will give meaning to your life?

I: Is it important in your life?
   What influence does it have on how you take care of yourself?
   How have your beliefs influenced your behavior during this illness?
   What role do your beliefs play in regaining your health?

C: Are you part of a spiritual or religious community?
   Is this of support to you and how?
   Is there a person or group of people you really love or who are really important to you?

A: How would you like me, your health care provider, to address these issues in your health care?

General recommendations when taking a spiritual history:

Consider spirituality as a potentially important component of every patient's physical well-being and mental health.
Address spirituality at each complete physical exam and continue addressing it at follow-up visits, if appropriate. In patient care, spirituality is an ongoing issue.
Respect a patient's privacy regarding spiritual beliefs; don't impose your beliefs on others.
Make referrals to chaplains, spiritual directors, or community resources as appropriate.
Be aware that your own spiritual beliefs will help you personally and will overflow in your encounters with those for whom you care to make the doctor–patient encounter a more humanistic one.

Abbreviations: FICA; Faith, Importance, Community, Address.
Source: Derived from Ref. 44.

simple screening tool and also gives the physician and patient an initial opportunity to discuss spiritual issues in a nonthreatening way. Anecdotal experience indicates that the FICA has a high acceptance by patients with ALS. However, health care providers should keep in mind that some patients may interpret their attempt to discuss spiritual issues as an indication of impending death. If so, patients may respond defensively, and such a situation requires particular sensitivity on the health professional's part. The assessment is therefore better if first performed early rather than late in the disease course, and repeated periodically as the disease progresses (Table 2).

Other assessment instruments relating to spiritual and existential issues in end-of-life care are available but have been used primarily for research purposes. Of these, the spiritual well-being scale has been used in a pilot study in ALS patients (45). Other scales include the Scales for the Evaluation of Life Quality in Tumor Patients—Modified (SELT-M) (46), the Spiritual Involvement and Beliefs Scale (SIBS) (47), and the Life Evaluation Questionnaire (48). In addition, the Schedule for the Evaluation of Individual Quality of Life (SEIQoL-DW) (49) may provide information on existential domains that are relevant for the individual patient's quality of life and may prove useful in clinical assessment as well (50). Finally, qualitative research may provide invaluable information on this highly personal dimension of quality of life.

Spirituality and Life Closure

A sense of reaching closure is a primary indicator of the patient's readiness for death. The concept of closure varies, but usually includes a life review—looking back as to what has been achieved or left behind. Achieving a feeling of completion is very important for the dying patient, as it is easier to leave a life when one has addressed spiritual, psychosocial, family, and financial issues. Regardless of a patient's religious beliefs or spirituality, closure is an integral part of the dying process and can begin either months before or in the minutes preceding the actual process of dying.

As Cicely Saunders, the founder of modern palliative care, has said, "It is not the worst thing for patients to find out that they have lived and are now going to die; the worst thing is to find out that they *haven't* lived and are now going to die." Obviously, no end-of-life care process can completely address such feelings. However, appropriate spiritual counseling may help the patient come to terms with missed opportunities. If counseling does not help, and the patient dies in despair, health care providers must remember that it is not their fault. Nor, conversely, is it their merit if some patients show an almost incredible serenity and acceptance of their disease and approaching death. The professionals' task is simply to remove all obstacles that might interfere with such acceptance, and facilitate it through gentle counseling when appropriate and desired by the patient. End-of-life care is similar to the task that midwives perform at the beginning of life: removing obstacles and allowing a natural process to unfold (51). In this respect, professionals involved in end-of-life care can and should consider themselves as "midwives for the dying."

BEREAVEMENT

Bereavement is most frequently considered in the context of death and focuses on the loss of an individual. However, one can also mourn the loss of physical function and independence, as occurs in ALS. Thus, bereavement affects both the patient with ALS patient and the family. Bereavement can affect many aspects of an individual's physical, social, and psychological health (42). Several terms are associated with bereavement, and they will be used interchangeably in this section. Bereavement is a process that begins when something is lost or someone dies. Grief is the feeling of sadness associated with the loss. Mourning is the expression of sorrow and grief. Recognizing that bereavement can encompass more than mourning the loss of life can help the patient, caregiver, and family members understand many of their feelings and emotions and may lessen distress.

Issues and Types of Grief in ALS

As grieving is experienced not just by survivors, but also by the patients as they reflect on their lost abilities, it is necessary to regard bereavement on a longer time scale, starting with the diagnosis, extending through the course of the disease, and lasting beyond the time of death. Further, the progressive nature of ALS allows family members to prepare for the death of their loved one. The bereavement process in ALS, therefore, differs from bereavement accompanying a sudden and unexpected death. Bereavement has been divided into stages (52), but it may be more practical to view the resolution of grief as a series of tasks: (i) accepting the reality of the loss, (ii) working through the pain of grief, (iii) adjusting to the loss, and (iv) relocating emotionally and moving on (42,53). Issues unique to chronic terminal illnesses such as ALS include the following.

Anticipatory grief can be significant in ALS. It often begins at diagnosis and may be magnified by imagination and inaccurate or limited knowledge concerning the manner of death in ALS. Bereavement may develop gradually, with the sense of loss growing as specific functional losses occur. Bereavement also may subside but then recur when the health care professional periodically evaluates the patient's loss of abilities. Anticipatory grief may help the family and caregiver prepare for the patient's death and may even lessen the intensity and duration of bereavement after death.

Final grief represents bereavement that starts at the time of death. As the progressive loss of the patient's functional abilities leads to a loss of the caregiver's independence, the intensity of final bereavement may be tempered by physical and emotional relief when the patient dies. On the other hand, the relief from the burden of care can cause the caregiver to feel resentful because his or her work and identity as a caregiver no longer exist (54).

The family context of bereavement includes previous intrafamily relationships and will influence anticipatory and final bereavement. The illness may bring family members together, leading to a mutually supportive environment. Attempts to reunite the family are an important part of preparing for the end-of-life process because the reunited family is likely to be stronger and will provide mutual support (54). Within a family, support may be greater when multiple generations are involved. For example, grandchildren can provide a sense of balance between aging and death, and youth and promise. Exposing a child to infirmities and death as natural aspects of life may help them cope in the future with deaths of family members and friends.

Cultural Differences and External Factors

Responses to death vary markedly among religions and cultures, and these differences may not be obvious to an outside observer. Health care providers should be willing to consider and respect the patient's customs and religious beliefs and should inquire about the patient's beliefs as a means of opening the initial discussion of bereavement. External factors, such as family financial and social resources, can have an impact on the bereavement process. Division of property can generate strife, and if the patient and family discuss in advance how property can be distributed, conflict may be reduced during bereavement. Monetary loss because of the illness can lead to financial struggles. Several studies have found that the financial burden of tracheostomy and ventilatory support in ALS can cause hardship, bitterness, and guilt (55,56).

Resources for the Patient and Family

Bereavement in ALS has been discussed primarily in the context of hospice care (57,58), but should be considered as a continuous process that starts at diagnosis and continues through the course of the disease and for an extended period after death. An approach that includes both unstructured and structured programs should be available to patients and their families.

Unstructured Programs

Informally, bereavement counseling can start with discussing how death is a consequence of living and that ALS gives the patient and family time to come to closure. Such a discussion can be initiated when one of the six triggers for discussing end-of-life issues is identified in the patient and family (Table 3; see also Mitsumoto et al. (2) and Chap. 36, 37).

Anticipating the Stages of Bereavement. Patients and families can gain adequate knowledge of the relationship between the tasks of bereavement and disease progression by reading, attending lectures, and engaging in discussions with other patients, families, and health care providers (53,59–61).

The actual manner in which the patient with ALS dies may be a major fear for the patient and family, and it is important to describe the dying process for them. A recent review of 171 patient deaths from ALS indicates that death was peaceful in almost all cases, without evidence of choking or pain (62), findings that were also shown in the ALS CARE Database study (63; see also Chap. 29). These fears surrounding the end of life may interfere in the family's and patient's attempts to deal with other emotional aspects of the disease and should be addressed before the patient is near death. This information may need to be repeated at various stages of the disease, particularly when the end-of-life is near.

It is essential that the patient and family are made to feel that they are not alone. In the past, a diagnosis of ALS was associated with abandonment by the health care profession because of the attitude concerning terminal diseases that "there is nothing that can be done, so no return appointment is necessary, and your affairs should be put in order." The development and proliferation of ALS clinics has changed this approach. Although the neurologist and ALS nurse may not provide formal psychosocial care, their ongoing therapeutic relationship with the patient and family is often close and supportive, and neither the provider, patient, nor family may be fully aware of the depth of this attachment.

The patient's death is a point at which health care providers can easily distance themselves or "step out" of the bereavement process if they are uncomfortable with the patient's death. However, this is the time when formal bereavement begins for the family, caregiver, and even for the health care providers. A personal phone call and follow-up card or letter to the family are extremely important, and their absence can leave a long-lasting emptiness (64). If health care professionals attend the funeral or memorial service, this provides a chance for the whole family to come to closure with the medical personnel as well as the medical aspects of the care and disease.

Table 3 Six Triggers for Initiating the End-of-Life Discussion

The patient or family asks, or "opens the door," for end-of-life information and/or interventions (elicited or spontaneous, verbal or nonverbal)
Severe psychological and/or social or spiritual distress or suffering
Pain requiring high dosages of analgesic medications
Dysphagia requiring feeding tube
Dyspnea or symptoms of hypoventilation, a forced vital capacity of 50% or less
Loss of function in two body regions (regions include bulbar, arms, and legs)

Source: From Ref. 2.

Structured Programs

Structured bereavement programs are important because a full spectrum of issues can be addressed comprehensively. Structured programs include written handouts, professional counseling, and support groups; counseling and support group participation can continue as long as necessary to meet an individual's needs.

Written material about death and bereavement can be helpful to the patient and family, particularly for family members who cannot attend clinic visits. The material should be written in language that is easy to understand. Handouts should include information that can raise awareness of feelings and fears about the dying process. The information should be discussed and questions answered at follow-up appointments.

The complexity of psychological processes in bereavement may not be clearly and fully recognized by health care providers who are not mental health professionals. Accordingly, social workers, psychologists, and psychiatrists can be very helpful to the patient and family. Formal bereavement support groups can help family members reach closure. They are usually directed by mental health professionals.

Continued involvement as volunteers in ALS clinics and support groups can be useful for some family members. Ongoing involvement may be important for family members who have been intensely involved with patient care because their routine comes to a stop when the patient dies, and these individuals may benefit by "winding down" their emotional and physical energy by helping other families with ALS. Receiving periodic ALS clinic newsletters is another method of staying in touch.

Bereavement Care for Health Care Providers

Providing health care to ALS patients and their families is emotionally taxing. Strong relationships and attachments to patients are not unusual in ALS. The care team at an ALS clinic may experience the deaths of several patients within a short period. The health care providers must also face their own mortality every time they prepare a patient and family for death. It is therefore important for providers to come to terms with their own feelings about loss of function, death, and grief, and to understand their emotional involvement with their patients. Mental health counselors can be of benefit, and providers should not hesitate to discuss these issues with them (54).

END-OF-LIFE CHOICES AND EXPECTATIONS

Initiating the end-of-life discussion with the patients and families is always difficult. Table 3 outlines six events, any one of which should serve as a trigger for the health care provider to begin discussing end-of-life issues. Among the most important decisions for patients with ALS are those concerning the initiation and discontinuation of life-prolonging measures such as invasive ventilation or percutaneous endoscopic gastrostomy. Ideally, these decisions are discussed in advance, before the onset of swallowing or respiratory failure, by the patient and family after they have received thorough education and counseling on the risks and benefits so that they are clearly comfortable with their decision. The results of the discussion should be set forth in an advance directive. See Chap. 37 for end-of-life decision making (65,66).

Making end-of-life decisions is not easy, and the process that patients and families go through is well documented (67). Most importantly, these decisions are not based only on the medical circumstances. Financial resources, caregiver support and resources, quality of life, and the patient's readiness for dying must all be considered. Open-ended questions can make the initial discussion more conversational, less threatening, and thus more apt to be continued in the future. For example, health care providers may initially ask questions such as:

- Have you ever experienced the death of others in your life?
- What was that like for you?
- Have you ever thought about your death before you became ill?
- What thoughts do you have now?

If the patient is able to articulate his decisions or feelings about his death, one should further explore the patient's decisions and document them in an advance directive. One should also provide positive feedback for having thought through and discussed this difficult topic. Once the health care provider has begun to explore choices with the patient regarding the end-of-life, it is important to encourage discussion of the patient's expectations of the end-of-life experience.

Regardless of whether patients choose life-extending measures or a natural death combined with palliative care, the care pathway at the end-of-life should be discussed. In the case of life-extending measures, the circumstances are more complex and require more advanced financial and caregiving planning. All patients should be educated about palliative care and the role of hospice in decreasing anticipatory anxiety, fear, and respiratory discomfort; be offered an introductory visit by a hospice service; and be referred to hospice when they meet eligibility criteria.

BEING "PRESENT" WITH THE DYING PATIENT

The care provider, whether a hospice nurse, physician, friend, or family member, may feel awkward and uncomfortable during the final period. It is important for the caregiver to slow down and be in the present moment with the patient. Often, making this shift depends on the patient's own realization and acknowledgment that he or she is dying. The death of the ALS patient is often "the most unexpected event," and therefore the patient's and family's lack of preparedness should not be underestimated. For families who are caring for the patient, making this change from a hectic and task-filled day to one that includes reflection and quiet support can be difficult. Health care professionals may experience the same problem, which manifests as continuing to address medical issues such as bowel function, blood pressure, and medication refills for an actively dying patient. When the patient begins to die, health care professionals and family caregivers should strive to:

- *Be yourself*: Relate to the person, not the illness. One should bring both one's strength and vulnerability to the bedside. People who are dying continue to need intimate, natural, and honest relationships. Health care providers should not use their role in a patient's death to downplay or avoid the patient's suffering. One should express one's feelings, give the patient permission to die, and express thanks for being able to care for and spend time with the patient.

- *Empathize*: The greatest gift we can offer one another is our undivided attention. Care providers should listen without judgment or an agenda, be aware of feelings the patient may have, and watch for nonverbal cues. It is important to respect personal truths that the dying person may be discovering. Being mindful of one's own inner experience and talking about it if the patient asks can be helpful.
- *Show kindness*: Details do matter—a cool cloth to the patient's perspiring brow, holding a patient's hand, listening to a lifetime of stories. When offered with caring attention, these ordinary activities convey caring and comfort. We need to trust our innate compassion and ability to embrace the suffering of another as our own.
- *Keep it simple*: As mentioned above, care providers and family should slow down and allow room for death to occur, as emotionally painful as this may be. During the final phase, the power of simple human presence should not be underestimated. Talking with patients even if they cannot reply can be comforting and calming. Importantly, even these ordinary acts can be an acknowledgment that the patient is dying.

Hospice team members normally visit the home daily while the patient is dying and should assure the family that the patient's neurologist is available by phone if needed. Also, although home is the principal environment for most ALS patients, it may not be the place the patient or family would like death to occur. It is important to be sensitive to this issue and openly discuss it either before the patient begins to die or early in the period so that alternative arrangements can be made. Hospice can make arrangements for a bed at a hospice facility, hospital, or continuing care nursing facility. The hospice can also have a nurse available at the patient's home on a continuous basis for up to 72 hours if more intensive medical management is needed.

PSYCHOLOGICAL ASPECTS OF WITHDRAWAL OF VENTILATION

The functional, ethical, juridical, and medical issues related to withdrawal of mechanical ventilation are well documented (68,69). In ALS, what is not so well understood is the patient's tolerance for living in the advanced stages of disease (55,70). However, physicians should not hesitate to offer mechanical ventilation because of the issues concerning withdrawal—attaining a good quality of life is possible with mechanical ventilation and should be explored with patients. What is unique in ALS is that the patient is competent to make the decision for ventilation and withdrawal, and thus can make a thoughtful decision long before intervention is required. The request for withdrawal may occur soon after intervention or after a number of years. As ALS continues to progress after mechanical ventilation is initiated, patients will decline functionally, making communication almost impossible. Thus, when mechanical support becomes necessary, health care providers should fully discuss the timing of withdrawal with patients (even if this has been done previously) to ensure that patients fully understand in the event that they cannot indicate when they want withdrawal. In addition, because withdrawal is more difficult if patients are geographically isolated from their medical providers, it is essential in such circumstances to maintain good contact with the health care team (71).

When the time has arrived that the patient no longer desires mechanical ventilation, assessment should be started immediately—initiation of withdrawal is crucial so neither the patient nor family suffers. First, the appropriateness of withdrawal should be assessed collaboratively by a neurologist and psychiatric specialist (preferably someone with experience in ALS and terminal disease). If, after meeting with the family, there is any question regarding the patient's or family's position on the withdrawal decision and plan, an ethicist should also assess the appropriateness of withdrawal. Assessing the patient for clinical depression and unrelieved suffering is critical because these issues may be implicated in the patient's decision. The meeting with the family should determine family consensus and detail the plan for withdrawal, how long withdrawal may take, and the possible physical symptoms that their loved one may experience. Special attention should be given to the cultural and religious backgrounds of those involved, rituals they may want to perform, and family dynamics before the patient's illness.

Regardless of whether the patient is at home, in a hospice, or hospitalized, a care pathway should be in place that adheres to the American Academy of Neurology position statement on withdrawal of mechanical ventilation (68,72). Withdrawal must be done in a peaceful and sensitive manner in which family, relatives, friends, clergy, the health care team, and others involved can be with the patient.

ACKNOWLEDGMENT

The authors are part of a national working group for promoting end-of-life care in ALS funded by the Robert Wood Johnson Foundation and ALS Association.

REFERENCES

1. McDonald ER, Wiedenfeld SA, Hillel A, Carpenter CL, Walter RA. Survival in amyotrophic lateral sclerosis. Arch Neurol 1994; 51:17–23.
2. Mitsumoto H, Bromberg M, Johnston W, Tandan R, Byock I, Lyon M, Miller RG, Appel SH, Benditt J, Bernat JL, Borasio GD, Carver AC, Clawson L, Del Bene ML, Kasarskis EJ, LeGrand SB, Mandler P, McCarthy J, Munsat T, Newman D, Sufit RL, Versenyi A. Promoting excellence in end-of-life care in ALS. Amyotrophr Later Scler Other Motor Neuron Disord, 2005. In press.
3. Mitsumoto H, Munsat TL. Amyotrophic Lateral Sclerosis: A Guide for Patients and Families. New York: Demos Medical Publishing, 2001.
4. Levine C, Zuckerman C. The trouble with families: toward an ethic of accommodation. Ann Int Med 1999; 130:148–152.
5. Bradley WG, Anderson F, Bromberg M, Gutmann L, Harati Y, Ross M, Miller RG. ALS CARE study group. Current management of ALS: comparison of the ALS CARE database and the AAN practice parameter. Neurology 2001; 57:500–504.
6. Krivickas LS, Shockley L, Mitsumoto H. Home care of patients with amyotrophic lateral sclerosis (ALS). J Neurol Sci 1997; 152(suppl 1):S82–S89.
7. Gelinas DF, O'Connor P, Miller RG. Quality of life for ventilator-dependent ALS patients and their caregivers. J Neurol Sci 1998; 160(suppl 1):S134–S136.
8. Kaub-Wittemer D, von Steinbüchel N, Wasner M, Laier-Groeneveld G, Borasio GD. Quality of life and psychosocial issues in ventilated patients with amyotrophic lateral sclerosis and their caregivers. J Pain Symptom Manage 2003; 26:890–896.
9. Goldstein LH, Adamson M, Jeffrey L, Down K, Barby T, Wilson C, Leigh PN. The psychological impact of MND on patients and carers. J Neurol Sci 1998; 160(suppl 1):S114–S1121.
10. Rabkin JG, Wagner GJ, Del Bene M. Resilience and distress among amyotrophic lateral sclerosis patients and caregivers. Psychosom Med 2000; 62:271–279.

11. Cobb AK, Reckling JB, Fernengel KJ. The ALS caregiver's experience: an impelled journey. In: Mitsumoto H, Norris FH Jr, eds. Amyotrophic Lateral Sclerosis. A Comprehensive Guide to Management. NewYork: Demos Medical Publishing, 1994:241–252.
12. Grand A, Grand-Filaire A, Bocquet H, Clement S. Caregiver stress: a failed negotiation? A qualitative study in South West France. Int J Aging Hum Dev 1999; 49:179–195.
13. Yates ME, Tennstedt S, Chang BH. Contributors to and mediators of psychological well-being for informal caregivers. J Gerontol B Psychol Sci Soc Sci 1999; 54:12–22.
14. Jepson C, McCorkle R, Adler D, Nuamah I, Lusk E. Effects of home care on caregivers' psychosocial status. Image J Nurs Sch 1999; 31:115–120.
15. Sisk RJ. Caregiver burden and health promotion. Int J Nurs Stud 2000; 37:37–43.
16. Schulz R, Beach SR. Caregiving as a risk factor for mortality: the caregiver health effects study. JAMA 1999; 282:2215–2219.
17. Yates P, Stetz KM. Families' awareness of and response to dying. Oncol Nurs Forum 1999; 26:113–120.
18. Allen SM, Goldscheider F, Ciambrone DA. Gender roles, marital intimacy, and nomination of spouse as primary caregiver. Gerontologist 1999; 39:150–158.
19. Williamson GM, Shaffer DR, Schulz R. Activity restriction and prior relationship history as contributors to mental health outcomes among middle-aged and older spousal caregivers. Health Psychol 1998; 17:152–162.
20. Kramer BJ, Lambert JD. Caregiving as a life course transition among older husbands: a prospective study. Gerontologist 1999; 39:658–667.
21. Dautzenberg MG, Diederiks JP, Philipsen H, Tan FE. Multigenerational caregiving and well-being: distress of middle-aged daughters providing assistance to elderly parents. Women Health 1999; 29(4):57–74.
22. Centers L. One day at a time: the experience of an ALS caregiver. In: Oliver D, Borasio GD, Walsh D, eds. Palliative Care in Amyotrophic Lateral Sclerosis. New York: Oxford University Press, 2000:183–187.
23. Houde SC. Predictors of elders' and family caregivers' use of formal home services. Res Nurs Health 1998; 21:533–543.
24. Braithwaite V. Institutional respite care: breaking chores or breaking social bonds? Gerontologist 1998; 38:610–617.
25. Hanson EJ, Tetley J, Clarke A. Respite care for frail older people and their family carers: concept analysis and user focus grup findings of a pan-European nursing research project. J Adv Nurs 1999; 30:1396–1407.
26. McNally S, Ben-Shlomo Y, Newman S. The effects of respite care on informal carers' well-being: a systematic review. Disabil Rehabil 1999; 21:1–14.
27. Emanuel EJ, Fairclough DL, Slutsman J, Emanuel LL. Understanding economic and other burdens of terminal illness: the experience of patients and their caregivers. Ann Intern Med 2000; 132:451–459.
28. Wahner-Roedler DL, Knuth P, Juchems RH. The german pflegeversicherung (long-term care insurance). Mayo Clin Proc 1999; 74:196–200.
29. Sevick MA, Bradham DD. Economic value of caregiver effort in maintaining long-term ventilator-assisted individuals at home. Heart Lung 1997; 26:148–157.
30. Chang BH, Noonan AE, Tennstedt SL. The role of religion/spirituality in coping with caregiving for disabled elders. Gerontologist 1998; 38:463–470.
31. Mitsumoto H, Chad D, Pioro EP. Comprehensive care. In: Mitsumoto H, Chad D, Pioro EP, eds. Amyotrophic Lateral Sclerosis. Contemporary Neurology Series No. 49, Philadelphia: FA Davis, 1998:305–320.
32. Wasner M, Bold U, Vollmer TC, Borasio GD. Sexuality in patients with amyotrophic lateral sclerosis and their partners. J Neurol 2004; 251:445–448.
33. Oliver D. Ethical issues in palliative care—An overview. Palliat Med 1993; 7:15–20.
34. Pernick E. Sexuality/intimacy/sensitivity of ALS patients. In: Mancall EL, ed. Current Concepts in Managing ALS. Philadelphia: ALS Association, 1994:129–134.

35. World Health Organization. Cancer pain relief and palliative care. Report of a WHO Expert Committee. Geneva: World Health Organization, 1990.
36. Murphy PL, Albert SM, Weber C, Del Bene ML, Rowland LP. Impact of spirituality and religiousness on outcomes in patients with ALS. Neurology 2000; 55:1581–1584.
37. Borasio GD. Meditation and ALS. In: Mitsumoto H, Munsat T, eds. Amyotrophic Lateral Sclerosis: A Comprehensive Guide to Management. New York: Demos Medical Publishing, 2001:271–276.
38. Doyle D. Have we looked beyond the physical and psychosocial? J Pain Symptom Manage 1992; 7:302–311.
39. Sykes N. End-of-life care in ALS. In: Oliver D, Borasio GD, Walsh D, eds. Palliative Care in Amyotrophic Lateral Sclerosis. Oxford: Oxford University Press, 2000:159–168.
40. Balducci L, Meyer R. Spirituality and medicine: a proposal. Cancer Control 2001; 8: 368–376.
41. Martin J, Turnbull J. Lasting impact, and ongoing needs, in families months to years after death from ALS. Amyotroph Lateral Scler Other Motor Neuron Disord 2000; 2:181–187.
42. McMurray A. Bereavement. In: Oliver D, Borasio GD, Walsh D, eds. Palliative Care in Amyotrophic Lateral Sclerosis. Oxford: Oxford University Press, 2000:169–8.
43. Ackerman GM, Oliver D. Psychosocial support in an outpatient clinic. Palliat Med 1997; 11:167–168.
44. Puchalski C, Romer AL. Taking a spiritual history allows clinicians to understand patients more fully. J Palliat Med 2000; 3:129–137.
45. Dal Bello-Haas V, Andrews-Hinders D, Bocian J, Mascha E, Wheeler T, Mitsumoto H. Spiritual well-being of the individual with amyotrophic lateral sclerosis. Amyotroph Lateral Scler Other Motor Neuron Disord 2000; 1:337–341.
46. van Wegberg B, Bacchi M, Heusser P, Helwig S, Schaad R, von Rohr E, et al. The cognitive-spiritual dimension—an important addition to the assessment of quality of life: validation of a questionnaire (SELT-M) in patients with advanced cancer. Ann Oncol 1998; 9:1091–1096.
47. Hatch RL, Burg MA, Naberhaus DS, Hellmich LK. The Spiritual Involvement and Beliefs Scale. Development and testing of a new instrument. J Fam Pract 1998; 46:476–486.
48. Salmon P, Manzi F, Valori RM. Measuring the meaning of life for patients with incurable cancer: the life evaluation questionnaire (LEQ). Eur J Cancer 1996; 32A:755–760.
49. Hickey AM, Bury G, O'Boyle CA, Bradley F, O'Kelly FD, Shannon W. A new short form individual quality of life measure (SEIQoL-DW): application in a cohort of individuals with HIV/AIDS. Br Med J 1996; 313:29–33.
50. Neudert C, Wasner M, Borasio GD. Patients' assessment of quality of life instruments: a randomised study of SIP, SF-36 and SEIQoL-DW in patients with amyotrophic lateral sclerosis. J Neurol Sci 2001; 191:103–109.
51. Vaughan C. Teach me to hear mermaids singing (Editorial). Br Med J 1996; 313:565.
52. Kubler-Ross E. On Death and Dying. New York: MacMillan, 1969.
53. Worden WJ. Grief Counseling and Grief Therapy: A Handbook for the Mental Health Practioner. London: Tavistock, 1982/1991.
54. Murphy NM. Mourning. In: Mitsumoto H, Munsat TL, eds. Amyotrophic Lateral Sclerosis. A Guide for Patients and Families. 2d ed. New York: Demos Medical Publishing, 2001:399–340.
55. Moss AH, Oppenheimer EA, Casey P, Gazzolli PA, Roos RP, Stocking CB, Siegler M. Patients with amyotrophic lateral sclerosis receiving long-term mechanical ventilation. Advance care planning and outcomes. Chest 1996; 10:249–255.
56. Bromberg MB, Forshew DA, Iaderosa S, McDonald ER. Ventilator dependency in ALS: management, disease progression, and issues of coping. J Neurol Rehabil 1996; 10:195–121.

57. Thompson B, Murphy NM. Hospice care. In: Mitsumoto H, Munsat TL, eds. Amyotrophic Lateral Sclerosis. A Guide for Patients and Families. 2d ed. New York: Demos Medical Publishing, 2001:373–398.

58. Oliver D, McMurray N. Bereavement—whose responsibility? Palliat Med 1993; 7(suppl 2): 73–76.

59. Curry CL. When Your Spouse Dies. Notre Dame, IN: Ave Maria Press, 1990.

60. Fitzgerald H. The Mourning Handbook. A Fireside Book. New York: Simon & Schuster, 1994.

61. James JW, Friedman R. The Grief Recovery Handbook. New York: Harper Perennial, 1998.

62. Neudert C, Oliver D, Wasner M, Borasio GD. The course of the terminal phase in patients with amyotrophic lateral sclerosis. ALS J Neurol 2001; 248:612–616.

63. Miller G, Anderson F, Bradley WG, et al. The ALS patient CARE program—North American patient CARE database. In: Mitsumoto H, Przedborski, Gordon P, eds. ALS, New York: Marcel Dekker, 2005.

64. Bedell SE, Cadenhead K, Graboys TB. The doctor's letter of condolence. N Engl J Med 2001; 344:1162–1164.

65. Borasio GD, Voltz R. Advance directives. In: Oliver D, Borasio GD, Walsh D, eds. Palliative Care in Amyotrophic Lateral Sclerosis (Motor Neurone Disease). Oxford: Oxford University Press, 2000:36–41.

66. Bromberg M. Life support and dilemma. In: Mitsumoto H, Munsat TL, eds. Amyotrophic Lateral Sclerosis. A Guide for Patients and Families. 2d ed. New York: Demos Medical Publishing, 2001:187–210.

67. Albert SM, Murphy PM, Del Bene ML, Rowland LP. A prospective study of preferences and actual treatment choices in ALS. Neurology 1999; 53:278–283.

68. Stillman MJ. Palliative care: the management of advanced disease. In: Mitsumoto H, Munsat TL, eds. Amyotrophic Lateral Sclerosis. A Guide for Patients and Families. 2d ed. New York: Demos Medical Publishing, 2001:359–372.

69. Borasio GD, Voltz R. Discontinuation of life support in patients with amyotrophic lateral sclerosis. J Neurol 1998; 245:717–722.

70. Hayashi H. Ventilatory support: Japanese experience. J Neurol Sci 1997; 152(suppl 1): S97–S100.

71. Schwarz J, Del Bene ML. Obstacles to carrying out the end-of-life wishes of a ventilator-dependent patient with amyotrophic lateral sclerosis. J Clin Ethics 2004; 15:282–290.

72. Bernat JL, Cranford RE, Kittredge FI, Rosenberg RN. Competent patients with advanced states of permanent paralysis have the right to forgo life-sustaining therapy. Neurology 1993; 43:224–225.

35
Palliative Care at the End of Life

Nigel P. Sykes
St. Christopher's Hospice and King's College, University of London, London, U.K.

THE PHILOSOPHY OF PALLIATIVE CARE—WHEN DOES PALLIATIVE CARE BEGIN?

In our present state of knowledge the whole of the management of amyotrophic lateral sclerosis (ALS) is palliative, in the sense that the disease remains incurable and our ability even to modify its progression is slight. Therefore, therapeutic efforts are directed toward maximizing the comfort and function, and hence the quality of life of people with ALS. Implicitly included in this work are the families and others close to the patient who very often will be shouldering much of the burden of care and who will in any case be affected emotionally by seeing the impact of ALS on the one they love and eventually by their death. This palliation is needed from the moment of diagnosis and is the responsibility of all physicians and other health care professionals involved in ALS care, whether specialists or not.

However, the purpose of this chapter is to look at the palliation of the very end of life, when death is recognized to be imminent or, at least, not far off. This is the time when specialist palliative care, if available, is most likely to be needed in order to meet the challenges of the patient's symptoms and the distress of those around them. Both will be much less, though, if this phase of care can be built on a foundation of competent palliation extending back over the prior course of the ALS condition. Therefore, it should not be supposed that what will be described here contains all that good palliative care is about, or that a person with ALS who receives such attention only as their life is drawing to a close has thereby received adequate palliation of their disease.

RECOGNIZING THE TERMINAL PHASE

Most people with ALS die as a result of respiratory failure (1). Consequently, the trajectory of decline in respiratory function is the key to anticipating the final stage of the illness. In general, the last two days of a terminally ill person's life are indicated by their being bedridden, barely able to take even fluids by mouth, and lapsing into semiconsciousness (2). However, because the specific effects of ALS often grossly impair mobility and swallowing well in advance of the person dying, being bedridden and having little or no oral intake are not useful indicators of impending death for this group. More significant are increasing breathlessness accompanied by a subjective impression of the person being globally less well, noticed characteristically by family or nursing staff, which shades into a reducing level of consciousness.

However, the onset of this stage, when it comes, is often rapid and ALS is a cause of sudden death. In a series of 124 ALS patients cared for until death, 40% deteriorated suddenly and died within 12 hours; a further 18% had died within 24 hours of a change in condition first being noticed (3). This rapidity has implications for the preparations the caring team must make in order to respond quickly to symptom changes, and particularly the guidance they must give patients' families in order to prepare them for what may appear to be a catastrophically sudden demise.

Alternatively, the character of end-of-life ALS care can be altered completely by the use of assisted ventilation in the presence of gastrostomy feeding. It has become clear that noninvasive ventilation (NIV) can extend life significantly (4) and that tracheostomy ventilation can do so for considerable periods to the extent that functional deterioration continues to the point of a locked-in state. The timing and nature of the terminal event are then the result of the availability of assisted ventilation within the prevailing health care system, whether tracheostomy ventilation is offered to a patient whose NIV is ceasing to be adequate and whether it is decided to withdraw tracheostomy ventilation at some point in the patient's disease progression.

It has to be noticed that the timing of respiratory crisis in a non-ventilated ALS patient or one who is receiving NIV is probably strongly influenced by otherwise benign intercurrent respiratory tract infections. The use of assisted cough techniques, including the mechanical aid of an insufflator–exsufflator machine, has been demonstrated to reduce significantly the need for hospitalization of ALS patients receiving NIV and, by implication, has contributed to their life extension (5). However, when respiratory failure does supervene in the face of NIV, the character and duration of the terminal phase do not seem generally to be much altered compared with patients who are not using NIV. On the other hand, a few patients appear to be sustained in a condition of virtual unrousability over several days, causing considerable distress to both family and health care staff. It may then be decided to conduct a ventilator withdrawal in the same way as the more familiar withdrawal of tracheostomy ventilation.

If death occurs suddenly in ALS it seems most often to happen at night, presumably as a result of an exacerbation of nocturnal hypoventilation, whether or not further compromised by respiratory tract infection. Where there are clinical changes that herald the terminal phase of the illness, these usually take the form of an increased sense of breathlessness, even in the face of NIV and despite adjustments to the ventilator settings, or the onset of a reduced level of consciousness associated with diminished respiratory effort. Medication changes can ease the distress associated with breathlessness, but as respiration fails transition is into loss of awareness and ultimately a state of unrousability. At this point the patient's condition is not significantly different from that seen in the end stage of cancer or other terminal diseases, but in ALS this period tends to last for a shorter time.

ETHICAL ISSUES

The ethical issues around care at the end of life for people with ALS primarily concern choice. One view of ALS is that it is an incurable, relentlessly progressive disease that culminates in the sufferer's death. At the opposite pole is the perception of ALS as a condition specifically affecting the nervous system that as a result leaves a person requiring increasing degrees of physical support. If such support is provided appropriately, their life can continue indefinitely as vital organs are not directly involved in the disease.

The practical working out of these two philosophies will give rise to very different life expectancies for the patients concerned. In the first case, the prognosis is likely to average around three years from diagnosis to death. In the second, the addition of feeding tubes and invasive ventilation may add another 25 years to the outlook. This is a stark difference and one that most people with ALS around the world do not have the opportunity to choose between. The choice is made for them by their health care systems, on the ethical basis of a just and equitable distribution of limited resources.

Paradoxically, even where tracheostomy ventilation and the attendant support are available, the patient still all too often does not get the choice, either because of the limitations of insurance-based funding or because initiation of ventilation happens as an emergency treatment for acute respiratory failure. The latter has been reported to account for most episodes of tracheostomy ventilation in the United States, Japan, and Germany (6). Patient and family are then left with the very difficult decision of whether, and if so when, to terminate this support. While communication channels can be kept open between physician and patient, a dialogue can continue in which the person with ALS is helped to weigh the benefits of continuing ventilation against the burdens of the disease. However, should the disease progress to the point of the patient becoming "locked in" it becomes impossible to know if their attitude to ventilation has altered.

Meanwhile, the majority of tracheostomy ventilated ALS patients rate their life quality highly. The same cannot necessarily be said of their caregivers, a reflection of the physical, emotional, and financial impact that maintenance of a severely dependent member can have on a family. NIV can delay the need for tracheostomy ventilation for several years in some cases and is far more likely to be started only after consultation with the patient and those close to them. It is also less stressful for caregivers (7). Although NIV may be the prelude to tracheostomy ventilation, there is a point of choice at which the person with ALS can decide not to follow this progression and for their life to end when NIV ceases to be adequate for their respiratory needs.

The pattern and trajectory of the end of life in ALS are therefore hugely influenced by availability and choices of life-sustaining treatments. Choice implies autonomy, a quality highly prized in Western culture and one of the four principles commonly held to be the basis of medical ethics (8); indeed, in medical decision making autonomy often appears to be held pre-eminent among these principles. Yet in fact, an autonomous choice is not the experience of most ALS patients entering respiratory failure.

However, there is also the matter of choice relating to life-terminating treatments. People with ALS are over-represented among groups applying for or receiving euthanasia or physician-assisted suicide (PAS), where these are legal. Prior to the legalization of assisted suicide in Oregon, 56% of a sample of ALS patients said they would opt for the procedure (9). In the United Kingdom, where neither euthanasia nor PAS are available, several ALS patients have been *causes celebres* in aid of pro-euthanasia pressure groups. The reasons for these are assumed to be negative perceptions of the symptoms of advanced ALS, with its loss of function leading to complete dependence, and the manner of dying. In particular, persistent media assertions of the inevitability of choking to death and of intractable pain have created a perception of unique unpleasantness about the end of life with ALS.

ALS is certainly a particularly terrible disease. However, the evidence from settings where adequate palliative care is available does not confirm the specific assertions of uncontrolled symptoms. In particular, pain was judged to be well controlled in 75% of an ALS group receiving inpatient hospice treatment and tolerably controlled in a further 18% (3). In the same series, only one patient was thought to have died as a result of choking, but even there, postmortem examination revealed that the airway was unobstructed. A more recent multicenter study of ALS patients at the end of life found no instance of death through choking and 98% of the group were perceived to have had peaceful deaths (10). Such information has ethical importance because a prerequisite for competent treatment consent or refusal is the possession of as full and accurate knowledge about the outcomes as possible. There are indications that in a sizeable number of cases neither ALS patients nor their doctors have such a level of knowledge when discussing disease outcomes and symptom management. Significantly, nearly half of Oregon physician-assisted suicide candidates withdrew their request if offered even one palliative intervention (11).

Advance directives (or "living wills") are a potential means of increasing patient choice through leaving a record of the patient's wishes into a time when illness prevents a contemporaneous choice being made. A person cannot demand an inappropriate treatment through an advance directive any more than face to face with their doctor, so these records have more the character of "advance refusals." The use of advance directives varies enormously between countries: 90% of 2018 patients recorded on the U.S. ALS CARE Database had advance directives (12), whereas these documents remain relatively rare in the United Kingdom. The reason for this discrepancy is unlikely to be simply a vastly greater emphasis on patient choice on one side of the Atlantic than the other. An ethically adequate process of drafting an advance directive in ALS entails confrontation with a full range of information about the likely course of the disease and its outcome so that the decisions that are enshrined in the directive are properly informed. To do this at an early stage of the condition as, given the high advance directive completion rate, is presumably quite often done is likely to be emotionally stressful for at least a proportion of patients. This suggests that the motivation for advance directives in this system lies elsewhere, perhaps, in issues such as cost containment, the reimbursement rules for hospice access, and the avoidance of litigation. An alternative U.S. view is that advance directives are inappropriate for people with ALS on the basis that they tend to be given inadequate information, particularly about options for NIV (13). This viewpoint seems to ignore the uneven availability of the full range of such options.

It might be argued that the most helpful approach to the care of a person with ALS, and the one most likely to satisfy the key principles of medical ethics, is the so-called "deliberative" model of the patient-physician relationship (which has equal applicability to the relationship between patient and nurse or other health care workers), in which the patient's values in relation to their illness and its management are the subject of ongoing discussion in order to achieve a shared perspective (14). This is different from an emphasis either on the patient's autonomy or on the doctor's paternalism. By agreement the process may result in a formal advance directive, or the modification of an existing one, or simply the recording of the outcome of different stages of the conversation in the clinical record.

In this way the patient can determine the pace at which information is received, and choices can be made in a timely fashion related to the patient's evolving experience of the illness and having consideration to the options that are available and immediately relevant. As a result, the risk of harm through incomplete or, on the other hand, unwanted information should be minimized, the autonomy of both patient and doctor is recognized, and it should be possible to demonstrate that the patient's best interests have been served in so far as justice within the prevailing health care resources allow. Requirements for a deliberative relationship model are a physician and accompanying health care team who are willing to work in this way and who are knowledgeable about the progression of ALS and the relevant supportive and palliative therapies.

The emergency institution of tracheostomy ventilation without prior consultation is clearly undesirable because of its invasiveness and major long-term implications, not only for the patient, but also their family. It is here that an advance directive, formulated through sensitive, well-informed discussion with the patient and, preferably, those close to them, may be particularly valuable—whichever view is taken of the procedure. However, most often a person with ALS will not end up in this position. Instead, they are likely to be experiencing a degree of distress from worsening respiratory failure either where no ventilation is available or when NIV is no longer sufficient. The ethical imperative is then to relieve their breathing and other distress.

This situation is morally challenging for some physicians and nurses. The principal drug classes that will provide relief from distressing breathlessness are opioids and sedatives. Both of these have the potential to depress respiration and hence precipitate death, particularly in someone already in respiratory failure. How, it is sometimes asked, does their use in this situation differ from euthanasia? The ethical defense often mounted is that of the Principle of Double Effect. Briefly put, this states that an action that has the incidental effect of shortening life may, even if this effect is foreseen, be morally legitimate provided that the intention was to produce a beneficial end and that death was not the necessary means to achieve that end. The use of the Principle of Double Effect has been criticized on the basis that it is very difficult to be sure of another person's intention or even of one's own (15). The evidence is that, in general, the competent use of opioids and sedatives in palliative care does not hasten death (16) and hence the Principle is simply not required. But in the specific instance of a patient facing death from respiratory failure within a few hours, or a day or two at most, the possibility of shortening this span even further is at its highest.

The key difference between an act intended to kill and one intended to provide relief is proportionality. An attempt must be made to use the lowest dose of medication consistent with the patient's previous experience of opioids and sedatives, pursuing a judicious titration of dose against response. The right dose is the one that gives acceptable relief of distress, not unconsciousness or death. Sometimes the result of relieving distress is that the patient relaxes, no longer puts sufficient effort into breathing, and rapidly dies. This is not always the case, though, and the aim is to find a point where distress is alleviated but breathing continues. Both the appropriateness of the starting dose in relation to the patient's previous opioid/sedative regime and the process of titration should subsequently provide evidence from the medication record of the treatment approach that has been used. The worst moral position of all would be to offer the person with ALS no way out of their fear and dyspnea.

SUPPORTING THE PATIENT

Quality of life can be thought of as resulting from the degree of agreement between hopes and expectations on the one hand and the reality of their achievement on the other (17). If there is a serious mismatch between activities a person regards as their principal source of satisfaction and their actual ability to pursue those activities, the results are frustration and a sense of meaninglessness. Caregivers have to work to help the patient to adjust their horizons and focus to achieve enjoyment and a sense of worth from activities that may be new or may previously have been discounted but which still lie within their capacity. This type of support is a major contribution of hospice day units or creative living centers. Naturally, the range of these activities becomes increasingly limited over time, but this aspect of care remains important right up to the onset of the terminal phase of the illness. It answers not only to the psychological needs of the individual but also the social and probably the spiritual as well.

By "spiritual" is meant the need to find within present existence a sense of meaning. How to define this is a matter for each person. It may, but often does not, involve a framework of religion and the idea of a God with whom it is possible to have a relationship. When religion is an important feature the clerical involvement might be appropriate, but caregivers also have to be ready for a person to prefer to talk to them as someone who is not an official representative of religion and is unlikely to have all the answers. Certainty, whether in the existence or the non-existence of God, appears to be associated with the lowest levels of anxiety in dying people (18). For those in between, there may be a need to talk through feelings of anger against the Creator for a condition as dreadful as ALS, or of apprehension about long-suppressed ideas of judgment.

Should religion not provide a context for meaning this must come out of a person's sense of relationship to others, the fulfillment they derive from favored activities, and their perception of personal autonomy and control. All three of these factors can be severely impaired by ALS, and as the disease progresses it is a particular challenge for the caregivers—professional, family, and friends—to demonstrate that the ill person still retains a valued place in a social setting, allow them the maximum practicable degree of personal control, and enable them to modify their sources of satisfaction. Not everyone has the same ability to make these adjustments and the necessary compromises for coexistence with a chronic, debilitating condition. From the lack of such reconciliations, from unresolved personal issues, from the awareness of present losses with more to come both of functions and relationships, comes the suffering that is an inevitable part of any terminal illness.

Only the ill person can achieve a resolution of their suffering. It cannot be relieved by medical therapeutics or nursing interventions. Nevertheless, the caring environment can either facilitate or hinder the individual's progress in reaching a resolution of suffering. It is especially for this reason that the context of care for patient and family must be a multiprofessional team. No one discipline is adequate to meet the whole need, but the mutually complementary skills of professionals who respect and communicate with each other provide the best resource to enable the person with ALS to approach the end of their life with dignity and tranquility.

ALS imposes huge burdens on those who develop it, and on their caregivers, resulting from the relentless increase in disability it brings about. The extent of non-respiratory disability is not necessarily a reliable guide to prognosis, especially in younger people, but it is claimed that the requirement for physical aids and adaptations marks approximately the halfway point of the disease career, with gastrostomy feeding at about 80% and ventilatory support at 80% to 90% (19). The ability of so many with ALS to adapt remarkably to the ravages of their condition is a source of admiration to those close to them, but the sense of physical disintegration, the loss of control and of a great deal of what previously made life worth living, mean that death is not necessarily seen as unwelcome by patients in the later stages of the disease.

It can be a consolation to someone greatly disabled by ALS, and whose respiratory function is deteriorating, to be told that their condition will not go on for much longer. Naturally, an exact prognosis is impossible to judge and if a time is asked for the answer has to be relatively imprecise. Yet simply to be told that time appears short is not enough without an assurance of continued support and symptom control, because there is also the issue of ongoing hope.

Some professionals find it very difficult to be asked by patients for an estimate of prognosis, not only because any attempt at accuracy is likely to be misplaced but also because they fear that the answer will cause the person to give up. Relatives are even more likely to take this view. There is evidence that the grounds for hope change as illness progresses (20). Because of the inexorable nature of ALS, this transition is perhaps less pronounced here than in other conditions encountered in palliative care. However, there may still be a change from hopes that the disease may be slower in its progression or relatively limited in its scope or that it may be contained by a therapeutic intervention, to the hope for relief of discomfort and for a peaceful end to life. Such change is likely to be facilitated by maintenance of an open and sensitively honest relationship between the caring team and not only the person with ALS but also their family, whose own emotional adjustment to the patient's condition will have a profound effect on the patient's quality of life and, indeed, quality of death (21).

For any ill person to be most comfortable they must feel esteemed and understood by their caregivers and confident in the ability of the involved professionals to respond appropriately to their needs for information and physical care. Esteem implies a personal warmth and trustworthiness on the part of caring staff that is more than a professional façade yet not an inappropriate emotional closeness. True understanding of the patient's situation can often be particularly hard to gain in ALS because of the radical degree of disability, and especially the impairment of communication. The fullest use of communication aids is needed, together with all the skills of empathy and patience the caregiver possesses. Empathy is the imaginative entering into the other person's situation, but not the premature and superficial assurance of "I understand how you feel" which distances and is the enemy of trust. Continuity of professional caregivers (without a burdensome reliance on a single "favored" individual) is often important in facilitating communication in advanced ALS, as much depends on knowledge of personality, facial expression, and patterns of speech.

Becoming aware that death is getting nearer can stimulate a desire for resolution of outstanding personal conflicts, even long standing ones, or for the tidying of personal affairs. Even for someone with intact speech it can be difficult to broach these topics and request help. There needs to be sensitivity on the part of the caring team to the possibility that such issues might lie behind an appearance of restlessness or anxiety, and a readiness to probe gently for the existence of "unfinished business." Appropriate help can make a radical difference to the closing days or weeks of a patient's life. Conversely, not everyone can identify, share, or resolve issues like this, and the resulting anxiety can be relieved only by pharmacological means.

It should be remembered that any persistent discomfort makes any other discomfort worse and is also mentally wearing. Hence attention to detail is important in symptom control, so that by the time end-of-life care dawns, a capacity for competent symptom control should have been demonstrated and maintained. There is much in ALS that cannot be fully alleviated, but patients and families usually accept that there are limits to what medicine can achieve as long as the physician shows a commitment to stay alongside them and keep trying. Whatever the problems earlier on, it should be possible for the promise to be made that at the end distress can be controlled and that death need be neither painful nor frightening. Provided that the correct drugs are available and are administered in the right doses and combinations, the promise can be fulfilled (3,10).

Many patients, and perhaps even more relatives, ask what will happen as ALS progresses and what dying is going to be like. Accurate information provided at the right time can be a great help in a person's ability to cope with the advance of disease, and particularly with the prospect of its end.

SUPPORTING SIGNIFICANT OTHERS

By family is meant those who are closest and most significant for the patient, whether relatives or friends. It is important, although not always easy, to identify who these are. This is not accomplished simply by obtaining details of the next of kin. A great help is to construct a genogram, or family tree, which allows the professional team to see at a glance who constitutes the family, where they are, and what other difficulties the family might be enduring at the moment (22). Around the edge of the genogram should be included particular friends and "significant others" including—sometimes—pets. Ideally this should have been done well before the terminal phase of the illness.

Being close to someone with ALS is hugely stressful. Family may be at greater risk of depression and social isolation than the patient (7). The progressive functional deterioration is apparent to all, but family members may not recognize how this links with shortening of the prognosis. In particular they may not realize that death from ALS can be sudden. When the end of life is considered, thoughts may be colored by unfounded apprehension about symptoms such as suffocation, choking, and pain. A family's need for accurate information is at least as great as that of the patient.

The paralysis and loss of speech associated with ALS produce a feeling of impotence in all who care for people with it. This sensation, which can be uncomfortable even for knowledgeable professionals, may be disabling and extremely distressing for lay caregivers. Without guidance as to what to expect as swallowing and respiration deteriorate, and how they can gain urgent help in a crisis, an episode of choking or breathlessness can be terrifying not only to patient but also to family. It has been noted previously that a high proportion of those with ALS who receive tracheostomy ventilation do so without prior discussion of the procedure. This is because it was initiated in the midst of a respiratory crisis to which the response had been to take the patient to the hospital emergency room. This is not the way to begin such an invasive technique with so many grave implications. Prior involvement of a multiprofessional team, preferably with 24 hours availability, can allow the making of informed choices in anticipation of the event and be a resource for advice and practical help in an emergency.

Such a team can also facilitate the continuing care of the patient at home, where most terminally ill people wish to be. As life becomes more difficult the proportion wishing to stay at home diminishes but still remains about 50% (23). Despite assistance from community nursing services, the brunt of home care is borne by the family. Respite admissions to a hospice, hospital, or nursing home can help caregivers to recuperate and resume their task, or additional respite nursing help may be available for limited periods, but for a significant number of families there comes a point when they feel they can no longer look after the patient at home. In this the patient himself may agree, or there may be divergence.

Even if all are in agreement that admission is needed, family members may still be left with a sense of failure and of guilt that they have let their relative down. This may be especially marked if the person with ALS dies soon after they have been admitted, leading to feelings that "if only we had kept going that little bit longer we could have looked after him to the end." It is important for their response in bereavement that families receive reassurance about the quality of their caring efforts prior to the admission, and the appropriateness of seeking inpatient care now. It is also important that there are the facilities and encouragement to enable them to remain with the patient as death approaches, if that would be helpful to them.

For some families it is important that their relative does not die in their home, because of the memories that would leave for the future. Any service caring for terminally ill patients at home needs to have conversations with patient and family about the preferred place of death if at all possible, so that in case of a difference there can be discussion and understanding, if not always agreement. Plans need to be made so that admission does not occur as an acute event in response to the distress of a family who has never been able to reveal their concerns about end-of-life care of their relative. Even when death does take place in a hospice or other inpatient unit, usually at least 80% of the patient's last year of life will have been spent at home, and afterwards the perception of families is that they have indeed cared for the person themselves (23).

Most bereaved people do not need specific bereavement care: they will work through the feelings of loss that are at some time part of every individual's experience by themselves with the support of their own network of family and friends. For a minority, perhaps up to 25%, their adjustment can be helped by specialist bereavement support, although this, unfortunately, is only unevenly available.

SUPPORTING THE PROFESSIONALS

Even for professionals committed to palliative care, ALS is perhaps particularly prone to producing a pervasive sense of helplessness and failure. The difficulties in communication are a considerable contributory factor, as is the prominence of an irreversible process of functional deterioration that may be in contrast to the patient's continued mental vigor—inwardly they seem "well" but their bodies inexorably weaken in a way the professionals can do little about. This leads to feelings of frustration and deskilling that can result in avoidance of the patient by caregivers unless the problem is recognized.

To some extent these tensions are eased in the terminal phase, as the end comes into view and the situation begins to resemble more closely that of people dying of cancer and other conditions. Afterwards, however, staff memories of the case may be influenced by feelings that persist from earlier stages of care. It is likely that they will have known an ALS patient for longer than the average for palliative care patients as a whole, and so the sense of personal loss might be stronger. These factors risk leaving a residue of distress, which might impair professionals' ability to look after people with ALS in the future. The situation is worsened by the relative rarity of

ALS, meaning that staff can find it difficult to gain and maintain confidence in their expertise in caring for those with this condition.

Therefore, it can be helpful if there is both a program of staff education covering the management of ALS and also the opportunity of staff as a multiprofessional group to meet for a sharing of views on how the care of a particular patient went. This session may well identify ways in which care could be improved in the future, but should in addition be a chance for congratulation on the ways in which things have gone well. It should be a managerial responsibility to identify staff members who have particular problems resulting from the experience of care, and without imparting a sense of inadequacy, enable them to talk through the important issues confidentially either on the ward or with an independent counselor.

SYMPTOM CONTROL AT THE END OF LIFE

The crucial issue in symptom control at the end of life is preparedness. It is a wholly inadequate response to the onset of a distressing symptom if control has to wait on a physician's order or the pharmacist's acquisition of the medication required. As respiratory capacity shows evidence of serious decline, a stock of key drugs should be made available on the ward or in the home ready for use. The following categories of drug should be on hand:

- Opioids
- Sedatives
- Anticholinergic agents

If the drugs are to be used at home, it is sometimes possible for family members to administer them in a crisis if the rectal, or particularly the gastrostomy route is available. Whether or not the family is willing to assume this responsibility following adequate guidance, locally agreed paperwork must be filled out to enable community nurses to give the drugs when needed.

Opioids

Morphine is effective in the management of pain, breathlessness, and nocturnal discomfort in ALS long before the terminal phase of the illness. Doses are widely variable and not usually high, with a median of 60 mg/day being reported (24). Even in its use for dyspnea there is no evidence that morphine shortens life when it is used competently: Oliver's study found a median length of use of 51 days and a maximum of 970 days (24). Dose stability has been noted over periods of years and it is not inevitable that dose escalation will be required in the terminal phase. However, the morphine dose may have to rise if new symptoms intervene or old symptoms worsen, in particular if breathlessness increases. In this case the dose should be titrated upward in the usual way, making increments of 20% to 50% of the preceding dose level with the aim of providing a noticeable therapeutic effect without causing excessive drowsiness. If morphine has not been used before it is appropriate to commence at 5 to 10 mg per four hours for pain, orally or by gastrostomy, or 2.5 mg per four hours for breathlessness.

It was noted previously that the final phase of ALS tends to be very rapid with the onset of respiratory failure. Despite this, many patients do not require changes in medication: death is sudden or takes the form of a tapering of respiratory effort with an accompanying progressive loss of consciousness. Conversely, some patients become acutely distressed as a consequence of increasing breathlessness and anxiety. Initiation or upward dose adjustment of morphine is likely to be helpful in this situation, but opioids are inefficient anxiolytics, and if anxiety and restlessness are prominent the use of a benzodiazepine in combination is indicated.

The relief of distress as the end-point of dose titration needs to be kept clearly in mind. In this circumstance a degree of sedation may be a necessary part of achieving comfort, but here we are dealing with a gravely ill person who is already entering terminal respiratory failure as a result of their ALS. Despite our best efforts at careful dose management there is a possibility that enough respiratory depression will occur that death appears to be hastened. Whether or not such hastening actually occurs can never truly be determined as the experiment of leaving a control group of dying ALS patients without any symptom control interventions would be unethical. Any shortening that does occur is certainly, given the trajectory of the dying phase of most ALS patients, of the order of only a few hours. The ethical imperative is to ease the distress of the person with ALS and, provided that a dose titration process has been followed, guided by symptom response as indicated by close monitoring of the patient, physicians and nurses should not confuse what they are doing with euthanasia.

If a gastrostomy is in situ the administration of medication can continue, as before, but without it many patients will require a change of route from oral to parenteral. This can be accomplished by subcutaneous injections (made less uncomfortable if a plastic cannula is left in place to avoid repeated needle sticks) or more conveniently, if the length of the prognosis appears to justify it, by a subcutaneous infusion delivered by a portable syringe driver. Intravenous infusion has a greater potential for morbidity and is not required for clinical effectiveness. Alternatively, morphine or some alternative strong opioids, such as hydromorphone, oxycodone (in the United Kingdom), or oxymorphone (in the United States) are available as rectal preparations. Fentanyl and the partial opioid agonist buprenorphine are formulated as patches for transdermal administration, but the nature of this route means that it is suitable only for a steady opioid requirement. Rapid dose titration—in either direction—in response to changing clinical needs is not possible owing to a lag of around 12 to 24 hours in establishing or re-establishing steady-state blood levels.

An important consideration if there is a change of route of an existing opioid is to make an appropriate calculation of the equivalent dose (Table 1). A change from oral (or per gastrostomy) morphine to subcutaneous morphine involves a halving of the daily dose and the same transition for hydromorphone a division of the daily dose by five. All such ratios are subject to individual variation and resulting doses

Table 1 Conversion Ratios from Oral Opioids to Subcutaneous Morphine

Oral opioid	To obtain dose of SC morphine divide by:
Morphine	2
Codeine	16
Oxycodone	1
Hydromorphone	Multiply by 3

Abbreviation: SC, subcutaneous.

may require upward or downward adjustment according to response. A change to the sublingual or rectal route of the same opioid does not require a change in dose except in the case of oxycodone, whose dose should be doubled in transferring from oral to rectal.

A patient who has gained particular analgesic benefit from a non-steroidal anti-inflammatory drug (NSAID) can have it continued by suppository (e.g., in the form of naproxen or ketoprofen) or syringe driver. Ketorolac will mix in a syringe with diamorphine but, if as is usually the case, other drugs are also required, it is more reliable to give the NSAID rectally.

Whether in cancer or ALS, pain is not generally a problem at the end of life if it has been adequately controlled previously. In a patient who can no longer indicate their feelings caregivers interpret nonverbal signs of distress—for instance, groaning, grimacing, or restlessness. Before increasing medication, it should be checked whether there are remediable causes of discomfort, particularly a full bladder or rectum.

Sedatives

A generalized restlessness, which may be due to pain but also to anxiety, has to be distinguished from focal myoclonic jerks as these may be worsened by opioids, especially in the presence of phenothiazines. Rather than persist with opioid medication for restlessness it is more appropriate to use a benzodiazepine, either instead or in addition, for its anxiolytic and muscle relaxant properties. This may take the form of diazepam suppositories rectally or diazepam liquid via a gastrostomy, given as required or b.i.d. = t.i.d., or midazolam subcutaneously. Midazolam combines satisfactorily with morphine, hydromorphone, oxycodone, or anticholinergic agents in a syringe driver. An initial midazolam dose is 2.5 mg stat or 10 mg/24 hr.

In ALS a principal role of benzodiazepines is in the control of breathlessness where theoretically their action is complementary to that of opioids, although controlled trial evidence is lacking (25). In an acute deterioration in breathing associated with failing respiratory function it is appropriate to give a combination of a strong opioid and diazepam/midazolam initially and then to titrate the doses of each. A phenothiazine can be used instead of the benzodiazepine, e.g., chlorpromazine or the more sedating levomepromazine. Both have an antiemetic effect, if this is important, and there is limited evidence that chlorpromazine can palliate breathlessness (26) but watch should be kept for myoclonic jerking. Levomepromazine can be given by subcutaneous infusion, but chlorpromazine causes too many skin reactions to be given by this route.

Midazolam is also an appropriate choice of drug when it is agreed by patient (if still conscious and capable of making such a decision), family, and professionals that life is now being prolonged by assisted ventilation to a degree that is intolerable. A dose of 2.5 to 5 mg SC (1–2 mg IV) stat, with morphine 5 to 10 mg SC (2–10 mg IV) should be given, or more if the patient is already receiving regular sedation or opioids. This should be supplemented by an anticholinergic agent if there have been difficulties with retention of secretions. A continuous infusion of about 50% of the bolus doses per hour should be set up and adjusted to achieve the required degree of comfort and sedation. The use of these drugs is also indicated if the patient appears comatose in order to guard against the onset of distress once ventilator settings are changed. Further bolus doses should be available throughout the procedure in case any distress occurs. This is not the place to discuss in detail the technique of ventilator withdrawal, but a process of weaning over 30 to 60 minutes allows prompt control of any distress that might appear after each adjustment of the ventilator without being unduly prolonged (27).

Antisecretory Drugs

In bulbar ALS retention of secretions in the upper airways is a frequent problem well before the terminal phase. However, any severely ill patient with reduced ability to cough can accumulate secretions in the upper airways, resulting in noisy breathing that, if not always a distress to the ill person, may well be to attending relatives. At the end of life it is best to anticipate this problem, as it is not easy to get rid of secretions that which have already gathered. If respiratory failure is associated with unsuccessful treatment of a chest infection, there are likely also to be purulent exudates present, which cannot be prevented, so that it is not possible to stop rattly breathing altogether. Hence, the first step in management is to explain to the patient's family the mechanism of the noisy breathing, what is being done and what the limitations of therapy are, and reassure them that by this stage of their illness the dying person is unlikely to be nearly as aware of the sounds as they are themselves.

If an anticholinergic agent is already being given by gastrostomy or subcutaneous patch it can be continued and the dose increased if secretion retention is worsening (28). Atropine tends to be arousing, though, and should dose titration be required it would at this stage be more appropriate to change to a more neutral drug, such as hyoscine butyl bromide or glycopyrronium bromide, or hyoscine hydrobromide, which is normally sedating. Any of these can be given subcutaneously by syringe driver in combination with morphine and midazolam or levomepromazine. In the United Kingdom, the first two are significantly cheaper than the third.

Dose ranges are:

- Hyoscine butylbromide: 20 mg stat SC; 60–240 mg/24 hr by SC infusion
- Glycopyrronium bromide: 0.2–0.4 mg stat SC; 0.6–1.2 mg/24 hr by SC infusion
- Hysocine hydrobromide: 0.4–0.8 mg stat SC; 1.2–2.4 mg/24 hr by SC infusion

SUMMARY

Adequate management of the final phase of ALS is more likely to be achieved if it is founded on good provision of palliation throughout the course of the illness. The most common cause of death in ALS is respiratory failure. Around 60% of ALS patients die within 24 hours of a deterioration in their clinical condition and a proportion die suddenly. The prognosis can be extended significantly by NIV and almost indefinitely by tracheostomy ventilation where these techniques are available. The formulation of an advance directive can assist in preventing tracheostomy ventilation being instituted in a crisis without prior consent from the patient, but the key to good care is an ongoing and open dialogue between the person living with ALS and the health care team.

It is important to realize that the grounds of hope can change for a person with a terminal illness and that gentle honesty is fundamental to a therapeutic relationship. Caring for someone with ALS, especially toward the end of life, is highly demanding and families need reliable support and guidance from a multiprofessional health and social care team if they are to continue with their task. Because the clinical changes that herald death in ALS can happen rapidly, it is important to have opioid, sedative, and anticholinergic drugs readily, available. Distress is most likely to arise from increasing breathlessness and accompanying anxiety. Medication doses should be titrated in proportion to the existing medication regime with an end-point of control of distress. Adequate sedation should be given before withdrawal of assisted ventilation and maintained throughout the procedure.

The quality of a patient's dying is a powerful memory for those left behind and good care at this time is crucial in shaping public attitudes toward disability and serious illness.

REFERENCES

1. Leigh PN, Ray-Chaudhuri K. Motor neurone disease. J Neurol Neurosurg Psychiatry 1994; 57:886–896.
2. Ellershaw JE, Sutcliffe JM, Saunders CM. Dehydration and the dying patient. J Pain Symptom Manage 1995; 10:192–197.
3. O'Brien T, Kelly M, Saunders C. Motor neurone disease: a hospice perspective. Br Med J 1992; 304:471–473.
4. Aboussouan LS, Khan SU, Banerjee M, Arroliga AC, Mitsumoto H. Objective measures of the efficacy of noninvasive positive pressure ventilation in amyotrophic lateral sclerosis. Muscle Nerve 2001; 24:403–409.
5. Bach JR. Noninvasive ventilation interventions and best practice: use of respiratory muscle aids to avoid respiratory failure and hospitalization. Amyotrophic Lateral Sclerosis 2000; 1(suppl 3):19.
6. Oppenheimer EA. Decision-making in the respiratory care of amyotrophic lateral sclerosis: should home mechanical ventilation be used? Pall Med 1993; 7:49–64.
7. Kaub-Wittemer D, von Steinbuchel N, Wasner M, Laier-Groeneveld G, Borasio GD. Quality of life and psychosocial issues in ventilated patients with amyotrophic lateral sclerosis and their caregivers. J Pain Symptom Manage 2003; 26:890–896.
8. Beauchamp TL, Childress JF. Principles of Biomedical Ethics. Oxford: Oxford University Press, 2001.
9. Ganzini L, Johnston WS, McFarland BH, Tolle SW, Lee MA. Attitudes of patients with Amyotrophic Lateral Sclerosis and their caregivers towards assisted suicide. N Eng J Med 1998; 339:967–973.
10. Neudert C, Oliver D, Wasner M, Borasio GD. The course of the terminal phase in patients with amyotrophic lateral sclerosis. J Neurol 2001; 248:612–616.
11. Horton R. Euthanasia and assisted suicide: What does the Dutch vote mean? Lancet 2001; 357:1221–1222.
12. Bradley WG, Anderson F, Bromberg M, Gutmann L, Harati Y, Ross M, Miller RG. Current management of ALS: comparison of the ALS CARE Database and the AAN Practice Parameter. Neurology 2001; 57:500–504.
13. Bach JR. Threats to "informed" advance directives for the severely physically challenged? Arch Phys Med Rehabil 2003; 84(suppl 2):S23–S28.
14. Ezekiel J Emmanuel, Emmanuel LL. Four models of the physician-patient relationship. JAMA 1992; 267:2221–2226.
15. Quill TE. The ambiguity of clinical intentions. New Eng J Med 1993; 329:1039–1040.
16. Sykes NP, Thorns A. The use of opioids and sedatives at the end of life. Lancet Oncol 2003; 4:312–318.
17. Calman KC. Quality of life in cancer patients—an hypothesis. J Med Ethics 1984; 10:124–127.
18. Hinton J. The physical and mental distress of the dying. Quar J Med 1963; 32:1–21.

19. Bromberg MN, Liow M, Forshew DA, Swenson M. A time line for predicting durable medical equipment needs for ALS/MND patients. Proceedings of 9th International Symposium on ALS/MND. International Alliance of ALS/MND Associations, Munich, 1998, 58.
20. Herth K. Fostering hope in terminally ill people. J Adv Nurs 1990; 15:1250–1259.
21. Centers LC. Beyond denial and despair: ALS and our heroic potential for hope. J Pall Care 2001; 17(4):259–264.
22. McGoldrick M, Gerson R. Genograms in Family Assessment. Norton: New York, 1985.
23. Hinton J. Which patients with terminal cancer are admitted from home care? Pall Med 1994; 8:197–210.
24. Oliver D. Opioid medication in the palliative care of motor neurone disease. Pall Med 1998; 12:113–115.
25. Leach RM. Palliative medicine and non-malignant, end-stage respiratory disease. In: Doyle D, Hanks G, Cherny N, Calman K, eds. Oxford Textbook of Palliative Medicine. 3rd ed. Oxford: Oxford University Press, 2004:895–916.
26. Ventafridda V, Spoldi E, De Conno F. Control of dyspnoea in advanced cancer patients. Chest 1990; 6:1544–1545.
27. Von Gunten C, Weissman DE. Ventilator withdrawal protocol (Part 1). J Pall Med 2003; 6:773–776.
28. Bennett M, Lucas V, Brennan M, Hughes A, O'Donnell V, Wee B. Using antimuscarinic drugs in the management of death rattle: evidence-based guidelines for palliative care. Pall Med 2002; 16:369–374.

36

Palliative Care: Family Perspective

Steven M. Albert
Department of Behavioral and Community Health Sciences, Graduate School of Public Health, University of Pittsburgh, Pittsburgh, Pennsylvania, U.S.A

Judith G. Rabkin
Department of Psychiatry, New York Psychiatric Institute, New York, New York, U.S.A.

Maura L. Del Bene
Department of Neurology, New York University School of Medicine, New York, New York, U.S.A.

INTRODUCTION

The World Health Organization (WHO) defines palliative care as "the active total care of patients and their families by a multiprofessional team when the patient's disease is no longer responsive to curative treatment" (1). This important definition needs revision in one regard: Lynn (2) has shown that an abrupt division between curative and palliative care is not true to good clinical practice and not in the best interest of patients. Indeed, multidisciplinary teams typically provide a mix of palliative and curative therapy throughout the course of chronic progressive disease, shifting the balance as death approaches. Yet the WHO definition is valuable nonetheless for its stress on families as well as patients. The patient and family form a single unit of care (3,4) and should be considered partners in any palliative care effort.

More recent guidelines in palliative care emphasize the centrality of the family to an even greater extent. Three of the four central principles in the *Clinical Practice Guidelines* proposed by the National Consensus Project for Quality Palliative Care involve family members. The *Guidelines* recommend that palliative care teams address psychosocial distress, spiritual issues, and practical needs in family members as well as patients; that family members participate in decision making and receive information about the benefits and burdens of treatment; and that "both patient and family are prepared for the dying process and for death, when it is anticipated" (5).

This said, it is curious that relatively little research is available on the experience of families who care for dying patients at home, and also that the few studies available rarely examine the impact of hospice care on families. Most studies are limited to cancer and Alzheimer's disease care and have relied on ethnographic interviews rather than population-based epidemiologic surveys. Very few have followed families prospectively to examine changes in caregiving relative to disease progression and the approach of death.

In this chapter, we examine available literature on family caregiving in the setting of ALS and palliative care, especially, hospice service. Hospice is only one element in the continuum of palliative care and marks the most intensive delivery of palliative care. Palliative care, as indicated earlier, really begins with recognition that a disease is progressive and in need of aggressive management. In the case of ALS, some forms of palliative care are appropriate at the point of diagnosis. As palliative need and challenges are greatest in the final months of life, however, we concentrate on the hospice period, recognizing that this period is only one element in a larger continuum of palliative care. We compare the ALS experience to reports from cancer caregivers, a more intensively investigated area, to see how the family caregiver experience of palliative care may differ across settings. We also ask how the caregiving experience may differ according to the stage of disease progression.

We supplement this literature review with our own experience following a cohort of ALS patients and their family caregivers over the final months of life, the Columbia University "Living with ALS" cohort. These 80 patients were recruited when patients' forced vital capacity (FVC) first dipped below 50%, an indicator of six-month survival (6,7), or when clinicians at our center determined that other changes in clinical status also indicated a life expectancy of about six months. Patients were recruited on a rolling basis over a three-year period. About two-thirds of patients approached in this effort agreed to join the study and provided informed consent. Family caregivers for 78 of these 80 patients were also enrolled (two patients had no caregiver; see below), and both patient and caregiver were interviewed every month until death or the end of the study. In the case of patients choosing tracheostomy, families were followed every month until tracheostomy and then every three months thereafter. For patients who died, we attempted to interview caregivers after the death.

Over the course of the study, two-thirds of the patients died, 15% opted for tracheostomy, 14% were alive at the end of the follow-up period, and 5% were lost to follow up. Among patients dying over the course of the study, the median duration of follow up was 130 days, with patients, on average, completing three research interviews. The median interval between the last research assessment and death was 32 days. Caregivers completed bereavement interviews for 76% of the patients who died. The median interval between death and caregiver bereavement interviews was 23 days.

PALLIATIVE CARE AND HOSPICE USE IN THE TERMINAL PERIOD

The majority of people with terminal ALS use hospice and die at home (8,9). This outcome represents a change from earlier decades (10,11). Increased availability of hospice through the Medicare hospice benefit in the United States, first authorized in 1983, has allowed greater opportunity for patients to die at home. In the United States, about 20% of American decedents are served by hospice, which includes both home hospice and hospice inpatient units (12), and about 20% of Americans die at home (13). These figures stand in sharp contrast to the experience of people with ALS. In the Columbia cohort, 35% were enrolled in hospice at baseline and 57% used hospice at some point over follow up. Of the 58 patients who died during the study, 83% used hospice. All but four of the patients who died were able to die at home. This rate of hospice use is higher than that reported in the national ALS CARE Database for 1996 to 1999, in which 47% of patients dying at home used hospice (14).

While the median length of stay on hospice nationally is currently 15.6 days [as reported in the National Home and Hospice Care Survey, 2000 (12)], among patients in the Columbia cohort the median length of stay was 110 days. Also, in our patients, all but two who died while on hospice used home hospice. Thus, for ALS patients entering the terminal phase of the disease at our center, relatively long periods of hospice care and death at home are modal. However, it should be noted that nearly one-third of the patients in the Columbia cohort who died spent less than two months on hospice, considered the minimum length of time required to benefit fully from hospice service (13).

FAMILY AS CAREGIVERS

"Natural caregivers," i.e., unpaid, non-medical helpers or care organizers (15), are involved in almost all cases of ALS end-of-life care. For example, in the Columbia cohort all but 2 of the 80 patients had family caregivers involved in daily care and decision making. The two patients without caregivers were highly atypical. They had neither spouses nor family living nearby, nor any close friends who stepped in to serve as caregivers.

Even with such heavy family involvement, it is important to recognize that a wide variety of family and nonfamily fill the caregiver role. In the Columbia cohort, spouses or partners (including one person who was divorced and no longer sharing a household) served as caregivers in about two-thirds of the cases. Parents (for young-onset patients) and adult children served as caregivers in about a quarter of the cases. The remainder of caregivers were either more remote family (6%) or friends and neighbors (9%). The latter are worth special mention, since they were often part of group efforts in which neighbors, friends, or members of a religious fellowship took on caregiving duties in a "Share the Care" arrangement. If not for friends or neighbors, these patients would not have had any natural caregivers.

We should also note that caregivers may relinquish the role during the course of ALS care. In the Columbia cohort, two family caregivers chose to step aside (in one case through divorce from the patient), and in both cases other family members stepped in to replace them. In fact, changes in family caregiver personnel, including exits and re-entry into caregiving, are common in the case of family care over long-term follow up (16).

Involvement of family caregivers in daily care also varies considerably, though meeting the needs of these patients is on the whole quite demanding. Upon enrollment, when patients were first noted to have a forced vital capacity (FVC)$\leq$50% and expected survival of less than six months, caregivers already spent a median of 18 hr/day (range 1–24) with patients and a median of 5 hr/day (range 0–24) providing hands-on help. Three-quarters also received help from paid personnel, who worked a median of 20 hr/wk in patients' homes. Given that one-third of patients had already begun hospice care at the time of enrollment, it is clear that family remain quite involved in care even after hospice admission.

The same situation holds for patients who enter skilled nursing care facilities (SNF), either for tracheostomy care, inpatient hospice, or rehabilitation after hospitalization. About 10% of patients in the end-of-life cohort had at least one SNF admission over the prior year before enrollment in the cohort, and 4% entered an SNF during follow up. Families continued to be very involved in care for these patients, typically visiting daily and continuing to provide feeding support and help with other activities of daily living.

DAILY CAREGIVING CHALLENGES IN END-OF-LIFE CARE

Family caregivers to patients receiving end-of-life care face a variety of challenges, all, for the most part, daunting. In the setting of cancer care, one report summarized the experience as "good days, bad days, crisis events, and miraculous rallies" (17). These day-to-day, event-to-event challenges make daily caregiving extremely stressful and introduce a high level of uncertainty among family members. Caregivers may find this period so challenging that they often do not know where to begin when asked what kind of help they need or what they find difficult. As one cancer caregiver recounted, "If anybody asks about something I only say that everything is ok; you cannot say anything else" (18). If patients seek comfort at this time, caregivers seek "security," reassurance regarding what is coming next and access to the support and resources they need to confront the next challenge (19,20).

ALS caregiving at the end of life is characterized first of all by the severe disability of patients. At the baseline assessment of the Columbia cohort, for example, more than half the patients were completely dependent in each of the instrumental (using telephone, taking medications, and handling finances) and basic (bathing, dressing, toileting, transferring between bed and chair, and feeding) activities of daily living (ADL). By the time of the last assessment, more than three-quarters were completely dependent in each task.

While a count of instrumental and basic ADL needs will certainly be correlated with indicators of caregiving challenge (how many hours caregivers provide help each day, how much burden and fatigue they report, and how long they continue to provide care at home), these correlations will only be moderate in size. Indeed, ADL status explains only a modest amount of the variance in caregiver reports of burden (21). One reason for such low correlations is the inability of ADL measures to capture the full context in which families provide care (22). What kinds of home modifications have family members made to facilitate caregiving? What kinds of care arrangements have families put in place to insure such care if they work or wish to travel or are themselves weak or ill? How much of a financial drain do these arrangements entail? These too will determine how challenging patient disability will be for any particular caregiver.

A second challenge to family caregivers is hands-on medical management in end-of-life care. For the ALS patient, this domain may include a feeding tube for management of nutrition, noninvasive ventilation for management of respiratory decline, pharmacologic interventions for management of pain and psychic suffering, general monitoring of patient health, and use of other medical equipment. Such complex nursing care is well described by Reinhard (21) in her survey of care for older adults. She points out that family caregivers are now expected to manage dressing changes, suctioning equipment, oxygen, feeding tubes, catheters, injections, and intravenous therapy—"things that make nursing students tremble."

In the case of these medical management challenges, family caregivers often face the same dilemmas as medical providers, but without the training and professional distance that come with formal training. In the setting of pain management, Ferrel reports that family caregivers "made difficult decisions on a daily basis regarding which medicines to give, how much, and when to give analgesics. Family members struggled with titration, when to increase the dose, how to balance relief with side effects, fear of overdosing, and fear of addiction. Family caregivers felt responsible for unrelieved pain" (23). We unfairly expect family caregivers, who usually lack any kind of formal medical or nursing training, to make difficult medical decisions and also to bear responsibility for the consequences of these decisions.

A third challenge to family caregivers is cognitive support, which includes remote and direct supervision, as well as measures to ensure safety, efforts to orient patients, and attempts to vary the environment to provide stimulation and engagement. Cognitive support may also include management of delirium, agitation, and the psychiatric sequelae of neurocognitive disorders. While the prevalence of dementia in ALS is unclear, recent research suggests that some forms of cognitive disability, such as disinhibition and executive dysfunction, may be more common than formerly believed (24). The final weeks of life are also associated with increased risk of delirium and cognitive dysfunction. In one study of cancer patients on hospice in the last weeks of life, only one-third could complete a personal interview because of cognitive dysfunction or fatigue (25).

Finally, as indicated earlier, caregiving requires a supportive environment. It is impossible to provide adequate help if family members cannot lift a patient, or if someone cannot be in the home throughout the day, or if the home lacks an essential piece of assistive equipment (such as a sliding board or Hoyer lift). "Care management" activities are no less burdensome or difficult than hands-on care. In-home care management tasks include home modification; hiring and supervision of paid home care workers; and purchase, maintenance, and instruction in the use of assistive devices. "Out-of-home" tasks include arranging medical care, processing insurance claims, arranging transportation, and putting financial statements together to qualify for entitlements and benefits related to medical disability.

These challenges are not all there is to caregiving. As we note below, caregivers commonly report positive mood despite the distress associated with end-of-life caregiving. Providing support, successfully meeting care needs, and becoming a partner in palliative care efforts also offer satisfaction to many family members. This component of end-of-life caregiving is less well studied. When asked about positive caregiving experiences, family members in the Columbia cohort often pointed to challenges they overcame, successful advocacy for services or medical care on the part of patients, and planning or alterations of environments that enabled patients to enjoy an activity or maintain a routine. This dimension of family caregiving at the end of life should not be underestimated if we wish to understand the experience fully and develop interventions that may enhance positive features of caregiving.

CAREGIVER BURDEN, DISTRESS, AND DEPRESSION

An elevated risk of depressive symptoms is a consistent finding in research on family caregivers (26,27). Although the vast majority of caregiving studies focus on caregivers to patients with dementia, caregivers to patients with other conditions, such as ALS (28), AIDS (29,30), brain injury (31), cancer (32,33), and heart transplant (34), also show high levels of caregiver distress, suggesting that caregiving in virtually any illness context leads to high levels of distress in the caregiver. Further, a recent comprehensive review of psychiatric morbidity among family caregivers shows a consistent gender difference; female caregivers report more distress than male caregivers (26). Given the prevalence of high levels of depressive symptomatology in both men and women, it is surprising that very few studies use diagnostic interviews to assess clinical depression in caregivers.

Little is known about the effects of patient depression on caregivers, or caregiver depression on patients. In our previous work, spouse caregivers of ALS patients were as likely as patients to be distressed, and distress levels were highly correlated between the two (28). The same association has been reported for caregivers to patients with cancer who face end-of-life challenges (35–37). Clearly, a patient's mental health can affect caregiver well-being, but there are few longitudinal studies of the relationship between caregiver and patient distress (37). Given patients' concerns about being a burden to caregivers (32,38), it is possible that patients may interpret caregiver distress as a sign of this feared burden, which in turn could affect patient mood.

In a cross-sectional study of baseline status in the Columbia cohort, we found disparities in patient and caregiver perceptions of the effects of the disease. These disparities did not occur in ratings of patient function, which were highly congruent, but rather regarding the impact of the disease. The disparity was systematic and skewed in a particular direction. In pairwise analyses, caregivers rated patient suffering higher than patients rated their own suffering, and patients viewed caregivers as more burdened than caregivers reported for themselves (39). Both parties exaggerated how negative the experience was for the other. This may be a sign of the mutual compassion that often governs relationships between patients and caregivers.

An important question is the degree to which caregiver competence or self-efficacy can mitigate the challenges of end-of-life caregiving. Do caregivers with strong personal resources have an easier time handling these challenges, and do patients with such caregivers have an easier time at the end of life? Studies of pain management in cancer care suggest an association between caregiver self-efficacy and both patient and caregiver outcomes. In one study, caregivers' perceptions of their efficacy in managing patient pain were associated with lower reported strain and better mood among caregivers (40). Thus, strong self-efficacy in pain management may help protect caregivers from distress associated with the many physical and emotional challenges of caregiving. In this study, caregiver ratings of efficacy in managing pain were not related to patient ratings of pain, but were associated instead with patient reports of physical well-being overall. The authors suggest that "caregivers who were confident that they could help the patient manage pain helped patients control the impact of their pain so that they were able to be more active" (40).

CAREGIVING AND POSITIVE MOOD

As mentioned earlier, positive mood and distress co-occur in caregiving. That is, it is possible for caregivers to report both high levels of distress and also positive experiences, such as satisfaction with caregiving tasks. In the Columbia cohort, measures of caregiver burden and satisfaction were not significantly correlated, suggesting that the two are distinct features of caregiver experience. Similar findings have been reported for caregivers to people with HIV (41). Positive mood is common among caregivers in the final weeks of care to the dying patient; and, as we discuss below, a majority of caregivers report positive mood in the bereavement period.

CAREGIVER RECOGNITION OF DYING AND THE END OF LIFE

"Sometimes I wonder, is this the end? And then I think, what will it be like? How will I know, and will I know? And what will happen? ...I get myself all braced up to ask [the hospice nurse], but when she actually comes, I just can't do it. Perhaps I don't really want to know" (42). This statement from a cancer caregiver summarizes many of the fears and anxieties family members face, even when concerted attempts are made to include them as members of a hospice team. Fear of the physical changes of death and lack of knowledge about the dying process is common and should not be surprising, given that the nonhealth professional may witness only one to two deaths first hand in a lifetime. It remains to be seen if an educational program designed to demystify death and dying, combined with appropriate palliative care, could reduce anticipatory grief and improve the dying experience for patients and caregivers.

DECISIONS TO USE HOME HOSPICE

The decision to provide palliative care at home appears to be most commonly made in the form of a promise to a patient (42). Patients express a wish to spend their last days at home, and caregivers, respecting the patient's wish, promise to do what they can to maintain the dying patient at home. Caregivers who experienced a death at home also recognized that privacy and self-determination were best ensured in a home rather than hospital death.

Because of its clear and relatively predictable course, opportunities for home deaths and planning at the end of life may be greater in ALS than in other diseases. However, research with the Columbia cohort suggests that hospice use can be suboptimal even with generally long and nearly universal use of hospice. Many, if not a majority, of ALS patients delay the use of hospice, do not use the full set of services offered by hospice, or fail to have frank discussions about end-of-life care even when on hospice. Ethnographic interviews with patients and caregivers in the cohort revealed that a quarter of our families, despite hospice admission, never discussed death and dying openly. This "collusion of silence" between patients, families, and sometimes even hospice staff may increase anxiety in patients and burden in caregivers. It makes planning for the end of life more difficult. Also, even when families discuss dying frankly, in some cases families did not speak to hospice personnel with a single voice. As one of our caregivers noted, "Things would be said or meds delivered, and we, the daughters, were caught unawares. Mom was communicating her needs to particular people only and the communications were not shared." In many cases, no single person coordinates care within the family. Finally, even when these two obstacles are surmounted, a majority of patients and their families still prefer to keep caregiving needs private and resist services until quite late in disease progression. Families in our study took as long as three months to decide to use hospice even after patients qualified and treating physicians authorized it.

MEDICAL PROFESSIONALS IN THE HOME

The benefits of home hospice—access to health professionals, medical equipment in the home, and time with the patient at the end of life—are also its liabilities. For families receiving home hospice, the presence of medical professionals may interrupt home life and introduce a new set of stresses. Caregivers may complain that they are losing control over their own home and must relinquish a great deal of privacy.

On the other hand, the reassurance of having access to hospice nurse expertise and the support of other health care professionals in the home is invaluable. In the Columbia cohort, virtually all family caregivers praised hospice without reserve or qualification.

Additional research on home hospice could profitably turn to specification of the ways caregivers might be included in hospice practice. Also, the effect of hospice and home death on other family members, especially young children, remains unclear.

The central question is the extent to which home hospice death may be superior to hospital death on such outcomes as caregiver adjustment after bereavement, quality of dying, and quality of life at the end-of-life. One systematic meta-analysis suggests that end-of-life care provided by palliative care teams is superior to non-hospice service in the areas of pain management and caregiver satisfaction with health care services (43). The authors conclude, "One of the most consistent effects was of improved satisfaction for caregivers and, to a lesser extent, for patients, when services were compared to conventional or non-hospice services. This finding was strongest for home care services" (43).

AFTER THE DEATH

Caregiving for a dying person and witnessing the death of a family member may sometimes lead to persistence or exacerbation of distress after the death. In the period following a family member's death, cancer caregivers in one study reported poor mental health relative to people of the same age who had not provided care (44). In the same study, dying at home was associated with better caregiver mental health after the death. Poor caregiver physical health and insufficient family support put caregivers at higher risk for poor mental health after the death (43,45).

Little research is available for ALS caregivers in the bereavement period. Initial results from the Columbia cohort suggest that one-third of the ALS caregivers who had witnessed a death had a difficult transition to the post-caregiving period.

These caregivers did not report relief that the dying process had ended and continued to report sadness, guilt, anxiety, and numbness. These reports do not appear to be strongly related to a caregiver's perception of the quality of the patient's death. That is, even when caregivers reported that the death was in accord with their own and the patient's wishes, they were still likely to endorse indicators of difficulty in reintegrating into the community and assuming a post-caregiver role. However, two-thirds of the caregivers did not experience elevated or persistent distress, a finding also observed among caregivers of men dying of AIDS (41).

Thus, while witnessing death may be stressful, effective palliative care and introduction of hospice service in the last months of life are likely to lower this distress through more effective treatment of end-of-life symptoms and increasing caregiving control over the dying process. In the subset of families in the Columbia cohort who were observed to begin hospice over follow up, we found significant increases among caregivers in perceived control over the disease and in positive mood (46).

CONCLUSION

Family care at the end of life for people with ALS may be more challenging than end-of-life care in other diseases. The severe disability typical of the disease and need for intensive caregiving support make the last months of life extremely demanding for family caregivers. On the other hand, the clear and undeniable course of the disease offers families the advantage of earlier use of hospice and perhaps greater opportunity for multidisciplinary management of the disease. ALS may also allow families more time to prepare for dying and a greater likelihood of a "good death" than other terminal diseases. At this point, however, comparative studies of family caregiving (e.g., differences by ethnicity), mental health in patients and caregivers, the dying period, and bereavement are still unavailable. While family are now acknowledged as key members of any palliative care effort, many gaps remain in research and service delivery that might benefit these mostly unacknowledged partners in life and death.

ACKNOWLEDGMENTS

Research supported by National Institute of Mental Health, MH62200. We are grateful to the many patients and family members from the Eleanor and Lou Gehrig MDA/ALS Center who have participated in our research.

REFERENCES

1. World Health Organization. Cancer pain relief and palliative care. Geneva: Technical Report Series, No. 804, 1990.
2. Lynn J. Perspectives on care at the close of life. Serving patients who may die soon and their families: the role of hospice and other services. JAMA 2001; 285:925–932.
3. Proot IM, Abu-Saad HM, Crebolder HFJM, Goldsteen M, Luker KA, Widdershoven GAM. Vulnerability of family caregivers in terminal palliative care at home: balancing between burden and capacity. Scand J Caring Sci 2003; 17:113–121.
4. Davies B. Family functioning and its implications for palliative care. J Palliat Care 1994; 10:29–36.
5. National Consensus Project for Quality Palliative Care. Clinical Practice Guidelines. New York, 2004. www.nationalconsensusproject.org.
6. Del Bene ML, Albert SM, Brandis M, Mitsumoto H. Can death be predicted in ALS? Amyotrophic Lateral Sclerosis and Other Motor Neuron Disorders. 2003; 4(suppl 1):40.
7. McCluskey L, Houseman G. Medicare hospice referral criteria for patients with amyotrophic lateral sclerosis: a need for improvement. J Palliat Care 2004; 20:47–53.
8. Albert SM, Murply PL, Del Bene ML, Rowland LP. Prospective study of palliative care in ALS: choice, timing, outcomes. J Neurol Sci 1999; 169:108–113.
9. Mandler RN, Anderson FA, Miller RG, Clawson L, Cudkowicz M, Del Bene ML, ALS CARE study group. The ALS patient care database: insights into end of life care in ALS. Amyotroph Lateral Scler Other Motor Neuron Disord 2001; 2:203–208.
10. Krivickas LS, Shockley L, Mitsumoto H. Home care of patients with amyotrophic lateral sclerosis. J Neurol Sci 1997; 152(suppl 1):S82–S89.
11. Carter GT, Bednar-Butler LM, Abresch RT, Ugalde VO. Expanding the role of hospice care in amyotrophic lateral sclerosis. Am J Hosp Palliat Care 1999; 16:707–710.
12. Haupt BJ. Characteristics of hospice care discharges and their length of service: United States, 2000. National Center for Health Statistics. Series 13, Data from the National Health Survey; No. 154, 2003.
13. Last Acts. Means to a better end: A report on dying in America today, 2002. www.lastacts.org.

14. Bradley WG, Anderson F, Bromberg M, Gutmann L, Harati Y, Ross M, Miller RG, ALS CARE study group. Current management of ALS: comparison of the ALS CARE database and the AAN practice parameter. Neurology 2001; 57:500–504.

15. Baillargeon L. Palliative care at home. Dying at home: an increasingly important trend. Can Fam Physician 2003; 49:1581–1582.

16. Dwyer JW, Henretta JC, Coward RT, Barton AJ. Changes in helping behaviors of adult children as caregivers. Res Aging 1992; 14:351–375.

17. Farber SJ, Egnew TR, Herman-Bertsch JL, Taylor TR, Guidin GE. Issues in end-of-life care: patient, caregiver, and clinician perceptions. J Palliat Med 2003; 6:19–31.

18. Broback G, Bartero C. How next of kin experience palliative care of relatives at home. Eur J Cancer Care 2003; 12:339–346.

19. Milberg A, Strang P, Carlsson M, Borjesson S. Advanced palliative home care: next-of-kin's perspective. J Palliat Med 2003; 6:749–756.

20. Hudson PL, Aranda S, Kristjanson LJ. Meeting the supportive needs of family caregivers in palliative care: challenges for health professionals. J Palliat Med 2004; 7:19–25.

21. Reinhard S. The work of caregiving: What do ADLs and IADLs tell us? In: Levine C, ed. Toward a New Job Description for Family Caregivers. New York: United Hospital Fund, 2004:70–98.

22. Albert SM. Beyond ADL/IADL: Recognizing the Full Scope of Family Caregiving. In: Levine C, ed. Toward a New Job Description for Family Caregivers. New York: United Hospital Fund, 2004:99–122.

23. Ferrel B. Pain observed: the experience of pain from the family caregivers perspective. Clin Geriatric Med 2001; 17(3):595–609.

24. Loman-Hoerth C, Murphy J, Langmore S, Kramer JH, Olney RK, Miller B. Are amyotrophic lateral sclerosis patients cognitively normal? Neurology 2003; 60:1094–1097.

25. Chochinov HM, Tataryn D, Clinch JJ, Dudgeon. Will to live in the terminally ill. Lancet 1999; 354:816–819.

26. Yee JL, Schulz R. Gender differences in psychiatric morbidity among family caregivers: a review and analysis. Gerontologist 2000; 40:147–164.

27. Schulz R, Quittner AL. Caregiving for children and adults with chronic conditions: introduction to the special issue. Health Psychol 1998; 17:107–111.

28. Rabkin JG, Wagner G, Del Bene ML. Resilience and distress among amyotrophic lateral sclerosis patients and caregivers. Psychosom Med 2000; 62:271–279.

29. Folkman S, Chesney MA, Cooke M, Boccellari A, Collette L. Caregiver burden in HIV-positive and HIV-negative partners of men with AIDS. J Consult Clin Psychol 1994; 62:746–756.

30. Wight RG, LeBlanc AJ, Aneshensel CS. AIDS caregiving and health among midlife and older women. Health Psychol 1998; 17:130–137.

31. Marsh NV, Kersel DA, Havill JH, Sleigh JW. Caregiver burden at 1 year following severe traumatic brain injury. Brain Injury 1998; 12:1045–1059.

32. Nijboer C, Triemstra M, Tempelaar R, Sanderman R, van den Bos GA. Determinants of caregiving experiences and mental health of partners of cancer patients. Cancer 1999; 86:577–588.

33. Hinton J. Can home care maintain an acceptable quality of life for patients with terminal cancer and their relatives? Palliat Med 1994; 8:183–196.

34. Dew MA, Kormos RL, Roth LH, Murali S, DiMartini A, Griffith BP. Early post-transplant medical compliance and mental health predict physical morbidity and mortality one to three years after heart transplantation. J Heart Lung Transplant 1999; 18:549–562.

35. Blanchard CG, Albrecht TL, Ruckdeschel JC. The crisis of cancer: psychological impact on family caregivers. Oncology 1997; 11:189–194.

36. Harding R, Higginson IJ, Donaldson N. The relationship between patient characteristics and carer psychological status in home palliative care. Support Care Cancer 2003; 11:638–643.

37. Murray SA, Kendall M, Worth A, Benton TF, Clausen H. Dying of lung cancer or cardiac failure: prospective qualitative interview study of patients and their carers in the community. Br Med J 2002; 325:929–934.

38. Redinbaugh EM, Baum A, Tarbell S, Arnold R. End-of-life caregiving: What helps family caregivers cope? J Palliat Med 2004; 6:901–909.

39. Adelman EE, Albert SM, Rabkin JG, Del Bene ML, Tider T, O'Sullivan I. Disparities in perceptions of distress and burden in ALS patients and family caregivers. Neurology 2004; 62:1766–1770.

40. Keefe FJ, Ahles TA, Porter LS, Sutton LM, McBride CM, Pope MS, McKinstry ET, Furstenberg CP, Dalton J, Bausom DH. The self-efficacy of family caregivers for helping cancer patients manage pain at the end of life. Pain 2003; 103:157–162.

41. Folkman S. Positive psychological states and coping with severe stress. Soc Sci Med 1997; 45:1207–1221.

42. Stajduhar KI. Examining the perspectives of family members involved in the delivery of palliative care at home. J Palliat Care 2003; 19:27–35.

43. Higginson IJ, Finlay IG, Goodwin DM, Hood K, Edwards AGK, Cook A, Douglas H-R, Normand CE. Is there evidence that palliative care teams alter end of-life experiences of patients and their caregivers? J Pain Symptom Manage 2003; 25:150–168.

44. Brazil K, Bedard M, Willison K. Correlates of health status for family caregivers in bereavement. J Palliat Med 2002; 5:849–855.

45. Ferrario SR, Cardillo V, Balzarini E, Zotti AM. Advanced cancer at home: caregiving and bereavement. Palliat Med 2004; 18:129–136.

46. Albert SM, Del Bene ML, Rabkin JG, Tider T, O'Sullivan I, Mitsumoto H. Hospice and mental health at the end of life: A prospective study of ALS patients. Neurology 2004; 62(suppl 5):A213.

37

End-of-Life Decision Making

Linda Ganzini
Department of Psychiatry, Oregon Health & Science University, Portland, Oregon, U.S.A.

Wendy Johnston
Neurology, University of Alberta, Alberta, Canada

INTRODUCTION

ALS is a relentlessly disabling neurological disorder that inevitably progresses to respiratory failure. Without respiratory support, the five year survival is between 10% and 20% (1). ALS is almost always the cause of death in individuals diagnosed with the illness. The nature of ALS and the limited options for treatment force those who suffer from it to face stark decisions about accepting or forgoing treatments that sustain life.

The spectrum of apparent choice for patients with ALS ranges from seemingly indefinitely postponing death with long-term assisted ventilation and gastrostomy feeding through hastening death by forgoing life-sustaining treatments, stopping all food and hydration, and, at times, physician-assisted suicide (PAS) and euthanasia. Whether by choice, chance, or lack of recourse, most patients with ALS die without availing themselves of either long-term ventilation or euthanasia, but as a consequence of disease progression. In the terminal stage, when palliative measures come to the forefront of care, clinicians' fear of hastening death may result in withholding sedatives and opioids necessary for adequate symptom management.

End-of-Life Decisions: ALS Compared to Other Terminal Conditions

ALS patients, compared to patients with more common terminal illnesses such as cancer and heart disease, are more likely to actively consider end-of-life medical decisions for several reasons. First, their physical decline is steady and inexorable, with less variability in the disease progression, and only rare remissions. It is difficult for each ALS patient to hope that decisions about life-sustaining interventions can be avoided. Second, unlike cancer or cardiovascular disease, medical interventions including nutritional and respiratory support can prolong life indefinitely (2). Finally, cognition and therefore decision-making capacity often remains intact, sometimes until the final days of life (3,4).

In diseases such as cancer, decisions to aggressively treat with the goal of extending life often results in decreased quality of life. For example, even if life is extended, ventilator support in a terminally ill cancer patient must take place in an intensive care unit, and often results in isolation, pain, agitated delirium, and poor symptom control. With further progression of cancer, ventilator care eventually becomes futile. Alternatively, when cancer patients choose hospice care they no longer receive life-sustaining treatments. Care for cancer patients in hospice focuses on symptom control, often in a home environment, and allows unlimited contact with family and friends, all resulting in better quality of life. These trade-offs between quality and quantity of life are common in many terminal illnesses.

In ALS patients, distinctions between treatments that extend life versus those that are palliative are less clear, especially at the time treatments are first started. For example, a percutaneous endoscopic gastrostomy (PEG) may improve quality of life by improving nutrition, lessening fatigue, alleviating the struggle and effort to eat, and lessening the fear of choking (5,6). The value of PEG in prolonging survival is less clear. The decision to stop gastrostomy feeding then may not reflect the burdens or medical futility of treatment, but an intolerable decrease in quality of life that treatment interventions no longer overcome. Similarly, noninvasive ventilation (NIV) is associated with longer survival, but also has an important role in palliating chronic hypoventilation. NIV improves sleep and mental health, and decreases shortness of breath, fatigue, and social isolation. This quality-of-life benefit persists from nine months to over a year (2). As such, stopping treatment among ALS patients often represents acceptance of death or even intent to die, as treatment can extend life but no longer improve life's unacceptable quality.

Ethical Principles in End-of-Life Care

Ethical principles guide clinicians in their collaboration with patients around end-of-life decisions. In Western cultures, especially the United States, it is universally agreed that competent patients have the right to forgo medical treatments, even if such a refusal may hasten death. Physicians may recommend treatments, including artificial food and hydration, and at times, may feel strongly that patients should receive them. The more important obligation, however, is to ensure that patients are informed about available choices, and are supported in their effort to choose the correct course for themselves based on their own personal goals and values. Physicians must communicate the diagnosis clearly and prognosticate honestly in order for a patient to make a competent decision. The right to refuse treatments is rooted both ethically in respect for autonomy and legally in the right to self-determination (7–9).

In the U.S. legal system, the right to refuse is conceptualized as the right to be free of unwanted burdensome treatments (9). In some situations, patients may forgo or stop treatments, not because of objections to their burdens, but because life's quality is unacceptable and they wish for death to come sooner. For patients who are depressed or lack decision-making capacity, these preferences may be suicidal equivalents. But for competent patients, the legal legitimacy of the request is not rendered invalid by the reason, though individual clinicians may find a patient's intent to die ethically problematic.

In addition, there is no ethical or legal difference between withdrawing a treatment and never starting one (7–9). Again, for some clinicians withdrawing a treatment feels more emotionally stressful than never starting one, as the latter is perceived as allowing a natural death (10,11). There are many potential advantages of a trial of treatment such as noninvasive ventilation and nutritional support, as these interventions may improve quality of life for some time.

Deliberately harming a patient is always unacceptable, under the principles of non-malfeasance (do not harm) and beneficence (provide good) (7,8). At times, clinicians cannot avoid all harm in order to achieve important patient-centered goals. Under the rule of double effect, physicians may prescribe medications to treat pain and dyspnea, even if these treatments may hasten death if the following conditions are met—the goal of treatment must be amelioration of symptoms; shortening of life is foreseen but not intended; and death cannot be the means of relieving suffering. This principle is widely accepted by philosophers and theologians and supports the use of narcotics and anxiolytic agents for symptom control in the final days of life (7).

There is much less agreement about whether patients have the right to hasten death through PAS or euthanasia. PAS describes a physician prescribing medication to cause death, which the patient self-administers, usually orally. Physicians commit active voluntary euthanasia when they administer a medication to a competent, requesting patient for the purpose of ending life. The ethical arguments against PAS and euthanasia include that there are limits to patient autonomy, and that clinician participation may undermine the integrity of the medical profession, leading down a slippery slope to nonvoluntary or involuntary euthanasia. Proponents counter that physician-assisted death (PAD) is consistent with autonomy and that the patient's goals and intentions may not differ between PAD and decisions to stop life-sustaining treatments (8). In addition to ethical arguments there are clinical, social, and political arguments for and against allowing these practices (7–9,12–15).

Voluntary refusal of food and fluids has been proposed as an alternative to euthanasia (16–18). The choice to stop eating and drinking in order to hasten death is legal in most jurisdictions and available to competent persons. A key issue for the clinician is to assure that the choice is voluntary, competent, and not coerced or unduly influenced by others. Like PAS, however, some clinicians believe that collaboration with a patient who intends to hasten death in this manner is morally impermissible (19).

The hegemony of autonomy is not as strong outside of the United States, Canada, and northwestern Europe. Ethnic minorities living in the western cultures may carry very different views of the patient's right to know and to make decisions, and the role of the family and the physician. For example, Silani and Borasio (20) report that a decade ago, only 20% of Japanese ALS patients were informed of their diagnosis (though this appears to be changing to more open disclosure). In some cultures disclosure of a terminal condition or planning around life's end is considered insensitive because discussing adverse outcomes is believed to increase their likelihood. Clinicians can explore with patients whether they wish to be informed of their illness and make decisions, or prefer to have other people, such as family members, assume this role. Consultation with an institutional ethics committee, community leaders, or spiritual counselors of the individual may be needed to resolve conflicts between patients and families.

Determination of Decision-Making Capacity

Competence, also called decision-making capacity, reflects the ability to make autonomous choices. The central abilities required are that the patient must be able to: (i) communicate a choice, (ii) understand the relevant information, (iii) appreciate the situation and its consequences, and (iv) manipulate the information rationally

(21). Communication itself is a challenge in ALS. Alternative and augmented communication techniques may be needed, requiring a substantial commitment of clinical time. In addition, communication about preferences for treatment is not an event but a process that occurs over time, and preferences may change as the patient experiences progression of disease. Patients must understand the relevant information, including the risks, benefits, and burdens of alternative courses of treatments available, including the risk of death. Patients "appreciate" their situation when they can apply information to themselves. For example, depressed patients may not be able to appreciate benefits of treatment if they are too hopeless to imagine that an intervention such as a gastrostomy tube might improve the quality of their life (22). Reasoning behind the decision must be logical and understandable, even when the clinician does not agree with the decision. Impairments in appreciation and rationality are most often found in patients with other major psychiatric disorders such as psychosis, mania, or depression (21).

Unlike patients with other terminal illnesses, ALS patients often retain decision-making capacity up until the final hours of life. Intact decision-making abilities cannot be assumed, however, in ALS patients. When patients lack decision-making capacity, the most common reasons are psychiatric disorders, such as delirium and depression, and cognitive impairments. Delirium is found in 90% of cancer patients in hospice during the final weeks of life and universally interferes with decision-making capacity (23). Family caregivers of 50 ALS patients who died reported that 26% were confused in the final month of life (Ganzini et al., unpublished data). Among ALS patients, dehydration, hypercarbia, infections, and other organ system dysfunction may all contribute to delirium. Medications commonly used at the end of life that may cause delirium include anticholinergics, benzodiazepines, and opioids (23). Ironically, at times, patients whose wishes are not known will require ventilation or hydration in order to recover capacity to make these decisions.

Frank dementia in ALS patients is not common, but recent research reveals that many ALS patients suffer from frontotemporal lobe impairments. In some studies, these impairments were found in half of the study participants (24,25). The relationship between these impairments and decision-making capacity in ALS patients has not been studied. But in other studies of patients with neuropsychiatric diseases such as schizophrenia and Alzheimer's disease, it is frontotemporal lobe dysfunction, even more than memory impairments or psychiatric symptoms, that are most associated with difficulties with capacity to make medical decisions (21,26–28). The frontal lobe is especially important in the ability to flexibly consider and weigh alternatives, to apply ones values and goals, and to appreciate the information. In ALS these impairments appear progressive, underscoring the importance of beginning discussions about values and goals early in the course of the illness.

Major depressive disorder can be diagnosed in approximately 10% of ALS patients (29,30). Symptoms of depression that have an impact on decision-making ability include hopelessness, pessimism, low self-esteem, and suicidal thoughts. In a previous study, we found that mild to moderate depression did not influence decisions; however, with effective treatment of severe depression, elderly patients were more likely, when presented hypothetical scenarios of illness, to prefer life-sustaining treatments. Patients with severe depression who would decline treatment were hopeless, overestimated the risks and burdens of treatment, and underestimated the benefits (22).

Patients accept or decline treatment through the process of informed consent. Choices must be voluntary and without undue influence from others. Clinicians must assure that patients have adequate and balanced information. There are two situations in which informed consent is not required. First, patients may waive their right to make an informed decision and ask that their decision be made by their family, or even that their physician. Second, informed consent is not required for emergencies (31). Failure, however, to determine and clearly document goals of care in advance will often result in emergent use of interventions. Even when patients have advance directives, these are overridden, ignored, or never communicated in emergency settings.

Patients Who Lack Decision-Making Capacity

Only competent patients are allowed to make decisions to start or stop medical treatment. When patients lack decision-making capacity, surrogates must make decisions for them. In the United States, most states authorize surrogates or proxies identified through durable power of attorney for health care (DPAHC) forms. The assigned health care agent's role is to make decisions based on previous communications from the patient (substituted judgment). In the absence of conversations, the surrogates should base their decisions on the patient's values and what they believe would be in the patient's best interest (9). Because determinations of best interest can be very subjective, substituted judgments are considered ethically superior. Clinicians caring for ALS patients should recommend that patients and families discuss preferences and document them before capacity is lost. Health care agents may authorize both withholding and withdrawing of life-sustaining treatments. In addition, patients may complete directives, often called living wills, with instructions that limit or support a variety of treatments should the patients be unable to communicate their preferences (3). The ALS CARE Database revealed that 90% of ALS patients had an advance directive before death and advance directives were honored in 97% of cases (32). In the absence of either an advance or proxy directive, involved family members may make decisions for incapacitated patients, though the extent of their authority to stop life-sustaining treatments differs from state to state. Most health care systems have ethics experts available for consultation in cases where there are conflicts or uncertainty regarding these decisions.

ALS Specialists' Views, Understanding, and Experiences in End-of-Life Care

The American Academy of Neurology (AAN) surveyed its members regarding knowledge of end-of-life care in 1999. The survey was sent to all 149 self-identified ALS specialists in the United States, who were AAN members; 77% responded. Ninety-eight percent of ALS specialists agreed that a competent patient has the right to refuse life-sustaining treatments, including hydration and nutrition, even if death results. Yet only 25% of physicians had discussed with ALS patients their wishes concerning "do not resuscitate" orders. Thirty-nine percent of respondents agreed with the incorrect statement that withdrawing treatment is ethically different from withholding or not starting one (33).

These ALS specialists expressed some confusion regarding the difference between the principle of double effect and euthanasia. Although 95% would, with consent, order intravenous morphine to reduce discomfort in an ALS patient and 70% thought it was an important part of proper palliative care, 24% indicated this action was the same as killing. Twenty-nine percent of ALS specialists believed incorrectly that it was illegal to give painkillers in doses that risk respiratory depression to the point of death (33).

The debate about the ethics of PAS and euthanasia center on interpretation of basic principles of medical practice that superficially do not conflict; the imperatives to relieve suffering, respect patient autonomy, and do no harm. Medical ethicists have written in support of PAS and euthanasia for patients with ALS (34) and in opposition (15,16). It is therefore not surprising that the AAN survey revealed a range of attitudes on PAS. Forty-eight percent of respondents supported that PAS should be made explicitly legal by statute for terminal patients, though more (66%) agreed that there should be no law making PAS explicitly illegal. Forty-one percent had received a request from an ALS patient for a lethal prescription to be used with the primary intention of ending life. One in five respondents would participate in PAS given the current legal constraints, and 47% would participate if PAS were legalized. Views on euthanasia were much less positive, with only 4% willing to participate under current conditions and 25% willing to participate if legalized (33). Similarly, Meier et al. (35) surveyed 239 U.S. neurologists and reported that 46% would participate in PAS and 32% in euthanasia if legalized.

Decisions About Life-Sustaining Treatments

The initial management of ALS is rehabilitation; overcoming or adapting to disability is the usual focus of care. From the time of diagnosis, maintaining quality of life should be emphasized. Dimensions beyond the physical domain must be recognized, including psychosocial, spiritual, and financial realms. With all the challenges facing those with ALS, it is tempting to delay or avoid altogether discussions about end of life care. Table 1 outlines three levels of interactions that can occur between the health care practitioner, patient, and family.

The principles of palliative care are applicable to the management of ALS from the time of diagnosis, but assume greater prominence as the disease progresses. Palliative care is the active, total care of patients whose disease is not responsive to curative treatments. The focus of care is to improve quality of life for the patient and the family (36). One goal of palliative care is a "good death" defined by the Institute of Medicine as one that is free from avoidable distress and suffering for patients and caregivers, in general accord with patient and family wishes, and reasonably consistent with clinical, cultural, and ethical standards (37). Much of palliative care is delivered in hospice. In the United States, hospice is a system of care, both

Table 1 Choice of Life-Sustaining Treatment

Passive
  No plan
Active planning for intervention
  Monitor swallowing, pulmonary symptoms, and function
  Offer PEG when comfort with eating or nutrition compromised or FVC 50% predicted
  Offer NIV (discuss LTV) when symptomatic or FVC 50% predicted
Active planning to forgo interventions
  Explicitly discuss symptoms and scenarios at end of life
  Plan hospice referral
  Involve proxy decision maker

Abbreviations: PEG, percutaneous endoscopic gastrostomy; FVC, forced expiratory vital capacity; NIV, noninvasive ventilation; LTV, long-term mechanical ventilation.

inpatient and outpatient, available for patients who have an estimated six months or less of life, and who are no longer receiving life-sustaining medical treatment. What constitutes the best end-of-life care and how it can be improved was the focus of the recent Robert Wood Johnson Foundation Promoting Excellence in End-of-Life Care ALS Peer Workgroup Project, which provided both a guide to current management and direction of research and policy development (38).

Advance care planning should be considered from the time of diagnosis. Each ALS patient should work with a health care practitioner to develop an individualized advance care plan, particularly addressing preferences for respiratory and nutritional support. The timing of the discussion of end-of-life issues and advance care planning with patients and their families must strike a balance between the desire to know on their part, and the need to make timely decisions about life-sustaining therapies. Six triggers to begin discussion of end-of-life choices were identified by the Robert Wood Johnson working group (Table 2).

Between 2% and 5% of ALS patients receive tracheotomies with long-term ventilator support (5,32,39–41). The ALS CARE Database, with information on 1458 U.S. and Canadian patients, reported that 2.1% of patients had used invasive mechanical ventilation, whereas approximately one in six had used noninvasive positive pressure ventilation (42). Patients who used NIV were more likely to be male and have a higher income. Attitudes about life-sustaining treatment appear relatively stable in ALS patients and predict subsequent choices. Albert et al. (5) followed 121 ALS patients for a median of 12 months. At the beginning of the study all patients received educational information and counseling regarding treatment choices. Between 6% and 12% of patients were certain or nearly certain that they would eventually have tracheostomies, and 28% stated they were in favor of gastrostomy placement. Preferences expressed earlier in the disease were strongly related to actual choices and timing of choices within the following year. Preferences for life-sustaining technologies were stronger in those with shorter duration and more rapid progression of disease, and greater attachment to life. Age, education, gender, depression, and hopelessness were not influential in choices. PEG use and tracheostomy are strongly correlated (5,43).

Murphy et al. (44) examined the effect of spirituality, religiousness, depression, hopelessness, attachment to life and attitudes toward death on life-sustaining treatment in 46 ALS patients. Patients who chose NIV support were more religious; however, highly spiritual patients were less likely to choose PEG. A preference for tracheostomy was associated with neither religiousness nor spirituality. Firm conclusions are limited in these studies because of the small numbers of participants.

Table 2 Triggers for Discussing End-of-Life Care

The patient or family asks
Severe psychological, social or spiritual distress, or suffering
Pain requiring high doses of analgesic medication
Dysphagia requiring feeding tube
Dyspnea or symptoms of hypoventilation, or FVC of 50% or less
Loss of function in two body regions

Abbreviation: FVC, forced expiratory vital capacity.
Source: From Robert Wood Johnson "Promoting Excellence in End-of-Life Care ALS Peer Workgroups," 2003 (37).

Despite the clinicians' best efforts, many patients will not be psychologically ready to participate in advanced care planning. Even with intensive education about ventilation using videotapes, up to half of ALS patients still cannot complete this item on health care directives. PEG is recommended soon after onset of dysphagia, when patients' vital capacity is still greater than 50%. Yet according to information from the ALS CARE Database, only 13% of patients with dysphagia received this intervention. Eighty percent of patients who never received a PEG declined it despite the fact that a physician discussed PEG at least once with 79% of patients (6).

Whether from the clinician's failure to address advance care planning or the patient's inability to participate, unplanned interventions are routine. Sixty-six percent of patients on long-term ventilation surveyed in Germany were not aware of their impending respiratory failure before emergency intubation (4) and 81% did not give informed consent for the procedure. Similarly, Moss et al. (39,45) reported that of 50 ALS patients on long-term mechanical ventilation, only three-quarters had discussed this possibility of respiratory failure before it developed. Though many tracheotomies occur emergently, patients appear satisfied with the decision to continue mechanical ventilation at least initially, and rate quality of life as high (45). In a study of 52 home-ventilated patients—32 with noninvasive ventilation and 21 with tracheostomy ventilation, both groups rated quality of life high (4). In another study of 19 ALS patients on home ventilation, 15 had discussed the option before developing respiratory failure, but only four had chosen it in advance. Ninety percent were glad they were receiving home ventilation and would do it again, though over one-third had considered stopping it at one point in the past (45). Seventeen percent of patients chose to stop ventilation over the next year (42). Kaub-Wittemer et al. (4) reported that very few patients who received noninvasive ventilation wished to have tracheostomy ventilation necessary to prolong life as the disease progresses.

Physicians' attitudes about mechanical ventilation influenced these rates. There is marked variability in use of PEG and ventilation across clinics. Physicians "frame" the discussion of mechanical ventilation in chronic lung diseases in either a positive or negative way depending on their perception of the patient's quality of life, ethical beliefs, and the potential reversibility of respiratory failure (46). Moss et al. (39) reported over a decade ago that 24% of neurologists believed home ventilation should not be discussed until respiratory failure occurs.

Sedation and Pain Relief for Terminally Ill Patients

ALS patients may suffer from a variety of symptoms that are most effectively treated with medications that may hasten death. Sedatives including benzodiazepines and narcotics may be required to effectively treat agitation, anxiety, shortness of breath, insomnia, and pain. In a Dutch study of 203 ALS deaths, the use of medications in doses that "probably shortened the patient's life" occurred in 24% and was probably the most frequent end-of-life decision (40). Given the context of the study, with categories that reflected the intention of the physician to end life explicitly, this category does not likely reflect intentional overdose, but may reflect concern on the part of the physician that the use of morphine and sedatives such as benzodiazepines would shorten life. Similar concerns were reflected in the survey of U.S. neurologists (33), where 39% equated the use of morphine in treating dyspnea sufficient to depress respiratory drive with euthanasia.

Even if pain or dyspnea is acute or severe enough that the doses required could result in clinically relevant respiratory suppression, the prevention of suffering is the more important goal under the principle of double effect, which is supported by most religious leaders, ethicists, and legal critics. The respiratory depressant effects of medications used for relief of pain and anxiety are susceptible to the development of tolerance; thus early and appropriate use of these medications can lead to doses that might be lethal to a naïve patient, but are better tolerated by well-palliated patients. Studies in terminal cancer patients, including those with lung involvement, have shown that morphine can relieve symptoms without altering respiratory parameters, even in the elderly (47). Among 1014 ALS deaths reported to the ALS CARE Database, 74% of patients received pain medications in the final days of life (48).

Insomnia was a significant symptom in the last month of life (48,49) and may reflect nocturnal hypoventilation (47). Symptomatic relief may be obtained initially with the use of nocturnal NIV. Reluctance to prescribe hypnotic sedation due to fear of respiratory depression may deprive these patients of a beneficial therapy. Tricyclic antidepressant medications (e.g., amitriptyline) may offer benefit, but anxiolytics may be required as well.

At times these treatments will occur when the patient is actively dying and receiving sedation to treat anxiety or agitation associated with delirium. At other times, these treatments may be initiated to treat potential suffering from air hunger when ventilation is stopped. Patients' preferences for these treatments can be elicited before the care is required. Family should also be involved to determine the goals of care and to reassure that there is no intent to hasten death.

Stopping Food and Hydration

Unlike euthanasia or PAS, the choice to stop food and hydration is legal for competent patients. For ALS patients this may include the choice to never start any type of feeding tube or, after starting, to stop hydration at some point. Oregon hospice nurses reported that deliberate hastening of death by voluntarily stopping food and fluids was almost twice as common as PAS since the latter was legalized. Eighty-five percent of patients who made this choice died within 15 days, and the quality of the death was good, with minimal suffering. Compared to PAS patients, hospice patients who stopped eating and drinking were more likely than PAS patients to have a terminal diagnosis of a neurological disease. Similar to Oregon patients who chose assisted suicide, patients chose to stop eating and drinking because of poor quality of life, difficulty in finding meaning, and wanting to stay in control (50). Good care of patients who stop hydration may include sedation and extensive oral care for thirst symptoms.

Physician-Assisted Suicide and Euthanasia

ALS patients have played prominent roles in the debate on euthanasia and assisted suicide. Court cases in Canada and Great Britain, widely viewed television broadcasts in the Netherlands and the United States, and personal accounts support that for many ALS patients consideration of death-hastening events is not rare, and may even be common.

Assisted suicide and euthanasia are allowed or tolerated in several jurisdictions—the state of Oregon, the Netherlands, Switzerland, and more recently Belgium. Oregon's Death with Dignity Act was passed by a slim majority in 1994, and implemented in 1997. This law allows a physician to prescribe a medication for a patient to self-administer for the purposes of causing death, if the patient is competent. A series of safeguards include a two-week waiting period during which the patient must make three separate requests, confirmation by a second physician that the patient is terminally ill (estimated less than six months of life), and assessment by a mental health professional if there is concern that the decision is influenced by depression. Euthanasia remains illegal in Oregon. Since implementation, approximately 0.1% of all deaths in Oregon are by legalized assisted suicide (51).

In the Netherlands both assisted suicide and euthanasia were not prosecuted for several decades, and both practices were formally legalized in 2001. Belgium legalized euthanasia, but not assisted suicide, in 2002. In both the countries euthanasia can only be performed by a physician, the patient request must be voluntary and well considered, the patient must have a poor medical prognosis, and suffering must be unbearable. In Belgium the request must be written, palliative care options explicitly outlined, and a second physician must be consulted if death is not expected in a short period of time. In both countries assisted deaths are reviewed by an independent board (52).

In Switzerland, assisted suicide is a crime only if the motive is selfish. Assisting suicide for altruistic reasons is legally condoned, physician involvement is not required, and the patient does not need to be terminally ill (53,54). As reported by a Swiss Right to Die Society, there are approximately 300 assisted suicides per year, constituting approximately 1 in 200 deaths (54). Exit Suisse Romande, one of three associations that assist with suicides, reports that of 48 assisted deaths in 2003, two patients had ALS (personal communication with Elizabeth Leresche, Exit Suisse Romande). Elsewhere in Europe the rates of administration of drugs with the explicit intention of hastened death ranges from less than 1% in Denmark, Italy, and Sweden, 1.8% in Belgium, and 3.4% in the Netherlands, with large variations in the degree to which these practices are discussed with patients, relatives, and caregivers (55). There is little information available on characteristics of patients in countries other than the Netherlands and Oregon.

In the survey of U.S. neurologists, 41% had received at least one request for PAD, with two-third occurring in the last six months of life (33). Data from the Netherlands and Oregon support that ALS is an important risk factor for interest in hastened death and completed physician-assisted suicide and euthanasia. About 3% of all ALS deaths are by assisted suicide, but ALS patients are 25 times more likely to die by PAS than all other deaths in Oregon. No other clinical or demographic factor is as strongly associated with completed PAS in Oregon as is ALS (56).

In the Netherlands between 1994 and 1998, 20% of deaths among 203 ALS patients were by PAS or euthanasia. In 36% of cases, patients had completed an advance directive indicating desire for PAD. As reported by physicians, PAD patients had less anxiety before death than non-PAD, but there were no other differences in symptom prevalence or severity. PAD patients were less religious and more likely to die at home, but there were no other demographic or care-related differences. Most euthanasia patients had advanced disease; physicians estimated that in 83% of cases life was shortened by less than one month (40).

Studies have examined the factors associated with ALS patients' interest in PAS and euthanasia. One hundred ALS patients in Oregon were asked about their interest in assisted suicide between 1995 and 1997. Their mean duration of illness was four years, and 24% were receiving hospice services (this low proportion in hospice reflects that most study patients were not in the last six months of life). Fifty-six percent indicated that they would consider PAS; they were more likely to be men, had higher educational levels, were more hopeless as measured by the Beck

Hopelessness Scale, were less likely to be religious, and rated their quality of life as lower than those who did not want PAS. Those who wanted assisted suicide were more likely to indicate they would refuse other life-sustaining treatments. For example, 80% who considered PAS favorably indicated they might refuse a feeding tube, compared to 41% who would never consider PAS. Similarly, those who favored PAS were more likely to indicate they would decline cardiopulmonary resuscitation and mechanical ventilation (29).

For many ALS patients, interest in PAS is sustained throughout the course of the disease. Fifty family caregivers of ALS patients, including 38 who had participated in the previously mentioned Oregon study, reported that loved ones' interest in PAS was associated with their worries about being a burden, pain, insomnia, and discomfort other than pain. Caregivers reported that one-third ($N = 16$) of the patients expressed a desire for PAS in the month before death, even though only one died of PAS. Among the 38 who had previously participated in the interview a median of 11 months before death, higher levels of hopelessness and previous interest in PAS strongly predicted persistent interest in PAS in the last month of life (49).

A study of ALS patients with advanced disease (58) revealed that 19% had a significant interest in hastening death. The preference to hasten dying was expressed consistently before death and was associated with poorer mood, more hopelessness and were less religious. Three patients hastened death. Neudert et al. (58) interviewed primary caregivers of 128 patients who died from ALS. Caregivers reported that 33 (26%) patients repeatedly wished to die and 10 (8%) repeatedly asked for voluntary active euthanasia. Seven of the ten patients were under the care of a palliative care service or a neurologist with training in palliative care.

The Approach to the Patient Who Wishes to Hasten Death

The approach to the patient who wishes to hasten death by any means includes comprehensive palliative care and the health care practitioner's attempts to understand and ameliorate sources of suffering. The health care provider should thoroughly explore the patient's reasoning, looking for opportunities to correct misperceptions and fears. Treatable psychiatric disorders including delirium, depression, and anxiety should be evaluated and aggressively treated. Referral to hospice or a palliative care team allows comprehensive evaluation by social workers, mental health practitioner, and chaplains.

Most requests for assisted suicide and euthanasia do not persist, but persistent requests are very challenging for physicians. Interviews with physicians in Oregon who received these requests demonstrated that they are emotionally difficult both for physicians who might participate in PAD as well as those who feel they cannot (59,60). The physician should be ready to listen thoroughly and assure the patient that no matter what the final decision, the physician is available to the patient through the illness, even if the physician cannot prescribe a lethal medication. Some physicians reported a sense of hopelessness and failure after receiving a request. At other times too much empathy and identification with the patient will lead to failure to thoroughly look for alternatives. In our experience, patients who persist in wanting assisted suicide have strong needs for control, negative views of the future, and strong dislike of being dependent on others—all areas in which ALS particularly effects patients. There is the risk that too much medical intervention may result in the patient feeling more dependent. Every effort to improve the patient's independence and avoid institutionalization should be made, even if safety in the home is not optimal (59).

REFERENCES

1. Howard RS, Orrell RW. Management of motor neurone disease. Postgrad Med J 2002; 78:736–741.
2. Bourke SC, Bullock RE, Williams TL, Shaw PJ, Gibson GJ. Non-invasive ventilation in ALS: Indications and effect on quality of life. Neurology 2003; 61:171–177.
3. Benditt JO, Smith TS, Tonelli MR. Empowering the individual with ALS at the end-of-life: Disease-specific advance care planning. Muscle Nerve 2001; 24:1706–1709.
4. Kaub-Wittemer D, Steinbuchel N, Wasner M, Laier-Groeneveld G, Borasio GD. Quality of life and psychosocial issues in ventilated patients with amyotrophic lateral sclerosis and their caregivers. J Pain Symptom Manage 2003; 26:890–896.
5. Albert SM, Murphy PL, Del Bene ML, Rowland LP. A prospective study of preferences and actual treatment choices in ALS. Neurology 1999; 53:278–283.
6. Mitsumoto H, Davidson M, Moore D, Gad N, Brandis M, Ringel S, Rosenfeld J, Shefner JM, Strong MJ, Sufit R, et al. ACS Group Percutaneous endoscopic gastrostomy (PEG) in patients with ALS and bulbar dysfunction. Amyotroph Lateral Sclero Other Motor Neuron Disord 2003; 4:177–185.
7. Beauchamp TL, Childress JF. Principles of Biomedical Ethics. New York: Oxford University Press Inc., 1994.
8. Jonsen AR, Siegler M, Winslade WJ. Clinical Ethics: A Practical Approach to Ethical Decisions in Clinical Medicine. New York: McGraw-Hill Health Professions Division, 1998.
9. Lo B. Resolving Ethical Dilemmas: A Guide for Clinicians. Baltimore: Williams & Wilkins, 1995.
10. Caralis PV, Hammond JS. Attitudes of medical students, housestaff, and faculty physicians toward euthanasia and termination of life-sustaining treatment. Crit Care Med 1992; 20:683–690.
11. Solomon MZ, O'Donnell L, Jennings B, Guilfoy V, Wolf SM, Nolan K, Jackson R, Koch-Weser D, Donnelley S. Decisions near the end-of-life: Professional views on life-sustaining treatments. Am J Public Health 1993; 83:14–23.
12. Faber-Langendoen K. Death by request: assisted suicide and the oncologist. Cancer 1998; 82:35–41.
13. American Geriatrics Society Ethics Committee. Physician-assisted suicide and voluntary active euthanasia. J Am Geriatr Soc 1995; 43:579–580.
14. Koenig HG. Legalizing physician-assisted suicide: Some thoughts and concerns. J Fam Pract 1993; 37:171–179.
15. Foley KM. Competent care for the dying instead of physician-assisted suicide. N Engl J Med 1997; 336:54–58.
16. Bernat JL, Gert B, Mogielnicki RP. Patient refusal of hydration and nutrition. An alternative to physician-assisted suicide or voluntary active euthanasia. Arch Intern Med 1993; 153:2723–2728.
17. Quill TE, Byock IR. Responding to intractable terminal suffering: The role of terminal sedation and voluntary refusal of food and fluids. Ann Intern Med 2000; 132:408–414.
18. Miller FG, Meier DE. Voluntary death: A comparison of terminal dehydration and physician-assisted suicide. Ann Intern Med 1998; 128:559–562.
19. Jansen LA, Sulmasy DP. Sedation, alimentation, hydration, and equivocation: Careful conversation about care at the end-of-life. Ann Intern Med 2002; 136:845–849.
20. Silani V, Borasio GD. Honesty and hope: Announcement of diagnosis in ALS. Neurology 1999; 53(8 suppl 5):537–539.
21. Appelbaum PS, Grisso T. The MacArthur treatment competence study I, II, III. Law Hum Behav 1995; 19:105–174.
22. Ganzini L, Lee MA, Heintz RT, Bloom JD, Fenn DS. The effect of depression treatment on elderly patients' preferences for life-sustaining medical therapy. Am J Psychiatry 1994; 151:1631–1636.

23. Goy ER, Ganzini L. Delirium, anxiety and depression. In: Morrison RS, Meier DE, Capello C, eds. Geriatric Palliative Care. Oxford: Oxford University Press Inc., 2003:286–303.

24. Lomen-Hoerth C, Murphy J, Langmore S, Kramer JH, Olney RK, Miller B. Are amyotrophic lateral sclerosis patients cognitively normal? Neurology 2003; 60:1094–1097.

25. Evdokimidis I, Constantinidis TS, Gourtzelidis P, Smyrnis N, Zalonis I, Zis PV, Andreadou E, Papageorgiou C. Frontal lobe dysfunction in amyotrophic lateral sclerosis. J Neurol Sci 2002; 195:25–33.

26. Palmer BW, Dunn LB, Appelbaum PS, Jeste DV. Correlates of treatment-related decision-making capacity among middle-aged and older patients with schizophrenia. Arch Gen Psychiatry 2004; 61:230–236.

27. Marson DC, Ingram KK, Cody HA, Harrell LE. Assessing the competency of patients with Alzheimer's disease under different legal standards. Arch Neurol 1995; 52:949–954.

28. Marson DC, Chatterjee A, Ingram KK, Harrell LE. Toward a neurologic model of competency: Cognitive predictors of capacity to consent in Alzheimer's disease using three different legal standards. Neurology 1996; 46:666–672.

29. Ganzini L, Johnston WS, McFarland BH, Tolle SW, Lee MA. Attitudes of patients with amyotrophic lateral sclerosis and their care givers toward assisted suicide. N Engl J Med 1998; 339:967–973.

30. Rabkin JG, Albert SM, Del Bene ML, O'Sullivan I, Tider T, Rowland LP, Mitsumoto H. Prevalence of depressive disorders and change over time in late stage ALS. Neurology 2005; 65:62–67.

31. Ganzini L, Volicer L, Nelson WA, Fox E, Derse AR. Ten myths about decision-making capacity. J Am Med Direct Assoc 2004; 5:1–5.

32. Bradley WG, Anderson F, Bromberg M, Gutmann L, Harati Y, Ross M, Miller RG, ALS Care Study Group. Current management of ALS: Comparison of the ALS CARE database and the AAN practice parameter. The American Academy of Neurology. Neurology 2001; 57:500–504.

33. Carver AC, Vickrey BG, Bernat JL, Keran C, Ringel SP, Foley KM. End-of-life care: A survey of US neurologists' attitudes, behavior, and knowledge. Neurology 1999; 53: 284–293.

34. Loyal L. The case for physician-assisted suicide and active euthanasia in amyotrophic lateral sclerosis. In: Brown RH, Meininger V, Swash M, eds. Amyotrophic Lateral Sclerosis. London: Martin Dunitz, 2000.

35. Meier DE, Emmons CA, Wallenstein S, Quill T, Morrison RS, Cassel CK. A national survey of physician-assisted suicide and euthanasia in the United States. N Engl J Med 1998; 338:1193–201.

36. WHO Expert Committee. Cancer Pain Relief and Palliative Care. Geneva: World Health Organization, 1990:11.

37. Field MJ, Cassel CK. Approaching Death: Improving Care at the End-of-Life. Washington, DC: National Academy Press, 1997.

38. Mitsumoto H, ALS Peer Workgroup Members. ALS: Completing the continuum of ALS care: A consensus document. Missoula, Montana: Promoting Excellence in End-of-Life Care, a national program of The Robert Wood Johnson Foundation, 2004.

39. Moss AH, Casey P, Stocking CB, Roos RP, Brooks BR, Siegler M. Home ventilation for amyotrophic lateral sclerosis patients: outcomes, costs, and patient, family, and physician attitudes. Neurology 1993; 43:438–443.

40. Veldink JH, Wokke JH, van der Wal G, Vianney de Jong JM, van den Berg LH. Euthanasia and physician-assisted suicide among patients with amyotrophic lateral sclerosis in the Netherlands. N Engl J Med 2002; 346:1638–1644.

41. Oppenheimer EA. Decision-making in the respiratory care of amyotrophic lateral sclerosis: should home mechanical ventilation be used? Palliat Med 1993; 7:49–64.

42. Lechtzin N, Wiener CM, Clawson L, Davidson MC, Anderson F, Gowda N, Diette GB, ALS Care Study Group. Use of non-invasive ventilation in patients with amyotrophic lateral sclerosis. Amyotroph Lateral Sclero Other Motor Neuron Disord 2004; 5:9–15.

43. Albert SM, Del Bene ML, Rabkin JG, Tider T, O'Sullivan I, Mitsumoto H. The decision to hasten death in people with ALS. Amyotroph Lateral Sclero Other Motor Neuron Disord 2003; 4(suppl 1):39.

44. Murphy PL, Albert SM, Weber CM, Del Bene ML, Rowland LP. Impact of spirituality and religiousness on outcomes in patients with ALS. Neurology 2000; 55:1581–1584.

45. Moss AH, Oppenheimer EA, Casey P, Cazzolli PA, Roos RP, Stocking CB, Siegler M. Patients with amyotrophic lateral sclerosis receiving long-term mechanical ventilation: advance care planning and outcomes. Chest 1996; 110:249–255.

46. Sullivan KE, Hebert PC, Logan J, O'Connor AM, McNeely PD. What do physicians tell patients with end-state COPD about intubation and mechanical ventilation? Chest 1996; 109:258–264.

47. Borasio GD, Lyall R, Kaub-Wittemer D. Respiratory symptoms. In: Voltz R, Bernat JL, Borasio GD, Maddocks I, Oliver D, Portenoy RK, eds. Palliative Care in Neurology. Oxford: Oxford University Press, 2004.

48. Mandler RN, Anderson FA Jr, Miller RG, Clawson L, Cudkowicz M, Del Bene M, ALS Care Study Group. The ALS Patient Care Database: insights into end-of-life care in ALS. Amyotroph Lateral Sclero Other Motor Neuron Disord 2001; 2:203–208.

49. Ganzini L, Silveira MJ, Johnston WS. Predictors and correlates of interest in assisted suicide in the final month of life among ALS patients in Oregon and Washington. J Pain Symptom Manage 2002; 24:312–317.

50. Ganzini L, Goy ER, Miller LL, Harvath TA, Jackson A, Delorit MA. Nurses' experiences with hospice patients who refuse food and fluids to hasten death. N Engl J Med 2003; 349:359–365.

51. Ganzini L, Harvath TA, Jackson A, Goy ER, Miller LL, Delorit MA. Experiences of Oregon nurses and social workers with hospice patients who requested assistance with suicide. N Engl J Med 2002; 347:582–588.

52. Deliens L, van der Wal G. The euthanasia law in Belgium and the Netherlands. Lancet 2003; 362:1239–1240.

53. Kapp C. Swiss allow assisted suicide, but what about euthanasia? Lancet 1999; 354:2059.

54. Hurst SA, Mauron A. Assisted suicide and euthanasia in Switzerland: allowing a role for non-physicians. BMJ 2003; 326:271–273.

55. van der Heide A, Deliens L, Faisst K, Nilstun T, Norup M, Paci E, van der Wal G, van der Maas PJ. Eureld Consortium. End-of-life decision-making in six European countries: descriptive study. Lancet 2003; 362:345–350.

56. Oregon Department of Human Services. http://www.ohd.hr.st.or.us/chs, 2003.

57. Albert SM, Rabkin JG, Del Bene ML, Tider T, O'Sullivan I, Rowland LP, Mitsumoto H. Wish to die in end-stage ALS. Neurology 2005; 45:68–74.

58. Neudert C, Wasner M, Borasio GD. Attitudes towards life-prolonging treatments and active euthanasia in German patients with amyotrophic lateral sclerosis. Amyotroph Lateral Sclero Other Motor Neuron Disord 2003; 4(suppl 1):41.

59. Ganzini L, Dobscha SK, Heintz RT, Press N. Oregon physicians' perceptions of patients who request assisted suicide and their families. J Palliat Med 2003; 6:381–390.

60. Dobscha SK, Heintz RT, Press N, Ganzini L. Oregon physicians' responses to requests for assisted suicide: A qualitative study. J Palliat Med 2004; 7:450–460.

Index

About the Editors

HIROSHI MITSUMOTO is the Wesley J. Howe Professor of Neurology at the Neurological Institute of New York and Columbia University Medical Center, New York, New York, and is Director of the Neuromuscular Division and the Elanor and Lou Gehrig MDA/ALS Research Center, Department of Neurology, Columbia University, New York, New York. He received the M.D. degree from Toho University School of Medicine, Japan, and completed residency training in neurology at Case Western Reserve University, Cleveland, Ohio, and a neuromuscular fellowship at Tufts New England Medical Center, Medford, Massachusetts. Dr. Mitsumoto has published and lectured extensively on the topic of ALS. He is a member of the MDA Medical Advisory Board, the ALS CARE Board of Directors, and serves on the editorial board of *Neurology*.

SERGE PRZEDBORSKI is the William Black Professor of Neurology and Professor of Pathology at the College of Physicians and Surgeons, Columbia University, New York, New York. He received the M.D. degree from the Université Libre de Bruxelles (ULB), Belgium; completed an internship and residency in neurology and psychiatry at the ULB-Erasme Medical Center, Belgium; and received the Ph.D. degree in neurological sciences from the ULB School of Medicine, Belgium.

PAUL H. GORDON is the Associate Medical Director of the Elanor and Lou Gehrig ADA/ALS Research Center at Columbia University, New York, New York. After graduating from the University of Arizona, he trained in neurology at the Neurological Institute at Columbia University, New York, New York. He is a member of the American Medical Association, the American Academy of Neurology, the American Academy of Electrodiagnostic Medicine, and the Movement Disorder Society, among other organizations.